CARDIOVASCULAR THROMBOSIS

Thrombocardiology and Thromboneurology

Second Edition

CARDIOVASCULAR THROMBOSIS
Thrombocardiology and Thromboneurology
Second Edition

Editors

Marc Verstraete, M.D., Ph. D.
Professor of Medicine
Founder and Director Emeritus of the
Center for Molecular and Vascular Biology
University of Leuven
Leuven, Belgium

Valentin Fuster, M.D., Ph.D.
Arthur M. and Hilda A. Master
Professor of Medicine
Director
Cardiovascular Institute
Dean for Academic Affairs
Mount Sinai Medical Center
New York, New York

Eric J. Topol, M.D.
Chairman
Department of Cardiology
Director
Joseph J. Jacobs Center for Thrombosis and Vascular Biology
Department of Cardiology
The Cleveland Clinic Foundation
Cleveland, Ohio

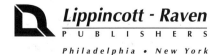

Lippincott - Raven
PUBLISHERS
Philadelphia • New York

Acquisitions Editor: Ruth W. Weinberg
Developmental Editor: Ellen DiFrancesco
Manufacturing Manager: Dennis Teston
Production Manager: Kathleen Bubbeo
Production Editor: Carolyn Foley
Cover Designer: Brian Crede/BC Graphics
Indexer: Susan Thomas
Compositor: Lippincott–Raven Electronic Production
Printer: Quebecor Kingsport

Printed in the United States of America

9 8 7 6 5 4 3 2 1

Library of Congress Cataloging-in-Publication Data
Cardiovascular thrombosis : thrombocardiology and thromboneurology / edited by Marc Verstraete, Valentin Fuster, Eric J. Topol. — 2nd ed.
        p. cm.
    Rev. ed. of: Thrombosis in cardiovascular disorders / edited by Valentin Fuster, Marc Verstraete. c1992.
    Includes bibliographical references and index.
    ISBN 0-397-58772-4
    1. Thrombosis. 2. Thrombolytic therapy. I. Verstraete, M. (Marc) II. Fuster, Valentin.
III. Topol, Eric J., 1954– IV Thrombosis in cardiovascular disorders.
    [DNLM: 1. Thrombosis—physiopathology. 2. Thrombosis—therapy. 3. Fibrinolytic Agents.
4. Heart Diseases—therapy. WG 300 C26789 1998]
RC694.3.C38 1998
616.1'35—dc21
DNLM/DLC
For Library of Congress   97-42477
                                                                        CIP

To the medical staff, fellows, research fellows, and alumni of our respective departments. Without their intellectual input, enthusiastic work, and constructive criticism, thrombocardiology and thromboneurology never would have matured to their respective positions.

Contents

Contributors

Ale Algra, M.D.
Associate Professor of Clinical Epidemiology
The Julius Center for Patient-Oriented Research
Department of Neurology
Utrecht University
Universiteitsweg 100
3584 CG Utrecht, The Netherlands

Walter Ageno, M.D.
Research Fellow
Department of Internal Medicine
McMaster University
Hamilton Civic Hospitals
237 Barton Street East
Hamilton, Ontario L8L 2X2, Canada

Maureen Andrew, M.D.
Professor of Pediatrics
McMaster University, Hamilton
1200 Main Street West
Hamilton, Ontario L8V 1C3, Canada

Jef Arnout, M.D.
Research Associate
The Center for Molecular and Vascular Biology
University of Leuven
Campus Gasthuisberg
Herestraat 49
B-3000 Leuven, Belgium

Juan Jose Badimon, Ph.D.
Associate Professor of Medicine
Cardiovascular Institute
Mount Sinai School of Medicine
One Gustave L. Levy Place
New York, New York 10029-6574

Lina Badimon, Ph.D.
Professor of Cardiovascular Research
Cardiovascular Research Center
CSIC Hospital Santa Cruz y San Pablo UAB
Jordi Girona 18-26
08034 Barcelona, Spain

Kenneth A. Bauer, M.D.
Associate Professor of Medicine
Harvard Medical School
Hematology-Oncology Section
Brockton-West Roxbury Veterans Administration
  Medical Center
1400 VFW Parkway
West Roxbury, Massachusetts 02132

Jill J. F. Belch, M.B.Ch.B., M.D. (Hon)
Professor of Vascular Medicine
Department of Medicine
Ninewells Hospital and Medical School
Dundee DD1 9SY, United Kingdom

Oscar Benavente, M.D.
Department of Neurology
University of Texas Health Science Center
7703 Floyd Curl Drive
San Antonio, Texas 78284-7883

David Bergqvist, M.D., Ph.D.
Professor of Vascular Surgery
Department of Surgery
University Hospital
S-75185 Uppsala, Sweden

Michel E. Bertrand, M.D.
Professor of Medicine
Division of Cardiology B
Hôpital Cardiologique
Boulevard Place Leclercq
59037 Lille, France

Henri Bounameaux, M.D.
Associate Professor of Medicine
Division of Angiology and Hemostasis
University Hospital of Geneva
Rue Micheli-du-Crest 24
CH-1211 Geneva 14, Switzerland

Ernest Briët, M.D.
Professor
Department of Internal Medicine, F4-119
Academic Medical Center
Meibergdreef 9
1105 AZ Amsterdam, The Netherlands

Lu Ann C. Brooker, R.T.
Department of Pediatrics
McMaster University
Hamilton Civic Hospitals Research Centre
711 Concession Street
Hamilton, Ontario L8V 1C3, Canada

Eric G. Butchart, M.B.
Director of Cardiothoracic Surgery
University Hospital of Wales
Heath Park
Cardiff CF4 4XW, United Kingdom

Christopher P. Cannon, M.D.
Assistant Professor of Medicine
Harvard Medical School;
Associate Physician
Cardiovascular Division
Brigham and Women's Hospital
75 Francis Street
Boston, Massachusetts 02115-6195

Luis Carreras
Instituto de Cardiologia y Cirugia Cardiovascular
Belgrado 1746
1093 Buenos Aires, Argentina

Cedric J. Carter, M.B.
Associate Professor of Pathology and Laboratory
  Medicine
University of British Columbia
2211 Westbrook Mall
Vancouver, British Columbia V6T 2B5, Canada

James H. Chesebro, M.D.
Professor of Research
Cardiovascular Institute
Mount Sinai School of Medicine
One Gustave L. Levy Place
New York, New York 10029-6574

Paul L. Cisek, M.D.
Clinical Fellow in Vascular Surgery
Section of Vascular Surgery
Temple University Hospital
Broad and Ontario Streets
Philadelphia, Pennsylvania 19140

Marc Cohen, M.D.
Professor of Medicine
Chief, Division of Cardiology
Allegheny University of the Health Sciences
Cath Lab MS 119
Broad and Vine Streets
Philadelphia, Pennsylvania 19102

Désiré Collen, M.D., Ph.D.
Professor of Medicine
The Center for Molecular and Vascular Biology
University of Leuven
Campus Gasthuisberg
Herestraat 49
B-3000 Leuven, Belgium

Anthony J. Comerota, M.D.
Professor of Surgery
Temple University School of Medicine
Broad and Ontario Streets
Philadelphia, Pennsylvania 19140

Jacqueline Conard, Ph.D.
Hematologist MCU-PH
Service d'Hématologie Biologique
Hotel Dieu University Hospital
Place du Parvis Notre Dame
75004 Paris, France

James McNiven Courtney, Ph.D.
Professor
University of Strathclyde
Bioengineering Unit
106 Rottenrow
Glasgow G4 0NW, United Kingdom

J. Andrew Davies, M.D.
Professor of Clinical Education
Consultant Physician
Division of Medicine
University of Leeds School of Medicine
G Floor Martin Wing
The General Infirmary
Leeds LS1 3EX, United Kingdom

Gregory J. del Zoppo, M.S., M.D.
Associate Professor
Department of Molecular and Experimental
  Medicine
The Scripps Research Institute
10550 North Torrey Pines Road, SBR-17
La Jolla, California 92037

Alexios P. Dimas, M.D.
Director of Interventional Cardiology
Hygeia Hospital
9 Trapezountos Street
171 24 Nea Smirni
Athens, Greece

Erling Falk, M.D., Ph.D.
Professor
Coronary Pathology Research
Aarhus University Hospital Skejby
8200 Aarhus N, Denmark

Jawed Fareed, Ph.D.
Professor of Pathology and Pharmacology
Loyola University Medical Center
2160 South First Avenue
Maywood, Illinois 60153

Garret A. FitzGerald, M.D.
Professor and Chair
Department of Pharmacology;
Director of the Center for Experimental
  Therapeutics and Clinical Research Center
University of Pennsylvania School of Medicine
153 Johnson Pavilion
Philadelphia, Pennsylvania 19104-6084

Charles D. Forbes, M.D., D.Sc.
Professor of Medicine
University of Dundee
Ninewells Hospital and Medical School
Dundee DD1 9SY, United Kingdom

Valentin Fuster, M.D., Ph.D.
Arthur M. and Hilda A. Master Professor of
  Medicine;
Director of Cardiovascular Institute;
Dean for Academic Affairs
Mount Sinai Medical Center
One Gustave L. Levy Place
New York, New York 10029-6574

Jeffrey S. Ginsberg, M.D.
Associate Professor
Department of Medicine
McMaster University
1200 Main Street West, HSC-3W11
Hamilton, Ontario L8N 3Z5, Canada

Samuel Z. Goldhaber, M.D.
Associate Professor of Medicine
Harvard Medical School;
Cardiovascular Division
Brigham and Women's Hospital
75 Francis Street
Boston, Massachusetts 02115

Steven Goldman, M.D.
Professor of Medicine
University of Arizona;
Chief of Cardiology
Tucson Veterans Administration Medical Center
3601 South Sixth Avenue
Tucson, Arizona 85723

Christopher B. Granger, M.D.
Assistant Professor of Medicine
Department of Medicine / Cardiology
Duke University Medical Center
2074 West Main Street, Bay A1
Durham, North Carolina 27705

Peter J. Grant, M.D.
Professor of Molecular Vascular Medicine
Leeds General Infirmary;
Unit of Molecular Vascular Medicine
University of Leeds School of Medicine
Division of Medicine
G Floor Martin Wing
Leeds LS1 3EX, United Kingdom

Werner Hacke, M.D., Ph.D.
Professor of Neurology
University of Heidelberg
Im Neuenheimer Feld 400
D69120 Heidelberg, Germany

Jonathan L. Halperin, M.D.
Robert and Harriet Heilbrunn Professor of Medicine
Cardiovascular Institute
Mount Sinai Medical Center
One Gustave L. Levy Place
New York, New York 10029-6574

Laurence A. Harker, M.D.
Blomeyer Professor of Medicine
Director of the Division of Hematology and
  Oncology
Emory University School of Medicine
1639 Pierce Drive, Room 1003
Atlanta, Georgia 30322

Robert G. Hart, M.D.
Professor of Medicine
Department of Medicine/Neurology
University of Texas Health Science Center
7703 Floyd Curl Drive
San Antonio, Texas 78284-7883

Patricia R. Hebert, M.D.
Associate Professor of Preventive Medicine and
  Medicine
Vanderbilt University School of Medicine
1129 MCN
Nashville, Tennessee 37232

Charles H. Hennekens, M.D., Dr.P.H.
Eugene Braunwald Professor of Medicine
Harvard Medical School;
Brigham and Women's Hospital
900 Commonwealth Avenue East
Boston, Massachusetts 02115-1204

Jack Hirsh, M.D.
Professor Emeritus
McMaster University;
Director of the Hamilton Civic Hospitals Research
  Centre
711 Concession Street
Hamilton, Ontario L8V 1C3, Canada

Russell D. Hull, M.Sc.
Professor of Medicine
Department of General Internal Medicine;
Co-Director of the Thrombosis Research Unit
University of Calgary/Foothills Hospital
1403-29 Street NW
Calgary, Alberta T2N 4N1, Canada

Beverley J. Hunt, M.B.Ch.B., M.D.
Consultant in Departments of Haematology and
  Rheumatology
Guys and St. Thomas' Trust, London;
Honorary Senior Lecturer
Department of Cardiothoracic Surgery
National Heart and Lung Institute
Imperial College School of Medicine
London SE1 7EH, United Kingdom

Kenneth B. Hymes, M.D.
Associate Professor of Medicine
Department of Hematology
New York University Medical Center
530 First Avenue
New York, New York 10016

Sara J. Israels, M.D.
Associate Professor
Department of Pediatrics and Child Health
University of Manitoba
100 Olivia Street
Winnipeg, Manitoba R3E OV9, Canada

Brigitte Kaiser, M.D.
Assistant Professor for Pharmacology and
  Toxicology
Center for Vascular Biology and Medicine
Friedrich Schiller University Jena
Nordhäuser Strasse 78
D-99089 Erfurt, Germany

Vijay V. Kakkar, M.D.
Director of the Thrombosis Research Institute
Emmanuel Kaye Building
Manresa Road
London SW3 6LR, United Kingdom

Simon Karpatkin, M.D.
Professor of Medicine
New York University Medical Center
550 First Avenue
New York, New York 10016

Sudhir S. Kushwaha, M.D.
Assistant Professor of Medicine
Department of Cardiology
Mount Sinai Medical Center
One Gustave L. Levy Place
New York, New York 10029-6574

C. Seth Landefeld, M.D.
Chief, Division of Geriatrics
University of California, San Francisco;
Veterans Administration Medical Center
4150 Clement Street
Box 111G
San Francisco, California 94121

Marcel M. Levi, M.D., Ph.D
Associate Professor
Department of Hemostasis, Thrombosis,
  Atherosclerosis, and Inflammation Research
Academic Medical Center
Meibergdreef 9
1105 AZ Amsterdam, The Netherlands

Roger H. Lijnen, Ph.D.
Professor and Adjunct Director
The Center for Molecular and Vascular Biology
University of Leuven
Campus Gasthuisberg
Herestraat 49
B-3000 Leuven, Belgium

Gordon D.O. Lowe, M.B.Ch.B., M.D.
Professor of Vascular Medicine
Royal Infirmary
10 Alexandra Parade
Glasgow G31 2ER, United Kingdom

Michael D. Malone, M.D.
Instructor of Surgery
Temple University Hospital
Broad and Ontario Streets
Philadelphia, Pennsylvania 19140

Kenneth G. Mann, Ph.D.
Professor of Biochemistry and Medicine
University of Vermont College of Medicine
Given Building, C-401
Burlington, Vermont 05405-0068

Pier M. Mannucci, M.D.
Professor of Medicine
Department of Internal Medicine
University of Milan
Via Pace 9
20127 Milano, Italy

Margaret McLaren, Ph.D.
Lecturer
Department of Medicine
Ninewells Hospital and Medical School
Dundee DD1 9SY, United Kingdom

Eugène P. McFadden, M.R.C.P., F.E.S.C.
Practicien Hospitalier
Division of Cardiology B
Hôpital Cardiologique
59037 Lille, France

Thomas W. Meade, D.M., D.R.C.P.
Professor
MRC Epidemiology and Medical Care Unit
St. Bartholomew's and the Royal London School of
*   Medicine and Dentistry*
Wolfson Institute of Preventive Medicine
Charterhouse Square
London EC1M 6BQ, United Kingdom

Piera Angelica Merlini, M.D.
Assistant Professor
Dipartimento Cardiologico De Gasperis
Ospedale Niguarda
Ca'Granda
20162 Milan, Italy

Saskia Middeldorp, M.D.
Department of Internal Medicine
Center of Thrombosis, Haemostasis, Atherosclerosis,
*   and Inflammation Research*
Academic Medical Center
Meibergdreef 9
1105 AZ Amsterdam, The Netherlands

George J. Miller, M.D.
MRC Epidemiology and Medical Care Unit
Northwick Park Hospital
Watford Road, Harrow
Middlesex HAQ 3UJ, United Kingdom

David J. Moliterno, M.D.
Assistant Professor of Medicine
Department of Cardiology
The Cleveland Clinic Foundation
9500 Euclid Avenue, F-25
Cleveland, Ohio 44195

David W. M. Muller, M.D.
Associate Professor of Medicine
Department of Cardiology
St. Vincent's Hospital
Victoria Street
Darlinghurst NSW 2010, Australia

Gert Müller-Berghaus, M.D.
Professor and Director
Department of Hemostaseology and Transfusion
*   Medicine*
Kerckhoff-Klinik
Sprudelhof 11
D-61231 Bad Nauheim, Germany

Karl-Ludwig Neuhaus, M.D.
Professor
Medizinische Klinik II
Städtische Kliniken Kassel
Mönchebergstrasse 41-43
D-34125 Kassel, Germany

Carlo Patrono, M.D.
Professor of Pharmacology
Department of Medicine and Aging
University of Chieti
G. D'Annunzio School of Medicine
Via dei Vestini 31
66013 Chieti, Italy

Kathelijne Peerlinck, M.D., Ph.D.
Associate Professor
The Center for Molecular and Vascular Biology
University of Leuven
Campus Gasthuisberg
Herestraat 49
B-3000 Leuven, Belgium

Palle Petersen, M.D., D.M.Sc.
Assistant Professor
Department of Neurology
Hvidovre Hospital
Kettegards Alle 30
DK-2650 Hvidovre, Denmark

Graham F. Pineo, M.D.
Professor of Medicine
Thrombosis Research Unit
University of Calgary/Foothills Hospital
601 South Tower
Calgary, Alberta T2N 2T9, Canada

Gary E. Raskob, M.Sc.
Associate Professor
Departments of Biostatistics, Epidemiology, and
*   Medicine*
University of Oklahoma Health Sciences Center
P.O. Box 26901
Oklahoma City, Oklahoma 73190

Paul M. Ridker, M.D., M.P.H.
Associate Professor of Medicine
Brigham and Women's Hospital
75 Francis Street
Boston, Massachusetts 02167

Robert D. Rosenberg, M.D., Ph.D.
Professor of Biology
Massachusetts Institute of Technology
77 Massachusetts Avenue
Building 68-480
Cambridge, Massachusetts 02139-4307

Frits R. Rosendaal, M.D.
Professor of Epidemiology
Departments of Clinical Epidemiology and
*   Haematology*
Leiden University Medical Center
P.O. Box 9600
2300 RC Leiden, The Netherlands

Philip A. Routledge, M.D.
Professor of Clinical Pharmacology
Departments of Pharmacology, Therapeutics, and
*   Toxicology*
University of Wales College of Medicine
Heath Park
Cardiff CF4 4XN, United Kingdom

Meyer M. Samama, M.D.
Professor of Hematology
Service d'Hématologie Biologique
Hotel Dieu University Hospital
Place du Parvis Notre Dame
75004 Paris, France

Prediman K. Shah, M.D.
Professor of Medicine
University of California, Los Angeles;
Division of Cardiology
Cedars-Sinai Medical Center
8700 Beverly Boulevard
Los Angeles, California 90048

David G. Sherman, M.D.
Professor of Medicine
Division of Neurology
University of Texas Health Science Center
7703 Floyd Curl Drive
San Antonio, Texas 78284-7883

Hamsaraj Gundal Mahabala Shetty, B.Sc.,
**   M.B.B.S.**
Consultant Physician
Department of Integrated Medicine
University Hospital of Wales
Heath Park
Cardiff CF4 4XN, United Kingdom

Maarten L. Simoons, M.D., Ph.D.
Professor of Cardiology
Erasmus University Rotterdam
Dr. Molewaterplein 40
30159 GD Rotterdam, The Netherlands

Pål J. Smith, M.D., Ph.D.
Department of Medicine
Baerum Hospital
N-13555 Baerum, Norway

Hervé Sors, M.D., M.Sc.
Professor of Medicine
Department Pneumology and Intensive Care
University of Paris V
Hôpital Laennec
42 Rue de Sèvres
75007 Paris, France

Anton Heinz Sutor, M.D.
Professor of Pediatric Hematology
Department of Pediatrics
University of Freiburg
Mathildenstrasse 2
D-79117 Freiburg, Germany

John W. Suttie, Ph.D.
Professor of Biochemistry
University of Wisconsin, Madison
420 Henry Mall
Madison, Wisconsin 53706-1569

Hugo ten Cate, M.D.
Internist and Research Associate
Department of Internal Medicine
Slotervaart Hospital
Louwesweg 6
1066 EC Amsterdam, The Netherlands

Jan W. ten Cate, M.D.
Professor of Vascular Medicine
Centre of Hemostasis, Thrombosis, and
*   Atherosclerosis Research*
Academic Medical Center F-4-211
Meibergdreef 9
1105 AZ Amsterdam, The Netherlands

Eric J. Topol, M.D.
Chairman of the Department of Cardiology;
Director of the Joseph J. Jacobs Center for
*   Thrombosis and Vascular Biology;*
The Cleveland Clinic Foundation
One Clinic Center
9500 Euclid Avenue, F-25
Cleveland, Ohio 44195

Alexander G. G. Turpie, M.D.
Professor of Medicine
McMaster University
237 Barton Street East
Hamilton, Ontario L8L 2X2, Canada

Eric Van Belle, M.D.
Division of Cardiology B
Hôpital Cardiologique
Boulevard Place Leclercq
59037 Lille, France

Jan van Gijn, M.D.
Professor
University Department of Neurology
University Hospital Utrecht
P.O. Box 85500
3508 GA Utrecht, The Netherlands

Frans J. Van de Werf, M.D., Ph.D.
Professor of Medicine
Department of Cardiology
University Hospital Gasthuisberg
Herestraat 49
B-3000 Leuven, Belgium

Raymond Verhaeghe, M.D.
Professor of Medicine
The Center for Molecular and Vascular Biology
University of Leuven
Campus Gasthuisberg
Herestraat 49
B-3000 Leuven, Belgium

Marc Verstraete, M.D., Ph.D.
Professor of Medicine
Founder and Director Emeritus of the Center for
*   Molecular and Vascular Biology*
University of Leuven
Campus Gasthuisberg
Herestraat 49
B-3000 Leuven, Belgium

David A. Vorchheimer, M.D.
Assistant Professor of Medicine;
Director of the Coronary Care Unit
Cardiovascular Institute
Mount Sinai Medical Center
One Gustave L. Levy Place, Box 1030
New York, New York 10029-6574

Jeanine M. Walenga, Ph.D.
Associate Professor of Thoracic-Cardiovascular
*   Surgery and Pathology*
Cardiovascular Institute
Loyola University Medical Center
2160 South First Avenue
Maywood, Illinois 60153

Harvey D. White, D.Sc.
Professor of Medicine
Department of Cardiology
Green Lane Hospital
Green Lane West, Epsom
Auckland 1003, New Zealand

Patrick L. Whitlow, M.D.
Director of Interventional Cardiology
Department of Cardiology, F25
The Cleveland Clinic Foundation
9500 Euclid Avenue
Cleveland, Ohio 44195

James T. Willerson, M.D.
Professor and Chairman
Department of Internal Medicine
University of Texas Medical School at Houston
Suite 1.150, 6431 Fannin
Houston, Texas 77030

Eliot C. Williams, M.D., Ph.D.
Associate Professor of Medicine
Departments of Medicine, Pathology, and
*   Laboratory Medicine*
University of Wisconsin Hospital and Clinics
600 Highland Avenue, H4/5I6
Madison, Wisconsin 53792-5156

Magdi H. Yacoub, M.D.
Professor of Cardiothoracic Surgery
National Heart and Lung Institute
Heart Science Center
Harefield Hospital
Harefield, Middlesex UB9 6JH, United Kingdom

Uwe Zeymer, M.D.
Medizinische Klinik II
Städtische Kliniken Kassel
Mönchebergstrasse 41-43
D-34125 Kassel, Germany

Pierre Zoldhelyi, M.D.
Director of the Wafic Said Molecular Cardiology
*   and Gene Therapy Research Laboratory*
Texas Heart Institute, Houston;
Assistant Professor
Divisions of Cardiology and Hematology
University of Texas Health Science Center
1101 Bates, MC 2-225
Houston, Texas 77030

Foreword

Progress in science and medicine is often greatest at the interface between what once were separate disciplines. Such hybrid fields include some of the most exciting scientific realms: physical chemistry, bioengineering, immunogenetics, astrophysics, neurobiology, and electrophysiology, to name just a few. Cardiovascular thrombosis, an area of growing importance, and the subject of *Cardiovascular Thrombosis: Thrombocardiology and Thromboneurology, Second Edition,* involves three specialties: cardiology, hematology, and neurology. Although the important role of thrombosis in the development of both chronic cardiovascular and neurovascular disease, as well as in acute, life-threatening complications, has been recognized for more than a century, critical developments in the last dozen years have helped to illuminate the pathophysiologic changes in thrombosis and have increased greatly our ability to modify this process. These advances are revolutionizing cardiovascular therapeutics. Among the relatively recent landmark events in this field are the following.

1. The observation—in the *living patient*—that coronary thrombosis is the proximate cause for most instances of acute transmural myocardial infarction and that it frequently plays a critical role in the development of unstable angina as well.
2. The unequivocal demonstration that thrombolytic therapy, when delivered in a timely and appropriate manner, substantially improves the immediate survival of patients with acute myocardial infarction and ischemic stroke, and that this improvement is sustained.
3. The successful completion of clinical trials demonstrating that aspirin—an inexpensive, readily-available drug—is effective in both the *primary* prevention of acute myocardial infarction, and in the *secondary* prevention of unstable angina pectoris, myocardial infarction, and stroke.
4. Advances in molecular biology and synthetic chemistry that allow the production of substances that exert profound effects on various aspects of the coagulation process. These advances include a variety of thrombolytic agents, novel antithrombotics, and potent antiplatelet agents.

To apply these and many other important developments to the clinical arena, physicians must have more than a nodding acquaintance with thrombosis and the many conditions and drugs that can affect the coagulation process. However, except for investigators and subspecialists who deal with disorders of coagulation and bleeding, most physicians (including cardiologists and neurologists) are uncomfortable with this complex field and have had difficulty understanding it. Therefore, this second edition comes at a most opportune time. *Cardiovascular Thrombosis* is among the first books written on this important subject, and I believe that it is both the most ambitious and the best. It is designed to aid physicians in all specialties as they apply recent information about the coagulation system to the care of patients with cardiovascular and neurovascular diseases.

The three editors are highly respected world leaders in this field whose backgrounds, formidable personal contributions, and deep knowledge of the subject complement each other remarkably. They have skillfully orchestrated the writing efforts of some of the most capable clinical investigators in this field on both sides of the Atlantic. The editorial decision to invite authors from different institutions and often different countries to collaborate in the preparation of many of the individual chapters was particularly insightful, as this adds balance and perspective to a field in which opinions are often polarized and emotions run high.

Cardiovascular Thrombosis provides clear explanations of the fundamental principles and theoretical underpinnings of the subject. At the same time, it is intensely practical and brings the unique knowledge and insights of the editors and authors to bear on the interpretation of the experimental and clinical observations in this rapidly expanding field. This book is as up-to-date as this month's journals—a tribute to the editors insistence on presenting as current a picture as possible, and the authors willingness to respond to this demand.

Although the first edition of this book *(Thrombosis in Cardiovascular Disorders)* was superb, the second edition is distinctly superior, something not uncommon with outstanding textbooks. Important new material has been incorporated and an even higher standard of excellence has been achieved. Eric J. Topol, M.D., an addition to the editorship, has made a strong and positive impact, which is clearly apparent.

In the foreword to the first edition, I suggested that this important new field at the interface between hematology and cardiology deserved its own name: *thrombocardiology.* I am pleased that the editors have included this term along with *thromboneurology* in the title of the second edition.

The recent advances in the study of coagulation have altered profoundly—and I believe permanently—the management of patients with cardiovascular and neurovascular disease, as well as of healthy persons at risk for such disease. We are just beginning to realize the benefits that accrue to patients from research at the interface between three medical specialties (hematology, cardiology, and neurology) and the physical interface between two tissues (the vascular wall and its contents). Armed with the information in the second edition, these benefits will become even clearer in the next few years. For these reasons, I look forward to the third edition of this splendid book.

Eugene Braunwald
Boston, Massachusetts

Foreword

As I predicted in my foreword to the first edition, this book has enjoyed remarkable success. Since its publication in 1992, developments in understanding, pharmacology, and management of cardiovascular thrombosis have occurred at such a rapid pace that the publication of this second edition, with 21 new chapters and very substantial updating of the original 31, appears quite timely.

The neologisms *thrombocardiology* and *thromboneurology,* which now complement the title, express the editors view that modern cardiologists, as well as neurologists, need expertise with a solid foundation in the field of thromboembolic disorders, a view that I share.

Marc Verstraete, Valentin Fuster, and Eric J. Topol should be congratulated for their wise and thorough selection of topics covered by the new chapters, and also for the clarity and depth of coverage to be found throughout.

Hopefully in the near future, we shall have a clearer understanding of when, why, and how thrombosis may occasionally become a tragic disease mechanism, rather than remaining as a useful process of physiologic repair. Until then, prevention of lysis of excess thrombus represents the main treatment of thromboembolic disorders. This volume provides state-of-the-art information about such treatments.

I believe that this second edition, like its predecessor, will prove invaluable to all investigators of thromboembolic disorders and will be a fundamental source of reference for cardiologists, neurologists, and internists wishing to make informed clinical decisions and choices when dealing with thromboembolic problems in their daily practice.

Attilio Maseri
Rome, Italy

Preface

For decades, the nonhematologist has been confused by the profusion and complexity of ideas on the mechanism of clotting. However, he may have lost sight of the simplest of all observations—the fact that normal blood does not clot in normal blood vessels. This is the result of a delicate balance between proteins favoring coagulation (procoagulants) and those opposing it (anticoagulants). For every patient who dies because of the failure of his blood to clot, many thousands of people die because of the failure of their blood to remain fluid in vital parts of their circulation. There is a growing appreciation that many disease states result from an imbalance between endogenous pro- and anticoagulants and from interaction between these proteins and an abnormal vascular wall.

Thrombosis occurs in different sites and organs, confronting doctors with an important clinical problem whether they are general physicians, internists, pediatricians, cardiologists, neurologists, surgeons, or, of course, hematologists. The awareness of the importance of arterial thrombosis in the pathogenesis of cardiovascular and neurovascular diseases creates a new paradigm: suddenly, cardiologists and neurologists look at things rather differently. Traditionally, scientists and specialists have communicated regularly with other workers in their particular discipline while remaining curiously isolated from those in other fields. To achieve an interdisciplinary approach, the three editors of this book (two American cardiologists and a European hematologist) recruited outstanding scientists and clinicians from diverse fields and from different geographical areas. More than 100 coauthors, all busy individuals of independent spirit, contributed to the 51 chapters. The editors purposely invited authors from different institutions and often different countries to collaborate in writing individual chapters. In doing so, the editors' hope was not to reach a consensus on all issues, but rather to present a volume of complementary and balanced views. By allowing for differences of opinion, *Cardiovascular Thrombosis: Thrombocardiology and Thromboneurology, Second Edition,* actually gives the reader a clearer understanding of thrombosis in medicine today.

The three editors independently and vigorously refereed each chapter. The chapters were then resubmitted in revised forms. The editors are most grateful to the forbearance of the coauthors who graciously acquiesced to this extensive peer review. There still remains a refreshing variation in emphasis and opinion among chapters, although some slight overlaps were unavoidable. Remembering that history does not repeat itself, the editors asked the authors to free themselves from the fetters of lengthy historical material. One should take the fire from the altar of the past, not the ashes.

Toward the end of the book the reader might agree that the greater the island of knowledge, the greater the shoreline of the unknown. However, the authors and editors hope that the reader will be left with a belief in the interconnectedness of facts and a better understanding of the subject at hand.

It is said that a preface is written last, printed first, and read the least. Hopefully the latter will not hold true, since the editors wish to thank here the authors, the real producers of this book, who have endured pressing demands, adhered to a tight schedule, and enthusiastically collaborated in a cost-ineffective undertaking. Their best reward would be that this book is avidly read, warmly received, and that it provides good competition for its rivals.

This book does not contain all the wisdom and truth the editors hope for. Perhaps one virtue can be claimed for human beings: as limited as we are, we can get at some truth as, in fact, we have a tropism for it.

Marc Verstraete
Valentin Fuster
Eric J. Topol

PART I

Fundamental Considerations

Cardiovascular Thrombosis: Thrombocardiology and Thromboneurology, Second Edition, edited by M. Verstraete, V. Fuster, and E. J. Topol, Lippincott–Raven Publishers, Philadelphia © 1998.

1

Thrombosis and Fibrinolysis

Laurence A. Harker and *Kenneth G. Mann

*Division of Hematology and Oncology, Emory University School of Medicine, Atlanta, Georgia 30322; and *Department of Biochemistry, University of Vermont College of Medicine, Burlington, Vermont 05405*

Blood constituents do not normally interact with undamaged vascular endothelium. This nonreactive endothelial interface between highly reactive components in blood and highly thrombogenic elements comprising nonendothelial vascular structures is maintained by multiple active and passive mechanisms (Fig. 1-1). Mechanical disruption of blood vessels initiates localized hemostatic responses involving vascular endothelium, platelets, coagulation, and fibrinolysis. Initially, tissue factor (TF) expressed on adventitial cells binds avidly with plasma factor VII/VIIa, leading to the local activation of both factor IX and factor X and the consequent thrombin generation via enzyme–cofactor complexes on phospholipid surfaces. Thrombin activates platelets and cleaves fibrinogen and factor XIII, giving rise to hemostatic plugs consisting of adherent and coherent platelets, insoluble fibrin, leukocytes, and entrapped red cells, stabilized by cross-linked fibrin. Hemostatic plugs undergo gradual lytic removal via plasmin-mediated fibrinolysis. Hemostasis is affected by functional changes in endothelium, platelets, coagulation or fibrinolysis (1–3).

Denuded endovascular or prosthetic flow surfaces initiate thrombogenesis involving deposited platelets, insoluble fibrin, leukocytes, and entrapped erythrocytes in variable flow-dependent patterns, resulting in mechanical masses that may occlude subtending vascular blood flow, or detach and embolize to occlude blood flow downstream (Fig. 1-2). Abnormalities in blood, blood flow, and blood vessels contribute to thrombus formation (Virchow's triad) (4). Arterial flow conditions produce platelet-rich ("white") thrombi, and static venous flow yields fibrin- and red cell–rich ("red") thrombi. Endogenous fibrinolysis gradually removes formed thrombus, and endothelial mechanisms limit the extent of thrombus propagation. The site, size, and composition of thrombi and thromboemboli are determined by mechanical hemodynamic blood flow effects, amount and thrombogenicity of nonendothelialized exposed surfaces, concentrations and reactivity of responding plasma and cellular blood constituents, and effectiveness of the physiologic protective mechanisms, particularly the protease inhibitor proteins, protein C anticoagulant pathway, and fibrinolysis. Mechani-

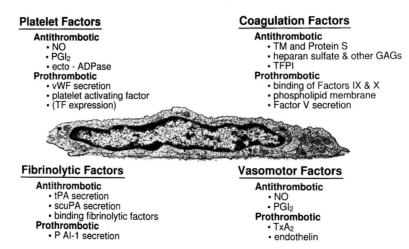

Platelet Factors

Antithrombotic
- NO
- PGI₂
- ecto - ADPase

Prothrombotic
- vWF secretion
- platelet activating factor
- (TF expression)

Coagulation Factors

Antithrombotic
- TM and Protein S
- heparan sulfate & other GAGs
- TFPI

Prothrombotic
- binding of Factors IX & X
- phospholipid membrane
- Factor V secretion

Fibrinolytic Factors

Antithrombotic
- tPA secretion
- scuPA secretion
- binding fibrinolytic factors

Prothrombotic
- P AI-1 secretion

Vasomotor Factors

Antithrombotic
- NO
- PGI₂

Prothrombotic
- TxA₂
- endothelin

FIG. 1-1. Endothelial regulation of hemostasis and thrombosis. The endothelium participates in both antithrombotic and prothrombotic mechanisms involving platelets, coagulation, fibrinolysis, and vasomotor responses. Endothelial antithrombotic mechanisms include (a) antiplatelet effects of NO and prostacyclin (PGI_2), together with the destruction of proaggregatory ADP by endothelial ecto-ADPase; (b) endothelial thrombomodulin (TM)-dependent conversion of protein C to APC and its subsequent inactivation of factor Va in the presence of its cofactor protein S, neutralization of thrombin via heparan sulfate-mediated covalent binding with antithrombin III, and the inactivation of both factor VIIa and factor Xa by complexing with TFPI in association with TF; (c) local endothelial secretion of tissue plasminogen activator (t-PA) and scu-PA and endothelial assembly of fibrinolytic factors (plasminogen, t-PA, and u-PA) leading to plasmin generation and accelerated local fibrinolysis; and (d) local enhancement of blood flow by endothelial production of the vasodilators NO and PGI_2. Endothelial prothrombotic mechanisms include (a) enhanced platelet attachment due to secretion of vWF and platelet-activating factor (PAF), and possibly the endothelial expression of TF, although this has only been demonstrated for cultured endothelial cells in vitro, not for nonmalignant endothelium in vivo; (b) serine protease complex formation on endothelium due binding of factors IXa, X, and V to endothelial phospholipid membranes, and endothelial secretion of factor V; (c) inactivation of plasminogen activators by PAI-1; and (d) vasoconstriction mediated by thromboxane A_2 (TxA_2) produced by forming thrombus, and endothelial secretion of endothelin.

cally damaged vascular tissues and ruptured atherosclerotic plaques initiate TF-dependent generation of thrombin that converts fibrinogen to fibrin and mediates platelet recruitment by cleaving G protein-coupled thrombin receptors (TRs), in the formation of fibrin-stabilized vascular thrombosis, producing thrombotic and thromboembolic occlusion of diseased arteries and resultant life-threatening heart attacks, strokes, or peripheral ischemia. Thrombo-occlusive complications also develop in patients undergoing interventional vascular procedures for symptomatic atherosclerotic vascular disease, including angioplasty, various types of atherectomies, endarterectomy, endovascular stent deployment, or implanted small-caliber vascular grafts.

Additionally, thrombotic reocclusion may compromise thrombolytic therapy for acute myocardial infarction. Venous thrombosis and thromboembolism also lead to serious disability and death (1–3).

The late vascular healing effects of mechanical or spontaneous vascular disruption involve the catalytic activation of TRs on platelets, leukocytes, vascular medial smooth muscle cells (SMCs), endothelium, and other mesenchymal cells. Medial SMCs proliferate and migrate to the intima, leading to SMC intimal proliferation and synthesis of extracellular matrix in the local formation of stenosing neointimal proliferative vascular lesions (5–10). This chapter summarizes the complex integrated reactions comprising hemostatic,

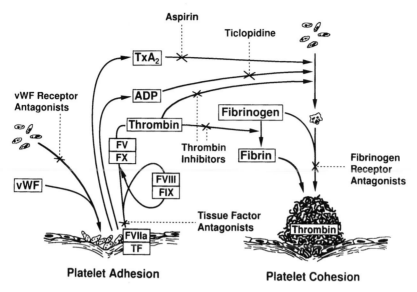

FIG. 1-2. Vascular thrombogenesis. Platelets undergo attachment to nonendothelialized surfaces by adherence, activation, and spreading and subsequent recruitment to form rapidly enlarging platelet thrombi. These processes involve platelet attachment to subendothelial connective tissue constituents, platelet activation, and inside-out expression of platelet membrane integrin receptors for fibrinogen and other adhesive proteins, initiation of the contractile processes leading to shape change and secretion of storage granule contents, platelet cohesion via interplatelet fibrinogen bridging, and self-amplifying platelet recruitment by outside-in signaling mediated by thrombin, adenosine diphosphate (ADP), and thromboxane A_2 (TxA$_2$), three independent but interactive physiologic agonists. Thrombin is rapidly generated in response to vascular injury, and plays the central role in platelet recruitment and in the formation of the stabilizing fibrin network.

thrombotic, and neointimal vascular processes and their regulation.

HEMODYNAMIC EFFECTS

Blood normally flows with characteristic streaming flow patterns involving concentric cylindrical layers of blood with minimal flow at the vessel wall and successively more rapid flow toward the central stream. The axial stream of red cells displaces the smaller, similarly charged platelets toward the vascular wall, with little tendency for inward radial migration. Developing platelet aggregates have extended residence times and greater likelihood of attaching to the wall in the formation of thrombus. When flow is disturbed—such as in the vortex patterns produced distal to sites of stenosis—activated species of platelets and coagulation factors, or factors that induce vascular damage, are concentrated and retained at the vessel wall. Platelet-rich thrombus forming at sites of arterial narrowing tends to embolize because of increased shear forces and dilutes activated species more quickly. Thus, occlusive thrombus is unlikely to form until blood flow is disturbed and retarded. After flow is arrested, thrombus formation is propagated into stagnant proximal and distal vascular segments (11,12).

In veins, flow is characteristically slow, and at times it is interrupted. Venous thrombi generally begin at sites of maximum stasis, often as platelet aggregates in the pockets of vein valves or in the intramuscular venous sinuses of the legs (13). When stasis is combined with focal vascular injury, venous thrombi readily form because of the consequent local activation of platelets and coagulation proteins. Impaired protective mechanisms also predispose to venous thrombotic events, as illustrated by increased venous thromboembolic events in patients with hereditary deficiencies of antithrombin III, protein C, protein S, factor V (resistance to activated protein C [APC]), and reduced fibrinolytic activity (14,15). Similarly, if stasis is associated with circulating prothrombotic species, as is the case with some malignancies (see Chapter 45) or with remote tissue damage, the likelihood of venous thrombosis increases substantially. By combining stasis with both local vessel injury and systemically activated platelets and coagulation factors, the development of venous thrombosis is predictable, as illustrated by the high probability of venous thrombosis complicating orthopedic surgery (16).

ENDOTHELIUM

By enveloping blood within the circulatory system, endothelium constitutes the structural and functional interface between blood and vascular systems, including the processes of hemostasis, thrombus formation, and atherogenesis (Fig. 1-1). Endothelial anatomic location, expansive interactive surface area, and magnitude of tissue mass contribute to its functional roles as a selectively permeable, blood-compatible, secretory membrane regulating inflammatory, vasomotor, growth factor, and hormonal responses (17–19).

Uncontrolled extension of thrombus throughout the vascular system is prevented by multiple, blood, and endothelial cell–dependent mechanisms designed to limit thrombus formation to the site of vascular injury. The efficacy of these endothelial cell–related mechanisms are greatest in the microcirculation because the ratio of endothelial surface area to blood volume is highest in capillaries. The luminal negative charge, nonreactive glycosaminoglycans, and endothelial glycocalyx largely insulate the vessel wall from blood elements. Intact endothelium also clears vasoactive amines and inactivates proaggregatory adenosine diphosphate (ADP) by membrane-bound ADPase (19).

The most important endothelial mechanisms for limiting thrombus extension are related to the inactivation of thrombin activity, the reduction in thrombin generation, and the thrombin-stimulated production of antithrombotic and vasodilating factors by intact endothelium (Fig. 1-1). Thrombin entering the circulation is directly inactivated by plasma protease inhibitors (20). Antithrombin III, a 58,000-dalton plasma protein (3 μmol/L), inhibits thrombin and factors XIa, Xa, and IXa (but not factor VIIa in the absence of TF) (Table 1-1). Whereas antithrombin III alone inactivates serine proteases slowly, the process is accelerated 3 orders of magnitude when antithrombin III is bound to heparin. Inactivation by antithrombin III is similarly facilitated by heparin-like glycosaminoglycans, particularly heparan sulfate and thrombomodulin on endothelial surfaces. The protection provided by antithrombin III is shown by the thrombotic predisposition of patients with heterozygous deficiency of plasma antithrombin III. Another endothelial-bound protein, tissue factor pathway inhibitor (TFPI), inactivates both factors VIIa and Xa by forming quaternary complexes (TFPI, TF, and factors VIIa and Xa) in the presence of phospholipid surfaces and calcium ions (21).

Thrombin stimulates endothelium to produce prostacyclin and nitric oxide (NO) (endothelial-derived relaxing factor [EDRF]), two highly potent local antiaggregatory vasodilators (19,22). These molecules contribute significant antithrombotic protection for microvascular beds distal to sites of thrombus formation. In addition, thrombin induces endothelial release of tissue-plasminogen activator (t-PA) and urokinase (u-PA) from adjacent intact endothelium (19,23,24). t-PA binds with the fibrin present in thrombus and forms a trimeric complex with bound or circulating plasminogen, resulting in the formation of plasmin and consequent increase in fibrinolysis. The endothelium provides the phospholipid surface for assembly of fibrinolytic activity giving rise to plasmin generation (25).

Thrombin also binds with thrombomodulin, a constitutive endothelial membrane protein (100,000 copies per endothelial cell), forming a termolecular complex with protein

TABLE 1-1. *Properties of human clotting factors*

Clotting factor	Molecular weight (No. of chains)	Normal plasma concentration (µmol/L)	Plasma half-life (days)
Intrinsic system			
Factor XII	80,000 (1)	0.4	
Prekallikrein	80,000 (1)	0.6	
High molecular weight kininogen	105,000 (1)	0.7	
Factor XI	160,000 (2)	0.03	3.0
Factor IX	68,000 (1)	0.09	1.0
Factor VIII	265,000 (1)	0.0007	0.4
vWF	1–15,000,000[a]		
Extrinsic system			
Factor VII	47,000 (1)	0.01	0.25
Tissue factor	46,000 (1)	0	Cell bound
Common pathway			
Factor X	56,000 (2)	0.17	1.25
Factor V	330,000 (1)	0.02	0.5
Prothrombin	72,000 (1)	1.4	2.5
Fibrinogen	340,000 (6)	7.0	5.0
Factor XIII	320,000 (4)	0.03	9–10
Anticoagulant pathway			
Protein C	56,000 (2)	0.06	0.25
Protein S	67,000 (1)	0.14	1.75
Thrombomodulin	35,000 (1)	0	Cell bound
Tissue factor pathway inhibitor (TFPI)		0.003	Endothelium bound

[a]Subunit molecular weight of factor VIII/vWF is approximately 220,000 with a series of multimers found in circulation.

C, that catalytically activates the natural antithrombotic zymogen protein C (26,27). Thrombomodulin comprising six epidermal growth factor (EGF)-like domains (EGF repeats 2 through 6 of thrombomodulin facilitate the activation of protein C by thrombin, and repeats 5 and 6 provide the site for thrombin binding). Protein C is a 56,000-dalton vitamin K–dependent plasma zymogen that circulates at a concentration of about 0.1 µmol/L (Table 1-1). Both protein C and APC possess γ-carboxyglutamic and β-hydroxyaspartic acid residues, thereby retaining the formed calcium-dependent complexes bound to endothelial cell surfaces. APC catalytically inactivates surface-bound factor Va (15,27). The importance of protein C activation in protecting against unwanted thrombus formation is evident from the life-threatening thrombotic consequences in newborns with homozygous deficiency and the predisposition to thrombosis in some kindreds with heterozygous individuals (15). Protein S is a biologically relevant but poorly understood cofactor for the activation of protein C on both platelets and endothelium. Protein S enhances the efficacy of APC-mediated inactivation of membrane-bound factor Va (and factor VIIIa) (27). Protein S circulates in the blood as the active free protein and in noncovalent association with a large, multisubunit protein of the complement system, C4bBP, in an inactive state. Patients with heterozygous hereditary deficiency states are predisposed to thrombotic events. Thus, the protein C/thrombomodulin/protein S pathway provides an important thrombin-dependent protective mechanism initiating negative feedback regulation for decreasing thrombin's own production.

PLATELETS

Platelets undergo attachment to nonendothelialized surfaces by adherence, activation, and spreading and subsequent recruitment to form rapidly enlarging platelet thrombi. These processes involve (a) platelet attachment to subendothelial connective tissue constituents; (b) platelet activation and inside-out signaling leading to expression of platelet membrane integrin receptors for fibrinogen and other adhesive proteins, as well as initiation of the contractile processes leading to shape change and secretion of storage granule contents; (c) platelet cohesion via interplatelet fibrinogen bridging; and (d) self-amplifying platelet recruitment by outside-in signaling mediated by thrombin, ADP, and thromboxane A_2 (TxA$_2$), three potent, independent but interactive agonists (Fig. 1-2) (1–3,28).

Platelet adhesion involves the diffusive transport of platelets to the reactive surface and the interaction of platelet surface glycoprotein (GP) receptors with injured wall or with adhesive proteins bound to the surface of biomaterials (12). Platelet-reactive subendothelial extracellular matrix adhesive proteins include von Willebrand factor (vWF), fibrinogen, fibronectin, laminin, vitronectin, and thrombospondin. The membrane GP receptors and their respective coupling extracellular ligand(s) capable of mediating platelet adhesion include (a) GPIb/IX–vWF; (b) GPIa/IIa–collagen; (c) GPIc/IIa–fibronectin; (d) GPIc/IIa–laminin; (e) vitronectin receptor–vitronectin/vWF/fibronectin/thrombospondin; (f) GPIIb/IIIa–fibronectin/thrombospondin/vitronectin; and (g) GPIV–thrombospondin/collagen (Table 1-2) (29–31).

Unactivated platelets adhere at sites of denuded vascular injury because matrix-bound or biomaterial-bound adhesive proteins (vWF, fibrinogen thrombospondin, laminin, fibronectin, and vitronectin) are expressed in a conformation capable of binding directly with platelet GPIb/IX receptors, particularly under high shear conditions, i.e., vWF, fibrinogen, and fibronectin. The GPIb/IX heterodimeric complex is the most prominent sialoglycoprotein of platelet membranes (25,000 copies per platelet) and contributes to their negative charge. GPIb/IX mediates platelet adhesion by serving as the receptor for vWF immobilized on exposed vascular subendothelium (Table 1-2). The cytoplasmic domain of GPIb/IX links the platelet membrane to actin-binding proteins that crosslink with the polymerizing actin filaments of the submembranous skeleton upon activation. Platelet attachment initiates intracellular platelet signaling leading to platelet spreading, expression of functional $\alpha_{IIb}\beta_3$ fibrinogen receptor (30) and platelet secretion (inside-out signaling). Patients who lack GPIb/IX (Bernard-Soulier disease) have a bleeding disorder caused by the dysfunctional platelets (large globular platelets that do not bind vWF and fail to form effective hemostatic plugs). Similarly, patients with reduced or dysfunctional vWF (von Willebrand's disease) manifest impaired hemostatic plug-forming capability. GPIV is the principal platelet receptor for thrombospondin and may be an alternative receptor for collagen (Table 1-2). It is a highly glycosylated major platelet surface GP that is also expressed by monocytes (assigned the cluster designation CD36) and endothelial cells (12,29).

The integrin receptors comprise a family of membrane GPs consisting of two subunits, α and β. The ligand-binding site of integrin receptors appears to be formed by sequences from both subunits and their cytoplasmic domains that connect with the cytoskeleton, thereby integrating the extracellular matrix reactions with the intracellular cytoskeletal responses (Table 1-2). $\alpha_{IIb}\beta_3$ integrin receptor (GPIIb/IIIa) is restricted to megakaryocytes and their platelet products, whereas the vitronectin receptor ($\alpha_v\beta_3$) is also expressed by macrophages and a broad range of non-hematopoietic cells (29,31).

Thrombin is the critically important activator of platelets in the processes of hemostatic plug formation, as shown by the lethal consequences of experimentally eliminating genes for its substrate, prothrombin, or other factors leading to its production (32). Thrombin is also the most important physiologic agonist in the process of recruiting platelets into thrombus forming after vascular injury.

Thrombin receptors are seven-transmembrane, G-protein–coupled molecules with relatively large amino-terminal extracellular domains that undergo activation by thrombin-mediated cleavage of the terminal peptides yielding neoaminoterminal peptide sequences

TABLE 1-2. *Platelet membrane glycoproteins and their function*

Platelet glycoprotein receptors	Adhesive glycoproteins	Platelet function
GP Ib-IX (CD42b,c)	vWF	Adhesion
Integrins $\alpha_1\beta_1$, $\alpha_2\beta_1$, $\alpha_3\beta_1$ I (GP Ia–IIa; VLA-2; CD49b/CD29)	Collagen type I–VI	Adhesion
Integrin $\alpha_5\beta_1$ (GP Ic–IIa; VLA-5; CD49e/CD29)	Fibronectin	Adhesion
Integrin $\alpha_6\beta_1$ (GP Ic–IIa; VLA-6; CD49/DC29)	Laminin	Adhesion
Integrin $\alpha_v\beta_3$ (CD51/CD61)	Vitronectin, fibrinogen, fibronectin, vWF, thrombospondin	Adhesion
GPIV (CD36)	Thrombospondin and collagen	Adhesion
Integrin $\alpha_{IIb}\beta_3$ (GPIIb–IIIa; CD41/61)	Fibrinogen, vWF, fibronectin, vitronectin, thrombospondin	Cohesion (aggregation)
P-selectin (GMP-140; CD62P)	Sialyl-Le^x	Platelet-leukocyte interaction

that activate the receptors as tethered ligands (Fig. 1-3) (33). The classical TR neoaminoterminus begins with the sequence Ser-Phe-Leu-Leu-Arg-Asn (SFLLRN), and the synthetic peptide SFLLRN initiates receptor-dependent signaling directly without protease activation and is referred to as thrombin receptor agonist peptide (TRAP) (34). Platelets have approximately 1,000 copies of classical TRs per platelet. This TR is also expressed by leukocytes, endothelium, and vascular smooth muscle cells. The catalytic mechanism for TR activation explains thrombin's potency as a platelet agonist and why high concentrations of antithrombin IIIs are required to prevent TR activation, i.e., a single catalytic interac-

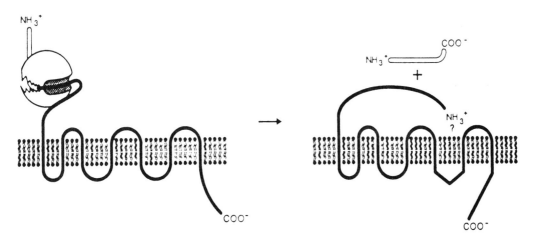

FIG. 1-3. TRs on platelets. TRs are seven-transmembrane G-protein–coupled molecules with amino-terminal extracellular domains that undergo activation by thrombin-mediated cleavage of the terminal peptides yielding neoaminoterminal peptide sequences that activate the receptors as tethered ligands. Single catalytic interaction with thrombin is sufficient to induce activation, and a single thrombin molecule may activate multiple receptors. The initially described TR neoaminoterminus begins with the sequence SFLLRN, and the synthetic peptide SFLLRN initiates receptor-dependent signaling directly without protease activation. A second platelet TR is structurally and functionally closely related, is expressed in a variety of tissues, including hematopoietic cells and peripheral blood platelets, and is catalytically activated by thrombin, yielding a neoaminoterminus with the sequence TFRGA, which initiates intracellular phosphoinositide-dependent signaling. Both TRs appear to participate in platelet activation by thrombin.

tion is sufficient to induce activation, and a single molecule of thrombin may activate multiple receptors. Because platelets from TR-null mice undergo normal activation by thrombin (35), the presence of a second related TR was sought, and recently was identified and characterized (36). The second platelet TR is designated as protease-activated receptor-3 (PAR-3) (36), discriminating it from the classical TR, known as PAR-1, and an analogous protease-activated receptor-2 (PAR-2) selectively activated by trypsin (37). PAR-3 is expressed in a variety of tissues, including hematopoietic cells and peripheral blood platelets, and is catalytically activated by thrombin, yielding a neoaminoterminus with the sequence Thr-Phe-Arg-Gly-Ala (TFRGA) that initiates intracellular phospho-inositide-dependent signaling (36). Both PAR-1 and PAR-3 contribute to platelet TR activities. Interestingly, the only TR antagonist preventing vascular thrombosis in vivo has been polyclonal antihuman TR (PAR-1) antibodies raised in rabbits, and evaluated in nonhuman primates (38). Presumably, the polyclonal anti-TR (PAR-1) antibodies were sufficiently cross-reacting with structurally related PAR-3 to block thrombin-induced activation of both PAR-1 and PAR-3 (36).

Platelet activation initiates intracellular signaling that conformationally reconfigures platelet membrane $\alpha_{IIb}\beta_3$ to create functional membrane receptors for fibrinogen and other adhesive proteins (29–31). Calcium-dependent interplatelet linkages may then form between the activation-expressed platelet receptors and bivalent fibrinogen, and to a lesser extent with vWF, fibronectin, vitronectin, and thrombospondin. von Willebrand factor may substitute for fibrinogen as the bridging ligand when fibrinogen is deficient or defective. However, receptor binding with fibronectin, thrombospondin, and vitronectin normally also appears to contribute toward the usual process of platelet recruitment.

Platelets generally contain about 50,000 copies of $\alpha_{IIb}\beta_3$ (1% to 2% of the total platelet protein) distributed randomly on the surface of resting platelets. The α_{IIb} subunit (molecu-

lar weight [M_r] 140,000 daltons) consists of a large chain (M_r = 125,000) linked by a disulfide bond to a light chain (M_r = 22,000). Only the light chain has a transmembrane domain. The β_3 subunit is a single polypeptide chain (M_r = 105,000) that contains a transmembrane domain and a 41-residue cytoplasmic tail. The extracellular portion of GPIIIa contains cysteine residues clustered in four tandemly repeated segments. The $\alpha_{IIb}\beta_3$ is a calcium-dependent heterodimer, noncovalently associated on the platelet surface. The heterodimer consists of a globular head and two rodlike tails extending from the globular domain (29,31).

The Arg-Gly-Asp (RGD) sequence is the integrin recognition sequence present in the adhesive proteins fibrinogen, vWF, fibronectin, thrombospondin, laminin, vitronectin, and collagen (39). The capability of $\alpha_{IIb}\beta_3$ to bind to many different adhesive proteins is due to the common presence of the RGD sequence. Fibrinogen contains RGD sequences in each α chain, one near the N-terminus (residues 95–97) and a second near the C-terminus (residues 572–574). An additional site on fibrinogen that binds to $\alpha_{IIb}\beta_3$ is the carboxyl-terminal dodecapeptide of each γ chain. This sequence is not found in other adhesive proteins and does not contain the RGD sequence. Peptides containing either RGD or dodecapeptide sequences inhibit platelet aggregation. A heterogeneous array of genetic defects affecting either α_{IIb} or β_3 or both subunits may cause the Glanzmann disease phenotype in patients, which is manifest as a disorder of platelet hemostatic plug formation with abnormal bleeding (29,31).

The conformational alterations in both α_{IIb} and β_3 are dependent on ligand occupancy and lead to clustering of the ligand-occupied receptors (30). The conformational change in $\alpha_{IIb}\beta_3$ is evidenced by the appearance of ligand-induced binding sites, as detected by monoclonal antibodies (30). The expression of $\alpha_{IIb}\beta_3$ fibrinogen-binding determinants are under intracellular control, being inhibited by increases in cytoplasmic cyclic adenosine monophosphate (cAMP).

The conformational changes in $\alpha_{IIb}\beta_3$ initiate intracellular signaling, as shown by (a) tyrosine-specific phosphorylation of threonine residues in β_3 and (b) linkage between $\alpha_{IIb}\beta_3$ and the cytoskeleton. The signal transduction induces metabolic activation within the cell, involving G protein–dependent phospholipase C activation, generation of inositol 1,4,5-triphosphate (IP_3) and diacylglycerol, protein kinase C activation, and intracellular release of cytosolic Ca^{2+} from the dense tubular system (40).

Importantly, these activation processes induce the production of two potent platelet agonists: TxA_2 (also a potent inducer of vasoconstriction), generated via arachidonic acid conversion to diacylglycerol and cyclic endoperoxides, and ADP, secreted through dense granule release. Through the release of TxA_2 and ADP, together with platelet-dependent production of thrombin, platelet recruitment becomes self-amplifying. Thrombin, ADP, and TxA_2 bind to specific receptors, initiate signaling, reduce cAMP activity, induce shape change, and activate platelet contractile elements to form irregular extending pseudopodia and to secrete granular contents, thereby perpetuating platelet recruitment (ADP, ATP, serotonin, and Ca^{2+} from dense granules, and adhesive proteins and coagulation factors from α granules). Although epinephrine and possibly serotonin are weaker platelet agonists at physiologic concentrations, they may promote platelet aggregation in combination with other stimulatory agents. Collagen and thrombin are clearly the most potent and relevant inducers of platelet activation (29–31,40).

COAGULATION

Thrombin is rapidly generated in response to vascular injury (Fig. 1-2) and plays a central role in platelet recruitment and in the formation of the associated insoluble fibrin network (41–43). The thrombotic response is localized, amplified, and modulated. Localized reactions of the blood coagulation cascade are achieved by the reversible binding of circulating coagulation proteins to damaged vascular cells, elements of the exposed subendothelium (especially collagen), platelets, and monocytes/macrophages (Table 1-1). These binding events lead to the assembly of enzyme complexes that rapidly deliver products locally, whereby small initiating stimuli become greatly amplified to yield high levels of terminal products (42,43). The formation of membrane-bound enzyme complexes, the membrane binding properties of the substrates, and the resistance of the bound complexes to potent inhibitory systems are important features of these localized amplification processes (Table 1-1).

Surface-dependent reactions convert the vitamin K–dependent zymogens to the respective serine protease (44). Each complex comprises a vitamin K–dependent serine protease and an accessory or cofactor protein in association with a membrane surface (Fig. 1-4). The presence of calcium is essential for the assembly and activity of these enzyme complexes. Although each enzyme complex exhibits discreet substrate and proteolytic specificity, the complexes share several common features: (a) the complex constituents are functionally and structurally homologous; (b) the complexes assemble in similar patterns; and (c) the assembled complexes greatly amplify the localized catalytic rates by regulating the conversion or expression of the membrane-bound proteins to their active forms. Included among these processes are the proteolytic activation of the cofactors Va and VIIIa to their active forms, the expression of the integral membrane protein cofactors TF and thrombomodulin, and the expression and function of the cellular membrane reactivity for these complex enzymes. Both thrombin and activated factor X (factor Xa) amplify their own formation rates by catalyzing the activation of factor VII to factor VIIa and the activation of factors V and VIII to factors Va and VIIIa, respectively. In addition, thrombin activates the expression of cellular binding sites for assembly of the vitamin K–dependent complexes.

Vitamin K–dependent zymogens are formed by the liver and are characterized by

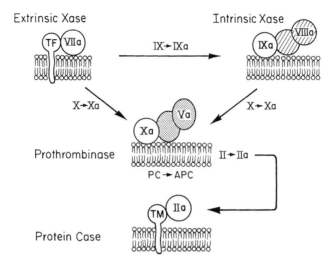

FIG. 1-4. Schematic representation of the vitamin K–dependent serine macromolecular protease complexes of coagulation. Surface-dependent reactions convert the vitamin K–dependent zymogens to the respective serine protease. Each complex comprises a vitamin K–dependent serine protease and an accessory or cofactor protein in association with a membrane surface. Factor VII/VIIa avidly binds with TF exposed on cellular membranes at sites of vascular disruption leading to the proteolytic activation of factor X and subsequent factor Xa–factor Va complex cleavage of prothrombin to produce thrombin on platelet phospholipid surfaces. TF also activates factor IX, which amplifies the formation of factor Xa by complexing with thrombin-activated factor VIIIa, thereby greatly magnifying thrombin generation. The shuttling of product between reaction centers appears to take place on the same membrane surface with channeling of products between assembled complexes without dissociating from the membrane surface.

(a) an amino-terminal Gla domain containing nine to 12 glutamic acid residues that undergo posttranslational γ carboxylation and mediate calcium-dependent binding to acidic phospholipid membranes, as well as (b) a carboxyl-terminal serine protease domain similar in general structure to chymotrypsin. Prothrombin also includes two "kringle" structural domains that facilitate its binding to factor Xa and Va constituents in the prothombinase complex. The other vitamin K–dependent zymogens factors VII, IX, and X, as well as protein C, substitute two EGF-like domains to mediate their unique binding properties in complex assembly. Prothrombin, factor VII, and factor IX are synthesized and circulate as single-chain proteins, whereas factor X and protein C circulate in plasma as two-chain proteins because of proteolytic cleavages during synthesis and secretion. During proteolytic activation, factor X, factor IX, and pro-tein C release specific activation peptides. Current findings indicate that factor VII is activated by limited proteolytic cleavage (at Arg[152] when complexed with the cofactor cell–bound TF), similar to other vitamin K–dependent enzyme precursors in blood.

Calcium-dependent binding of the vitamin K–dependent factors to acidic phospholipid membranes involves conformational transition of the aminoterminal residues 1 to 35 (see Chapter 16). This conformational reconfiguration depends on the posttranslational γ carboxylation of the glutamate sites. Interruption of this carboxylation process by either dietary deficiency of vitamin K or by the administration of vitamin K antagonists such as warfarin produces molecules that are unable to interact with membranes and eliminates their participation in the formation of enzyme complexes. The kinetic properties of the vitamin K–dependent proteins are presented in Table 1-1.

Of the four proteins providing coagulant complex cofactor activity, factors V and VIII circulate as inactive plasma proteins, whereas TF and thrombomodulin are integral membrane proteins anchored via transmembrane domains in adherent cells. TF is an integral membrane protein and does not require activation (45,46). It consists of a cysteine-containing cytoplasmic domain, transmembrane domain and extracellular macromolecular ligand binding-domain. TF is abundant on extravascular cells and also may be expressed on blood monocytes and possibly endothelial cells when stimulated by chemicals, cytokines, and endotoxin, although TF expression by endothelial cells has not been documented directly in vivo (47). TF is an important trigger for initiating coagulation in ruptured arterial atheromatous lesions because of its abundant presence in these intimal plaques and exposure to blood after disruption of the vascular intima (48).

Factors V and VIII are homologous proteins sharing a common structural configuration of triplicated A domains and duplicated C domains with structurally divergent B domains connecting the A2 and A3 domains (43). Factor V circulates in plasma as a single-chain protein at a concentration of 20 nmol/L. Factor V is also present in the α granule of the platelet, and approximately 20% of the factor V in clotting blood is contributed by platelet secretion during the coagulation process (49). Secretion of this platelet compartment appears to be essential in the maintenance of normal hemostasis (50,51). Factor VIII circulates in a multiplicity of fragmented species in a tightly associated complex with vWF at a concentration of 1 nmol/L (Table 1-2). During activation by thrombin or factor Xa, the B domains are excised, leading to the association of A_1A_2 with $A_3C_1C_2$ domains. In the case of factor Va, the active species is a heterodimer composed of aminoterminal-derived heavy chains (A_1A_2) and carboxyl-terminal–derived light chains ($A_3C_1C_2$) that interact tightly and noncovalently in the presence of divalent cations. In contrast, thrombin acts on factor VIII, resulting in the removal of a peptide at the NH_2 terminal of the A_3 domain and the release from vWF (52). Factor VIII activation occurs by a cleavage between the A1 and A2 domains, resulting in the unstable heterotrimeric factor VIIIa molecule. Both factors Va and VIIIa bind tightly to membranes that contain acidic phospholipids. The binding site appears to reside in the A_3 and C_2 domains, which are in the light chains of the molecules. Although the heavy chain of factor Va is responsible for binding prothrombin, factor Xa binding depends on both the heavy and light chains of the factor Va molecule. Both factors Va and VIIIa may be inactivated by plasmin, forming polydisperse smaller peptides, and by APC by cleaving factor Va at two sites and factor VIIIa at a single site to produce inactive proteins (27).

The formation of the prothombinase complex on membrane surfaces initially involves the independent binding of factor Va and Xa to the membrane. This is followed by surface-facilitated complexing of the membrane-bound and oriented proteins and leads to a tight complex with a dissociation constant of about 1 nmol/L. This membrane reaction affinity constant is three orders of magnitude greater than that observed for the solution phase reaction between factors Va and Xa. This enhancement may be due to a conformational change in the two proteins' orientation or the reduction in the permissible orientations of the reacting molecules, or all of the above. The intrinsic factor IX and X activation complexes also appear to assemble and function in a facilitated and coordinated fashion (53,54). The addition of cofactors and the assembly of the appropriate membrane-bound enzyme complex leads to profound enhancement of reaction rates. For example, the activation of prothrombin by factor Xa is enhanced nearly 300,000-fold by the addition of saturating concentrations of factor Va and acidic phospholipid membranes (43).

The membrane-bound prothombinase complex initially cleaves Arg^{323}, producing the intermediate meizothrombin, followed by cleavage of Arg^{274} to yield α-thrombin (42). Meizothrombin remains membrane bound through the retained Gla domain linkage and activates protein C, but lacks some procoagulant properties, including the capacity to activate platelets and cleave fibrinogen.

For the sequentially linked reactions comprising the coagulation cascade, it has been hypothesized that the shuttling of product between reaction centers appears to take place on the same membrane surface with channeling of products between assembled complexes without dissociating from the membrane surface. This type of mechanism would increase the efficiency of the interactions by several orders of magnitude. Moreover, single-membrane channeling protects critical intermediate products from the inactivating effects of potent plasma inhibitors (antithrombin III, heparin cofactor II, α-2 macroglobulin, α-1 antitrypsin, etc.), the inactivating effects of APC (see below), and the

rapid and inactivating dissociation of the unstable cofactor VIIIa as well as from dilution by blood flow over the generating thrombus.

The final phase of thrombus formation in vivo involves the generation of a stable fibrin network that provides the structural support for the blood cellular elements comprising the thrombus and the scaffolding for subsequent cellular remodeling (Fig. 1-5). In this process, thrombin cleaves fibrinopeptides A and B from soluble circulating fibrinogen, producing fibrin monomers that multimerize to form soluble fibrillar strands of fibrin. This process is followed by an orderly fibrillar assembly, branching, lateral association, and covalent cross-linking to form the mature fibrin network (Fig. 1-6). Thrombin-activated factor XIII (factor XIIIa) stabilizes fibrin by forming covalent bonds through transamidation between adjacent fibrin strands.

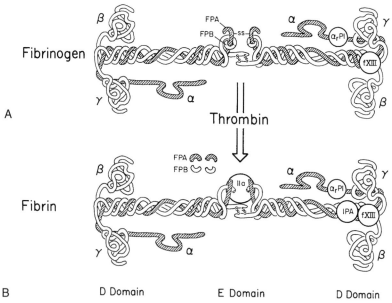

FIG. 1-5. Schematic model of fibrinogen and fibrin. Fibrinogen consists of three pairs of polypeptide chains—Aα, Bβ, and γ—joined by disulfide bonds to form a symmetric dimeric structure **(A)**. The NH_2-terminal regions of all six chains form the central domain (E domain) of the molecule containing FPA and FPB sequences that are cleaved by thrombin during enzymatic conversion to fibrin. Enzymatic conversion of fibrinogen to fibrin **(B)** by thrombin cleavage results in release of FPA and FPB. A binding site for thrombin is present in the central domain of α,β-fibrin and depends largely on the presence of the β15 to 42 sequence. Binding sites for thrombin, t-PA, factor XIII, and $α_2$-PI, respectively, are indicated on the fibrinogen or fibrin molecule.

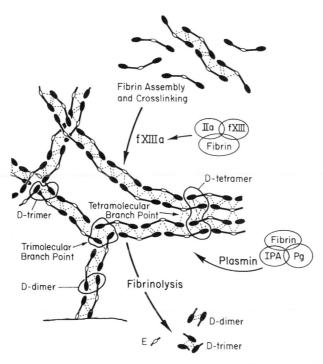

FIG. 1-6. Schematic model of fibrin assembly, cross-linking, and fibrinolysis. Fibrin molecules are represented by trimolecular structures having a central E domain and two outer D domains. After enzymatic conversion of fibrinogen to fibrin, fibrin monomeric units assemble in a staggered overlapping manner by noncovalent interactions between the E and D domains to form two-stranded fibrils. Polymerization of α-fibrin forms similar fibrils. The fibrils undergo noncovalent lateral associations to form thicker fibers, as well as trimolecular and tetramolecular branch points to form a three-dimensional matrix. In the presence of factor XIIIa, assembled fibrin undergoes covalent cross-linking by formation of epsilon γ glutamyl-lysl isopeptide bonds, mainly between γ chains and α chains. When cross-linked fibrin undergoes fibrinolysis, the peptides joining the D and E domains are cleaved, leading to generation of fragment E(E), fragment E– and D–containing fragments (DY), and fragment D–containing products containing cross-linked multimeric D domains that reflect the type of γ-chain cross-linking that has occurred (D dimer, D trimer, D tetramer).

Fibrinogen is a tridomainal disulfide-bridged molecule comprising two symmetric half molecules, each consisting of one set of three different polypeptide chains termed Aα, Bβ, and γ (Fig. 1-5). The two half molecules are joined in the central amino-terminal domain in an antiparallel manner by three interchain disulfide bridges, two of which are between γ chains at positions 8 and 9 and the other at Aα 28. Release of fibrinopeptide A (FPA) and fibrinopeptide B (FPB) exposes binding sites in the amino-terminal regions of the fibrin monomer that function cooperatively in the self-assembly process. FPA release exposes a polymerization site in the central region of the molecule (E domain) that subsequently aligns with a complementary site in the outer region (D domain) of another molecule to form staggered overlapping two-stranded fibrils (Fig. 1-6). The slower FPB release also exposes an independent polymerization site that is used in a similar complementary alignment of the fibrin polymer. Polymerization of the A chains involves the peptide sequences Aα 17 to 20 and a second sequence in the amino-terminal region of the Bβ chain near the thrombin cleavage site at position 14. Thus, fibrin polymer assembly begins with the formation of double-stranded fibrils through noncovalent intermolecular interactions between outer D and central E domains in a staggered overlapping manner

(Fig. 1-6). Subsequently, lateral association of fibrils occurs, increasing fiber thickness. The branching structures consist of laterally associated double-stranded fibrils that form a four-stranded fiber.

Structural stability and integrity of the fibrin network is achieved through covalent cross-linking. Fibrin molecules undergo interchain linkages in the presence of factor XIIIa and calcium ions by forming covalent epsilon-(γ-glu)lys isopeptide bonds. Intermolecular γ chain cross-linking within fibrils forms γ dimers, which occur as reciprocal bridges between lysine at position 406 of one γ chain and glutamine at position 398 of another γ chain. Slower cross-linking among α chains and between γ and α chains also creates covalent polymers. In addition, γ trimers and tetramers have been identified.

Thrombin binds with fibrin through its exosite and the central molecular domain of fibrin. The fibrin-bound thrombin retains its catalytic coagulant and platelet-activating capabilities. Moreover, the fibrin-bound thrombin is protected from inactivation by heparin–antithrombin III complexes (55). Thus, in arterial thrombi, thrombin bound to fibrin continues to mediate platelet-dependent thrombus formation despite heparin or thrombolytic therapies.

The overall process of thrombin generation by the coagulation system occurs in two discrete phases: an initiation phase in which tiny amounts of factors IXa and Xa are produced and nearly quantitative cleavage of factors VIII and V occurs. During the initiation phase, thrombin-dependent platelet activation also occurs, with approximately half the platelets activated. Subsequently, a propagation phase of thrombin generation occurs, leading to the near quantitative activation of prothrombin. Poised versus the procoagulant system are stoichiometric inhibitors, TFPI, antithrombin III, and APC generated as a consequence of thrombin-thrombomodulin activation of the zymogen protein C. TFPI appears to be most effective in quenching the initiation phase of the reaction by its inhibition of the intrinsic factor X activating complex, whereas anti–thrombin III appears to provide a primary function, extinguishing the proteases generated during the propagation phase of the reaction (56). Once some thrombin is generated, the APC sequence proceeds to quench catalyst generation by proteolytic inactivation of factor Va (57). The overall effect of this interplay between activation and inhibition processes is to lead to the establishment of stimulation thresholds in which sufficient levels of initiating activity (TF expression) must be achieved for significant thrombin generation to occur. The combination of activation and inhibition processes collectively produce a switch that either permits or resists significant thrombin generation.

It is instructive to identify the extent of the activation processes that are required for quantitative fibrin formation. Studies conducted with TF-induced coagulation of minimally altered whole blood show that clotting occurs after the generation of only 15 mmol/L thrombin, which is produced by 7 pmol/L prothrombinase (Fig. 1-4). These concentrations correspond to 1% and 0.04% of the potential concentration of these two catalysts (58). The major fraction of the thrombin generated occurs after the clot has been formed. This postclot thrombin generation may be most significant in understanding the pathology of thrombotic and hemorrhagic diseases.

FIBRINOLYSIS

Fibrinolysis plays an important role in the dissolution of thrombi and in maintaining the vascular system patent, as illustrated by the clinical occurrence of thrombosis in patients with constitutive or acquired hypofibrinolysis (19,23) and gene deletion studies in mice (59,60). The fibrinolytic system removes thrombi by proteolytically degrading fibrin into soluble fragments (Fig. 1-6). In this process, the serine protease plasmin is formed from the zymogen plasminogen by the action of either t-PA (61) or urokinase-type plasminogen activator (u-PA) (62). Plasmin cleaves fibrin to produce progressively smaller degradation products, typically containing two D domains (D-dimer), each from different monomers of fibrin that are covalently linked through factor XIIIa–mediated transamidation during the stabilization of fibrin, and therefore resistant to lysis by plasmin. Physiologic inhibition of fibrinolysis may occur at the level of the t-PA and u-PA by specific plasminogen activator inhibitors (PAI-1 and PAI-2), or at the level of plasmin, by α_2-antiplasmin. Some of the properties of this system are outlined in Table 1-3.

Plasminogen, a 92,000-dalton molecule, exhibits four functional domains: (a) the carboxyl-terminal serine protease domain, (b) the amino-terminal finger domain (homologous to the finger domains in fibronectin), (c) the EGF domain (homologous to growth factors), and (d) the domain containing the five triple-looped sulfide-bonded kringle structures. Native plasminogen has an amino-terminal glutamic acid. Limited proteolysis at Arg^{67} may convert it to the more reactive Lys-plasminogen. Plasminogen binds specifically to fibrin through the lysine binding sites contained in the first three kringles, particularly with the first kringle structure. Its activation involves the cleavage of Arg^{560}, creating the two-chain proteolytically active plasmin. Intrinsic activation involves contact factor complex formation (factor XII, prekallikrein, and high molecular weight kininogen). This pathway may be involved in single-chain u-PA (scu-PA) activation, but its physiologic importance is uncertain.

Tissue plasminogen activator is a 70,000-dalton molecule comprising a carboxyl-terminal serine protease domain, an amino-terminal finger domain, an EGF domain, and two kringle domains (61). It is synthesized mainly by endothelium and circulates at a concentration of about 1 nmol/L. Plasmin quickly converts t-PA to a two-chained molecule. Binding of t-PA to fibrin is essential for effective plasmin generation. The binding is mediated via the finger and second kringle domains. Fibrin provides a surface on which t-PA and plasminogen absorb in a sequential and ordered way, yielding a ternary complex. Since the plasmin formed on fibrin retains its lysine binding sites, plasmin generally remains bound and therefore resists inactivating complex formation with α_2-antiplasmin. However, when plasmin ultimately degrades fibrin, lysis may be enhanced because of increased binding by both t-PA and plasminogen.

Single-chain u-PA is a 54,000 dalton protein exhibiting an amino-terminal EGF domain and a single kringle domain with a carboxyl-terminal catalytic domain (62). scu-PA (as opposed to the two-chain urokinase type plasminogen activator) has significant fibrin specificity, which is due to neutralization by fibrin of components in plasma that impair plasminogen activation. Alternatively, scu-PA has been claimed to be inactive toward circulating plasminogen but active toward conformationally altered plasminogen bound to partially digested fibrin. It circulates at about 1 nmol/L and is synthesized by many cells of different origin.

Platelets promote fibrinolysis (63). Plasminogen binds with platelets, facilitating the conversion of plasminogen to plasmin by plasminogen activators; this binding is en-

TABLE 1-3. *Properties of the fibrinolytic system*

Component	Catalytic triad	Reactive site	Molecular weight ($\times 10^3$)	Plasma concentration (mg/ml)
Plasminogen	—	—	92	200
Plasmin	His^{602}, Asp^{645}, Ser^{740}	—	85	—
t-PA	His^{322}, Asp^{371}, Ser^{478}	—	68	0.005
scu-PA	His^{204}, Asp^{255}, Ser^{356}	—	54	0.008
α_2-antiplasmin	—	Arg^{364}-Met^{365}	70	70
PAI-1	—	Arg^{346}-Met^{347}	52	0.05
PAI-2	—	Arg^{358}-Thr^{359}	60,47	<0.005

The numbering of amino acid residues is usually based on these initially determined incorrect values.

hanced by thrombin activation. scu-PA also binds with platelet receptors, and plasmin induces platelet aggregation and release.

α_2-Antiplasmin, a 70,000-dalton protein present in plasma at a concentration of about 1 μmol/L, belongs to the serpin family of inhibitors and is a potent and rapid inhibitor of unbound plasmin. PAI-1 and PAI-2 are also serpin-type inhibitors.

In general, plasmin generation occurs locally and is confined to the vicinity of the thrombotic mass without significant plasmin escape into the systemic circulation (19,23, 63). The mechanisms to ensure that plasmin does not act systemically include (a) the local release of plasminogen activators from intact adjacent endothelial cells by the action of thrombin; (b) the activation of plasminogen activators within thrombi due to affinity for fibrin in the case of t-PA and by some less well understood mechanism for scu-PA; and (c) the inactivation of free plasmin in the circulation by antiplasmin, and the inhibition of t-PA and scu-PA by PAI-1 and PAI-2.

An important linkage between the procoagulant response and fibrinolysis has recently been elucidated. The plasmin lysis of clots is a consequence of enhanced catalytic efficiency and protection of plasmin from inhibition by antiplasmin. Both of these processes are associated with the fibrin binding qualities of this enzyme. These qualities are associated with the carboxyl-terminal lysine residues, which are formed during the initial cleavage of fibrin. An activity termed "thrombin activatable fibrinolysis inhibitor" (TAFI) has been identified as the plasma procarboxypeptidase B zymogen (64–66). This protein is activated by thrombin thrombomodulin (67). The resulting carboxypeptidase B cleaves terminal lysyl residues from the fibrin fragments and, as a consequence, slows fibrinolysis.

VASCULAR LESION FORMATION

Denuding vascular injury initiates TF-dependent thrombin production, platelet recruitment, platelet secretion of storage-granule platelet-derived growth factor (PDGF) (9,68, 69), fibrin formation, accumulation of mononuclear blood leukocytes (70,71), and subsequent vascular lesion formation (9,10, 72) (Fig. 1-7). There are several lines of evidence indicating that thrombin initiates the molecular and cellular interactions leading to the formation of neointimal vascular lesions at sites of vascular injury by catalytic activation TRs. First, thrombin mediates vascular thrombosis, as shown by the interruption of vascular thrombogenesis by administering the potent and specific direct antithrombin III hirudin (73–75), TR antagonist (38), or inhibitors of thrombin generation (76–80). Second, thrombin is a potent chemokine and mitogen mediating the intimal migration and proliferation of vascular SMCs (9,81,82). Third, thrombin modulates the effects of other growth factors, including PDGF (83–85). Fourth, thrombin moderates inflammatory responses involving neutrophils, monocytes, and the corresponding endothelial counter receptors (70,86–89). Moreover, neutrophils, monocytes, and endothelium stimulated by other agonists express TR in vitro and in vivo (90). The inhibition of thrombin activity or its production reduces these thrombin-sensitive inflammatory pathways.

CONCLUSION: REGULATION OF THROMBUS FORMATION

In conclusion, vascular damage initiates a localized, amplified, and regulated assembly of localized insoluble thrombus that physiologically prevents excessive blood loss caused by invasive injuries without impairing blood's fluidity. In disease states, the formation of occlusive thrombi or thromboemboli in veins or diseased arteries threatens the viability of dependent tissues. Initial localization is achieved by the focal deposition of platelets. Amplification is dependent on the assembly of highly efficient interactive enzyme–cofactor complexes on the membrane surfaces of deposited cells and is modulated by the expression of membrane binding activity, cofactor activation, and zymogen acti-

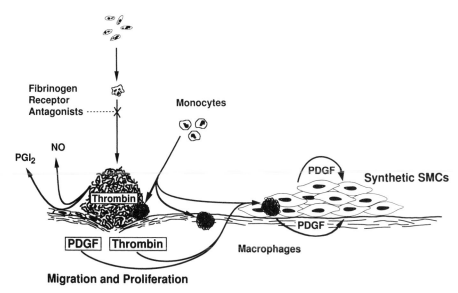

Migration and Proliferation

FIG. 1-7. Neointimal vascular lesion formation. The late vascular healing effects of mechanical or spontaneous vascular disruption involve the catalytic activation of TRs on leukocytes, vascular medial SMCs, endothelium, and other mesenchymal cells. Medial SMCs proliferate and migrate to the intima, leading to SMC intimal proliferation and synthesis of extracellular matrix in the local formation of stenosing neointimal proliferative vascular lesions. Neointimal stenosis complicates all interventional vascular procedures used in the treatment of symptomatic atherosclerotic arterial disease, including angioplasty, atherectomy, endarterectomy, stent deployment, use of indwelling cardiovascular devices and vascular graft implantation. Those factors affecting vascular lesion formation include hemodynamic variables, platelet deposition and secretion of growth factors, thrombin generation, monocyte/macrophage accumulation, autocrine/paracrine growth factor production and secretion by proliferating SMCs or intimal mononuclear leukocytes, and other promoters and inhibitors of cell growth.

vation. Regulation is mediated by (a) inactivation and removal as inhibitor–enzyme complexes, (b) destruction of membrane cofactor activities by APC, (c) thrombin-induced release of antithrombotic products (prostacyclin, nitric oxide, and t-PA), and (d) enhanced fibrinolysis. Resolution proceeds by fibrinolysis and healing. In recent years our understanding of thrombosis and its pathogenesis, detection, evaluation, prevention, and management has greatly expanded (1–3).

REFERENCES

1. Colman RW, Hirsh J, Marder V, Salzman EW. *Hemostasis and Thrombosis: Basic Principles and Clinical Practice.* Philadelphia: Lippincott, 1994.
2. Bloom AL, Thomas DP. *Haemostasis and Thrombosis.* New York: Churchill Livingstone, 1994.
3. Loscalzo J, Schafer AI. *Thrombosis and Hemorrhage.* Boston: Blackwell, 1994;1–1337.
4. Virchow R. Phlogose und Thrombose in Gefass-system. In: Virchow R (ed). *Gesammlte Abhandelungen zur Wissenschaftlichen Medizin.* Frankfurt: von Meidinger Sohn, 1856;458–636.
5. Davies MJ. Mechanisms of thrombosis in atherosclerosis. In: Colman RW, Hirsh J, Marder VJ, Salzman EW (eds). *Hemostasis and Thrombosis.* Philadelphia: Lippincott, 1994;1224–1237.
6. George BS, Voorhees WD III, Roubin GS, et al. Multicenter investigation of coronary stenting to treat acute or threatened closure after percutaneous transluminal coronary angioplasty: clinical and angiographic outcomes. *J Am Coll Cardiol* 1993;22:135–143.
7. Topol EJ, Leya F, Pinkerton CA, et al. CAVEAT Study Group. A comparison of directional atherectomy with coronary angioplasty in patients with coronary artery disease. *N Engl J Med* 1993;329:221–227.
8. King SBI, Lembo NJ, Weintraub WS, et al. Emory angioplasty versus surgery trial (EAST). A randomized

trial comparing coronary angioplasty with coronary bypass surgery. *N Engl J Med* 1994;331:1044–1050.

9. Ross R. The pathogenesis of atherosclerosis: a perspective for the 1990's. *Nature* 1993;362:801–809.

10. Dzau VJ, Gibbons GH, Cooke JP, Omoigui N. Vascular biology and medicine in the 1990s: scope, concepts, potentials, and perspectives [Review]. *Circulation* 1993; 87:705–719.

11. Goldsmith HL, Turitto VT. Rheological aspects of thrombosis and haemostasis: basic principles and applications. *Thromb Haemost* 1986;55:415.

12. Turitto VT, Baumgartner HR. Initial deposition of platelets and fibrin on vascular surfaces in flowing blood. In: Colman RW, Hirsh J, Marder VJ, Salzman EW (eds). *Hemostasis and Thrombosis.* Philadelphia: Lippincott, 1994;805–822.

13. Sevitt S. The structure and growth of valve-pocket thrombi in femoral veins. *J Clin Pathol* 1974;27: 517–528.

14. Hirsh J, Prins MH, Samama M. Approach to the thrombophilic patient for hemostasis and thrombosis: basic principles and clinical practice. In: Colman RW, Hirsh J, Marder VJ, Salzman EW (eds). *Hemostasis and Thrombosis.* Philadelphia: Lippincott, 1994;1543–1561.

15. Dahlback B. Inherited thrombophilia: resistance to activated protein C as a pathogenic factor of venous thromboembolism. *Blood* 1995;85:607–614.

16. Dalen JE, Hirsh J. Fourth ACCP consensus conference on antithrombotic therapy. *Chest* 1995;108(suppl):225–522.

17. Gimbrone MA Jr. *Vascular Endothelium in Hemostasis and Thrombosis.* Edinburgh: Churchill Livingstone, 1986;1–250.

18. Schwartz SM, Majesky MW. Structure and function of the vessel wall. In: Colman RW, Hirsh J, Marder VJ, Salzman EW (eds). *Hemostasis and Thrombosis: Basic Principles and Clinical Practice.* Philadelphia: Lippincott, 1994;705–717.

19. Jaffe EA. Biochemistry, immunology, and cell biology of endothelium. In: Colman RW, Hirsh J, Marder VJ, Salzman EW (eds). *Hemostasis and Thrombosis: Basic Principles and Clinical Practice.* Philadelphia: Lippincott, 1994;718–744.

20. Rosenberg RD, Bauer KA. The heparin-antithrombin system: a natural anticoagulant mechanism. In: Colman RW, Hirsh J, Marder VJ, Salzman EW (eds). *Hemostasis and Thrombosis: Basic Principles and Clinical Practice.* Philadelphia: Lippincott, 1994;837–860.

21. Broze GJ Jr. The tissue factor pathway of coagulation. In: Loscalzo J, Schafer AI (eds). *Thrombosis and Hemorrhage.* Boston: Blackwell, 1994;57–86.

22. Smith JA, Henderson AH, Randall MD. Endothelium-derived relaxing factor, prostanoids and endothelins. In: Bloom AL, Forbes CD, Thomas DP, Tuddenham EGD (eds). *Haemostasis and Thrombosis.* Edinburgh: Churchill Livingstone, 1994;183–197.

23. Collen D, Lijnen HR. Molecular and cellular basis of fibrinolysis. In: Hoffman R, Benz EJ Jr, Shattil SJ, Furie B, Cohen HJ (eds). *Hematology: Basic Principles and Practice.* New York: Churchill Livingstone, 1991; 1232–1242.

24. Shatos M, Orfeo T, Doherty JM, Penar PL, Collen DJ, Mann KG. α-thrombin stimulates urokinase production and DNA synthesis in cultured human cerebral microvascular endothelial cells. *Arterioscler Thromb Vasc Biol* 1995;15:903–911.

25. Bu G, Warshawsky I, Schwartz AL. Cellular receptors for the plasminogen activators. *Blood* 1994;83: 3427–3436.

26. Esmon CT. Molecular events that control the protein C anticoagulant pathway. *Thromb Haemost* 1993;70:29–35.

27. Dahlback B, Stenflo J. A natural anticoagulant pathway: proteins C, S, C4b-binding protein and thrombomodulin. In: Bloom AL, Forbes CD, Thomas DP, Tuddenham EGD (eds). *Haemostasis and Thrombosis.* Edinburgh: Churchill Livingstone, 1994;671–698.

28. Kashiwagi H, Eigenthaler M, Ginsberg MH, Shattil SJ. Affinity modulation of the platelet fibrinogen receptor by ₃-endonexin, a selective binding partner of the ₃ integrin cytoplasmic tail [Abstract]. *Blood* 1996;88:140.

29. Nurden AT. Human platelet membrane glycoproteins. In: Bloom AL, Forbes CD, Thomas DP, Tuddenham EGD (eds). *Haemostasis and Thrombosis.* Edinburgh: Churchill Livingstone, 1994;115–165.

30. Ginsberg MH, Frelinger AL, Lam SC-T. Analysis of platelet aggregation disorders based on flow cytometric analysis of membrane glycoprotein IIb-IIIa with conformation-specific monoclonal antibodies. *Blood* 1990; 76:2017–2023.

31. Ware JA, Coller BS. Platelet morphology, biochemistry, and function. In Beutler E, Lichtman MA, Coller BS, Kipps TJ (eds). *Hematology.* New York: McGraw–Hill, 1995;1161–1201.

32. Cui J, O'Shea KS, Purkayastha A, Saunders TL, Ginsburg D. Fatal hemorrage and incomplete block to embryogenesis in mice lacking coagulation factor V. *Nature* 1996;384:66–68.

33. Vu T-KH, Hung DT, Wheaton VI, Coughlin SR. Molecular cloning of a functional thrombin receptor reveals a novel proteolytic mechanism of receptor activation. *Cell* 1991;64:1057–1068.

34. Coughlin SR, Vu T-KH, Hung DT, Wheaton VI. Characterization of a functional thrombin receptor. Issues and opportunities. *J Clin Invest* 1992;89:351–355.

35. Connolly AJ, Ishihara H, Kahn ML, Farese RV Jr, Coughlin SR. Role of the thrombin receptor in development and evidence for a second receptor. *Nature* 1996; 381:516–519.

36. Ishihara H, Connolly AJ, Zeng D, et al. Protease-activated receptor 3 is a second thrombin receptor in humans. *Nature* 1997;386:502–506.

37. Santulli RJ, Derian CK, Darrow AL, et al. Evidence for the presence of a protease-activated receptor distinct from the thrombin receptor in human keratinocytes. *Proc Natl Acad Sci U S A* 1995;92:9151–9155.

38. Cook JJ, Sitko GR, Bednar B, et al. An antibody against the exosite of the cloned thrombin receptor inhibits experimental arterial thrombosis in the African green monkey. *Circulation* 1995;91:2961–2971.

39. Doolittle RF, Watt KWK, Cottrell BA, Strong DD, Riley M. The amino acid sequence of the α-chain of human fibrinogen. *Nature* 1979;280:464–467.

40. Brass LF. The biochemistry of platelet activation. In: Hoffman R, Benz EJ Jr, Shattil SJ, Furie B, Cohen HJ (eds). *Hematology: Basic Principles and Practice.* New York: Churchill Livingstone, 1991;1176–1197.

41. Mann KG, Nesheim ME, Church WE, Haley P, Krishnaswamy S. Surface-dependent reactions of the vitamin K-dependent enzyme complexes. *Blood* 1990;76:1–16.

42. Bovill EG, Tracy RP, Hayes TE, Jenny RJ, Bhushan FH, Mann KG. Evidence that meizothrombin is an interme-

diate product in the clotting of whole blood. *Arterioscler Thromb Vasc Biol* 1995;15:754–758.

43. Mann KG, Gaffney D, Bovill EG. Molecular biology, biochemistry, and lifespan of plasma coagulation factors. In: Beutler E, Lichtman MA, Coller BS, Kipps TJ (eds). *Hematology*. New York: McGraw–Hill, 1995;1206–1226.

44. Furie B, Furie BC. Molecular and cellular biology of blood coagulation. *N Engl J Med* 1992;326:800–806.

45. Morrissey JH, Fakhrai H, Edgington TS. Molecular cloning of the cDNA for tissue factor, the cellular receptor for the initiation of the coagulation protease cascade. *Cell* 1987;50:129–135.

46. Spicer EK, Horton R, Bloem L. Isolation of cDNA clones coding for human tissue factor: primary structure of the protein and cDNA. *Proc Natl Acad Sci U S A* 1987;84:5148.

47. Krishnaswamy S, Field KA, Edgington TS, Morrissey JH, Mann KG. Role of the membrane surface in the activation of human coagulation factor X. *J Biol Chem* 1992;267:26110–26120.

48. Wilcox JN, Smith KM, Schwartz S, Gordon D. Localization of tissue factor in the normal vessel wall and in the atherosclerotic plaque. *Proc Natl Acad Sci U S A* 1989;86:2839–2843.

49. Tracy PB, Eide LL, Bowie JW, Mann KG. Radioimmunoassay of factor V in human plasma and platelets. *Blood* 1982;60:59–63.

50. Tracy PB, Giles AR, Mann KG, Eide LL, Hoogendoorn H, Rivard GE. Factor V (Quebec): a bleeding diathesis associated with a qualitative platelet factor V deficiency. *J Clin Invest* 1984;74:1221–1228.

51. Nesheim ME, Nichols WL, Cole TL. Isolation and study of an acquired inhibitor of human coagulation factor V. *J Clin Invest* 1986;77:405–415.

52. Lollar P, Parker CG. Subunit structure of thrombin-activated porcine factor VIII. *Biochemistry* 1989;28:666.

53. Mutucumarana VP, Duffy EJ, Lollar P, Johnson AE. The active site of factor IXa is located far above the membrane surface and its conformation is altered upon association with factor VIIIa: a fluorescence study. *J Biol Chem* 1992;267:17012–17021.

54. Brandstetter H, Bauer M, Huber R, Lollar P, Bode W. X-ray structure of clotting factor IXa: active site and module structure related to Xase activity and hemophilia B. *Proc Natl Acad Sci U S A* 1995;92:9796–9800.

55. Weitz JI, Hudoba M, Massel D, Maraganore J, Hirsh J. Clot-bound thrombin is protected from inhibition by heparin-antithrombin III but is susceptible to inactivation by antithrombin III–independent inhibitors. *J Clin Invest* 1990;86:385–391.

56. Van't Veer C, Mann KG. Regulation of tissue factor initiated thrombin generation by the stoichiometric inhibitors tissue factor pathway inhibitor, antithrombin-III, and heparin cofactor II. *J Biol Chem* 1997;272:4367–4377.

57. Van't Veer C, Golden NJ, Kalafatis M, Mann KG. Inhibitory mechanism of the protein C pathway on tissue factor-induced thrombin generation: synergistic effect in combination with tissue factor pathway inhibitor. *J Biol Chem* 1997;12:7983–7994.

58. Rand MD, Lock JB, Van't Veer C, Gaffney DP, Mann KG. Blood clotting in minimally altered whole blood. *Blood* 1997;88:3432–3445.

59. Carmeliet P, Stassen JM, Schoonjans L, et al. Plasminogen activator inhibitor-1 gene-deficient mice: II. Effects on hemostasis, thrombosis and thrombolysis. *J Clin Invest* 1993;92:2756.

60. Carmeliet P, Schoonjans L, Kieckens L, et al. Physiological consequences of loss of plasminogen activator gene function in mice. *Nature* 1994;368:419–424.

61. Pennica D, Holmes WE, Kohr WJ, et al. Cloning and expression of human tissue-type plasminogen activator cDNA in *E. coli. Nature* 1983;301:214–221.

62. Holmes WE, Permica D, Blaber M. Cloning and expression of the gene for prourokinase in *Escherichia coli. Biotechniques* 1985;3:923–929.

63. Coller BS. Platelets and thrombolytic therapy. *N Engl J Med* 1990;322:33–42.

64. Bajzar L, Manuel R, Nesheim ME. Purification and characterization of TAFI, a thrombin-activable fibrinolysis inhibitor. *J Biol Chem* 1995;270:14477–14484.

65. Eaton DL, Malloy BE, Tsai SP, Henzel W, Drayna D. Isolation, molecular cloning, and partial characterization of a novel carboxypeptidase B from human plasma. *J Biol Chem* 1991;266:21833–21838.

66. Hendriks D, Wang W, Scharpe S, Lommaert M, van Sande M. Purification and characterization of a new arginine carboxypeptidase in human serum. *Biochim Biophys Acta* 1990;1034:86–92.

67. Bajzar L. TAFI, or plasma procarboxypeptidase B, couples the coagulation and fibrinolytic cascades through the thrombin-thrombomodulin complex. *J Biol Chem* 1996;271:16603–16608.

68. Fingerle J, Johnson R, Clowes AW, Majesky MW, Reidy MA. Role of platelets in smooth muscle cell proliferation and migration after vascular injury in rat carotid artery. *Proc Natl Acad Sci U S A* 1989;86:8412–8416.

69. Ferns GA, Raines EW, Sprugel KH, Motani AS, Reidy MA, Ross RR. Inhibition of neointimal SMC accumulation after angioplasty by an antibody to PDGF. *Science* 1991;253:1129–1132.

70. Harlan JM. Leukocyte-endothelial interactions. *Blood* 1985;65:513–525.

71. Majesky MW, Reidy MA, Bowen-Pope DF, Hart CE, Wilcox JN, Schwartz SM. PDGF ligand and receptor gene expression during repair of arterial injury. *J Cell Biol* 1990;111:2149–2158.

72. Dobrin PB. *Intimal Hyperplasia*. Austin, TX: RG Landes, 1994;1–355.

73. Hanson SR, Harker LA. Interruption of acute platelet-dependent thrombosis by the synthetic antithrombin D-phenylalanyl-L-prolyl-L-arginyl chloromethylketone. *Proc Natl Acad Sci U S A* 1988;85:3184–3188.

74. Kelly AB, Marzec UM, Krupski W, et al. Hirudin interruption of heparin-resistant arterial thrombus formation in baboons. *Blood* 1991;77:1006–1012.

75. Kelly AB, Maraganore JM, Bourdon P, Hanson SR, Harker LA. Antithrombotic effects of synthetic peptides targeting different functional domains of thrombin. *Proc Natl Acad Sci U S A* 1992;89:6040–6044.

76. Waxman L, Smith DE, Arcuri KE, Vlasuk GP. Tick anticoagulant peptide (TAP) is a novel inhibitor of blood coagulation factor Xa. *Science* 1990;248:593–596.

77. Nutt EM, Jain D, Lenny AB, Schaffer L, Siegl PK, Dunwiddie CT. Purification and characterization of recombinant antistasin: a leech-derived inhibitor of coagulation factor Xa. *Arch Biochem Biophys* 1991;285:37–44.

78. Lindahl AK, Wildgoose P, Lumsden AB, et al. Active site-inhibited factor VIIa blocks tissue factor activity

and prevents arterial thrombus formation in baboons [Abstract]. *Circulation* 1993;88(suppl I):I-417.

79. Jang Y, Guzman LA, Lincoff AM, et al. Influence of blockade at specific levels of the coagulation cascade on restenosis in a rabbit ahterosclerotic femoral artery injury model. *Circulation* 1995;92:3041–3050.

80. Pawashe AB, Golino P, Ambrosio G, et al. A monoclonal antibody against rabbit tissue factor inhibits thrombus formation in stenotic injured rabbit carotid arteries. *Circ Res* 1994;74:56–63.

81. Rosenberg RD. Vascular smooth muscle cell proliferation: basic investigations and new therapeutic approaches [Review]. *Thromb Haemost* 1993;70:10–16.

82. Fager G. Thrombin and proliferation of vascular smooth muscle cells [Review]. *Circ Res* 1995;77:645–650.

83. Okazaki H, Majesky MW, Harker LA, Schwartz SM. Regulation of platelet-derived growth factor ligand and receptor gene expression by α-thrombin in vascular smooth muscle cells. *Circ Res* 1992;71:1285–1293.

84. Vouret-Craviari V, Van Obberghen-Schilling E, Rasmussen UB, Pavirani A, Lecocq J-P, Pouyssegur J. Synthetic α-thrombin receptor peptides activate G protein-coupled signaling pathways but are unable to induce mitogenesis. *Mol Biol Cell* 1992;3:95–102.

85. Wilcox JN, Rodriguez J, Subramanian R, et al. Characterization of thrombin receptor expression during vascular lesion formation. *Circ Res* 1994;75:1029–1038.

86. Geng JG, Bevilacqua MP, Moore KL, et al. Rapid neutrophil adhesion to activated endothelium mediated by GMP-140. *Nature* 1990;343:757–760.

87. Huber AR, Schall TJ, Ellis SE. Thrombin induction of VCAM-1 and Rantes/SIS expression and monocyte invasion in an in vitro model of the vessel wall through a specific endothelial thrombin-receptor, G-protein coupled pathway [Abstract]. *Blood* 1992;80(suppl 1):251.

88. Wilcox JN, Harker LA. Molecular and cellular mechanisms of atherogenesis: studies of human lesions linked with animal modelling. In: Bloom AL, Forbes CD, Thomas DP, Tuddenham EGD (eds). *Haemostasis and Thrombosis*. Edinburgh: Churchill Livingstone, 1994; 1139–1152.

89. Kling D, Fingerle J, Harlan JM, Lobb RR, Lang F. Mononuclear leukocytes invade rabbit arterial intima during thickening formation via CD18- and LVA-4-dependent mechanisms and stimulate smooth muscle migration. *Circ Res* 1995;77:1121–1128.

90. Wilcox JN, Subramanian RR, Runge M, Ellis SE, Huber AR. Synthesis of thrombin receptors by activated neutrophils in vitro and in vivo after denuding vascular injuries [Abstract]. *Circulation* 1993;88(suppl I):I-619.

*Cardiovascular Thrombosis: Thrombocardiology
and Thromboneurology, Second Edition,*
edited by M. Verstraete, V. Fuster, and E. J. Topol,
Lippincott–Raven Publishers, Philadelphia © 1998.

2

Pathogenesis of Thrombosis

Lina Badimon, *Juan Jose Badimon, and *Valentin Fuster

*Cardiovascular Research Center, CSIC Hospital Santa Cruz y San Pablo UAB, 08034 Barcelona,
Spain; and *Cardiovascular Institute, Department of Medicine, Mount Sinai School of Medicine,
New York, New York 10029*

Although coronary thrombotic occlusion causing acute myocardial infarction was suspected at the turn of the century (1,2), only over the last few years have clinical and pathologic observations and experimental investigation led to a better understanding of how a coronary thrombus forms and of its incidence in acute ischemic coronary events. Thrombus is usually found secondary to atherosclerotic plaque disruption in the acute coronary syndromes (3–12). In addition, there is clear evidence indicating that mural thrombosis, also at the site of plaque rupture, is an important mechanism in the progression of atherosclerosis even when symptoms are absent.

MURAL THROMBUS AND THROMBOGENIC RISK FACTORS

Numerous pathologic and angiographic (3–14) and several angioscopic (15–18) reports have documented the presence of intraluminal thrombi both in unstable angina and in acute myocardial infarction. In contrast with the very high incidence of thrombi in acute myocardial infarction, the incidence in unstable angina varied significantly among different studies, related in part to the interval between the onset of symptoms and the angiographic study (19–23). Accordingly, when cardiac catheterization was delayed for weeks, the incidence of thrombi was low; on the other hand, angiography early after the onset of anginal symptoms showed the presence of thrombi in approximately two thirds of cases. Presumably, the thrombus is occlusive at the time of anginal pain and later may become subocclusive and slowly lysed or digested. Local and systemic thrombogenic risk factors at the time of coronary plaque disruption may favor the degree and time length of thrombus deposition and so the different pathologic and clinical syndromes.

Severity of Vessel Wall Damage

To investigate the dynamics of platelet deposition and thrombus formation after vascular damage and to study the influence of various biochemical and physical factors, we developed and characterized a sensitive and specific computer-assisted nuclear scintigraphic method with an extracorporeal perfusion system to study the process of platelet deposition on various degrees of vascular stenosis and injury in both in vitro and in vivo perfusion conditions (24–27) (Fig. 2-1). Exposure of de-endothelialized vessel wall (thus mimicking mild vascular injury) to pig blood at high shear rate (mimicking a stenosed coronary artery) induced platelet deposition to the exposed vessel. The deposition of platelet reached a maximum within 5 to 10 minutes of exposure. However, the thrombi could be dislodged from the substrate by the flowing blood, suggesting that the platelet-rich thrombus was labile. Exposure of fibrillar collagen (thus mimicking a deeper injury into the vessel wall) to blood produced platelet deposition of more than two orders of magnitude greater than on the subendothelium (25). Even at high shear rate, platelet thrombus formed was not dislodged but remained adherent to the surface. Similar experimental quantitative information on the importance of the degree of vascular damage on the degree and stability of thrombus formation has now been documented by varying degrees of stenosis (26,27) and the different components of an atherosclerotic plaque (28).

Foam cell–rich matrix (obtained from fatty streaks), collagen-rich matrix (from sclerotic plaques), collagen-poor matrix without cholesterol crystals (from fibrolipid plaques), atheromatous core with abundant cholesterol crystals (from atheromatous plaques), highly cellular plaque (hyperplastic), and segments of normal intima derived from human aortas at necropsy were comparatively studied (Fig. 2-2). Specimens were mounted in the Badimon chamber placed within an ex vivo extracorporeal perfusion system and exposed to heparinized porcine blood (activated partial thromboplastin time ratio 1.5 ± 0.04) for 5 minutes at high shear rate conditions mimicking medium-grade stenosis. Thrombus was quantitated by measurement of indium-labeled platelets and morphometric analysis. Under similar conditions, substrates were perfused with heparinized human blood (2 IU/ml) in an in vitro system, and thrombus formation was similarly evaluated. Thrombus formation on atheromatous core was up to sixfold greater than on other substrates, including collagen-rich matrix, in both heterologous and homologous systems (Fig. 2-3). Although the atheromatous core had a more irregular exposed surface and thrombus formation tended to increase with increasing roughness, the atheromatous core remained the most thrombogenic substrate when the substrates were normalized by the degree of irregularity as defined by the roughness index. The atheromatous core is the most thrombogenic component of human atherosclerotic plaques; therefore, plaques with a large atheromatous core content are at high risk to lead to acute coronary syndromes after spontaneous or mechanically induced rupture (28). Importantly, exposed thromboplastin or tissue factor (29) seems to significantly contribute to the increased thrombogenicity when deep or severe injury occurs.

Human arterial segments (foam cell–rich, collagen-rich, lipid-rich atherosclerotic lesions, and normal, nonatherosclerotic segments) were exposed to heparinized blood at high shear rate conditions in the Badimon perfusion chamber. The thrombogenicity of the arterial specimens was assessed by ^{111}In-labeled

---

FIG. 2-1. Diagram of the experimental setting **(top and middle)** and the Badimon flow perfusion device **(bottom)**. The longitudinal general external view of the chamber **(A)** and a cross-sectional view **(B)** are depicted.

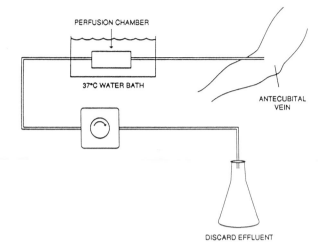

PERFUSION CHAMBER

37°C WATER BATH

ANTECUBITAL VEIN

DISCARD EFFLUENT

PERISTALTIC PUMP

FLOW METER

JUGULAR VEIN

PERFUSION CHAMBER

37°C WATER BATH

CAROTID ARTERY

DRUGS

PERISTALTIC PUMP

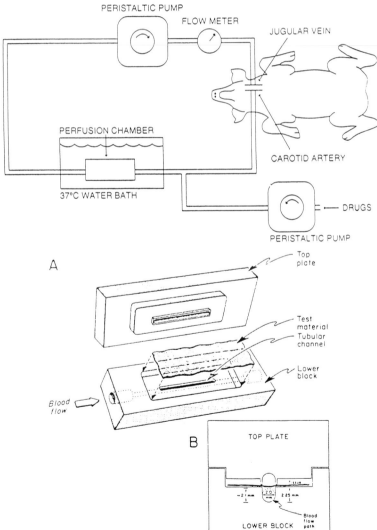

A

Top plate

Test material

Tubular channel

Lower block

Blood flow

B

TOP PLATE

~2.1 mm   2.0 mm   2.25 mm

Blood flow path

LOWER BLOCK

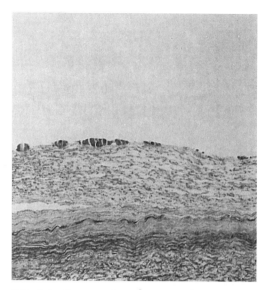 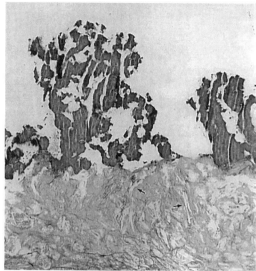

FIG. 2-2. Comparative mural thrombus triggered by a fibrolipid plaque **(left)** and an atheromatous core with cholesterol crystals **(right)** from human aorta perfused in the Badimon perfusion chamber for 5 minutes at a shear rate typical of a medium grade coronary stenosis. (From Fernández-Ortiz et al., ref. 28, with permission.)

platelets. After perfusion, specimens were stained for tissue factor using an in situ binding assay for factor VIIa. Tissue factor in specimens was semiquantitatively assessed on a scale of 0 to 3. Platelet deposition on the lipid-rich atheromatous core was significantly higher than on all other substrates. The lipid-rich core also exhibited the most intense tissue factor staining compared with other arterial components (Fig. 2-4). Comparison of all specimens showed a positive correlation between quantitative platelet deposition and tissue factor staining score. These results show that tissue factor is present in lipid-rich human atherosclerotic plaques and suggest that it is an important determinant of the thrombogenicity of human atherosclerotic lesions after spontaneous or mechanical plaque disruption (29).

Vessel characteristics also regulate fibrin(ogen) deposition kinetics; a significantly different outcome in fibrin(ogen) deposition (^{125}I–fibrinogen) kinetics is observed on mildly and severely damaged vessel wall (30). Fibrin(ogen) deposition to damaged vascular wall was studied at a constant laminar flow typical of unobstructed medium size arteries. Mildly damaged (subendothelial) and severely damaged (below internal elastic lamina) vascular wall were studied as triggers of thrombosis. Fibrin deposition per surface area as well as longitudinal axial dependence of

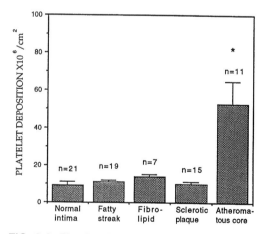

FIG. 2-3. Platelet deposition on human atherosclerotic plaque components evaluated by perfusing blood with radiolabeled platelets. Depicted results were obtained by perfusing citrated human blood for 5 minutes over the substrates (as in Fig. 2-2). (From Fernández-Ortiz et al., ref. 28, with permission.)

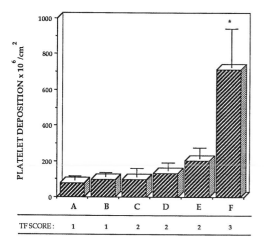

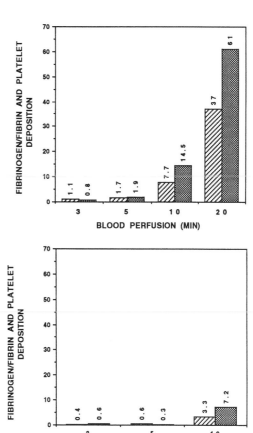

FIG. 2-4. Platelet deposition and tissue factor (TF) activity score. Platelet deposition data are expressed as mean ± SE. TF staining intensity was calculated as the average of scores assigned by the independent observers. Note the positive correlation between platelet thrombus formation and TF score on the exposed human substrates (p < 0.01). *A:* Normal intima. *B:* Collagen-rich matrix. *C:* Foam cell–rich matrix. *D:* Tunica media. *E:* Adventitia. *F:* Lipid-rich core. *p = 0.0002, ANOVA (29).

FIG. 2-5. Fibrin(ogen) (μg/mm^2) *(striped bars)* and platelet (P $\times$ 10^5/mm^2) *(shaded bars)* deposition were measured on severely **(top)** and mildly **(bottom)** injured vessels with 80% stenosis. Deposition was measured up to 20 minutes of blood perfusion. Substrate effects on deposition kinetics are highly significant.

fibrin deposition and its relationship to platelet deposition were studied by segmental analysis of the substrates exposed in the flow chamber placed in an extracorporeal shunt. Autologous ^{111}In-labeled platelets and ^{125}I-labeled fibrinogen (a marker for both fibrinogen and fibrin deposition on the vessel wall) were injected into the pig and studies were performed with nonanticoagulated and heparinized blood (heparin levels = 0.147 IU/ml). Fibrin(ogen) deposition was similar in nonanticoagulated and heparinized bloods in acute perfusions and significantly higher on severely damaged vessels than on mildly damaged vessels (Fig. 2-5). Segmental dependence analysis showed a significant decrease in fibrin(ogen) deposition with distal location on both types of lesions. The ratio of fibrin(ogen) to platelet deposition was similar at all perfusion times on mild injury, whereas on severe injury a higher ratio was found at short perfusion times. That is, fibrin deposition is higher in the thrombus layers closest to

the vessel wall on severe injury. Even under low shear conditions of arterial thrombosis, fibrin deposition and fibrin to platelet ratio are highly dependent on the degree of vascular damage (30).

Overall, it is likely that when injury to the vessel wall is mild, the thrombogenic stimulus is relatively limited, and the resulting thrombotic occlusion is transient, as occurs in unstable angina. On the other hand, deep vessel injury secondary to plaque rupture or ulceration results in exposure of substrates that may lead to relatively persistent thrombotic occlusion and myocardial infarction (11).

Influence of Stenosis

Using the same above-mentioned computer-assisted extracorporeal perfusion system in which the rheology of the blood flow can be controlled and varying degrees of stenosis can be produced on severely damaged vessel wall, it was observed (26,27) that platelet deposition increased significantly with a higher stenosis, indicating a shear-induced cell activation (Fig. 2-6). In addition, analysis of the axial distribution of platelet deposition indicated that the apex, and not the flow recirculation zone distal to the apex, was the segment of greatest platelet accumulation. These data suggest that the severity of the acute platelet response to plaque disruption depends in part on the sudden changes in degree of stenosis following the rupture.

The kinetics of fibrin(ogen) deposition on an arterial thrombus triggered by a damaged stenotic (80%) vessel wall were studied when triggered by mildly (subendothelial) and severely damaged (below the internal elastic lamina) vessel wall. The study was performed in pigs treated with low-dose heparin which was previously shown not to affect platelet deposition (heparin plasma levels, 0.12 IU/ml) and surgically instrumented for carotid artery–jugular vein extracorporeal circulation with ex vivo analysis of the perfused substrates exposed in the flow chamber. Fibrin(ogen) deposition and platelet depositon, were studied using ^{125}I–fibrinogen and ^{111}In platelets. Fibrin(ogen) deposition was significantly higher in stenotic than poststenotic (flow recirculation) areas of severely injured sites, and it was similar (but lower) in stenotic and poststenotic areas of mildly damaged sites. In these mildly damaged vessels, the flow recirculation area had a higher fibrin/platelet ratio than did the apex, whereas for severe injury the ratios were similar in both areas. Therefore, fibrin(ogen) deposition increases over time and is markedly greater in stenotic than poststenotic segments in severely injured sites but not in mildly injured vessels (31).

The effects of an eccentric severe stenosis on fibrin(ogen) deposition on severely damaged vessel wall in relation to platelet deposition were further investigated by our group (32). Fibrin(ogen) and platelet deposition were maximal at the apex of the stenosis, where shear rate is extremely high, and parallel streamlines are deformed (Fig. 2-7). Nevertheless, fibrin(ogen) deposition seems to be significantly less dependent on high shear rate than platelet deposition, and the pattern is not influenced by time. Finally, fibrin(ogen) deposition seems to be predominant in the thrombus layers adjacent to a severely damaged vessel wall, regardless of the local shear stress levels and flow conditions (32). We have studied by immunohistochemistry whether the higher ratio of deposition of fibrin(ogen) over platelets could be observed on the layer closest to the substrate, and a clear layer of fibrin is evident covering the injured severely damaged vessel (33).

Thrombogenicity of Residual Thrombus

Spontaneous lysis of thrombus does occur, not only in unstable angina (34), but also in acute myocardial infarction (35,36). In these patients, as well as in those undergoing thrombolysis for acute infarction, the presence of a residual mural thrombus predisposes to recurrent thrombotic vessel occlusion (37–40). Two main contributing factors for the development of rethrombosis have been identified.

First, a residual mural thrombus may encroach into the vessel lumen, resulting in increased shear rate, which facilitates the activation and deposition of platelets on the lesion. As mentioned previously, using an experimental animal model of ex vivo perfusion, it has been shown that platelet deposition is higher with increasing degrees of vessel stenosis (26,27).

Second, the presence of a fragmented thrombus appears to be one of the most powerful thrombogenic surfaces. This also was evaluated in the ex vivo perfusion model, where platelet deposition was assessed by continuous scintigraphic imaging of ^{111}In-la-

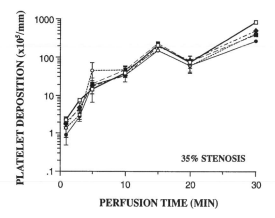

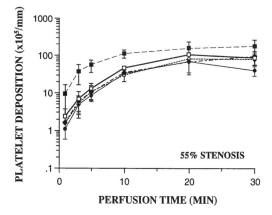

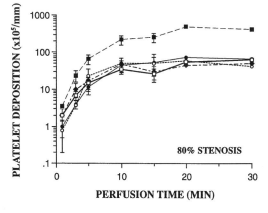

FIG. 2-6. Platelet deposition on severely injured vessel wall with an eccentric 80% stenosis. Maximal deposition occurs at the apex of the stenosis (area 4) and not at the flow recirculation zone next to the apex (areas 5 and 6). Differences in deposition on the apex versus the other areas become significant at stenosis >35%. Areas 2 and 3 correspond to laminar flow zones prestenosis.

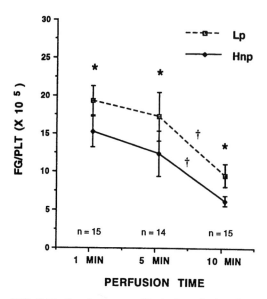

FIG. 2-7. Graph shows effect of perfusion time on fibrin(ogen)/platelet ratio (FG/PLT, $\times 10^5$) at different shear rates and flow conditions (Hnp and Lp). Data are means ± SEM. Hnp indicates high-shear, nonparallel streamlines; Lp indicates low-shear, parallel streamlines. *Significances between Hnp and Lp. †Significances in perfusion time. (From Mailhac et al., ref. 32, with permission.)

beled platelets (27). A gradual increase in platelet deposition in the area of maximal stenosis was observed, followed by an abrupt decrease, probably owing to spontaneous thrombus embolization or platelet disaggregation. This was immediately followed by a rapid increase in platelet deposition, suggesting that the remaining thrombus was markedly thrombogenic. In fact, platelet deposition is increased two to four times on residual thrombus compared with a deeply injured arterial wall (26), and thrombus continues to grow during heparin therapy but is inhibited by r-hirudin, a specific thrombin inhibitor (41,42). Supporting the observations of a highly thrombogenic surface and the role played by thrombin, Fitzgerald and Fitzgerald (43) reported that the reocclusion of a recanalized artery in a canine model of coronary thrombolysis was mainly related to the high local thrombin activity on the surface of the fragmented thrombus. Indeed, in vitro,

when thrombus breaks, the thrombin bound to fibrin becomes exposed (44).

Because residual mural thrombus on a severely damaged arterial wall is very thrombogenic, we tested the hypothesis that direct thrombin inhibition would block thrombus growth on fresh thrombus better than indirect thrombin inhibition, cyclooxygenase inhibition, or both (45). A fresh mural thrombus was formed by directly perfusing blood for 5 minutes over a severely damaged arterial wall at a high shear rate, mimicking stenotic conditions in the perfusion system. The average platelet and fibrinogen deposition achieved in 5 minutes over the triggering vessel was recorded and the thrombus secondary growth on the performed mural thrombus was quantitated separately. Treatment included recombinant hirudin as a probe for thrombin, aspirin as a platelet inhibitor of cyclooxygenase, in two doses as an indirect thrombin inhibitor, and heparin plus aspirin. Thrombus growth was mildly but not significantly reduced by aspirin compared with baseline. Inhibition of thrombus growth with heparin was dose dependent. A regression analysis showed an inverse correlation of platelet fibrinogen deposition with mean plasma heparin concentrations. Recombinant hirudin led to a profound inhibition of secondary thrombus growth, which was significant compared with all groups, even the highest dosage of heparin. Specific thrombin inhibition markedly inhibited platelet and fibrinogen deposition onto fresh mural thrombus at high shear rate. Aspirin alone or in combination with heparin had little effect on evolving thrombosis. Heparin dose dependently reduced thrombus growth, but even the highest dosage was less effective than hirudin. Thrombin appeared to be the primary agonist for platelets in thrombus growth on preformed thrombi (45).

Thus, after lysis of thrombus, thrombin may become exposed to the circulating blood, leading to platelet and clotting activation, and further thrombosis. The antithrombin activity of heparin is limited for three main reasons (42–46) First, a residual thrombus contains active thrombin bound to fibrin, which is thus poorly accessible to the heparin–antithrombin III complexes; second, a platelet-rich arterial thrombus releases large amounts of platelet factor 4, which inhibits heparin; third, fibrin II monomer, formed by the action of thrombin on fibrinogen, also inhibits heparin. Conversely, molecules of hirudin and other specific antithrombins are at least 10 times smaller than the heparin–antithrombin III complex, have no natural inhibitors, and therefore have greater accessibility to thrombin bound to fibrin. Finally, aside from the clot itself being the source for active thrombin, recent studies have suggested that platelet or thrombin activity is enhanced by the effects of the thrombolytic agents themselves (i.e., plasmin). These observations were based on the presence of increased plasma and urinary metabolites of thromboxane A_2 (47), an increase in fibrinopeptide A (48), which results from the action of thrombin on fibrinogen, and, most importantly, an increase in thrombin–antithrombin III complexes.

These experimental results clarify the clinical observations in patients with acute myocardial infarction undergoing thrombolysis, which have shown that residual stenosis is in part related to residual nonlysed thrombus (49–51). Such residual stenosis or intracoronary thrombi are associated with an increased risk of thrombotic reocclusion.

Systemic Thrombogenic Risk Factors

Focal thrombosis may lead to a local hypercoagulable or thrombogenic state of the circulation that may favor progression or recurrence of the thrombi. In addition, there is increasing experimental and clinical evidence that a primary hypercoagulable or thrombogenic state of the circulation exists that can favor focal thrombosis. Thus, experimentally, platelet aggregation and the generation of thrombin may be activated by circulating catecholamines (52,53); this interrelationship could be of importance in humans because it may be a link between conditions of emotional stress or circadian variation (early morning hours) (54) with catecholamine ef-

fects (55–57) and the development of myocardial infarction. Of importance is the increasing evidence of enhanced platelet reactivity in cigarette smokers (58,59), which may or may not be related to catecholamine stimulus (60); indeed, in agreement with the thrombogenic role of cigarette smoking, after discontinuation of smoking it has been observed that there is a sharp decrease in acute vascular events most often associated with thrombosis (61–63).

Of no less importance is the increasing clinical and experimental evidence of hypercoagulability (fibrinogen, factor VII, von Willebrand factor [vWF], and reduced fibrinolysis) in patients with progressive coronary disease (64) and of enhanced platelet reactivity at the site of vascular damage in experimental hypercholesterolemia (65), which supports previous clinical observations (66,67); in addition, enhanced platelet reactivity also has been documented in young patients with a strong family history of coronary disease, related or not to hyperlipidemia (59). Within this context of metabolic abnormalities in young patients with coronary disease, high plasma levels of homocysteine after methionine loading and of lipoprotein(a) are also beginning to be identified as powerful thrombogenic risk factors. Homocystinemia in its heterozygous trait is now being identified as an important risk factor for atherosclerotic disease in young individuals with a strong family history of coronary disease (68,69). Lipoprotein(a), which is very similar to low-density lipoproteins in its configuration (70), has been shown to be an important risk factor for ischemic heart disease, presumably for thrombotic occlusion and particularly in familial hypercholesterolemia (71,72).

A deficient fibrinolysis also may be considered as a thrombogenic risk factor in coronary disease patients. One of the parameters of the fibrinolytic system is plasminogen activator inhibitor-1 (PAI-1); some studies suggest high levels of PAI-1 as a risk factor for ischemic heart disease (73,74) and myocardial infarction (75,76). Finally, aside from the possibility that true defective fibrinolysis with high PAI-1 levels is a thrombogenic risk factor, other hemostatic parameters, specifically fibrinogen, vWF, and factor VII levels, also have been clearly involved (77–79).

PATHOPHYSIOLOGY OF THROMBUS FORMATION

In the initial stages of endothelial injury, with functional alterations but without major morphologic changes, no significant platelet deposition or thrombus formation can be demonstrated. A few scattered platelets may interact with such subtly injured endothelium and contribute, by the release of growth factors, to very mild intimal hyperplasia. In contrast, with endothelial denudation and mild intimal injury, one to a few layers of platelets may deposit on the lesion, with or without mural thrombus formation. The release of platelet growth factors may contribute significantly to an accelerated intimal hyperplasia as it occurs in the coronary vein graft within the first postoperative year. In severe injury, with exposure of components of deeper layers of the vessel, as in spontaneous plaque rupture or in angioplasty, marked platelet aggregation with mural thrombus formation follows. Vascular injury of this magnitude also stimulates thrombin formation through both the intrinsic (surface-activated) and extrinsic (tissue factor–dependent) coagulation pathways, in which the platelet membrane facilitates interactions between clotting factors. This concept of vascular injury as a trigger of the platelet coagulation response is important in understanding the pathogenesis of various vascular diseases associated with atherosclerosis and coronary artery disease (80,81).

Growing thrombi may locally occlude the arterial lumen, or embolize and be washed away by the blood flow to occlude distal vessels. However, thrombi may be physiologically and spontaneously lysed by mechanisms that block thrombus propagation. Thrombus size, location, and composition is regulated by hemodynamic forces (mechanical effects), thrombogenicity of exposed substrate (local molecular effects), relative concentration of fluid phase and cellular blood components (local cellular effects), and the efficiency of the physiologic mechanisms of control of the system, mainly fibrinolysis (82,83).

Platelet Activation

Exposed collagen from the vessel wall and thrombin generated by the activation of the coagulation cascade as well as circulating agonists may be powerful platelet activators.

Most platelet aggregation agonists seem to act through the hydrolysis of platelet membrane phosphatidylinositol by phospholipase C, which results in the mobilization of free calcium from the platelet-dense tubular system. Exposed matrix from the vessel wall and thrombin generated by the activation of the coagulation cascade as well as circulating epinephrine are powerful platelet agonists. Adenosine diphosphate (ADP) is a platelet agonist that may be released from hemolyzed red cells in the area of vessel injury. Each agonist stimulates the discharge of calcium from the platelet-dense tubular system and promotes the contraction of the platelet, with the subsequent release of its granule contents. Platelet-released ADP and serotonin stimulate adjacent platelets, further enhancing the process of platelet activation. Arachidonic acid (AA), which is released from the platelet membrane by the stimulatory effect of collagen, thrombin, ADP, and serotonin, is another platelet agonist. AA is converted to thromboxane A_2 by the sequential effects of cyclooxygenase and thromboxane synthase. Thromboxane A_2 not only promotes further platelet aggregation, but is also a potent vasoconstrictor (Fig. 2-8).

Signal transduction mechanisms initiated upon binding of agonists to membrane-spanning receptors on the platelet surface have been partially elucidated (84). Agonist binding triggers cascades of intracellular second messengers, including inositol 1,4,5-triphosphate (IP_3) and diacylglycerol (DG). IP_3 releases Ca^{2+} from the platelet dense tubular system, raising the cytosolic free Ca^{2+} con-

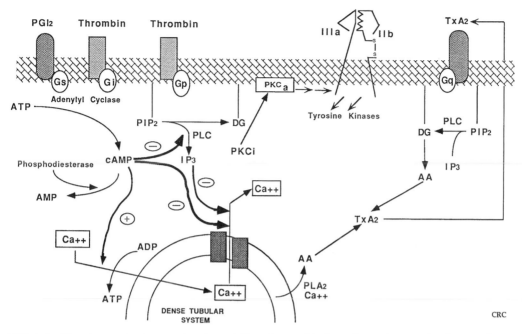

FIG. 2-8. Signal transduction mechanisms initiated upon binding of agonists to platelet membrane receptors. Binding activates G proteins and triggers intracellular second messengers (IP$_3$, DG). The final outcome is the activation of platelet secretion, IIb/IIIa receptor exposure, and aggregation. PGI$_2$, prostacyclin; TxA$_2$, thromboxane A$_2$; PIP$_2$, phosphoinositol diphosphate; PLC, phospholipase C; PKC and PKCa, protein kinase C inactivated and activated, respectively; DG, diacylglycerol; IP$_3$, inositol 1,4,5-triphosphate; AA, arachidonic acid; PLA$_2$, phospholipase A$_2$; Gs, Gi, Gp, Gq, guanine nucleotide-binding regulatory proteins; IIb/IIIa, glycoprotein receptor for adhesive ligands, which supports platelet aggregation.

centration. DG activates the serine/threonine kinase protein kinase C, translocating it to the plasma membrane and triggering granule secretion and fibrinogen receptor exposure (glycoprotein [GP]IIb–IIIa complex). At the same time, the rising cytosolic free Ca^{2+} concentration facilitates AA release from phospholipids by phospholipase A$_2$, a process that may occur at both the plasma membrane and the dense tubular system membrane. AA is metabolized to thromboxane A$_2$ (TxA$_2$), which diffuses out of the cell, interacts with receptors on the platelet surface, and causes further platelet activation. At some point during this process, tyrosine kinases, including members of the src (protein product of the first retroviral oncogene discovered, v-*src*, which causes sarcoma) family of nonreceptor protein tyrosine kinases, are activated in platelets and cause the phosphorylation on tyrosine of multiple

platelet proteins, most of which have not been identified. Tyrosine kinase activation in platelets appears to occur predominantly as a consequence of fibrinogen receptor expression and platelet aggregation, but can also occur as an early step in platelet activation. In many cases, the interactions between agonists and the enzymes responsible for second messenger generation are mediated by a guanine nucleotide-binding regulatory protein (G protein). In platelets, G proteins have been shown to regulate phosphoinositide hydrolysis and cyclic adenosine monophosphate formation, and are probably involved in the activation of phospholipase A$_2$. Phospholipase C (presumably phospholipase C$_b$) is activated in a pertussis toxin–sensitive manner by the still unidentified G protein G$_p$, as well as in a pertussis toxin-resistant manner by the G protein G$_q$. Adenylylcyclase is stimulated by the G protein G_s and inhibited by the G protein G_i. The G protein that regulates phospholipase A_2 activity remains to be characterized. Platelet receptors for thrombin, epinephrine, thromboxane A_2, and platelet activating factor have been cloned and shown to resemble other G protein–coupled receptors with a characteristic structure composed of a single polypeptide with seven transmembrane domains. The low molecular weight guanosine triphosphate (GTP)-binding protein rap1B has recently been shown to form a complex with phospholipase C_g and ras-GAP, supplying a potential mechanism for regulating phospholipase C_g activity. Other low molecular weight GTP-binding proteins may be involved in the regulation of vesicular transport and granule secretion in platelets (84–86).

The initial recognition of damaged vessel wall by platelets involve (a) adhesion, activation, and adherence to recognition sites on the thromboactive substrate (extracellular matrix proteins; e.g., vWF, collagen, fibronectin, vitronectin, laminin); (b) spreading of the platelet on the surface; and (c) aggregation with each other to form a platelet plug or white thrombus. The efficiency of the platelet recruitment depends on the underlying substrate and local geometry. A final step of recruitment of other blood cells also occurs; erythrocytes, neutrophils, and occasionally monocytes are found on evolving mixed thrombus (Fig. 2-9).

Platelet function depends on adhesive interactions and most of the glycoproteins on the platelet membrane surface are receptors for adhesive proteins. Many of these receptors have been identified, cloned, sequenced, and classified within large gene families that mediate a variety of cellular interactions (87,88) (Table 2-1). The most abundant is the integrin family, which includes GPIIb–IIIa, GPIa–IIa, GPIc–IIa, the fibronectin receptor, and the vitronectin receptor, in decreasing order of magnitude. Another gene family present in the platelet membrane glycocalix is the leucine-rich glycoprotein family represented by the GPIb–IX complex, receptor for vWF on unstimulated platelets that mediates adhe-

sion to subendothelium and glycoprotein V (GPV). Other gene families include the selectins (such as GMP-140) and the immunoglobulin domain protein (HLA class I antigen and cell adhesion molecule–related platelet endothelial cell adhesion molecule-1 [PECAM-1]). Unrelated to any other gene family is the GPIV (IIIa) (87) (Table 2-1).

The GPIb–IX complex consists of two disulfide-linked subunits (GPIbα and GPIbβ) tightly (not covalently) complexed with GPIX in a 1:1 heterodimer. GPIbβ and GPIX are transmembrane glycoproteins and form the larger globular domain. The elongated, protruding part of the receptor corresponds to GPIbα. The major role of GPIb–IX is to bind immobilized vWF on the exposed vascular subendothelium and initiate adhesion of platelets. GPIb does not bind soluble vWF in plasma; apparently it undergoes a conformational change upon binding to the extracellular matrix and then exposes a recognition sequence for GPIb–IX. The vWF binding domain of GPIb–IX has been narrowed to amino acids 251 to 279 on GPIbα (89). The GPIbα binding domain of vWF resides in a tryptic fragment extending from residue 449 to 728 of the subunit that does not contain an RGD-sequence (Arg-Gly-Asp) (90). The cytoplasmic domain of GPIb–IX has a major function in linking the plasma membrane to the intracellular actin filaments of the cytoskeleton and functions to stabilize the membrane and to maintain the platelet shape (91,92).

Randomly distributed on the surface of resting platelets are about 50,000 molecules of GPIIb–IIIa. The complex is composed of one molecule of GPIIb (disulfide-linked large and light chains) and one of GPIIIa (single polypeptide chain). It is a Ca^{2+} dependent heterodimer, noncovalently associated on the platelet membrane (93). Calcium is required for maintenance of the complex and for binding of adhesive proteins. On activated platelets, the GPIIb–IIIa is a receptor for fibrinogen, fibronectin, vWF, vitronectin, and thrombospondin (94). The receptor recognition sequences are localized to small peptide sequences (Arg-Gly-Asp [RGD]) in the adhe-

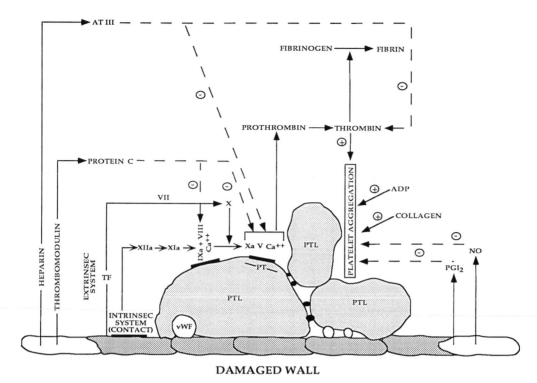

FIG. 2-9. Simplified diagram of platelet-vessel wall, platelet-platelet interaction and coagulation enzymes. Platelet adhesion to recognition sites occurs in lesioned areas of the endothelium. Adhesion spreading and aggregation of newly arriving platelets contributes to mural thrombosis. Aggregation is enhanced by agonists present in the microenvironment *(arrows with + signs)*, whereas there are spontaneous pathways of inhibition *(arrows with − signs)* derived from neighboring normal endothelium (TF, tissue factor; AT III, antithrombin III; NO, nitric oxide; PT, prothrombinase complex; vWF, von Willebrand factor).

sive proteins (95). Fibrinogen contains two RGD sequences in its α chain, one near the N-terminus (residues 95 to 97) and a second near the C-terminus (residues 572 to 574) (96). Fibrinogen has a second site of recognition for GPIIb–IIIa that is the 12–amino acid sequence located at the carboxyl-terminus of the γ chain of the molecule (97). This dodecapeptide is specific for fibrinogen and does not contain the RGD sequence, but competes with RGD-containing peptides for binding to GPIIb–IIIa (87,98,99).

TABLE 2-1. *Platelet membrane glycoprotein receptors*

Glycoprotein receptor	Ligand	Function
GPIIb–IIIa ($\alpha IIb\beta_3$)	Fg, vWF, Fn, Ts, Vn	Aggregation, adhesion at high shear rate
Receptor Vn ($\alpha_v\beta_3$)	Vn, vWF, Fn, Fg, Ts	Adhesion
GPIa–IIa (VLA-2, $\alpha_2\beta_1$)	C	Adhesion
GPIc–IIa (VLA-5, $\alpha_5\beta_1$)	Fn	Adhesion
GPIc′–IIa (VLA-6, $\alpha_6\beta_1$)	Ln	Adhesion
GPIb–IX	vWF, T	Adhesion
GPV	Substrate T	Unknown
GPIV (GPIIIB)	Ts, C	Adhesion
GMP-140 (PADGEM)	Unknown	Interaction with leukocytes
PECAM-1 (GPIIa)	Unknown	Unknown

Fg, fibrinogen; Fn, fibronectin; Ts, thrombospondin; Vn, vitronectin; C, collagen; Ln, laminin; T, thrombin.

Thrombin plays an important role in the pathogenesis of arterial thrombosis. It is one of the most potent known agonists for platelet activation and recruitment. The thrombin receptor has 425 amino acids with seven-trans-membrane domains and a large NH_2-terminal extracellular extension that is cleavaged by thrombin to produce a "tethered" ligand that activates the receptor to initiate signal transduction (100,101). Thrombin is a critical enzyme in early thrombus formation, it cleaves fibrinopeptide A and B from fibrinogen to yield insoluble fibrin which effectively anchors the evolving thrombus. Both free and fibrin-bound thrombin are able to convert fibrinogen to fibrin, allowing propagation of thrombus at the site of injury.

Therefore, platelet activation triggers intracellular signaling and expression of platelet membrane receptors for adhesion and initiation of cell contractile processes that will induce platelet shape change and secretion of the granular contents. The expression of the integrin IIb–IIIa ($\alpha IIb\beta_3$) receptors for adhesive glycoprotein ligands (mainly fibrinogen and vWF) in the circulation initiate platelet-to-platelet interaction. The process is perpetuated by the arrival of passing platelets. Most of the glycoproteins in the platelet membrane surface are receptors for adhesive proteins or mediate cellular interactions.

The receptor-mediated mechanisms related to platelet interaction in the thrombotic process around a vascular stenosis have not been directly studied as yet; however, in laminar parallel flow conditions, platelet glycoprotein Ib is necessary for normal platelet adhesion to subendothelium at high shear rates (102,103), through its interaction with vWF (103,104). vWF has been shown to bind to platelet membrane glycoproteins in both adhesion (platelet–substrate interaction) and aggregation (platelet–platelet interaction), leading to thrombus formation in perfusion studies conducted at high shear rates (102,105–109). The present consensus is that, at high shear rate conditions, platelet glycoproteins Ib and IIb–IIIa both appear to be involved in the events of platelet adhesion, whereas glycoprotein IIb–IIIa may be involved predominantly in platelet–platelet interaction. The specific plasma proteins that are predominantly involved in platelet–platelet interactions under various shear conditions and triggering atherosclerotic substrates remain to be determined. The absence of platelet aggregation in thrombasthenia (observed using low shear and nonflow systems) has been ascribed to the inability of platelets to bind fibrinogen because platelets are known to require fibrinogen for aggregation in plasma or buffer; however, this requirement is not absolute. In perfusion studies, platelet attachment or aggregate build-up (thrombus formation) on subendothelium was shown to be normal in afibrinogenemia under a wide variety of shear conditions (103,110). Antibodies to fibrinogen, even when added to afibrinogenemic blood in order to remove any small trace of residual fibrinogen, did not inhibit platelet interaction with the vessel wall (111), although they did reduce aggregation with ADP and collagen when tested in an aggregometer.

Blocking the glycoprotein IIb–IIIa receptor site on platelets with either an antibody (LJ-CP8) that blocks the general binding of adhesive proteins or with various peptides that simulate the sequence Arg-Gly-Asp (RGD) inhibits both platelet adhesion and thrombus formation in flowing blood at high shear rates. These findings reinforce the importance of the glycoprotein IIb–IIIa site in platelet–vessel wall interaction and suggest that fibrinogen is not always a necessary component for such interactions. Moreover, diverse studies have demonstrated the relative low importance of fibrinogen in favor of vWF in both platelet–platelet and platelet–vessel wall interactions at certain rheologic conditions (112). Pigs that have normal fibrinogen levels but are congenitally deficient in vWF showed a significantly reduced ability to deposit platelets in subendothelium, severely damaged vessel walls, and collagen type I bundles using a variety of in vivo and in vitro perfusion conditions at high and low local shear rates in native (nonanticoagulated) and anticoagulated blood (112).

The use of platelet biologic response modifiers has reached the clinical arena. The monoclonal antibody 7E3 anti GPIIb–IIIa has shown clinical benefits in blocking platelet function in diverse trials (113–115). The field is rapidly evolving, and new molecules—peptide-mimetics or nonpeptide mimetics—have been introduced and are in their clinical development phase (116). Development of oral IIb–IIIa antagonists that may overcome the inconveniences of intravenous delivery are also in progress (117). However, more research is needed to ascertain the basic mechanisms of platelet receptor function and thrombus formation to be able to properly target medication.

Activation of the Coagulation System

During plaque rupture, in addition to platelet deposition in the injured area, the clotting mechanism is activated by the exposure of the de-endothelialized vascular surface and the release of tissue factor. The activation of the coagulation cascade leads to the generation of thrombin which, as mentioned before, is a powerful platelet activator that also catalyzes the formation and polymerization of fibrin. Fibrin is essential in the stabilization of the platelet thrombus and allows it to resist removal by high intravascular pressure and shear rate. These basic concepts have clinical relevance in the context of the acute coronary syndromes where plaque rupture exposes components, which activates platelets and the coagulation system and results in the formation of a fixed and occlusive platelet-fibrin thrombus.

The efficacy of fibrinolytic agents pointedly demonstrates the importance of fibrin-related material in the thrombosis associated with myocardial infarction (118). It is quite plausible to suspect that flow may have direct effects on certain enzyme or polymerization kinetics involved in thrombosis, in addition to the well-defined effect that flow has in enhancing transport of reactants and products to and from the vessel wall (119). Such effects of flow on immobilized enzymes have

been observed occasionally but never have been studied with respect to coagulative processes (120). The influence of flow on procoagulant activity both in laminar or nonparallel streamline conditions has been described before (30–32). We have shown that under the same blood conditions, local fibrin formation on the damaged vessel wall is dependent on the severity of the damage. The exposure of deep layers of the vessel wall to blood will stimulate local fibrin formation even in the presence of heparin (1 to 2 IU heparin/ml plasma) (121).

MURAL THROMBUS AND ITS CONTRIBUTION TO THE PROGRESSION OF ATHEROSCLEROSIS

After plaque rupture or vascular damage, it has been postulated that platelets, releasing platelet-derived growth factor (PDGF) and other mitogenic factors, play a role in the myofibrotic response of atherosclerosis (80,82). Pigs with homozygous von Willebrand's disease have shown a reduced tendency to develop thrombosis as well as resistance to atherosclerosis (112). In the pig and rat model of carotid balloon injury models, three phases in the process of myofibrosis have been distinguished (122–124). Phase 1 is characterized by platelet deposition, which occurs within minutes and reaches a stable state within 24 hours. At approximately 24 hours, smooth muscle cell proliferation in the media, as detected by increased DNA synthesis, begins. Phase 2 is characterized by the onset of smooth muscle cell migration from the media to the intima and is initiated at approximately day 4; smooth muscle cells continue to migrate and then to proliferate up until day 14, at which point the cell population number has reached its maximum. During phase 3 (day 14 to 3 months) intimal thickening progresses, but this progression is due entirely to accumulation of extracellular matrix, which contributes to the fibrotic organization and configuration of the thrombi (Fig. 2-10).

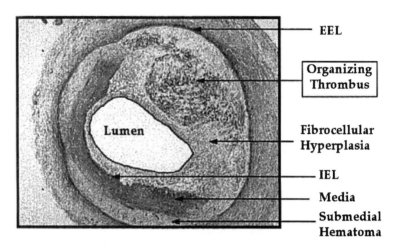

EEL

Organizing
Thrombus

Fibrocellular
Hyperplasia

IEL

Media

Submedial
Hematoma

Lumen

FIG. 2-10. Postangioplasty specimen (28 days). Vascular lesion developed 28 days after coronary angioplasty in the porcine model (Mason's trichrome staining).

Because the initiation of medial smooth muscle proliferation occurs within hours of platelet deposition at the site of injury, it has been suspected that the primary role of the platelet is the induction of such medial smooth muscle cell replication. Platelets have been considered important in the formation of vascular lesions in that they stimulate cell migration into the intima. That is, platelets may induce smooth muscle migration by secreting PDGF, which is known to have chemotactic as well as mitogenic activities (125). Thus, it is reasonable to think that PDGF released at the luminal surface by platelets would better establish the concentration gradient necessary to direct movement of smooth muscle cells from the media to the intima. As in the early medial smooth muscle cell proliferation, smooth muscle cells (after their migration to the intima) may be involved in a non–platelet-dependent autocrine pathway of intimal proliferation. It has been demonstrated that there is a tenfold increase in the production of PDGF-like proteins by smooth muscle cells isolated from arterial intima 2 weeks after balloon injury, compared with cells derived from noninjured media (126). In addition, using the sensitive technique of in situ hybridization, Wilcox et al. (127) demonstrated the presence of PDGF messenger RNA in mesenchymal-appearing cells localized within thrombus material undergoing fibrotic organization at the surface of human carotid plaques removed by endarterectomy. Furthermore, this capacity to produce endogenous, potentially self-stimulating growth factors has been demonstrated in smooth muscle cells isolated from atheroma (128).

The above-mentioned non–platelet-dependent early medial and late intimal smooth muscle cell proliferative response and other stages of the myofibrotic reaction can be related in part to the original thrombus, specifically, to the enzyme thrombin. This experimental evidence suggests that alphathrombin, which has a central bioregulatory function in hemostasis and is generated at high concentrations during blood clotting, is able to bind specifically to the subendothelial extracellular matrix where it remains functionally active, localized, and protected from inactivation by its major circulating inhibitor, antithrombin III (129). Incorporated in the extracellular matrix or into clots (130), thrombin may be released gradually in active form during spontaneous fibrinolysis, or during the stages of thrombus organization. Surface-bound fibrin in particular may act as a reservoir for enzymatically active thrombin (130,131). A reservoir of slowly released thrombin, with its known ability to bind to platelet membrane receptors and produce platelet activation, may help explain how, after significant vascular damage, platelets come to be involved in the relatively delayed process of smooth muscle cell migration. In addition, adjunctive to autocrine or self-stimulating processes, such thrombin–platelet interaction may play a role in the subsequent intimal smooth muscle proliferation. In addition, thrombin has been shown to be a potent activator of multiple growth-related signals in smooth muscle cells, including the expression of the c-*fos* oncogene, which may be related to the significant increase in protein synthesis and hypertrophy (132). Such hypertrophy of the smooth muscle cells may be important in the early stages of medial smooth muscle cell activation, but most importantly may be one of the triggers for the synthesis and secretion of the late intimal extracellular matrix of thrombus organization. In fact, such formation of fibrous tissue in the arteries contributes significantly to the composition of the growing atherosclerotic plaques (133). The elements that make up this fibrous tissue are collagen, proteoglycans, elastin, and glycoproteins.

Disruption of small atherosclerotic plaques, with subsequent mural thrombosis and fibrotic organization of the thrombus, seems to contribute to the progression of atherosclerosis. Although at the present time it is unknown how prevalent this process is, it has potential clinical significance because of its possible inhibition.

ARTERIAL THROMBOSIS: A COMPLICATION OF ATHEROSCLEROTIC VASCULAR DISEASE

Atherosclerotic disease in the coronary artery system may manifest in the form of stable or unstable angina, acute myocardial infarction, or sudden cardiac death. Atherosclerotic disease in the cerebral arterial system (including the intracranial and extracranial arteries) can manifest in the form of transient ischemic attack (TIA) and cerebral ischemic infarction. In contrast to that of acute coronary syndromes, the pathophysiologic process leading to acute cerebral ischemia is less well

defined but appears to involve multiple etiologic mechanisms. Atherosclerotic disease of the abdominal or leg arteries can result in acute and chronic ischemia of the extremities and usually involves thrombosis or embolism or both originating from atherosclerotic plaques. Later chapters address thrombosis and its treatment in the acute coronary syndromes, thrombosis in cerebrovascular disease, thrombosis in peripheral arterial disease, and thrombosis in the cardiac chambers.

VENOUS THROMBOSIS

Although arterial thrombi are predominantly formed by platelets, venous thrombi are intravascular deposits composed predominantly of fibrin and red cells, with a variable platelet and leukocyte component (134). These thrombi usually form in regions of slow or disturbed flow and begin as small deposits that frequently arise in large venous sinuses in the calf, in valve cusp pockets either in the deep veins of the calf or thigh, or in venous segments that have been exposed to direct trauma. The major predisposing factors to venous thrombosis are activation of blood coagulation and venous stasis, whereas vascular wall damage is much less important than in arterial thrombosis. Nevertheless, wall damage may predispose to venous thrombosis in special circumstances. Venous thrombosis and its pathogenesis and clinical complications are addressed in later chapters.

CONCLUSION

There is clear evidence indicating that mural thrombosis, at the site of atherosclerotic plaque disruption, is an important mechanism in the onset of acute coronary syndromes and progression of atherosclerotic disease.

Platelet–vessel wall interactions and thrombus formation are modulated by the interplay of vascular factors, systemic factors, and local rheology. Vascular factors are related to the severity of the arterial injury and the nature of the exposed substrate (lipid versus collagen-rich plaques, residual thrombus, etc.). Among the systemic factors, we should include hyperlipidemia, Lp(a), catecholamine levels, smoking, and diabetes, as well as prothrombotic states (fibrinogen, vWF, factor VII plasma levels) and poor fibrinolytic states. When blood flows over disrupted plaques at high shear rate conditions (i.e., stenosed arteries), the thrombus formed is always larger and more stable than those formed at low shear rate conditions (i.e., patent arteries).

Platelet activation and aggregation are associated with the release of PDGF and other mitogenic factors. Thus, it is reasonable to think that the acute mural thrombus formed after native plaque disruption and coronary interventions, by releasing platelet-PDGF, may contribute to the activation and migration of medial smooth muscle cells, organization of the native thrombus, and restenosis after angioplasty.

REFERENCES

1. Herrick JB. Clinical features of sudden obstruction of the coronary arteries. *JAMA* 1912;59:2015–2020.
2. Benson RL. The present status of coronary arterial disease. *Arch Pathol* 1926;2:876–916.
3. Constantinides P. Plaque fissures in human coronary thrombosis. *J Atheroscler Res* 1966;6I:1–17.
4. DeWood MA, Spores J, Notske R, et al. Prevalence of total coronary occlusion during the early hours of transmural myocardial infarction. *N Engl J Med* 1980;303:897–902.
5. DeWood MA, Stifter WF, Simpson CA, et al. Coronary arteriographic findings soon after non-Q wave myocardial infarction. *N Engl J Med* 1986;315:417–423.
6. Falk E. Plaque rupture with severe pre-existing stenosis precipitating coronary thrombosis. Characteristics of coronary atherosclerotic plaques underlying fatal occlusive thrombi. *Br Heart J* 1983;50:127–134.
7. Falk E. Morphologic features of unstable atherothrombotic plaques underlying acute coronary syndromes. *Am J Cardiol* 1989;63:1114E–1120E.
8. Falk E. Unstable angina with fatal outcome, dynamic coronary thrombosis leading to infarction and/or sudden death: autopsy evidence of recurrent mural thrombosis with peripheral embolization culminating in total vascular occlusion. *Circulation* 1985;71:699–708.
9. Richardson PD, Davies MJ, Born GVR. Influence of plaque configuration and stress distribution on fissuring of coronary atherosclerotic plaques. *Lancet* 1989;2:941–944.
10. Davies MJ, Bland MJ, Hartgartner WR, et al. Factors influencing the presence or absence of acute coronary thrombi in sudden ischemic death. *Eur Heart J* 1989;10:203–208.
11. Davies MJ. A macro and micro view of coronary vascular insult in ischemic heart disease. *Circulation* 1990;82(suppl II):38–46.
12. Davies MJ, Thomas AC. Plaque fissuring—the cause of acute myocardial infarction, sudden ischemic death and crescendo angina. *Br Heart J* 1985;53:363–373.
13. Rentrop P, Blanke H, Karsch KR, Kaiser H, Kostering H, Leitz K. Selective intracoronary thrombolysis in acute myocardial infarction and unstable angina pectoris. *Circulation* 1981;63:307–317.
14. Rehr R, Disciascio G, Vetrovec G, Crowley M. Angiographic morphology of coronary artery stenoses in prolonged rest angina: evidence of intracoronary thrombosis. *J Am Coll Cardiol* 1989;14:1429–1435.
15. Sherman CT, Litvak F, Grundfest W, et al. Coronary angioscopy in patients with unstable angina. *N Engl J Med* 1986;315:913–919.
16. Ramee SR, White CJ, Collins TJ, Mesa JE, Murgo JP. Percutaneous angioscopy during coronary angioplasty using a steerable microangioscope. *J Am Coll Cardiol* 1991;17:100–105.
17. Uchida Y, Tomaru T, Nakamura F, Furuse A, Fujimori Y. Percutaneous coronary angioscopy in patients with ischemic heart disease. *Am Heart J* 1987;1114:1216–1222.
18. Uchida Y. Percutaneous coronary angioscopy by means of a fiberscope with steerable guidewire. *Am Heart J* 1989;117:1153–1155.
19. Ambrose JA, Winters SL, Stern A, et al. Angiographic morphology and the pathogenesis of unstable angina pectoris. *J Am Coll Cardiol* 1985;5:609–616.
20. Vetrovec GW, Cowley MJ, Overton H, Richardson DW. Intracoronary thrombus in syndromes of unstable angina myocardial ischemia. *Am Heart J* 1981;102:1202–1208.
21. Mandelkorn JB, Wolf NM, Singh S, et al. Intracoronary thrombus in non-transmural myocardial infarction and in unstable angina pectoris. *Am J Cardiol* 1983;52:1–6.
22. Capone G, Wolf NM, Meyers B, Meister SG. Frequency of intracoronary filling defects by angiography in unstable angina pectoris at rest. *Am J Cardiol* 1985;56:403–406.
23. Gotoh K, Minamino T, Hatoh O, et al. The role of intracoronary thrombus in unstable angina: angiographic assessment and thrombolytic therapy during ongoing anginal attacks. *Circulation* 1988;77:526–534.
24. Badimon L, Badimon JJ, Galvez A, Chesebro JH, Fuster V. Influence of arterial damage and wall shear rate on platelet deposition. Ex vivo study in swine model. *Arteriosclerosis* 1986;6:312–320.
25. Badimon L, Badimon JJ, Turitto VT, Vallabhajosula S, Fuster V. Platelet thrombus formation on collagen type I. A model of deep vessel injury-influence of blood rheology, von Willebrand factor and blood coagulation. *Circulation* 1988;78:1431–1442.
26. Badimon L, Badimon JJ. Mechanism of arterial thrombosis in non-parallel streamlines: platelet grow at the apex of stenotic severely injured vessel wall. Experimental study in the pig model. *J Clin Invest* 1989;84:1134–1144.
27. Lassila R, Badimon JJ, Vallabhajosula S, Badimon L. Dynamic monitoring of platelet deposition on severely

damaged vessel wall in flowing blood. Effects of different stenosis on thrombus growth. *Arteriosclerosis* 1990;10:306–315.

28. Fernández-Ortiz A, Badimon JJ, Falk E, et al. Characterization of the relative thrombogenicity of atherosclerotic plaque components: implications for consequences of plaque rupture. *J Am Coll Cardiol* 1994;23: 1562–1569.

29. Toschi V, Gallo R, Lettino M, et al. Tissue factor modulates the thrombogenicity of human atherosclerotic plaques. *Circulation* 1997;95:594–599.

30. Badimon JJ, Fuster V, Chesebro JH, Badimon L. Effect of depth of arterial injury on kinetics of fibrinogen deposition in arterial thrombosis. *Thromb Haemost* 1993;69:796.

31. Badimon L, Fuster V, Chesebro JH, Badimon JJ. Kinetics of fibrinogen deposition on stenotic damaged vessel wall in arterial thrombosis. *Thromb Haemost* 1993;69: 813.

32. Mailhac A, Badimon JJ, Fallon JT, et al. Effect of an eccentric severe stenosis on fibrin(ogen) deposition on severely damaged vessel wall in arterial thrombosis. Relative contribution of fibrin(ogen) and platelets. *Circulation* 1994;90:988–996

33. Pueyo C, Royo T, Berrozpe M, Badimon JJ, Gaffney P, Badimon L. A fibrin (Bβ chain) monolayer precedes platelets in the thrombotic response to atherosclerotic plaque rupture. *Circulation* 1995;92:I-555.

34. Fuster V, Chesebro JH. Mechanisms of unstable angina. *N Engl J Med* 1986;315:1023–1025.

35. Rentrop KP, Feit F, Blanke H, Sherman W, Thornton JC. Serial angiographic assessment of coronary artery obstruction and collateral flow in acute myocardial infarction. *Circulation* 1989;80:1166–1175.

36. Van de Werf F, Arnold AER, European Cooperative Study Group for Recombinant Tissue-Type Plasminogen Activator (rt-PA). Effect of intravenous tissue plasminogen activator on infarct size, left ventricular function and survival in patients with acute myocardial infarction. *Br Med J* 1988;297:374–379.

37. Van Lierde, De Geest H, Verstraete M, et al. Angiographic assessment of the infarct-related residual coronary stenosis after spontaneous or therapeutic thrombolysis. *J Am Coll Cardiol* 1990;16:1545–1549.

38. Fuster V, Stein B, Badimon L, Badimon JJ, Ambrose JA, Chesebro JH. Atherosclerotic plaque rupture and thrombosis: evolving concepts. *Circulation* 1990;82 (suppl II):47–59.

39. Davies SW, Marchant B, Lyon JP, et al. Coronary lesion morphology in acute myocardial infarction: demonstration of early remodeling after streptokinase treatment. *J Am Coll Cardiol* 1990;16: 1079–1086.

40. Gulba DC, Barthels M, Westhoff-Bleck M, et al. Increased thrombin levels during acute myocardial infarction. Relevance for the success of therapy. *Circulation* 1991;83:937–944.

41. Badimon L, Badimon J, Lassila R, Heras M, Chesebro JH, Fuster V. Thrombin inhibition by hirudin decreases platelet thrombus growth on areas of severe vessel wall injury [Abstract]. *J Am Coll Cardiol* 1989; 13:145.

42. Weitz JI, Hudoba M, Massel D, Maragamore J, Hirsh J. Clot-bound thrombin is protected from inhibition by heparin-antithrombin III but is susceptible to inactivation by antithrombin III–independent inhibitors. *J Clin Invest* 1990;86:385–391.

43. Fitzgerald DJ, FitzGerald GA. Role of thrombin and thromboxane A₂ in reocclusion following coronary thrombolysis with tissue-type plasminogen activator. *Proc Natl Acad Sci U S A* 1989;86:7585.

44. Francis CW, Markham RE, Barlow GH, Florack TM, Dobrzynski DM, Marder VJ. Thrombin activity of fibrin thrombi and soluble plasmic derivatives. *J Lab Clin Med* 1983;102:220–230.

45. Meyer BJ, Badimon JJ, Mailhac A, et al. Inhibition of growth of thrombus on fresh mural thrombus: targeting optimal therapy. *Circulation* 1994;90:2432–2438.

46. Hogg PJ, Jackson CM. Fibrin monomer protects thrombin from inactivation by heparin-antithrombin III: implications for heparin efficacy. *Proc Natl Acad Sci U S A* 1989;86:3619–3623.

47. Fitzgerald DJ, Catella F, Roy L, et al. Marked platelet activation in vivo after intravenous streptokinase in patients with acute myocardial infarction. *Circulation* 1988;77:142–150.

48. Eisenberg PR, Sherman LA, Jaffe AS. Paradoxic elevation of fibrinopeptide A after streptokinase: evidence for continued thrombosis despite intense fibrinolysis. *J Am Coll Cardiol* 1987;10:527–529.

49. Brown GB, Gallery CA, Badger RS, et al. Incomplete lysis of thrombus in the moderate underlying atherosclerosis lesion during intracoronary infusion of streptokinase for acute myocardial infarction: quantitative angiographic observation. *Circulation* 1986;73:653–661.

50. Waller BF, Rothbaum DA, Pinkerton CA, et al. Status of the myocardium and infarct-related coronary artery in 19 necropsy patients with acute recanalization using pharmacologic (streptokinase, r-tissue plasminogen activator), mechanical (percutaneous transluminal coronary angioplasty) or combined types of reperfusion therapy. *J Am Coll Cardiol* 1987;9:785–801.

51. Badger RS, Brown BG, Kennedy JW, et al. Usefulness of recanalization to luminal diameter of 0.6 millimeter or more with intracoronary streptokinase during acute myocardial infarction in predicting "normal" perfusion status, continued arterial patency and survival at one year. *Am J Cardiol* 1987;59:519–522.

52. Rowsell HC, Hegardt B, Downie HG, Mustard JF, Murphy EA. Adrenaline and experimental thrombosis. *Br J Haematol* 1966;12:66–73.

53. Haft JI, Fani K. Intravascular platelet aggregation in the heart induced by stress. *Circulation* 1973;47:353–358.

54. Mueller JE, Stone PH, Turi ZG, et al. The MILIS Study Group. Circadian variation in the frequency of onset of acute myocardial infarction. *N Engl J Med* 1985;313:1315–1322.

55. Willich SN, Linderer T, Wegscheider K, et al. Increased morning incidence of myocardial infarction in the ISAM study: absence with prior β-adrenergic blockade. *Circulation* 1989;80:853–858.

56. Hjalmarson A, Gilpin EA, Nicod P, et al. Differing circadian patterns of symptoms onset in subgroups of patients with acute myocardial infarction. *Circulation* 1989;80:267–275.

57. Tofler GH, Brezinski D, Schafer AI, et al. Morning increase in platelet response to ADP and epinephrine: association with the time of increased risk of myocardial infarction and sudden cardiac death. *N Engl J Med* 1987;316:1514–1518.

58. Levine PH. An acute effect of cigarette smoking on platelet function: a possible link between smoking and arterial thrombosis. *Circulation* 1973;48:619–623.

59. Fuster V, Chesebro JH, Frye RL, Elveback L. Platelet survival and the development of coronary artery disease in the young adult: effects of cigarette smoking, strong family history and medical therapy. *Circulation* 1981;63:546–551.

60. Winniford MD, Wheelan KR, Kremers MS, et al. Smoking-induced coronary vasoconstriction in patients with atherosclerotic coronary artery disease: evidence for adrenergically mediated alterations in coronary artery tone. *Circulation* 1986;73:662–667.

61. Cullen JW, McKenna JW, Massey MM. International control of smoking and the US experience. *Chest* 1986;89(suppl):206–218.

62. Buhler FR, Vesanen K, Watters JT. Impact of smoking on heart attacks, strokes, blood pressure control, drug dose, and quality of life aspects in the International Prospective Primary Prevention Study in Hypertension. *Am Heart J* 1988;115:282–288.

63. Paul O. Background of the prevention of cardiovascular disease. II. Arteriosclerosis, hypertension and selected risk factors. *Circulation* 1989;80:206–214.

64. Hunt BJ. The relation between abnormal hemostatic function and the progression of coronary disease. *Curr Op Cardiol* 1990;5:758–765.

65. Badimon JJ, Badimon L, Turitto VT, Fuster V. Platelet deposition at high shear rates is enhanced by high plasma cholesterol levels. In vivo study in the rabbit model. *Arteriosclerosis* 1991;11:395–402.

66. Carvalho ACA, Colman RW, Lees RS. Platelet function in hyperlipoproteinemia. *N Engl J Med* 1974;290:434–438.

67. Stuart MJ, Gerrard JM, White JG. Effect of cholesterol on production of thromboxane B_2 by platelets in vitro. *N Engl J Med* 1980;302:6–10.

68. Boers GHJ, Smals AGH, Trijbels FJM, et al. Heterozygosity for homocystinuria in premature peripheral and cerebral occlusive arterial disease. *N Engl J Med* 1985;313:709–715.

69. Murphy-Chutorian DR, Wexman MP, Grieco AJ, et al. Methionine intolerance: a possible risk factor for coronary artery disease. *J Am Coll Cardiol* 1985;6:725–730.

70. Berg K. A new serum system in man-the LP system. *Acta Pathol Microbiol Scand* 1963;59:369–382.

71. Dahlen GH, Guyton JR, Attar M, et al. Association of levels of lipoprotein Lp(a), plasma lipids, and other lipoproteins with coronary artery disease documented by angiography. *Circulation* 1986;74:758–765.

72. Seed M, Hoppichler F, Reaveley D, et al. Relation of serum lipoprotein(a) concentration and apolipoprotein(a) phenotype to CHD patients with familial hypercholesterolemia. *N Engl J Med* 1990;332:1494–1499.

73. Paramo JA, Colucci M, Collen D. Plasminogen activator inhibitor in blood of patients with coronary artery disease. *Br Med J* 1985;291:573–574.

74. Olofsson BO, Dahlen G, Nilsson TK. Evidence for increased levels of plasminogen activator inhibitor and tissue plasminogen activator in plasma of patients with angiographically verified coronary artery disease. *Eur Heart J* 1989;10:77–82.

75. Hamsten A, Wilman B, de Faire U, Blombäck M. Increased plasma levels of a rapid inhibitor of tissue plasminogen activator in young survivors of myocardial infarction. *N Engl J Med* 1980;303:897–902.

76. Barbash GI, Hanoch H, Roth A, et al. Correlation of baseline plasminogen activator inhibitor activity with patency of the infarct artery after thrombolytic therapy in acute myocardial infarction. *Am J Cardiol* 1989;64:1231–1235.

77. Conlan MG, Folsom AR, Finch A, et al. Associations of factor VIII and von Willebrand factor with age, race, sex, and risk factors for atherosclerosis. *Thromb Haemos* 1993;70:380–385.

78. Cortellaro M, Boschetti C, Confrancesco E, et al. The PLAT Study: hemostatic function in relation to atherothrombotic ischemic events in vascular disease patients:principal results. *Arterioscler Thromb* 1992;12:1063–1070.

79. Thompson SG, Kienast J, Pyke SDM, Haverkate F, Van de Loo JCW for the European Concerted Action on Thrombosis and Disabilities Angina Pectoris Study Group. Hemostatic factor and the risk of myocardial infarction or sudden death in patients with angina pectoris. *N Engl J Med* 1995;332:635–641.

80. Fuster V, Badimon L, Badimon JJ, Chesebro JH. The pathogenesis of coronary artery disease and the acute coronary syndromes (Part I). *N Engl J Med* 1992;326:242–250.

81. Badimon JJ, Fuster V, Chesebro JH, Badimon L. Coronary atherosclerosis. *Circulation* 1993;87(suppl II):3–16.

82. Fuster V, Badimon L, Badimon JJ, Chesebro JH. The pathogenesis of coronary artery disease and the acute coronary syndromes (Part II). *N Engl J Med* 1992;326:310–318.

83. Badimon L, Chesebro JH, Badimon JJ. Thrombus formation on ruptured atherosclerotic plaques and rethrombosis on evolving thrombi. *Circulation* 1992;86(suppl III):74–85.

84. Marcus A, Safier LB. Thromboregulation: multicellular modulation of platelet reactivity in hemostasis and thrombosis. *FASEB J* 1993;7:516–522.

85. Kroll MH, Schafer AI. Biochemical mechanisms of platelet activation. *Blood* 1989;74:1181–1195.

86. Brass LF. In: Hoffman R, Benz EJ Jr, Shattil SJ, Furie B, Cohen HJ (eds). *Hematology. Basic Principles and Practice.* New York: Churchill Livingstone, 1991;1176–1197.

87. Kieffer N, Phillips DR. Platelet membrane glycoproteins: functions in cellular interactions. *Annu Rev Biol* 1990;6:329–357.

88. Kunicki TJ. Organization of glycoproteins within the platelet plasma membrane. In: George JN, Nurden AT, Philips DR (eds). *Platelet Membrane Glycoproteins.* New York: Plenum, 1985;87–101.

89. Vicente V, Houghten RA, Ruggeri ZM. Identification of a site in the a chain of platelet glycoprotein Ib that participates in von Willebrand factor binding. *J Biol Chem* 1990;265:274–280.

90. Fujimura Y, Titani K, Holland LZ, et al. von Willebrand factor. A reduced and alkylated 52/48-kDa fragment beginning at amino acid residue 449 contains the domain interacting with platelet glycoprotein Ib. *J Biol Chem* 1986;261:381–385.

91. Fox JEB, Boyles JK, Berndt MC, Steffen PK, Anderson LK. Identification of a membrane skeleton in platelets. *J Cell Biol* 1988;106:1525–1538.

92. Meyer D, Girma JP. von Willebrand factor: structure and function. *Thromb Haemost* 1993;70:99–104.
93. Fitzgerald LA, Phillips DR. Calcium regulation of the platelet membrane glycoprotein IIb-IIIa complex. *J Biol Chem* 1985;260:11366–11376.
94. Plow EF, Ginsberg MH, Marguerie GA. Expression and function of adhesive proteins on the platelet surface. In: Phillips DR, Shuman MA (eds). *Biochemistry of Platelets*. New York: Academic, 1986;225–256.
95. Ruoslahti E, Pierschbacher MD. New perspectives in cell adhesion: RGD and integrins. *Science* 1987;238:491–497.
96. Doolittle RF, Watt KWK, Cottrell BA, Strong DD, Riley M. The amino acid sequence of the α-chain of human fibrinogen. *Nature* 1979;280:464–467.
97. Kloczewiak M, Timmons S, Lukas TJ, Hawiger J. Platelet receptor recognition site on human fibrinogen. Synthesis and structure-function relationship of peptides corresponding to the carboxyterminal segment of the γ chain. *Biochemistry* 1984;23:1767–1774.
98. Ginsberg MH, Xiaoping D, O'Toole TE, Loftus JC, Plow EF. Platelet integrins. *Thromb Haemost* 1993;70:87–93.
99. Shattil SJ. Regulation of platelet anchorage and signaling by integrin $\alpha IIb\beta_3$. *Thromb Haemost* 1993;70:224–228.
100. Vu TH, Hung DT, Wheaton VI, Coughlin SR. Molecular cloning of a functional thrombin receptor reveals a novel proteolytic mechanism of receptor activation. *Cell* 1991;64:1057–1068.
101. Coughlin SR. Thrombin receptor structure and function. *Thromb Haemost* 1993;70:184–187.
102. Sakariassen KS, Nievelstein PF, Coller BS, Sixma JJ. The role of platelet membrane glycoproteins Ib and IIb/IIIa in platelet adherence to human artery subendothelium. *Br J Haematol* 1986;63:681–691.
103. Weiss HJ, Turitto VT, Baumgartner HR. Effect of shear rate on platelet interaction with subendothelium in citrated and native blood. I. Shear rate-dependent decrease of adhesion in von Willebrand's disease and the Bernard-Soulier syndrome. *J Lab Clin Med* 1978;92:750–754.
104. Turitto VT, Baumgartner HR. In: Colman R, Hirsh J, Marder V, Salzman E (eds). *Hemostasis and Thrombosis, Basic Principles and Clinical Practice* (2nd ed). New York: Lippincott, 1987;555–571.
105. Sakariassen K, Bolhuis PA, Sixma J. Human blood platelet adhesion to artery subendothelium is mediated by factor VIII-von Willebrand factor bound to the subendothelium. *Nature* 1979;636–638.
106. Badimon L, Badimon JJ, Turitto VT, Fuster V. Platelet deposition in von Willebrand factor deficient vessel wall. *J Lab Clin Med* 1987;110:634–647.
107. Badimon L, Badimon JJ, Chesebro JH, Fuster V. Inhibition of thrombus formation: blockage of adhesive glycoprotein mechanisms versus blockage of the cyclooxygenase pathway [Abstract]. *J Am Coll Cardiol* 1988;11:30.
108. Badimon L, Badimon JJ, Turitto VT, Fuster V. Platelet interaction to vessel wall and collagen. Study in homozygous von Willebrand's disease associated with abnormal collagen aggregation in swine. *Thromb Haemost* 1989;61:57–64.
109. Badimon L, Badimon JJ, Turitto VT, Fuster V. Role of von Willebrand factor in mediating platelet-vessel wall interaction at low shear rate; the importance of perfusion conditions. *Blood* 1989;73:961–967.
110. Weiss HJ, Turitto VT, Vicic WJ, Baumgartner HR. Fibrin formation, fibrinopeptide A release, and platelet thrombus dimensions on subendothelium exposed to flowing native blood: greater in factor XII and XI than in factor VIII and IX deficiency. *Blood* 1984;63:1004–1014.
111. Weiss HJ, Hawiger J, Ruggeri ZM, Turitto VT, Thiagarajan I, Hoffman T. Fibrinogen-independent interaction of platelets with subendothelium mediated by glycoprotein IIb-IIIa complex at high shear rate. *J Clin Invest* 1989;83:288–297.
112. Badimon L, Badimon JJ, Chesebro JH, Fuster V. von Willebrand factor and cardiovascular disease. *Thromb Haemost* 1993;70:111–118.
113. The EPIC Investigators. Use of a monoclonal antibody directed against the platelet glycoprotein IIb/IIIa receptor in high-risk coronary angioplasty. *N Engl J Med* 1994;330:956–961.
114. Topol EJ, Califf RM, Weisman HF, et al. Randomised trial of coronary intervention with antibody against platelet IIb/IIIa integrin for reduction of clinical restenosis :results at six months. *Lancet* 1994;343:881–886.
115. Tcheng JE. Glycoprotein IIb/IIIa receptor inhibitors: putting the EPIC, IMPACT II, RESTORE, and EPILOG trials into perspective. *Am J Cardiol* 1996;78:35–40
116. Pueyo C, Badimon JJ, Royo T, Feigen LP, Badimon L. A mimetic of the RGDF-peptide (arginine-glycine-aspartic acid-phenylalanine) blocks aggregation and flow-induced thrombosis on severely injured stenotic arterial wall. Effects on different animal models and in humans. *Thromb Res* 1996;81:101–112.
117. Badimon JJ, Meyer B, Feigen LP, et al. Thrombosis triggered by severe arterial lesions is inhibited by oral administration of a glycoprotein IIb/IIIa antagonist. *Eur J Clin Invest* 1997;27:568–574.
118. Rentrop KP, Feit F, Blanke H, et al. Effects of intracoronary streptokinase and intracoronary nitroglycerin infusion on coronary angiographic patterns and mortality in patients with acute myocardial infarction. *N Engl J Med* 1984;311:1457–1463.
119. Goldsmith HL, Turitto VT. Rheological aspects of thrombosis and haemostasis: basic principles and applications. *Thromb Haemost* 1986;55:415–436.
120. Charm SE, Wong BL. Enzyme inactivation with shearing. *Biotechnol Bioeng* 1970;12:1103–1109.
121. Badimon L, Badimon JJ, Lassila R, Heras M, Chesebro JH, Fuster V. Thrombin regulation of platelet interaction with damaged vessel wall and isolated collagen type I at arterial flow conditions in a porcine model. Effects of hirudins, heparin and calcium chelation. *Blood* 1991;78:423–434.
122. Steele PM, Chesebro JH, Stanson AW, et al. Balloon angioplasty: natural history of the pathophysiologic response to injury in a pig model. *Circ Res* 1985;57:105–112.
123. Clowes AW, Clowes MM, Fingerle J, Reidy MA. Regulation of smooth muscle cell growth in injured artery. *J Cardiovasc Pharmacol* 1989;14(suppl 6):12–15.
124. Fuster V, Falk E, Fallon J, Badimon L, Chesebro JH, Badimon JJ. The three processes leading to post PTCA

restenosis: dependence on the lesion substrate. *Thromb Haemost* 1995;74:552–559.

125. Fingerle J, Johnson R, Clowes A, Majesky M, Reidy MA. Role of platelets in smooth muscle cell proliferation and migration after vascular injury in rat carotid artery. *Proc Natl Acad Sci U S A* 1989;86: 8412–8416.

126. Walker LN, Bowen-Pope DF, Ross R, Reidy MA. Production of platelet-derived growth factor-like molecule by cultured arterial smooth muscle cells accompanied proliferation after arterial injury. *Proc Natl Acad Sci U S A* 1986;83:7311–7315.

127. Wilcox JN, Smith KM, Williams CT, Schwartz JM, Gordon D. Platelet-derived growth factor mRNA detection in human atherosclerotic plaques by in-situ hybridization. *J Clin Invest* 1988;82:1134–1143.

128. Libby P, Warner SJC, Salomon RN, Birinyi LK. Production of platelet-derived growth factor-like mitogen by smooth muscle cells from human atheroma. *N Engl J Med* 1988;318:1493–1498.

129. Bar-Shavit R, Amiram E, Vlodavsky I. Binding of thrombin to subendothelial extracellular matrix. Pro-

tection and expression of functional properties. *J Clin Invest* 1989;84:1096–1104.

130. Weitz JI, Hudoba M, Massel D, Maraganore J, Hirsh J. Clot-bound thrombin is protected from inhibition by heparin-antithrombin III but is susceptible to inactivation by antithrombin III-independent inhibitors. *J Clin Invest* 1990;86:385–391.

131. Wilner GD, Danitz MP, Mudd MS, Hsieh KH, Fenton JW. Selective immobilization of alpha-thrombin by surface bound fibrin. *J Lab Clin Med* 1981;97:403–411.

132. Berk BC, Taubman MB, Griendling KK, Cragoe E, Fenton J. Thrombin-stimulated events in cultured vascular smooth muscle cells. *J Biol Chem* 1990;265: 17334–17340.

133. Schwartz SM, Reidy MA, O'Brien ERM. Assessment of factors important in atherosclerotic occlusion and restenosis. *Thromb Haemost* 1995;74:541–551.

134. Hirsh J, Salzman EW. Pathogenesis of venous thromboembolism. In: Colman RW, Hirsh J, Marder VJ, Salzman EW (eds). *Thrombosis and Hemostasis: Basic Principles and Clinical Practice*. Philadelphia: Lippincott, 1987;1199–1207.

Cardiovascular Thrombosis: Thrombocardiology and Thromboneurology, Second Edition,
edited by M. Verstraete, V. Fuster, and E. J. Topol,
Lippincott–Raven Publishers, Philadelphia © 1998.

3

Interrelationship Between Atherosclerosis and Thrombosis

Erling Falk, *Valentin Fuster, and †Prediman K. Shah

Coronary Pathology Research, Aarhus University Hospital Skejby, 8200 Aarhus N, Denmark;
**Cardiovascular Institute, Department of Medicine, Mount Sinai School of Medicine, New York, New*
York 10029; and †Division of Cardiology, Cedars-Sinai Medical Center, Los Angeles, California 90048

Atherosclerosis is the most frequent underlying cause of ischemic heart disease (IHD) and cerebrovascular disease and is thus the leading cause of death in Western societies. However, atherosclerosis by itself is rarely fatal. The serious and potentially lethal consequences of atherosclerosis such as acute coronary syndromes (unstable angina, acute myocardial infarction, and many cases of sudden death) and ischemic stroke are usually caused by acute thrombosis superimposed on a chronic atherosclerotic plaque with a disrupted or eroded surface (1–3). If these thrombotic complications could be prevented, atherosclerosis would be a much less menacing disease. Because of these pathophysiologic considerations, factors that determine the vulnerability of plaques to undergo disruption or superficial erosion and the factors that determine the thrombotic consequences of plaque disruption become relevant in as far as our ability to prevent the lethal manifestations of atherosclerosis is concerned.

CORONARY ATHEROSCLEROSIS

Plaque Heterogeneity and Risk Factors

Patients with IHD generally have many atherosclerotic plaques in their coronary arteries, which vary considerably in their composition. Although coronary angiography may show only one or a few stenotic lesions, many more plaques are observed on intravascular ultrasound examination in living patients and at autopsy in deceased patients (4,5). Only a minority of plaques protrude into and compromise the lumen because of compensatory abluminal vascular enlargement (remodeling) during plaque growth (6–9). Thus, the lumen may remain normal despite build-up of large volumes of atherosclerotic plaque in the vessel wall. Several studies have demonstrated that plaque composition, rather than stenosis severity, is a major determinant of the risk for disruption and subsequent thrombosis. A recent pathoanatomic study of 160 mature and nondisrupted coronary plaques identified no simple relationship between plaque type, plaque size, and stenosis severity, thereby highlighting the shortcomings of angiography for identification of vulnerable and rupture-prone plaques; many vulnerable plaques do not produce a significant stenosis and are thus missed by angiography (10).

Although many phenotypic, genotypic, and environmental characteristics, known as risk factors, are associated with an increased risk for development of IHD, little is known about a specific relationship between risk factors for clinical disease and composition of the plaque in the vessel wall (11–14). For pathologists interested in atherothrombosis, it has been particularly frustrating to realize the extreme diversity in plaque composition in the same individual; many plaques are collagen rich and stable, few are lipid rich and unstable, but most plaques contain a variable amount of collagen and other types of extracellular matrix (hard components), as well as the soft lipid-rich core. Nevertheless, a few studies have identified significant associations between some plaque features and individual risk factors. In coronary arteries, plaque calcification increases with age and the overall plaque burden (15–17), but apparently not with the degree of luminal obstruction (15). Interestingly, culprit lesions responsible for unstable angina (15) and myocardial infarction (18) are less calcified, indicating that calcium might stabilize plaques against disruption and thrombosis. Based on an autopsy study of 113 sudden coronary death cases (men only), Burke et al. concluded that abnormal serum cholesterol concentrations, particularly elevated ratios of total cholesterol to high-density lipoprotein cholesterol, predispose to rupture of vulnerable plaques, whereas cigarette smoking predisposes to acute thrombosis (19). Davies reported his experience from rather similar studies of sudden death due to coronary thrombosis; in 134 men without diabetes, plaque rupture (versus erosion) accounted for 84% of thrombi, whereas in 27 women without diabetes, rupture was found in 59% (20). In 41 patients with diabetes (men and women), only 34% of thrombi were attributable to plaque rupture (20).

Plaque Composition and Vulnerability

As the term "atherosclerosis" implies, mature plaques consist typically of two main components resulting from two different processes: atherosis and sclerosis. The atheromatous plaque component is lipid rich and soft (Greek *athere,* gruel), whereas the sclerotic plaque component is collagen rich and hard (Greek *skleros,* hard). Generally, the sclerotic component is the most voluminous, constituting more than 70% of an average stenotic coronary plaque (21,22). A thick fibrous cap in collagen and other components of extracellular matrix appears to confer resistance to disruption, whereas the presence of a large soft atheromatous component is associated with vulnerability to disruption and subsequent thrombosis (23). Accordingly, a significant atheromatous component is usually present in culprit lesions responsible for the thrombus-mediated acute coronary syndromes (24,25).

Pathoanatomic studies have identified several features that appear to be associated with plaque disruption (Figs. 3-1 and 3-2): (a) a large pool of extracellular lipid (lipid core); (b) thinning of the fibrous cap with an underlying active inflammatory and immune response characterized by increased density of activated macrophages, T-lymphocytes, and mast cells; and (c) a relative paucity of smooth muscle cells (SMCs) in the fibrous cap with evidence of reduced collagen content (26); it has been implied by a number of pathologists that increased plaque revascularization also may contribute to plaque disruption. Plaque disruption may thus evolve when extrinsic triggers, such as sudden mechanical and/or hemodynamic stresses (trig-

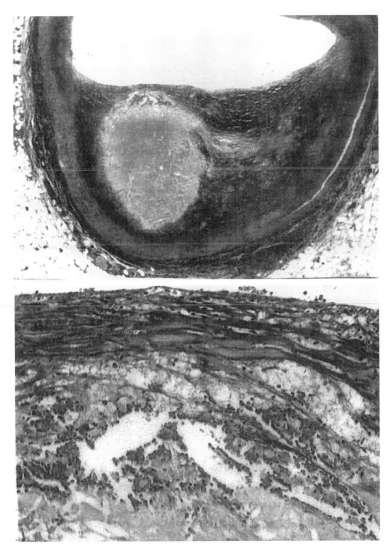

FIG. 3-1. Photomicrographs illustrating composition and vulnerability of coronary plaques. A vulnerable plaque, containing a core of soft atheromatous gruel (devoid of collagen) that is separated from the vascular lumen by a thin cap of fibrous tissue. The fibrous cap is infiltrated by foam cells that can be clearly seen at high magnification, indicating ongoing disease activity. Such a thin and macrophage-infiltrated cap is probably weak and vulnerable, and it was indeed disrupted nearby, explaining why erythrocytes can be seen in the gruel just beneath the macrophage-infiltrated cap. (From Falk et al., ref. 26, with permission.)

gers), interact with vulnerable plaques or with long-term repetitive cyclic stresses that gradually weaken the fibrous cap and ultimately lead to mechanical fatigue failure, culminating in sudden and unprovoked (i.e., untriggered) disruption of the plaque surface (27).

Lipid Accumulation

The atheromatous core is totally devoid of supporting collagen (25), is avascular (28,29) and hypocellular (except at its periphery, where macrophage foam cells are frequently found) (29–31), and is rich in extracellular

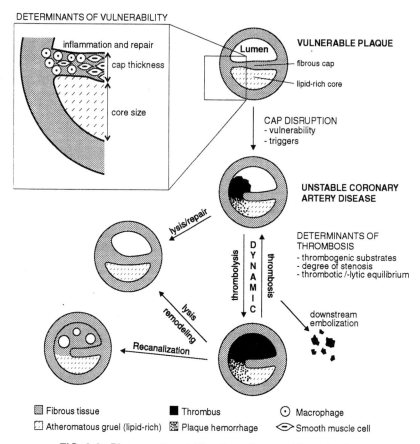

FIG. 3-2. Plaque vulnerability, disruption, and thrombosis.

lipids, consisting mainly of cholesterol and its esters (32,33). The size of such a soft lipid core appears to influence the vulnerability to disruption. At autopsy, Gertz and Roberts noted that the lipid core occupied 32% of volume in plaques that had disrupted compared with 5% to 12% of the volume in nondisrupted plaques (28). Similarly, Davies et al. found that aortic plaques containing a lipid core occupying 40% or more of the plaque area were most often the ones that had undergone disruption with superimposed thrombosis (34).

Not only the size but also the consistency of the lipid-rich core is important for the stability of a plaque (35). Liquid cholesteryl esters soften the core, whereas the solid cholesterol crystals are believed to have the opposite effect (32,33). At room temperature post-

mortem, the atheromatous gruel usually has a consistency like toothpaste, and it is even softer at body temperature in vivo. Based on animal experiments (32,36), lipid-lowering therapy in humans is expected to deplete plaque lipid with an overall reduction in the liquid and mobile cholesteryl esters and a relative increase in the solid and inert crystalline cholesterol, theoretically resulting in a stiffer and more stable plaque (35).

Recent studies using immunohistochemical and tunel staining techniques have identified macrophage-specific antigens and apoptotic nuclear fragments within the lipid-core, indicating that lipid and other cell constituents released from dead lipid-laden macrophage foam cells could contribute significantly to the formation and growth of the lipid core, emphasizing the inflammatory origin of this destabilizing core (37–40). Thus, the lipid core may be aptly labeled as the "graveyard" of dead macrophages. However, other studies have suggested that direct trapping of blood-derived lipoproteins within the extracellular matrix, without prior uptake by macrophages, also may play an important role in extracellular lipid accumulation, particularly in the early stage of core formation (41,42).

Inflammation, Matrix Dysregulation, and Cap Thinning

Inflammation and immune responses appear to play an important role in both the early as well as advanced stages of atherogenesis (43,44). Hypercholesterolemia and other risk factors for atherosclerosis are associated with increased endothelial permeability, increased transcytosis and intimal retention of lipoproteins, and endothelial activation with focal expression of vascular cell adhesion molecule type 1 and chemotactic molecules such as macrophage-chemoattractant-protein (MCP)-1, eventually leading to monocyte and T-lymphocyte recruitment into the subendothelial space. Within intima, the monocytes differentiate into macrophages, probably under the influence of cytokines such as monocyte colony-stimulating factor (M-CSF). The macrophages ingest oxidatively modified low-density lipoproteins, probably via their scavenger receptor, leading to the formation of lipid-filled foam cells. These inflammatory cells constitute by far the major part of the early fatty streak lesion, with a ratio of approximately 1:10 to 1:50 between T cells and macrophages, and they probably play a significant role in the progression of fatty streaks to mature atherosclerotic plaques (44). The presence of activated macrophages and T cells strongly suggest that an immunologic reaction is taking place in the atherosclerotic plaque. The antigens that elicit this response are not yet known, and both autoantigens (i.e., against oxidized low-density lipoprotein) and microorganisms (i.e., *Chlamydia pneumoniae*) have been proposed to play a role (44).

Disrupted fibrous caps are usually heavily infiltrated by macrophage foam cells (45–47), and recent observations have shown that such rupture-related macrophages are activated, indicating ongoing inflammation at the site of plaque disruption (48). For eccentric plaques, the shoulder regions are sites of predilection for both active inflammation (endothelial activation and macrophage infiltration) and disruption (49,50), and mechanical testing of aortic fibrous caps indicate that foam cell infiltration indeed weakens caps locally, reducing their tensile strength (51). van der Wal et al. identified superficial macrophage infiltration in plaques beneath all 20 coronary thrombi examined, regardless of whether the underlying plaque was disrupted or just eroded (48), although a more recent study of coronary thrombi responsible for sudden coronary death could not confirm that observation (52). Using an immunohistochemical technique, van der Wal et al. found that macrophages and adjacent T-lymphocytes were activated, indicating ongoing disease activity (48). Comparable results were obtained by the same group in a study of coronary atherectomy specimens, showing an inverse relationship between the extent of inflammatory activity in culprit lesions and the clinical stability of the ischemic syndrome (53). However, there was considerable overlap between groups, indicating that not all patients with clinically stable angina have histologically stable plaques (53). These observations confirmed a previous study of coronary atherectomy specimens from culprit lesions responsible for stable angina, unstable rest angina, or non–Q-wave infarction (54). Culprit lesions responsible for the acute coronary syndromes (unstable rest angina or non–Q-wave infarction) contained significantly more macrophages than did lesions responsible for stable angina pectoris (14% versus 3% of plaque tissue occupied by macrophages) (54).

Macrophages are capable of degrading extracellular matrix by phagocytosis or by secreting proteolytic enzymes such as plasminogen activators and a family of matrix metalloproteinases (MMPs)—collagenases (MMP-1), gelatinases (MMP-2 and MMP-9), strome-olysins (MMP-3), and matrilysin (MMP-7)—which may digest the matrix component of the fibrous cap, leading to its thinning and predisposing it to rupture (55,56). The MMPs are secreted in a latent zymogen form requiring extracellular activation, after which they are capable of degrading virtually all components of the extracellular matrix. The ability of MMPs to induce matrix degradation is tightly regulated in part by cosecretion of tissue inhibitors of MMPs (TIMPS) that neutralize the effects of MMP, as well as their secretion in a zymogen precursor form that requires extracellular activation. This activation of pro-MMPs can be produced by plasmin (produced by macrophages), tryptase and chymase (produced by activated mast cells), oxidant stress, and exposure to oxidized LDL. In addition, a novel transmembrane MMP (membrane type MMP [MT-MMP]) that can activate pro-MMP-2, originally identified in tumor cells, recently was identified in cultured human macrophages and human atherosclerotic plaques. Thus, the milieu in the atherosclerotic plaque is conductive to activation of pro-MMPs, thereby facilitating net matrix degradation (55). Collagen confers stability to plaques, and human monocyte–derived macrophages grown in culture are indeed capable of degrading the old and mature collagen present in advanced aortic plaques (57). Simultaneously, they express MMP-1 and induce MMP-2 activity in the culture medium (57). Besides macrophages, a wide variety of cells may produce MMPs (56). Activated mast cells may secrete powerful proteolytic enzymes such as tryptase and chymase that can activate pro-MMPs secreted by other cells (i.e., macrophages), and mast cells are actually present in shoulder regions of mature plaques and at sites of disruption, although at very low density (58,59). Neutrophils also can destroy tissue by secreting proteolytic enzymes, but they are rare in intact plaques (44,48). Cell culture studies have suggested that activated T-lymphocytes can markedly upregulate MMP-9 production by macrophages via a nonsecreted membrane-to-membrane signaling pathway.

Plaque Repair: Vascular Smooth Muscle Cells

Obviously, the thickness and collagen content of the fibrous cap is important for its strength and stability; the thinner the cap, the weaker it is and the more vulnerable is the plaque to rupture (60). Ruptured aortic caps contain fewer SMCs and less collagen than do intact caps (34,61), and SMCs are usually missing at the actual site of disruption (48,59).

Collagen is responsible for the mechanical strength of the fibrous cap, and it is synthesized by the intimal SMCs. SMC proliferation and matrix synthesis may protect plaques against disruption, whereas local loss of SMCs or impaired SMC function may be deleterious, leading to gradual plaque destabilization due to impaired healing and repair. It is unknown why SMCs are lacking at sites of disruption, but apoptotic cell death could play an important role (37,39). Recently, preliminary information from a number of laboratories suggest that macrophages in tissue culture, as well as in the atherosclerotic plaque, induced apoptosis in vascular SMCs, raising the possibility that macrophages may contribute to SMC loss in the atherosclerotic plaque.

Plaque Disruption

Rupture of vulnerable plaques occurs frequently. It is probably the most important mechanism underlying the sudden and rapid progression of coronary lesions seen by serial angiographic examination. Rupture of the plaque surface is followed by a variable amount of luminal thrombosis and/or hemorrhage into the soft gruel, causing rapid growth of the lesion (24). Autopsy data indicate that 9% of healthy persons harbor disrupted plaques (without superimposed thrombosis) in their coronary arteries, increasing to 22% in persons with diabetes or hypertension (62). In fatal IHD, two or more disrupted plaques, with or without superimposed thrombosis, are usually present in the coronary arteries (45,63).

Disruption of the plaque surface occurs most often where the cap is thinnest and most heavily infiltrated by macrophages and therefore weakest, namely at the cap's shoulders (26,49). However, the weak shoulder regions are also points where biomechanical and hemodynamic forces acting on plaques often are concentrated (49,64). Thus, plaque disruption is probably the result of a dynamic interaction between intrinsic plaque changes (vulnerability) and extrinsic forces imposed on the plaque (triggers) (26); the former predispose a plaque to rupture, whereas the latter may precipitate it. Because the presence of a vulnerable plaque is a prerequisite for plaque disruption, plaque vulnerability is probably more important than rupture triggers in determining the risk of a future heart attack. If no vulnerable plaque is present in the coronary arteries, there is no rupture-prone substrate for a potential trigger to function on.

CORONARY THROMBOSIS

Detailed microscopic examination of coronary thrombi using serial sectioning technique has revealed that plaque disruption is responsible for two thirds to three fourths of all fatal thrombi, whereas superficial plaque erosions usually are found beneath the rest of the thrombi (3,19,20). However, in diabetic patients and in women, plaque erosion appears to occur with higher frequency (20,25, 52). There is no general agreement on what the term "plaque erosion" includes, other than that it indicates the presence of nondisruptive plaque changes (i.e., no cap rupture/core exposure) beneath a thrombus. Some investigators always find activated macrophages (i.e., ongoing inflammation) superficially in eroded plaques beneath thrombi (48), whereas others believe that intimal SMCs and plaque matrix constitute the most important local thrombogenic substrate in erosion-induced thrombosis (52). Another matter of controversy is the role played by stenosis severity; Davies and his colleagues found more severe pre-existing atherosclerotic stenosis in thrombosis on eroded (versus disrupted) plaques (25), whereas Virmani's group reported just the opposite finding (52).

Thrombogenic Factors

Coronary thrombosis is the result of a dynamic interaction between the arterial wall and the flowing blood (Table 3-1). There are three major determinants for the thrombotic response to plaque disruption/erosion (1,79): (a) character and extent of exposed plaque components (local thrombogenic substrate); (b) degree of stenosis and surface irregularities (local flow disturbances); and (c) thrombotic–thrombolytic equilibrium at the time of plaque disruption/erosion (systemic thrombotic tendency).

Local Thrombogenic Substrate

Recently, the thrombogenicity of different plaque components was evaluated using the Badimon perfusion chamber (Fig. 3-3). The atheromatous gruel (lipid core) was five-fold more thrombogenic than any other plaque components, including collagen, which is known to be very thrombogenic (23). Therefore, the lipid-rich atheromatous gruel is not only associated with plaque disruption, but it is also the most thrombogenic component of the disrupted plaque. The enhanced thrombogenicity of the lipid core is most likely due to its high tissue factor content and procoagulant activity derived from activated macrophages (38,65–69). Tissue factor antigen and activity (using a factor Xa generation assay) were sig-

TABLE 3-1. *Thrombogenic risk factors, 1997[a]*

Local factors
  Degree of plaque disruption (i.e., fissure, ulcer)
  Degree of stenosis (i.e., change in geometry)
  Tissue substrate (i.e., lipid-rich plaque)
  Surface of residual thrombus (i.e., recurrence)
  Vasoconstriction (i.e., platelets, thrombin)
Systemic factors
  Catecholamines (i.e., smoking, stress, cocaine)
  Cholesterol, Lp(a) and other metabolic states
    (i.e., homocysteinemia, diabetes)
  Fibrinogen, impaired fibrinolysis (i.e., PAI-1),
    activated platelets, and clotting (i.e., Factor VII,
    thrombin generation [F1 + 2] or activity [FPA])

[a]High risk, occlusive acute coronary syndromes (ACS); low risk, mural (progression).
Data from Fuster et al., ref. 79, and Burke et al., ref. 19.

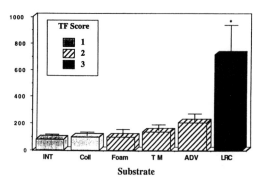

FIG. 3-3. Platelet deposition and tissue factor activity. Platelet deposition data are expressed as means ± SEM; TF staining intensity is expressed as the average of the independent observers. Note the positive correlation between platelet-thrombus formation and TF score on the exposed human substrates (p < 0.01). INT, normal intima; COLL, collagen-rich matrix; FOAM, foam cell-rich matrix; TM, normal tunica media; ADV, adventitia; LRC, lipid-rich core (*p = 0.0002, ANOVA). (From Wilcox et al., ref. 66, with permission.)

nificantly higher in culprit lesions obtained by coronary atherectomy from patients with unstable angina and myocardial infarction than in those from patients with stable angina (67,69).

When thrombosis occurs without frank plaque disruption and with only a superficial plaque erosion, the critical thrombogenic plaque components are more in question. Tissue factor, expressed by activated macrophages or SMCs, could be important, but matrix components (i.e., collagen and proteoglycans) probably play a more important thrombogenic role in superficial plaque erosion (48,52).

In patients with thrombus-mediated unstable angina pectoris, early antithrombotic therapy with heparin and platelet glycoprotein IIb/IIIa receptor blockers improve the short-term prognosis (70). However, the initial benefit obtained during treatment is often lost soon after treatment due to rebound, reactivation, or persistency of the thrombogenic substrate (70). Obviously, antithrombotic therapy does not affect the mechanisms underlying plaque disruption and plaque thrombogenicity. To improve the prognosis in unstable angina, we need also

to target the plaque directly, i.e., reducing the thrombogenicity of the culprit lesion. If the local plaque thrombogenicity is mediated via tissue factor, which seems likely, a vital question is: What turns tissue factor on in plaques? Preliminary results from a pilot study of oral roxithromycin, an antichlamydial antibiotic, in unstable coronary artery disease suggests that in some high-risk patients active infection with *Chlamydia pneumoniae* could play a decisive role in plaque disruption and thrombosis (71). *Chlamydia* has been identified in coronary plaques, it contains lipopolysaccharide (LPS) in the cell wall, and LPS is a well-known strong inducer of many enzymes, including matrix metalloproteinases and tissue factor (72–74).

Local Flow Disturbances

The severity of stenosis and surface irregularities at the site of plaque disruption may disturb local rheology and influence the thrombotic response. The tighter the stenosis and the rougher the surface, the more platelets are activated and deposited (23,45,75,76). A platelet thrombus may form and grow within a severe stenosis where the blood velocity and shear forces are highest, probably due to shear-induced platelet activation (77,78). It may explain the clinical observation that the more obstructive a plaque is at baseline angiographic examination, the higher risk of subsequent progression to occlusion or to culprit for myocardial infarction (26). However, because less obstructive plaques by far outnumber severely obstructive plaques, most coronary occlusions and myocardial infarctions originate from plaques that were only mildly to moderately obstructive just before the acute event (Fig. 3-4) (26).

Systemic Thrombotic Tendency

Systemic thrombogenic factors are summarized in Table 3-1 (79,80). In addition, a transient or persistent hypercoagulable state, probably partly mediated by activated monocytes in the peripheral blood, can be identified in many patients with acute coronary syndromes

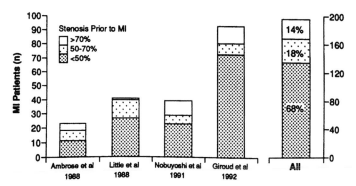

FIG. 3-4. Bar graph showing stenosis severity and associated risk of myocardial infarction (MI). MI evolves most frequently from plaques that are only mildly to moderately obstructive months to years before infarction. (The bar graph is constructed from data published by Ambrose et al., ref. 16; Little et al., ref. 17; Nobuyoshi et al., ref. 95; and Giroud et al., ref. 96.)

(81,82). The importance of the actual thrombotic–thrombolytic equilibrium at the time of plaque disruption is clearly documented by the protective effect of antiplatelet agents and anticoagulants against myocardial infarction and coronary death in patients with IHD (79,80).

Thrombosis: Platelets and Fibrin

The thrombotic response to plaque disruption is a dynamic process; thrombosis and thrombolysis occur simultaneously in many patients with acute coronary syndromes, with or without concomitant vasospasm, causing intermittent flow obstructions (1–3,83) (Fig. 3-5). The initial flow obstruction is usually caused by platelet aggregation, but fibrin is important for subsequent stabilization of the early and fragile platelet thrombus (83). Therefore, both platelets and fibrin play a role in the evolution of a persisting coronary thrombus.

If the white platelet-rich thrombus at the rupture site occludes the lumen totally, the blood proximal and distal to the occlusion will stagnate and may coagulate, giving rise to a secondarily formed venous-type, red stagnation thrombosis (3). Proximal thrombus propagation may pass side branches, but usually does so without occluding them. In contrast, distal thrombus propagation may occlude side branches, particularly in the right coronary

artery with its relatively few major side branches. The amount of thrombus formed (thrombotic burden) probably depends to some extent on the available collateral flow. If there is no collateral flow, the blood will stagnate and it may coagulate. Although the secondarily formed venous-type thrombus is probably more easily lyzed than the primary platelet-rich thrombus at the rupture site, a huge clot may contribute significantly to the overall thrombotic burden and thus hamper thrombolysis. Extensive stagnation thrombosis seems to be a problem particularly in coronary vein grafts because, compared with native coronary arteries, their caliber is larger and they have no side branches. Clinical experiences indicate that coronary vein grafts generally are difficult to open rapidly by intravenous thrombolytic therapy, probably because of their larger thrombotic burden (84).

CLINICAL MANIFESTATIONS

The occurrence and course of coronary atherosclerosis and IHD are largely unpredictable (85). For individuals with the same number and degree of stenoses evaluated angiographically, some live for years without any symptoms, whereas others are severely handicapped by angina pectoris, experience acute coronary syndromes, or die suddenly and unexpectedly. Plaque vulnerability and

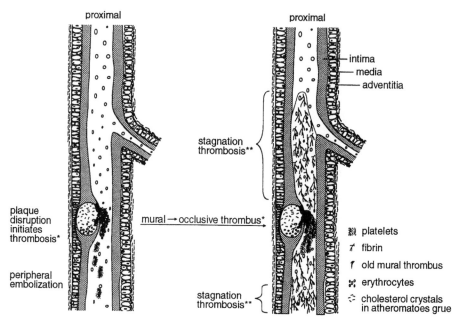

FIG. 3-5. Coronary thrombosis: plaque, flow, and blood.

Local thrombogenic substrate	**plaque disruption : 60 - 80%** **plaque erosion : 20 - 40%**
Local flow disturbances	**stenosis causing high shear surface irregularities**
Systemic thrombotic tendency	**platelet hyperaggregability hypercoagulability impaired fibrinolysis**
Thrombus at site of injury	**platelet-rich, stabilized by fibrin dynamic obstruction**
Thrombus propagation	**blood stagnation causing coagulation**

thrombogenicity rather than plaque size or stenosis severity are most important for event-free survival in IHD (26).

Stable Angina

Hangartner et al. categorized the plaque type in 54 men with stable angina and found that 60% of the plaques were fibrous and 40% were lipid-rich (86). More interestingly, all the plaques were fibrous in 15% of the patients, and not a single plaque with a large lipid pool was found in as many as one third of the patients. Apparently, many patients with stable angina lack the appropriate pathoanatomic substrate for plaque disruption and may, consequently, be at low risk of an acute coronary syndrome. However, it should be noted that in the same patient, individual plaques usually differ significantly, and the composition of one plaque does not predict the composition of a nearby plaque in the same artery.

Silent Plaque Disruption

Plaque disruption itself is asymptomatic, and the associated rapid plaque growth is usually clinically silent. It is probably the most important mechanism responsible for the unpredictable, sudden, and nonlinear progression of coronary lesions frequently observed angiographically (87).

Acute Coronary Syndromes

After plaque disruption, hemorrhage into the plaque, luminal thrombosis, and/or vasospasm may cause sudden flow obstruction, giving rise to new or changing symptoms. The culprit lesion is frequently dynamic, causing intermittent flow obstruction, and the clinical presentation and the outcome depend on the severity and duration of myocardial ischemia. A nonocclusive or transiently occlusive thrombus most frequently underlie primary unstable angina with pain at rest and non–Q-wave infarction (often, but not always subendocardial), whereas a more stable and occlusive thrombus is most frequently seen in Q-wave infarction (often, but not always transmural), modified overall by vascular tone and collateral flow (79). The lesion responsible for out-of-hospital cardiac arrest or sudden death is often similar to that of unstable angina: a disrupted plaque with superimposed nonocclusive thrombosis (63,79,88).

Triggering of Disease Onset

Onset of acute coronary syndromes does not occur at random (89). Myocardial infarction occurs at increased frequency in the morning, particularly within the first hour after awakening, on Mondays, during winter months and on colder days the year around, during emotional stress, and during vigorous exercise (89–94). The pathophysiologic mechanisms responsible for the nonrandom and apparently often triggered onset of myocardial infarction are unknown, but possibly are: (a) plaque disruption, likely due to surges in sympathetic activity with a sudden increase in blood pressure, pulse rate, heart contraction, and coronary blood flow; (b) thrombosis, occurring on previously disrupted or intact plaques when the systemic thrombotic tendency is high (Table 3-1) because of platelet activation, hypercoagulability, and/or impaired fibrinolysis; and (c) vasoconstriction, generalized or occurring locally around a coronary plaque.

CONCLUSION

Coronary atherosclerosis is by far the most frequent cause of IHD, but atherosclerosis alone is rarely fatal. Most acute coronary syndromes are caused by sudden plaque disruption with superimposed thrombosis, with or without concomitant vasospasm. For event-free survival, the vital question is not why atherosclerosis develops but rather why atherosclerosis, after years of indolent growth, suddenly becomes complicated by life-threatening thrombosis. Atherosclerosis would be a much more benign disease if plaque disruption and thrombosis could be prevented.

Therefore, we must focus on plaque vulnerability to rupture and plaque thrombogenicity, rather than on plaque size and stenosis severity. The challenge of today is to find and treat the dangerous vulnerable plaques responsible for the life-threatening coronary events; to find and treat only stenotic angina-producing lesions is not enough. Culprit lesion-based interventions usually eliminate anginal pain but do not substantially improve the long-term outcome because myocardial infarction and death depend more on coexisting asymptomatic vulnerable plaques than on the stenotic angina-producing lesions. For effective prevention and treatment, a systemic approach that addresses all coronary plaques and not only the stenotic ones will prove to be most rewarding.

REFERENCES

1. Fuster V, Badimon L, Badimon J, Chesebro JH. The pathogenesis of coronary artery disease and the acute coronary syndromes. *N Engl J Med* 1992;326:242–250, 310–318.
2. Shah PK. Pathophysiology of unstable angina. *Cardiol Clin* 1991;9:11–26.
3. Falk E. Coronary thrombosis: pathogenesis and clinical manifestations. *Am J Cardiol* 1991;68(suppl B): 28B–35B.
4. Ge J, Erbel R, Gerber T, et al. Intravascular ultrasound imaging of angiographically normal coronary arteries: a prospective in vivo study. *Br Heart J* 1994;71:572–578.
5. Roberts WC. Diffuse extent of coronary atherosclerosis in fatal coronary artery disease. *Am J Cardiol* 1990;65: 2F–6F.
6. Glagov S, Weisenberd E, Zarins C, Stankunavicius R, Kolettis G. Compensatory enlargement of human atherosclerotic coronary arteries. *N Engl J Med* 1987;316: 1371–1375.
7. Ge J, Erbel R, Zamorano J, et al. Coronary artery remodeling in atherosclerotic disease: an intravascular ultrasound study in vivo. *Coronary Artery Dis* 1993;4: 981–986.
8. Losordo DW, Rosenfield K, Kaufmann J, Pieczek A, Isner JM. Focal compensatory enlargement of human atherosclerotic coronary arteries in response to progressive atherosclerosis: in vivo documentation using intravascular ultrasound. *Circulation* 1994;89:2570–2577.
9. Mintz GS, Kent KM, Pichard AD, Satler LF, Popma JJ, Leon MB. Contribution of inadequate arterial remodeling to the development of focal coronary artery stenoses. An intravascular ultrasound study. *Circulation* 1997;95:1791–1798.
10. Mann JM, Davies MJ. Vulnerable plaque. Relation of characteristics to degree of stenosis in human coronary arteries. *Circulation* 1996;94:928–931.
11. Kragel AH, Roberts WC. Composition of atherosclerotic plaques in the coronary arteries in homozygous familial hypercholesterolaemia. *Am Heart J* 1991;121: 210–211.
12. Gertz SD, Malekzadeh S, Dollar AL, Kragel AH, Roberts WC. Composition of atherosclerotic plaques in the four major epicardial coronary arteries in patients ≤90 years of age. *Am J Cardiol* 1991;67:1228–1233.
13. Dollar AL, Kragel AH, Fernicola DJ, Waclawiw MA, Roberts WC. Composition of atherosclerotic plaques in coronary arteries in women <40 years of age with fatal coronary artery disease and implications for plaque reversibility. *Am J Cardiol* 1991;67:1223–1227.
14. Mautner SL, Lin F, Roberts WC. Composition of atherosclerotic plaques in the epicardial coronary arteries in juvenile (type I) diabetes mellitus. *Am J Cardiol* 1992; 70:1264–1268.
15. Mintz GS, Pichard AD, Popma JJ, Kent KM, Satler LF, Bucher TA, Leon MB. Determinants and correlates of target lesion calcium in coronary artery disease: a clinical, angiographic and intravascular ultrasound study. *J Am Coll Cardiol* 1997;29:268–274.
16. Rumberger JA, Simons B, Fitzpatrick LA, Sheedy PF, Schwartz RS. Coronary artery calcium area by electron-beam computed tomography and coronary atherosclerotic plaque area. A histopathologic correlative study. *Circulation* 1995;92:2157–2162.
17. Wexler L, Brundage B, Crouse J, et al. Coronary artery calcification: pathophysiology, epidemiology, imaging methods, and clinical implications. A statement for health professionals from the American Heart Association. *Circulation* 1996;94:1175–1192.
18. Khurana S, Schreiber TL, Nino CL, Dooris M, Sachs D, Safian RD. Does coronary calcification influence plaque stability? *Circulation* 1994;90(suppl I):I-438.
19. Burke AP, Farb A, Malcom GT, Liang YH, Smialek J, Virmani R. Coronary risk factors and plaque morphology in men with coronary disease who died suddenly. *N Engl J Med* 1997;336:1276–1282.
20. Davies MJ. The composition of coronary-artery plaques. *N Engl J Med* 1997;336:1312–1314.
21. Kragel AH, Reddy SG, Wittes JT, Roberts WC. Morphometric analysis of the composition of atherosclerotic plaques in the four major epicardial coronary arteries in acute myocardial infarction and in sudden coronary death. *Circulation* 1989;80:1747–1756.
22. Kragel AH, Reddy SG, Wittes JT, Roberts WC. Morphometric analysis of the composition of coronary arterial plaques in isolated unstable angina pectoris with pain at rest. *Am J Cardiol* 1990;66:562–567.
23. Fernandez-Ortiz A, Badimon JJ, Falk E, et al. Characterization of the relative thrombogenicity of atherosclerotic plaque components: implications for consequences of plaque rupture. *J Am Coll Cardiol* 1994;23:1562–1569.
24. Falk E. Morphologic features of unstable atherosclerotic plaques underlying acute coronary syndromes. *Am J Cardiol* 1989;63(suppl E):114E–120E.
25. Davies MJ. Stability and instability: two faces of coronary atherosclerosis. The Paul Dudley White Lecture 1995. *Circulation* 1996;94:2013–2020.
26. Falk E, Shah PK, Fuster V. Coronary plaque disruption. *Circulation* 1995;92:657–671.
27. MacIsaac AI, Thomas JD, Topol EJ. Toward the quiescent coronary plaque. *J Am Coll Cardiol* 1993;22:1228–1241.
28. Gertz SD, Roberts WC. Hemodynamic shear force in rupture of coronary arterial atherosclerotic plaques. *Am J Cardiol* 1990;66:1368–1372.
29. Friedman M. The coronary thrombus: its origin and fate. *Hum Pathol* 1971;2:81–128.
30. Guyton JR, Klemp KF. The lipid-rich core region of human atherosclerotic fibrous plaques. Prevalence of small lipid droplets and vesicles by electron microscopy. *Am J Pathol* 1989;134:705–717.
31. Stary HC. Evolution and progression of atherosclerotic lesions in coronary arteries of children and young adults. *Arteriosclerosis* 1989;9(suppl I):I-19–I-32.
32. Small DM. Progression and regression of atherosclerotic lesions. Insights from lipid physical biochemistry. *Arteriosclerosis* 1988;8:103–129.
33. Lundberg B. Chemical composition and physical state of lipid deposits in atherosclerosis. *Atherosclerosis* 1985;56:93–110.
34. Davies MJ, Richardson PD, Woolf N, Katz DR, Mann J. Risk of thrombosis in human atherosclerotic plaques: role of extracellular lipid, macrophage, and smooth muscle cell content. *Br Heart J* 1993;69:377–381.
35. Loree HM, Tobias BJ, Gibson LJ, Kamm RD, Small DM, Lee RT. Mechanical properties of model atherosclerotic lesion lipid pools. *Arterioscler Thromb* 1994; 14:230–234.
36. Wagner WD, St. Clair RW, Clarkson TB, Connor JR. A study of atherosclerosis regression in Macaca mulatta.

III. Chemical changes in arteries from animals with atherosclerosis induced for 19 months and regressed for 48 months at plasma cholesterol concentrations of 300 or 200 mg/dl. *Am J Pathol* 1980;100:633–650.

37. Geng Y-J, Libby P. Evidence for apoptosis in advanced human atheroma. *Am J Pathol* 1995;147:251–266.

38. Ball RY, Stowers EC, Burton JH, Cary NRB, Skepper JN, Mitchinson MJ. Evidence that the death of macrophage foam cells contributes to the lipid core of atheroma. *Atherosclerosis* 1995;114:45–54.

39. Björkerud S, Björkerud B. Apoptosis is abundant in human atherosclerotic lesions, especially in inflammatory cells (macrophages and T cells), and may contribute to the accumulation of gruel and plaque instability. *Am J Pathol* 1996;149:367–380.

40. Witztum JL. The oxidation hypothesis of atherosclerosis. *Lancet* 1994;344:793–795.

41. Wight TN. Cell biology of arterial proteoglycans. *Arteriosclerosis* 1989;9:1–20.

42. Guyton JR, Klemp KF. Development of the atherosclerotic core region: chemical and ultrastructural analysis of microdissected atherosclerotic lesions from human aorta. *Arterioscler Thromb* 1994;14:1305–1314.

43. Libby P. Molecular bases of the acute coronary syndromes. *Circulation* 1995;91:2844–2850.

44. Hansson GK. Immune responses in atherosclerosis. In: Hansson GK, Libby P (eds). *Immune Functions of the Vessel Wall.* Amsterdam: Harwood Academic, 1996.

45. Falk E. Plaque rupture with severe pre-existing stenosis precipitating coronary thrombosis. Characteristics of coronary atherosclerotic plaques underlying fatal occlusive thrombi. *Br Heart J* 1983;50:127–134.

46. Friedman M. The coronary thrombus: its origin and fate. *Hum Pathol* 1971;2:81–128.

47. Constantinides P. Plaque fissures in human coronary thrombosis. *J Atheroscler Res* 1966;6:1–17.

48. van der Wal AC, Becker AE, van der Loos CM, Das PK. Site of intimal rupture or erosion of thrombosed coronary atherosclerotic plaques is characterized by an inflammatory process irrespective of the dominant plaque morphology. *Circulation* 1994;89:36–44.

49. Richardson PD, Davies MJ, Born GVR. Influence of plaque configuration and stress distribution on fissuring of coronary atherosclerotic plaques. *Lancet* 1989;2:941–944.

50. Poston RN, Haskard DO, Coucher JR, Gall NP, Johnson-Tidey RR. Expression of intercellular adhesion molecule-1 in atherosclerotic plaques. *Am J Pathol* 1992;140:665–673.

51. Lendon CL, Davies MJ, Born GVR, Richardson PD. Atherosclerotic plaque caps are locally weakened when macrophages density is increased. *Atherosclerosis* 1991;87:87–90.

52. Farb A, Burke AP, Tang AL, et al. Coronary plaque erosion without rupture into a lipid core: a frequent cause of coronary thrombosis in sudden coronary death. *Circulation* 1996;93:1354–1363.

53. van der Wal AC, Becker AE, Koch KT, et al. Clinically stable angina pectoris is not necessarily associated with histologically stable atherosclerotic plaques. *Heart* 1996;76:312–316.

54. Moreno PR, Falk E, Palacios IF, Newell JB, Fuster V, Fallon JT. Macrophage infiltration in acute coronary syndromes: implications for plaque rupture. *Circulation* 1994;90:775–778.

55. Galis ZS, Sukhova GK, Lark MW, Libby P. Increased expression of matrix-metalloproteinases and matrix degrading activity in vulnerable regions of human atherosclerotic plaques. *J Clin Invest* 1994;94:2493–2503.

56. Matrisian LM. The matrix degrading metalloproteinases. *Bioessays* 1992;14:455–463.

57. Shah PK, Falk E, Badimon JJ, et al. Human monocyte-derived macrophages induce collagen breakdown in fibrous caps of atherosclerotic plaques. Potential role of matrix-degrading metalloproteinases and implications for plaque rupture. *Circulation* 1995;92:1565–1569.

58. Kaartinen M, Penttilä A, Kovanen PT. Accumulation of activated mast cells in the shoulder region of human coronary atheroma, the predilection site of atheromatous rupture. *Circulation* 1994;90:1669–1678.

59. Kovanen PT, Kaartinen M, Paavonen T. Infiltrates of activated mast cells at the site of coronary atheromatous erosion or rupture in myocardial infarction. *Circulation* 1995;92:1084–1088.

60. Loree HM, Kamm RD, Stringfellow RG, Lee RT. Effects of fibrous cap thickness on peak circumferential stress in model atherosclerotic vessels. *Circ Res* 1992; 71:850–858.

61. Burleigh MC, Briggs AD, Lendon CL, Davies MJ, Born GV, Richardson PD. Collagen types I and III, collagen content, GAGs and mechanical strength of human atherosclerotic plaque caps: span-wise variations. *Atherosclerosis* 1992;96:71–81.

62. Davies MJ, Bland JM, Hangartner JRW, Angelini A, Thomas AC. Factors influencing the presence or absence of acute coronary artery thrombi in sudden ischaemic death. *Eur Heart J* 1989;10:203–208.

63. Davies MJ, Thomas A. Thrombosis and acute coronary-artery lesions in sudden cardiac ischemic death. *N Engl J Med* 1984;310:1137–1140.

64. Cheng GC, Loree HM, Kamm RD, Fishbein MC, Lee RT. Distribution of circumferential stress in ruptured and stable atherosclerotic lesions. A structural analysis with histopathological correlation. *Circulation* 1993;87: 1179–1187.

65. Toschi V, Gallo R, Lettino M, et al. Tissue factor modulates the thrombogenicity of human atherosclerotic plaques. *Circulation* 1997;85:594–599.

66. Wilcox JN, Smith KM, Schwartz SM, Gordon D. Localization of tissue factor in the normal vessel wall and in the atherosclerotic plaque. *Proc Natl Acad Sci U S A* 1989;86:2839–2843.

67. Moreno PR, Bernardi VH, López-Cuéllar J, et al. Macrophages, smooth muscle cells, and tissue factor in unstable angina. Implications for cell-mediated thrombogenicity in acute coronary syndromes. *Circulation* 1996;94:3090–3097.

68. Thiruvikraman SV, Guha A, Roboz J, Taubman MB, Nemerson Y, Fallon JT. In situ localization of tissue factor in human atherosclerotic plaques by binding of digoxigenin-labeled factors VIIa and X. *Lab Invest* 1996;75: 451–461.

69. Ardissino D, Merlini PA, Ari'ns R, Coppola R, Bramucci E, Mannucci PM. Tissue-factor antigen and activity in human coronary atherosclerotic plaques. *Lancet* 1997;349:769–771.

70. Wallentin L. Unstable coronary artery disease—need for long term antithrombotic treatment. Aspirin alone is not sufficient, I would associate an anticoagulant. *Cardiovasc Res* 1997;33:292–294.

71. Gurfinkel E, Bozovich G, Doroca A, et al. ROXIS Study Group. Randomised trial of roxithromycin in non-Q-wave coronary syndromes: ROXIS pilot study. *Lancet* 1997;350:404–407.

72. Muhlestein JB, Hammond EH, Carlquist JF, et al. Increased incidence of Chlamydia species within the coronary arteries of patients with symptomatic atherosclerotic versus other forms of cardiovascular disease. *J Am Coll Cardiol* 1996;27:1555–1561.

73. Ramirez JA. Isolation of *Chlamydia pneumoniae* from the coronary artery of a patient with coronary atherosclerosis. *Ann Intern Med* 1996;125:979–982.

74. Gupta S, Leatham EW. The relation between *Chlamydia pneumoniae* and atherosclerosis. *Heart* 1997;77: 7–8.

75. de Cesare NB, Ellis SG, Williamson PR, Deboe SF, Pitt B, Mancini GB. Early reocclusion after thrombolysis is related to lesion length and roughness. *Coronary Artery Dis* 1993;4:159–166.

76. Folts J. An in vivo model of experimental arterial stenosis, intimal damage, and periodic thrombosis. *Circulation* 1991:83(suppl IV):IV-3–IV-14.

77. Badimon L, Badimon JJ. Mechanism of arterial thrombosis in non-parallel streamlines: platelet thrombi grow on the apex of stenotic severely injured vessel wall. *J Clin Invest* 1989;84:1134–1144.

78. Ruggeri ZM. Mechanisms of shear-induced platelet adhesion and aggregation. *Thromb Haemost* 1993;70: 119–123.

79. Fuster V, Lewis A. Connor Memorial Lecture: mechanisms leading to myocardial infarction: insights from studies of vascular biology. *Circulation* 1994;90: 2126–2146.

80. Fuster V, Fallon JT, Nemerson Y. Coronary thrombosis. *Lancet* 1996;348(suppl: coronary heart disease):7–10

81. Jude B, Agraou B, McFadden EP, et al. Evidence for time-dependent activation of monocytes in the systemic circulation in unstable angina, but not in acute myocardial infarction or in stable angina. *Circulation* 1994;90: 1662–1668.

82. Merlini PA, Bauer KA, Oltrona L, et al. Persistent activation of coagulation mechanism in unstable angina and myocardial infarction. *Circulation* 1994;90:61–68.

83. Falk E. Unstable angina with fatal outcome: dynamic coronary thrombosis leading to infarction and/or sudden death. Autopsy evidence of recurrent mural thrombosis with peripheral embolization culminating in total vascular occlusion. *Circulation* 1985;71:699–708.

84. Grines CL, Booth DC, Nissen SE, et al. Mechanism of acute myocardial infarction in patients with prior coronary artery bypass grafting and therapeutic implications. *Am J Cardiol* 1990;65:1292–1296.

85. Tavazzi L, Volpi A. Remarks about postinfarction prognosis in light of the experience with the Gruppo Italiano per lo Studio della Sopravvivenza nell Infarto miocardico (GISSI) trials. *Circulation* 1997;95:1341–1345.

86. Hangartner JRW, Charleston AJ, Davies MJ, Thomas AC. Morphological characteristics of clinically significant coronary artery stenosis in stable angina. *Br Heart J* 1986;56:501–508.

87. Bruschke AVG, Kramer JR, Bal ET, Haque IU, Detrano RC, Goormastic M. The dynamics of progression of coronary atherosclerosis studied in 168 medically treated patients who underwent coronary arteriography three times. *Am Heart J* 1989;117:296–305.

88. Spaulding CM, Joly L-M, Rosenberg A, et al. Immediate coronary angiography in survivors of out-of-hospital cardiac arrest. *N Engl J Med* 1997;336:1629–1633.

89. Muller JE, Abela GS, Nesto RW, Tofler GH. Triggers, acute risk factors and vulnerable plaques: the lexicon of a new frontier. *J Am Coll Cardiol* 1994;23:809–813.

90. Mittleman MA, Maclure M, Tofler GH, Sherwood JB, Goldberg RJ, Muller JE. Triggering of acute myocardial infarction by heavy physical exertion: protection against triggering by regular exertion. *N Engl J Med* 1993;329: 1677–1683.

91. Willich SN, Lewis M, Löwel H, Arntz H-R, Schubert F, Schröder R. Physical exertion as a trigger of acute myocardial infarction. *N Engl J Med* 1993;329:1684–1690.

92. Mittleman MA, Maclure M, Sherwood JB, et al. Triggering of acute myocardial infarction onset by episodes of anger. *Circulation* 1995;92:1720–1725.

93. Muller JE, Mittleman A, Maclure M, Sherwood JB, Tofler GH. Triggering myocardial infarction by sexual activity. Low absolute risk and prevention by regular physical exertion. *JAMA* 1996;275:1405–1409.

94. Leor J, Poole WK, Kloner RA. Sudden cardiac death triggered by an earthquake. *N Engl J Med* 1996;334: 413–419.

95. Nobuyoshi M, Tanaka M, Nosaka H, et al. Progression of atherosclerosis: is coronary spasm related to progression? *J Am Coll Cardiol* 1991;18:904–910.

96. Giroud D, Li JM, Urban P, Meier B, Rutishauser W. Relation of the site of acute myocardial infarction to the most severe coronary arterial stenosis at prior angiography. *Am J Cardiol* 1992;69:729–732.

Cardiovascular Thrombosis: Thrombocardiology and Thromboneurology, Second Edition,
edited by M. Verstraete, V. Fuster, and E. J. Topol,
Lippincott–Raven Publishers, Philadelphia © 1998.

4

Familial Thrombophilia

Saskia Middeldorp, Ernest Briët, and *Jacqueline Conard

*Department of Internal Medicine, Academic Medical Center, Amsterdam, The Netherlands; and
Service d'Hématologie Biologique, Hotel Dieu University Hospital, 75004 Paris, France

The occurrence of venous thromboembolism within certain families has been observed for many decades (1–3). These thrombophilic families have been a great source for gaining insight into the pathophysiologic mechanisms of venous thrombosis by recognizing different inborn abnormalities in the coagulation cascade or its regulatory mechanisms that cause the tendency for venous thromboembolism.

In this chapter we discuss the definition of familial thrombophilia, including epidemiologic aspects and clinical manifestations. For the established abnormalities, we elaborate on pathophysiologic mechanisms, diagnosis, epidemiology, and clinical presentation. Furthermore, we tentatively propose guidelines for management and screen-ing indications. Finally, we give a short overview of the possible candidate risk factors for venous thromboembolism.

DEFINITION OF THROMBOPHILIA: GENETIC RISK FACTORS

For any abnormality to be considered a risk factor, the association between the defect and a disease must be established. For venous thromboembolism this is not always easy because the disease becomes manifest episodically with long asymptomatic periods in between. Furthermore, the manifestations may differ from superficial phlebitis to fatal pulmonary embolism. In inherited abnormalities leading to an increased tendency for venous thromboembolism, a dose-response relation-

TABLE 4-1. *Risk factors for venous thromboembolism*

Risk factors	Remarks and key references
Well established inherited risk factors	
Antithrombin deficiency	See text (3)
Protein C deficiency	See text (16)
Protein S deficiency	See text (17,18)
FV:Q^{506} mutation (APC resistance)	See text (6)
Hyperhomocysteinaemia	See text: multifactorial etiology; relationship between identified genetic defects and thrombotic risk unclear (8–13)
Hereditary dysfibrinogenemia	Very rare, not discussed in text (19)
Candidate risk factors	
Prothrombin mutation	Association between defect and thrombotic risk (RR ≈ 3); awaiting confirmation from other studies (20)
Thrombomodulin mutations	Four mutations identified; relationship with thrombotic risk not firmly established (21,22)
Elevated factor VIII levels	Risk factor for deep vein thrombosis; no confirmation from other studies or reports on hereditability and etiology (165)
Plasminogen deficiency	Conflicting data of association between low plasminogen levels and thrombotic risk (23,24)
Elevated histidine-rich glycoprotein levels	Reports of thrombophilic families only; no case-control studies to confirm relationship between abnormality and thrombotic risk (25,26)
Heparin cofactor II deficiency	Reports of thrombophilic families; no confirmation in case control studies (27,28,165)
β2 glycoprotein I deficiency	Probably not a risk factor for thrombosis (29)
Factor XII deficiency	Probably not a risk factor for thrombosis (conflicting data) (30,31)
Tissue factor pathway inhibitor	No mutations found (Reitsma PH and Bertina R; unpublished observations)
Thrombin-activated fibrin inhibitor	No reports yet

ship is often found, in the sense that a homozygous abnormality leads to more frequent occurrence of venous thromboembolism than the heterozygous trait.

The relationship between a number of acquired conditions and venous thromboembolism is well established. Examples of these conditions or situations are surgery, trauma and immobilization, malignancy, antiphospholipid antibodies, and exposure to estrogens. These acquired risk factors will not be discussed further.

Familial thrombophilia was originally defined as a tendency toward recurrent venous thromboembolism, usually at a young age and in the absence of the above mentioned conditions, occurring sometimes at unusual sites, and affecting several members of a family. In many of these families, genetic defects have been detected that explain the thrombotic tendency. However, it is important to note that in-

herited prothrombotic factors have a variable clinical penetrance and do not always cause familial thrombophilia. If the family history is strongly positive for venous thromboembolism, it may favor the presence of an inherited thrombophilic factor in an individual thrombosis patient. On the other hand, a negative family history is not very helpful unless the pedigree is large and detailed information is available (4).

Currently, a genetic risk factor can be detected in approximately 50% of patients with a first episode of venous thromboembolism. Well-established genetic risk factors for venous thromboembolism comprise deficiencies or functional abnormalities in two natural anticoagulant pathways: the antithrombin–heparin sulphate pathway (antithrombin deficiency) and the protein C pathway, in which protein S serves as a cofactor (protein C deficiency, protein S deficiency, and resistance to activated protein C) (3,5–7). Hyperhomocys-teinemia has been shown to be a prevalent risk factor for venous thrombosis (8–11). Although elevated homocysteine levels are shown to be familial in many patients (8,10), this is often not due to well-defined genetic abnormalities (12–14). Furthermore, several candidate genetic risk factors have been or are now under investigation. Table 4-1 summarizes both established and less well defined risk factors for inherited or familial thrombophilia (6,8–13,15–31).

NATURAL ANTICOAGULANT PATHWAYS

The coagulation abnormalities that are associated with inherited thrombophilia are found in two natural anticoagulant pathways.

In the antithrombin–heparin sulphate pathway, antithrombin is the primary inactivator of thrombin and factor Xa, but it also inhibits other activated coagulation factors. Antithrombin forms an irreversible complex with the activated coagulation factors. Heparin and heparinlike proteoglycans associated with the vessel wall markedly accelerate the inhibition of serine proteinases by antithrombin (32).

In the protein C pathway, activated protein C, after complex formation with free protein S, selectively inactivates cofactors Va and VIIIa, thereby regulating the formation of thrombin. First, protein C needs activation by thrombin, a reaction that is accelerated by binding of thrombin to thrombomodulin, a protein that is present on the endothelium (33,34). Factor Va is inactivated by activated protein C, with primary cleavage at Arg^{506}, followed by cleavage at Arg^{306} and Arg^{679} (35).

Antithrombin, protein C, protein S, and factor V are synthesized in the liver; protein S and factor V are also present in megakaryocytes, and protein S is also synthesized in endothelial cells and Leydig cells. The genes, coding for antithrombin (36,37), protein C (38), protein S (39), and factor V (40) have been completely elucidated.

HOMOCYSTEINE METABOLISM

Homocysteine is an amino acid derived from the metabolic conversion of methionine. Homocysteine is either remethylized to methionine or transsulfurated to cysteine. One remethylation pathway is catalyzed by methionine synthetase and methylenetetrahydrofolate reductase, in which methyltetrahydrofolate donates the methyl group and cobalamine (vitamin B_{12}) acts as a cofactor. The other remethylation pathway is catalyzed by betaine-homocysteine methyltransferase, in which betaine is the methyl group donor. The transsulfuration pathway to cysteine is catalyzed by cystathionine-β-synthase, and pyridoxine (vitamin B_6) acts as a cofactor. In plasma, homocysteine is oxidized to disulfides and exists both in free and protein-bound forms.

TYPES OF DEFICIENCIES

In general, two types of deficiencies of antithrombin, protein C and protein S, are distinguished. In type I deficiency, levels of both antigen and activity are reduced. In type II deficiency, antigen levels are normal, but one or more functional defects of the molecule lead to a decreased activity.

For type II antithrombin and protein C deficiency, different subtypes are recognized, depending on the location of the functional defect. For antithrombin type II deficiency, defects are found in the reactive site or the heparin-binding site; multiple, pleiotropic defects also may be found. A database of mutations in the gene coding for antithrombin is available and updated on a regular basis (41,42). For protein C type II deficiency, abnormalities can occur on sites of substrate binding, thrombomodulin interaction, or calcium binding. A database of mutations in the gene coding for protein C is available and updated on a regular basis (43,44).

For protein S deficiency, three types are distinguished. In type I, total and free antigen and the protein S activity are reduced. In type II, concentrations of both total and free antigen are normal, but the protein S activity is reduced. In type III, total antigen is normal, but the concentrations of free antigen and the protein S activity are reduced. A database of mutations in the protein S gene was recently published (45).

Resistance of factor Va to the proteolytic action of activated protein C (APC resistance) was first described in 1993 (6,46), and in the majority of individuals this resistance is caused by a single point mutation at the first cleavage site of factor Va, where Arg^{506} is substituted by Gln (47–51). By lacking this cleavage site, the inactivation of factor Va is markedly decreased (52,53). The mutant factor V also has been named factor V Leiden (47). So far, the factor V–Arg→Gln^{506} ($FV:Q^{506}$) mutation is the only genetic defect identified as a cause of resistance to activated protein C. Similar mutations in the gene coding for factor VIII have not been found (54). In vitro, APC ratios are lower in women as compared with men, in oral contraceptive users (55), and in pregnant women (56–58).

Hyperhomocysteinemia is a heterogeneous disorder, caused by both inherited and acquired conditions. Mutations in the cystathionine–β-synthase gene as well as in the methylenetetrahydrofolate reductase gene have been reported to be associated with hyperhomocysteinemia (13,59–62). Severe hyperhomocysteinemia (referred to as homocysteinuria) with plasma levels over 100 μmol/L is caused by homozygous deficiency of cystathionine–β-synthase in the majority of cases (63). A minority is caused by homozygous deficiency of methylenetetrahydrofolate reductase (64). Mild or moderate hyperhomocysteinemia (plasma levels between 16 and 100 μmol/L) may be caused by genetic defects such as heterozygous deficiency of cystathionine–β-synthase and homozygosity for a thermolabile mutant of methylenetetrahydrofolate reductase (13), although the relationship of these genetic abnormalities to the occurrence of venous thromboembolism is probably weak or absent (14). More frequent causes of hyperhomocysteinemia are acquired deficiencies of

cobalamin, folate, and pyridoxine (65,66), as well as chronic renal insufficiency, inflammatory bowel disease, and medication interfering with folate or cobalamine metabolism (67,68).

LABORATORY DIAGNOSIS OF FAMILIAL THROMBOPHILIA

To investigate the presence or absence of an inherited thrombophilic abnormality, some aspects have to be taken into consideration.

It is important to time the collection of blood samples properly. Antithrombin levels are lowered by the use of heparin (69), and the levels of protein C and protein S are reduced by oral anticoagulants (70) Furthermore, the levels of antithrombin, protein C, and protein S can be influenced by different acquired conditions, for example, liver disease, disseminated intravascular coagulation, and acute inflammatory events (including acute venous thromboembolism) but also by pregnancy and estrogen therapy (71–74).

Laboratory testing for antithrombin, protein C, and protein S deficiency, as well as for APC resistance, should be performed when the patient is not treated with anticoagulant drugs and preferably some time after the acute thrombotic event. When a test result is abnormal, it is important to confirm the finding in an independent sample before diagnosing a patient as having a deficiency (of antithrombin, protein C, or protein S) and to confirm APC resistance by DNA testing for the $FV:Q^{506}$ mutation (because there is no complete concordance between APC resistance and the $FV:Q^{506}$ mutation). Furthermore, family studies may be indicated to confirm the hereditary nature, especially for the anticoagulant factor deficiencies.

Homocysteine is measured in plasma after an overnight fast. Measurement 6 to 8 hours after a methionine load of 0.1 mg/kg body weight, while the patient is on a low-protein diet, is indicated to gain optimal sensitivity (10,75–77). However, the nuissant low-protein diet appears not to be necessary (78). Methionine loading is contraindicated in individuals who are suspected to have the severe form of homocysteinuria, which is rare.

For the diversity of assays and methods that are available for testing the different abnormalities of familial thrombophilia, we refer the reader to recent reviews (79–81).

CLINICAL MANIFESTATIONS

Deficiencies of Antithrombin, Protein C, and Protein S and the FV:Q[506] Mutation

In heterozygous individuals with a deficiency of antithrombin, protein C, or protein S and in heterozygous carriers of the FV:Q[506] mutation, the usual manifestations are venous thrombosis of the lower limbs or pulmonary embolism. However, venous manifestations range from superficial thrombophlebitis to thrombosis at unusual sites, such as in the arm or mesenteric veins. In general, it is thought that heterozygosity for the FV:Q[506] mutation is associated with a lower tendency toward venous thromboembolism than the classical anticoagulant deficiencies, although this is based on a limited number of studies (82,83). There is debate whether recurrent venous thromboembolism occurs more frequently in carriers of this mutation, as compared with noncarriers (84–87). In Table 4-2 we summarize estimated annual incidences for first and recurrent episodes of venous thromboembolism for the different abnormalities (15,86,88–94).

It is important to emphasize that these hereditary thrombophilic defects are not associated with an increased risk of arterial thrombosis (83,92,95,96). The rare exception to this rule is provided by two patients, homozygous for type I antithrombin deficiency (97).

Homozygous protein C and protein S deficiency are associated with neonatal purpura fulminans shortly after birth (98,99), and adult patients are prone to skin necrosis after the initiation of coumarin therapy (100–102).

It was recently reported that women with antithrombin, protein C, or protein S deficiency or heterozygosity for the FV:Q[506] mutation have a somewhat higher risk of fetal loss than do women without these abnormalities, possibly due to placental thromboembolic disease (103,104).

Hyperhomocysteinemia

Severe hyperhomocysteinemia or homocystinuria caused by either homozygous cystathionine–β-synthase deficiency or, less frequently, homozygous deficiency of methylenetetrahydrofolate reductase, leads to a clinical picture of skeletal abnormalities (Marfan-like stature), ectopic lens, mental retardation, and severe premature arterial and venous thromboembolism (63,64). These findings have led to several studies concerning mild forms of hyperhomocysteinemia. It appears that this condition is also associated with both premature venous and arterial venous thromboembolism (8–11). The venous thromboembolic manifestations do not differ from those occurring in other thrombophilic defects.

GENERAL EPIDEMIOLOGIC CONSIDERATIONS: PREVALENCE AND THROMBOTIC RISK

Venous thromboembolism is a frequent disease in the general population, with an annual incidence of one to two per 1,000 in

TABLE 4-2. *Estimated annual incidence of a first episode and recurrent episode of venous thromboembolism above the age of 15 years*

Type of deficiency	First episode (%)	Recurrent episode (%)
General population [86,88,89]	0.16	2–4
Antithrombin (15,90–92)	3	6
Protein C (15,90–92)	3	6
Protein S (15,90–92)	3	6
FV:Q[506] mutation (93,94)	0.5–1.9	5–10

Western populations (88). Its incidence increases with age from approximately 0.05 per 1,000 person years in adolescents to approximately eight per 1,000 in individuals over 80 years of age (88).

As can be expected, the reported prevalences of inherited coagulopathies depend a great deal on the selection of the patients for the study population. The first data on familial thrombophilia were derived from families that were selected because of a severe tendency for venous thromboembolism, as well as from individual patients with thrombosis at a very young age or with several recurrent episodes. In these studies, family members with and without the genetic defect were compared with respect to the occurrence of venous thromboembolism, usually excluding the propositus from the analysis. These studies provide us with disease-free survival curves and give some idea of the life-time thrombotic risk of individuals, albeit selected, from thrombophilic families. Another frequently used approach is the case-control analysis, in which patients with a history of venous thromboembolism are compared with healthy, population-derived controls. These studies render an odds ratio for the occurrence of venous thromboembolism in carriers of a thrombophilic defect, as compared with healthy controls. Neither the family studies nor the case-control studies give an estimate of the absolute incidence of venous thromboembolism in carriers of a thrombophilic defect in the general population. These incidence figures are much needed, but we await the results of long-term follow-up studies in unselected individuals. Despite the above-mentioned uncertainties, Table 4-2 summarizes the presently known estimates of absolute annual incidences of first and recurrent episodes of venous thromboembolism in the different types of thrombophilia.

A first episode of venous thromboembolism appears to be a risk factor for a recurrent episode (89) so that it is important to know whether the individuals studied were symptomatic or asymptomatic carriers of a defect.

The first three known causes of familial thrombophilia—antithrombin, protein C, and protein S deficiency—could only be detected in 8% of unselected thrombosis patients, whereas it occurred in 2% of control patients without thrombosis (105). Resistance of factor V to activated protein C, caused by the $FV:Q^{506}$ mutation, is found in approximately 20% of unselected thrombosis patients and in up to 50% of patients selected for (familial) thrombophilia (7,51,82). Hyperhomocysteinemia is found in approximately 20% of patients with venous thromboembolism (8–11).

Increasingly, combined thrombophilic defects are recognized, especially with the relatively prevalent $FV:Q^{506}$ mutation, and these appear to be associated with a more severe tendency for venous thromboembolism (20, 106–115).

Antithrombin Deficiency

The prevalence of antithrombin deficiency is estimated to be approximately 0.3% in the general population (116,117) and 1% to 5% in patients with venous thromboembolism (105,118). Data on the risk of venous thromboembolism are based on family studies. Antithrombin deficiency appears to carry a greater risk for the occurrence of venous thromboembolism than the other established inherited risk factors, especially during pregnancy and the puerperium (92,119), although the reason for the difference has not been elucidated. It has been estimated that approximately half of the deficient members of reported families experience a first episode of venous thromboembolism by the age of 25 (15,91), but it should be noted that these figures were found in selected, thrombophilic families. Although some members of thrombophilic families with antithrombin deficiency have died from fatal venous thromboembolism, historic pedigree analysis has not shown any excess overall mortality as compared with the general population (120,121).

Protein C Deficiency

The prevalence of protein C deficiency is estimated to be approximately 0.5% in the general population (122–124). In cohorts of unselected thrombosis patients, the prevalence of protein C was found to be between 3% and 5% (105,125). Studies of selected families have shown that heterozygous individuals have a 50% chance of experiencing a first venous thromboembolic event by the age of 45 (15,91). In population-based case-control studies, the relative risk for the occurrence of a first episode of venous thromboembolism is estimated to be between 8 and 11 (15,126). Historic pedigree analyses did not show any excess in total mortality in patients with protein C deficiency (127).

Protein S Deficiency

For the general population, the prevalence of protein S deficiency is not known. In cohorts of unselected thrombosis patients, the prevalence of protein S deficiency is found to be approximately 2% (105,128). The relative risk for venous thromboembolism is estimated to be approximately 10 (15). There are no data available on a possible excess mortality in individuals with protein S deficiency, but considering the findings in protein C and antithrombin deficiency, excess overall mortality is unlikely.

Factor V:Q^{506} Mutation

The prevalence of the FV:Q^{506} mutation is high in the general population and is estimated to be between 2% and 10% in the Western world (82,83,129). In cohorts of unselected patients with venous thrombosis, the prevalence of the FV:Q^{506} mutation is approximately 20%, and up to 50% in selected patients (7,82,83). It is the most frequent genetic risk factor for venous thromboembolism that

is known at this moment. The risk for venous thromboembolism seems to be lower than in antithrombin, protein C, and protein S deficiency. A study that combined members from thrombophilic families and consecutive patients with thrombosis has shown that heterozygous individuals have a 25% chance of experiencing a first venous thromboembolic event by the age of 50 (7). In population-based case-control studies, the relative risk for the occurrence of a first episode of venous thromboembolism in heterozygous carriers was estimated to be between 3 and 7 (82,83). Curiously, a study of unselected patients presenting with symptoms of pulmonary embolism did not find a different prevalence of APC resistance in patients with and without an objective diagnosis of pulmonary embolism (130), which is not understood. The relative risk of venous thrombosis in homozygous individuals is estimated to be approximately 10-fold higher than in heterozygous carriers, and about 90-fold higher than in individuals without the FV:Q^{506} mutation (131). However, homozygosity for the FV:Q^{506} mutation has a variable clinical penetrance and does not seem to lead to the severe thrombotic syndrome seen in homozygous protein C or protein S deficiency (132).

Hyperhomocysteinemia

Homocysteinuria or severe hyperhomocysteinemia is a rare disease with an estimated prevalence between 1:200,000 and 1:335,000. It is estimated that 50% of patients experience a first episode of venous or arterial thromboembolism (or both) before the age of 30 (63,64).

The prevalence of mild and moderate hyperhomocysteinemia is estimated to be approximately 5% in the general population. It was first noticed that the prevalence of hyperhomocysteinemia in young selected patients with venous thromboembolism was relatively high (10% to 20%) (8,10), which was later confirmed in unselected thrombosis patients (9,11). As yet, no data are available on the thrombosis-free survival of individuals with hyperhomocysteinemia, or on recurrence rates. The clinical relevance of the identified enzyme defects leading to hyperhomocysteinemia with respect to the risk for venous thromboembolism is uncertain (14).

GUIDELINES FOR MANAGEMENT

Prophylaxis of Venous Thromboembolism in Relation to Concomitant Risk Factors

General Considerations

Thus far, only coumarin derivates are available for long-term anticoagulant prophylaxis. This seems to be highly effective in all genetic thrombophilic abnormalities (92,133), even though, interestingly, it aggravates the deficiency of protein C and protein S. Coumarin treatment is associated with a risk of bleeding. The incidence of major bleeding is found to be between 2% and 10% per treatment year, with fatal bleedings of approximately 0.5% per treatment year, depending on the intensity of anticoagulation, age, and other underlying diseases (134–137).

In order to balance the risks and benefits of anticoagulant prophylaxis, information on the thrombotic risk with its associated morbidity and mortality in carriers of the different abnormalities is necessary. In the next paragraphs we will discuss some considerations that are helpful in clinical decision making. Because appropriate data are frequently lacking, the management of a thrombophilic patient should be guided by common sense, allowing for individual judgment of the risk of venous thromboembolism in a particular person. Different risk factors for venous thromboembolism—proven previous episode of thrombosis, acquired prothrombotic states, combined inherited defects, or homozygosity for one defect—combined in one patient seem to call for a more vigorous prophylactic approach, even though clinical studies are not available.

Asymptomatic Carriers

Lifelong Prophylaxis?

In asymptomatic individuals with an inherited thrombophilic defect, anticoagulant pro-

phylaxis of venous thromboembolism could be considered. These individuals are usually identified through family screening of a known proband who experienced a thromboembolic episode.

However, it should be noted that approximately half of the episodes of venous thromboembolism in carriers of thrombophilic defects occur spontaneously (88,94). The annual incidence of a first episode of venous thromboembolism in individuals with antithrombin, protein C, or protein S deficiency is approximately 3% (Table 4-2) (15,90), which appears to be lower than or equal to the bleeding risks of long-term anticoagulant prophylaxis. In carriers of the FV:Q^{506} mutation, the annual incidence of venous thromboembolism is estimated to be between 0.5% and 0.9% (93,94). Therefore, lifelong coumarin prophylaxis in all asymptomatic individuals with this defect would do more harm than good.

Prophylaxis During High-Risk Situations?

Anticoagulant prophylaxis during high-risk situations, such as surgery, pregnancy, and the puerperium, would theoretically prevent approximately half of the episodes of venous thromboembolism in carriers of a hereditary thrombophilic defect.

Perioperative Prophylaxis

There are several reports on the risk of thromboembolic complications after surgery in subjects with antithrombin, protein C, or protein S deficiency (approximately 30%), but it should be noted that available studies often included patients with previous episodes of venous thromboembolism, and different perioperative prophylactic regimens were used (90–92,138). Therefore, one should be cautious in extrapolating these study results to thromboembolic risks for asymptomatic carriers. Oral anticoagulant prophylaxis or therapeutic dosages of (low molecular weight) heparin during surgery or immobilization is often given to asymptomatic individuals with known antithrombin, protein C, or protein S deficiency. Retrospective studies have shown that this strategy is highly effective in preventing venous thromboembolism in carriers of thrombophilic defects (92). However, no large prospective studies are available that have balanced the risks and benefits of such an approach. In one prospective study, the nowadays routine administration of a prophylactic dose of low molecular weight heparin perioperatively appeared to be as effective in preventing perioperative venous thromboembolism, although the number of patients studied was small (90). The optimal prophylactic strategy in asymptomatic carriers of the FV:Q^{506} mutation is unknown. One retrospective study reported a low risk of perioperative venous thromboembolism (4% of reported episodes of surgery or immobilization, partly using standard thromboprophylaxis) in asymptomatic carriers of the FV:Q^{506} mutation (94).

For practical purposes, we suggest using the same approach in known asymptomatic carriers of the different types of thrombophilia. During surgery and strict immobilization, we propose using standard anticoagulant prophylaxis with low molecular weight heparin.

Prophylaxis in Pregnancy and Puerperium

The risk of venous thromboembolism related to pregnancy in women with antithrombin deficiency was reported to vary between 12% and 48% per pregnancy; in protein C the reported risk varies between 2% and 20%; in women with protein S deficiency it is estimated to be 14% (90,138–141); and in women with the FV:Q^{506} mutation and a history of thrombosis the risk is reported to be as high as 28% (142). However, a study of asymptomatic carriers of the FV:Q^{506} mutation only showed a frequency of venous thromboembolism in 2% of the pregnancies (94), illustrating the disadvantages of studies in selected patient groups. Most of the pregnancy-related episodes of venous thromboembolism occur during the puerperium or third trimester (94,140,141).

Again, we suggest using the same approach in known asymptomatic carriers of the differ-

ent types of thrombophilia. For known carriers of thrombophilic defects, we propose installing prophylaxis with coumarin during the 6 weeks postpartum and consider the use of low molecular weight heparin during the third trimester (141). However, these guidelines are subject to debate due to the lack of clinical management studies. Therefore, an approach of "watchful waiting" also seems to be justified. This strategy consists of periodic ultrasound imaging of the leg veins to detect deepvein thrombosis early and careful instruction of the patient to seek immediate medical assistance when symptoms of venous thromboembolism occur. The prophylactic approach of choice can be made based on balancing the nuissance of anticoagulant prophylaxis and the fear of thrombosis or embolism individually. It is clear that further studies in this area are urgently needed.

Use of Oral Contraceptives

The use of oral contraceptives increases the risk of venous thromboembolism, and it has been shown that this is also the case in women with inherited thrombophilic defects, particularly in women with antithrombin deficiency or the FV:Q^{506} mutation (143,144). There is debate whether this should lead to denying asymptomatic carriers oral contraceptives because the absolute risk for venous thromboembolism is low (145,146).

Symptomatic Carriers

Carriers of thrombophilic defects who have experienced one or more episode(s) of venous thromboembolism have a high risk for recurrence (Table 4-2). No studies are available on the optimal duration of anticoagulant therapy after a first episode of thrombosis, although it is known that a longer duration of anticoagulants reduces the recurrence rate in patients with previous thrombosis (147,148). This might be particularly true for individuals with an inherited thrombophilic defect, for the recurrence rates in these patients appear to be higher (85,86,149). Large trials to assess the optimal benefit risk ratio in the duration of anticoagulation treatment are warranted. After a second or third episode of thrombosis, many clinicians decide to treat their thrombophilic patients life-long, although it is unsure whether the considerable bleeding risks of anticoagulants outweigh the risk for recurrent venous thromboembolism.

In thrombophilic patients with a previous episode of venous thromboembolism, adequate prophylaxis during subsequent high-risk situations is necessary. However, the selected regimen should take into account the circumstances under which the earlier thrombosis occurred, as well as its severity. A choice can be made from a prophylactic dosage of low molecular weight heparin up to therapeutic heparin or coumarin dosages. During pregnancy, it is important to note that coumarins are potentially teratogenic (150,151) and should be replaced by (low molecular weight) heparin at least during the first trimester and 4 weeks before delivery (151–155).

Although no studies on recurrence rates during oral contraceptive use are available, it is generally accepted that in women who have experienced thrombosis, alternative methods of contraception are preferred. This is especially the case when starting with the pill was the trigger for the thrombotic episode (within the first 6 months). It should be emphasized that oral contraceptives are indicated, not contraindicated, in women who are using long-term anticoagulation. First, the teratogenicity of coumarins calls for adequate contraception, and second, the protective effect of coumarins against thrombosis effectively abolishes the prothrombotic effect of the contraceptives.

Management of Hyperhomocysteinemia

Because mild hyperhomocysteinemia has been identified only recently as a risk factor for venous thromboembolism, hardly any data on how to manage this disorder are available. Supplementation of vitamins such as folic acid and pyridoxine, but also cobalamin, lowers the elevated plasma homocysteine level, irrespective of the initial vitamin levels (156). It is unknown whether this treatment decreases the thrombotic risk in individuals with mild hyperhomocysteinemia, but it is generally recommended in patients with hyperhomocysteinemia who have experienced venous thrombosis. Although no particular combination of vitamin supplement therapy has proved to be more effective than the other, the usual recommendation is to supply folic acid and, if no decrease of homocysteine levels is observed, to add pyridoxine.

The incidence of first or recurrent episodes of venous thromboembolism in individuals with mild or moderate hyperhomocysteinemia is unknown, as is its relationship with concomitant high-risk situations. Therefore, we suggest using standard prophylaxis perioperatively. There is no evidence to promote thromboprophylaxis during pregnancy or puerperium in women with hyperhomocysteinemia.

Acute Episodes of Venous Thromboembolism

As for all patients, a clinically suspected episode of venous thromboembolism should be confirmed by objective diagnostic methods. In case of deep-vein thrombosis of the lower extremities, compression ultrasound or venography are indicated, and in case of suspected pulmonary embolism, a ventilation-perfusion scan (followed by pulmonary angiography when the ventilation-perfusion scan is inconclusive) should be performed (157).

In general, treatment of acute thromboembolic events is the same for patients with as for patients without a genetic thrombophilic defect. Initial therapy consists of intravenously administered heparin or low molecular weight heparin given subcutaneously (158). Heparin therapy should be maintained for a minimum of 5 days and can be stopped after the prothrombin time is within the target range (International Normalized Ratio [INR] between 2.0 and 3.0). Oral anticoagulants can be safely commenced within the first 24 hours (158,159).

Thrombolytic therapy should only be considered in patients with massive, life-threatening pulmonary embolism.

In antithrombin-deficient patients, replacement therapy with antithrombin concentrates is not more effective than standard therapy with heparin and coumarin (160). In our opinion, replacement therapy with antithrombin concentrates is hardly ever indicated.

In protein C deficiency, skin necrosis after installment of coumarin therapy is a rare but potentially serious complication (100–102,161). If a patient with venous thromboembolism is known or highly suspected to be protein C deficient, coumarins should not be started until the patient is fully heparinized. The dose of coumarin should be started without the usual loading dose and increased gradually until the INR is in the therapeutic range (162,163). When a patient started with oral anticoagulants develops skin necrosis, discontinuation of the coumarin is immediately warranted, vitamin K should be administered, and therapeutic heparinization should be installed. If the skin necrosis progresses despite these measures, the administration of protein C concentrate should be considered. In patients with protein C deficiency and a history of coumarin-induced skin necrosis, successful treatment with protein C concentrate or fresh frozen plasma appears to provide protection against recurrent skin necrosis until a stable level of anticoagulation is achieved (161).

In homozygous protein C deficiency, the occurrence of neonatal purpura fulminans has been reported. Treatment with either fresh frozen plasma or protein C concentrate should be installed until the purpura heal. Long-term coumarin treatment or protein C replacement therapy is necessary in these children (164).

SCREENING FOR INHERITED THROMBOPHILIA

Should all patients with an acute episode of venous thromboembolism be screened for an inherited thrombophilic defect? Because venous thromboembolism is a common disease, this would have a large impact on the community resources. The purpose of screening thrombosis patients for inherited defects would be to modify prophylaxis in identified carriers because as yet there is no evidence that treatment of acute events should differ.

Therefore, it is generally recommended that some index of suspicion for a patient to have an inherited thrombophilic defect should be present before testing is initiated, for example: a positive family history (but this instrument should be used critically) (4), a first episode at a young age (under 45 years of age), recurrent episodes, life-threatening thromboembolism, or thrombosis at unusual sites. When acquired conditions predisposing to venous thromboembolism were present at the time of diagnosis, further investigation is generally not warranted. The FV:Q^{506} mutation, which of course is more prevalent than the classical coagulation inhibitor defects, has been shown to be related to primary venous thromboembolism at older age as well (82,83,93).

When an inherited defect in a proband is diagnosed, usually family screening is recommended to identify asymptomatic carriers who might benefit from prophylaxis of venous thrombosis during high-risk situations. However, whether this is always necessary, especially with the FV:Q^{506} mutation, is subject to investigation and debate (94). It should be noted that for asymptomatic individuals the knowledge of carrying an inherited defect, which has no direct clinical consequences, may induce psychological stress as well as problems with obtaining insurances and social security benefits.

OTHER CANDIDATE RISK FACTORS

Several, sometimes genetic, abnormalities are possibly associated with an increased risk of venous thromboembolism. However, firm evidence is lacking or reports are premature with respect to the number of observed patients.

A recently described mutation in the prothrombin gene, which leads to increased levels of prothrombin, was reported to be a relatively prevalent risk factor for venous thromboembolism (20) and needs confirmation by other studies. We have summarized our views on each of these candidate risk factors in Table 4-1 (20–31).

CONCLUSION

Many aspects of inherited thrombophilia are still uncertain. There is a need for more precise estimates of the risk for venous thromboembolism in unselected individuals with genetic abnormalities, as well as the risk for recurrent thromboembolism in these patients. Large clinical trials are warranted to assess the optimal balance between the benefits and hazards of anticoagulant treatment in symptomatic individuals. Especially for the newly elucidated and prevalent FV:Q^{506} mutation, this should lead to valuable tools in clinical decision making when confronted with a patient with venous thromboembolism and an inherited thrombophilic defect, with respect to management, screening, and counseling. For hyperhomocysteinemia, clinical trials with vitamin supplementation to study outcome are indicated.

One of the major challenges for the future is to find new genetically determined risk factors. Finally, there is still a need for more sophisticated anticoagulant drugs that do not have the serious side effects of bleeding. Until then, it should become clear whether less intensive anticoagulation with lower INRs is still effective in preventing recurrent thromboembolism with lower bleeding risks.

REFERENCES

1. Briggs JB. Recurrent phlebitis of obscure origin. *Johns Hopkins Hosp Bull* 1905;16:228–233.
2. Jordan FLJ, Nandorff A. The familial tendency in thrombo-embolic disease. *Acta Med Scand* 1956;156:267–275.
3. Egeberg O. Inherited antithrombin III deficiency causing thrombophilia. *Thromb Diath Haemorrh* 1965;13:516–530.
4. Briët E, van der Meer FJ, Rosendaal FR, Houwing-Duistermaat JJ, van Houwelingen HC. The family history and inherited thrombophilia. *Br J Haematol* 1994;87:348–352.
5. Esmon CT. The protein C anticoagulant pathway. *Arterioscler Thromb* 1992;12:135–145.
6. Dahlback B, Carlsson M, Svensson PJ. Familial thrombophilia due to a previously unrecognized mechanism characterized by poor anticoagulant response to activated protein C: prediction of a cofactor to activated

7. protein C. *Proc Natl Acad Sci U S A* 1993;90:1004–1008.
8. Svensson PJ, Dahlback B. Resistance to activated protein C as a basis for venous thrombosis. *N Engl J Med* 1994;330:517–522.
9. Falcon CR, Cattaneo M, Panzeri D, Martinelli I, Mannucci PM. High prevalence of hyperhomocyst(e)inemia in patients with juvenile venous thrombosis. *Arterioscler Thromb* 1994;14:1080–1083.
10. den Heijer M, Blom HJ, Gerrits WB, et al. Is hyperhomocysteinaemia a risk factor for recurrent venous thrombosis? *Lancet* 1995;345:882–885.
11. Fermo I, Vigano D'Angelo S, Paroni R, et al. Prevalence of moderate hyperhomocysteinemia in patients with early-onset venous and arterial occlusive disease. *Ann Intern Med* 1995;123:747–753.
12. den Heijer M, Koster T, Blom HJ, et al. Hyperhomocysteinemia as a risk factor for deep-vein thrombosis. *N Engl J Med* 1996;334:759–762.
13. Kluijtmans LA, van den Heuvel LP, Boers GH, et al. Molecular genetic analysis in mild hyperhomocysteinemia: a common mutation in the methylenetetrahydrofolate reductase gene is a genetic risk factor for cardiovascular disease. *Am J Hum Genet* 1996;58:35–41.
14. Frosst P, Blom HJ, Milos R, et al. A candidate genetic risk factor for vascular disease: a common mutation in methylenetetrahydrofolate reductase. *Nat Genet* 1995;10:111–113.
15. Kluijtmans LA, den Heijer M, Reitsma PH, Heil SG, Blom HJ, Rosendaal FR. Thermolabile methylenetetrahydrofolate reductase and factor V Leiden in the risk of deep-vein thrombosis. *Thromb Haemost* 1998, in press.
16. van den Belt AGM, Prins MH, Huisman MV, Hirsh J. Familial thrombophilia: a review analysis. *Clin Appl Thromb Hemost* 1996;2:227–236.
17. Griffin JH, Evatt B, Zimmerman TS, Kleiss AJ, Wideman C. Deficiency of protein C in congenital thrombotic disease. *J Clin Invest* 1981;68:1370–1373.
18. Comp PC, Esmon CT. Recurrent venous thromboembolism in patients with a partial deficiency of protein S. *N Engl J Med* 1984;311:1525–1528.
19. Schwarz HP, Fischer M, Hopmeier P, Batard MA, Griffin JH. Plasma protein S deficiency in familial thrombotic disease. *Blood* 1984;64:1297–1300.
20. Haverkate F, Samama M. Familial dysfibrinogenemia and thrombophilia. Report on a study of the SSC Subcommittee on Fibrinogen. *Thromb Haemost* 1995;73:151–161.
21. Poort SR, Rosendaal FR, Reitsma PH, Bertina RM. A common genetic variation in the 3'-untranslated region of the prothrombin gene is associated with elevated plasma prothrombin levels and an increase in venous thrombosis. *Blood* 1996;88:3698–3703.
22. Ohlin AK, Marlar RA. The first mutation identified in the thrombomodulin gene in a 45-year-old man presenting with thromboembolic disease. *Blood* 1995;85:330–336.
23. Ohlin AK, Marlar RA. Mutations in the thrombomodulin gene associated with thromboembolic disease [Abstract]. *Thromb Haemost* 1995;73:1096.
24. Dolan G, Greaves M, Cooper P, Preston FE. Thrombovascular disease and familial plasminogen deficiency: a report of three kindreds. *Br J Haematol* 1988;70:417–421.

24. Sartori MT, Patrassi GM, Theodoridis P, Perin A, Pietrogrande F, Girolami A. Heterozygous type I plasminogen deficiency is associated with an increased risk for thrombosis: a statistical analysis in 20 kindreds. *Blood Coagul Fibrinolysis* 1994;5:889–893.

25. Engesser L, Kluft C, Briët E, Brommer EJ. Familial elevation of plasma histidine-rich glycoprotein in a family with thrombophilia. *Br J Haematol* 1987;67: 355–358.

26. Castaman G, Ruggeri M, Burei F, Rodeghiero F. High levels of histidine-rich glycoprotein and thrombotic diathesis. Report of two unrelated families. *Thromb Res* 1993;69:297–305.

27. Blinder MA, Andersson TR, Abildgaard U, Tollefsen DM. Heparin cofactor II Oslo. Mutation of Arg-189 to His decreases the affinity for dermatan sulfate. *J Biol Chem* 1989;264:5128–5133.

28. Simioni P, Lazzaro AR, Coser E, Salmistraro G, Girolami A. Hereditary heparin cofactor II deficiency and thrombosis: report of six patients belonging to two separate kindreds. *Blood Coagul Fibrinolysis* 1990;1: 351–356.

29. Bancsi LF, van der Linden IK, Bertina RM. Beta 2-glycoprotein I deficiency and the risk of thrombosis. *Thromb Haemost* 1992;67:649–653.

30. Halbmayer WM, Mannhalter C, Feichtinger C, Rubi K, Fischer M. THe prevalence of factor XII deficiency in 103 orally anticoagulated outpatients suffering from recurrent venous and/or arterial thromboembolism. *Thromb Haemost* 1992;68:285–290.

31. Koster T, Rosendaal FR, Briët E, Vandenbroucke JP. John Hagemann's factor and deep-vein thrombosis: Leiden thrombophilia Study. *Br J Haematol* 1994;87: 422–424.

32. Griffith MJ. Kinetic analysis of the heparin-enhanced antithrombin III/thrombin reaction. Reaction rate enhancement by heparin-thrombin association. *J Biol Chem* 1979;254:12044–12049.

33. Esmon CT. Protease inhibitors of human plasma. Protein C. *J Med* 1985;16:285–301.

34. Clouse LH, Comp PC. The regulation of hemostasis: the protein C system. *N Engl J Med* 1986;314:1298–1304.

35. Kalafatis M, Rand MD, Mann KG. The mechanism of inactivation of human factor V and human factor Va by activated protein C. *J Biol Chem* 1994;269: 31869–31880.

36. Bock SC, Harris JF, Balazs I, Trent JM. Assignment of the human antithrombin III structural gene to chromosome 1q23-25. *Cytogenet Cell Genet* 1985;39:6 7–69.

37. Olds RJ, Lane DA, Chowdhury V, De Stefano V, Leone G, Thein SL. Complete nucleotide sequence of the antithrombin gene: evidence for homologous recombination causing thrombophilia. *Biochemistry* 1993;32: 4216–4224.

38. Foster DC, Yoshitake S, Davie EW. The nucleotide sequence of the gene for human protein C. *Proc Natl Acad Sci U S A* 1985;82:4673–4677.

39. Lundwall A, Dackowski W, Cohen E, et al. Isolation and sequence of the cDNA for human protein S, a regular of blood coagulation. *Proc Natl Acad Sci U S A* 1986;83:6716–6720.

40. Jenny RJ, Pittman DD, Toole JJ, et al. Complete cDNA and derived amino acid sequence of human factor V. *Proc Natl Acad Sci U S A* 1987;84:4846–4850.

41. Lane DA, Ireland H, Olds RJ, Thein SL, Perry DJ, Aiach M. Antithrombin III: a database of mutations. *Thromb Haemost* 1991;66:657–661.

42. Lane DA, Olds RJ, Boisclair M, et al. Antithrombin III mutation database: first update. For the Thrombin and its Inhibitors Subcommittee of the Scientific and Standardization Committee of the International Society on Thrombosis and Haemostasis. *Thromb Haemost* 1993;70:361–369.

43. Reitsma PH, Poort SR, Bernardi F, et al. Protein C deficiency: a database of mutations. For the Protein C & S Subcommittee of the Scientific and Standardization Committee of the International Society on Thrombosis and Haemostasis. *Thromb Haemost* 1993;69:77–84.

44. Reitsma PH, Bernardi F, Doig RG, et al. Protein C deficiency: a database of mutations, 1995 update. On behalf of the Subcommittee on Plasma Coagulation Inhibitors of the Scientific and Standardization Committee of the ISTH. *Thromb Haemost* 1995;73:876–889.

45. Gandrille S, Borgel D, Ireland H, et al. Protein S deficiency: a database of mutations. For the Plasma Coagulation Inhibitors Subcommittee of the Scientific and Standardization Committee of the International Society on Thrombosis and Haemostasis. *Thromb Haemost* 1997;77:1201–1214.

46. Griffin JH, Evatt B, Wideman C, Fernandez JA. Anticoagulant protein C pathway defective in majority of thrombophilic patients. *Blood* 1993;82:1989–1993.

47. Bertina RM, Koeleman BP, Koster T, et al. Mutation in blood coagulation factor V associated with resistance to activated protein C. *Nature* 1994;369:64–67.

48. Voorberg J, Roelse J, Koopman R, et al. Association of idiopathic venous thromboembolism with single point-mutation at Arg506 of factor V. *Lancet* 1994; 343:1535–1536.

49. Greengard JS, Sun X, Xu X, Fernandez JA, Griffin JH, Evatt B. Activated protein C resistance caused by Arg506Gln mutation in factor Va. *Lancet* 1994;343: 1361–1362.

50. Zoller B, Dahlback B. Linkage between inherited resistance to activated protein C and factor V gene mutation in venous thrombosis. *Lancet* 1994;343: 1536–1538.

51. Zoller B, Svensson PJ, He X, Dahlback B. Identification of the same factor V gene mutation in 47 out of 50 thrombosis-prone families with inherited resistance to activated protein C. *J Clin Invest* 1994;94:2521–2524.

52. Rosing J, Hoekema L, Nicolaes GA, et al. Effects of protein S and factor Xa on peptide bond cleavages during inactivation of factor Va and factor VaR506Q by activated protein C. *J Biol Chem* 1995;270: 27852–27858.

53. Griffin JH, Heeb MJ, Kojima Y, et al. Activated protein C resistance: molecular mechanisms. *Thromb Haemost* 1995;74:444–448.

54. Roelse JC, Koopman MM, Buller HR, et al. Absence of mutations at the activated protein C cleavage sites of factor VIII in 125 patients with venous thrombosis. *Br J Haematol* 1996;92:740–743.

55. Henkens CM, Bom VJ, Seinen AJ, van der Meer J. Sensitivity to activated protein C; influence of oral contraceptives and sex. *Thromb Haemost* 1995;73: 402–404.

56. Cumming AM, Tait RC, Fildes S, Yoong A, Keeney S, Hay CR. Development of resistance to activated pro-

tein C during pregnancy. *Br J Haematol* 1995;90: 725–727.

57. Mathonnet F, de Manzancourt P, Bastenaire B, et al. Activated protein C sensitivity ratio in pregnant women at delivery. *Br J Haematol* 1996;92:244–246.

58. Cumming AM, Tait RC, Fildes S, Hay CR. Diagnosis of APC Resistance during pregnancy. *Br J Haematol* 1996;92:1026–1027.

59. de Franchis R, Kozich V, McInnes RR, Kraus JP. Identical genotypes in siblings with different homocystinuric phenotypes: identification of three mutations in cystathionine beta-synthase using an improved bacterial expression system. *Hum Mol Genet* 1994;3: 1103–1108.

60. Sebastio G, Sperandeo MP, Panico M, et al. The molecular basis of homocystinuria due to cystathionine beta-synthase deficiency in Italian families, and report of four novel mutations. *Am J Hum Genet* 1995;56: 1324–1333.

61. Goyette P, Frosst P, Rosenblatt DS, Rozen R. Seven novel mutations in the methylenetetrahydrofolate reductase gene and genotype/phenotype correlations in severe methylenetetrahydrofolate reductase deficiency. *Am J Hum Genet* 1995;56:1052–1059.

62. Goyette P, Sumner JS, Milos R, et al. Human methylenetetrahydrofolate reductase: isolation of cDNA mapping and mutation identification. *Nat Genet* 1994; 7:551.

63. Mudd SH, Skovby F, Levy HL, et al. The natural history of homocystinuria due to cystathionine beta-synthase deficiency. *Am J Hum Genet* 1985;37:1–31.

64. Malinow MR. Homocyst(e)ine and arterial occlusive diseases. *J Intern Med* 1994;236:603–617.

65. Stabler SP, Lindenbaum J, Savage DG, Allen RH. Elevation of serum cystathionine levels in patients with cobalamin and folate deficiency. *Blood* 1993;81: 3404–3413.

66. Ubbink JB, Vermaak WJ, van der Merwe A, Becker PJ. Vitamin B-12, vitamin B-6, and folate nutritional status in men with hyperhomocysteinemia. *Am J Clin Nutr* 1993;57:47–53.

67. Ueland PM, Refsum H. Plasma homocysteine, a risk factor for vascular disease: plasma levels in health, disease, and drug therapy. *J Lab Clin Med* 1989;114: 473–501.

68. Moelby L, Rasmussen K, Rasmussen HH. Serum methylmalonic acid in uraemia. *Scand J Clin Lab Invest* 1992;52:351–354.

69. Marciniak E, Gockerman JP. Heparin-induced decrease in circulating antithrombin III. *Lancet* 1977;2: 581–582.

70. Vigano D'Angelo S, Comp PC, Esmon CT, D'Angelo A. Relationship between protein C antigen and anticoagulant activity during oral anticoagulation and in selected disease states. *J Clin Invest* 1986;77:416–425.

71. Marlar RA, Endres-Brooks J, Miller C. Serial studies of protein C and its plasma inhibitor in patients with disseminated intravascular coagulation. *Blood* 1985;66: 59–63.

72. Rodeghiero F, Mannucci PM, Vigano S, et al. Liver dysfunction rather than intravascular coagulation as the main cause of low protein C and antithrombin III in acute leukemia. *Blood* 1984;63:965–969.

73. Faught W, Garner P, Jones G, Ivey B. Changes in protein C and protein S levels in normal pregnancy. *Am J Obstet Gynecol* 1995;172:147–150.

74. Granata A, Sobbrio GA, D'Arrigo F, et al. Changes in the plasma levels of proteins C and S in young women on low-dose oestrogen oral contraceptives. *Clin Exp Obstet Gynecol* 1991;18:9–12.

75. Fowler B, Sardharwalla IB, Robins AJ. The detection of heterozygotes for homocystinuria by oral loading with L-methionine. *Biochem J* 1971;122:23–24.

76. Boers GJH, Fowler B, Smals AGH. Improved identification of heterozygotes for homocystinuria due to cystathionine synthase deficiency by the combination of methionine loading and enzyme determination in cultured fibroblasts. *Hum Genet* 1985;69:164–169.

77. Andersson A, Brattstrom L, Israelsson B, Isaksson A, Hamfelt A, Hultberg B. Plasma homocysteine before and after methionine loading with regard to age, gender, and menopausal status. *Eur J Clin Invest* 1992;22: 79–87.

78. den Heijer M, Bos GM, Brouwer IA, Gerrits WB, Blom HJ. Variability of the methionine loading test: no effect of a low protein diet. *Ann Clin Biochem* 1996; 33:551–554.

79. De Stefano V, Finazzi G, Mannucci PM. Inherited thrombophilia: pathogenesis, clinical syndromes, and management. *Blood* 1996;87:3531–3544.

80. Lane DA, Mannucci PM, Bauer KA, et al. Inherited thrombophilia: part 1. *Thromb Haemost* 1996;76: 651–662.

81. Lane DA, Mannucci PM, Bauer KA, et al. Inherited thrombophilia: part 2. *Thromb Haemost* 1996;76: 824–834.

82. Koster T, Rosendaal FR, de Ronde H, Briët E, Vandenbroucke JP, Bertina RM. Venous thrombosis due to poor anticoagulant response to activated protein C: Leiden Thrombophilia Study. *Lancet* 1993;342: 1503–1506.

83. Ridker PM, Hennekens CH, Lindpaintner K, Stampfer MJ, Eisenberg PR, Miletich JP. Mutation in the gene coding for coagulation factor V and the risk of myocardial infarction, stroke, and venous thrombosis in apparently healthy men. *N Engl J Med* 1995;332: 912–917.

84. Rintelen C, Pabinger I, Knobl P, Lechner K, Mannhalter C. Probability of recurrence of thrombosis in patients with and without factor V Leiden. *Thromb Haemost* 1996;75:229–232.

85. Ridker PM, Miletich JP, Stampfer MJ, Goldhaber SZ, Lindpaintner K, Hennekens CH. Factor V Leiden and risks of recurrent idiopathic venous thromboembolism. *Circulation* 1995;92:2800–2802.

86. Simioni P, Prandoni P, Lensing AW, et al. The risk of recurrent venous thromboembolism in patients with an Arg506/Gln mutation in the gene for factor V (Factor V Leiden). *N Engl J Med* 1997;336:399–403.

87. Eichinger S, Pabinger I, Stümpflen A, et al. The risk of recurrent venous thromboembolism in patients with and without Factor V Leiden. *Thromb Haemost* 1997; 77:624–628.

88. Nordstrom M, Lindblad B, Bergqvist D, Kjellstrom T. A prospective study of the incidence of deep-vein thrombosis within a defined urban population. *J Intern Med* 1992;232:155–160.

89. Prandoni P, Lensing AW, Cogo A, et al. The long-term clinical course of acute deep venous thrombosis. *Ann Intern Med* 1996;125:1–7.

90. Pabinger I, Kyrle PA, Heistinger M, et al. The risk of thromboembolism in asymptomatic patients with pro-

tein C and protein S deficiency: a prospective cohort study. *Thromb Haemost* 1994;71:441–445.

91. Pabinger I, Schneider B. Thrombotic risk in hereditary antithrombin III, protein C, or protein S deficiency. A cooperative, retrospective study. Gesellschaft fur Thrombose- und Hamostaseforschung (GTH) Study Group on Natural Inhibitors. *Arterioscler Thromb Vasc Biol* 1996;16:742–748.

92. De Stefano V, Leone G, Mastrangelo S, et al. Clinical manifestations and management of inherited thrombophilia: retrospective analysis and follow-up after diagnosis of 238 patients with congenital deficiency of antithrombin III, protein C, protein S. *Thromb Haemost* 1994;72:352–358.

93. Ridker PM, Glynn RJ, Miletich JP, Goldhaber SZ, Stampfer MJ, Hennekens CH. Age-specific incidence rates of venous thromboembolism among heterozygous carriers of factor V Leiden mutation. *Ann Intern Med* 1997;126:528–531.

94. Middeldorp S, Henkens CMA, Koopman MMW, et al. The incidence of venous thromboembolism in family members of patients with the FV:Q506 mutation and venous thrombosis. *Ann Intern Med* 1998, in press.

95. Demers C, Ginsberg JS, Hirsh J, Henderson P, Blajchman MA. Thrombosis in antithrombin-III–deficient persons. Report of a large kindred and literature review. *Ann Intern Med* 1992;116:754–761.

96. Demarmels Biasiutti F, Merlo C, Furlan M, et al. No association of APC resistance with myocardial infarction. *Blood Coagul Fibrinolysis* 1995;6:456–459.

97. Chowdhury V, Lane DA, Mille B, et al. Homozygous antithrombin deficiency: report of two new cases (99 Leu to Phe) associated with arterial and venous thrombosis. *Thromb Haemost* 1994;72:198–202.

98. Branson HE, Katz J, Marble R, Griffin JH. Inherited protein C deficiency and coumarin-responsive chronic relapsing purpura fulminans in a newborn infant. *Lancet* 1983;2:1165–1168.

99. Mahasandana C, Suvatte V, Marlar RA, Manco-Johnson MJ, Jacobson LJ, Hathaway WE. Neonatal purpura fulminans associated with homozygous protein S deficiency. *Lancet* 1990;335:61–62.

100. Broekmans AW, Bertina RM, Loeliger EA, Hofmann V, Klingemann HG. Protein C and the development of skin necrosis during anticoagulant therapy. *Thromb Haemost* 1983;49:251.

101. Conard J, Horellou MH, van Dreden P, et al. Homozygous protein C deficiency with late onset and recurrent coumarin-induced skin necrosis. *Lancet* 1992;339:743–744.

102. Locht H, Lindstrom FD. Severe skin necrosis following warfarin therapy in a patient with protein C deficiency. *J Intern Med* 1993;233:287–289.

103. Sanson BJ, Friederich PW, Simioni P, et al. The risk of abortion and stillbirth in antithrombin-, protein C-, and protein S-deficient women. *Thromb Haemost* 1996;75:387–388.

104. Preston FE, Rosendaal FR, Walker ID, et al. Increased fetal loss in women with heritable thrombophilia. *Lancet* 1996;348:913–916.

105. Heijboer H, Brandjes DP, Buller HR, Sturk A, ten Cate JW. Deficiencies of coagulation-inhibiting and fibrinolytic proteins in outpatients with deep-vein thrombosis. *N Engl J Med* 1990;323:1512–1516.

106. van Boven HH, Reitsma PH, Rosendaal FR, et al. Factor V Leiden (FV R506Q) in families with inherited antithrombin deficiency. *Thromb Haemost* 1996;75:417–421.

107. Koeleman BP, van Rumpt D, Hamulyak K, Reitsma PH, Bertina RM. Factor V Leiden: an additional risk factor for thrombosis in protein S deficient families? *Thromb Haemost* 1995;74:580–583.

108. Brenner B, Zivelin A, Lanir N, Greengard JS, Griffin JH, Seligsohn U. Venous thromboembolism associated with double heterozygosity for R506Q mutation of factor V and for T298M mutation of protein C in a large family of a previously described homozygous protein C-deficient newborn with massive thrombosis. *Blood* 1996;88:877–880.

109. Simioni P, Scudeller A, Radossi P, et al. "Pseudo homozygous" activated protein C resistance due to double heterozygous factor V defects (factor V Leiden mutation and type I quantitative factor V defect) associated with thrombosis: report of two cases belonging to two unrelated kindreds. *Thromb Haemost* 1996;75:422–426.

110. Formstone CJ, Hallam PJ, Tuddenham EG, et al. Severe perinatal thrombosis in double and triple heterozygous offspring of a family segregating two independent protein S mutations and a protein C mutation. *Blood* 1996;87:3731–3737.

111. Beauchamp NJ, Daly ME, Cooper PC, Makris M, Preston FE, Peake IR. Molecular basis of protein S deficiency in three families also showing independent inheritance of factor V Leiden. *Blood* 1996;88:1700–1707.

112. Brenner B, Vulfsons SL, Lanir N, Nahir M. Coexistence of familial antiphospholipid syndrome and factor V Leiden: impact on thrombotic diathesis. *Br J Haematol* 1996;94:166–167.

113. Gandrille S, Greengard JS, Alhenc-Gelas M, et al. Incidence of activated protein C resistance caused by the ARG 506 GLN mutation in factor V in 113 unrelated symptomatic protein C-deficient patients. The French Network on the behalf of INSERM. *Blood* 1995;86:219–224.

114. Zoller B, Berntsdotter A, Garcia de Frutos P, Dahlback B. Resistance to activated protein C as an additional genetic risk factor in hereditary deficiency of protein S. *Blood* 1995;85:3518–3523.

115. Koeleman BP, Reitsma PH, Allaart CF, Bertina RM. Activated protein C resistance as an additional risk factor for thrombosis in protein C-deficient families. *Blood* 1994;84:1031–1035.

116. Tait RC, Walker ID, Davidson JF, Islam SI, Mitchell R. Antithrombin III activity in healthy blood donors: age and sex related changes and prevalence of asymptomatic deficiency. *Br J Haematol* 1990;75:141–142.

117. Tait RC, Walker ID, Perry DJ, et al. Prevalence of antithrombin deficiency in the healthy population. *Br J Haematol* 1994;87:106–112.

118. Pabinger I, Brucker S, Kyrle PA, et al. Hereditary deficiency of antithrombin III, protein C and protein S: prevalence in patients with a history of venous thrombosis and criteria for rational patient screening. *Blood Coagul Fibrinolysis* 1992;3:547–553.

119. Finazzi G, Barbui T. Different incidence of venous thrombosis in patients with inherited deficiencies of antithrombin III, protein C and protein. *Thromb Haemost* 1994;71:15–18.

120. Rosendaal FR, Heijboer H, Briët E, et al. Mortality in hereditary antithrombin-III deficiency—1830 to 1989. *Lancet* 1991;337:260–262.

121. van Boven HH, Olds RJ, Thein SL, et al. Hereditary antithrombin deficiency: heterogeneity of the molecular basis and mortality in Dutch families. *Blood* 1994;84:4209–4213.

122. Miletich J, Sherman L, Broze G Jr. Absence of thrombosis in subjects with heterozygous protein C deficiency. *N Engl J Med* 1987;317:991–996.

123. Tait RC, Walker ID, Islam SI, et al. Protein C activity in healthy volunteers—influence of age, sex, smoking and oral contraceptives. *Thromb Haemost* 1993;70: 281–285.

124. Tait RC, Walker ID, Reitsma PH, et al. Prevalence of protein C deficiency in the healthy population. *Thromb Haemost* 1995;73:87–93.

125. Koster T, Rosendaal FR, Briët E, et al. Protein C deficiency in a controlled series of unselected outpatients: an infrequent but clear risk factor for venous thrombosis (Leiden Thrombophilia Study). *Blood* 1995;85: 2756–2761.

126. Allaart CF, Poort SR, Rosendaal FR, Reitsma PH, Bertina RM, Briët E. Increased risk of venous thrombosis in carriers of hereditary protein C deficiency defect. *Lancet* 1993;341:134–138.

127. Allaart CF, Rosendaal FR, Noteboom WM, Vandenbroucke JP, Briët E. Survival in families with hereditary protein C deficiency, 1820 to 1993. *Br Med J* 1995;311:910–913.

128. Briët E, Engesser L, Brommer EJP, Broekmans AW, Bertina RM. Thrombophilia: its causes and a rough estimate of its prevalence. *Thromb Haemost* 1987; 58:39.

129. Rees DC, Cox M, Clegg JB. World distribution of factor V Leiden. *Lancet* 1995;346:1133–1134.

130. Desmarais S, de Moerloose P, Reber G, Minazio P, Perrier A, Bounameaux H. Resistance to activated protein C in an unselected population of patients with pulmonary embolism. *Lancet* 1996;347:1374–1375.

131. Rosendaal FR, Koster T, Vandenbroucke JP, Reitsma PH. High risk of thrombosis in patients homozygous for factor V Leiden (activated protein C resistance). *Blood* 1995;85:1504–1508.

132. Greengard JS, Eichinger S, Griffin JH, Bauer KA. Brief report: variability of thrombosis among homozygous siblings with resistance to activated protein C due to an Arg→Gln mutation in the gene for factor V. *N Engl J Med* 1994;331:1559–1562.

133. Finazzi G, Barbui T. A retrospective study on oral anticoagulant prophylaxis in 103 Italian patients with hereditary thrombophilia and thrombosis. Ad hoc Study Group. *Ric Clin Lab* 1990;20:245–252.

134. Launbjerg J, Egeblad H, Heaf J, et al. Bleeding complications to oral anticoagulant therapy: multivariate analysis of 1010 treatment years in 551 outpatients. *J Intern Med* 1991;229:351–355.

135. Landefeld CS, Goldman L. Major bleeding in outpatients treated with warfarin: incidence and prediction by factors known at the start of outpatient therapy. *Am J Med* 1989;87:144–152.

136. van der Meer FJ, Rosendaal FR, Vandenbroucke JP, Briët E. Bleeding complications in oral anticoagulant therapy. An analysis of risk factors. *Arch Intern Med* 1993;153:1557–1562.

137. van der Meer FJ, Rosendaal FR, Vandenbroucke JP, Briët E. Assessment of a bleeding risk index in two cohorts of patients treated with oral anticoagulants. *Thromb Haemost* 1996;76:12–16.

138. De Stefano V, Leone G, Mastrangelo S, et al. Thrombosis during pregnancy and surgery in patients with congenital deficiency of antithrombin III, protein C, protein S. *Thromb Haemost* 1994;71:799–800.

139. Vicente V, Rodriguez C, Soto I, Fernandez M, Moraleda JM. Risk of thrombosis during pregnancy and post-partum in hereditary thrombophilia. *Am J Hematol* 1994;46:151–152.

140. Conard J, Horellou MH, van Dreden P, Lecompte T, Samama M. Thrombosis and pregnancy in congenital deficiencies in AT III, protein C or protein S: study of 78 women. *Thromb Haemost* 1990;63:319–320.

141. Friederich PW, Sanson BJ, Simioni P, et al. Frequency of Pregnancy-related venous thromboembolism in anticoagulant factor-deficient women: implications for prophylaxis. *Ann Intern Med* 1996;125:955–960.

142. De Stefano V, Mastrangelo S, Paciaroni K, et al. Thrombotic risk during pregnancy and puerperium in women with APC-resistance—effective subcutaneous heparin prophylaxis in a pregnant patient. *Thromb Haemost* 1995;74:793–794.

143. Pabinger I, Schneider B. Thrombotic risk of women with hereditary antithrombin III-, protein C- and protein S-deficiency taking oral contraceptive medication. The GTH Study Group on Natural Inhibitors. *Thromb Haemost* 1994;71:548–552.

144. Vandenbroucke JP, Koster T, Briët E, Reitsma PH, Bertina RM, Rosendaal FR. Increased risk of venous thrombosis in oral-contraceptive users who are carriers of factor V Leiden mutation. *Lancet* 1994;344: 1453–1457.

145. Dahlback B. Are we ready for factor V Leiden screening? *Lancet* 1996;347:1346–1347.

146. Vandenbroucke JP, van der Meer FJ, Helmerhorst FM, Rosendaal FR. Factor V Leiden—should we screen oral contraceptive users and pregnant women? *Br Med J* 1996;313:1127–1130.

147. Schulman S, Rhedin AS, Lindmarker P, et al. A comparison of six weeks with six months of oral anticoagulant therapy after a first episode of venous thromboembolism. Duration of Anticoagulation Trial Study Group. *N Engl J Med* 1995;332:1661–1665.

148. Schulman S, Granqvist S, Holstrom M, et al. The duration of oral anticoagulant therapy after a second episode of venous thromboembolism. *N Engl J Med* 1997;336:393–398.

149. van den Belt AGM, Sanson BJ, Simioni P, et al. Recurrence of venous thromboembolism in patients with familial thrombophilia. *Arch Intern Med* 1997;157: 2227–2232.

150. Iturbe-Alessio I, Fonseca MC, Mutchinik O, Santos MA, Zajarias A, Salazar E. Risks of anticoagulant therapy in pregnant women with artificial heart valves. *N Engl J Med* 1986;315:1390–1393.

151. Ginsberg JS, Hirsh J, Turner DC, Levine MN, Burrows R. Risks to the fetus of anticoagulant therapy during pregnancy. *Thromb Haemost* 1989;61:197–203.

152. Hall JA, Pauli RM, Wilson KM. Maternal and fetal sequelae of anticoagulation during pregnancy. *Am J Med* 1980;68:122–140.

153. Ginsberg JS, Kowalchuk G, Hirsh J, Brill-Edwards P, Burrows R. Heparin therapy during pregnancy. Risks to

the fetus and mother. *Arch Intern Med* 1989;149: 2233–2236.

154. Lecuru F, Desnos M, Taurelle R. Anticoagulant therapy in pregnancy. Report of 54 cases. *Acta Obstet Gynecol Scand* 1996;75:217–221.

155. Ginsberg JS, Hirsh J. Use of antithrombotic agents during pregnancy. *Chest* 1995;108(suppl):305–311.

156. Naurath HJ, Joosten E, Riezler R, Stabler SP, Allen RH, Lindenbaum J. Effects of vitamin B12, folate, and vitamin B6 supplements in elderly people with normal serum vitamin concentrations. *Lancet* 1995;346: 85–89.

157. Ginsberg JS. Management of venous thromboembolism. *N Engl J Med* 1996;335:1816–1828.

158. Brandjes DP, Heijboer H, Buller HR, de Rijk M, Jagt H, ten Cate JW. Acenocoumarol and heparin compared with acenocoumarol alone in the initial treatment of proximal-vein thrombosis. *N Engl J Med* 1992;327: 1485–1489.

159. ten Cate JW, Koopman MM, Prins MH, Buller HR. Treatment of venous thromboembolism. *Thromb Haemost* 1995;74:197–203.

160. Schulman S, Tengborn L. Treatment of venous thromboembolism in patients with congenital deficiency of antithrombin III. *Thromb Haemost* 1992; 68:634–636.

161. Schramm W, Spannagl M, Bauer KA, et al. Treatment of coumarin-induced skin necrosis with a monoclonal antibody purified protein C concentrate. *Arch Dermatol* 1993;129:753–756.

162. Samama M, Horellou HH, Soria J, Conard J, Nicolas G. Successful progressive anticoagulation in a severe protein C deficiency and previous skin necrosis at the initiation of oral anticoagulant treatment. *Thromb Haemost* 1984;51:132–133.

163. Enzenauer RJ, Berenberg JL, Campbell J. Progressive warfarin anticoagulation in protein C deficiency: a therapeutic strategy. *Am J Med* 1990;88:697–698.

164. Marlar RA, Montgomery RR, Broekmans AW. Report on the diagnosis and treatment of homozygous protein C deficiency. Report of the Working Party on Homozygous Protein C Deficiency of the ICTH-Subcommittee on Protein C and Protein S. *Thromb Haemost* 1989;61:529–531.

165. Koster T, Blann AD, Briët E, Vandenbroucke JP, Rosendaal FR. Role of clotting factor VIII in effect of von Willebrand factor on occurrence of deep-vein thrombosis. *Lancet* 1995;345:152–155.

166. Bertina RM, van der Linden IK, Engesser L, Muller HP, Brommer EJ. Hereditary heparin cofactor II deficiency and the risk of development of thrombosis. *Thromb Haemost* 1987;57:196–200.

Cardiovascular Thrombosis: Thrombocardiology and Thromboneurology, Second Edition,
edited by M. Verstraete, V. Fuster, and E. J. Topol,
Lippincott–Raven Publishers, Philadelphia © 1998.

5

Characteristics Associated with the Risk of Arterial Thrombosis

Thomas W. Meade, *George J. Miller, and †Robert D. Rosenberg

*MRC Epidemiology and Medical Care Unit, St. Bartholomew's and the Royal London School of Medicine and Dentistry, Wolfson Institute of Preventive Medicine, London EC1M 6BQ, United Kingdom; *Northwick Park Hospital, Middlesex HAQ 3UJ, United Kingdom; and †Massachusetts Institute of Technology, Cambridge, Massachusetts 02139*

General recognition of the thrombotic component of clinically manifest ischemic heart disease (IHD) is comparatively recent. With the advent of thrombolytic therapy and the need to establish the rationale for its use and effects, angiography demonstrated the high frequency of total coronary occlusion during myocardial infarction (MI) (1), and there is now no doubt about the significance of thrombosis in transmural MI (2). Thrombosis is probably also involved in subendocardial infarction, although the evidence on this point is less clear (2). When the results of a series of particularly careful autopsy studies became available in the 1980s—the best example being the work of Davies and Thomas (3)—the almost universal occurrence of at least a degree of thrombosis in sudden coronary death was recognized.

On the epidemiologic side, however, there had been much earlier recognition of a thrombotic component, even though its detailed characteristics had not been fully clarified. Thus, it was Morris (4) who first drew attention to the involvement of a major process other than atherogenesis through his analysis of postmortem findings at the London Hospital. There was no increase (if anything a decrease) in the prevalence of advanced atheroma over a period during which mortality from IHD had increased many times, suggesting a relatively short-term, acute effect rather than a longer term influence. The rapid initial decline in the risk of IHD in ex-smokers (5) is another observation that implies modification of an acute process.

In 1953, Morris and his colleagues (6) began their series of publications showing the protective effect of physical activity at work against clinically manifest IHD. In 1958, Morris and Crawford (7) complemented these findings with pathologic data. The National Necropsy Survey was based on simple, standardized

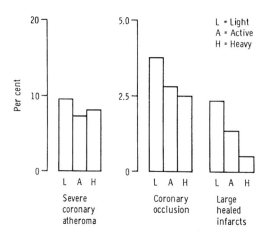

FIG. 5-1. National Necropsy Survey results showing relationship between physical activity of work and different pathological manifestations of ischemic heart disease.

recordings from 206 (85%) of the pathology departments in the British National Health Service, each of these departments contributing their findings in a total of 3,800 deaths from causes other than IHD. Figure 5-1 summarizes the clear results. There was no relationship between physical activity of occupation and atheroma of the coronary artery walls. There was some relationship between activity and coronary artery lumen occlusion. The strongest relationship was with large healed infarcts. The findings suggest that the effect of exercise, or of its absence, on occlusive episodes and infarction itself is mediated through some pathway other than atherogenesis. The epidemiologic studies discussed later show relationships of several hemostatic variables with the incidence of IHD that also provide a major stimulus to the concept and definition of "hypercoagulability" and the "prethrombotic state."

Given a major thrombotic contribution to IHD, an obvious question for the clinician or epidemiologist is the extent to which those at risk of IHD can be characterized on account of a thrombotic tendency. A major part of the answer depends on the results of studies that include measures of hemostatic function and relate these to the subsequent onset (incidence) of IHD.

HYPERCOAGULABILITY

Attempts to link hemostatic variables with the development of IHD implicitly assume that increased activity of coagulation proteins or platelets might serve as a marker of, or directly contribute to, the critical thrombotic component of this disease. It is epidemiologic studies of coagulation proteins that have so far been most rewarding with regard to this hypothesis, although the central role of platelets in thrombogenesis is acknowledged.

The coagulation mechanism is composed of a series of linked proteolytic reactions (8), illustrated schematically in Fig. 5-2. At each stage, a zymogen is converted to its corresponding serine protease (designated by the letter "a" after each specific factor, e.g., IXa), which activates the next zymogen in the cascade, ultimately leading to thrombin generation. This blood clotting enzyme is able to convert fibrinogen to fibrin and thereby initiate thrombus formation. In most steps, protein cofactors such as factors V and VIII are activated by blood-clotting enzymes, bind different pairs of zymogen-serine proteases to cell surfaces, and accelerate generation of the next proteolytic enzyme within the pathway. Thus, the coagulation mechanism can be pictured as a series of reactions in which a zymogen, a cofactor, and a converting enzyme interact to form a multimolecular complex on a natural surface. All the various reactants must be present if conversion of the zymogen is to take place at a significant rate. These transformations are suppressed if the converting enzyme is inhibited, the protein cofactor destroyed, or the surface receptors essential for the macromolecular complex sequestered.

The direct measurement of coagulation enzymes would be especially informative with regard to the detection of the hypercoagulable state in humans. Unfortunately, this approach has been unsuccessful because of the extremely short half-life of these enzymes within the circulation due to natural anticoagulant mechanisms. However, the transition of zymogens to serine proteases at separate stages in the coagulation mechanism occurs in concert with the

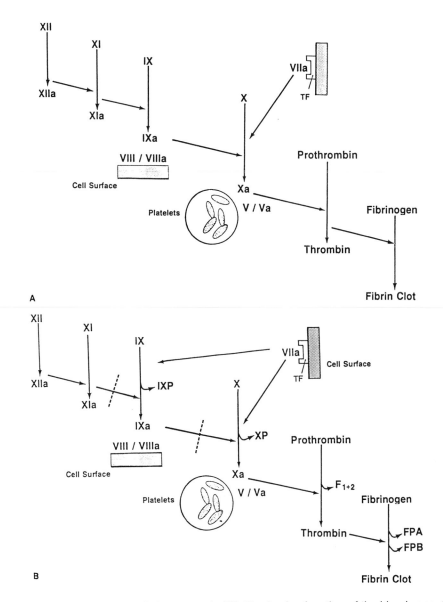

FIG. 5-2. The classical blood coagulation cascade **(A)**. The in vivo function of the blood coagulation cascade **(B)**. The dotted lines represent functional blocks that are removed during hemostasis/thrombosis.

release of an activation peptide, and thrombin-dependent production of fibrin also involves liberation of two small fragments of fibrinogen. Thus, the plasma concentrations of factor IX activation peptide (F1Xp), factor X activation peptide (FXp), prothrombin activation peptide (F1+2), and fibrinopeptide A (FPA) can be accurately quantitated by radioimmunoassay and used to monitor the generation of specific blood-clotting enzymes (9–12).

These peptide activation assays have allowed examination of the basal in vivo functioning of the blood coagulation mechanism (Fig. 5-2). This has been accomplished by measuring the concentrations of the activation peptides in patients with congenital deficiencies of factors VII, VIII, and IX before and immediately after normalization with purified or recombinant proteins (10,11,13). These and other studies demonstrate that the factor VII–tissue factor pathway serves as the major driving force to establish the basal activity of the coagulation mechanism. The intrinsic pathway is dormant with regard to thrombin generation, probably due to the inability of factor IXa produced by the factor VII–tissue factor pathway to act on factor X because of the absence of circulating factor VIIIa or activated platelets. It is surmised that vessel wall injury raises the thrombin concentration above basal levels via the factor VII–tissue factor pathway, which then converts small amounts of factor VIII to factor VIIIa and possibly activates platelets with resultant amplification of thrombin production by the action of existing factor IXa on factor X. Factor VII is produced by the liver as a single-chain zymogen, which can be cleaved to a two-chain species without release of an activation peptide upon exposure to factor XIIa, factor IXa, factor Xa, and thrombin (14,15). Current biochemical data indicate that factor VIIa is able to activate factors IX and X when coupled with tissue factor, but significant controversy exists about the ability of the zymogen to carry out the same reactions albeit at a greatly reduced level (16–18). Thus, elevated plasma levels of factor VII activity in hypercoagulable individuals would most likely be due to increased conversion of factor VII to factor VIIa. The increased production of F1+2 that occurs during the hypercoagulable state also might induce augmented levels of factor VII as well as other vitamin K–dependent coagulation factors, which could further elevate the apparent plasma levels of factor VII activity (19).

The blood coagulation cascade should probably be conceptualized as a set of zymogen conversion events that are individually regulated by several potent natural anticoagulant mechanisms (20). The heparan sulfate–antithrombin III mechanism of the blood vessel wall is responsible for the neutralization of circulating factor IXa, factor Xa, and thrombin (21,22). The protein C–thrombomodulin mechanism of the blood vessel wall captures thrombin, which then generates activated protein C that destroys activated cofactors VIIIa and Va, used in the production of factor Xa and thrombin, respectively (23). The last few years have seen increasing interest in a polymorphism for the gene coding for factor V, factor V-Leiden, and the ensuing resistance to activated protein C (24). It seems likely that the clinical consequences of the thrombophilic tendency induced are for venous rather than arterial disease in men (25), whereas the polymorphism may increase the risk of myocardial infarction in younger women (26). The fibrinolytic system can prevent fibrin deposition by transforming fibrin 1 (removal of fibrinopeptide A) to a fragment of fibrinogen via a plasmin-dependent cleavage of the Bβ chain, which suppresses conversion to insoluble fibrin II (removal of fibrinopeptide B) (27).

The hypercoagulable state exists between the extremes of normal basal coagulation system function and the augmented generation of serine proteases that takes place during thrombus formation. This prethrombotic state is operationally defined by small elevations of serine protease generation and fibrin deposition as measured by peptide activation assays which show that coagulation system activity is exceeding the inhibitory threshold of the natural anticoagulant mechanisms.

Elevated plasma concentrations of fibrinogen also might play a role in the hypercoagulable state because they might be expected to result in a large thrombus for an equivalent amount of thrombin generated.

The importance of the hypercoagulable state in IHD is presently at an interesting transitional stage with regard to clinical and epidemiologic studies. The past investigations have used classical coagulation assays to show strong associations of plasma factor VII activity and levels of fibrinogen with cardiovascular disease, as outlined below. The application of activation peptide assays now provides a technique for more directly assessing the relationship between coagulation system activity and IHD as well as monitoring preventive anticoagulant therapy.

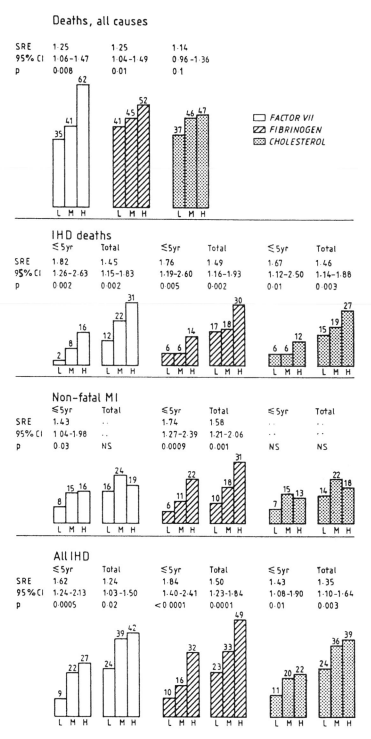

FIG. 5-3. Main results of the Northwick Park Heart Study. Numbers of events within 5 years and for total follow-up period by low (L), middle (M), and high (H) thirds of distributions. Standardized regression effects (SRE) show increases in risk of ischemic heart disease for a standard deviation increase in the variable concerned; e.g., SRE of 1.5 indicates that for a standard deviation rise, risk increases by 50%.

EPIDEMIOLOGIC EVIDENCE

There is still no generally accepted measure of platelet function that has been shown to be associated with the later onset of IHD in those so far free of clinical disease, although spontaneous platelet aggregation (28) and large platelet volume (29) may well be associated with recurrence.

The levels of factor VII coagulant (VIIc) activity and plasma fibrinogen are the two aspects of the hemostatic system that have so far been particularly highlighted by the results of prospective studies. (Factor VIIc is used to denote factor VII coagulant activity in a biologic assay. Factor VIIa [see also previous section] refers to the active, two-chain form of factor VII.) Factor VIIc was measured in the Northwick Park Heart Study using a semiautomated one-stage bioassay sensitive to VIIa (30,31).

Northwick Park Heart Study

In 1980, Meade et al. (32) showed preliminary results in 1,510 middle-aged white men, suggesting that high levels of factor VIIc and of plasma fibrinogen, and possibly also of factor VIII activity, were associated with mortality from cardiovascular disease, principally IHD. The main results of the Northwick Park Heart Study (NPHS) (33) are summarized in Fig. 5-3. High levels of factor VIIc and fibrinogen were associated with mortality from all causes, reflecting the predominance of IHD as a cause of death. The relationships of factor VIIc and fibrinogen with the incidence specifically of IHD within 5 years of recruitment were, if anything, stronger than for cholesterol, although the latter relationship, as expected, was also demonstrated. There was no clear relationship between factor VIIc or fibrinogen and the incidence of cancer, so the findings appear to be specific for vascular disease. The association of factor VIIc with IHD in the NPHS (34), also reported in a German prospective study (35), is largely confined to fatal episodes.

Göteborg Study

In 1984, Wilhelmsen et al. (36) showed a relationship in a study of 792 men born in

1913 between high fibrinogen levels and the incidence of both IHD and, in particular, stroke. For stroke, the data suggested an interaction between fibrinogen and systolic blood pressure, men with high levels of both being at considerably greater risk than might have been expected from the sum of the two effects separately, although the relatively small number of events on which this analysis was based must be taken into account.

Leigh Study

In 1985, Stone and Thorp (37) reported an association between high fibrinogen levels and IHD incidence in a group of 297 men 40 to 69 years of age who were observed for up to 20 years. The relationship was stronger than for cholesterol, blood pressure, or smoking. In this study, too, there was suggestive evidence of an interaction between fibrinogen and blood pressure. Thus, men whose systolic blood pressure and plasma fibrinogen levels were in the top third of the respective distributions experienced 12 times the incidence of IHD compared with those whose levels were in the low third.

Framingham Study

In 1985, Kannel et al. (38) reported an association between high fibrinogen levels and the incidence of cardiovascular disease in 554 men and 761 women 47 to 79 years of age who had not previously experienced a cardiovascular event, cardiovascular disease being defined as the sum of IHD, stroke, heart failure, and peripheral arterial disease. Subsequent publications (39,40) established a clear relationship between fibrinogen and the incidence of IHD in both men and women and between fibrinogen and stroke in men, although less clearly for stroke in women.

Caerphilly Study

The results of this study (41,42) also show a strong relationship between not only fibrinogen but also viscosity and the incidence of IHD. As Fig. 5-4 shows, these effects are independent, indicating that fibrinogen predisposes to IHD through pathways besides (although

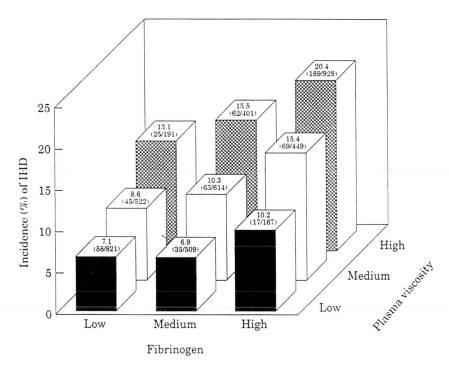

FIG. 5-4. Ten-year incidence of ischemic heart disease (IHD) jointly in relation to both fibrinogen and plasma viscosity. (Reproduced from Sweetnam et al., ref. 42, with permission.)

certainly including) viscosity, i.e., as a cofactor for platelet aggregation, through the amount of fibrin formed, by impairing clot deformability, and in contributing to atheroma (43,44).

NPHS also has reported an association of raised factor VIII activity and von Willebrand factor (vWF) levels with IHD (45). The apparently low incidence of IHD in hemophilia (46) is in agreement with this finding. Factor VIII activity and vWF are higher in those with deep vein thrombosis than in controls (47), a setting in which vessel wall pathology is not a major feature and which therefore suggests a direct, thrombogenic effect of intrinsically high levels.

A good clinical example of the potential value of the new activation peptides is the demonstration of a habitually increased state of hypercoagulability in patients with IHD, shown in high F1+2 values, suggesting increased thrombin production and manifesting itself as increased thrombin activity as indicated by FPA levels at the time of infarction (48).

As a whole, these studies suggest that the biochemical disturbance leading to IHD lies at least as much in the coagulation system as in the metabolism of cholesterol.

The potential defense mechanisms against thrombosis include antithrombin III. Yue et al. (49) found a gradient of increasing antithrombin III values from those at low risk of IHD via those at intermediate risk or with chronic IHD to those with acute myocardial infarction. Findings at recruitment to the Northwick Park Heart Study (43) also suggested higher rather than lower values in those who had previously experienced IHD. By contrast, other investigators (50–52) have reported lower levels in patients with a history of infarction or other manifestations of arterial disease. These apparently contradictory findings could be explained in part by postulating that antithrombin III levels, for example, tend not to be elevated in individuals who are at low risk of arterial disease and who do not therefore need to make an antithrombotic response. In those at high risk, on the other hand, antithrombin III levels may be low or high. Inability to increase antithrombin III levels in some individuals may directly contribute to subsequent events in which high procoagulatory clotting factor levels are involved, whereas levels in others may increase as a compensatory defense mechanism. NPHS data (53) suggest that both low and high levels may be associated with increased risk. Low antithrombin III levels are associated with an increased incidence of major thrombotic episodes in patients with angina (54).

High fibrinogen levels are also associated with the progression or recurrence of arterial disease at all three main sites, i.e., heart (55), brain (56), and peripheral circulation (57).

FIBRINOLYSIS

Altered fibrinolytic activity (FA) also has been shown in prospective (as well as cross-sectional) studies to be associated with an increased incidence of IHD in both men and women (58–60) and of stroke in men (61). Two of these studies used tissue plasminogen activator (t-PA) antigen in nested case-control studies based on the U.S. Physicians Health Study (58,61), and risk of IHD or stroke increased with t-PA antigen, which seems counterintuitive. However, it is likely that t-PA antigen, as distinct from t-PA activity, is indirectly measuring plasminogen activator inhibitor type 1 (PAI-1), in which case the interpretation is that the risk of IHD and stroke increases with increasing inhibition of FA. The other prospective reports come from the Northwick Park Heart Study using the dilute blood clot lysis time (DCLT) as a more "global" measure of FA and reflecting the balance of activation and inhibition. Low FA was associated with IHD incidence in both men and women (59,60). High PAI-1 levels are associated with recurrent IHD in young men (62).

However, association does not necessarily imply causation. Besides prospective studies, other types of evidence also have to be considered in establishing whether levels of factor VIIc, fibrinogen, and perhaps other hemostatic variables are associated with the subsequent incidence of IHD because they are causally involved or simply because they are markers of some other process. The results of randomized controlled trials are particularly valuable in this context, providing unbiased evidence on the consequences of altering clotting factor activities.

CLINICAL TRIALS

Overviews of the evidence from long-term trials (63) and short-term trials (64) established a 20% reduction in mortality attributable to oral anticoagulants after infarction. This observation and a larger reduction in recurrent nonfatal events were confirmed in the Dutch Sixty Plus trial (65), in the WARIS trial (66), and in the ASPECT trial (67). Warfarin reduces the activity levels of the other procoagulatory clotting factors besides factor VII (i.e., factors II, IX, and X), as well as the anticoagulatory factors protein C and protein S. It is therefore not possible to explain the effects of warfarin solely in terms of factor VIIc, although it is reasonable to conclude that decreasing the general level of coagulability prevents recurrent episodes. There are two sources of trial evidence involving fibrinogen. One is the World Health Organization clofibrate trial (68). This trial was based on the relationship between cholesterol (not fibrinogen) and IHD and was performed in men with hyperlipidemia, based on the cholesterol-lowering property of clofibrate. There was a significant reduction (about 20%) in the incidence of MI attributable to clofibrate, but there was also an increase in deaths from a variety of causes for reasons that are still unclear but that preclude the general use of clofibrate. However, it is clear that clofibrate also lowers fibrinogen levels (69). Furthermore, the beneficial effect of clofibrate against infarction appears to have been confined to heavy smokers who were also hypertensive. The heavy smokers will have had high fibrinogen levels. Current trials are establishing the value of bezafibrate (70), a newer member of this class of agents, which also lowers fibrinogen and may not have clofibrate's unwanted effects. The other source of evidence is a series of studies (71) in both humans and animals showing that ancrod, a defibrinating agent, reduces thrombosis and improves clinical function in immune kidney disease.

SMOKING, DIET, AND OTHER CHARACTERISTICS

Another useful if more circumstantial component of the epidemiologic evidence is the extent to which levels of the clotting factors associated with IHD alter according to personal and environmental characteristics associated with the disease. Probably of greatest interest are the relationships of smoking with fibrinogen and dietary fat intake with factor VIIc.

Smoking

Uniformly, all the large-scale studies already mentioned (and other, smaller studies) have found the highest fibrinogen levels in smokers, intermediate levels in ex-smokers, and lowest levels in nonsmokers (72). There is a dose-response relationship between the number of cigarettes smoked and the fibrinogen level (73). Figure 5-5, from data at entry to the NPHS, shows a rapid initial decline in fibrinogen on stopping, but levels remain above those for nonsmokers for up to 5 and perhaps 10 years after discontinuation, a time course that closely mirrors the decline in the risk of IHD itself after smoking cessation (5). This effect also has been shown prospectively (72). Thus, over the 6-year follow-up period in the NPHS, fibrinogen levels increased (over and above the increase with age) in those who started or resumed smoking and decreased in those who discontinued smoking. However, it is important to remember that high levels are associated with an increased risk of IHD in nonsmokers as well as in smokers.

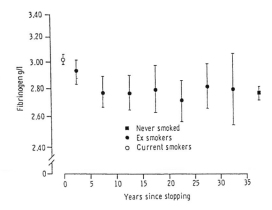

FIG. 5-5. Plasma fibrinogen (age adjusted) by time since stopping smoking in ex-smokers and in current and nonsmokers (log scale; bars show 95% confidence intervals).

Dietary Fat Intake

Experimental studies in healthy adults have shown a significant positive association between day-to-day variation in total fat intake and factor VIIc (74). Indeed, the influence of fat consumption on factor VIIc is sufficiently rapid for there to be an association between the diurnal variation in plasma triglyceride concentration induced by the meal pattern and the diurnal fluctuation in factor VIIc (75). The diurnal rhythm in factor VIIc lags behind that in plasma triglyceride by approximately 2 to 3 hours. The increase in factor VIIc postprandially has been shown to be a consequence of factor VII activation (76,77). By contrast, no association appears to exist between diurnal fluctuations in factor VII antigen concentration and plasma triglyceride (75). The mechanism linking dietary fat consumption with factor VII activation is incompletely understood but appears to involve the induction of an appreciable chylomicronemia after absorption of long-chain fatty acids (76), lipolysis of the triglyceride-rich lipoprotein (78), and activation of factor IX as intermediate steps (77).

The associations between factor VIIc and total dietary fat intake can be observed in the general community. The demonstration of such a relationship is handicapped by the dif-

ficulty in measurement of fat intake in the habitual diet, a problem that has thwarted most
attempts to show an association between fat
intake and serum cholesterol concentration
within communities. Nevertheless, a significant positive correlation with factor VIIc has
been demonstrated in middle-aged men when
fat intake was expressed relative to body size
(because it is overconsumption rather than absolute intake that is important for factor VIIc)
(79).

Two experimental studies, one lasting 7
days (75) and one 14 days (80), examined the
effects of dietary fat composition on factor
VIIc. Unlike total fat intake, the ratio of
polyunsaturated fatty acid to saturated fatty
acid in the diet had no demonstrable effect on
factor VIIc.

Many clinical conditions in which there is a
hyperlipidemia are associated with an increase
in factor VIIc, for example the primary hyper-
lipoproteinemias (81,82), pregnancy (83), and
diabetes mellitus (84). Reduction of plasma
lipid levels, particularly triglyceride, is associated with a decrease in factor VIIc (85). When
plasma lipid concentrations tend to be low, as
in vegetarians, factor VIIc is also reduced (86).

CONCLUSION

The risk of IHD can be modified either
pharmacologically or via life-style changes.

Life-style changes can be encouraged by
central policies affecting dietary habits or tobacco advertising, for example, and directed at
populations as a whole, or they can be adopted
through individual choice. They have almost
certainly been responsible for much of the
striking decline in IHD incidence in many
countries over the past 25 years. However,
their acceptance and implementation take
time. Many individuals find the recommended
changes difficult or impossible to follow; in
some individuals the changes are ineffective.
Therefore, pharmacologic intervention may be
required. Before considering this in further detail, however, there are some lessons for prevention through life-style changes that are
emerging from the recognition of the thrombotic component in IHD and its characteristics. Although this new information alters no
general principles, in some respects it enables
their sharper application. First, the independent relationship between high fibrinogen levels and the risk of IHD is sufficiently strong to
warrant the addition of the fibrinogen level to
the definition of the high-risk profile. Second,
the similarity of the time course for the decrease in fibrinogen and in the risk of IHD itself in ex-smokers emphasizes the importance
of not overlooking the considerable period of
time during which an ex-smoker remains at increased risk or the thrombotic contribution to
this risk. Turning to diet, the very rapid effect
of changes in fat intake on coagulability provides a sound basis for the adoption of dietary
measures at any age and argues strongly
against any remaining belief that these will
only succeed if they are adopted in early life
(although doing so then may well influence
atherogenesis as well).

Where pharmacologic measures for primary prevention are necessary, it is of course
with the modification of platelet aggregation
and fibrin formation that antithrombotic measures are concerned. The value of aspirin in
primary prevention is still unclear. The trial in
American doctors (87) suggested a reduction
in the incidence of MI of 44%, but no effect
on death from all vascular causes; the trial in
British doctors (88) showed no apparent benefit against MI. An overview of the two trials
suggests a significant reduction of 32% (89),
although there is marginally significant heterogeneity between the two trials in this respect, and an increase of 18% in nonfatal
stroke, which is not significant and contrasts
with the obvious reduction in stroke due to aspirin in the secondary prevention trials.
Therefore, there is a need for further information from primary prevention trials of aspirin,
including the effects of aspirin doses in the
range of 40 to 80 mg daily. A fairly consistent
finding in secondary prevention trials has so
far been a somewhat greater benefit due to
oral anticoagulants than aspirin, although this
conclusion is mainly based on indirect comparisons. Thus, the reduction in mortality at-

tributable to anticoagulants is, at 35% to 40%, somewhat more than the typical figures of 15% to 20% for aspirin. Similarly, anticoagulants reduce recurrent MI between a third and a half compared with a reduction of 25% or 30% in the case of aspirin.

If there truly is a more than marginal advantage of anticoagulants over aspirin, the greater complexity of anticoagulant treatment should not automatically rule it out in what is a common condition in which even small differences in effectiveness may be reflected in many lives saved and events avoided. A second consideration for the potential value of anticoagulants is the growing conviction that their benefit may perhaps be achieved at lower than conventional levels of anticoagulation. There would also be less bleeding and less need for monitoring. There is also the real possibility that the simultaneous modification of platelet function and fibrin formation may be more effective than the modification of either process on its own. A striking demonstration of this possibility comes from the ISIS-2 trial (90), in which the combination of aspirin and streptokinase was more effective than either active agent on its own, although each also reduced cardiovascular mortality. Another example comes from the value of adding aspirin to oral anticoagulation after heart valve surgery (91).

REFERENCES

1. DeWood MA, Spores J, Notske R, et al. Prevalence of total coronary occlusion during the early hours of transmural myocardial infarction. *N Engl J Med* 1980;303: 987–902.
2. Davies MJ. Thrombosis in myocardial infarction and sudden death. In: Mehta JL, Conti CR, Brest AN (eds). *Thrombosis and Platelets in Myocardial Ischemia.* Philadelphia: FA Davis, 1987;151–159.
3. Davies MJ, Thomas A. Thrombosis and acute coronary artery lesions in sudden cardiac ischemic death. *N Engl J Med* 1984;310:1137–1140.
4. Morris JN. Recent history of coronary disease. *Lancet* 1951;1:1–7.
5. Cook DG, Shaper AG, Pocock SJ, Kussick SJ. Giving up smoking and the risk of heart attacks. *Lancet* 1986;2: 1376–1380.
6. Morris JN, Heady JA, Raffle PAB, Roberts CG, Parks JW. Coronary heart disease and physical activity or work. *Lancet* 1953;2:1053–1057,1111–1120.
7. Morris JN, Crawford MD. Coronary heart disease and

physicial activity of work. Evidence of a national necropsy survey. *Br Med J* 1958;2:1485–1496.
8. Furie B, Furie BC. The molecular basis of blood coagulation. In: Hoffman R, Benz EJ Jr, Shattil SJ, Furie B, Cohen HJ (eds). *Hematology: Basic Principles and Practices.* New York: Churchill Livingstone, 1995; 1566–1587.
9. Teitel JM, Bauer KA, Lau HK, Rosenberg RD. Studies of the prothrombin blood activation pathway utilizing radioimmunoassay for the F2/F1-2 fragment and thrombin-antithrombin complex. *Blood* 1982;59:1086–1097.
10. Bauer KA, Kass BL, ten Cate H, Bednarek MA, Hawiger JJ, Rosenberg RD. Detection of Factor X activation in humans. *Blood* 1989;74:2007–2015.
11. Bauer KA, Kass BL, ten Cate H, et al. Factor IX is activated in vivo by the tissue factor mechanism. *Blood* 1990;76:731–736.
12. Nossel HL, Yudelman I, Canfield RE, et al. Measurement of fibrinopeptide A in human blood. *J Clin Invest* 1974;54:43–53.
13. Bauer KA, Mannucci PM, Gringeri A, et al. Factor IXa-factor VIIIa-cell surface complex does not contribute to the basal activation of the coagulation mechanism. *Blood* 1992;79:2039–2047.
14. Zur M, Radcliffe RD, Oberdick J, Nemerson Y. The dual role of factor VII in blood coagulation. *J Biol Chem* 1982;257:5623–5631.
15. Bach R, Oberdick J, Nemerson Y. Immunoaffinity purification of bovine factor VII. *Blood* 1984;63:393–398.
16. Rao LVM, Rapaport SI, Bajaj SP. Activation of human factor VII in the initiation of tissue factor-dependent coagulation. *Blood* 1986;68:695–691.
17. Williams EB, Krishnaswamy S, Mann KG. Zymogen/enzyme discrimination using peptide chloromethyl ketones. *J Biol Chem* 1989;264:7536–7545.
18. Wildgoose P, Berkner KL, Kisiel W. Synthesis, purification and characterization of an Arg 152-Glu site-directed mutant of recombinant human blood clotting factor VII. *Biochemistry* 1990;29:3413–3420.
19. Mitropoulos KA, Esnouf MP. The prothrombin activation peptide regulates synthesis of the vitamin K-dependent proteins in the rabbit. *Thromb Res* 1990;57:541–549.
20. Rosenberg RD, The biochemistry and pathophysiology of the prethrombotic state. *Ann Rev Med* 1987;38: 493–508.
21. Marcum JA, Atha DH, Fritze LMS, Nawroth P, Stern D, Rosenberg RD. Cloned bovine aortic endothelial cells synthesize anticoagulantly active heparan sulfate proteoglycan. *J Biol Chem* 1986;261:7507–7517.
22. Marcum JA, McKenney JB, Rosenberg RD. Acceleration of thrombin-antithrombin complex formation in rat hindquarters via naturally occurring heparin-like molecules bound to the endothelium. *J Clin Invest* 1984;74: 341–350.
23. Esmon NL, Owen WG, Esmon CT. Isolation of a membrane bound cofactor for thrombin-catalyzed activation of protein C. *J Biol Chem* 1982;257:859–864.
24. Kalafatis M, Mann KG. Factor V Leiden and thrombophilia. *Arterioscler Thromb Vasc Biol* 1997;17: 620–627.
25. Ridker PM, Hennekens CH, Lindpaintner K, Stampfer MJ, Eisenberg PR, Miletich JP. Mutation in the gene coding for coagulation factor V and the risk of myocardial infarction, stroke, and venous thrombosis in apparently healthy men. *N Engl J Med* 1995;332:912–917.

26. Rosendaal FR, Siscovick DS, Schwartz SM, et al. Factor V Leiden (resistance to activated protein C) increases the risk of myocardial infarction in young women. *Blood* 1997;89:2817–2821.

27. Nossel HL. Relative proteolysis of the fibrinogen B beta chain by thrombin and plasmin as a determinant of thrombosis. *Nature* 1981;291:165–167.

28. Trip MD, Cats VM, van Capelle FJL, Vreeken J. Platelet hyper-reactivity and prognosis in survivors of myocardial infarction. *N Engl J Med* 1990;322:1549–1554.

29. Martin JF, Bath PM, Burr ML. Influence of platelet size on outcome after myocardial infarction. *Lancet* 1991; 338:1409–1411.

30. Brozovic M, Stirling Y, Harricks C, North WRS, Meade TW. Factor VII in an industrial population. *Br J Haematol* 1974;28:381–391.

31. Miller GJ, Stirling Y, Esnouf MP, et al. Factor VII-deficient substrate plasmas depleted of protein C raise the sensitivity of the factor VII bio-assay to activated factor VII an international study. *Thromb Haemost* 1994;71: 38–48.

32. Meade TW, North WRS, Chakrabarti R, Stirling Y, Haines AP, Thompson SG. Haemostatic function and cardiovascular death: early results of a prospective study. *Lancet* 1980;1:1050–1054.

33. Meade TW, Mellows S, Brozovic M, et al. Haemostatic function and ischaemic heart disease: principal results of the Northwick Park Heart Study. *Lancet* 1986;2: 533–537.

34. Ruddock V, Meade TW. Factor VII activity and ischaemic heart disease: fatal and non- fatal events. *Q J Med* 1994;87:403–406.

35. Assmann G, Cullen P, Heinrich J, Schulte H. Hemostatic variables in the prediction of coronary risk: results of the 8 year follow-up of healthy men in the Münster Heart Study PROCAM. *Isr J Med Sci* 1996;32:364–370.

36. Wilhelmsen L, Svardsudd K, Korsan-Bengtsen K, Welin L, Tibblin G. Fibrinogen as a risk factor for stroke and myocardial infarction. *N Engl J Med* 1984;311:501–505.

37. Stone MC, Thorp JM. Plasma fibrinogen—a major coronary risk factor. *J R Coll Gen Pract* 1985;35:565–569.

38. Kannel WB, Castelli WP, Meeks SL. Fibrinogen and cardiovascular disease. Abstract of paper for 34th Annual Scientific Session of the American College of Cardiology, March 1985, Anaheim, California.

39. Kannel WB, Wolf PA, Castelli WP, D'Agostino RB. Fibrinogen and risk of cardiovascular disease. *JAMA* 1987;114:918–925.

40. Kannel WB. Hypertension and other risk factors in coronary heart disease. *Am Heart J* 1987;114;918–925.

41. Yarnell JWG, Baker IA, Sweetnam PM, et al. Fibrinogen viscosity and white blood cell count are major risk factors for ischemic heart disease. The Caerphilly and Speedwell Collaborative Heart Disease Studies. *Circulation* 1991;83:836–844.

42. Sweetnam PM, Thomas HF, Yarnell JWG, Beswick AD, Baker IA, Elwood PC. Fibrinogen, viscosity and the 10-year incidence of ischaemic heart disease. The Caerphilly and Speedwell Studies. *Eur Heart J* 1996;17: 1814–1820.

43. Meade TW. The epidemiology of atheroma, thrombosis and ischaemic heart disease. In: Bloom AL, Forbes CD, Thomas DP, Tuddenham EGD (eds). *Haemostasis and Thrombosis.* Vol. 2, 3rd ed. Edinburgh: Churchill Livingstone, 1994;1199–1227.

44. Scrutton MC, Ross-Murphy SB, Bennett GM, Stirling Y, Meade TW. Changes in clot deformability—a possible explanation for the epidemiological association between plasma fibrinogen concentration and myocardial infarction. *Blood Coagul Fibrinolysis* 1994;5:719–723.

45. Meade TW, Cooper JC, Stirling Y, Howarth DJ, Ruddock V, Miller GJ. Factor VIII, ABO blood group and the incidence of ischaemic heart disease. *Br J Haematol* 1994;88:604–607.

46. Rosendaal FR, Varekamp I, Smit C, et al. Mortality and causes of death in Dutch haemophiliacs, 1973–86. *Br J Haematol* 1989;71:71–76.

47. Koster T, Blann AD, Briët E, et al. Role of clotting factor VIII in effect of von Willebrand factor on occurrence of deep-vein thrombosis. *Lancet* 1995;345:152–155.

48. Merlini PA, Bauer KA, Oltrona L, et al. Persistent activation of coagulation mechanisms in unstable angina and myocardial infarction. *Circulation* 1994:90:61–8.

49. Yue R, Gertler M, Starr T, Koutrouby R. Alterations of plasma antithrombin III levels in ischemic heart disease. *Thromb Haemost* 1976;35:598–606.

50. Banerjee R, Sahni A, Kumar V, Arya M. Antithrombin III deficiency in maturity onset diabetes mellitus and atherosclerosis. *Thromb Diathesis Haemorrhagica* 1974;31:339–345.

51. O'Brien J, Etherington M, Jamieson S, Lawford P, Lincoln S, Alkjaersig N. Blood changes in atherosclerosis and long after myocardial infarction and venous thrombosis. *Thromb Diathesis Haemorrhagica* 1975;34: 483–497.

52. Innerfield I, Goldfischer J, Reichter-Reiss H, Greenberg J. Serum antithrombins in coronary artery disease. *Am J Clin Pathol* 1976;65:64–68.

53. Meade TW, Cooper J, Miller GJ, Howarth DJ, Stirling Y. Antithrombin III and arterial disease. *Lancet* 1991;337: 850–851.

54 Thompson SG, Fechtrup C, Squire E, Heyse U, Breithardt G, van de Loo JCW. Antithrombin III and fibrinogen as predictors of cardiac events in patients with angina pectoris. *Arterioscler Thromb Vasc Biol* 1996;16: 357–362.

55. Thompson SG, Kienast J, Pike SDM, et al. Hemostatic factors and the risk of myocardial infarction or sudden death in patients with angina pectoris. *N Engl J Med* 1995;332:635–641.

56. Qizilbash N, Jones L, Warlow C, Mann J. Fibrinogen and lipid concentrations as risk factors for transient ischaemic attacks and minor ischaemic strokes. *Br Med J* 1991;303:605–609.

57. Banerjee AK, Pearson J, Gilliland EL, et al. A six year prospective study of fibrinogen and other risk factors associated with mortality in stable claudicants. *Thromb Haemost* 1992;68:261–263.

58. Ridker PM, Vaughan DE, Stampfer MJ, et al. Endogenous tissue-type plasminogen activator and risk of myocardial infaction. *Lancet* 1993;341:1165–1168.

59. Meade TW, Howarth DJ, Cooper J, MacCallum PK, Stirling Y. Fibrinolytic activity and arterial disease. *Lancet* 1994;343:1442.

60. Meade TW, Cooper JA, Chakrabarti R, Miller GJ, Stirling Y, Howarth DJ. Fibrinolytic activity and clotting factors in ischaemic heart disease in women. *Br Med J* 1996;312:1581.

61. Ridker PM, Hennekens CH, Stampfer MJ, Manson JE, Vaughan DE. Prospective study of endogenous tissue

plasminogen activator and risk of stroke. *Lancet* 1994; 343:940–943.

62. Hamsten A, de Faire U, Wallius G,et al. Plasminogen activator inhibitor in plasma: risk factor for recurrent myocardial infarction. *Lancet* 1987;2:3–9.

63. International Anticoagulant Review Group. Collaborative analysis of long-term anticoagulant administration after acute myocardial infarction. *Lancet* 1970;1:203–209.

64. Chalmers TV, Matta RJ, Smith H, Kunzler A-M. Evidence favoring the use of anticoagulants in the hospital phase of acute myocardial infarction. *N Engl J Med* 1977;297:1091–1096.

65. Sixty-Plus Reinfarction Study Research Group. A double-blind trial to assess long-term oral anticoagulant therapy in elderly patients after myocardial infarction. *Lancet* 1980;2:989–994.

66. Smith P, Arnesen H, Holme I. The effect of warfarin on mortality and reinfarction after myocardial infarction. *N Engl J Med* 1990;323:147–152.

67. Anticoagulants in the Secondary Prevention of Events in Coronary Thrombosis (ASPECT) Research Group. Effect of long-term oral anticoagulant treatment on mortality and cardiovascular morbidity after myocardial infarction. *Lancet* 1994;343:499–503.

68. Co-operative trial in the primary prevention of ischaemic heart disease using clofibrate. *Br Heart J* 1978;40: 1069–1118.

69. Green KG, Heady A, Oliver MF. Blood pressure, cigarette smoking and heart attack in the WHO co-operative trial of clofibrate. *Int J Epidemiol* 1989;18:355–360.

70. Ericsson C-G, Hamsten A, Nilsson J, Grip L, Svane B, de Faire U. Angiographic assessment of effects of bezafibrate on progression of coronary artery disease in young male postinfection patients. *Lancet* 1996;347: 849–853.

71. Becker GL. Ancrod in glomerulonephritis. *Q J Med* 1988;69:849–850.

72. Meade TW, Imeson JD, Stirling Y. Effects of changes in smoking and other characteristics on clotting factors and the risk of ischaemic heart disease. *Lancet* 1987;2: 986–988.

73. Wilkes HC, Kelleher C, Meade TW. Smoking and plasma fibrinogen. *Lancet* 1988;1:307–308.

74. Miller GJ, Martin JC, Webster J, et al. Association between dietary fat intake and plasma factor VII coagulant activity—a predictor of cardiovascular mortality. *Atherosclerosis* 1986;60:269–271.

75. Miller GJ, Martin JC, Mitropoulos KA, et al. Plasma factor VII is activated by post-prandial triglyceridaemia irrespective of dietary fat composition. *Atherosclerosis* 1991;86:163–171.

76. Sanders TAB, Miller GJ, de Grassi T, Yahia N. Postprandial activation of coagulant factor VII by long-chain dietary fatty acids. *Thromb Haemost* 1996;76:369–371.

77. Miller GJ, Martin JC, Mitropoulos KA, et al. Activation of factor VII during alimentary lipemia occurs in healthy adults and patients with congenital factor XII deficiency or factor XI deficiency, but not in patients with factor IX deficiency. *Blood* 1996;87:4187–4196.

78. Mitropoulos KA, Miller GJ, Watts GF, Durrington PN. Lipolysis of triglyceride-rich lipoproteins activates coagulant factor XII: a study in familial lipoprotein-lipase deficiency. *Atherosclerosis* 1992;95:119–125.

79. Miller GJ, Cruickshank JK, Ellis LJ, et al. Fat consumption and factor VII coagulant activity in middle-aged men. An association between a dietary and thrombogenic coronary risk factor. *Atherosclerosis* 1989;78: 19–24.

80. Marckmann P, Sandstrom B, Jespersen J. Effects of total fat content and fatty acid composition in diet on factor VII coagulant activity and blood lipids. *Atherosclerosis* 1990;80:227–233.

81. Constantino M, Merskey C, Kudzma DJ, Zucker MB. Increased activity of vitamin K-dependent clotting factors in human hyperlipoproteinaemia-association with cholesterol and triglyceride levels. *Thromb Haemost* 1977;38:465–474.

82. Carvalho de Sousa J, Bruckert E, Giral P, et al. Plasma factor VII, triglyceride concentration and fibrin degradation products in primary hyperlipidemia: a clinical and laboratory study. *Haemostasis* 1989;19:83–90.

83. Stirling Y, Woolf L, North WRS, Seghatchian MJ, Meade TW. Haemostasis in normal pregnancy. *Thromb Haemost* 1984;52:176–182.

84. Fuller JH, Keen H, Jarrett RJ, et al. Haemostatic variables associated with diabetes and its complications. *Br Med J* 1979;2:964-966.

85. Simpson HCR, Mann JI, Meade TW, Chakrabarti R, Stirling Y, Woolf L. Hyper- triglyceridaemia and hypercoagulability. *Lancet* 1983;1:786–790.

86. Haines AP, Chakrabarti R, Fisher D, Meade TW, North WRS, Stirling Y. Haemostatic variables in vegetarians and non-vegetarians. *Thromb Res* 1980;19:139–148.

87. Physicians' Health Study Research Group. Final report on the aspirin component of the ongoing Physicians' Health Study. *N Engl J Med* 1989;321:129–135.

88. Peto R, Gray R, Collins R, et al. Randomised trial of prophylactic daily aspirin in British male doctors. *Br Med J* 1988;296:313–316.

89. Hennekens CH, Buring JE, Sandercock P, Collins R, Peto R. Aspirin and other antiplatelet agents in the secondary and primary prevention of cardiovascular disease. *Circulation* 1989;80:749–756.

90. ISIS-2 (Second International Study of Infarct Survival) Collaborative Group. Randomised trial of intravenous streptokinase, oral aspirin, both, or neither among 17,187 cases of suspected acute myocardial infarction: ISIS-2. *Lancet* 1988;2:349–360.

91. Turpie AGG, Gent M, Laupacis A, et al. A comparison of aspirin with placebo in patients treated with warfarin after heart valve replacement. *N Engl J Med* 1993;329: 524–529.

Cardiovascular Thrombosis: Thrombocardiology and Thromboneurology, Second Edition,
edited by M. Verstraete, V. Fuster, and E. J. Topol,
Lippincott–Raven Publishers, Philadelphia © 1998.

6

Characteristics Associated with the Risk of Venous Thrombosis

Cedric J. Carter and *Meyer M. Samama

*Department of Laboratory Medicine, University of British Columbia, Vancouver, British Columbia V6T 2B5, Canada; and *Service d'Hématologie Biologique, Hotel Dieu University Hospital, Paris 75004, France*

Venous thrombosis is a relatively rare disease in the general population with an incidence of approximately 100 per 100,000 per annum (1–3). In contrast, venous thrombosis is a common complication of major trauma and particularly trauma to the lower limbs. It was the problem of hospital-associated venous thrombosis that provided the initial impetus for studies that identified specific risk factors for venous thrombosis. More recently these investigations have been expanded to the ambulant population.

There are a variety of reasons for developing risk factor profiles for venous thrombosis. With limited medical resources a key issue is the identification of individuals who are likely to benefit from antithrombotic prophylaxis. Currently all prophylaxis methods either incur direct side effects such as hemorrhage in the case of anticoagulants or involve logistic problems such as availability as in the case of pulsatile stockings. In addition, in view of the thoughts about the need for long-term prophylaxis in some conditions, there are cost considerations to the patient or the health-care paymaster. Related to the above is the fact that prophylaxis against venous thrombosis is never completely effective, and lack of adequate prophylactic efficacy may need to be factored into planned surgeries or other procedures. The relevance of such issues to situations such as orthopedic surgery is obvious.

A less intense but important area of risk factor development is in the general population. An example of this is in contraception planning. For the appropriate individual the oral contraceptive has high efficacy and minimal side effects. The net result is millions of prescriptions per day. This means that although oral contraceptive–associated thrombosis is rare in terms of cases per recipient, the total impact of thrombosis is considerable for an age group in whom the basal rate of thrombosis is exceedingly low.

DEVELOPMENT OF RISK FACTOR PROFILES

The development of risk profiles for venous thrombosis involves the application of discrete yet related methodologies. These include sample selection, diagnostic or endpoint detection, and study architecture.

Population Sampling

The first task is to define the population of interest. This is not as straightforward as it may appear and involves a decision as to which population is likely to be the eventual target of the application of risk profiles. The population sample can be defined in many ways. Sample definition may be very general, for example, sex, broad age ranges, or ethnicity, or may be highly specific and relate to a particular surgical procedure or medication. The application of predictive risk factors is entirely dependent on the comparability of the target population with that of the population from which the risk factors were derived. This is the concept of the generalizability of the data, which although usually used in terms of diagnosis or therapy is equally applicable to predictive risks.

Diagnostic Tests or Endpoint Selection

An important decision that has to be made in investigation and development of risk predictors is the threshold of determination of the extent or degree of venous thrombosis. This is a spectrum with autopsy-proven fatal pulmonary embolism at one end down to ra-diofibrinogen leg scan positivity restricted to the distal lower limbs at the other. The latter is clearly a surrogate marker for a more clinically significant thrombosis. The issue then becomes how often and in what circumstances does calf radiofibrinogen positivity develop into proximal vein thrombosis, with its clinically significant complication such as the postphlebitic syndrome, as well as fatal and nonfatal pulmonary emboli. This issue is relevant to early European reports of leg scan positivity in surgical conditions. An extremely low threshold of sensitivity may not be a good disease predictor. Conversely, the frequency of fatal emboli makes this almost too insensitive as a marker for risk factor detection unless an enormous study is involved. Tied in with this concept is the question of the primary diagnostic characteristics of the detection test. An example of this would be the quality of information derived from clinical diagnosis of deep venous thrombosis (DVT) versus high-quality ascending venography.

Study Architecture

This is the third component of the triad needed to develop risk profiles. Even if endpoints and population sampling are optimal, weak study architecture will greatly decrease the applicability of any predictive information. In general, risk factors are developed on the basis of fairly simple observational studies. As such, they are derived from second-class information, and because venous thrombosis is a multifactorial pathologic process, it is difficult to ascertain the contribution of individual putative risk factors. An example of this would be DVT after hip surgery. The patients tend to be old and slow to mobilize, have poor cardiovascular reserve, and are receiving a major anesthetic. All of these factors are concomitant to the primary trauma of the surgery. In these complex situations, one records the distribution of putative risk factors and tries to analyze them initially as univariate risk factors using regression analysis or its equivalent. If one has a sufficient number of subjects, this can be expanded to a multiple regression or linear logistic type of analysis. Factors derived in this manner can be analyzed as odds ratios or similar predictive integers, and a strength of association can be derived. Risk factors that are likely to be causal should have a high odds ratio that can also be demonstrated in multiple studies. The other end of the spectrum is where one can directly intervene in respect to a specific risk factor and observe in a randomized experiment the relative outcomes. An example of this would be the use of antithrombin concentrates in antithrombin-deficient pregnancies or surgeries. In practice, such opportunities are rare, and the usual issue is to try to derive the maximum useful information for structurally weak studies.

In descriptive studies, factors will emerge that may have a causal relationship to thrombosis, although this cannot be directly proven from these studies, or they may only be fellow travelers in a causal sense. It should be noted that although the latter factors may not have a direct biologic relationship to thrombosis they may still be predictive risk factors.

There are a few situations where one can use a predictive cohort approach to defining the clinical relevance of a risk factor. Examples of this would include some of the defined biochemical hypercoagulable markers where one identifies subjects with and without the specific defect, then compares thrombotic outcomes of either spontaneous thrombosis or secondary thrombosis. A typical example would be thrombosis rates in factor V Leiden positive and negative users of the oral contraceptive.

COMMUNITY-BASED SURVEYS AS A SOURCE OF THROMBOTIC CHARACTERISTICS

The study of risk factors in the general population has posed a series of logistic problems. Unlike inpatient-based studies on thrombotic risk factors, where primary documentation of health status and exact circumstances are clear, and objective tests are usually mandatory, community studies often

have been ill defined. The first issue is whether the sample is a true community sample or actually a subsample due to referral patterns. A second issue is quality of documentation. In many communities this has been of poor or inconsistent quality. A third issue is the documentation of putative risk factors. In the first place one has to pose the direct question to the patient of events such as whether they have had surgery in the previous few months. The second component of this is that any reply should be adequately recorded in such a fashion that it can be retrospectively retrieved with some degree of accuracy. Such issues are often not perceived as a primary part of health care; as such, information is limited.

Despite some of the problems mentioned above, general risk patterns can be developed but not with the same degree of predictive accuracy as hospital-based prospective investigations, such as randomized trials of antithrombotic prophylaxis. It should be noted that community-based studies, although they may at first appear to relate to mainly ambulant cases, actually overlap with hospital series based on inpatient observations. Current reports do not usually make this distinction entirely clear.

One of the earlier studies was from the community of Tucumseh, Michigan (1). Coon et al. looked at observations recorded over an 11-year period. The study clearly suffers from several methodologic problems, such as a relative paucity of objective diagnostic testing, but the overall trends are probably valid. This study identified female gender as a risk factor for venous thrombosis but also indicated an interaction between sex and age. The female patients tended to be younger, and their cases appeared to relate in part to childbirth. Irrespective of sex, an increase in venous thrombosis was noted in later life and became marked after the sixth decade. This may relate to some form of age effect on coagulation physiology but also may represent confounding factors such as an increasing incidence of surgery in these age groups. This type of analysis was not provided.

A second U.S. study was published 20 years later (2). This study from Worcester, Massachusetts, had the advantage of an 82% rate of objective diagnosis. Due to a linked system of health records, it appears to be reasonably representative of its community. This frequency of the traditional risk factors was ascertained in the 405 cases of venous thromboembolic disease. As can be seen from Table 6-1, age, cancer, obesity, surgery, and congestive heart failure in that order were the outstanding associations. This information represents the difference between individual risk assignation versus the community impact of the presence of such factors, and should be borne in mind when analyzing specific conditions in hospital-based studies.

A third community-based study was from Malmo, Sweden (3). This study was unique in that it used formal ascending contrast dye venography for diagnosis. This quality of diagnostic information is not available in North America, where ultrasound has become the dominant diagnostic method. In addition, this study had a captive population in that the central hospital controlled all diagnostic investigation for the area. Again, the outstanding risk factors appeared to be age and the presence of malignancy. The difficulty of interpreting these data is similar to that of the other studies: cancer, heart failure, and similar risk factors are age related and, in the absence of a huge data base with a powerful statistical strategy such as linear logistic modeling, the relative contribution of the various risk factors cannot be determined.

In conclusion, community-based studies provide a broad overview and estimate of impact of risk factors. This information is useful for health-care planning but is not as useful as specific hospital studies for the development of individual risk profiles for a particular patient.

HOSPITAL-BASED STUDIES FOR THE DEVELOPMENT OF RISK FACTOR CHARACTERISTICS

Hospital-based studies can take some of the general risk factors observed in the community-based studies and refine them so that specific information for patients undergoing a particular procedure can be examined. This more direct sort of information is critical for the planning of prophylaxis regimens, particularly in situations where side effects such as hemorrhage are an issue.

Hospital-based studies span three decades of investigation. This is important in relating any findings of risk factors to present day conditions. Diagnostic methods have evolved, although not necessarily for the better. Early studies, particularly from the United Kingdom, used radiofibrinogen leg scanning as the initial screen. Certainly for distal thrombosis this technique is exquisitely sensitive but will also generate some false-positive results. In some studies confirmatory ascending venography was a diagnostic sequel to leg scan positivity but not in all studies. Many small radiofibrinogen thrombi will resolve without deleterious complications. This means estimates of incidence using this diagnostic technique may represent an overcall in terms of clinical importance but does not negate it as a sensitive indicator of potential risk. Ascending venography remains the most useful test, although it is invasive. In general, the more recent studies involving randomized trials have retained this diagnostic modality. The information obtained from this technique should be regarded as reliable and allows a

TABLE 6-1. *Risk factors in 405 patients with an initial episode of deep-vein thrombosis and/or pulmonary embolism (PE)*

Risk Factors	DVT (n = 274)	PE (n = 131)
Age ≥40 yr	85%	89%
Cancer	32%	27%
Congestive heart failure	15%	31%
Chronic obstructive pulmonary disease	18%	34%
Diabetes	14%	15%
Fracture	13%	11%
Myocardial infarction	3%	9%
Obesity	39%	38%
Stroke	2%	8%
Surgery	19%	19%
Trauma	1%	3%

distinction between proximal and calf thrombi. The most recent trend has been to use duplex ultrasound as a substitute for venography as a screening test. In its current form, diagnostic accuracy is insufficient for asymptomatic screening. Irrespective of the specifics of diagnostic modality, certain clinical procedures and conditions are recognized as being the source of significant venous thromboembolic disease. These will summate with the more general risk factors such as advancing age. For hospital-based surveys, a hierarchy is apparent, ranging from the most high-risk category of major orthopedic surgery down to minor abdominal surgery. Analysis within these specific groups gives further insight into the processes that relate to the risk of thrombosis. This information can be applied in a general predictive sense to individual patients.

ORTHOPEDIC AND TRAUMA STUDIES

Trauma to the lower limbs remains the most hazardous for thrombotic risk. Knee replacement often carries a thrombotic risk in the region of 50% (4–6). These figures in the absence of aggressive prophylaxis have not materially changed over 20 years. It had been postulated that improved perioperative care in terms of fluid balance, better anesthesia, shortened operating time, and early mobilization would impact on thrombosis rates. In the few remaining studies where there was a true placebo arm, the high thrombotic rate has persisted (7). Widespread application of antithrombotic prophylaxis will curtail this flow of informative data.

Hip replacement and fracture are also high-risk situations (8,9). Hip-related thrombosis together with knee surgery cases provides some clues as to the pathologic process. A common feature to this type of surgery is direct trauma to vessels. The localization of the thrombi support this as a primary risk factor (8,9). In the case of hip fractures, the degree of trauma also seems to be a predictive factor. Subcapital fractures appear to have a lower thrombosis rate than peritrochanteric fractures (10). It should be noted that these specific thrombotic risk factors occur against a background of more general risk factors, such as immobility and age. Related to this is the appreciable incidence of calf vein thrombosis in the nonoperated limb. This may reflect a less localized and general prothrombotic diathesis such as probably occurs in general surgery. The age effect noted in the community-based studies also can be examined in the orthopedic milieu. Most reconstructive orthopedic treatment is undertaken in elderly patients with advanced osteoarthritis, but a subset of patients with rheumatoid arthritis are younger and appear to have a lower thrombosis rate (11).

On the basis of the above data, it was assumed that other forms of trauma such as that seen in motor vehicle accidents would also have a high incidence of thrombosis. For some reason this issue was not directly addressed until recently, when a large Canadian study confirmed clinicians' suspicions. The overall venous thrombosis rate was almost 60%, with a third of these thrombi in the proximal venous system (12).

ABDOMINAL AND PELVIC SURGERY

Abdominal and pelvic surgeries span a wide range of procedures and interact with more general risk factors such as age and malignancy. In general, the thrombosis rates are not as high as those seen in major orthopedic procedures. This may be related in part to the absence of direct trauma to the vessels of the lower limbs. The range of reported frequencies is huge and depends to a certain extent on the diagnostic modality and individual case series. For general abdominal surgery, rates of 10% to 20% seem to be representative (13).

Major pelvic surgery shows a similar frequency of thrombosis, and in some ways it is surprising that thrombosis rates are not higher, given that in some surgeries there may be trauma to the pelvic veins. The relatively low rate in these circumstances may relate to hemodynamic considerations or may even be artifactually low because pelvic veins are difficult to completely visualize via routine venography.

Both gynecologic surgery and prostatic surgery provide some support for the concept that the extent of surgical trauma is an independent risk factor for venous thrombosis. In gynecologic surgery, abdominal hysterectomy had a thrombosis rate of 12% compared with vaginal hysterectomy, a less extensive procedure, at 7% (14). Of course, the surgeries were not randomly assigned, so there may have been unrecognized confounding factors. In a similar pattern, transurethral prostatectomy had a thrombosis rate of 10% versus 40% for the transvesical procedure (15,16).

Most of the above abdominopelvic studies used radiofibrinogen leg scanning as at least the initial diagnostic test. Data from these studies were used to look at both univariate and multivariate analyses of individual risk factors in the broad surgical groups (17). Because risk factors were not procedure specific, they are discussed under General Risk Factors below.

PREGNANCY AND THE PUERPERIUM

Pregnancy has been traditionally regarded as a period of increased risk for venous thrombosis. This association was noted prior to objective testing, and some of the symptoms of leg swelling may not have been due to venous thrombosis. Even allowing for the vagaries of clinical diagnosis, reanalysis of the published data suggested that much of the pregnancy risk was in fact postpartum (18). These relatively soft data received support from a Swedish venography study, which confirmed the low incidence of venous thrombosis in pregnancy with only 11 cases of DVT in a 5-year study of 15,000 women, and nine of these cases occurred postpartum (19). The other traditional concept of risk was that antepartum the risk increased with the gestation period. A recent international study that managed to accrue 60 cases of DVT in pregnancy showed no statistical difference among the three trimesters (20). An additional finding

was that all of the cases of DVT involved the left leg, with two cases also having a concomitant right DVT. This finding, at least in pregnancy, lends some support to the concept of physiologic compression of the left iliac vein by the right femoral artery.

There have been no studies that have directly compared vaginal and cesarian deliveries as risk factors for thrombosis, although national mortality certificates of fatal emboli suggest that cesarian section, as one might expect, carries a higher thromboembolic rate (21).

MEDICAL CONDITIONS

The intense interest in the very high-risk surgical situations for venous thromboembolism has obscured the fact that some medical conditions, including cardiac and some neurologic disease, show a similar risk profile. This is probably due to the general risk factors such as prolonged immobilization as discussed below. These general risk factors are common to both surgical and medical cases.

Cardiac Disease

Early reports on venous thrombosis in cardiac disease as diagnosed by radiofibrinogen leg scanning showed a surprisingly high incidence. For myocardial infarction and congestive failure, rates in the region of 30% occurred (22,23). It is unlikely that this reflects the current situation. Myocardial infarction used to be managed using bed rest. Intercurrent use of fibrinolytics and anticoagulants was unusual, and the general supportive therapies, particularly in the case of congestive failure, were not well developed. Nevertheless, there are no recent studies on venous thrombosis in cardiac patients, and from the clinical perspective (unlike, e.g., as in orthopedics) there are insufficient adverse venous events to stimulate such studies.

Neurologic Disease

Neurologic paresis of the lower limbs results in a very high incidence of leg scan positivity. This is particularly marked in the case of hemiplegia, where rates of up to 70% have been observed (24). The number of venographically confirmed thrombi is somewhat less but still of sufficient frequency to support mandatory prophylaxis. Paraplegia and hemiplegia provide an interesting practical example as to the importance of immobilization. In paraplegia the interlimb thrombosis rate is approximately equal (25). In hemiplegia there is a tenfold increase of thrombosis in the plegic limb (24).

GENERAL RISK FACTORS

In the course of the study of thrombosis rates for specific disease conditions there will clearly be factors common to many clinical situations. From a demographic perspective, factors such as age and ethnicity need to be considered. From a pathophysiologic point of view, factors such as immobility and malignancy are relevant. In addition there are the acquired and congenital deficiencies of the natural anticoagulants. These are described in detail in Chapter 4 and will not be elaborated on here except to stress that venous thrombi are of multifactorial pathogenesis and any general risk factor such as immobilization will interact with the underlying biochemical abnormality.

Much of the work on venous thrombosis risk factors was performed 20 years ago. This means that detailed information on the levels of natural anticoagulants was not available. What was available were the more general demographic data, specific disease conditions as discussed above, and both continuous and discontinuous variables (26). Examples of continuous variables would include the degree of immobilization, body weight, duration of anesthesia, and similar factors. Discontinuous or discrete variables would include type of anesthesia, the presence of cancer, a history of previous thrombosis, familial thrombosis, and exposure to prothrombotic medications.

The practical problem is to take a diverse group of cases of thrombosis and identify factors that show a statistical association. As discussed above, an association that is not necessarily causally related may still be predictive, but strong consistent associations often tend to be causal, and their presence is certainly an impetus to investigate pathophysiologic mechanisms.

The selection of variables to be examined is often determined by previous clinical observations and an understanding of coagulation physiology. The analysis of the associations depend on the nature of the variable. The presence or absence of a putative risk factor can be analyzed by χ^2 statistics or their variants such as the Mantel-Haenzel test. Continuous variables are usually analyzed by some form of regression. Initial analysis is usually achieved via the univariate method. This method generates the most likely candidate factors for multivariate analysis. The latter is used to try to discern the relative contributions of partially linked potential risk factors. This step is important when trying to demonstrate apparent causal associations.

Age

As discussed in the community-based studies, age appeared to correlate with the venous thrombosis rate (1–3). The obvious flaw in accepting this as a direct and possible causal factor is that age correlates with most of the specific prothrombotic clinical conditions such as hip replacement and stroke. However, age as an independent risk factor did receive support in the multivariate analysis of a large series of abdominopelvic thrombosis cases (17).

Malignancy

All large series of venous thrombosis cases show an excess of patients with malignancy. In particular, adenocarcinomas are frequent. This observation has recently received some support from the demographic mix of patients in the recent multicenter trials of treatment of DVT by low molecular weight heparin. At the biochemical level, procoagulant substances can be extracted from carcinomas (27).

Somewhat surprisingly, the large multivariate analysis that has proven so useful for the identification of other risk factors was not able to show malignancy as an independent risk factor for venous thrombosis (17). Two more recent studies used an alternative methodologic approach. One study measured the rate of development of malignancy in two large cohorts of DVT-positive and -negative cases over a period of approximately 2 years (28). In the patients under the age of 50, malignancy was strikingly over-represented. The interpretation was that these cases of malignancy were predetectable, at least at the clinical level, at the time of the initial DVT. The second study used yet another approach. Patients with DVT who were free of cancer at the time of their DVT diagnosis were classified into idiopathic and secondary DVT cases (29). It was postulated that if occult cancer had a significant association with DVT, then upon observation it would most likely manifest itself in the primary DVT group. In this study 105 cases of secondary thrombosis (excluding cancer) were compared with 145 idiopathic DVT cases. On follow-up the development of cancer in the idiopathic cases at 7.6% was four times more common than in the secondary cases. In addition, 35 of the 145 idiopathic cases experienced a recurrence of DVT in follow-up, and cancer was present in six (15%) of these cases.

The above studies and various descriptive series strongly supports a linkage between cancer for both initial DVT and recurrence of DVT. An aging population and more aggressive, if sometimes still palliative, therapy for cancer makes this group of patients an increasingly larger component of thrombosis practice.

Obesity

Obesity as defined by body weight in excess of 20% of the population median poses an interesting methodologic problem. Traditional clinical dogma plus the standard textbooks list obesity as an important determinant for postsurgical thrombosis. Univariate analysis supports this view. When one uses multivariate analysis, the picture changes somewhat in that it cannot be shown to be an independent risk factor (19). The suspicion is that it is closely linked to other deleterious aspects of surgery and its impact obscured in moderate size studies. This issue is somewhat semantic in that risk factors need not have a causal relationship and obesity may be acting as a surrogate marker for one or several risk factors. This hypothesis really needs to be tested prospectively in large studies, where the effects of multiple risk factors can be evaluated. In the absence of this sort of hard data, it appears to be reasonable to include obesity as a risk factor even if the mechanistic nature of the contribution is not understood.

Previous Venous Thrombosis and Family History

This area has rapidly evolved with the advent of modern biochemical markers of hypercoagulability. Before the development of these methods, clinical studies analyzed by both univariate and multivariate techniques identified previous thrombosis as a predictor of subsequent events (17). More recently, papers addressing the question of recurrence of DVT and the question of duration of anticoagulation have indicated that the recurrence rate of idiopathic DVT in the first 2 years is at least 10% (30,31). There is no formal control group for this figure, but it is clearly greater than the population incidence. The same logic holds for family history.

The modern approach would be to take the previous or family history at face value and then try to document biochemical markers as described in Chapter 4. The attraction of this approach is that if a factor is identified, then the risk can be described to the family members with the defect rather than empirically to all close relatives.

Immobilization

This aspect has been addressed in some detail in respect to neurologic disease and clearly is a major risk factor. Alternative evidence is supplied by the results of pneumatic compression devices and their reduction in various types of postsurgical venous thrombosis (32). Clinical practice places great emphasis on the effects of prolonged automobile journeys or plane trips. The hard objective evidence to support these as risk factors on the basis of immobilization is not available.

Anesthesia

One feature of general anesthesia is a decrease in venous return with venous pooling (33). The latter is regarded as part of the basic pathophysiology of the development of DVT. On this basis it was suggested that local anesthetic procedures including spinal anesthesia would be associated with a lower incidence of DVT. Despite some impressive descriptive series, the data are inconsistent. In general, the results of formal randomized trials have been less impressive and in many cases show no benefit (34).

Blood Groups

In the field of coagulation there has been an interest in linkage between particular blood groups and both hemorrhagic and thrombotic conditions. Historical observations suggested that blood group A showed an association with DVT. The reason for this fairly consistent finding has never made much biologic sense, although the relatively higher levels of von Willebrand factor in group A individuals has been cited. In the recent Swedish Community Study, DVT patients were typed as 47% group A compared with 44% in routine blood donors, suggesting that if there is a linkage phenomenon it is not of sufficient magnitude to be a major determinant in advising patients on antithrombotic prophylactic regimens (3). A recent publication and review of this topic used blood group A:O ratios, but because these two blood groups account for most of the white population, there is an inverse relationship between them in terms of frequency, and the use of ratios will mathematically enhance any apparent association with thrombosis without affecting the biologic relationship (35).

Oral Contraception and Estrogen Replacement Therapy

The role of oral contraception in DVT and its sequelae continues to cause concern. Early descriptive studies led to innumerable case control studies. Without exception, these supported an association between oral contraception and both primary and secondary DVT. On the basis that prospective studies were required, there has been one randomized trial of oral contraception versus other methods (36). For logistic reasons this trial was not interpretable. There also have been three major cohort analytic studies, the Royal College of General Practitioners (RCGP) study from the United Kingdom, the Oxford Family Planning Association study from the United Kingdom, and a study from Walnut Creek, California (37–39). All studies reached similar conclusions that the oral contraceptive was associated with an increased risk of DVT, thus confirming the earlier case control studies and supporting some later studies.

The RCGP study remains the most substantive general study on the thrombotic complications of oral contraception. The original cohorts have been followed over the years, and new information, particularly on the arterial side, has been retrieved. Contrary to some reviews on the RCGP studies, most patients were on a 50-μg or less estrogen contraceptive. Subsequent descriptive reports suggested that the oral contraceptive in its second generation form with 30-μg doses of estrogen had negligible thrombogenicity, but further studies have not substantiated these claims (40,41). The story took an interesting twist more recently. For practical purposes it was thought that a further major decrease in estrogen, the component of the combined oral contraceptive that traditionally was thought to relate to venous thrombogenicity, would lead to loss of efficacy. On the other hand, the progestogen portion had adverse effects on both lipid and glucose metabolism, so a third generation of oral contraceptive was formulated with new and putatively safer progestogens but still combined with 20 to 30 μg of ethanol estradiol or its equivalent. Three new case control articles published in late 1995 and early 1996 created great consternation when it appeared that the new "safer" third-generation oral contraceptives had double the venous thrombotic risk (at least as derived from a relative odds ratio compared with their second-generation counterparts) (42–44). This made little biologic sense, and it should be noted that these data were nonexperimental. In early 1997, an extensive reanalysis of the above studies addressed the question of confounding variables and demonstrated that increased age of third-generation oral contraceptive users relative to second-generation oral contraceptive users could explain the apparent differences (45). What appeared to have happened was that because the third-generation oral contraceptives were perceived by physicians to have favorable pharmacologic profiles, they had been preferentially prescribed for cases considered as high risk for the second-generation oral contraceptive preparations.

The other area that has been the subject of recent controversy is estrogen replacement therapy for menopausal or postoophorectomy cases. Until recently, most estrogen replacement therapy (ERT) used natural estrogens. The most common type was extracted from the urine of pregnant mares. These natural estrogens were a semi-standardized mix of multiple estrogen components. As such, the equivalent estrogen dosage relative to ethanol estradiol was difficult to assess, but it has been assumed that the overall estrogen dose from natural hormonal replacement estrogens was less than oral contraceptive levels. Most studies supported a positive effect for natural estrogens on cardiovascular mortality. This appeared to be due to protective effects on arterial function. Despite a widely held misconception that natural estrogens were high-dose estrogen preparations, and the resulting belief that they caused venous thrombosis, case control studies from as recently as 1992 showed no excess of DVT in ERT cases (46). This reassuring data was the basis of permitting ERT usage in patients who would not have been considered eligible for conventional oral contraceptive doses of estrogen.

This interpretation is now challenged by three recent back-to-back articles published in late 1996 by one British and two U.S. groups. The study architecture of the Oxford Study was a traditional case control design, and they reported their results as odds ratios (47). The two U.S.-based studies identified cases but also looked at longitudinal exposure, and their findings were expressed as relative risks (48,49). Notwithstanding different study methodologies, the conclusions were similar in that a three- to fourfold increased risk of DVT or pulmonary embolism was demonstrated. This somewhat alarming statistic has to be interpreted in the light of the fact that the basal DVT risk in this patient group is low and that in theory arterial disease benefits should outweigh any venous risk. This rationalization of course applies to long-term general usage but for specific risk periods such as surgery it may be prudent to discontinue HRT therapy before the procedure.

Other Thrombosis Risks

There are a variety of relatively rare medical conditions that carry a significant thrombosis risk. These include paroxysmal nocturnal hemoglobinuria, Behçet's disease, myeloproliferative syndromes, and collagen vascular diseases. The latter include frank lupus erythematosus. Related to this are the antiphospholipid syndromes manifesting themselves as permutations of antiphospholipid antibodies, in some cases with the so-called lupus anticoagulant, sometimes together with positive autoimmune serology such as positive antinuclear antibodies. A diagnosis of these conditions should be pursued in someone presenting with unexplained venous thrombosis, but these investigations would not be part of routine presurgical thrombosis risk assessment.

CONCLUSION

Risk profiles for venous thrombosis have evolved from clinical impressions through descriptive studies, case control studies, and eventually via prospective studies. In general, the studies have been noninterventional in that one cannot randomize for variables such as age and malignancy. Further study in the area of risk definition is confounded by the earlier information. This has resulted in antithrombotic prophylaxis regimens. Unfortunately, in some instances the application of the prophylaxis regimens has preceded an understanding of the natural history of the condition. Such an example would be determining the risk of subsequent DVT in pregnancy after an earlier event.

Ideally, composite risk profiles incorporating the various risk factors described above should have been prospectively applied to patients at apparent risk and the importance of factors such as age, malignancy, previous thrombosis, and similar factors evaluated. This has only been done in a limited fashion. Most clinicians use either their personal impression of the overall risk factor profile or are guided by one of the published risk profiles such as that presented in the ACCP Consensus Conference (32). The latter recommendations were largely derived from retrospective analyses. They have never been formally validated but do provide a framework for decision making.

Conventional risk factor assessment interacts with any of the underlying congenital predisposition described in Chapter 4. The gene frequencies of antithrombin, protein C, and protein S deficiencies are sufficiently low that measurement of these proteins would not be a routine part of presurgery thrombotic risk assessment. The recent description and frequency of the factor V Leiden genotype does raise the question of whether this risk factor should be included in preoperative planning, although to date there has been no information suggesting that such individuals will behave differently than their normal cohort with respect to response to antithrombotic prophylaxis.

An ideal addition to a predictive composite of risk factors would be some form of blood test that would give a net balance between pro- and antithrombotic regulation of the coagulation system along the lines of a dynamic marker of Xa or thrombin generation, together with the fibrinolytic counterpart. This might help select individuals for more extreme antithrombotic prophylaxis. To date this type of technology has not been developed.

REFERENCES

1. Coon WW, Willis PW, Keller JB. Venous thromboembolism and other venous disease in the Tecumseh Community Health Study. *Circulation* 1973;48:839–846.
2. Anderson FA, Wheeler HB, Goldberg RJ, et al. A population-based perspective of the hospital incidence and case-fatality rates of deep vein thrombosis and pulmonary embolism. The Worcester DVT Study. *Arch Intern Med* 1991;151:933–938.
3. Nordstrom M, Lindblad B, Berqvist D, Kjellstrom T. A prospective study of the incidence of deep-vein thrombosis within a defined urban population. *J Intern Med* 1992;232:155–160.
4. Hjelmstedt A, Bergvall U. Incidence of thrombosis in patients with tibial fractures. *Acta Chir Scand* 1968; 134:209–218.
5. Cohen SH, Ehrlich GE, Kaufman MS, et al. Thrombophlebitis following knee surgery. *J Bone Joint Surg* 1973;55:106–111.
6. Hull R, Delmore TJ, Hirsh J, et al. Effectiveness of an intermittent pulsatile elastic stocking for the prevention of calf and thigh vein thrombosis in patients undergoing elective knee surgery. *Thromb Res* 1979;16:37–45.
7. Leclerc J, Desjardins L, Geerts W, et al. A randomized trial of enoxaparin for the prevention of deep vein thrombosis after knee surgery. *Thromb Haemost* 1991; 65(suppl):753.
8. Hull RD, Raskob GE. Prophylaxis of venous thromboembolic disease following hip and knee surgery. *J Bone Joint Surg* 1986;68:146–150.
9. Evarts C, Feil E. Prevention of thromboembolic disease after elective surgery in the hip. *J Bone Joint Surg [Am]* 1971;53:1271–1280.
10. Field ES, Nicolaides AN, Kakkar VV, et al. Deep-vein thrombosis in patients with fractures of the femoral neck. *Br J Surg* 1972;59:377–379.
11. Buchanan RRC, Kraag G. Is there a lower incidence of deep venous thrombosis after joint replacement in rheumatoid arthritis. *J Rhematol* 1980;7:551–554.
12. Geerts EH, Code KI, Jay RM, Chen E, Szalai JP. A prospective study of venous thrombosis after major trauma. *N Engl J Med* 1994;331:1601–1606.
13. Bergqvist D. Frequency of thromboembolic complications. In: Bergqvist D (ed). *Post-operative Thromboembolism: Frequency, Etiology, Prophylaxis.* Berlin: Springer-Verlag, 1983;12–13.
14. Walsh JJ, Bonnar J, Wright FW. A study of pulmonary embolism and deep vein thrombosis after major gynaecological surgery using labelled fibrinogen-phlebography and lung scanning. *J Obstet Gynaecol Br Commonw* 1974;81:311–316.
15. Nicolaides AN, Field ES, Kakkar VV, et al. Prostatectomy and deep-vein thrombosis. *Br J Surg* 1972;59: 487–488.
16. Mayo M, Halil T, Browse NL. The incidence of deep vein thrombosis after prostatectomy. *Br J Urol* 1971; 43:738–742.
17. Nicolaides AN, Irving D. Clinical factors and the risk of deep venous thrombosis. In: Nicolaides AN (ed).

Thromboembolism: Aetiology, Advances in Prevention and Management. Lancaster, England: MTP Press, 1975;193–204.

18. Carter CJ, Gent M, Leclerc JR. The epidemiology of venous thrombosis. In: Colman RW, Hirsh J, Marder VJ, Salzman EW (eds). *Hemostasis and Thrombosis.* 2nd ed. Philadelphia: Lippincott, 1987;1185–1198.

19. Kierkegaard A. Incidence and diagnosis of deep vein thrombosis associated with pregnancy. *Acta Obstet Gynecol Scand* 1983;62:239–243.

20. Ginsberg JS, Brill-Edwards P, Burrows RF, et al. Venous thrombosis during pregnancy: Leg and trimester of presentation. *Thromb Haemost* 1992;67:519–520.

21. Department of Health, Welsh Office, Scottish Home and Health Department and Department of Health and Social Services, Northern Ireland. *Report on Confidential Enquiries into Maternal Deaths in the United Kingdom 1985–87.* London: HMSO, 1991.

22. Maurer BJ, Wray R, Shillingford JP. Frequency of venous thrombosis after myocardial infarction. *Lancet* 1971;2:1385–1387.

23. Kotilainen M, Ristola P, Ikkala E, et al. Leg vein thrombosis diagnosed by ^{125}I-fibrinogen test after acute myocardial infarction. *Ann Clin Res* 1973;5:365–368.

24. Warlow C, Ogston D, Douglas AS. Deep venous thrombosis of the legs after strokes. *Br Med J* 1976;1:1178–1181.

25. Bors E, Conrad CA, Massell TB. Venous occlusion of the lower extremities in paraplegic subjects. *Surg Gynecol Obstet* 1954;99:451–454.

26. Coon WW. Epidemiology of venous thromboembolism. *Ann Surg* 1977;186:149–164.

27. Gordon SG, Cross BA. A factor X-activating cysteine protease from malignant tissue. *J Clin Invest* 1981;67:1665–1671.

28. Goldberg RJ, Seneff M, Gore JM, et al. Occult malignant neoplasms in patients with deep venous thrombosis. *Arch Intern Med* 1987;147:251–253.

29. Prandoni P, Lensing AWA, Buller HR, et al. Deep vein thrombosis and the incidence of subsequent symptomatic cancer. *N Engl J Med* 1992;327:1128–1133.

30. Research Committee of the British Thoracic Society. Optimum duration of anticoagulation for deep vein thrombosis and pulmonary embolism. *Lancet* 1992;340:873–876.

31. Levine MN, Hirsh J, Gent M, et al. Optimal duration of oral anticoagulant therapy: a randomized trial comparing four weeks with three months of warfarin in patients with proximal deep vein thrombosis. *Thromb Haemost* 1995;74:606–611.

32. Clagett GP, Anderson FA, Heit J, Levine MN, Wheeler HB. Prevention of venous thromboembolism. *Chest* 1995;108(suppl):312–334.

33. Polkolainen E, Hendolin H. Effects of lumbar epidural analgesia and general anaesthesia on flow velocity in the femoral vein and post operative deep vein thrombosis. *Acta Chir Scand* 1983;149:361–364.

34. Hjortso NC, Neumann P, Frosig F, et al. A controlled study on the effect of epidural analgesia with local anaesthetics and morphine on morbidity after abdominal surgery. *Acta Anaesth Scand* 1985;29:790–796.

35. Lourenco DM, Mirandaq F, Lopes LH. ABO blood groups as risk factors for thrombosis. *Clin Appl Thromb Haemost* 1996;2:196–199.

36. Fuertes-De La Haba A, Curet JO, Pelegrina I, et al. Thrombophlebitis among oral and nonoral contraceptive users. *Obstet Gynecol* 1971;38:259–263.

37. Royal College of General Practitioners' Oral Contraception Study. Oral contraceptives, venous thrombosis, and varicose veins. *J R Coll Gen Pract* 1978;28:393–399.

38. Vessey MP, McPherson K, Johnson B. Mortality among women participating in the Oxford Family Planning contraceptive study. *Lancet* 1977;2:731–733.

39. Petitti DB, Pellegrin F, Ramcharan S. Risk factors of vascular disease in women: smoking, oral contraceptives, non contraceptive estrogens, and other factors. *JAMA* 1979;242:1150–1154.

40. Bottinger LE, Boman G, Eklund G, et al. Oral contraceptives and thromboembolic disease: effects of lowering oestrogen content. *Lancet* 1980;1:1097–1101.

41. Kierkegaard A. Deep vein thrombosis and the oestrogen content in oral contraceptives-an epidemiological analysis. *Contraception* 1985;31:29–41.

42. Jick H, Jick SS, Gurewicgh V, Myers MW, Vasilakis C. Risk of idiopathic cardiovascular disease and non fatal venous thromboembolism in women using oral contraceptives with differing prostetagen content. *Lancet* 1995;346:1589–1593.

43. World Health Organization Collaborative Study of Cardiovascular Disease and Steroid Hormone Contraception. Venous thromboembolic disease and combined oral contraceptives: results of international multicentre case-control study. *Lancet* 1995;346:1575–1581.

44. Spitzer WO, Lewis MA, Heinemann LAJ, Thorogood M, MacRae KD. On behalf of the Transnational Research Group on Oral Contraceptive and the Health of Young Women: third generation oral contraceptives and risk of venous thromboembolic disorders: an international case control study. *Br Med J* 1996;312:83–87.

45. Farmer RDT, Lawrenson RA, Thompson TR, Kennedy JD, Hambleton IR. Population-based study of risk of venous thromboembolism associated with various oral contraceptives. *Lancet* 1997;349:83–88.

46. Devor M, Barrett-Connor E, Renvall M, et al. Estrogen replacement therapy and the risk of venous thrombosis. *Am J Med* 1992;92:275–282.

47. Daly E, Vessey MP, Hawkins M, Carson J, Gough P, Marsh M. Risk of venous thromboembolism in users of hormone replacement therapy. *Lancet* 1996;348:977–980.

48. Jick H, Derby LE, Myers MW, Vasilakis C, Newton KM. Risk of hospital admission for idiopathic venous thromboembolism among users of postmenopausal oestrogens. *Lancet* 1996;348:981–983.

49. Grodstein F, Stampfer MJ, Goldhaber SZ, et al. Prospective study of exogenous hormones and risk of pulmonary embolism in women. *Lancet* 1996;348:983–987.

Cardiovascular Thrombosis: Thrombocardiology and Thromboneurology, Second Edition,
edited by M. Verstraete, V. Fuster, and E. J. Topol,
Lippincott–Raven Publishers, Philadelphia © 1998.

7

Laboratory Detection of the Prethrombotic State

Piera Angelica Merlini, *Kenneth A. Bauer, and †Pier M. Mannucci

*Dipartimento Cardiologico De Gasperis, Ospedale Niguarda, 20162 Milan, Italy; *Harvard Medical School, Brockton-West Roxbury Veterans Administration Medical Center, West Roxbury, Massachusetts 02132; and †Department of Internal Medicine, University of Milan, 20127 Milan, Italy*

Blood coagulation is a highly integrated and regulated system that under normal conditions functions by maintaining a substantial procoagulant/anticoagulant balance. The procoagulant drive involves a number of zymogens and cofactors that, once activated by limited proteolysis, are able to generate thrombin that, in turn, converts fibrinogen into fibrin; the anticoagulant drive consists of powerful inhibitory systems, such as heparan sulfate–antithrombin III, protein C–thrombomodulin/protein S, and tissue factor pathway inhibitor. The importance of maintaining a balance between these two forces is demonstrated by the fact that defects in the procoagulant component of the coagulation system cause a bleeding tendency, whereas deficiencies of inhibitors may lead to a thrombotic tendency.

OVERVIEW OF THE COAGULATION SYSTEM

Coagulation consists of a series of proteolytic reactions, at each step of which a zymogen, a cofactor, and a converting enzyme assemble in a multimolecular complex on cell membranes of platelets or endothelial cells. The membrane binding sites for these complexes include negatively charged phospholipids. The coagulation proteins circulating in the blood include the zymogens such as factors VII, XII, XI, IX, X, and prothrombin, cofactors such as factor V and VIII, and fibrinogen, which is the substrate of the last step of the cascade. The main function of the coagulation system is to transform fibrinogen into fibrin at the sites of vascular injury (Fig. 7-1).

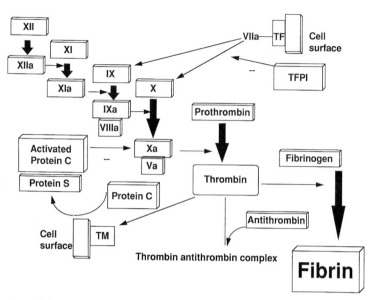

FIG. 7-1. Overview of the coagulation cascade. TM, thrombomodulin; TF, tissue factor; TFPI, tissue factor pathway inhibitor.

The main drives of the coagulation system are traditionally considered to be the extrinsic and intrinsic pathways, which were thought to be functionally independent. The initiation of the intrinsic system is triggered by damage to the endothelium and the consequent exposure of subendothelial components that activate the contact factors (factor XII, prekallikrein, high molecular weight kininogen, factor XI); this leads to the generation of factor XIa, which acts on factor IX to form activated factor IX (IXa), which is then assembled on cell surfaces with its cofactor, factor VIIIa, in order to activate factor X. The extrinsic pathway is triggered when blood comes into contact with tissue factor, a glycoprotein that is constitutively expressed by the subendothelial components of the vessel wall; the interaction of tissue factor with activated factor VII (VIIa) forms the factor VIIa–tissue factor complex that directly activates factor X. The activated factor X (Xa) that is generated by either of these two pathways can then convert prothrombin to thrombin by binding to factor Va on activated cell membranes.

Based on data from in vivo studies using markers of coagulation activation, it has been demonstrated that, under basal conditions (i.e., in the absence of vascular injury or thrombotic stimuli), the factor VIIa–tissue factor complex is the main trigger for coagulation activation. This complex not only leads directly to the generation of factor Xa, but also activates factor IX to factor IXa (1). The factor IXa–factor VIIIa complex amplifies factor Xa generation, and it has been hypothesized that this pathway is recruited only when sufficient amounts of thrombin (formed through the prevailing stimulus of the factor VIIa–tissue factor complex) convert factor VIII to factor VIIIa and, perhaps, also factor XI to factor XIa (2). This amplification is necessary for blood coagulation under normal circumstances, as demonstrated by the fact that patients with hemophilia A and B, who are deficient in factor IX and VIII, respectively, have severe hemorrhagic problems.

The formation of thrombin requires the assembly of the prothrombinase complex (consisting of factor Xa, factor Va, and calcium on a platelet membrane surface), which converts prothrombin to thrombin. During this process, the amino-terminus of the prothrombin molecule is released as the inactive fragment 1+2

(Fig. 7-2). The generated thrombin converts fibrinogen into fibrin by releasing fibrinopeptides A and B, or may be inhibited by the endogenous heparan sulfate–antithrombin III mechanism to form thrombin–antithrombin III complexes. Alternately, thrombin binds to thrombomodulin on endothelial cells, and this leads to the activation of protein C. Together with protein S, activated protein C is a circulating anticoagulant that inactivates factor Va as well as factor VIIIa.

For many years, clinicians have sought blood tests that might be used to monitor the level of activation of the coagulation cascade, to confirm or exclude the presence of thrombosis, and to predict thrombotic events. To this end, various approaches are possible that are based on the measurement of plasma levels the following components.

Coagulation Substrates

The measurement of plasma concentrations of coagulation zymogens (such as factor IX, factor X, and prothrombin), cofactors (factor V and VIII), or substrates (fibrinogen) has been proposed. Prospective cohort studies of healthy individuals have shown that elevated plasma levels of factor VII coagulant activity predict the development of ischemic heart disease or cardiac death (3), and that high fibrinogen levels are associated with an increased risk of developing nonfatal myocardial infarction or cardiac death in normal individuals (3,4) and patients with angina pectoris (5) (see Chapter 5). These data broadly indicate that an increase in the plasma concentrations of coagulation proteins favors the development of ischemic cardiac events. Furthermore, data from other studies suggest that an imbalance due to a reduction in natural anticoagulant potential or defective fibrinolysis is also associated with an increased risk of cardiac events (4–6). Although this approach has provided information concerning the role of hypercoagulability in arterial thrombosis, the attempt to monitor arterial thrombotic or prethrombotic states by measuring the circulating levels of zymogens, inhibitors, or substrate have thus far been of limited clinical utility. This is attributable to the fact that these species exist in a large excess in plasma, and only a small percentage are converted to their active form in vivo.

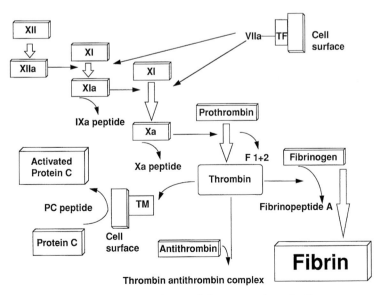

FIG. 7-2. Markers of coagulation cascade activation.

TABLE 7-1. *Laboratory markers of coagulation activation*

Biochemical step	Marker	Half-life
Factor VII → factor VIIa	Factor VIIa	150 min
Factor XII → factor XIIa	Factor XIIa	Unknown
Factor IX → factor IXa	Factor IX activation peptide	15 min
Factor X → factor Xa	Factor X activation peptide	30 min
Prothrombin → thrombin	Prothrombin fragment 1+2	90 min
Thrombin inhibition by antithrombin III	Thrombin–antithrombin complex	15 min
Protein C → activated protein C	Protein C activation peptide	5 min
	Activated protein C–protein C inhibitor	40 min
	Activated protein C–α1 antitrypsin complex	140 min
	Activated protein C	20 min
Fibrinogen → fibrin	Fibrinopeptide A	3–5 min

Coagulation Enzymes

The measurement of plasma levels of coagulation enzymes generated as a result of the activation of zymogens is another possible approach. Most enzymes cannot be measured in plasma because they are rapidly neutralized by naturally occurring inhibitors or bound to cell receptors. However, assays have been developed to measure two coagulation enzymes that have relatively long half-lives in the circulation: factor VIIa and factor XIIa (7,8). Activated protein C, the anticoagulant enzyme that is central to one of the major regulatory systems, also can be measured (9).

Activation Peptides or Enzyme–Inhibitor Complexes

The measurement of plasma levels of peptides released from zymogen molecules when these are activated to enzymes, or enzyme–inhibitor complexes (Fig. 7-2), is very promising. Unlike their corresponding enzymes, both activation peptides and enzyme–inhibitor complexes have relatively long plasma half-lives and can therefore be measured. The assays developed and in vivo half-lives of some of the species are listed in Table 7-1.

MARKERS OF COAGULATION ACTIVATION

Fibrinopeptide A

Nossel and colleagues (10,11) developed a sensitive radioimmunoassay for measuring fibrinopeptide A, a 16–amino acid peptide that is cleaved from the alpha chain of fibrinogen by thrombin. It therefore represents a sensitive biochemical marker of thrombin activity and fibrin formation. The finding that fibrinopeptide A was measurable in small amounts, even in the plasma of healthy individuals, suggested the physiologic existence of ongoing low-level coagulation activation and fibrin formation, thereby indicating that the hemostatic balance is in dynamic equilibrium. The concentration of fibrinopeptide A can be determined by means of commercially available radioimmunoassays or immunoenzymatic assays, using antibodies with significant, but not absolute, specificity for fibrinopeptide A over fibrinogen. Before performing these assays, it is therefore necessary to use simple procedures to remove fibrinogen from plasma samples, without altering peptide levels. Unfortunately, the usefulness of fibrinopeptide A is limited by the fact that the test is highly susceptible to in vitro artifacts occurring during blood sampling and often yields spuriously high values, which make it difficult to interpret the results. Furthermore, fibrinopeptide A has a short half-life (3–5 min), so it is only capable of providing insights into the activation of the coagulation system that relate to the brief period before blood sampling. To overcome these problems, some investigators have proposed measuring fibrinopeptide A in urine. Approximately 70% of the total fibrinopeptide A produced is proteolytically degraded by intravascular and extravascular peptidases, but only 0.2% to 0.5% is excreted in urine. Twenty-four hour urinary fibrinopeptide A levels correlate with plasma levels in normal subjects, and spot urinary fibrinopeptide A levels correlate with those concomitantly obtained in plasma (12,13). However, a major limitation of this measurement is the wide intrasubject variability in fibrinopeptide A catabolism, which may offset its potential advantages.

Prothrombin Activation Fragment 1+2

More recently, assays have been developed to measure prothrombin activation fragment 1+2, which is released from prothrombin when the zymogen is activated by the prothrombinase complex to yield thrombin (14,15) (Fig. 7-2). Measurement of this polypeptide provides information concerning upstream activation of the coagulation cascade, in contrast with fibrinopeptide A, which reflects a more distal step (thrombin activation of fibrinogen). Normal individuals manifest finite plasma levels of prothrombin fragment 1+2, and its half-life of about 90 minutes makes it a less transient index of coagulation activation than fibrinopeptide A. This coagulation marker also has the advantage that the assay results are less susceptible to artefacts in vitro from faulty blood sampling than fibrinopeptide A, although precautions must still be taken during venipuncture and plasma preparation (16). In addition to the original double-antibody liquid-phase radioimmunoassay, enzyme-linked immunosorbent assay (ELISA) kits are now commercially available (17). However, the correlations between the different methods, in terms of individual values as well as the classification of values as normal or abnormal (18), are poor. Thus laboratories can only compare results that are obtained using the same method and must ensure the presence of an age- and sex-matched control population in order to establish a local normal range of values.

Factor IX and X Activation Peptides

Radioimmunoassays have been developed that measure the activation peptides of both factor X (19) (an indicator of the increased enzymatic activity of factor IXa-factor VIIIa-cell surface complex and the factor VIIa–tissue factor complex) and factor IX (1,2) (an indicator of the increased enzymatic activity of factor XIa and the factor VIIa–tissue factor complex). These assays can provide information on coagulation activation at an even earlier step of the coagulation system than prothrombin fragment 1+2. Although the use of these markers has clarified the role of the extrinsic pathway in activating blood coagulation activation in vivo under basal conditions (i.e., in the absence of vascular injury or thrombotic stimuli) (1,2,20), their clinical utility in defining a hypercoagulable state has not yet been validated.

Protein C Activation Peptide

Another activation marker is protein C activation peptide, the fragment released when protein C is transformed into activated protein C. Measurements of this marker have provided important mechanistic information concerning the physiologic role of protein C and activated protein C. Protein C is a vitamin K–dependent zymogen that is activated by thrombin bound to endothelial cell thrombomodulin and then inactivates the thrombin-activated cofactors of the coagulation cascade (factor Va and factor VIIIa); this is one of the major anticoagulant drives of the hemostatic mechanism. Plasma levels of the protein C activation peptide can be taken as an indicator of thrombin/thrombomodulin function and can be measured by means of radioimmunoassay (21). In asymptomatic individuals with heterozygous protein C deficiency, plasma protein C activation peptide levels are reduced to about 50% of normal, and plasma prothrombin fragment 1+2 levels are increased, thus indicating increased thrombin generation (22). In patients with homozygous protein C deficiency, plasma protein C activation peptide and prothrombin fragment 1+2 levels can be normalized by administering monoclonal antibody–purified protein C concentrate (23). This demonstrates that an increase in the activity of the protein C anticoagulant pathway can inhibit prothrombin activation in vivo and that the activation of protein C by the thrombin–thrombomodulin complex is a tonically active mechanism in the regulation of coagulation activation.

Thrombin–Antithrombin III Complex

An additional assay of thrombin generation and thrombin neutralization is measurement of thrombin–antithrombin III complexes. Because the thrombin–antithrombin complex is stable and has a half-life of approximately 15 minutes (24), immunologic methods have been developed for its quantitation in plasma. The original radioimmunoassay used a liquid-phase double-antibody method (25), whereas the commercially available method is a solid-phase ELISA (26). The plasma levels of the complex are increased in a number of conditions associated with the activation of the co-agulation cascade, such as venous throm-boembolism (27), promyelocytic leukemia (28), and endotoxin infusion (29). An intriguing difference between the two methods is that the range of normal values differ by a factor of 100: with the radioimmunoassay the average normal concentration is 2 nmol/L; with the immunoenzymatic method, it is around 0.02 nmol/L. In stoichiometric terms, the enzymatic activation of 1 nmol of prothrombin will yield 1 nmol of thrombin and 1 nmol of prothrombin fragment 1+2. Assuming that all of the formed thrombin associates with antithrombin III, 1 nmol of thrombin will bind 1 nmol of antithrombin, thus leading to the formation of 1 nmol of complex. Because the half-life of the complex is one sixth that of prothrombin fragment 1+2, the plasma levels of thrombin–antithrombin complex should be less than those of prothrombin fragment 1+2, around 0.2 to 0.3 nmol/L. However, because these theoretical values differ considerably from those obtained using either of the methods, the biologic significance of the measured values must be interpreted with caution until the reasons for these discrepancies are elucidated. The binding of thrombin to receptors on cells and its internalization may contribute in part to this discrepancy.

DEFINITION OF A BIOCHEMICAL HYPERCOAGULABLE STATE

A hypercoagulable state can be defined biochemically if there is heightened activation of the blood coagulation mechanism in the absence of thrombosis (30). The laboratory detection of this condition, which can occur before overt thrombosis is apparent, is potentially important in order to identify subjects who are at greatest risk for developing thrombotic events and might benefit from prophylaxis. Studies in which simultaneous plasma measurements of prothrombin fragment 1+2 and fibrinopeptide A have been performed have facilitated a definition of one type of biochemical hypercoagulability. High fragment 1+2 concentrations in the presence of increased fibrinopeptide A levels signify heightened production of factor Xa, which is capable of generating sufficient free thrombin to initiate thrombus formation, i.e., a condition of overt thrombosis. However, high fragment 1+2 concentrations in the presence of normal or only slightly increased fibrinopeptide A levels signify enhanced production of factor Xa, which is unable to generate sufficient free thrombin to initiate thrombus formation, and represents a hypercoagulable state in biochemical terms. This condition of increased thrombin generation without fibrin formation may predispose affected individuals to develop overt thrombotic events in response to relatively minor prothrombotic stimuli. Theoretically this transition from a prethrombotic state to a thrombotic event occurs if there are small increases in the generation of coagulation enzymes that exceed the inhibitory threshold of an individual's endogenous anticoagulant mechanisms. Because the activity of the blood coagulation mechanism in these individuals is closer to the level at which the normal inhibitory processes are overwhelmed, thrombotic stimuli may induce the generation of slightly more thrombin via the factor VII–tissue factor pathway. This thrombin could then ignite the dormant intrinsic cascade by activating the factor IXa–factor VIIIa–cell surface complex, and thus lead to the generation of increased amounts of free thrombin and the development of arterial or venous thrombosis.

The validity of markers of coagulation activation in documenting the presence of a hypercoagulable state clinically has been investigated in various models. The following sections will review data regarding the ability of coagulation activation markers to identify biochemical hypercoagulability and its significance in cardiovascular diseases. Markers of platelet activation and fibrinolysis will not be addressed here.

ACUTE CORONARY SYNDROMES

The majority of patients with acute myocardial infarction and unstable angina have high plasma levels of fibrinopeptide A (31–34). The levels of fibrinopeptide A in spot urine samples as well as 24-hour urine collections from these patients also have been found to be elevated (12,13). These findings are consistent with the results of angiographic, angioscopic, and pathologic studies, which have clearly shown that intracoronary thrombosis plays a pivotal role in the pathogenesis of these coronary syndromes (35,36). Abnormally high plasma fragment 1+2 or fibrinopeptide A levels are found in nearly 50% of patients during the acute phase of the disease (34), their prevalence being higher in those with acute unstable angina or angiographic evidence of intracoronary thrombosis (12,13). No difference in the levels of these peptides has been observed between patients with unstable angina and those with acute myocardial infarction (34). This may indicate that plasma fragment 1+2 and fibrinopeptide A levels are not dependent on the characteristics of the thrombus (which is subocclusive and platelet rich in unstable angina, but occlusive and fibrin rich in myocardial infarction) (37), but rather reflect a systemic condition of hypercoagulability.

The degree of coagulation activation in the acute phase of unstable angina or myocardial infarction seems to be related to prognosis. Ardissino et al. (38) measured both plasma and urinary fibrinopeptide A levels in patients with unstable angina on hospital admission and found that elevated plasma levels were associated with a higher risk of developing primary (death or myocardial infarction) or secondary (refractory angina requiring emergency coronary revascularization) clinical endpoints during hospitalization. Granger et al. (39) found that higher baseline levels of fragment 1+2 were associated with an increased likelihood of death or myocardial reinfarction during a 30-day follow-up period in patients with myocardial infarction receiving thrombolytic therapy.

The serial measurement of coagulation activation peptides over time has provided interesting information concerning the pathophysiology of acute coronary syndromes. Merlini et al. (34) measured fragment 1+2 and fibrinopeptide A plasma levels in patients with unstable angina or acute myocardial infarction during the acute phase and 6 months after their initial acute presentation. Levels of fragment 1+2 and fibrinopeptide A were both elevated during the acute ischemic episode, thereby reflecting the presence of an intracoronary thrombosis. However, in patients with an uneventful clinical course at 6 months, fibrinopeptide A levels had returned to the normal range, whereas fragment 1+2 levels remained high (Fig. 7-3). This observation of a decrease in plasma levels of fibrinopeptide A, without substantial change in fragment 1+2, indicates that increased thrombin generation persists after initial coronary ischemic episodes, but is not sufficient to initiate fibrin formation and deposition. It is not known whether the presence of such a biochemical hypercoagulability state is a risk factor for the occurrence (or recurrence) of coronary events, but studies are currently ongoing to address this question in both normal populations without prior cardiac events as well as in patients with recent prior coronary events. Miller et al. (40) showed that men who were clinically free of cardiovascular disease had levels of factor IX activation peptide, fragment 1+2, fibrinopeptide A, factor VII antigen, factor VII coagulant activity, and fac-

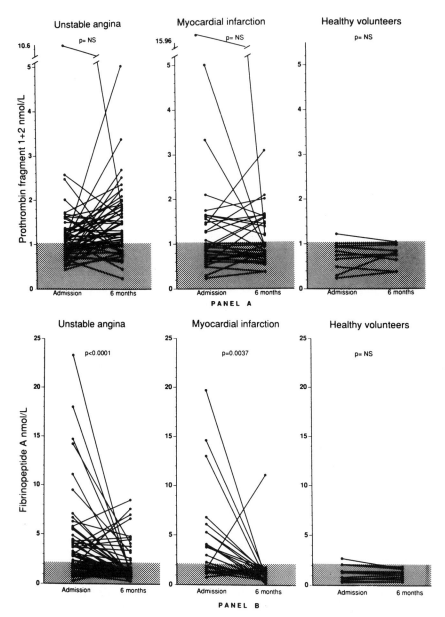

FIG. 7-3. Plots of plasma concentrations of prothrombin fragment 1+2 (F1+2) and plasma levels of fibrinopeptide A (FPA) in 57 patients with unstable angina and 23 patients with myocardial infarction at hospital admission. All patients had an uneventful clinical course, and follow-up determinations were obtained at 6 months. In 12 healthy blood donors, plasma concentration of F1+2 and FPA were evaluated at baseline (admission) and after 6 months. The top of the shaded area indicates the up-per limit of the normal range for each measurement (95th percentile of the distribution for the con-trol group of 32 healthy individuals matched for age and sex with the study population). (From Merlini et al., ref. 34.)

tor VIIa that were all positively and significantly correlated with higher risk scores for fatal coronary artery disease.

Coronary angioplasty mechanically causes plaque disruption that may evoke a thrombotic response, and abrupt coronary artery occlusion still represents one of the major complications of the procedure. Tearing of the atherosclerotic plaque might induce cap rupture that exposes the procoagulant matrix of the plaque itself to blood flow, giving rise to thrombosis. Marmur et al. (41) measured arterial blood fragment 1+2 and fibrinopeptide A during uncomplicated coronary angioplasty. Although no changes occurred in the majority of patients, seven of 32 showed an increase in fragment 1+2, which was associated with an increase in fibrinopeptide A in four. These data show that the majority of patients do not experience heightened coagulation system activation during uncomplicated coronary angioplasty under antithrombotic treatment with heparin; a minority do, however, and this could be due to the biochemical characteristics of the plaque itself (42) or to deeper trauma of the vessel wall induced by the angioplasty procedure. In another series of patients undergoing mechanical revascularization, Oltrona et al. (43) showed that a failure to normalize fibrinopeptide A levels during the interventional procedure (heparin resistance) was associated with a higher risk of complications, and this further emphasizes the possibility that useful prognostic information may be provided by the measurement of coagulation activation markers in the angioplasty setting.

ATRIAL FIBRILLATION

Chronic atrial fibrillation predisposes to thromboembolism (44), and cardioversion itself is also associated with cerebral, systemic, and pulmonary embolic events (45). The mechanism underlying the occurrence of embolic episodes after the restoration of sinus rhythm in these patients is poorly understood. The reduction in the incidence of cardioversion-related embolic events induced by the administration of warfarin (46,47) has led to

the widespread recommendation that anticoagulation should be prescribed for several weeks before and after cardioversion in patients with chronic atrial fibrillation (48,49). However, the use of anticoagulants is not recommended in patients with acute atrial fibrillation lasting less than 48 hours who undergo cardioversion, although definitive data regarding the risk of postcardioversion embolism in these patients are scanty. The recent finding of atrial thrombosis in 14% of patients with recent-onset atrial fibrillation suggests that these individuals are also at risk for developing embolic events (50). Oltrona et al. (51) measured the plasma concentrations of thrombin–antithrombin complex and fibrinopeptide A in a series of patients with acute nonvalvular atrial fibrillation and found a significant increase in the plasma concentrations of both markers early after pharmacologic cardioversion as compared with hospital admission; the levels decreased toward baseline values 1 month after restoration of sinus rhythm. This finding of a hypercoagulable state early after cardioversion in patients with recent-onset atrial fibrillation thus raises the important question as to whether prophylactic antithrombotic treatment also should be adopted for these patients.

ANTITHROMBOTIC THERAPY

Intravenous heparin, frequently used in the treatment of patients with acute coronary syndromes, acts by inhibiting thrombin and activated factors X, IX, XI, and XII (52). The anticoagulant action of heparin is primarily due to its ability to bind antithrombin III, thereby accelerating the rate of inhibition of the major coagulation enzymes, particularly thrombin (see Chapter 11). Biochemical studies of patients with acute coronary syndromes have clearly demonstrated that intravenous heparin rapidly inhibits the action of thrombin on fibrinogen and lowers plasma fibrinopeptide A levels to within the normal range (53–55). Heparin is also capable of inhibiting other serine proteases, such as activated factors XII, XI, IX, and, above all, X. Merlini et al. (56)

showed that intravenous heparin at doses giving an activated partial thromboplastin time within the therapeutic range (greater than twice the baseline level) reduced plasma fibrinopeptide A levels (Fig.7-5) but did not lower plasma prothrombin fragment fragment 1+2 levels in the majority of patients (Fig. 7-4). Recent studies also have shown that hirudin, a high-affinity direct thrombin inhibitor, does not decrease thrombin generation in patients with stable angina or acute coronary syndromes (57,58). Because thrombin plays a critical role in the amplification of the coagulation cascade by activating factor V (59) and factor VIII (60), persistent thrombin generation may partly contribute to the persistent thrombotic risk that exists despite anticoagulation. Plasma levels of both fibrinopeptide A and fragment 1+2 have been found to be higher in patients developing infarction, reinfarction, or refractory ischemia, suggesting that the presence of a persistent hypercoagulable state in patients with acute coronary syndromes, notwithstanding heparin therapy at the usual dose, may still be associated with an unfavorable outcome (39,56).

The measurement of coagulation peptides after the discontinuation of heparin or hirudin has shown the presence of a so-called rebound phenomenon. Gallino et al. (54) have shown that, although there is a decrease in plasma fibrinopeptide A levels during heparin infusions, a sharp increase occurs once the infusion is over, which suggests a reactivation of coagulation system activity. This finding has been confirmed by Granger et al. (61), who found the same phenomenon for fragment 1+2 and activated protein C levels (which also in part reflect increased thrombin generation). A similar effect has been observed after the discontinuation of argatroban (62). It is tempting to speculate that the increase in clinical events that is observed after the cessation of heparin or argatroban therapy is linked to this rebound in coagulation activation (62,63).

The failure to achieve reperfusion and the occurrence of subsequent reocclusion after successful thrombolysis are major limitations of thrombolytic therapy in acute myocardial infarction. The measurement of coagulation activation markers during thrombolytic therapy has demonstrated the prothrombotic effect of thrombolysis (64). In patients receiving streptokinase or recombinant tissue plasminogen activator, there is an increase in the plasma levels of fibrinopeptide A, the thrombin–an-

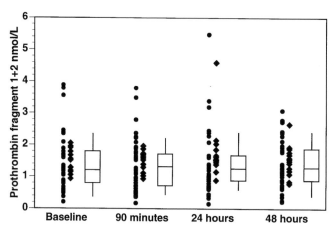

FIG. 7-4. Plots of plasma prothrombin fragment 1+2 levels in 40 patients with unstable angina and 14 patients with acute myocardial infarction who received intravenous heparin. Solid circles indicate patients with unstable angina, and solid squares indicate patients with myocardial infarction. The samples were obtained at hospital admission (baseline) and 90 minutes, 24 hours, and 48 hours after the start of heparin therapy. Plot boxes with median, 25th, 75th, 10th, and 90th percentiles refer to the whole study population.

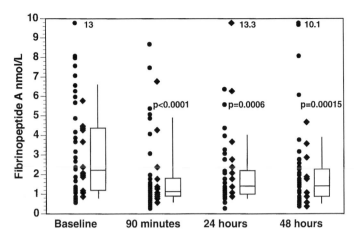

FIG. 7-5. Plots of plasma fibrinopeptide A levels in 40 patients with unstable angina and 14 patients with acute myocardial infarction who received intravenous heparin. Solid circles indicate patients with unstable angina, and solid squares indicate patients with myocardial infarction. The samples were obtained at hospital admission (baseline) and 90 minutes, 24 hours, and 48 hours after the start of heparin therapy. Plot boxes with median, 25th, 75th, 10th, and 90th percentiles refer to the whole study population. Probability values are versus baseline.

tithrombin III complex, and fragment 1+2 (65–68). Although the concomitant administration of heparin prevents fibrinopeptide A levels from increasing (69), fragment 1+2 levels increase in the majority of the patients regardless of the associated anticoagulant therapy (70). These findings raise the question of the role of hypercoagulability in the pathogenesis of the failure of reperfusion or postthrombolytic reocclusions. In patients receiving thrombolytic therapy, the behavior of coagulation activation markers after treatment seems to be predictive of outcome. Gulba et al. (71) have shown that patients in whom plasma thrombin–antithrombin complex levels increase 90 minutes after the start of thrombolytic therapy are those with no reperfusion or in whom reocclusion occurrs. Granger et al. (39) have assessed the relationship of fibrinopeptide A and fragment 1+2 levels with subsequent reinfarction and death in patients who received either recombinant tissue plasminogen activator or streptokinase; higher levels of fibrinopeptide A or fragment 1+2 after 12 hours were associated with a higher likelihood of subsequent reinfarction.

In patients with unstable angina receiving thrombolytic therapy, Merlini et al. (72) measured the plasma concentrations of fragment 1+2 and fibrinopeptide A. The patients were randomized to receive placebo alone, streptokinase 1,500,000 IU over 1 hour followed by a 48-hour placebo infusion, or streptokinase 250,000 over 1 hour followed by a continuous infusion of 100,000 IU per hour over 48 hours. All of the patients received intravenous heparin for 72 hours. The plasma levels of the different markers were measured at baseline, 90 minutes, and 24 and 48 hours after the start of therapy. In comparison with placebo, an increase in plasma prothrombin fragment 1+2 and fibrinopeptide A was observed after 90 minutes in the two groups receiving thrombolysis. After 24 and 48 hours, the prothrombin fragment 1+2 levels remained significantly higher only in the patients receiving the 48-hour streptokinase infusion (Fig. 7-6). The distribution of adverse outcome events (myocardial infarction, symptomatic or asymptomatic persistent myocardial ischemia) over the 72-hour study period in the three treatment groups (Fig. 7-7) showed that there was a clustering of ischemic episodes in the first 24 hours in the acute streptokinase group, as well as in the first 48 hours in the prolonged streptokinase group (when hemostatic system function is actually increased); in the placebo group, the events were evenly distributed throughout the 72 hours of the study period.

PANEL A

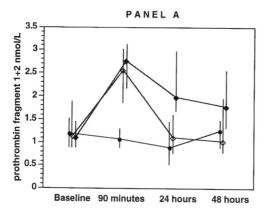

PANEL B

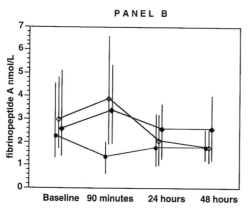

FIG. 7-6. Median plasma concentrations of pro-thrombin fragment 1+2 **(A)** and fibrinopeptide A **(B)** at baseline and 90 minutes, 24 hours, and 48 hours in patients with unstable angina receiving thrombolytic therapy. Solid circles indicates the placebo group, open squares the group receiving streptokinase 1,500,000 U over 1 hour, and solid squares the group receiving 250,000 U over 1 hour followed by 100,000 U per hour for 48 hours. Plot boxes with median, 25th, 75th, 10th, and 90th percentiles of the whole population are shown.

The median fibrinopeptide A levels measured in the plasma sample drawn before the occurrence of an adverse outcome event were higher than the median fibrinopeptide A levels measured in the plasma sample drawn at the corresponding time point in the patients who did not develop an event. These data suggest that the hypercoagulable state induced by thrombolytic therapy may be detrimental in the setting of the subocclusive thrombosis typical of

unstable angina and could explain the unfavorable results of this therapy both in a large clinical trial (73) and during interventional procedures (74).

Therapy with coumarin derivatives suppresses prothrombin activation in vivo as measured by the sharp decrease in plasma fragment 1+2 levels. In patients with thrombotic histories and high fragment 1+2 levels, Conway et al. (75) demonstrated that moderately intense stable anticoagulation (as reflected by International Normalized Ratios of 2.5 to 3.5) leads to a five- to tenfold reduction in the extent of prothrombin activation; the mean values decrease in parallel with the intensity of oral anticoagulant therapy. These investigators have thus surmised that the dosage of warfarin may be adjusted on the basis of factor 1+2 concentrations (76). In a cross-sectional study, Mannucci et al. (77) measured fragment 1+2 levels in patients stabilized on oral anticoagulants and found that there was a close relationship between the factor 1+2 concentrations and the intensity of anticoagulation.

On the basis of these data, clinical studies have been performed in situations in which the monitoring of coagulation system function by standard methods has been unsatisfactory, e.g., the prophylaxis of subacute thrombosis after stent implantation. The main problem of intracoronary stenting is subacute thrombosis, which often occurs unpredictably even in conditions of optimal anticoagulation according to classical standard coagulation tests. It has been shown that an increase in fragment 1+2 levels despite optimal anticoagulation is a very sensitive indicator of subacute thrombosis (78,79). In a case-control study (80), a study population on oral anticoagulants was investigated using fragment 1+2 measurements as well as classical coagulation tests and compared with a control population in which only the classical tests were used to monitor the level of anticoagulation. It was found that the incidence of subtotal occlusion was 3.5% in the study group, but 17% in the control group. For elective and nonelective stenting, the monitoring of fragment 1+2 levels may therefore be associated with a reduced rate of subacute thrombosis (80).

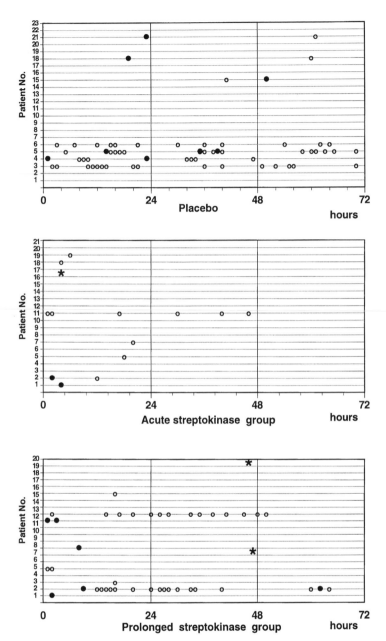

FIG. 7-7. Distribution of adverse outcome events during the 72-hour study period in patients with unstable angina receiving thrombolytic therapy. Each horizontal line represents a patient. Asterisks denote myocardial infarction, black circles symptomatic ischemic episodes, and open circles asymptomatic ischemic episodes. (From Merlini et al., ref. 72.)

CONCLUSION

1. The laboratory detection of a biochemical hypercoagulable state has been made possible by the development of new assays that allow the different steps of the coagulation cascade to be monitored. The information provided by coagulation activation markers has been useful for improving our understanding of the mechanisms of disease.

2. Clinical studies using these markers indicate that a biochemical imbalance between procoagulant and anticoagulant mechanisms can be detected in the blood of individuals before the appearance of a thrombotic disorder.

3. Cohort studies are in progress that will determine whether these techniques will enable us to, first, identify biochemically those individuals who are at highest risk of a thrombotic event, and therefore to intervene with appropriate therapy before the onset of the thrombotic disorder itself.

REFERENCES

1. Bauer KA, Kass BL, ten Cate H, Hawiger JJ, Rosenberg RD. Factor IX is activated in vivo by a tissue factor mechanism. *Blood* 1990;76:731–736.
2. Bauer KA, Mannucci PM, Gringeri A, et al. Factor IXa–factor VIIIa–cell surface complex does not contribute to the basal activation of the coagulation mechanism in vivo. *Blood* 1992;79:2039–2047.
3. Meade TW, Mellows S, Brozovic M, et al. Haemostatic function and ischemic heart disease: principal results of the Norwick Park Heart Study. *Lancet* 1986;2:533–537.
4. Heinrich J, Balleisen L, Schulte H, Assmann G, van de Loo J. Fibrinogen and factor VII in the prediction of coronary risk. Results from the PROCAM study in healthy men. *Arterioscler Thromb* 1994;14:54–59.
5. Thompson SG, Kienast J, Pyke SD, Haverkate F, van de Loo JC. Hemostatic factors and the risk of myocardial infarction or sudden death in patients with angina pectoris. The European Concerted Action on Thrombosis and Disabilities Angina Pectoris Study Group. *N Engl J Med* 1995;332:635–641.
6. Meade TW, Cooper J, Miller GJ, Howarth D, Stirling Y. Antithrombin III and arterial disease: an unexpected relationship. *Lancet* 1991;337:850–851.
7. Morrissey JH, Macik BG, Neuenschwander PF, Comp PC. Quantification of activated factor VII levels in plasma using a tissue factor mutant selectively deficient in promoting factor VII activation. *Blood* 1993;81:734–744.
8. Boisclair MD, Lane DA, Philippou H, et al. Mechanism of thrombin generation during surgery and cardiopulmonary bypass. *Blood* 1993;82:3350–3357.
9. Gruber A, Griffin J. Direct detection of activated protein C in blood from normal subjects. *Blood* 1992;79:2340–2348.
10. Nossel HL, Yudelman I, Canfield RE, et al. Measurement of fibrinopeptide A in human blood. *J Clin Invest* 1974;54:43–53.
11. Nossel HL, Ti M, Kaplan KL, Spanondis K, Soland T, Butler VP Jr. The generation of fibrinopeptide A in clinical blood samples. Evidence for thrombin activity. *J Clin Invest* 1976;58:1136–1144.
12. Wilensky RL, Bourdillon PD, Vix VA, Zeller JA. Intracoronary artery thrombus formation in unstable angina: a clinical, biochemical and angiographic correlation. *J Am Coll Cardiol* 1993;21:692–699.
13. Ardissino D, Gamba MG, Merlini PA, et al. Fibrinopeptide A excretion in urine: a marker of cumulative thrombin activity in stable versus unstable angina patients. *Am J Cardiol* 1991;68:58B–63B.
14. Teitel JM, Bauer KA, Lau HK, Rosenberg RD. Studies of the prothrombin activation pathway utilizing radioimmunoassays for the F2/F1+2 fragment and thrombin-antithrombin complex. *Blood* 1982;59:1086–1097.
15. Lau HK, Rosenberg JS, Beeler DL, Rosenberg RD. The isolation and characterization of a specific antibody population directed against the prothrombin activation fragments F2 and prothrombin fragment 1+2. *J Biol Chem* 1979;254:8751–8761.
16. Miller GJ, Bauer KA, Barzegar S, et al. The effect of quality and timing of venipuncture on markers of blood coagulationin in healthy middle-aged men. *Thromb Heamost* 1995;73:82–86.
17. Pelzer H, Schwarz A, Stuber W. Determination of human prothrombin activation fragment 1+2 in plasma with an antibody against a synthetic peptide. *Thromb Haemost* 1991;65:153–159.
18. Tripodi A, Chantarangkul V, Bottasso B, Mannucci PM. Poor comparability of prothrombin fragment 1+2 values measured by two commercial ELISA methods: influence of different anticoagulants and standards. *Thromb Haemost* 1994;71:605–608.
19. Bauer KA, Kass BL, ten Cate H, Bednarek MA, Hawinger JJ, Rosenberg RD. Detection of factor X activation in humans. *Blood* 1989;74:2007–2015.
20. ten Cate H, Bauer KA, Levi M, et al. The activation of factor X and prothrombin by recombinant factor VIIa in vivo is mediated by tissue factor. *J Clin Invest* 1993;92:1207–1212.
21. Bauer KA, Kass BL, Beeler DL, Rosenberg RD. Detection of protein C activation in humans. *J Clin Invest* 1984;74:2033–2041.
22. Bauer KA, Broekmans AW, Bertina RM, et al. Hemostatic enzyme generation in the blood of patients with hereditary protein C deficiency. *Blood* 1988;71:1418–1426.
23. Conard J, Bauer KA, Gruber A, et al. Normalization of markers of coagulation activation with a purified protein C concentrate in adults with homozygous protein C deficiency. *Blood* 1993;82:1159–1164.
24. Shifman MA, Pizzo SV. The in vivo metabolism of antithrombin III and antithrombin III complexes. *J Biol Chem* 1982;257:3243–3248.
25. Lau HK, Rosenberg RD. The isolation and characterization of a specific antibody population directed against the thrombin-antithrombin complex. *J Biol Chem* 1980;255:5885–5893.

26. Peltzer H, Schwarz A, Heimburger N. Determination of human thrombin–antithrombin III complex in plasma with an enzyme-linked immunosorbent assay. *Thromb Haemost* 1988;59:101–106.

27. Blanke H, Praetorius G, Leschke M, Seitz R, Egbring R, Strauer BE. Significance of the thrombin-antithrombin III complex in the diagnosis of pulmonary embolism and deep vein thrombosis: comparison with fibrinopeptide A, platelet factor 4 and beta-thromboglobulin. *Klin Wochenschr* 1987;65:757–763.

28. Bauer KA, Rosenberg RD. Thrombin generation in acute promyelocytic leukemia. *Blood* 1984;64:791–796.

29. van Deventer SJH, Buller HR, tenCate JW, Aarden LA, Hack E, Sturk A. Experimental endotoxinemia in humans: analysis of cytokine release and coagulation fibrinolytic and complement pathway. *Blood* 1990;76: 2520–2526.

30. Bauer KA, Rosenberg RD. The pathophysiology of the prethrombotic state in humans: insight gained from studies using markers of hemostatic system activation. *Blood* 1987;70:343–350.

31. Neri Serneri GG, Gensini GF, Abbate R, Laureano R, Parodi O. Is raised plasma fibrinopeptide A a marker of acute coronary insufficiency? *Lancet* 1980;2:982–983.

32. Theroux P, Latour JG, Leger-Gautier C, De Lara J. Fibrinopeptide A plasma levels and platelet factor 4 levels in unstable angina pectoris. *Circulation* 1987;75: 156–162.

33. van Hulsteijn H, Kolff J, Briët E, van der Laarse A, Bertina R. Fibrinopeptide A and beta thromboglobulin in patients with angina pectoris and acute myocardial infarction. *Am Heart J* 1984;107:39–45.

34. Merlini PA, Bauer KA, Oltrona L, et al. Persistent activation of the coagulation mechanism in unstable angina and myocardial infarction. *Circulation* 1994;90: 61–68.

35. Fuster V, Badimon L, Badimon JJ, Chesebro JH. Mechanism of disease: the pathogenesis of coronary artery disease and the acute coronary syndromes. *N Engl J Med* 1992;326:242–250.

36. Fuster V, Badimon L, Badimon JJ, Chesebro JH. Mechanism of disease: the pathogenesis of coronary artery disease and the acute coronary syndromes. *N Engl J Med* 1992;326:310–318.

37. Mizuno K, Satumora K, Miyamoto A, et al. Angioscopic evaluation of coronary artery thrombi in acute coronary syndromes. *N Engl J Med* 1992;326:287–291.

38. Ardissino D, Merlini PA, Gamba G, et al. Thrombin activity and early outcome in unstable angina pectoris. *Circulation* 1996;93:1634–1639.

39. Granger CB, Becker R, Tracy RP, et al. for the GUSTO Hemostasis Substudy Group. Thrombin generation, inhibition, and clinical outcomes in patients with acute myocardial infarction treated with thrombolytic therapy and heparin: results from the GUSTO trial. (Submitted.)

40. Miller GJ, Bauer KA, Barzegar S, Cooper JA, Rosenberg RD. Increased activation of the hemostatic system in men at high risk of fatal coronary artery disease. *Thromb Haemost* 1996;75:767–771.

41. Marmur JD, Merlini PA, Sharma SK, et al. Thrombin generation in human coronary arteries after percutaneous transluminal balloon angioplasty. *J Am Coll Cardiol* 1994;24:1484–1491.

42. Ardissino D, Merlini PA, Ariens R, Coppola R, Bramucci E, Mannucci PM. Tissue factor antigen and activity of human coronary atherosclerotic plaques. *Lancet* 1997;349:769–771.

43. Oltrona L, Eisenberg PR, Lasala JM, Sewall DJ, Shelton ME, Winters KJ. Association of heparin-resistant thrombin activity with acute ischemic complications of coronary interventions. *Circulation* 1996;94:2064–2071.

44. Goldman MJ. The management of atrial fibrillation: indications for and method of conversion to sinus rhythm. *Prog Cardiovasc Dis* 1969;2:465–479.

45. Wolf PA, Dawber TR, Thomas E Jr, Kannel WB. Epidemiological assessment of chronic atrial fibrillation and risk of stroke: the Framingham Study. *Neurology* 1978;28:973–977.

46. Bjerkelund CJ, Orning OM. The efficacy of anticoagulant therapy in preventing embolism related to DC electrical conversion of atrial fibrillation. *Am J Cardiol* 1969;23:208–216.

47. Weinberg DM, Mancini GBJ. Anticoagulation for cardioversion of atrial fibrillation. *Am J Cardiol* 1989;63: 745–746.

48. Laupacis A, Albers G, Dunn M, Feinberg W. Antithrombotic therapy in atrial fibrillation. *Chest* 1992; 102(suppl):426–433.

49. Prystowsky EN, Benson W, Fuster V, et al. Management of patients with atrial fibrillation. *Circulation* 1996;93: 1262–1277.

50. Stoddard MF, Dawkins PR, Prince CR, Ammash NM. Left atrial appendage thrombus is not uncommon in patients with acute atrial fibrillation and a recent embolic event: a transesophageal echocardiographic study. *J Am Coll Cardiol* 1995;25:452–459.

51. Oltrona L, Broccolino M, Merlini PA, Spinola A, Pezzano A, Mannucci PM. Activation of the hemostatic mechanism following pharmacological cardioversion of acute nonvalvular atrial fibrillation. *Circulation* 1997; 95:2003–2006.

52. Rosenberg RD. Actions and interactions of antithrombin and heparin. *N Engl J Med* 1975;292:146–151.

53. Mombelli G, Hof I, Haeberli A, Straub PW. Effect of heparin on plasma fibrinopeptide A in patients with acute myocardial infarction. *Circulation* 1984;69:684–689.

54. Gallino A, Haeberli A, Hess T, Mombelli G, Straub PW. Fibrin formation and platelet aggregation in patients with acute myocardial infarction: effect of intravenous and subcutaneous low-dose heparin. *Am Heart J* 1986;112:285–290.

55. Neri Serneri GG, Gensini G, Poggesi L, et al. Effect of heparin, aspirin, or alteplase in reduction of myocardial ischemia in refractory unstable angina. *Lancet* 1990; 335:615–618.

56. Merlini PA, Ardissino D, Bauer KA, et al. Persistent thrombin generation durin heparin therapy in acute coronary syndromes. *Arterioscler Thromb Vasc Biol* 1997;17:1325-1330.

57. Zoldhelyi P, Bichler J, Owen WG, et al. Persistent thrombin generation in humans during specific thrombin inhibition with hirudin. *Circulation* 1994;90:2671–2678.

58. Kottke-Marchant K, Zoldhelyi P, Zaramo C, Brooks L, Cianciolo C, Janssens S. The effect of desirudin vs. heparin on hemostatic parameters in acute coronary syndromes: the Gusto IIb hemostasis substudy. *Circulation* 1996;94:I–742.

59. Nesheim ME, Mann KG. Thrombin catalyzed activation of single-chain bovine factor V. *J Biol Chem* 1979;254:1326–1334.

60. Hoyer LW, Trabold NC. Effect of thrombin on human factor VIII: cleavage of the factor VIII procoagulant protein during activation. *J Lab Clin Med* 1989;97: 50–64.

61. Granger CB, Miller JM, Bovill EG, et al. Rebound increase in thrombin generation and activity after cessation of intravenous heparin in patients with acute coronary syndromes. *Circulation* 1995;92:1929–1935.

62. Gold HK, Torres FW, Garaberian HD, et al. Evidence for a rebound coagulation phenomenon after cessation of a 4-hour infusion of a specific thrombin inhibitor in patients with unstable angina pectoris. *J Am Coll Cardiol* 1993;21:1039–1047.

63. Theroux P, Waters D, Lam J, Juneu M, McCans J. Reactivation of unstable angina after discontinuation of heparin. *N Engl J Med* 1992;327:141–145.

64. Eisenberg PR, Sherman LA, Jaffe AS. Paradoxic elevation of fibrinopeptide A after streptokinase: evidence of continued thrombosis despite intense fibrinolysis. *J Am Coll Cardiol* 1987;10:527–529.

65. Owen J, Friedman KD, Grossman BA, Wilkins C, Berke AD, Powers ER. Thrombolytic therapy with tissue-type plasminogen activator or streptokinase induced transient thrombin activity. *Blood* 1988;72:616–620.

66. Baglin TP, Luddington R, Jennings I, Richards EM. Thrombin generation and myocardial infarction during infusion of tissue-plasminogen activator. *Lancet* 1993; 1:504–505.

67. Genser N, Mair J, Maier J, Dienstl F, Puschendorf B, Lechleitner P. Thrombin generation during infusion of tissue-type plasminogen activator [Letter]. *Lancet* 1993; 1:1038.

68. Merlini PA, Cattaneo M, Spinola A, Ardissino D, Belli C, Mannucci PM. Activation of the hemostatic system during thrombolytic therapy. *Am J Cardiol* 1993;72: 59G–65G.

69. Rapold HJ, deBono D, Arnold AER, et al. Plasma fibrinopeptide A levels in patients with myocardial infarction treated with alteplase. *Circulation* 1992;85: 928–34.

70. Merlini PA, Bauer K, Oltrona L, et al. Thrombin generation and activity during thrombolysis and concomitant heparin therapy in patients with acute myocardial infarction. *J Am Coll Cardiol* 1995;25:203–209.

71. Gulba DC, Barthels M, Westhoff-Bleck M, et al. Increased thrombin levels during thrombolytic therapy in acute myocardial infarction. *Circulation* 1991;83: 937–944.

72. Merlini PA, Ardissino D, Bauer K, et al. Activation of the hemostatic mechanism during thrombolysis in patients with unstable angina pectoris. *Blood* 1995;86: 3327–3332.

73. The TIMI IIIB Investigators. Effect of tissue plasminogen activator and a comparison of early invasive and conservative strategies in unstable angina and non-Q wave myocardial infarction. *Circulation* 1994;89:1545–1556.

74. Ambrose JA, Almeida OD, Sharma S, et al. Adjunctive thrombolytic therapy during angioplasty for ischemic rest angina. Results of the TAUSA trial. TAUSA Investigators. Thrombolysis and Angioplasty in Unstable Angina trial. *Circulation* 1994;90:69–77.

75. Conway EM, Bauer KA, Barzegar S, Rosenberg RD. Suppression of hemostatic system activation by oral anticoagulants in the blood of patients with thrombotic diatheses. *J Clin Invest* 1987;80:1535–1544.

76. Millenson MM, Bauer KA, Kistler JP, Barzegar S, Tulin L, Rosenberg RD. Monitoring "mini-intensity" anticoagulation with warfarin: comparison of prothrombin time using a sensitive thomboplastin with prothrombin fragment F1+2 levels. *Blood* 1992;79:2034–2038.

77. Mannucci PM, Bottasso B, Tripodi A. Prothrombin fragment 1+2 and intensity of treatment with oral anticoagulant [Letter]. *Thromb Haemost* 1991;66:741.

78. Swars H, Hafner G, Erbel R, et al. Prothrombin fragment and thrombotic occlusion of coronary stents [Letter]. *Lancet* 1991;337:59.

79. Hafner G, Swars H, Erbel R, et al. Monitoring prothrombin fragment 1+2 during initiation of oral anticoagulant therapy after intracoronary stenting. *Ann Haematol* 1992;65:83–87.

80. Haude M, Hafner G, Jablonka A, et al. Guidance of anticoagulation after intracoronary implantation of Palmaz-Schatz stents by monitoring prothrombin and prothombin fragment 1+2. *Am Heart J* 1994;130:228–238.

PART II

Antithrombotic and Thrombolytic Drugs

Cardiovascular Thrombosis: Thrombocardiology
and Thromboneurology, Second Edition,
edited by M. Verstraete, V. Fuster, and E. J. Topol,
Lippincott–Raven Publishers, Philadelphia © 1998.

8

Antiplatelet Drugs

Garret A. FitzGerald and *Carlo Patrono

*Department of Pharmacology, University of Pennsylvania School of Medicine,
Philadelphia, Pennsylvania 19104; and *Department of Medicine and Aging,
G. D'Annunzio School of Medicine, 66013 Chieti, Italy*

PLATELET CYCLOOXYGENASE INHIBITORS

Aspirin and other nonsteroidal anti-inflammatory drugs (NSAIDs) inhibit the cyclooxygenase activity of the enzyme prostaglandin (PG) H-synthase, which catalyzes the conversion of arachidonic acid and oxygen to PGH_2, the first committed step in prostanoid biosynthesis (1). Two isozymes are known, called PGHS-1 or COX-1 and PGHS-2 or COX-2. They are both homodimeric, heme-containing, glycosylated proteins with two catalytic activities. The enzymes catalyze both a cyclooxygenase (bis-oxygenase) reaction, in which arachidonic acid is converted to PGG_2, and a peroxidase reaction, in which PGG_2 undergoes a two-electron reduction to PGH_2.

PGHS-1 is constitutively expressed in virtually all cells of the human body, including platelets. In contrast, PGHS-2 is undetectable in most mammalian tissues, but its expression can be induced rapidly in monocytes, endothelial cells and other specialized cells in response to various inflammatory and mitogenic mediators (e.g., cytokines, tumor promoters, and growth factors) (1).

In human platelets, the product of PGHS-1, PGH_2, is largely metabolized to thromboxane $(TX)A_2$ by a specific isomerase called TX-synthase. TXA_2 provides a mechanism for amplifying the activation signal, by virtue of its being synthesized and released in response to a variety of platelet agonists (e.g., collagen, adenosine diphosphate [ADP], and thrombin) and in turn inducing irreversible platelet aggregation (2). Inhibition of the cyclooxygenase activity of platelet PGHS-1 is associated with inhibition of TXA_2-dependent platelet function and a reduced risk of platelet-dependent vascular occlusion.

Aspirin

Acetylsalicylic acid, synthesized by the German chemist Felix Hoffmann at Bayer AG in 1897, was introduced into medicine in 1899 under the name of aspirin. The drug has a number of pharmacologic effects that are characterized by markedly different dose-response relationships in humans. Thus, although an antiplatelet effect has been demonstrated with doses as low as 30 to 75 mg, the analgesic and antipyretic effects require at least 300 mg, and an anti-inflammatory effect can be obtained only at daily doses in excess of 2,000 mg and may require 4,000 to 5,000 mg. Moreover, these diverse pharmacologic effects of aspirin show a remarkably different duration, from as short as a few hours to as long as a few days. This is reflected in the drug being used once daily, as an antiplatelet agent, and four to six times daily when used as an analgesic/anti-inflammatory remedy. Such a different dose- and time-dependence of the effects of aspirin is rather unusual and largely related to its unique mechanism of action and short half-life in the human circulation.

Mechanism of Action

Aspirin induces a long-lasting functional defect in platelets, detectable clinically as a prolongation of the bleeding time. This appears to be related primarily, if not exclusively, to permanent inactivation by aspirin of platelet PGHS-1.

Aspirin selectively acetylates the hydroxyl group of a single serine residue at position 529 (Ser^{529}) within the polypeptide chain of human platelet PGHS-1 (3–5). X-ray crystallographic analysis (6) of the aspirin-acetylated enzyme has established that when Ser^{529} is acetylated by aspirin, the acetyl group protrudes into the cyclooxygenase channel at a critical site for arachidonic acid interaction with the tyrosine residue responsible for initiating catalysis (Fig. 8-1). As a consequence of O-acetylation of Ser^{529} by aspirin, the cyclooxygenase activity is permanently lost, whereas the hydroperoxidase activity is unaffected (Fig. 8-2). Aspirin also inhibits the cyclooxygenase activity of PGHS-2, although at higher concentrations than required for inhibition of PGHS-1. This may account in part for the different dose requirement for the analgesic/anti-inflammatory versus antiplatelet effects of the drug as noted above. The recent characterization of two rotameric states of the acetyl-serine side chain that block the cyclooxygenase channel to different extents may explain the dissimilar effects of aspirin on the two PGHS isoforms (6).

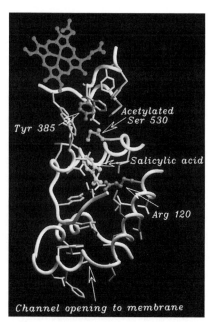

FIG. 8-1. Crystal structure of the active site of aspirin-acetylated ovine PGHS-1. The carboxylic moiety of the salicylic acid interacts reversibly with Arg^{120}, a common docking site for all NSAIDs. This creates a local pool of acetylating moiety just beneath Ser^{530} thereby explaining selective acetylation of this particular serine residue by aspirin. Acetylated Ser^{530} occupies a strategic position within the cyclooxygenase channel directly below Tyr^{385}, a key residue for initiating cyclooxygenase catalysis. Any arachidonic acid diffusing up the channel would be prevented from interacting with Tyr^{385} by steric hindrance introduced by this adduct. (Courtesy of Dr. P. Loll, Department of Pharmacology, University of Pennsylvania School of Medicine.)

Reduced formation of various eicosanoids (i.e., TXA$_2$ as well as PGE$_2$ and PGI$_2$) in different tissues can probably account for the variety of pharmacologic effects of aspirin that form the basis for both its therapeutic use and its toxicity (7). Because inactivation of PGH-synthases by aspirin is irreversible, de novo synthesis of the enzyme is required in order to restore normal eicosanoid formation. This occurs within hours in nucleated cells but cannot adequately take place in platelets that derive from fragmentation of the megakaryocyte cytoplasm and have a negligible capacity for protein synthesis. Thus, the duration of

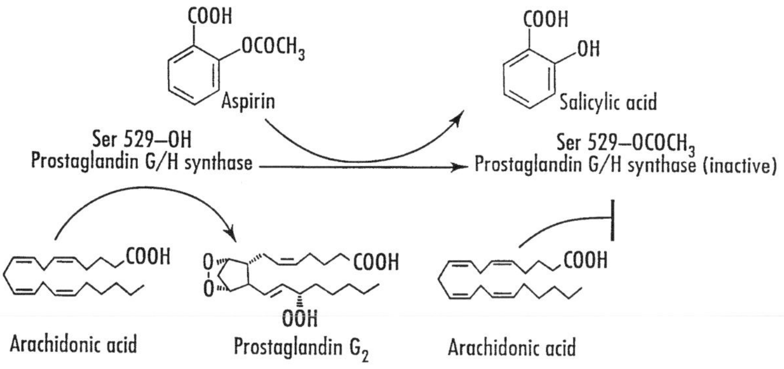

FIG. 8-2. Mechanism of the antiplatelet action of aspirin. Aspirin acetylates the hydroxyl group of a serine residue at position 529 (Ser[529]) in the polypeptide chain of human platelet prostaglandin G/H synthase, resulting in the inactivation of its cyclooxygenase catalytic activity. Aspirin-induced blockade of prostaglandin G_2 synthesis will result in decreased biosynthesis of prostaglandin H_2 and thromboxane A_2. (Adapted from Patrono, ref. 8, with permission.)

platelet and extraplatelet effects of a single dose of the drug varies considerably, ranging from several days to a few hours, respectively.

Alternative mechanisms have been proposed to explain the protective effect of aspirin against thrombosis (8). Thus, aspirin can acetylate other proteins, including the lysine residues of fibrinogen, although at higher concentrations and over longer time periods than required for acetylation of PGH-synthase. N-acetylated fibrinogen facilitates plasminogen activation and is much less effective in supporting platelet aggregation than unmodified fibrinogen. Moreover, it has been suggested that aspirin inhibits thrombin generation by acetylating macromolecules of the platelet membrane and/or prothrombin (9). However, both the dose-response relationship and the clinical relevance of these additional effects of the drug remain to be established.

Pharmacokinetics

Orally ingested aspirin is absorbed rapidly, partly from the stomach but mostly from the upper small intestine. This occurs primarily by passive diffusion of the nondissociated lipid-soluble aspirin across gastrointestinal membranes. Aspirin is also hydrolyzed by gastric and jejunal esterases and is therefore absorbed, in part, as salicylate. Such presystemic metab-

olism contributes to variable systemic bioavailability, as a function of fluid and food ingestion. Systemic bioavailability of regular aspirin tablets is on the order of 40% to 50%, in a range of doses from 20 to 1,300 mg (10). A considerably lower bioavailability has been reported for enteric-coated tablets and sustained-release, microencapsulated preparations. Thus, different pharmaceutical formulations may deliver little or no measurable aspirin to the systemic circulation. Because of acetylation of platelet PGH-synthase in the presystemic circulation (10), the antiplatelet effect of aspirin is largely independent of systemic bioavailability. Both a controlled-release formulation (11) and a transdermal patch (12) of aspirin with very low systemic bioavailability have been developed, in an attempt to achieve selective inhibition of platelet TXA_2 production without suppressing systemic PGI_2 synthesis. However, the clinical relevance of varying degrees of biochemical selectivity remains to be established.

The absorbed ester is rapidly hydrolyzed to salicylate in plasma, the liver, the lungs, and erythrocytes. The plasma half-life of aspirin is approximately 15 minutes; that for salicylate is dose dependent and ranges between 2 and 12 hours.

Salicylate is further metabolized to salicyluric acid (the glycine conjugate), to the ether or phenolic glucuronide, and to the ester or acyl glucuronide. In addition, a small fraction is oxidized to 2,3-dihydroxybenzoic, 2,5-dihydroxybenzoic (gentisic acid), and 2,3,5-trihydroxybenzoic acids. With the possible exception of gentisic acid, no pharmacologic effects have been ascribed to these metabolites.

Salicylates are excreted mainly by kidneys. The pharmacokinetics of aspirin have been approximated by an open, two-compartment model with first-order absorption and elimination and metabolism from the central compartment.

Effects of Aspirin on Platelet Biochemistry and Function

The dose dependence and time dependence of the antiplatelet effect of aspirin have been investigated by measuring three distinct indices of platelet biochemistry and function: cyclo-oxygenase activity (13,14), aggregation in response to various agonists (15), and the forearm template bleeding time (16). A large number of studies assessing aspirin pharmacodynamics in humans have relied on measurements of serum TXB_2, as a reflection of thrombin-induced platelet TXA_2 production during whole blood clotting (13). This relatively simple method evaluates the capacity of platelets to synthesize TXB_2 in response to virtually maximal stimulation and by no means reflects the actual production rate of TXB_2 in vivo, which is several orders of magnitude lower (17).

When given orally to healthy subjects, aspirin inhibits TXA_2 production and TXA_2-dependent platelet function in a dose- and time-dependent fashion (18,19). A log-linear inhibition of platelet cyclooxygenase activity is found after single doses in the range of 10 to 100 mg. Moreover, such a dose-response relationship is similar in healthy subjects and in patients with atherosclerosis, when assessed ex vivo by the same technique of determination of TXB_2 production in whole blood. No consistent gender-related difference in the antiplatelet effect of aspirin has been described. After oral administration, serum TXB_2 is significantly reduced as early

as 5 minutes after dosing. In as much as no aspirin can be detected in peripheral venous blood at this time, acetylation of PGHS-1 during the first 5 minutes is likely to occur by exposure of platelets to the drug in the presystemic circulation (10). Serum TXB_2 is maximally suppressed 30 to 60 minutes after oral aspirin and remains stable thereafter up to 24 hours, reflecting irreversible enzyme inactivation. Evidence has been presented that the recovery of unacetylated platelet PGHS-1 (20) and enzyme activity (18), after a single dose of aspirin, does not occur for approximately 48 hours. The 2-day lag in the return of functioning enzyme to the circulation has been interpreted as evidence that aspirin acetylates PGHS-1 in the megakaryocyte.

Because of irreversible enzyme inactivation and lack of de novo enzyme synthesis in platelets, acetylation of platelet PGHS-1 and consequent inhibition of TXA_2 production by low-dose aspirin is cumulative on repeated dosing (18,20). A log-linear relationship also exists between the oral dose of aspirin and the inhibition of platelet TXB_2 production, measured at steady-state upon repeated daily dosing (21). When comparing this dose-response relationship with that based on measurements performed after single dosing, an eightfold shift is apparent, with the $ID_{50}s$ (the dose required to inhibit enzyme activity by 50%) approximating 3 and 26 mg, respectively (21). This finding suggests that the fractional dose of aspirin necessary for achieving a given level of acetylation of the enzyme by virtue of cumulative effects (or for maintaining it after a full acetylating dose) approximately equals the fractional daily platelet turnover, i.e., 10% to 15% in healthy subjects (21). Thus, for a given dose of the drug, both the rate at which cumulative acetylation occurs and its maximal extent would essentially depend on the rate of platelet turnover and the dosing interval.

Given the greater variability of platelet aggregation measurements, relatively few studies have attempted to correlate changes in platelet functional responses to variable degrees of TXA_2 inhibition as a function of aspirin dosage. In the study of FitzGerald et al. (19), five healthy subjects received aspirin in daily doses of 20, 40, 80, 160, 325, 650, 1,300, and 2,600 mg. Each dose was given for 7 days, and ascending doses were administered in consecutive weeks. During this extended dose-ranging study, the aggregation response to ADP (T^{max} at 2.5, 5.0, and 10.0 μmol/L) was measured as a marker of the platelet-inhibiting effect of aspirin. T^{max} to ADP was reduced in the early weeks of the study, with the most pronounced changes in platelet response being observed at 20 to 80 mg per day. However, in the final 2 weeks of the study (at 1,300 and 2,600 mg per day) the aggregation response returned to control values despite continuing inhibition of TXA_2 biosynthesis (19). Although this was not a controlled study, this trend was evident at all doses of ADP used and in all volunteers. FitzGerald et al. have suggested that acetylation of platelet membrane proteins other than PGHS-1 may render platelets more liable to aggregate during long-term aspirin therapy at high doses (19).

De Caterina et al. (22,23) have conducted a randomized, double-blind, placebo-controlled study of 3-week therapy with aspirin at 30, 50, or 324 mg per day in 20 patients surviving an acute myocardial infarction. The secondary wave of ADP-induced aggregation, the epinephrine- and arachidonate-induced platelet aggregation, were maximally suppressed with respect to both basal and placebo measurements. No statistically significant differences were observed in platelet aggregation among the three doses of aspirin, concomitant with 93% to 99% inhibition of serum TXB_2 levels (22,23).

Given the limitations inherent to repeated measurement of the bleeding time in the same subjects, it is not surprising that the dose- and time-dependence of aspirin effects on this parameter have not been examined with the same degree of accuracy. The studies were performed in relatively small groups of subjects (n = 4 to 20) and rarely had sufficient statistical power to detect small differences in bleeding time between different aspirin doses, if they indeed existed. The vast majority of these studies did find a statistically significant increase in the bleeding time, ranging from 30% to approximately a doubling of the control measurements. These changes were obtained with single doses as low as 80 mg and, upon repeated daily dosing, with as low as 20 mg (19) of aspirin, coincident with greater than 90% suppression of serum TXB_2 levels. In the study of De Caterina et al. (23), the daily administration of 50 mg aspirin to patients with coronary artery disease was associated with biochemical and functional changes that were indistinguishable from those achieved with 324 mg daily, upon reaching steady-state suppression of platelet cyclooxygenase activity. Thus, the measurable ex vivo (i.e., inhibition of TXA_2-dependent platelet aggregation) and in vivo (i.e., prolongation of the bleeding time) effects of a standard dose of aspirin can be fully reproduced by a dose of the drug reducing platelet cyclooxygenase activity by greater than 95%. The only difference is related to the different rate at which such a maximal effect is achieved, over several days rather than instantaneously. Such a potential disadvantage of low-dose aspirin can be overcome by a loading dose (e.g., 120 mg) followed by a daily maintenance dose (e.g., 30 to 50 mg) (21,22). Lesser degrees of inhibition would not be expected adequately to prevent TXA_2-dependent platelet activation, because substantial TXA_2 biosynthesis in vivo may occur in the face of conventionally important (e.g., 80% to 90%) but incomplete suppression of the platelet biosynthetic capacity (24).

The Aspirin Dose Issue

There are both theoretical and practical reasons to choose the lowest effective dose of aspirin (Table 8-1). The gastrointestinal side effects of aspirin appear to be dose-dependent (8,25), and for secondary prevention, treatment with aspirin is recommended for an indefinite period. There are also theoretical reasons to select a dose of aspirin that inhibits TXA_2 synthesis without inhibiting the vascular synthesis of PGI_2. Thus, it has been speculated that a low dose (e.g., 30 mg daily) might be more antithrombotic because it inhibits

TABLE 8-1. Vascular disorders for which aspirin has been shown to be effective and minimum effective dose

Disorder	Minimum effective daily dose (mg)
Stable angina	75
Unstable angina	75
Acute myocardial infarction	160
Transient cerebral ischemia and minor ischemic stroke	50
Acute ischemic stroke	160

PGI_2 synthesis to a lesser degree than a high dose. However, attempts to identify a dosage (or dosing regimen) of aspirin that blocks TXA_2 production without inhibiting PGI_2 synthesis have yielded conflicting results, largely depending upon the ex vivo versus in vivo type of assessment of PGI_2 production (25). The clinical relevance of the so-called aspirin dilemma probably has been overemphasized. It seems likely that substantial PGI_2 production is maintained in vivo in the face of once-daily regimens of aspirin, because of the 24-hour dosing interval allowing recovery of COX-1 activity in vascular endothelial cells, and possibly because of endothelial COX-2 induction in response to platelet activation (26). On the other hand, it is possible that differences in the inhibitory effects of the doses of aspirin that were studied (30 to 1,300 mg daily) were too small to test the hypothesis that inhibition of vascular PGI_2 synthesis is clinically relevant (25). Recent experience with mice deficient in the gene encoding the PGI_2 receptor (IP) supports the importance of this eicosanoid in the regulation of both thrombosis and inflammation in vivo (27).

It has been claimed that the dose of aspirin needed to suppress fully platelet aggregation may be higher in patients with cerebrovascular disease than in healthy subjects and may vary from time to time in the same patient. Terms such as "aspirin failure" or "aspirin resistance" have been used in these studies (27,28) to designate less than complete inhibition of platelet aggregation. One important caveat in the interpretation of these measurements of platelet function is represented by the uncon-

trolled nature of the studies, which does not recognize the contribution of (a) intrasubject variability of the aggregation measurements, (b) lack of compliance with study medication, or (c) drug interactions potentially preventing acetylation of platelet PGHS-1 by aspirin (29). The latter may be particularly relevant to elderly patients who are often on NSAIDs because of arthritic problems and may require low-dose aspirin for cardiovascular prophylaxis. Because selective acetylation of Ser[529] of PGHS-1 by aspirin is probably due to a low-affinity, reversible binding of its carboxyl group to Arg[120], creating a local high concentration of the acetylating moiety in close proximity with Ser[529] (6) (Fig. 8-1), the concurrent administration on another NSAID docking at the same binding site on Arg[120] may interfere with the acetylation process. Certainly, questions about the effectiveness of aspirin therapy in blocking platelet and nonplatelet sources of prostanoid synthesis should continue to be raised. For example, enhanced TXB_2 metabolite excretion has been described in some patients with unstable angina while on an intravenous low-dose aspirin regimen (30). This may reflect the contribution of extraplatelet sources of TXA_2 biosynthesis, including the inducible expression of PGHS-2 in monocytes/macrophages (31).

To date, mutations in either PGHS isoform that render the enzyme immune to inactivation by aspirin have not been described. The functional importance, if any, of a common polymorphism in the human PGHS-2 sequence (32) remains to be elucidated.

Lack of Dose Dependence in the Antithrombotic Effect of Aspirin

Inhibition of TXA_2-dependent platelet function by aspirin may lead to prevention of thrombosis as well as to excess bleeding. The balance between the two depends critically on the absolute thrombotic versus hemorrhagic risk of the patient. Thus, in individuals at low risk for vascular occlusion, a small absolute benefit may be the offset by exposure of large numbers of healthy subjects to undue bleeding complications (Fig. 8-3). As the risk of experiencing a major vascular event increases, so does the absolute benefit of antiplatelet prophylaxis with aspirin (Fig. 8-3) for a number of clinical settings where the efficacy of the drug has been tested in randomized clinical trials. Based on the results of over 50 such trials, which are discussed elsewhere in this volume, the antithrombotic effect of aspirin does not appear to be dose related in a wide range of daily doses (30 to 1,300 mg), consistent with saturability of platelet cyclooxygenase inhibition at very low doses (8). In contrast, gastrointestinal toxicity of the drug does appear to be dose related, consistent with dose-dependent and dosing interval–dependent inhibition of PGHS-1 activity in the nucleated cell lining of the gastrointestinal mucosa. Thus, the lowest effective dose of the drug should be used for long-term prophylaxis. This ranges between 50 and 100 mg daily for most clinical indications (Table 8-1).

Other Cyclooxygenase Inhibitors

A variety of NSAIDs can inhibit TXA_2-dependent platelet function through competitive, reversible inhibition of PGHS-1. In general, these drugs, when used at conventional anti-inflammatory dosage, only incompletely inhibit platelet cyclooxygenase activity by 70% to 85%. This level of inhibition may be insufficient to block adequately platelet aggregation in vivo because of the very substantial biosynthetic capacity of human platelets to produce TXA_2 (17,24).

The only reversible cyclooxygenase inhibitors that have been tested in randomized clinical trials for their antithrombotic efficacy are sulfinpyrazone, indobufen, and triflusal. Sulfinpyrazone is a uricosuric agent structurally related to the anti-inflammatory agent phenlybutazone. When used at the highest approved dosage of 200 mg four times daily, the drug inhibits platelet cyclooxygenase activity by approximately 60%, after conversion from an inactive sulfoxide to an active sulfide metabolite (33). The conflicting or negative results obtained in randomized clinical trials of sulfinpyrazone (25) in patients with myocardial infarction or unstable angina, respectively, are not surprising in light of the drug being a weak cyclooxygenase inhibitor with no other established antiplatelet mechanism of action.

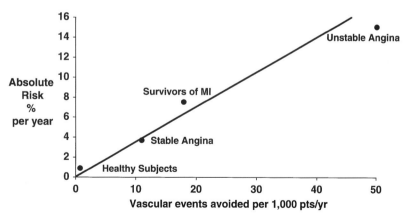

FIG. 8-3. The absolute risk of vascular complications is the major determinant of the absolute benefit of antiplatelet prophylaxis. Data are plotted from placebo-controlled aspirin trials in different clinical settings. For each category of patients, the ordinate denotes the absolute risk of experiencing a major vascular event as recorded in the placebo arm of the trial(s). The absolute benefit of antiplatelet treatment is reported on the abscissa as the number of important vascular events (non-fatal MI, non-fatal stroke, or vascular death) actually prevented by treating 1,000 patients with aspirin for 1 year. (Data from the Antiplatelet Trialists' Collaboration, ref. 54.)

In contrast, indobufen is an effective inhibitor of platelet cyclooxygenase activity and has biochemical, functional, and clinical effects that are comparable with those of a standard dose of aspirin. Thus, at therapeutic plasma levels achieved after oral dosing of 200 mg twice daily, indobufen inhibits serum TXB_2 by greater than 95% throughout the dosing interval (34) and reduces urinary thromboxane metabolite excretion to an extent comparable with aspirin (35). The finding that indobufen is as effective as aspirin in preventing coronary graft occlusion in two randomized trials (25) is mechanistically consistent with the concept of platelet cyclooxygenase inhibition, largely accounting for the antithrombotic effect of aspirin, as discussed above.

Triflusal, a salicylic acid derivative, reversibly inhibits platelet cyclooxygenase activity after conversion to a long-lived metabolite, 2-hydroxy-4-trifluoromethyl-benzoic acid (36). Although the half-life of the parent compound is only about 30 minutes, that of the deacetylated metabolite approximates 2 days. Although triflusal is claimed to have negligible effects on vascular PGI_2 production, this is likely to reflect the experimental conditions used for the assessment of PGI_2 production ex vivo. None of these reversible cyclooxygenase inhibitors is approved as an antiplatelet drug in the United States.

THROMBOXANE-SYNTHASE INHIBITORS AND THROMBOXANE RECEPTOR ANTAGONISTS

Thromboxane-synthase is the enzyme that catalyzes the synthesis of TXA_2 from its immediate precursor, PGH_2. Selective inhibitors of this enzyme have at least two theoretical advantages over cyclooxygenase inhibitors as potential antithrombotic agents (37). They do not prevent further metabolism of PGH_2 via other isomerases to form putatively beneficial eicosanoids, such as PGI_2 in the vasculature, gastric mucosa, and renal cortex, as well as PGE_2 in the gastric mucosa and renal medulla. Secondly, PGH_2 that accumulates in

platelets due to blockade of TX-synthase may be transferred to endothelial PGI_2-synthase at the site of platelet-vessel wall interaction, a process described as "endoperoxide steal" or transcellular metabolism (38). In fact, selective inhibition of TXA_2 biosynthesis coincident with enhanced PGI_2 formation in vivo has been demonstrated after short-term administration of dazoxiben and CGS 13080 to healthy subjects (37).

Despite these attractive features and the efficacy of selective TX-synthase inhibitors in short-term animal models of thrombosis, the results of limited phase II clinical studies have been largely disappointing and have led most pharmaceutical companies to stop clinical development of these compounds. Several factors may have contributed to such failures, including (a) the clinical endpoints of the studies being not necessarily related to TXA_2-dependent phenomena (e.g., restenosis after angioplasty), (b) inadequate pharmacokinetic features of the compounds tested resulting in substantial recovery of TXA_2 synthesis during the dosing interval, and (c) substitution for the biologic effects of TXA_2 by PGH_2 at the shared platelet and vascular receptors (37). Given that selective inhibition of platelet TXA_2 formation can be achieved with novel aspirin formulations (see above), the value of TX-synthase inhibitors is dependent on enhancing vascular PGI_2 production, the clinical significance of which remains to be established.

The TXA_2/PGH_2 receptor (TP) is a G protein–coupled receptor that, on ligand stimulation, results in activation of phospholipase C and subsequent increase in inositol 1,4,5-trisphosphate, diacylglycerol, and intracellular Ca^{2+} concentrations. The human TP cDNA was originally cloned from placenta and a platelet-like megakaryocyte cell line (39). A second form of the TP has recently been cloned from human umbilical vein endothelial cells (40). The endothelial isoform, termed $TP\beta$, and the platelet/placental receptor, termed $TP\alpha$, are derived by an alternative splicing mechanism; they are identical for the first 328 amino acids, but differ in their carboxyl-terminal cytoplasmic tails. Although endothelial cells contain only the TPβ, both TPα and TPβ are expressed in placental tissues and in platelets (40).

Potent (Kd in the low nanomolar range) and long-lasting (half-life more than 20 hours) TP antagonists have been developed, including GR 32191, BMS-180291 (ifetroban), and BM 13.177 (sulotroban). Despite the antithrombotic activity demonstrated in various animal species and the interesting "cardioprotective" activity demonstrated in dogs and ferrets (41), these compounds have yielded disappointing results in phase II/III clinical trials (42–44). Before drawing definitive conclusions on the apparent failure of this pharmacologic approach, it should be mentioned that these studies suffer from severe limitations, such as (a) unrealistic hypotheses of risk reduction being tested (e.g., a 50% reduction in the late clinical failure rate after successful coronary angioplasty); (b) heterogeneous endpoints being pooled together, including "clinically important restenosis," for which no evidence of TXA_2-dependence was obtained by earlier aspirin trials; and (c) an antischemic effect being tested in patients with unstable coronary syndromes treated with standard therapy, including aspirin.

Clinical development of GR 32191 and sulotroban has been discontinued, based on these disappointing, although largely predictable, results. It would be interesting to see the clinical development of at least one such compound being completed up to phase III trials with adequate endpoints and a realistic sample size. The potential advantages that potent TP antagonists might have vis-à-vis low-dose aspirin are related to the recent discovery of aspirin-insensitive agonists of the platelet receptor, such as TXA_2 derived from monocyte PGHS-2 and the F_2-isoprostane, 8-epi-$PGF_{2\alpha}$, a product of free radical–catalyzed peroxidation of arachidonic acid (45). The latter can synergize with subthreshold concentrations of other platelet agonists to evoke a full aggregatory response, thus providing an amplification mechanism of platelet activation in those clinical settings associated with enhanced lipid peroxidation (46).

Molecules that combine TX-synthase inhibition with TP antagonism also have been developed, based on experimental evidence suggesting a synergistic interaction between the two approaches (47,48). The only such molecule tested in clinical studies, ridogrel, is far from having the desirable balance of the two activities and, perhaps not surprisingly, has not lived up to its expectations (49).

DIPYRIDAMOLE

Dipyridamole is a pyrimidopyrimidine derivative with vasodilator and antiplatelet properties. Dipyridamole inhibits platelet aggregation in whole blood at lower concentrations than in plasma (50). The mechanism of action of dipyridamole as an antiplatelet agent has been a subject of controversy (51). Both inhibition of cyclic nucleotide phosphodiesterase (the enzyme that degrades cyclic adenosine monophosphate [cAMP] to 5′-AMP, resulting in the intraplatelet accumulation of cAMP) and blockade of the uptake of adenosine (which acts at A_2 receptors for adenosine to stimulate platelet adenylyl cyclase) have been suggested. Moreover, direct stimulation of PGI_2 synthesis and protection against its degradation have been reported, although the dipyridamole concentrations required to produce these effects far exceed the low micromolar plasma levels achieved after oral administration of conventional doses (100 to 400 mg daily).

The absorption of dipyridamole from conventional formulations is variable and may result in low systemic bioavailability of the drug. A modified-release formulation of dipyridamole with improved bioavailability has been developed recently in association with a low dose of aspirin (52). Dipyridamole is eliminated primarily by biliary excretion as a glucuronide conjugate and is subject to enterohepatic recirculation. A terminal half-life of 10 hours has been reported. This is consistent with the most recent twice-daily regimen used in clinical studies.

Although the clinical efficacy of dipyridamole, alone or in combination with aspirin, has been questioned on the basis of earlier randomized trials (51), the whole issue has been reopened by the results of the recently published European Stroke Prevention Study 2 (53). This study has been criticized for the continued inclusion of a placebo arm after the place of aspirin in the secondary prevention of stroke (54) had been established to the satisfaction of most authorities. Whether the favorable results obtained in this trial reflect the higher dose (400 versus 225 mg daily) and improved systemic bioavailability of modified-release dipyridamole (52) vis-à-vis conventional formulations and/or the large sample size and statistical power of the study remains to be established.

TICLOPIDINE AND CLOPIDOGREL

Ticlopidine and clopidogrel are structurally related thienopyridines with platelet-inhibitory properties. Both drugs selectively inhibit ADP-induced platelet aggregation with no direct effects on arachidonic acid metabolism (55). Although ticlopidine and clopidogrel also can inhibit platelet aggregation induced by collagen and thrombin, these inhibitory effects are abolished by increasing the agonist concentration and therefore are likely to reflect blockade of ADP-mediated amplification of the response to other agonists.

Neither ticlopidine nor clopidogrel affect ADP-induced platelet aggregation when added in vitro, up to 500 μmol/L, thus suggesting that in vivo hepatic transformation to an active metabolite(s) is necessary for their antiplatelet effects. However, the molecular characterization of these metabolites has remained elusive. Nor has the molecular target of thienopyridine derivatives been clearly elucidated. Several lines of evidence suggest that clopidogrel, and most likely, also ticlopidine, induces irreversible alterations of a putative platelet ADP receptor mediating the inhibition of stimulated adenylyl cyclase activity by ADP (56). The inhibition of platelet function by clopidogrel is associated with a selective reduction in the number of ADP binding sites,

with no consistent change in the binding affinity (56). Permanent modification of a putative ADP receptor by thienopyridines is consistent with time-dependent cumulative inhibition of ADP-induced platelet aggregation upon repeated daily dosing and with slow recovery of platelet function upon drug withdrawal (57).

Up to 90% of a single oral dose of ticlopidine is rapidly absorbed in humans (55). Peak plasma concentrations occur 1 to 3 hours after a single oral dose of 250 mg. These concentrations increase by approximately threefold because of drug accumulation upon repeated twice-daily dosing over 2 to 3 weeks. Greater than 98% of ticlopidine is reversibly bound to plasma proteins, primarily albumin. Ticlopidine is metabolized rapidly and extensively. A total of 13 metabolites have been identified in humans. Of these, only the 2-keto derivative of ticlopidine is more potent than the parent compound in inhibiting ADP-induced platelet aggregation (55).

The apparent elimination half-life of ticlopidine is 24 to 36 hours after a single oral dose and up to 96 hours after 14 days of repeated dosing (55). The recommended regimen of ticlopidine is 250 mg twice daily, although it is unclear how a twice-daily regimen is related to the pharmacokinetic and pharmacodynamic features noted above. A delayed antithrombotic effect was noted in at least one open clinical trial of ticlopidine, in patients with unstable angina, with no apparent protection during the first 2 weeks of drug administration (58).

A synergistic effect of ticlopidine and aspirin has been described in rats, both in terms of ADP-induced platelet aggregation ex vivo and in several experimental models of platelet-dependent thrombosis (59). Interestingly, the ticlopidine/aspirin combination was reported to produce only additive effects on the tail bleeding time prolongation (59). The mechanism(s) underlying these findings remains speculative. Ticlopidine is roughly equivalent to aspirin in the secondary prevention of stroke (54). However, the association of ticlopidine therapy with hypercholesterolemia and neutropenia and its comparative expense has reduced enthusiasm for this therapy as an alternative to aspirin in most situations (60). More recently, the combination of aspirin with ticlopidine has gained popularity as adjuvant therapy for patients undergoing pecutaneous transluminal coronary angioplasty (PTCA) with placement of stents (61). These issues are discussed in detail elsewhere in this volume.

The pharmacokinetics of clopidogrel are somewhat different from those of ticlopidine. Thus, after administration of single oral doses (up to 200 mg) or repeated doses (up to 100 mg daily), unchanged clopidogrel was not detectable in peripheral venous plasma (57). Concentrations of 1 to 2 ng/ml were measured in the plasma of patients receiving clopidogrel 150 mg per day (twice as much as the dose used in the CAPRIE [clopidogrel versus aspirin in patients at risk of ischaemic events] study and likely to be approved) for 16 days. The main systemic metabolite of clopidogrel is the carboxylic acid derivative SR 26334. Based on measurements of circulating levels of SR 26334, it has been inferred that clopidogrel is rapidly absorbed and extensively metabolized (57). The plasma elimination half-life of SR 26334 is approximately 8 hours. As noted above, clopidogrel, inactive in vitro, is metabolically transformed by the liver into a short-lived platelet inhibitor of unknown structure (56).

ADP-induced platelet aggregation was inhibited in a dose-dependent fashion with an apparent ceiling effect (40% inhibition) at 400 mg after single oral doses of clopidogrel administered to healthy volunteers. Inhibition of platelet aggregation was detectable at 2 hours after oral dosing of 400 mg and remained relatively stable up to 48 hours (57). Upon repeated daily dosing of 50 to 100 mg of clopidogrel to healthy volunteers, ADP-induced platelet aggregation was inhibited from the second day of treatment (25% to 30% inhibition) and reached a steady-state (50% to 60% inhibition) after 4 to 7 days. Such a level of maximal inhibition was comparable with that achieved with ticlopidine (500 mg daily),

although the latter showed a slower onset of the antiplatelet effect as compared with clopidogrel. No appreciable differences in the inhibitory effects of 50, 75, and 100 mg of clopidogrel were noted in this study, suggesting that 50 mg daily may be at or close to the top of the dose-response curve. It is interesting to note that 50 mg is only about 12% of the dose of clopidogrel necessary to achieve maximal inhibition of ADP-induced platelet aggregation, after single dosing. Given the short half-life of the putative active metabolite of clopidogrel, this is unlikely to accumulate to any substantial extent upon repeated daily dosing of the parent compound.

The best available interpretation of the above findings is that, upon repeated daily administration of low doses, the active metabolite of clopidogrel has a pharmacodynamic pattern similar to that of aspirin in causing cumulative inhibition. As in the case of aspirin, platelet function returned to normal 7 days after the last dose of clopidogrel. Both the cumulative nature of the inhibitory effects and the slow rate of recovery of platelet function are consistent with the active moieties of aspirin (acetylsalicylic acid) and clopidogrel (metabolite X), causing a permanent defect in a platelet protein, that cannot be repaired during the 24-hour dosing interval and can only be replaced as a function of platelet turnover. This also justifies the once daily regimen of both drugs, despite their short half-life in the human circulation.

Bleeding time measurements performed in the same multiple dose study of clopidogrel described above showed a comparable prolongation (by 1.5- to 2.0-fold over control) at 50 to 100 mg daily or ticlopidine 500 mg daily (57).

Clopidogrel has undergone an unusual clinical development, with limited phase II studies and a single, very large phase III trial (CAPRIE) to test its efficacy and safety at 75 mg daily vis-à-vis aspirin 325 mg daily (62). The overall results of this pivotal study indicate that the two drugs are equally effective in preventing major vascular complications in patients with a recent myocardial infarction or

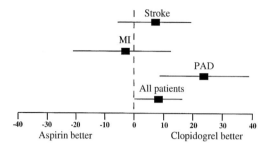

FIG. 8-4. Relative risk reduction and 95% confidence interval by disease subgroup in the CAPRIE study. A test of heterogeneity of these three treatment effects was statistically significant (p = 0.042). MI, myocardial infarction; PAD, peripheral arterial disease. A randomized, blinded, trial of clopidogrel versus aspirin in patients at risk of ischaemic events (CAPRIE). (Adapted from the CAPRIE Steering Committee, ref. 62, with permission.)

ischemic stroke (Fig. 8-4). However, clopidogrel seems more effective than aspirin in patients enrolled in the study because of symptomatic peripheral arterial disease (62). This interesting, and perhaps unexpected, finding would suggest varying pathophysiologic importance of TXA_2 and ADP in different clinical settings and may warrant further mechanistic studies exploring combined strategies based on the two best characterized approaches to antiplatelet therapy.

The safety of clopidogrel appears to be definitely superior to that of ticlopidine and comparable with that of medium-dose aspirin (62).

GLYCOPROTEIN IIb/IIIa ANTAGONISTS

Given the redundancy of discrete pathways leading to platelet aggregation, it is not surprising that the clinical efficacy of aspirin, ticlopidine, and clopidogrel is only partial. These drugs, although inhibiting TXA_2- or ADP-mediated platelet aggregation, leave the activity of other platelet agonists, such as thrombin, largely unaffected. After recognition that the expression of functionally active glycoprotein IIb/IIIa (GPIIb/IIIa) ($\alpha IIb\beta3$) on the platelet surface is the final common pathway of platelet aggregation, regardless of the initi-

ating stimulus, this glycoprotein has become the target of novel antiplatelet drugs (63,64). The inhibitors of GPIIb/IIIa include monoclonal antibodies against the receptor, naturally occurring RGD-containing peptides isolated from snake venoms, synthetic RGD- or KGD-containing peptides, as well as peptidomimetic and nonpeptide RGD mimetics that compete with fibrinogen for occupancy of its platelet receptor. The mechanism of action of these compounds is illustrated in Fig. 8-5.

Coller and colleagues demonstrated that blockade of the fibrinogen receptor could essentially induce a functional thrombasthenic phenotype by developing murine monoclonal antibodies against platelet GPIIb/IIIa (65). Approximately 40,000 antibody molecules bind to the surface of platelets, indicating that there are probably 40,000 to 80,000 GPIIb/IIIa receptors per platelet (64). Platelet aggregation is significantly inhibited at antibody doses that decrease the number of available receptors to less than 50% of normal. Platelet aggregation is nearly completely abolished at approximately 80% receptor blockade, although the bleeding time is only mildly affected. It is only with more than 90% receptor blockade that the bleeding time becomes extremely prolonged (64). Because of concerns about immunogenicity of the original 7E3 antibody, a mouse/human chimeric 7E3 Fab (abciximab) was created for clinical development. After bolus injection of abciximab, dose-dependent inhibition of ADP-induced platelet aggregation ex vivo was recorded in patients judged to be at moderate to high risk of PTCA-associated ischemic complications (66). A bolus dose of 0.25 mg/kg was found to result in blockade of more than 80% of platelet receptors and reduce platelet aggregation in response to 20 μmol/L ADP to less than 20% of baseline. A steep dose-response relationship was apparent in this study (66). Peak effects on receptor blockade, platelet aggregation, and bleeding time were observed at the first sampling time of 2 hours after bolus administration of 0.25 mg/kg. Gradual recovery of platelet function then occurred over time, with bleeding times returning to near normal values by 12 hours (66). The ad-

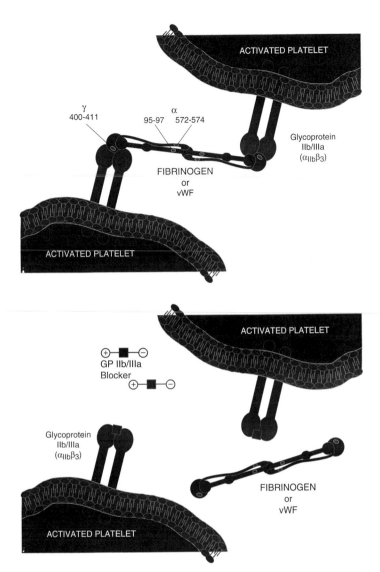

FIG. 8-5. Mechanism of action of GPIIb/IIIa antagonists. The upper portion of the figure illustrates fibrinogen binding to GPIIb/IIIa receptors expressed on the surface of two adjacent activated platelets. The sites of fibrinogen interaction with GPIIb/IIIa receptors have a positive charge separated from a negative charge within the primary amino acid sequence. This pattern is best characterized by the RGD sequence of fibrinogen. Compounds that mimic this RGD sequence form the basis for the development of GPIIb/IIIa antagonists (lower part of the figure). (From Dr. R.J. Gould, Department of Pharmacology, Merck & Co., West Point, PA, with permission.)

ministration of a 0.25 mg/kg bolus dose of abciximab followed by a 10 µg/min infusion for 12 hours demonstrated that receptor blockade, inhibition of platelet aggregation and prolongation of bleeding time could be maintained throughout the duration of the infusion (66).

This regimen was chosen for the pivotal phase III trial (EPIC) that demonstrated both short-term and long-term clinical efficacy of abciximab, added to conventional antithrombotic therapy, in reducing the incidence of ischemic events in patients undergoing PTCA.

These results formed the basis for approval by the U.S. Food and Drug Administration (FDA) of abciximab (ReoPro, Lilly, Indianapolis, IN) as adjunctive therapy for patients undergoing high-risk PTCA and atherectomy. Subsequently, it has been found that a reduction in the dosage of concomitant heparin can greatly reduce the bleeding complications attendant to abciximab administration (67). Further judicious study of the interaction of GPIIb/IIIa inhibitors with the newer, specific inhibitors of thrombin seems merited (68,69).

Although the efficacy of abciximab in preventing vascular occlusion by suppressing platelet aggregation is likely to be the major mechanism for its beneficial effects, it is quite possible that the potent inhibition of thrombus formation by this antibody may result in decreased thrombin formation (70). In fact, abciximab produced dose-dependent inhibition of tissue factor–induced thrombin generation, reaching a plateau of 45% to 50% inhibition at concentrations of at least 15 µg/ml (70). Whether the inhibition of thrombin generation by abciximab contributes to its immediate antithrombotic effect and/or to its alleged effects on long-term vascular restenosis (71) remains to be established.

Several RGD-containing low-molecular weight peptides that compete with fibrinogen for GPIIb/IIIa binding have been isolated from the venom of several species of the viper family. These peptides, known as "disintegrins," include trigramin, bitistatin, echistatin, kistrin, and applagin (72). The amino acid sequence of 25 different disintegrins is known (72).

Although these peptides have provided interesting insight into the structural requirements for GPIIb/IIIa antagonism, their potential clinical application is hampered by their immunogenicity and propensity to cause transient thrombocytopenia. Moreover, RGD-containing disintegrins are not integrin specific and inhibit the adhesive functions of many other RGD-dependent integrins. The unique disintegrin peptide, barbourin, containing a conservative amino acid substitution

of Lys (K) for Arg (R) in the RGD sequence, is highly specific for GPIIb/IIIa.

Integrin specificity can be mimicked by small, conformationally restrained peptides containing the KGD sequence (73). In addition to natural antagonists, a variety of RGD- or KGD-containing GPIIb/IIIa inhibitors have been synthesized. When in a cyclical configuration, these synthetic peptides show a markedly increased affinity for GPIIb/IIIa, quite comparable with that of the naturally occurring antagonists. Agents in this group include MK-852 and integrilin (eptifibatide). The latter drug causes very rapid and profound (more than 80%) suppression of ADP-induced platelet aggregation in patients undergoing PTCA, who were already receiving aspirin and heparin (74). Unfortunately, technical difficulties in phase II may have precluded selection of the optimal dose of eptifibatide for evaluation in phase III (75). A randomized, placebo-controlled evaluation of the drug in more than 4,000 patients undergoing elective, urgent, or emergency coronary intervention failed to establish a dose-response relationship or to influence the primary endpoint of the study (76), leading to a failure of the FDA to approve its usage (77). A preliminary report at the XIXth Congress of the European Society of Cardiology indicated that a higher dose of eptifibatide reduced death or myocardial infarct for 15.7% to 14.2% (p = 0.042) in patients with acute ischemic syndromes.

Whether the higher degree of specificity for GPIIb/IIIa receptors (perhaps in their activated form) on platelets, shorter half-life, and lower immunogenicity of the synthetic antagonists vis-à-vis abciximab will translate into improved efficacy and/or safety remains to be demonstrated. In fact, it has been argued that blockade of the $\alpha_v\beta_3$-vitronectin receptor in vascular cells by abciximab may have contributed to an effect on clinical restenosis (71). More recently, nonpeptide mimetics of the RGD sequence have been developed. These include lamifiban, tirofiban, fradafiban, roxifiban, orbofiban, and xemilofiban. Both lamifiban and tirofiban have undergone extensive clinical testing in phase II dose-ranging studies (78,79). Similarly to abciximab, these compounds inhibit ADP-induced platelet aggregation and prolong bleeding time with a steep dose-response relationship, encompassing only a three- to fivefold increase in dose and plasma concentrations. Tirofiban has recently been reported to reduce myocardial (re)infarction and death by 25% in 3,200 low-risk patients with unstable angina or non–Q-wave myocardial infarction, when compared with heparin alone (80), and in 1,500 patients on heparin who suffered unstable angina/non–Q-wave infarction and were undergoing acute intervention. Abciximab also has been shown recently to reduce the incidence of thrombotic complications in patients with refractory unstable angina (81).

Several of these nonpeptide GPIIb/IIIa inhibitors are orally active and have the potential to be given long term (82). However, a number of issues remain unsolved. These include the uncertainty as to the optimal degree of GPIIb/IIIa receptor blockade compatible with superior efficacy vis-à-vis aspirin (and most preferably clopidogrel) and acceptable bleeding risk during long-term administration; the inadequacy of currently available surrogate markers for efficacy (ADP-induced platelet aggregation) and safety (skin bleeding time), on which dose-finding studies are based; the steep dose-response curve noted above; and the potential need for dose titration and monitoring. In fact, there seems to be a large discrepancy between the state-of-the-art technology deployed in the design and clinical development of these novel an-

tiplatelet drugs and the somewhat antiquated methodology used to assess their functional effects in humans. Although the analytical measurement of mechanism-related biochemical endpoints has played a crucial role in defining the dose dependence and time dependence of the antiplatelet effects of aspirin in humans, no such development has occurred in the field of these novel antiplatelet agents.

OTHER DRUGS WITH ANTIPLATELET EFFECTS

A variety of other drugs have been shown to possess antiplatelet effects in vitro and/or ex vivo. These are listed in Table 8-2. Although at some stage they were considered potential candidates for new drug development by several pharmaceutical companies, none has actually reached the market with a specific labeling as an antiplatelet agent (with the possible exception of Japan), and emphasis in drug development has shifted toward other, more promising approaches.

A number of natural prostanoids (e.g., PGE_1 and PGI_2) and prostanoid analogs (iloprost, beraprost, cicaprost, ciprostene) can elevate platelet cAMP levels and inhibit platelet aggregation. A serious limitation to their use as antiplatelet agents is represented by concomitant, peripheral vasodilation as well as their short half-life in the systemic circulation. However, preliminary experience with oral prostacyclin analogs in primary pulmonary hypertension appears promising (83). Nitric oxide donors can potentially inhibit platelet activation by virtue of their effects in

TABLE 8-2. *Other drugs with antiplatelet effects*

Products	Mechanism of the antiplatelet action	Vascular effects
Adenylyl-cyclase activators (e.g., PGI₂ analogs)	↑ cAMP	Vasodilation
Guanylyl-cyclase activators (e.g., NO donors)	↑ cGMP	Vasodilation
Phosphodiesterase III inhibitors (e.g., cilostazol)	↑ cAMP	Vasodilation
5HT₂-antagonists (e.g., ketanserin)	↓ serotonin-induced aggregation	Vasodilation
PAF antagonists	↓ PAF-induced aggregation	Variable
Omega-3 fatty acids	Changes in membrane composition?	Slight decrease in blood pressure
Vitamin E	PKC-dependent mechanism?	Prevents endothelial dysfunction

elevating cyclic guanosine monophosphate (cGMP) levels. They represent a diverse group of agents with unique chemical structures and biochemical requirements for generation of NO (84). Preliminary evidence for an in vivo effect of the nitric oxide donor S-nitrosoglutathione in inhibiting platelet activation has been reported recently, in patients with severe preeclampsia (85) and in patients with acute coronary syndromes (86). However, this was associated with detectable hemodynamic changes. Potent inhibitors of phosphodiesterase III also have been developed as potential antithrombotic agents. A representative of this class, cilostazol, was approved in Japan for the treatment of peripheral arterial disease. However, the spectrum of pharmacologic effects of this compound is quite wide and includes bronchodilator and bronchoprotective effects in vivo (87), as well as suppression of mitogenesis of rat mesangial cells in vitro (88).

Ketanserin, a $5HT_2$ antagonist, has been developed as a potential antithrombotic agent up to a phase III evaluation in patients with peripheral vascular disease, which gave largely negative results (89). Another $5HT_2$ antagonist, Sarpogrelate (Mitsubishi), has been approved for the treatment of peripheral arterial disease in Japan, whereas other compounds are being developed for other indications such as migraine or anxiety.

Several potent and selective platelet activating factor (PAF) antagonists also have been developed, although their primary indication so far is in the treatment of asthma.

Omega-3 polyunsaturated fatty acids modulate a wide range of cellular responses, including platelet and vascular function (90–93). However, grams of fish oil suppress platelet activation less impressively than a single dose of aspirin (90), and convincing evidence that they influence the atherogenic process, other than by substituting for saturated fats in the diet, remains to be provided (94).

Finally, platelet incorporation of α-tocopherol at levels attained with oral supplementation is associated with inhibition of platelet aggregation via a protein kinase C-dependent mechanism (95). This may represent one potential mechanism for the observed beneficial effects of vitamin E supplementation in preventing myocardial infarction in patients with ischemic heart disease (96). However, pharmacologic doses of vitamin E can affect platelet as well as endothelial function through other mechanisms, possibly related to its ability to inhibit low-density lipoprotein oxidation. The development of analytical methods assessing lipid peroxidation in vivo, such as the measurement of urinary F_2-isoprostanes, should help in defining the dose-response relationship for the antioxidant effects of vitamin E as a rational basis for future trials in the cardiovascular area (45).

CONCLUSION

Given the very solid evidence for efficacy and safety combined with low cost, aspirin is likely to remain the mainstay of antiplatelet therapy. The results of a large head-to-head comparison of clopidogrel and aspirin suggest that a thienopyridine-sensitive ADP receptor and aspirin-sensitive TXA_2 biosynthesis may contribute equally to the amplification of the hemostatic response to plaque destabilization. This in turn provides a rationale for exploring the efficacy and safety of an aspirin/clopidogrel combination for secondary prevention.

A number of oral GPIIb/IIIa blockers are currently being developed for long-term antiplatelet prophylaxis, based on the encouraging results of the short-term use of parenteral agents in high-risk settings. Whether substantially improved efficacy will be obtained at acceptable levels of safety, compliance, and cost, vis-à-vis aspirin or aspirin plus clopidogrel, represents an interesting question for clinical trials of the next millennium.

ACKNOWLEDGMENTS

This work was supported by grants from the National Institutes of Health (HL54500 and HL57847) and from the Consiglio Nazionale Delle Ricerche (CNR) (Progetto

Strategico Infarto 96.05268ST74). The expert editorial assistance of Andre Harris and Esther Stuart is gratefully acknowledged.

REFERENCES

1. Smith WL, Garavito M, DeWitt DL. Prostaglandin endoperoxide H synthases (cyclooxygenases)-1 and -2. *J Biol Chem* 1996;271:33157–33160.

2. FitzGerald GA. Mechanisms of platelet activation: thromboxane A₂ as an amplifying signal for other agonists. *Am J Cardiol* 1991;68:11B–15B.

3. Roth GJ, Stanford N, Majerus PW. Acetylation of prostaglandin synthetase by aspirin. *Proc Natl Acad Sci U S A* 1975;72:3073–3076.

4. DeWitt DL, Smith WL. Primary structure of prostaglandin G/H-synthase from sheep vesicular gland determined from the complementary DNA sequence. *Proc Natl Acad Sci U S A* 1988;85:1412–1416.

5. Funk C, Funk LB, Kennedy M, Pong A, FitzGerald GA. Human platelet/erythroleukemia cell PGG/H synthase: cDNA cloning, expression, mutagenesis and gene chromosomal assignment. *FASEB J* 1991;5:2304–2312.

6. Loll PJ, Picot D, Garavito RM. The structural basis of aspirin activity inferred from the crystal structure of inactivated prostaglandin H₂ synthase. *Nature Struct Biol* 1995;2:637–643.

7. Vane JR. Inhibition of prostaglandins as a mechanism of action for aspirin-like drugs. *Nature* 1971;231:232–235.

8. Patrono C. Aspirin as an antiplatelet drug. *N Engl J Med* 1994;330:1287–1294.

9. Szczeklik A, Krzanowski M, Gora P, Radwan J. Antiplatelet drugs and generation of thrombin in clotting blood. *Blood* 1992;80:2006–2011.

10. Pedersen AK, FitzGerald GA. Dose-related kinetics of aspirin. Presystemic acetylation of platelet cyclooxygenase. *N Engl J Med* 1984;311:1206–1211.

11. Clarke RJ, Mayo G, Price P, FitzGerald GA. Suppression of thromboxane A₂ but not systemic prostacyclin by controlled-release aspirin. *N Engl J Med* 1991;325:1137–1141.

12. McAdam B, Keimowitz RM, Maher M, Fitzgerald DJ. Transdermal modification of platelet function: an aspirin patch system results in marked suppression of platelet cyclooxygenase. *J Pharmacol Exp Ther* 1996;277:559–564.

13. Patrono C, Ciabattoni G, Pinca E, et al. Low dose aspirin and inhibition of thromboxane B₂ production in healthy subjects. *Thromb Res* 1980;17:317–327.

14. Thorngreen M, Shafi S, Born GVR. Thromboxane A₂ in skin bleeding-time blood and in clotted venous blood before and after administration of acetylsalicyclic acid. *Lancet* 1983;1:1075–1078.

15. Born GVR. Aggregation of blood platelets by adenosine diphosphate and its reversal. *Nature (Lond)* 1962;194:927–929.

16. Harker LA, Slichter SJ. The bleeding time as a screening test for evaluation of platelet function. *N Engl J Med* 1972;287:155–159.

17. Patrono C, Ciabattoni G, Pugliese F, Pierucci A, Blair IA, FitzGerald GA. Estimated rate of thromboxane secretion into the circulation of normal humans. *J Clin Invest* 1986;77:590–594.

18. Patrignani P, Filabozzi P, Patrono C. Selective cumulative inhibition of platelet thromboxane production by low-dose aspirin in healthy subjects. *J Clin Invest* 1982;69:1366–1372.

19. FitzGerald GA, Oates JA, Hawiger J, et al. Endogenous biosynthesis of prostacyclin and thromboxane and platelet function during chronic administration of aspirin in man. *J Clin Invest* 1983;71:676–688.

20. Burch JW, Stanford N, Majerus PW. Inhibition of platelet prostaglandin synthetase by oral aspirin. *J Clin Invest* 1978;61:314–319.

21. Patrono C, Ciabattoni G, Patrignani P, et al. Clinical pharmacology of platelet cyclooxygenase inhibition. *Circulation* 1985;72:1177–1183.

22. De Caterina R, Giannessi D, Bernini W, et al. Low-dose aspirin in patients recovering from myocardial infarction: evidence for a selective inhibition of thromboxane-related platelet function. *Eur Heart J* 1985;6:409–417.

23. De Caterina R, Giannessi D, Boem A, et al. Equal antiplatelet effects of aspirin 50 or 324 mg/day in patients after acute myocardial infarction. *Thromb Haemost* 1985;54:528–532.

24. Reilly IAG, FitzGerald GA. Inhibition of thromboxane formation in vivo and ex vivo: implications for therapy with platelet inhibitory drugs. *Blood* 1987;69:180–186.

25. Hirsh J, Dalen JE, Fuster V, Harker LB, Patrono C, Roth G. Aspirin and other platelet-active drugs. The relationship among dose, effectiveness, and side effects. *Chest* 1995;108(suppl):247–257.

26. Barry OP, Praticò D, Lawson JA, FitzGerald GA. Transcellular activation of platelets and endothelial cells by bioactive lipids in platelet microparticles. *J Clin Invest* 1997;99:2118–2127

27. Murata T, Ushikubi F, Matsuoka T, et al. Altered pain perception and inflammatory response in mice lacking prostacyclin receptor. *Nature* 1997;388:678–682.

28. Helgason CM, Bolin KM, Hoff JA, et al. Development of aspirin resistance in persons with previous ischemic stroke. *Stroke* 1994;25:2331–2336.

29. Patrono C, Roth GJ. Aspirin in ischemic cerebrovascular disease. How strong is the case for a different dosing regimen? *Stroke* 1996;27:756–760.

30. Vejar M, Fragasso G, Hackett D, et al. Dissociation of platelet activation and spontaneous myocardial ischemia in unstable angina. *Thromb Haemost* 1990;63:163–168.

31. Cipollone F, Patrignani P, Greco A, et al. Differential suppression of thromboxane biosynthesis by indobufen and aspirin in patients with unstable angina. *Circulation* 1997;96:1109–1116.

32. Jones DA, Carlton DP, McIntyre TM, Zimmerman GA, Prescott SM. Molecular cloning of human prostaglandin endoperoxide synthase type II and demonstration of expression in response to cytokines. *J Biol Chem* 1993;268:9049–9054.

33. Pedersen AK, FitzGerald GA. Cyclooxygenase inhibition, platelet function and drug metabolite formation during chronic administration of sulfinpyrazone in man. *Clin Pharmacol Ther* 1985;37:36–42.

34. Rebuzzi AG, Natale A, Bianchi C, Mariello F, Coppola E, Ciabattoni G. Effects of indobufen on platelet thromboxane B₂ production in patients with myocardial infarction. *Eur J Clin Pharmacol* 1990;39:99–100.

35. Davì G, Patrono C, Catalano I, et al. Inhibition of

thromboxane biosynthesis and platelet function by indobufen in type II diabetes mellitus. *Arterioscler
Thromb* 1993;13:1346–1349.

36. Ramis J, Torrent J, Mis R, et al. Pharmacokinetics of triflusal after single and repeated doses in man. *Int J Clin
Pharmacol Ther Toxicol* 1990;28:344–349.

37. FitzGerald GA, Reilly IAG, Pedersen AK. The biochemical pharmacology of thromboxane synthase inhibition in man. *Circulation* 1985;72:1194–1201.

38. Marcus AJ, Weksler BB, Jaffe EA, Broekman MJ. Synthesis of prostacyclin from platelet derived endoperoxides by cultured human endothelial cells. *J Clin Invest*
1980;66:979–984.

39. Hirata M, Hayashi Y, Ushikubi F, et al. Cloning and expression of the cDNA for a human thromboxane A_2 receptor gene. *Nature* 1991;349:617–619.

40. Raychowdhury MK, Yukawa M, Collins LJ, McGrail
SH, Kent KC, Ware JA. Alternative splicing produces a
divergent cytoplasmic tail in the human endothelial
thromboxane A_2 receptor. *J Biol Chem* 1994;269:
19256–19260 (erratum in *J Biol Chem* 1995;270:7011).

41. Gomoll AW, Grover GJ, Ogletree ML. Myocardial salvage efficacy of the thromboxane receptor antagonist
ifetroban in ferrets and dogs. *J Cardiovasc Pharmacol*
1994;24:960–968.

42. Serruys PW, Rutsch W, Heyndrickx GR, et al. Prevention of restenosis after percutaneous transluminal coronary angioplasty with thromboxane A_2-receptor blockade. *Circulation* 1991;84:1568–1580.

43. Savage MP, Goldberg S, Bove AA, et al. Effect of
thromboxane A_2 blockade on clinical outcome and
restenosis after successful coronary angioplasty: Multi-
Hospital Eastern Atlantic Restenosis Trial (M-HEART
II). *Circulation* 1995;92:3194–3200.

44. Remme WJ. Prevention of ischaemic cardiac events in
unstable angina and non-Q infarction. PRINCE, a
placebo controlled trial with Ifegatran-thromboxane A_2
receptor antagonist. Presented at the XVIIIth Congress
of the European Society of Cardiology, Birmingham,
UK, August 25–29, 1996.

45. Patrono C, FitzGerald GA. Isoprostanes: potential
markers of oxidant stress in atherothrombotic disease.
Arterioscler Thromb Vasc Biol (in press).

46. Praticò D, Smyth EM, Violi F, FitzGerald GA. Local
amplification of platelet function by 8-epi prostaglandin
F_{2a} is not mediated by thromboxane receptor isoforms.
J Biol Chem 1996;271:14916–14924.

47. Gresele P, Arnout J, Deckmyn H, et al. Role of proaggregatory and antiaggregatory prostaglandins in hemostasis. Studies with combined thromboxane synthase inhibition and thromboxane receptor antagonism. *J Clin
Invest* 1987;80:1435–1445.

48. Fitzgerald DJ, Fragetta J, FitzGerald GA. Prostaglandin
endoperoxides modulate the response to thromboxane
synthase inhibition during coronary thrombosis. *J Clin
Invest* 1988;82:1708–1713.

49. The RAPT Investigators. Randomized trial of Ridogrel,
a combined thromboxane A_2 synthase inhibitor and
thromboxane A_2/prostaglandin endoperoxide receptor
antagonist, versus aspirin as adjunct to thrombolysis in
patients with acute myocardial infarction. The Ridogrel
versus Aspirin Patency Trial (RAPT). *Circulation* 1994;
89:588–595.

50. Gresele P, Arnout J, Deckmyn H, Vermylen J. Mecha-

nism of the antiplatelet action of dipyridamole in whole
blood: modulation of adenosine concentration and activity. *Thromb Haemost* 1986;55:12–18.

51. FitzGerald GA. Dipyridamole. *N Engl J Med* 1987;316:
1247–1257.

52. Müller TH, Su CAPF, Weisenberger H, Brickl R,
Nehmiz G, Eisert WG. Dipyridamole alone or combined with low-dose acetylsalicylic acid inhibits platelet
aggregation in human whole blood ex vivo. *Br J Clin
Pharmacol* 1990;30:179–186.

53. Diener HC, Cunha L, Forbes C, Sivenius J, Smets P,
Lowenthal A. European Stroke Prevention Study 2:
dipyridamole and acetylsalicylic acid in the secondary
prevention of stroke. *J Neurol Sci* 1996;143:1–13.

54. Antiplatelet Trialists' Collaboration. Collaborative
overview of randomized trials of antiplatelet therapy: I.
Prevention of death, myocardial infarction, and stroke
by prolonged antiplatelet therapy in various categories
of patients. *Br Med J* 1994;308:81–106.

55. Ito MK, Smith AR, Lee ML. Ticlopidine: a new platelet
aggregation inhibitor. *Clin Pharm* 1992;11:603–617.

56. Savi P, Heilmann E, Nurden P, et al. Clopidogrel: an antithrombotic drug acting on the ADP-dependent activation pathway of human platelets. *Clin Appl Thromb Hemost* 1996;2:35–42.

57. Herbert JM, Frehel D, Vallee E, et al. Clopidogrel, a
novel antiplatelet and antithrombotic agent. *Cardiovasc
Drug Rev* 1993;11:180–198.

58. Balsano F, Rizzon P, Violi F, et al. Studio della Ticlopidina nell' Angina Instabile Group: antiplatelet treatment with ticlopidine in unstable angina: a controlled
multicenter clinical trial. *Circulation* 1990;82:17–26.

59. Herbert JM, Bernat A, Samama M, Maffrand JP. The
antiaggregating and antithrombotic activity of ticlopidine is potentiated by aspirin in the rat. *Thromb
Haemost* 1996;76:94–98.

60. FitzGerald GA. Ticlopidine in unstable angina: a more
expensive aspirin? *Circulation* 1990;82:296–298.

61. More RS, Chauhan A. Antiplatelet rather than anticoagulant therapy with coronary stenting. *Lancet* 1997;349:
146–147.

62. CAPRIE Steering Committee. A randomised, blinded,
trial of clopidogrel versus aspirin in patients at risk of ischaemic events (CAPRIE). *Lancet* 1996;348:1329–1339.

63. Lefkovits J, Plow EF, Topol EJ. Platelet glycoprotein
IIb/IIIa receptors in cardiovascular medicine. *N Engl J
Med* 1995;332:1553–1559.

64. Coller BS. Platelet GPIIb/IIIa antagonists: the first anti-
integrin receptor therapeutics. *J Clin Invest* 1997;99:
1467–1471.

65. Coller BS, Peerschke EL, Scudder LE, Sullivan CA. A
murine monoclonal antibody that completely blocks
the binding of fibrinogen to platelets produces a thrombasthenic-like state in normal platelets and binds to
glycoproteins IIb and/or IIIa. *J Clin Invest* 1983;72:
325–338.

66. Tcheng JE, Ellis SG, George BS, et al. Pharmacodynamics of chimeric glycoprotein IIb/IIIa integrin antiplatelet antibody Fab 7E3 in high-risk coronary angioplasty. *Circulation* 1994;90:1757–1764.

67. The EPILOG Investigators. Platelet glycoprotein
IIb/IIIa receptor blockade and low-dose heparin during
percutaneous coronary revascularization. *N Engl J Med*
1997;336:1689–1696.

68. Shetler TJ, Crowe VG, Bailey BD, Jackson CV. Antithrombotic assessment of the effects of combination therapy with the anticoagulants efegatran and heparin and the glycoprotein IIb-IIIa platelet receptor antagonists 7E3 in a canine model of coronary artery thrombosis. *Circulation* 1996;94:1719:1725.

69. Praticò D, Murphy NP, Fitzgerald DJ. Interaction of a thrombin inhibitor and a platelet GPIIb/IIIa antagonist in vivo: evidence that thrombin mediates platelet aggregation and subsequent thromboxane A$_2$ formation during coronary thrombolysis. *J Pharmacol Exp Ther* 1997;281:1178–1185.

70. Reverter JC, Béguin S, Kessels H, Kumar R, Hemker HC, Coller BS. Inhibition of platelet-mediated, tissue factor-induced thrombin generation by the mouse/human chimeric 7E3 antibody: potential implications for effect of c7E3 Fab treatment on acute thrombosis and "clinical restenosis." *J Clin Invest* 1996;98:863–874.

71. Topol EJ, Califf RM, Weisman HF, et al. Randomised trial of coronary intervention with antibody against platelet IIb/IIIa integrin for reduction of clinical restenosis: results at six months. *Lancet* 1994;343:881–886.

72. Niewiarowski S, McLane MA, Kloczewiak M, Stewart GJ. Disintegrins and other naturally occurring antagonists of platelet fibrinogen receptors. *Semin Hematol* 1994;31:289–300.

73. Scarborough RM, Naughton MA, Teng W, et al. Design of potent and specific integrin antagonists: peptide antagonists with high-specificity for glycoprotein IIb/IIIa. *J Biol Chem* 1993;268:1066–1073.

74. Harrington RA, Kleiman NS, Kottke-Marchant K, et al. Immediate and reversible platelet inhibition after intravenous administration of a peptide glycoprotein IIb/IIIa inhibitor during percutaneous coronary intervention. *Am J Cardiol* 1995;76:1222–1227.

75. Catella-Lawson F, FitzGerald GA. Confusion in reperfusion. Problems in the clinical development of antithrombotic drugs. *Circulation* 1997;95:793–795.

76. The IMPACT-II Investigators. Randomised placebo-controlled trial of effect of eptifibatide on complications of percutaneous coronary intervention: IMPACT-II. *Lancet* 1997;349:1422–1428.

77. Roden DM. Cardiovascular and Renal Advisory Panel of the US Food and Drug Administration considers four drugs. *Circulation* 1997;95:2335–2337.

78. Théroux P, Kouz S, Roy L, et al. Platelet membrane receptor glycoprotein IIb/IIIa antagonism in unstable angina. The Canadian Lamifiban Study. *Circulation* 1996;94:899–905.

79. Kereiakes DJ, Kleiman NS, Amborse J, et al. Randomized, double-blind, placebo-controlled dose-ranging study of tirofiban (MK-383) platelet IIb/IIIa blockade in high risk patients undergoing coronary angioplasty. *J Am Coll Cardiol* 1996;27:536–542.

80. White HD. The PRISM Study. 46th Annual Scientific Session of the American College of Cardiology, March 1997, Anaheim, CA.

81. The CAPTURE Investigators. Randomised placebo-controlled trial of abciximab before and during coronary intervention in refractory unstable angina: the CAPTURE study. *Lancet* 1997;349:1429–1435.

82. Simpfendorfer C, Kottke-Marchant K, Lowrie M, et al. First chronic platelet glycoprotein IIb/IIIa integrin blockade. A randomized, placebo-controlled study of xemilofiban in unstable angina with percutaneous coronary interventions. *Circulation* 1997;96:76–81.

83. Okano Y, Yoshioka T, Shimouchi A, Satoh T, Kuneida T. Orally active prostacyclin analogue in primary pulmonary hypertension. *Lancet* 1997;349:1365–1368.

84. Hanson SR, Hutsell TC, Keefer LK, Mooradian DL, Smith DJ. Nitric oxide donors: a continuing opportunity in drug design. *Adv Pharmacol* 1995;34:383–398.

85. Lees C, Langford E, Brown AS, et al. The effects of S-nitrosoglutathione on platelet activation, hypertension, and uterine and fetal Doppler in severe preeclampsia. *Obstet Gynecol* 1996;88:14–19.

86. Langford EJ, Wainwright RJ, Martin JF. Platelet activation in acute myocardial infarction and unstable angina is inhibited by nitric oxide donors. *Arterioscler Thromb Vasc Biol* 1996;16:51–55.

87. Fujimura M, Kamio Y, Saito M, Hashimoto T, Matsuda T. Bronchodilator and bronchoprotective effects of cilostazol in humans in vivo. *Am J Resp Crit Care Med* 1995;151:222–225.

88. Matousovic K, Grande JP, Chini CC, Chini EN, Dousa TP. Inhibitors of cyclic nucleotide phosphodiesterase isozymes type-III and type-IV suppress mitogenesis of rat mesangial cells. *J Clin Invest* 1995;96:401–410.

89. PACK Trial group. Prevention of atherosclerotic complications: controlled trial of ketanserin. *Br Med J* 1989;298:424–430.

90. Knapp HR, Reilly IAG, Alessandrini P, FitzGerald GA. In vivo indexes of platelet and vascular function during fish-oil administration in patients with atherosclerosis. *N Engl J Med* 1986;314:937–943.

91. Knapp HR, FitzGerald GA. The anti-hypertensive effects of fish oil: a controlled study of polyunsaturated fatty acid supplements in essential hypertension. *N Engl J Med* 1989;320:1037–1043.

92. De Caterina R, Cybulsky MI, Clinton SK, Gimbrone MA Jr, Libby P. The omega-3 fatty acid docosahexaenoate reduces cytokine-induced expression of proatherogenic and proinflammatory proteins in human endothelial cells. *Arterioscler Thromb* 1994;14:1829–1836.

93. Leaf A, Weber P. Cardiovascular effects of n-3 fatty acids. *N Engl J Med* 1988;318:549–557.

94. Barbeau ML, Klemp KF, Guyton JR, Rogers KA. Dietary fish oil. Influence on lesion regression in the porcine model of atherosclerosis. *Arterioscler Thromb Vasc Biol* 1997;17:688–694.

95. Freedman JE, Farhat JH, Loscalzo J, Keaney JF Jr. α-Tocopherol inhibits aggregation of human platelets by a protein kinase C-dependent mechanism. *Circulation* 1996;94:2434–2440.

96. Stephens NG, Parsons A, Schofield PM, et al. Randomised controlled trial of vitamin E in patients with coronary disease: Cambridge Heart Antioxidant Study (CHAOS). *Lancet* 1996;347:781–786.

Cardiovascular Thrombosis: Thrombocardiology and Thromboneurology, Second Edition, edited by M. Verstraete, V. Fuster, and E. J. Topol, Lippincott–Raven Publishers, Philadelphia © 1998.

9

Specific Thrombin Inhibitors

Marc Verstraete, *Pierre Zoldhelyi, and †James T. Willerson

*The Center for Molecular and Vascular Biology, University of Leuven, B-3000 Leuven, Belgium; *Divisions of Cardiology and Hematology, University of Texas Health Science Center, Houston, Texas 77030; and †Department of Internal Medicine, University of Texas Medical School at Houston, Houston, Texas 77030*

Thrombin represents the culmination of the coagulation cascade as it converts fibrinogen to clottable fibrin by releasing fibrinopeptides A and B. Thrombin itself is responsible for its own nonlinear generation caused by positive feedback activation, whereby thrombin enhances neoformation of thrombin (Fig. 9-1). In addition, thrombin is a pivotal molecule for numerous other functions. By binding to its receptor and subsequent cleaving, thrombin is the most potent known platelet activator. The action of thrombin on platelets results in the release of platelet factor V exteriorization and the transbilayer movement of its inner membrane surface (flip-flop reaction). Thrombin activates three of the four cofactor or helper proteins (factors V and VIII, thrombomodulin, but not tissue factor). Thrombin further-

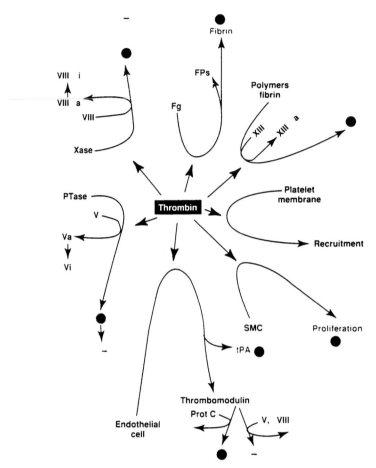

FIG. 9-1. Role of thrombin in the pathogenesis of arterial thrombosis. Positive signs (+) indicate reactions stimulated by thrombin, whereas negative signs (-) indicate reactions inhibited by it. In addition to its effects on the activation of coagulation factors and fibrin formation and stabilization, thrombin activates platelets, induces proliferation of smooth muscle cells (SMC), and contributes to the activation of the spontaneous anticoagulant pathway of normal endothelium. Fps, fibrinopeptides; Fg, fibrinogen. (From Badimon and Badimon, ref. 79, with permission.)

more activates factor XIII, which increases the strength and renders the fibrin more resistant to thrombolysis.

Thrombin also may prevent coagulation by a negative feedback mechanism. When thrombin binds thrombomodulin on endothelial cells, it cleaves and activates protein C, a natural anticoagulant, which in turn inactivates factors Va and VIIa. Protein S specifically accelerates the degradation of factor V catalyzed by activated protein C.

Thrombin in association with intact endothelium induces the production and release from the vascular endothelial cells of two highly potent local antiaggregatory vasodilators: prostacyclin and nitric oxide (endothelium-derived relaxing factor). These molecules are thought to provide significant antithrombotic protection for microcirculatory beds adjacent to sites of thrombus formation.

In vivo thrombin receptor expression was also demonstrated by macrophages and vascular smooth muscle cells in atherosclerotic lesions and in endarterectomy specimens. Exposure of selectins at the endothelial cell surface is stimulated by thrombin and plays a role in the incursion of monocytes and neutrophils to an injured vessel wall. In addition, thrombin has a direct chemotactic effect on monocytes and has apparent mitogenic effects on lymphocytes and vascular smooth muscle cells.

Considering the pivotal role of thrombin in the coagulation system, substantial research is focused on specific inhibitors of thrombin. What they all have in common is that unfortunately no specific antidote is presently available.

DESULFATOHIRUDIN

Biochemistry and Experimental In Vivo Studies

Several natural hirudin variants (isoinhibitors), with different N-terminal amino acids, are produced by the salivary gland of the European leech, *Hirudo medicinalis,* and are the prototype of direct antithrombins (1,2). Natural desirudin is a 65-residue polypeptide with three intramolecular disulfide bonds and a

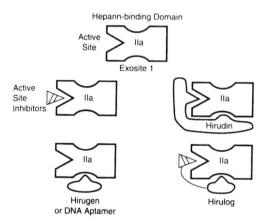

FIG. 9-2. Interaction of direct thrombin inhibitors with thrombin. In addition to the active site of thrombin (IIa), there are two distinct positively charged domains located at opposite poles of the enzyme. The first, known as anion-binding exosite 1, serves as the substrate recognition site, whereas the second, which has been designated exosite 2, contains the heparin-binding domain. Active-site inhibitors (e.g., D-Phe-Pro-Arg CH2 Cl and its derivatives) block the active site of thrombin, whereas hirugen and the thrombin-binding DNA aptamer bind to exosite 1, thereby preventing the enzyme from interacting with its substrates. In contrast, hirudin and hirulog bind both with the active site and with exosite 1. (From Weitz, ref. 80, with permission.)

sulfated tyrosine residue in position 63. It has a molecular weight of approximately 7 kDa and binds thrombin with extraordinary tightness (dissociation constant [K_D] 2×10^{-15} mol/L) and specificity (3,4), which is the result of 212 close (< 4 A°) contacts between inhibitor and enzyme (4). Hirudin binds thrombin with 1:1 stoichiometry. The highly negatively charged C-terminus of hirudin interacts with the anion-binding exosite of thrombin, whereas its apolar domain (residue 1–48), stabilized by the three disulfide bridges, interacts with a region adjacent to the amidolytic center of thrombin (Fig. 9-2). Multiple nonpolar contacts contribute to the exceptional affinity of the thrombin–hirudin complex (2). Recombinant desirudin is produced in *Escherichia coli* and yeast and lacks the sulfate residue on tyrosine-63, with the consequence that its affinity toward thrombin is decreased by one order of magnitude (to K_D 2×10^{-13} mol/L) relative to the natural sulfated form (Table 9-1) (5). Nonetheless, with the exception of natural hirudin, desirudin has by far the highest affinity toward thrombin of all known antithrombins.

The efficacy of hirudin was believed until recently to be based on direct thrombin inhibition and especially on the interruption of thrombin generation by inhibiting the positive feedback that thrombin exerts through multiple mechanisms on its own generation. When assembled on lipid (e.g., platelet membranes), the prothrombinase complex generates thrombin 280,000 times faster than when each component is present in solution. Self-amplifica-

TABLE 9-1. *Affinity for thrombin of experimental antithrombins*

Inhibitor	K_D of thrombin-inhibitor complex (mol/L)
r-Hirudin	2.0×10^{-13}
DuP 714	4.1×10^{-11}
Hirulog	2.3×10^9
PPACK[a]	3.7×10^8
Argatroban	3.9×10^8
Hirugen	1.5×10^7

[a]Thrombin and PPACK (D-Phe-Pro-ArgCH2Cl) form an irreversible, covalent bond after initial, reversible association in a complex with the indicated K_D (dissociation constant).

tion of thrombin through activation of platelets and factors V, VIII, and X is thought to be critical for the generation of thrombin in concentrations necessary for effective hemostasis and thrombosis (6,7). Heparin (8) and the specific antithrombins (7) are thought to block thrombin generation through interruption of this positive feedback. However, doubt has been cast on this latter mechanism by the demonstration that thrombin generation in vivo proceeds relentlessly in the presence of desirudin and other antithrombins in animals (9) and in humans with stable and unstable coronary artery disease (10–12).

The effects of natural hirudin on the platelet-rich thrombus have been studied for over 60 years (13). Like all direct antithrombins, hirudin inhibits thrombin without the need for additional cofactors. The notion that thrombin may play a pivotal role in the formation of platelet thrombi was suggested by several and disparate early observations: the studies with crude hirudin preparations and heparin in an ex vivo arteriovenous shunt model of "white thrombi" by Shionoya in late 1927 (13), the observation that thrombin may initiate platelet aggregation in vitro at lower concentrations than those required for fibrinogen cleavage (14), and in flow-modeling experiments, where thrombin reached platelet-active concentrations significantly more rapidly compared with the thromboxane A$_2$ analogue U-46619 (15). More recently, in the porcine carotid injury model, specific thrombin inhibition with desirudin completely prevented formation (16), and accelerated lysis (17), of platelet-rich thrombi. In this model of platelet-rich occlusive thrombus after deep carotid artery injury, desirudin, at activated partial thromboplastin times (APTT) two to three times baseline, was found to be significantly more effective than heparin (at APTT more than fivefold baseline) in accelerating lysis by t-PA, suggesting that thrombosis after deep arterial injury was thrombin dependent. Aspirin in this model was ineffective as adjunctive to t-PA (17). In a coronary electric injury study in the dog, desirudin, at APTT values only 1.5 to 2.0 times control, was also significantly more effective than as-

pirin or heparin and prevented coronary occlusion in six of six animals (18). Desirudin also prevented thrombus deposition in extracorporeal Dacron-grafted arteriovenous shunts (19). Comparing the amount of desirudin required for thrombus prevention in different thrombosis models (20), it appears that the plasma concentration of desirudin required to totally prevent thrombus may be proportional to the amount of thrombin generated in these models, where an increasing gradient of thrombin generation (from models of venous stasis and mild arterial injury to deep arterial injury by angioplasty in the pig) was noted (20). Like heparin (21,22), desirudin is an effective inhibitor of fibrin deposition at concentrations that do not affect platelet deposition. Thus, during disseminated coagulation in a rat model, a plasma desirudin concentration of 0.1 μg/ml was sufficient to inhibit fibrinogen deposition, whereas a concentration of 0.5 μg/ml was required to prevent deposition of platelets (23).

Pharmacodynamics and Dose-Finding Studies in Humans

In healthy young volunteers, the terminal half-life of desirudin was found to be 50 to 65 minutes, and the halflife on the APTT was 2 hours (24,25). In contrast, in older patients with stable coronary artery disease and normal renal function (serum creatinine ≤1.0 ± 0.2 mg/dl), both plasma half-life and the half-life of the APTT prolongation was found to be 2 to 3 hours (26). In these patients, plateau/baseline APTT ratios were 1.5, 2.0, 2.3, 2.7, and 2.9, respectively, with desirudin infused without initial bolus at 0.02, 0.05, 0.1, 0.2, and 0.3 mg/kg/hr. Interestingly, 62% to 77% of the plateau (3 to 6 hours) effect on the APTT was reached within 30 minutes of the start of the maintenance infusion. Plasma concentration of desirudin correlated well with both the APTT/baseline ratio (r = 0.88) and the activated clotting time (ACT) (r = 0.80), although there was a considerable overlap between baseline ACT and ACT at plasma desirudin concentrations of less than 1 μg/ml. Prothrombin times (PT) were insensitive to plasma desirudin levels, with an international normalized ratio (INR) of 2.3 observed only with the highest (0.3 mg/kg/hr) dose. Thrombin times (TT) were beyond the upper range (600 seconds) in nearly all patients. Bleeding times were not significantly prolonged in this study and only mildly prolonged in another trial (26). From these studies, the APTT emerged as the best test to evaluate the anticoagulant effect of desirudin.

Immunogenicity

Desirudin has very low immunogenic potential. In repeated administration of recombinant desirudin to 263 healthy volunteers, including 12% who had a history of previous allergy and 18% with high levels of total immunoglobulin E, no signs or symptoms directly attributable to desirudin were noted, and only three of 200 volunteers exposed to a second course of desirudin showed an allergic reaction. In all but one patient with a pruritic erythema, a causative role for desirudin was excluded (27). In the same study, specific antibodies directed against desirudin were detected in only one of the 263 subjects. Thus, repeated doses of desirudin can be considered safe. Similarly, antibody formation against desirudin was not observed in an older study of volunteers (28) or in the aforementioned study in older patients with stable coronary artery disease (26).

Clinical Trials of Desirudin

Trials of Desirudin in Patients Undergoing Percutaneous Transluminal Coronary Angioplasty for Stable or Unstable Angina

In a double-blind pilot trial, van den Bos et al. randomized 113 low-risk patients with stable angina pectoris undergoing percutaneous transluminal coronary angioplasty (PTCA) to a 24-hour infusion of either desirudin (Revasc™, Novartis) or heparin (29). All patients received 250 to 500 mg aspirin for at least 4 weeks beginning on the day of PTCA. Desirudin was given as a 20-mg bolus followed by an infusion of 0.16 mg/kg/hr, whereas heparin was administered as a

10,000-IU bolus followed by 12 IU/kg/hr. The two trial drugs were adjusted to a target APTT of 85 to 120 seconds. At the end of the infusion period, an angiography was performed to assess vessel patency. Acute closure, leading to myocardial infarction and/or coronary artery bypass graft (CABG), occurred in 10.3% of patients randomized to heparin but in only 1.4% of patients randomized to desirudin. Four desirudin patients (5%) developed major bleeding at the arterial puncture site versus none in the heparin group, in which one episode of cerebral infarction occurred. Immediately and 24 hours after PTCA, TIMI grade 3 flow was present in all desirudin-treated patients and, respectively, in 92% and 91% of heparin-treated patients. None of the differences in this small pilot trial reached statistical significance, in part because of low event rates and the small numbers of patients. Desirudin provided more predictable APTT prolongations with more patients in the target APTT range. Although the prothrombin fragment 1.2 levels (an indicator of prothrombin generation) were below the upper limit of normal in both groups, they tended to be higher in the desirudin group (29).

Based on the results of this pilot trial, it was concluded that desirudin can be administered safely to patients undergoing PTCA for stable angina pectoris.

Experimental animal studies had suggested that a short-term administration of desirudin may inhibit restenosis at 1 month from angioplasty (30). This hypothesis was tested in the large Helvetica study of 1,141 patients with unstable angina in which a higher dose of desirudin than in the pilot study was used (31). Desirudin was given as a 40-mg bolus and a 24-hour infusion at 0.2 mg/kg/hr followed by either subcutaneous (s.c.) desirudin (40 mg twice daily) or placebo for three consecutive days. The heparin dose was a bolus of 10,000 IU followed by an intravenous (i.v.) infusion of 15 IU/kg/hr over 24-hour infusion and two s.c. placebo injections per day for 3 days. The incidence of early (96 hours) ischemic events was reduced significantly by desirudin versus heparin (relative risk reduction in the combined desirudin groups, 0.61; 95% confidence interval [CI], 0.41 to 0.90, p = 0.023), which was particular evident for those patients with angina at rest: early event rate 21.6% in the heparin versus 5.3% in patients receiving both i.v. plus s.c. desirudin (relative risk reduction 0.41; 95% CI, 0.21 to 0.78, p = 0.006). There was no difference in the incidence of major or minor bleeding complications. Prothrombin fragments 1.2 levels immediately after angioplasty were decreased by heparin but not by desirudin (31). Seven-month event-free survival (freedom from death, nonfatal myocardial infarction or revascularization procedure within 7 months from PTCA) was 67.3% in the heparin group, 63.5% in the hirudin i.v. group, and 68.0% in the patients treated with i.v. plus s.c. hirudin (p = NS). Minimal lumen diameters at 6 months' follow-up angiography were 1.54 mm, 1.46 mm, and 1.56 mm, respectively, in the three treatment groups. In conclusion, compared with heparin, desirudin in this trial in unstable angina patients treated with angioplasty reduced acute events but neither improved cardiac events at 7 months nor produced changes, compared with heparin, in the minimal luminal diameter at angiographic follow-up.

Desirudin in Acute Coronary Syndromes

Pilot Trials of Desirudin in Unstable Angina without PTCA

In a multicenter open-label pilot trial, 166 patients with unstable angina and angiographic thrombus were randomized to a 72- to 120-hour infusion of heparin (50 patients) or desirudin (116 patients) at 0.05 mg/kg/hr to 0.3 mg/kg/hr (32). Heparin was adjusted to an APTT of 65 to 90 seconds (28 patients) or 90 to 110 seconds (22 patients), whereas desirudin was not adjusted to APTT prolongation. APTT prolongations with desirudin at 0.2 and 0.3 mg/kg/hr were not significantly different. Upon repeat angiography at 72 to 120 hours, patients assigned to desirudin (compared with heparin) had an improved cross-sectional area of the culprit vessel (p = 0.08) and a larger minimum cross-sectional area (p = 0.028), whereas the improvement in TIMI flow grade was not significant (p =

0.44). Equal angiographic benefit was seen with desirudin at 0.1 and 0.3 mg/kg/hr, suggesting a plateau effect for desirudin at 0.1 mg/kg/hr. Clinical outcomes at 30 days were not significantly different. Myocardial infarction (MI) developed in 2% of desirudin and 8% of heparin patients (p = 0.11). No patients died, and none had intracerebral bleeding or another major spontaneous bleed. No rebound activation of angina was observed after withdrawal of desirudin (32).

OASIS-1 (Organization to Assess Strategies for Ischemic Syndromes) is a relatively large pilot study in 368 patients with unstable angina or suspected myocardial infarction without PTCA (33). Patients were randomized to one of two doses of desirudin (0.2 mg/kg bolus, 0.1 mg/kg/hr over 72 hours; and 0.4 mg/kg bolus, 0.15 mg/kg/hr over 72 hours) or heparin (5,000 IU bolus, 1,200 U/hr infusion over 72 hours) (14). Overall, 96% of the patients received aspirin. From an efficacy standpoint, at 7 days there was a trend toward lower event rates in the desirudin groups, particularly in the higher hirudin dose. When the two desirudin groups were combined, there was a significant decrease in the combined incidence of death, myocardial infarction, and revascularization at 7 days. No cerebral hemorrhages occurred in the study. There was no significant increase in major bleeding events with desirudin, but the incidence of minor bleeding events was higher with desirudin, particularly in the higher dose group.

These promising initial results need to be confirmed with longer follow-up and in much larger randomized studies. Such a study is OASIS-2, which is a 2 × 2 factorial design testing the effects of a single regimen of hirudin versus heparin and warfarin versus placebo in 8,000 patients with unstable angina. The endpoints are death, myocardial infarction, and refractory angina.

Pilot Trials of Desirudin as Adjunct to Thrombolysis in Myocardial Infarction

In the open-label TIMI 5 pilot study of acute myocardial infarction treated with front-loaded t-PA, aspirin, and either heparin or desirudin, 162 patients received a 5-day infusion of escalating desirudin dosage (0.05 to 0.2 mg/kg/hr). Eighty-four received heparin adjusted to 65 to 90 seconds (34). Although, the difference in TIMI grade 2 and 3 flow was not significantly different between desirudin and heparin at 90 minutes (82.1% versus 78.6%, respectively), it reached significance at 18 to 26 hours (97.8% versus 89.2%, respectively, p < 0.01) due to a decrease in reocclusion rates (1.6% versus 6.7%, respectively, in patients receiving desirudin and heparin, p < 0.07) and a higher rate of reperfusion in the desirudin group. Major spontaneous hemorrhage occurred in 4.7% of heparin-treated versus 1.2% of desirudin-treated patients. Intracranial hemorrhage occurred in one heparin patient (34).

Patients in the TIMI-6 pilot trial were randomized to streptokinase (SK), aspirin, and desirudin or heparin. Desirudin appeared as safe as heparin, but the higher doses of desirudin (0.3 mg/kg bolus followed by 0.1 mg/kg/hr) was associated with a trend toward lower rates of death, reinfarction, cardiogenic shock, and congestive heart failure (35).

Large-Scale Randomized Multicenter Trials with Desirudin in Patients with Acute Myocardial Infarction

Results of the GUSTO-IIa, TIMI-9A and HIT-III Trials

Because the phase II pilot trials suggested that desirudin and heparin, at the doses tested, were safe, two large-scale heparin controlled studies—TIMI-9A (36) and GUSTO-IIa (37)—were started in patients with acute myocardial infarction with the same brand name of desirudin (Revasc™) and in a third trial coded HIT-III (38) with another recombinant hirudin (Lepirudin™). In the first two, desirudin was administered as a 0.6 mg/kg i.v. bolus followed by a fixed-dose infusion of 0.2 mg/kg/hr for 96 hours (TIMI-9A) or for 72 to 120 hours (GUSTO-IIa). All patients received aspirin. In the much smaller HIT-III trial, pa-

tients were randomized to a 48- to 72-hour infusion of desirudin (HBW023, Lepirudin™) at a dose of 0.4 mg/kg i.v. bolus, followed by an infusion of 0.15 mg/kg/hr or a bolus of 70 IU heparin/kg followed by 15 IU/kg/hr. A front-loaded alteplase protocol was used, and all patients received aspirin; 15% of patients in TIMI-9A received SK. In HIT-III, but not in GUSTO-IIa or TIMI-9A, the dose of desirudin was adjusted to achieve APTT values two to 3.5 times baseline.

When 2,564 patients with acute myocardial infarction had been enrolled in GUSTO-IIa, the trial was halted because intracranial bleeding rates of 0.9% and 1.9% with alteplase (with heparin or desirudin) and the astonishingly high rates of 2.7% and 3.2% with SK (with heparin or desirudin) were up to two times greater than GUSTO-1 (0.7%). Similarly, when 757 had been enrolled in TIMI-9A, this trial was suspended because of a high rate of cerebral bleeding (1.9% and 1.7% in patients given alteplase with heparin or desirudin, respectively).

Intracranial bleeding rates in the HIT-III trial were 3.4% in the 154 patients receiving recombinant hirudin but none in the group receiving heparin (38). All hemorrhagic strokes in HIT-III occurred within 24 hours of the start of treatment. In TIMI-9A and HIT-III trials, patients with major bleeding treated with desirudin tended to have higher median APTT values 12 hours after the start of treatment than did those without major bleeding.

In HIT-III, but not in GUSTO-IIa or TIMI-9A, adjustment of the study drug to an APTT prolongation of two to 3.5 times baseline was recommended. In addition to front-loaded t-PA (or SK in 15% of TIMI-9a patients), all patients in these three trials received aspirin. In contrast to GUSTO-1, where 50% of patients had an APTT below the target range of 60 to 85 seconds, a weight-adjusted heparin regimen was used in GUSTO-IIa and TIMI-9A (patients weighting less than 80 kg and ≥80 kg, respectively, 1,000 and 1,300 IU/hr) with titration to a target range of 60 to 90 seconds. This strategy resulted in a 20% increase in the total amount of heparin given. Heparin in HIT-III was weight adjusted (70 IU/kg followed by 15 IU/kg/hr). In TIMI-9A, major spontaneous noncerebral hemorrhage occurred in 7.0% and 3.0%, respectively (p < 0.02). A baseline creatinine of more than 1.5 mg/day, older age, lower body weight, and a higher APTT (100 seconds versus 86 seconds in nonstroke patients) were associated with bleeding in desirudin patients, suggesting that reduced renal clearance of desirudin could have contributed to the higher bleeding risk. In GUSTO-IIa, there was a trend toward increased intracerebral bleeding with age, female sex, and greater APTT prolongation (12-hour APTT 110 and 87 seconds, respectively, in patients with and without stroke, p = 0.031). This contrasted with the hemorrhagic stroke rates in GUSTO-1 (0.57% with i.v. heparin plus SK and 0.7% with i.v. heparin plus t-PA). The incidence of hemorrhagic stroke in GUSTO-IIa patients not receiving thrombolytic treatment was also relatively high (0.3%, all of which were patients randomized to desirudin). Stroke on thrombolytics occurred at a median time of 8 hours after start with desirudin and after 17 hours with heparin (p = NS).

HIT-III was also stopped when an imbalance in the incidence of hemorrhagic stroke became apparent. The incidence of confirmed cardiac rupture was 2% in desirudin versus 0.6% in heparin patients. Overall, spontaneous bleeding (other than intracranial) occurred in 2.7% of desirudin versus 1.3% of heparin patients. All hemorrhagic strokes (all on desirudin) occurred within the first 24 hours after treatment start. HIT-III patients bleeding on desirudin had a median APTT of 106 seconds versus 76 seconds in those who did not bleed. The early plasma desirudin levels produced by the 0.6 mg/kg bolus appeared to be in excess to what has been predicted in a phase I trial of patients with stable coronary artery disease and normal serum creatinine (39).

Rationale of the Reduced Desirudin and Heparin Doses in GUSTO-IIb and TIMI-9B

In view of these results and of the observation that infusion of desirudin at a dose of 0.1 mg/kg/hr was apparently as effective as higher doses in both unstable angina and myocardial infarction in pilot studies (32–35), GUSTO-IIb (40) and TIMI-9B (41) were restarted comparing low anticoagulant doses of desirudin (0.1 mg/kg i.v. bolus of desirudin, followed by 0.1 mg/kg/hr) or heparin (1,000 IU/hr not adjusted to body weight). In addition, both heparin infusion and desirudin infusion were adjusted to a reduced target APTT range of 55 to 85 seconds (TIMI-9B) (instead of 60 to 90 seconds) and 60 to 85 seconds (GUSTO-IIb) (instead of 60 to 90 seconds) because APTT values above 100 seconds clearly were associated with increased risk of intracerebral hemorrhage. It was expected that down-titration of desirudin and adjustment to APTT values to only two to three times baseline may take better advantage of the lower anticoagulant/antithrombotic ratio of desirudin compared with heparin. This had been clearly established in preclinical studies in which desirudin was more effective than heparin at APTT ratios several times lower than those achieved with high-dose heparin (16,17,19). Perhaps more important for the investigators, the American unstable angina multicenter trial also had suggested a plateau effect for the desirudin doses of 0.1 mg/kg/hr (32).

Results of GUSTO-IIb and TIMI-9B

The results of GUSTO-IIb on 12,142 patients were disappointing. The primary combined endpoint of death or nonfatal myocardial infarction or reinfarction at 30 days was similar in desirudin-treated patients (8.9%) as in the heparin group (9.8%, p = 0.06). However, at 24 hours the same endpoint was significantly different in favor of desirudin (1.3% versus 2.1%, p = 0.001), but this difference did not persist up to 30 days. There were no significant differences in the incidence of serious bleeding (1.2% versus 1.1%, p = 0.43), but intracranial bleeding occurred more often in desirudin-treated patients (0.3% versus 0.2%, p = 0.24). Desirudin therapy was associated with a significantly higher incidence of moderate bleeding (8.8% versus 7.7%, p = 0.03).

The same desirudin brand and dose was used in the 3,002 patients enrolled in TIMI-9B as in GUSTO-IIb. Intravenous desirudin or heparin were administered for 96 hours. The primary endpoint was a 30-day incidence of death, myocardial infarction, congestive heart failure, and shock. In contrast to the results of the GUSTO-IIb trial, there was no significant difference in TIMI-9B in the primary endpoint between either desirudin (12.8%) or heparin (11.8%) or in the incidence of death and myocardial infarction (9.6% versus 9.3%). Similarly, there was no significant difference in major bleeding events (4.6% versus 5.3%) between treatment groups. Intracranial bleeding occurred in 0.4% of the desirudin patients and 0.9% of the heparin patients.

Combined analysis of the results of both megatrials suggests a modest but significant reduction of 13% (p = 0.026) in the (re)infarction incidence with desirudin at 30 days (corresponding to an absolute reduction of nine events per 1,000 patients treated) without a striking effect on mortality. Among the 12,142 patients in GUSTO-IIb, 3,457 (28.5%) were treated with thrombolytics. Among them, 3,289 had presented with ST-segment elevation at the time of enrollment. They were treated at the investigator's discretion with either t-PA (2,274 patients) or SK (1,015 patients) and randomized to receive either heparin or hirudin as guided by the main GUSTO-IIb randomization. For the 1,015 patients receiving SK, a marked 40% reduction in the primary endpoint, death/reinfarction at 30 days, was demonstrated in patients treated with hirudin (8.6%) compared with heparin (14.4%) (odds ratio [OR] = 1.78, 95% CI = 12.0 to 2.66, p = 0.004). For the patients receiving t-PA (n = 2,274), there was only a minor (5.5%) reduction in the primary endpoint (30-day death/myocardial infarction) for accelerated t-PA reduced from 10.9% with heparin to 10.3% with hirudin (OR = 1.06, 95% CI = 0.81 to 1.38; p = 0.68, for treatment heterogeneity, χ^2 = 4.45, p = 0.03), suggesting a significant treatment effect in outcomes specific for SK-treated patients who were randomized to hirudin rather than heparin (42). Thus, a favorable treatment interaction of SK, but not t-PA, with hirudin, was demonstrated. These findings, coupled with recent trials combining SK and direct thrombin inhibitors, provide support for the importance of thrombin activity after therapy with this plasminogen activator.

Lessons Learned from the Large-Scale Trials with Desirudin in Patients with Acute Myocardial Infarction

The set dose of desirudin was obviously too high in GUSTO-IIa and TIMI-9A. This could possibly have been predicted from the dose-ranging TIMI-5 trial, where the highest dose of desirudin (0.6 mg/kg bolus followed by 0.2 mg/kg/hr infusion for 120 hours) was associated with a significant risk for major hemorrhage (29.4%) compared with lower desirudin doses (10.9%) (34). Also in TIMI-6 the same high dose of desirudin resulted in a higher rate of major bleeding (29%) compared with the lower doses of desirudin (13%, p = 0.007). This highest dose tested in phase II trials was probably selected in GUSTO-2a and TIMI-9A in view of the lack of a dose-response relationship in the three phase II pilot trials.

This decision was also based on the finding in GUSTO-I and in other trials that subtherapeutic anticoagulation was associated with lower infarct-related coronary patency. Indeed, weight-adjusted heparin (more than 80 kg: 1,300 IU/hr) was used in GUSTO-2a and TIMI-9A because approximately 50% of patients receiving i.v. heparin in GUSTO-I had APTTs below the predefined range of 60 to 85 seconds, with the majority of these patients weighing more than 80 kg. Considering the high incidence of cerebral bleeding, the heparin dose also was decreased in GUSTO-IIb and TIMI-9B to lower APTT target values and was not weight adjusted further. Moreover, the infusion of desirudin instead of being fixed was now adapted to the same APTT target values as for heparin (60 to 85 seconds), a range that is lower than in GUSTO-Ia and TIMI-9A (60 to 90 seconds).

The bolus dose of desirudin was drastically decreased from 0.6 mg/kg (in GUSTO-IIa and TIMI-9a) to 0.1 mg/kg in GUSTO-IIb and

TIMI-9B because 39% of the major hemorrhagic events occurred within 24 hours of initiation of thrombolysis and study drug treatment in the former studies; moreover, desirudin-treated patients experience major bleeding earlier in the course of treatment than heparin-treated patients in TIMI-9A (mean 8 hours versus 17 hours). It is possible that the dose of hirudin in GUSTO-IIb and TIMI-9B has been reduced too much to obtain therapeutic efficacy in the clinical endpoints. Of note, in the subsequently reported but not fully published OASIS trial using an intermediate dose of desirudin (a bolus of 0.4 mg/kg followed by an infusion of 0.15 mg/kg/hr), the incidence of bleeding was twice as high in the desirudin group as in the heparin group (43). The latter trial was conducted in another group of patients (unstable angina and suspected myocardial infarction), with another brand of recombinant hirudin (HBW 023) and in the absence of thrombolytic treatment. This suggests that there is a narrow therapeutic window for recombinant hirudin.

Another explanation for the disappointing therapeutic results of GUSTO-IIb and TIMI-9B could be the short duration of hirudin infusion. In TIMI-9B all the beneficial results were evident within the first 24 hours; beyond that point, the event-rate curves neither diverge nor converge. For equivalent fibrinopeptide A levels (reflecting thrombin activity), a greater reduction in prothrombin fragment 1+2 (F1+2) levels (reflecting thrombin generation) is seen with heparin compared with desirudin, even at high doses (2,39,43,44). In contrast, for equivalent F1+2 levels, a greater reduction in fibrinogen peptide A (FPA) levels is seen with hirudin compared with heparin (45). Thus, hirudin at medium and high doses has a relatively smaller effect than heparin in the feedback-amplifying mechanisms leading to prothrombinase generation and thrombin formation. The accumulation of thrombin at a thrombogenic surface (ruptured coronary plaque) may have detracted from the ability of desirudin to inhibit the activity of thrombin. Although the proposal of a longer infusion of desirudin is attractive, the lack of clinical benefit observed in the TIMI-9A trial, in which anticoagulation was administered an average of 30% longer than in TIMI-9B (120 hours versus 96 hours), makes this possibility less probable.

A third possibility is the rebound hypercoagulability noted after cessation of antithrombotic therapy in patients with coronary syndromes as observed after withdrawal of argatroban, heparin, bivalirudin, and desirudin.

A fourth possiblity is that mixing patients with and without ST elevation may not be appropriate because the mortality rate in patients without ST elevation at 24 hours is about one quarter of that of patients with ST-elevation.

Because of the worse performance of high-dose desirudin, compared with heparin, as inhibitor of thrombin generation (10–13,42,45) and its failure to inhibit the wave of thrombin generation triggered by thrombolytics (44), additional interventions blocking thrombin generation, including heparin itself, factor Xa inhibitors, or inhibitors of tissue factor, may be required to further address this issue. Nonetheless, as earlier mentioned, the potential for the direct thrombin inhibitors to reduce activation of protein C may represent another inherent limitation of all members of this class of drugs. Furthermore, the IIb/IIIa platelet receptor antagonist does induce a moderate inhibition of thrombin generation as reflected, in the case of abciximab (ReoPro, Eli Lilly and Company, Indianapolis, IN), in a prolongation of the ACT by about 35 seconds when used during percutaneous revascularization procedures (46). To a mild degree this is also true of aspirin (47). Experimental evidence also indicates that combined administration of relatively low doses of platelet receptor and thrombin inhibitors may be efficacious (48). Whether such combinations will be tested in clinical trials in the future remains to be seen, especially in view of the low recurrent event rates with present antithrombotic regimens of thrombin inhibitors (both heparin and desirudin), aspirin, and plasminogen activators.

Desirudin in Deep Vein Thrombosis

Recombinant desirudin has been used for the prevention and treatment of venous thromboembolism.

Desirudin was evaluated in two consecutive studies performed in patients having total hip replacement. The aim was first to find the optimal dose of desirudin (10, 15 or 20 mg s.c. twice daily) in comparison with unfractionated heparin (5,000 IU s.c. three times daily) (49) and second to investigate whether the efficacy and safety of desirudin (15 mg s.c. twice daily) could compete with a low molecular weight heparin (enoxaparin, 40 mg daily) in patients undergoing total hip replacement. Both trials were prospective, randomized, and double-blind and all regimens were started preoperatively and trial drugs administered s.c. for 8 to 12 days. The main efficacy parameter was the presence of deep venous thrombosis verified by mandatory bilateral phlebography at the end of the prophylaxis period. The phlebography was evaluated centrally. Safety was mainly evaluated by blood loss and transfusion requirements. In the first study the rates of proximal deep venous thrombosis in 1,120 patients were 19.6% for unfractionated heparin and 8.5%, 3.1%, and 2.4% for desirudin 10 mg, 15 mg, and 20 mg, respectively ($p < 0.01$).

The 15-mg dose of desirudin provided the best benefit/risk ratio and was selected for the next investigation in 2,079 patients with total hip replacement. The incidence of proximal deep venous thrombosis was 7.5% and 4.5% in the enoxaparin and the desirudin groups, respectively ($p < 0.02$) with a relative risk reduction of 40%. The safety profiles of the regimens were comparable. The results from this trial shows that the desirudin provides a benefit/risk ratio superior to that of low-molecular-weight heparin.

Two small pilot trials of desirudin for the treatment of established deep vein thrombosis failed to show significant changes in lower limb venography after 5 days of treatment (50,51). The performance of desirudin versus low molecular weight heparin in the prevention and treatment of thromboembolism has not been tested in clinical trials.

Desirudin in Heparin-Induced Thrombocytopenia

Immune-mediated heparin-induced thrombocytopenia, an uncommon and severe complication of heparin therapy, may be associated with venous and arterial thromboembolism. Desirudin has been used in a small trial of heparin-induced thrombocytopenia as an alternative to heparin, with resolution of thrombocytopenia and clinical complications (52).

Neutralization of Desirudin

Bleeding with hirudin should prompt immediate arrest of the desirudin infusion, and consideration should be given to the administration of DDAVP, a vasopressin analogue. Experimentally, DDAVP shortens the APTT and bleeding time prolonged by desirudin (53–55). In human volunteers, DDAVP, when given over 15 minutes in a dose of 0.3 µg/kg, has been shown to reduce the prolongation of APTT after desirudin administration (56). Prothrombin complex concentrate has been shown to reduce the bleeding response to desirudin, but cannot be recommended at this time. When bleeding is life threatening, consideration should be given to hemodialysis.

HIRUGEN

Modelled on the C-terminal fragment of hirudin, hirugen is a synthetic dodecapeptide comprising the 12 terminal residues of hirudin that block the fibrinogen binding site (the anion-binding exosite) of thrombin; the molecule contains sulfated tyrosine to increase its thrombin affinity (Fig. 9-2). Hirugen (BG 8863) inhibits thrombin, forming an inhibitor complex of substantially lower affinity (about 50 times) compared with hirudin (K_D of 1.5×10^{-7} mol/L versus 0.2×10^{-12}

mol/L for r-hirudin). In vitro, hirugen competitively inhibits thrombin-mediated fibrinogen cleavage and platelet activation (57,58). Because it does not block the active site of thrombin, hirugen does not block thrombin mediated by dialysis of low molecular weight synthetic substrates.

In experiments with exteriorized arteriovenous shunts in baboons, hirugen prevented ex vivo platelet deposition in low-shear flow chambers connected to chronic arteriovenous shunts of baboons but failed to affect ex vivo platelet deposition on collagen type I–coated tubing at a dose of 75 mg/kg (APTT fourfold baseline) (59).

Presently, no clinical studies with hirugen are underway because its antithrombotic activity is much less potent compared with hirudin and with the follow-up molecule hirulog.

BIVALIRUDIN

Coupling of peptides that mimic the carboxyterminal of hirudin to peptides that are specific for inhibition of the catalytic site of thrombin (D-Phe-Pro-Arg) has led to the development of a chimeric molecule termed bivalirudin (BG 8967, brandname Hirulog, Biosen, Cambridge, MA), in which the amino-terminus consists of the catalytic site-directed tetrapeptide, whereas the carboxy-terminus consists of the 12 terminal residues of hirudin. The two moieties are linked together by a bridge of glycine residues of variable length, and the whole molecule comprises 20 amino acids (60,61). Thus, bivalirudin inhibits thrombin by binding to both its catalytic site and its anion-binding exosite, conferring specificity to these molecules for thrombin. Its K_D toward thrombin is 2.3×10^{-9} mol/L (Fig. 9-2). Bivalirudin is a direct and specific inhibitor of free (fluid phase) and clot-bound thrombin. The hirulog–thrombin complex is only transient because thrombin, once complexed, can slowly cleave the Arg_3-Pro_4 bound on the N-terminal extension with catalytic rate constant (k_{cat}) = 0.012 seconds-1. This metabolic cleavage contributes to its short half-life on the APTT

of about 23 to 36 minutes (62,63). Only 20% of hirulog is excreted in the urine, indicating an extensive hepatic catabolism or proteolysis at other sites. Newer noncleavable bivalirudins have been synthesized containing a β-homoarginine at the scissile bond. As for other direct thrombin inhibitors, there is no antidote for bivalirudin.

In animal models of venous thrombosis, arterial thrombosis, and thrombolysis, bivalirudin demonstrated greater antithrombotic activity than heparin (64–68).

Pharmacodynamics and Dose-Finding Studies

Phase I studies in healthy volunteers showed a dose-dependent prolongation of the APTT with a 15-minute i.v. infusion of bivalirudin at 0.05 to 0.6 mg/kg, resulting in APTTs from 1.7 ± 0.08 to 2.8 ± 0.55 times baseline (3). When 0.3 mg/kg/hr of bivalirudin was infused during 12 or 24 hours, peak APTT ratios were 2.1 to 2.5. There was a good, although not linear, correlation between APTT and bivalirudin plasma concentrations. In turn, there is a linear relationship of total bivalirudin dose administered to the effect area for its anticoagulant activity. Thrombin times (too sensitive) and prothrombin times (not sensitive enough) were not useful in titrating the dose of bivalirudin. After i.v. infusion, the half-life was 24 minutes with a volume of distribution of 13.0 and a clearance rate of 419 ± 37 ml/min (63). There is no measurable effect of aspirin on bivalirudin anticoagulant activity, and bivalirudin does not alter the effect of aspirin on template bleeding time.

In a dose-finding study in 45 patients undergoing routine cardiac catheterization, a good correlation was confirmed between the APTT and plasma bivalirudin levels (r = 0.77) (69). The APTT was prolonged to 1.8 and 2.2 times baseline, respectively, 15 minutes after starting i.v. bivalirudin at 0.05 mg/kg (bolus) followed by 0.2 mg/kg/hr and 0.15 mg/kg (bolus) followed by 0.6 mg/kg/hr. No major hematoma or thrombotic complications occurred at both doses. FPA levels were suppressed during the hirulog administration at doses that, compared with heparin, caused less elevation in APTT, PT, and ACT.

In a dose-escalating pilot study, Lidon et al. (70) evaluated bivalirudin in 55 patients with unstable angina who also received aspirin and triple antiischemic therapy. Bivalirudin was administered in escalating dosages of 0.02 to 0.5 mg/kg/hr, increased every 30 minutes for 72 hours. With dosages up to 1 mg/kg/hr, only one patient of 20 experienced recurrent chest pain. The APTT in angina-free patients averaged 55.6 ± 6 seconds. Plasma FPA levels were suppressed at dosages of 0.25 to 0.5 mg/kg/hr. The APTTs decreased to baseline 4 hours after discontinuation of hirulog. There was no rebound elevation of FPA at that time. Neither interaction with i.v. nitrates nor a cumulative effect were noted when bivalirudin was administered for up to 5 days.

The TIMI-7 pilot trial was designed to evaluate whether a dose response existed in the efficacy of bivalirudin in conjunction with aspirin in patients with unstable angina (71). Four hundred ten such patients were randomized to receive i.v. bivalirudin 0.02, 0.25, 0.5, or 1 mg/kg/hr for 72 hours, in addition to oral aspirin (325 mg/day). There were no significant differences between the different dose levels for the occurrence of the primary efficacy composite endpoint "unsatisfactory outcome" (death, nonfatal myocardial infarction, recurrent ischemia pain at rest with ECG changes, or rapid clinical deterioration necessitating emergency angiography/revascularization within 72 hours), which occurred in 6.2% to 11.4% of patients in each group. However, nonfatal myocardial infarction or death during hospitalization occurred in significantly fewer patients who received one of the three higher doses of bivalirudin compared with those who received 0.02 mg/kg/hr (3.2% versus 10% of patients, respectively), this difference being still present at 6 months' follow-up. Bivalirudin was investigated as an adjunct to thrombolysis with the goals of accelerating drug-induced thrombolysis and to prevent thrombus progression and vessel reocclusion. Lidon et al. (72) randomized 45 patients to bivalirudin (0.5 mg/kg/hr without prior bolus, reduced to 0.1 mg/kg/hr after 12 hours) or heparin (1,000 IU/hr) added to SK. At 90 and 120 min, TIMI grade 2 and 3 flow was observed in 77% and 87% of patients treated with bivalirudin, respectively. TIMI grade 3 flow was present at 120 min in 77% of bivalirudin versus 40% of heparin patients. In patients receiving heparin plus SK, the corresponding rates of TIMI 2 and 3 flow were 47% for both time points (p < 0.05 for the 90-minute point and p < 0.01 for the 120-minute point). Bleeding complications occurred in 12% of bivalirudin recipients versus 27% of heparin recipients (no significant difference). There was only one intracerebral hemorrhage, which occurred in the heparin group. APTTs peaked at three and four times baseline, respectively, with bivalirudin and heparin, probably secondary to the fibrinolytic effect of SK, as plasma drug levels were not higher than predicted from phase I studies.

In another pilot study, angiographic patency of the culprit coronary artery lesion was assessed 90 and 120 minutes after the initiation of SK and aspirin and again after 4 ± 2 days in 68 patients with acute myocardial infarction (73). Patients were randomized to bivalirudin 0.5 mg/kg/hr for 12 hours followed by 0.1 mg/kg/hr (low dose), bivalirudin 1 mg/kg/hr for 12 hours then placebo (high dose), or to heparin 5,000 IU bolus then 1,000 IU/hr titrated to an APTT two to 2.5 times control after 12 hours. At 90 minutes, TIMI grade 2 or 3 was observed in 96% of low-dose bivalirudin recipients versus 79% of high-dose bivalirudin and 46% of heparin recipients (p = 0.006). Respective TIMI 3 flow grade rates were 85%, 61%, and 31% of patients (p = 0.008). At 120 minutes, respective TIMI 2 or 3 rates were 100%, 82%, and 62% (p = 0.046), and TIMI 3 rates were 92%, 68%, and 46% (p = 0.014). At 90 minutes the relative risk for restoring TIMI flow grade 3 was 2.77 with low-dose bivalirudin compared with heparin (p < 0.001) and 1.4 compared with high-dose bivalirudin (p = 0.04). Patients who received a placebo infusion after 12 hours experienced more clinical events and reocclusion during the following 4 days than did patients in the other groups. In this trial, bivalirudin yielded higher patency rates when used in conjunction with SK and aspirin in the early phase of acute myocardial infarction. High bivalirudin doses are unnecessary and may be less effective than lower doses. This suggests that too much thrombin inhibition may be harmful.

Therapeutic Trials in Patients Undergoing PTCA

In a multicenter trial, Topol et al. evaluated bivalirudin in 291 patients undergoing elective angioplasty and pretreated with aspirin (74). After bolus administration, a 4-hour infusion of bivalirudin at 0.6 to 2.2 mg/kg/hr was given. The results show a dose-dependent effect of bivalirudin toward reduction of acute complications (death, fatal evidence for abrupt closure) in that patients receiving one of the three lower doses had 10.2% acute complications compared with 3.3% in patients receiving the two higher doses of bivalirudin. Although there was a trend toward a dose-related increase in APTT prolongation, there was a wide overlap between APTT of different doses. No statistically significant ACT level was associated with complete prevention of acute coronary closure. There was no prolongation of the bleeding time, and no patient developed life-threatening bleeding. Acute closure within 24 hours was inversely related to the hirulog dose and was 3.9% for the 1.8- and 2.2-mg/kg/hr dose combined.

In a much larger Hirulog Angioplasty Study, bivalirudin at high dose (1.0 mg/kg i.v. bolus followed by a 4-hour infusion at 2.5 mg/kg/hr and a 14- to 20-hour infusion at 0.2 mg/kg/hr) was compared with heparin (1,750 U/kg bolus followed by an 18- to 24-hour infusion of 15 IU/kg/hr) during coronary angioplasty for unstable or postinfarction angina in 4,098 patients, all on aspirin (75). Bivalirudin did not significantly reduce the incidence of the primary composite study endpoint (death, in-hospital death, myocardial infarction, abrupt vessel closure, or rapid deterioration of cardiac origin) (11.4% versus 12.2% for he-

parin) but did result in a lower incidence of bleeding (3.8% versus 9.8%, p < 0.001). In a prospectively stratified subgroup of 704 patients with postinfarction angina, bivalirudin therapy resulted in a lower incidence of the primary endpoint (9.1% versus 14.2%, p = 0.04) and a lower incidence of bleeding (3.0% versus 11.1%, p < 0.001), but in a similar cumulative rate of death, myocardial infarction, and repeated revascularization in the 6 months after angioplasty (20.5% versus 25.1%, p = 0.17).

Of the 4,098 patients of this trial, 573 had angiographic evidence of coronary thrombus (filling defect, ulcerations, or occlusion). Patients with thrombus had higher rates of abrupt closure (13.4% versus 8.4%, p < 0.001) and myocardial infarction (5.1% versus 3.2%, p = 0.03) than did those without thrombus. The incidence of myocardial infarction and abrupt vessel closure was identical with both anticoagulants in patients with thrombus-containing lesions (76). This clinical analysis suggests that the direct thrombin inhibitor bivalirudin is equivalent to high-dose heparin for thrombus-containing lesions assessed by angiography.

The Hirulog Early Reperfusion/Occlusion (HERO) trial evaluated two doses of bivalirudin with heparin in 412 patients with acute myocardial infarction treated with SK (43). Heparin, 5,000 IU bolus followed by 1,000 to 1,200 IU/hr titrated to APTT, or low-dose bivalirudin (0.125 mg/kg bolus followed by 0.25 mg/kg/hr for 12 hours then 0.125 mg/kg/hr) or high-dose bivalirudin (0.25 mg/kg/hr followed by 0.5 mg/kg/hr for 12 hours then 0.25 mg/kg/hr) were administered in a random fashion. TIMI grade 3 flow at 90 to 120 minutes was achieved in 35% of the heparin patients and in 48% of the high-dose bivalirudin patients (p = 0.03). Of patients who presented within 6 hours of symptom onset, 40% achieved a TIMI-3 flow at 90 minutes, 49% with low-dose bivalirudin, and 56% with high-dose bivalirudin. Among those treated within 3 hours of symptom onset, death, cardiogenic shock, or recurrent myocardial infarction had occurred in 17.9% of the heparin patients and 14% of the low-dose bivalirudin patients at 35 days. Major bleeding occurred in 28% of heparin patients, 14% of low-dose bivalirudin patients, and 19% of high-dose bivalirudin patients. A large-scale randomized trial is now planned.

Thus, high-dose bivalirudin is just as effective as high-dose heparin in preventing ischemic complications in patients who underwent PTCA for unstable angina, but it carries a 60% lower risk of bleeding. Bivalirudin, as compared with heparin, reduces significantly the risk of immediate ischemic complications after PTCA in patients with postinfarction angina, but this difference was no longer apparent after 6 months. Bivalirudin appears to be more effective than heparin in promoting early patency in myocardial infarction patients treated with SK, without increase in risk of bleeding.

Trials for the Prevention and Treatment of Deep Venous Thrombosis

The effect of bivalirudin on the production of prothrombin fragments 1 and 2 was studied in patients with calf vein thrombosis. A single injection, either 1 mg/kg s.c. or 0.6 mg/kg as a 15-minute i.v. infusion induced an incomplete and temporary suppression of prothrombin F1+2 (77). Five dosage regimens of s.c. bivalirudin were tested in the prevention of postoperative venous thrombosis after hip or knee surgery: 0.3 mg/kg every 12 hours, 0.6 mg/kg every 12 hours, 1.0 mg/kg every 12 hours for 3 days followed by 0.6 mg/kg every 12 hours for up to 11 days, 1.0 mg/kg every 12 hours, and 1.0 mg/kg every 8 hours (78). One hundred seventy-seven patients who had technically adequate bilateral venography or objectively documented pulmonary embolism were included in the primary analysis of efficacy. The highest dosage regimen (1.0 mg/kg every 8 hours) provided the lowest rates of total (17%) and proximal deep vein thrombosis (2%), both of which were significantly lower (p = 0.010 and p = 0.023, respectively) than the pooled rates of total (43%) and proximal (20%) deep vein thrombosis seen with the first four regimens. Bleeding rates were low (less than 5%) with all regimens. This study demonstrates that 1.0 mg/kg bivalirudin every 8 hours started postoperatively is potentially efficacious and safe for the prevention of deep vein thrombosis after major hip or knee surgery.

HIRUNORM

Several peptide analogues of bivalirudin have been synthesized addressing the very issue of metabolic stability through modification of the amino acid composition of the spacer arm or of the NH_2-terminus, and by rendering nonhydrolyzable the critical peptide bond. In vitro activity and stability data for these compounds have been published (81,82). This novel class of specific thrombin inhibitors termed "hirunorms" is the result of a different strategy to the same target, that is, to imitate as far as possible hirudin's tridimensional approach to the sites on thrombin surface avoiding the characteristics of a partial substrate proper to hirulog-1 and analogues (83).

Hirunorm is a 26–amino acid computer-modeled synthetic peptide (84). It is equipotent to bivalirudin and 1/30 as potent as desirudin in blocking α-thrombin amidolytic activity (IC_{50} = 10 ± 2, 15 ± 1, and 0.3 ± 0.1 nmol/L, respectively), but it does not affect trypsin, plasmin, and t-PA activities at 10 μmol/L. Hirunorm inhibits clot-bound thrombin to clots prepared by thrombin hydrolysis of purified fibrinogen in buffer. Hirunorm and hirulog show similar species-dependent potency in doubling basal in vitro clotting times of human, rat, and rabbit plasma (EC200 varied 70 to 200 nmol/L for TT, 0.7 to 16 μmol/L for APTT, and 0.8 to 17 μmol/L for PT), whereas desirudin was always at least three times more active. Hirunorm was stable against α-thrombin and plasma hydrolases, but it was catabolized by rat liver and kidney enzymes.

Venous thrombosis was produced in anesthetized rats by vena cava ligation after a procoagulant serum injection. Intravenous and subcutaneous hirunorm inhibits venous thrombosis at doses (≥0.3 mg/kg) three times higher than those of r-hirudin. Bivalirudin was as active as hirunorm only after i.v. infusion. Arterial thrombosis was obtained in the anesthetized rat by chemical ($FeCl_2$) stimulation of a common carotid; an i.v. infusion of hirunorm (1 to 3 mg/kg/30 min) inhibited it dose-dependently; desirudin was partly active only at 3 mg/kg, but hirulog was inactive at either dose. Full antithrombotic doses of hirunorm did not affect the bleeding time as measured from punctured mesenteric vessels in anesthetized rats. This compound appears to be a potent peptide thrombin inhibitor endowed with antithrombotic activity in models of venous and arterial thrombosis.

ARGATROBAN

Argatroban (Argipidine, MD-805), a small-molecule derivative of the amino acid L-arginine, was designed to inhibit thrombin directly. Its molecular weight (circa 526 daltons) is considerably smaller than hirudin (circa 7,000 daltons) and low molecular weight heparins (4,500 to 6,500 daltons). This arylsulfonylarginine interacts selectively with serine and the basic pocket of the catalytic site of thrombin along with an adjacent hydrophobic site known as the apolar region of thrombin (Fig. 9-2); concentrations three to four orders of magnitude higher are required to inhibit other serine proteases (Table 9-1). This binding of argatroban to thrombin is rapid at a diffusion controlled rate (85). In contrast with the binding to thrombin of hirudin, which is extremely tight and irreversible (dissociation constant $K_D = 2.3 \times 10^{-13}$ mol/L), the binding of argatroban to thrombin is fully reversible (dissociation constant $K_i = 3.9 \times 10^{-8}$ mol/L) (86).

Argatroban (brandname Novastan or Slonnon) is a 64:36 mixture of 21-(R) and 21-(S) diastereoisomers, with the latter being approximately twice as potent as the former in an in vitro coagulation assay but considerably less soluble in aqueous buffer (87).

TABLE 9-2. *Inhibition of serine proteases by argatroban*

For enzyme	K_D (µM)
Thrombin (human)	0.039
Thrombin (bovine)	0.019
Trypsin	5.0
Factor-Xa	210
Plasmin	800
Kallikrein	1,500

K_D, dissociation constant.

In Vivo Antithrombotic Studies in Experimental Models

Argatroban has been shown to be superior to heparin in erythrocyte-rich and platelet-rich thrombosis in several species of arterial thrombosis when administered as an i.v. bolus or as continuous i.v. infusion (88). Compared with heparin, argatroban is significantly more effective in the prevention of platelet-rich thrombi after vascular injury and was effective at APTTs of only two to three times baseline control (89).

In a whole-blood thrombolysis study with stenosed femoral arteries in the rabbit, argatroban (100 µg/kg/min, APTT 2.5- to 3.0-fold baseline) accelerated reperfusion compared with heparin (200 IU/kg, APTT more than fivefold baseline) to the extent of causing a significant leftward shift of the t-PA dose-response curve. Addition of aspirin did not accelerate thrombolysis by either argatroban or heparin (89).

In a whole-blood clot thrombus model in stenotic canine coronaries, pretreatment with argatroban at 200 µg/kg/min (APTTs of six to 7.6 times control) significantly reduced the time to lysis by alteplase to 23 minutes compared with 40 minutes in the aspirin group. Addition of aspirin to argatroban did not shorten time to lysis but reduced the incidence of reocclusion by platelet-rich thrombi from 75% to 20% relative to argatroban alone (90). Argatroban was as effective in this model as abciximab in inhibiting the platelet glycoprotein (GP)IIb/IIIa receptor.

In a platelet-rich coronary thrombus model after endothelial injury created by electric current, acceleration of lysis by alteplase was observed in dogs pretreated with argatroban at a lower dose (41 µg/kg/min). However, abolition of cyclic flow reductions due intermittent platelet aggregates required the addition of a thromboxane A$_2$/prostaglandin endoperoxide receptor antagonist (91). Of note, in an open-chest canine model of unstable angina, both argatroban and heparin were equally efficacious at abolishing cyclic flow reductions caused by the formation or dislodgement of platelet-rich, fibrin-poor thrombi in the absence of platelet inhibitors (92,93).

The dose of argatroban that doubled the bleeding time (rat-tail transection) was five times greater than for heparin (11 versus 2.2 µg/kg/min) (94).

Overall, in experimental models of arterial thrombosis, argatroban achieves in vivo antithrombotic efficacy comparable with that of heparin, but with less systemic anticoagulation (APTT) and hemorrhagic potential.

In the Wessler venous thrombosis model (thromboplastin plus stasis of the left jugular vein) and arteriovenous shunt models in rabbits, argatroban was less active on a weight basis than heparin (95).

Pharmacokinetics and Pharmacodynamics

In rabbits and dogs, radiolabeled argatroban is cleared from the plasma in a biphasic manner, with α and β elimination half-lives of 3 to 6 minutes and 20 to 86 minutes, respectively (96). In normal volunteers, the elimination half-live is around 30 minutes. The majority of the drug is excreted fecally, indicating hepatic metabolism and biliary excretion (96). The metabolism is hydroxylation and aromatization of the 3-methyltetrahydroquinoline ring (97).

Compared with heparin, bolus doses of argatroban showed a slowly increasing dose-response effect in normal subjects, with an eightfold increase in dose (30 to 240 µg/kg) resulting in only a twofold increase in peak APTT (43 to 82 seconds). However, heparin showed a pronounced, rapidly rising effect on APTT, with a twofold increase in dose (15 to 30 IU/kg) doubling the peak APTT value (68 to 269 seconds) and with doses ≥30 IU/kg often associated with APTT values of more than 400 seconds, which is above the assay detection limits (98).

Figure 9-3 compares the effects of 4-hour infusions of various doses of argatroban or heparin on APTT. Over a twofold increase in dose, heparin displayed a steep dose-response curve; argatroban, however, displayed a gently rising, predictable response over an eight-fold range in infusion dose (98).

Figure 9-4 compares the time course of a combined bolus and continuous i.v. infusion regimen (4-hour duration) for argatroban (250-µg/kg bolus and 10-µg/kg/min infusion) and heparin (125-U/kg bolus and 0.3-U/kg/min infusion) on HemoTec ACT (98). Both drugs rapidly induced increases in ACT over baseline values. Argatroban maintained the ACT values at steady levels for 4 hours; the response with heparin, however, decreased during the infusion, likely a result of

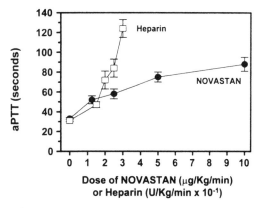

FIG. 9-3. Pharmacodynamic effects of continuous infusions (4-hr duration) of heparin *(open squares)* and argatroban *(filled circles)* on the mean APTT (± SEM) in nine normal subjects. The doses used were as follows: argatroban, 1.25, 2.5, 5.0, and 10.0 µg/kg/min; heparin, 0.15, 0.20, 0.25, and 0.30 IU/kg/min. (From Schwartz et al., ref. 98, with permission.)

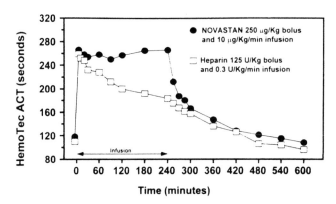

FIG. 9-4. Comparative effects of combined bolus injection continuous infusion (4-hr duration) of heparin *(open squares)* or agratroban *(filled circles)* on the mean HemoTec ACT for nine normal subjects. (From Schwartz et al., ref. 98, with permission.)

the release of platelet factor 4 from activated platelets, which interferes with the binding of heparin to antithrombin III.

The effects of renal impairment, age, and gender on the pharmacodynamics of argatroban have been studied. No significant effects were observed, but there was a trend toward an increased risk for bleeding events in patients with an APTT of more than 90 seconds, particularly in elderly, low body weight patients (especially female patients), and patients with renal impairment (99,100).

Clinical Development

The first clinical pilot study with argatroban (Novastan, Mitsubishi Kasai Corp., Midori-ku, Yokohama, Japan) was in 43 patients with unstable angina/non–Q wave myocardial infarction. Argatroban was infused over 4 hours (0.5 to 5.0 µg/kg/min), which resulted in a dose-dependent increase in APTT and effectively prevented recurrences of ischemic episodes, in the absence of aspirin (101). However, it was reported that cessation of therapy was associated with "rebound" thrombin generation (as measured by levels of plasma thrombin–antithrombin complex (TAT) and with an early dose-related recurrence of unstable angina. One should remember that abrupt termination of a thrombin inhibitor increases thrombin activity (as measured by FPA formation) but not thrombin

generation (as measured by the formation of either TAT or prothrombin fragment F1.2). The short duration of the argatroban infusion (4 hours) may be criticized for a condition in which the tendency toward thrombosis remains for days (102). No decrease in plasma TAT concentration was observed during the argatroban infusion, questioning whether the TAT increase observed after cessation of argatroban therapy is artifactual and no elevation in plasma FPA was observed after cessation of therapy, as would be expected in a hypercoagulable state (103). However, it is also possible that the dissociation of the drug from thrombin (argatroban is a competitive inhibitor) allowed regeneration and a rebound of thrombin (104). It remains to be established in larger trials whether argatroban offers a favorable clinical profile in unstable angina and non–Q wave myocardial infarction.

There is limited published experience with argatroban in PTCA patients. In order to define the optimal dose, 30 patients undergoing PTCA for stable or unstable angina were studied at four different dose regimens (105). Study endpoints were the occurrence of clinical cardiac events, bleeding complications, coagulation tests, and qualitative angiogram interpretation. All patients underwent control angiography 18 to 24 hours after PTCA. The group with the highest argatroban dosage received 250 µg/kg i.v. bolus followed by a 4-hour infusion of 15 µg/kg/min. At 4 hours the infusion rate was lowered to 3.8 µg/kg/min and continued for 68 hours. TT, APTT, and PT were significantly related to argatroban plasma levels (R-square 0.64, 0.71, 0.84 by regression analysis, respectively). F1+2 and TAT did not relate to argatroban plasma levels. Five patients experienced a cardiac event, and there were two cases of prolonged bleeding at a puncture site, one false aneurysm, and one epistaxis occurring under heparin and acenocoumaron 3 days after stopping argatroban requiring transfusion. This pilot trial identified an apparent safe and adequate dose regimen that is presently being evaluated in a double-blind, 2:1 randomized comparative trial versus heparin (Argaplasty trial).

In a pilot trial, i.v. argatroban was assessed versus unfractionated heparin as adjunctive therapy to the accelerated regimen of alteplase in 112 patients with acute myocardial infarction (106). Argatroban was given as a bolus of 100 µg/kg before the start of thrombolytic therapy followed by an infusion of 3 µg/kg/min. Heparin was administered as a bolus of 5,000 IU followed by an infusion of 1,000 IU/hr titrated against APTT. The TIMI grade 3 patency rate at 90 min was 56% in the argatroban group and 67% in the heparin group, a nonstatistical difference. Larger trials are required to decide the optimal dosage of argatroban and to assess its angiographic and clinical efficacy compared with unfractionated heparin.

Two multicenter, randomized, blinded, controlled clinical trials are assessing the efficacy and safety of argatroban as adjunctive therapy to thrombolytic agents in the treatment of acute myocardial infarction. The Argatroban in Myocardial Infarction (AMI) study has enrolled 400 patients with a diagnosis of myocardial infarction within the first 6 hours of onset of symptoms. All patients received aspirin and SK and were randomized to receive either high-dose argatroban (3.0 µg/kg/min), low-dose argatroban (1.0 µg/kg/min), or placebo for 48 to 72 hours. The dose of argatroban is to be titrated downward if the APTT exceeds 90 seconds. Patients were followed for 30 days to assess the incidence of death, acute myocardial infarction, recurrent angina,

need for coronary revascularization procedures (PTCA or CABG surgery), and new-onset congestive heart failure. In a substudy of an additional 180 patients, patency of the culprit coronary artery was assessed angiographically at 90 and 120 minutes after initiation of therapy.

A second trial, the Myocardial Infarction with Novastan and t-PA (MINT) Study was terminated. One hundred twenty patients were enrolled with the same diagnostic criteria as in the AMI trial. All patients received aspirin and accelerated t-PA and were randomized to one of three groups: (a) high-dose argatroban (3.0 µg/kg/min), (b) low-dose argatroban (1.0 µg/kg/min), or (c) heparin for 48 to 72 hours. As in the AMI study, patency of the culprit coronary artery was assessed angiographically at 90 and 120 minutes after initiation of therapy.

One pivotal multicenter trial investigating the safety and efficacy of argatroban in patients with heparin-induced thrombocytopenia (HIT) has been completed.

EFEGATRAN

Efegatran sulfate (GYKI 14766, LY 294468), a tripeptide aldehyde (mePhe-Pro-Arg-H) is an arginal catalytic-site inhibitor of thrombin (107). It is a reversible, competitive, tight-binding inhibitor (108). No time-dependent effects were observed for interactions of efegatran with thrombin, suggesting that there are no slow-binding interactions of practical consequence.

Table 9-3 shows that a concentration of 20 ng/ml of efegatran is required to double the TT, but over 1,000 ng/ml is required to prolong the PT and APTT. The functional anticoagulant selectivity for an inhibitor can be estimated by a ratio of the concentrations that prolong by twofold the APTT and the TT; such APTT/TT effect ratios are shown in Table 9-3. For efegatran the APTT/TT ratio is 55, which means that 55-fold higher concentrations are required for APTT prolongation (109).

These data suggest that hirudin and efegatran, although both are direct-acting inhibitors of thrombin, act differently on the APTT

TABLE 9-3. *Human plasma anticoagulant concentration for two-fold prolongation of thrombin time, prothrombin time, and APTT*

	Thrombin time		Prothrombin time (ng/ml)	APTT (ng/ml)	Ratio of APTT/TT
	ng/ml	nmol/L			
Efegatran	19 ± 2	33	1,360	1,050	55
Native hirudin	109 ± 4	16	1,800	280	2.5
Recombinant hirudin	126 ± 17	18	3,600	340	2.7

Control TT, 32 seconds; control PT, 18 seconds; control APTT, 32 seconds. From Smith et al., ref. 109, with permission.

pathway, possibly by inhibiting a different APTT element in addition to thrombin inhibition, or by differently affecting a thrombin-mediated function in the APTT pathway. Hypothetically, different effects on the thrombin feedback activation of factor V or factor VIII could cause the observed anticoagulant differences. More speculatively, if thrombin activation of protein C should prove to be an element of the APTT pathway and clotting rate, then different inhibition of this process by hirudin and efegatran could cause the observed APTT/TT selectivity differences. However, the observed anticoagulant functional difference is apparently exclusive to the APTT pathway because such functional differences between hirudin and efegatran were not observed in their respective effects on the PT pathway and no different effects of efegatran and hirudin could be found in the inhibition of other protease clotting factors (109–111). Therefore, the anticoagulant functional selectivity difference found between efegatran (APTT/TT ratio in the range of 30 to 55) and hirudin (APTT/TT ratio about 2 to 3) remains unexplained. The practical result of the mechanistic difference is that upon increasing doses of efegatran in vitro, in animal studies and in clinical use, the TT will become progressively and markedly prolonged without initially affecting the APTT.

In Vivo Studies in Animal Thrombosis Models

Efegatran, given in a constant infusion, was tested in a canine model of coronary artery thrombosis. Efegatran produced dose-depen-

dent anticoagulant effects in the anesthetized dog (112,113). Efegatran at a median dose of 1.0 mg/kg/hr caused a more than 10-fold increase in TT, but only a 1.7-fold increase in APTT. Peak APTT changes were 1.1 ± 0.03, 1.5 ± 0.07, 1.6 ± 0.1, 2.4 ± 0.2, and 3.3 ± 0.2-fold with 0.25, 0.5, 1.0, 2.0, and 4.0 mg/kg/hr efegatran, respectively. When the infusion of efegatran was stopped, APTT and TT returned to normal within the 2-hour washout period. All doses produced significant prolongations in time to total thrombotic occlusion. The dose-response curve resembled more of an "all or none" profile with 0.5 mg/kg/hr efegatran producing a time to occlusion of 205 ± 23 min compared with 213 ± 14 min for the 4.0 mg/kg/hr efegatran dose group. Template bleeding times were significantly increased only at the high dose of 4.0 mg/kg/hr efegatran. Baseline template bleeding times in efegatran-treated groups were 144 ± 5, 139 ± 5, 133 ± 10, and 126 ± 8 seconds for 0.25, 0.5, 1.0, 2.0, and 4.0 mg/kg/hr, respectively.

In the same dog model of coronary artery thrombosis, the combination therapy with minimum effective doses of efegatran enhanced the antithrombotic efficacy compared with heparin (114).

Efegatran was an effective anticoagulant when used as an adjunct during SK-induced thrombolysis in the anesthetised dog (113). A dose-dependent anticoagulant effect in the presence of SK was observed on TT and APTT. Peak TT increases were 526 ± 66 seconds and 793 ± 85 seconds versus baseline values of 37 ± 1 and 36 ± 1 seconds with 0.5 and 1.0 mg/kg/hr efegatran, respectively. Peak APTT increases were 76 ± 6 and 125 ± 4 seconds versus baseline values of 34 ± 1 and 35 ± 1 seconds with 0.5 and 1.0 mg/kg/hr efegatran, respectively. Time to reperfusion in response to SK-induced thrombolysis was 46 ± 10 minutes, whereas control dogs had no reperfusion. All animals receiving SK with either efegatran or ASA alone, or the combination of efegatran and ASA demonstrated reperfusion of their coronary artery. In the groups receiving SK alone and SK and 0.5 mg/kg/hr efegatran, all vessels that reperfused, reoccluded. The time to reocclusion for the SK alone group was 89 ± 23 minutes. Even though all animals receiving 0.5 mg/kg/hr efegatran reoccluded their coronary artery, the time to reocclusion was significantly longer (156 ± 19 min, p < 0.05) when compared with the SK alone group. In the group receiving 1.0 mg/kg/hr efegatran, the time to reocclusion was significantly prolonged (198 ± 12 minutes). In the group receiving SK and ASA, the time to reocclusion was 141 ± 32 min, not significantly different from the SK-treated group. The best antireocclusive efficacy was observed in the group receiving SK, 0.5 mg/kg/hr efegatran, and ASA. All vessels exposed to this regimen were patent at the end of the experiment (4 hours).

Thrombolytic therapy with SK in the dog produced a significant increase in template bleeding time (316 ± 50 sec versus 140 ± 10 sec, p < 0.05) (114). Anticoagulant and/or antiplatelet therapy with efegatran and ASA had no significant additive effect on template bleeding time beyond that induced by SK alone.

Studies in Human Volunteers

With a 15-minute i.v. infusion of efegatran in human volunteers, a dose of approximately 0.025 mg/kg was required to double the TT value. TT was a specific and extremely sensitive measure of the anticoagulant activity of efegatran. The upper limit of quantification for TT (120 seconds for the automated method chosen) was exceeded at doses above 0.1 mg/kg, making interpretation of the anti-

coagulant effect of efegatran, in terms of TT prolongation, more difficult. At higher dose levels of efegatran (0.225 mg/kg to 0.3 mg/kg), APTT values were prolonged in a dose-dependent fashion. Immediately before the termination of the 15-minute efegatran infusion of 0.3 mg/kg, APTT prolongation ranged from 175% to 238% of baseline. The offset of anticoagulant effect (measured by prolongation of APTT) after cessation of drug infusion was rapid, with a pharmacologic half-life for efegatran of approximately 30 minutes.

Prolonged i.v. administration of efegatran (0.2, 0.4, 0.6, and 0.8 mg/kg/hr) produced dose-related anticoagulant activity with no accumulation of effect. For all infusion rates, except 0.2 mg/kg/hr, the TT was prolonged to greater than the 120-second limit of the automated technique used; however, dose-related prolongations of APTT were observed. The anticoagulant effect of efegatran, measured by APTT prolongation as a percentage of baseline values, correlated in a linear fashion (p < 0.001) with the rate of infusion of efegatran, irrespective of the duration of infusion.

The template bleeding time was used in healthy male subjects as a surrogate assessment of bleeding risk. Bleeding times fell within the reference range for the method (2 to 10 minutes), irrespective of the dose level or duration of infusion of efegatran studied. In a few individuals, sporadic prolonged bleeding time measurements were recorded, without clear evidence of a dose-response relationship to efegatran. Prolonged bleeding times had returned to baseline by the time a follow-up assessment was made 6 hours post-termination of infusion.

Clinical Studies

The preclinical and clinical pharmacology of efegatran was recently reviewed (115).

Safety and anticoagulant properties of efegatran were studied at three dose levels in 36 patients with unstable angina (116). Three groups of 10 patients have been treated with a loading dose of 0.1 mg/kg in combination with a 48-hour infusion of 0.10, 0.32, and 0.63 mg/kg/hr, respectively. Six patients were randomly allocated to receive APTT-adjusted unfractionated heparin (5,000-IU bolus followed by 1,000 IU/hr). In contrast to treatments with heparin, no APTT overshoot at 0.5 hour was apparent.

At these dose levels, efegatran has been clinically well tolerated. One patient at the highest dose received 2 U packed cells for a hematoma after cardiac catheterization. Recurrent ischemia during infusion occurred in four, one, and four patients receiving efegatran at the respective dosages indicated above, as well as in three patients receiving heparin. No clinically significant prolongations of bleeding time have been recorded in any of the patients treated through dosages of 0.84 mg/kg/hr. The estimated clinically effective dosage is 0.63 mg/kg/hr.

APTT measurements show that efegatran produces a dose-dependent prolongation of APTT as predicted from both preclinical and human volunteer data. The APTT effect correlates linearly with efegatran plasma concentration. The i.v. half-life of APTT effect and efegatran plasma concentration was 35 minutes, and clearance from plasma was rapid (0.4 L/hr/kg). Eighty-five percent of the steady-state concentrations were achieved 2 hours after starting a constant rate infusion. There is no evidence of accumulation of anticoagulant effect over time.

Whether efegatran given for 72 to 96 hours and adjusted to APTT can reduce the patency lag associated with SK was studied in 247 patients with acute myocardial infarction in the randomized, open-label, dose-finding ESCALAT study (117). The combination of efegatran and SK was compared to t-PA and i.v. heparin using angiographic and clinical endpoints. The study has been completed but not reported. In a second dose ranging trial, heparin or escalating dosages of efegatran (0.3 to 1.2 mg/kg/hr) were compared in 330 patients with acute myocardial infarction (118). This trial was also completed but not

reported in detail. Further clinical trials with efegatran are not being pursued.

NAPSAGATRAN

Napsagatran (RO 46-6240) is a cyclopropyl derivative of a novel class of thrombin inhibitors bearing a 3-(aminomethyl)-1-amidinopiperidine as an arginine side chain mimetic. An attached L-aspartic acid serves as template to reach two hydrophic pockets near the active site of the enzyme (119).

Napsagatran is a selective, potent, competitive, and reversible inhibitor of thrombin of low molecular weight (559 daltons). It inhibits the catalytic activity of thrombin toward fibrinogen or the chromogenic substrate S-2238 at picomolar concentrations. In these tests the compound is approximately two orders of magnitude more potent than argatroban. This activity is also evident in clotting tests performed in human plasma such as the TT, PT, and APTT (120).

Many enzymes of the coagulation system are closely related to thrombin. Napsagatran represents one of the most specific synthetic thrombin inhibitors of small molecular weight known today. Specificity for thrombin is an important parameter for an antithrombotic compound because interference with most of the related enzymes is undesirable. To estimate the selectivity of napsagatran, inhibition of several serine proteases from different physiologic systems was determined. The selectivity ratio of napsagatran for trypsin was indicated by the ratio of K_i for trypsin/K_i for thrombin and amounts to 7140 (119–121). The selectivity ratios for plasmin, t-PA, kallikrein, C1-esterase, elastase and chymotrypsin range from 8,600 to 250,000.

Napsagatran inhibits clot-bound thrombin and thrombin in solution with equal potency, whereas hirudin is less active against clot-bound than against fluid-phase thrombin (122). It remains to be seen whether this interesting experimental property of napsagatran will translate into an increased therapeutic benefit in clinical situations of a preexisting clot.

Napsagatran efficiently inhibits fibrin deposition on tissue factor expressed by human endothelial cells. The procoagulant activity of tumor necrosis factor-α–stimulated monolayers of human endothelial cells was studied in a flow system with human venous blood using desirudin, napsagatran, and heparin. Under venous blood flow conditions (at wall shear rates of 65 seconds-1), these compounds inhibited fibrin deposition by 50% at concentration of 14, 28, and 412 ng/ml, respectively (123).

The shear rate–dependent and perfusion time–dependent effect of napsagatran at 100 μg/kg/min on thrombogenesis induced by subendothelium of rabbit aorta were studied using an ex vivo perfusion chamber system (124). The deposition of fibrin on subendothelium was completely abolished at shear rates of 100, 650, and 2,600 seconds-1 after 5- and 30-minute perfusions. In contrast, a significant effect on thrombus formation after a 5-minute perfusion could be observed only at a shear rate of 100 seconds-1, whereas after a 30-minute perfusion thrombus formation was reduced at all three shear rates. These results show that thrombin-mediated mechanisms are important in the latter phase of thrombus growth in this thrombosis model.

In Vivo Experimental Thrombosis Models

Napsagatran was compared with heparin in a canine model of coronary thrombosis (121). Occlusive thrombosis of the left circumflex coronary artery was induced by electrical injury. In parallel, arterial subendothelium was exposed to native blood using an annular perfusion chamber for 5, 10, and 20 minutes at a wall shear rate of 650/sec. Dogs received saline, heparin (40 and 70 IU/kg/hr), or napsagatran (3 and 10 μg/kg/min). Heparin (40 IU/kg/hr) and napsagatran (3 μg/kg/min) delayed or prevented in vivo thrombotic occlusion, but only napsagatran (10 μg/kg/min) significantly decreased the intracoronary

thrombus when compared with saline. High-dose unfractionated heparin (70 IU/kg/hr) or napsagatran (10 μg/kg/min) decreased the platelet-rich thrombus after a 20-minute chamber perfusion. Neither heparin nor napsagatran decreased the thrombus volume after a 5-minute perfusion. Heparin (70 IU/kg/hr) and napsagatran (10 μg/kg/min) prolonged the APTT differently (more than six-fold and 1.4-fold, respectively, $p < 0.01$), whereas the ACT was prolonged equally (2.5-fold). Thus, napsagatran in this dog model shows arterial antithrombotic effects similar to those of heparin.

In a guinea pig model of arterial thrombosis, cyclic variations of blood flow (CFV) in the carotid artery were monitored after mechanical damage of the vessel. These CFVs indicated build-up and embolization of platelet-rich thrombotic masses. Napsagatran, desirudin, and heparin applied as an i.v. bolus followed by a continuous i.v. infusion prevented the occurrence of CFVs in a dose-related manner (120). Thus, at a dosage of 30, 50, and 67 μg/kg/min, respectively, the compounds significantly inhibited the occurrence of CFVs without prolonging the bleeding time.

The antithrombotic effect of napsagatran was also evaluated in an acute in vivo venous stasis thrombosis model (Wessler model) in the rat (121). Napsagatran completely inhibited the appearance of a clot at a dosage of 3 μg/kg/min (ID_{100}). A partial inhibition was observed at 1 μg/kg/min. At these dosages the APTT was prolonged 1.6- to 2.5-fold in comparison with controls. As expected, recombinant hirudin was also fully effective and overall about three times as potent as napsagatran. In contrast, as compared with napsagatran, about five times more heparin was needed for a full inhibition ($ID_{100} = 20$ μg/kg/min) and this dose of heparin prolonged the APTT 12-fold.

Clinical Studies

Napsagatran is currently in phase II clinical trials to establish its efficacy and safety for preventing postoperative thrombosis as well as treating established venous thrombosis.

INOGATRAN

Inogatran (H314/27) is a synthetic dipeptide with a molecular weight of 439 daltons (125). Inogatran selectively, rapidly, and competitively binds thrombin. In vitro it doubles the plasma TT at a concentration of 23 nmol/L and the APTT at 1.1 μmol/L. Thrombin-induced platelet aggregation is inhibited at an IC_{50} of 17 nmol/L.

Inogatran was evaluated in three rat models of thrombosis. In the venous thrombosis model, inogatran dose-dependently inhibited thrombus formation with a more than 80% antithrombotic effect at a plasma concentration of 0.45 μmol/L-1 (126). In an arterial thrombosis model, inogatran dose-dependently inhibited thrombus formation and preserved vessel patency and the mean blood flow. Acetylsalicylic acid potentiated the effects of low plasma concentrations of inogatran in the arterial thrombosis model. In a model of rt-PA–induced thrombolysis of a thrombus in the carotid artery, the patency time and the cumulative blood flow improved more in the presence of inogatran during the 2-hour thrombolysis period than with rt-PA alone. At a high therapeutic plasma concentration of inogatran, there was only a moderate prolongation of bleeding time compared with the control value. A study was designed to examine the modulation of coronary artery reocclusion by inogatran with or without aspirin (127). Twenty-two dogs with electrically induced occlusive intracoronary thrombus were treated with saline or different doses of inogatran (up to 0.25 mg/kg bolus followed by 0.6 mg/kg/hr for 2 hours). rt-PA was infused for 20 minutes starting 2 minutes after the bolus in all dogs. Coronary artery blood flow was monitored for 120 minutes after rt-PA administration. Reperfusion rates were similar in all groups, but the time to reperfusion was the longest and the reocclusion rate the lowest in the high-dose inogatran group. Aspirin did not potentiate the effect of suboptimal doses of inogatran.

Studies in Healthy Male Volunteers

Inogatran was studied in healthy male human volunteers with regard to tolerability, pharmacokinetics, and effects on hemostasis. It was given i.v. as a bolus in doses up to 0.48 mg/kg body weight. The highest peak plasma concentration observed was 7 μmol/L, corresponding to an APTT prolongation of three times. The drug was also given as a constant i.v. infusion over 4 hours at a dosage of 0.32 mg/kg/hr, which resulted in a mean plasma concentration at steady state of 1.9 μmol/L and an APTT prolongation of 2.3 times. The drug was well tolerated and without side effects with the exception of a slightly increased bleeding tendency at the blood sampling site. Inogatran had a volume of distribution of 0.26 ml/kg and a total plasma clearance of 6.1 ml/min/kg, resulting in a terminal half-life of about 1 hour. The drug was not metabolized and it was excreted unchanged with the elimination evenly distributed between urine and feces. Ex vivo the TT was linearly correlated to the plasma concentration while the APTT-concentration curve was nonlinear. At the highest plasma concentrations a slight prolongation of the capillary bleeding time was seen in some subjects. Markers of thrombin activity (thrombin–antithrombin complex and prothrombin F1+2) decreased during the constant infusion of the drug. There was no effect on fibrinolysis (PAI-1 and t-PA activities) or protein C.

Clinical Development

In an open-design study, 37 patients with unstable angina or non–Q-wave infarction were treated within 72 hours of symptoms with aspirin and other standard treatment and were allocated consecutively to groups receiving a 4-hour infusion with one of three doses of inogatran (bolus of 0.035, 0.07, and 0.105 mg/kg followed by a 4-hour infusion of 0.063, 0.126, and 0.189 mg/kg/hr) (128). There was a predictable dose-response relationship between inogatran concentration and APTT. Thrombin generation (prothrombin F1+2) was suppressed after 4 hours of treatment compared with baseline, but thrombin activity (fibrinopeptide A) was not suppressed. There were no adverse hemodynamic or other effects. Minor bleeding was noted in 37% of the patients. During the first 4 hours after inogatran treatment, thrombin activity and episodes of ischemia were increased compared with the inogatran infusion period.

Three doses of inogatran were studied in 1,209 patients with unstable angina or non–Q-wave myocardial infarction in a randomized double-blind study (129). After a bolus of inogatran (1.10, 2.75, or 5.50 mg/kg) or heparin, infusions continued for 3 days with a low (2.0 mg/kg/hr), medium (5.0 mg/kg/hr), or high (10.0 mg/kg/hr) dosage of inogatran (resulting in APTT prolongations of 1.3, 1.5, and 1.8 times baseline at 24 hours, respectively) or heparin (1,200 IU/hr). A composite endpoint of death, myocardial infarction, or refractory or recurrent angina at 3, 7, and 30 days did not show differences between the groups. Thus, inogatran at the doses used was no better than heparin in preventing ischemic coronary events. There was no dose-effect relationship concerning inogatran. After cessation of infusion, hypercoagulability was noted in both the heparin and the inogatran groups.

Further clinical development of inogatran has been stopped.

OTHER DIRECT ANTITHROMBINS

A variety of other antithrombins have been synthesized but no clinical trials have been planned. Among them the peptide PPACK (d-Phe-Pro-Arg-CH$_2$Cl) (RWJ-27755) was found to be a highly potent irreversible inhibitor of thrombin by alkylating the active center site histidine (130–132). There is a rapid loss of activity of this compound due to reactions with other plasma components (133). Notwithstanding its antithrombotic effect at high doses in different arterial thrombosis models in the rat, dog, and pig, its alkylating properties have considerably tempered the enthusiasm for its clinical development. Boroarginine derivatives (DuP714) are potent

antithrombins with a potential for oral bioavailability (134). Unfortunately, their boron constituent induces liver toxicity. CVS-1123 (or CH$_3$CH$_2$CH$_2$)$_2$-CH-CO-Asp(OCH$_3$)-Pro-Arg-CHO) is a synthetic peptidometric of small molecular weight (575 daltons). It is a slow, competitive inhibitor of the amidolytic activity of thrombin as well as a potent anticoagulant in plasma in vitro. CVS-1123 has been shown in an anesthetized porcine model to be effective in preventing arterial thrombus formation (135). The oral antithrombotic efficacy of this compound, administered for 24 hours, has been demonstrated in the conscious canine dog to prevent primary thrombus formation after deep arterial coronary wall injury (136).

Other antithrombins still in development are hirudisin–hirudin derivatives combining blocking of the platelet IIb/IIIa receptor and direct thrombin inhibition. In the hirudisins, residues 32 to 35 of hirudin have been replaced by the integrin motif RGDS and KGDS, obtaining a potent thrombin inhibitor (K_D 0.16 to 0.26 × 10^{-12} mol/L compared with 0.2 × 10^{-12} mol/L for desirudin) with additional disintegrin activity (137). In addition to inhibiting GPIIb/IIIa receptor–dependent platelet interactions, the platelet-binding integrin motif is expected to target the antithrombin action of hirudin to platelets, possibly allowing lower and safer doses of desirudin in the treatment of thrombotic disease (138). Similarly, desirudin targeted to fibrin by coupling them to Fab′ portions of antibodies directed against platelet GPIIb/IIIa receptor or fibrin β-chain (139,140) may allow for highly efficient antithrombosis at doses lower than presently required for desirudin.

Aptamers are oligonucleotides (double- or single-stranded DNA or single-stranded RNA) some of which bind directly to thrombin with binding affinities in the range of 20 to 200 nmol/L (e.g., a single-stranded, 15-nucleotide DNA aptamer) (141). This potent aptamer with rapid onset of action and short half-life has been found to interact with the anion-binding exosite of thrombin, so that it competes with substrates that interact with that specific site, such as fibrinogen and thrombin platelet receptors (142). This aptamer has been shown to reduce arterial platelet thrombus formation in an animal model, as well as to inhibit clot-bound thrombin in an in vitro system (143).

Recently, there has been a report of a novel synthetic thrombin inhibitor, CVS #995, comprised of 19 amino acids, in which recognition sequences for the catalytic and primary exosite binding domains of thrombin have been linked by a transition state analogue (144). Catalytic inhibition of thrombin is obtained in the picomolar range for this slow and tightly binding thrombin inhibitor. When compared with bivalirudin, this agent was superior at inhibiting platelet aggregation and venous thrombosis in a rat model.

A number of lysyl α-ketocarbonyl derivatives were found to be as potent (on a weight basis) as hirudin when evaluated in a rat arterial thrombosis model (145). Their modest oral bioavailability (10% to 19%) suggests the possibility that α-keto amide containing thrombin inhibitors may have utility as orally active antithrombotic agents.

The main platelet receptor for thrombin (Fig. 9-5) was recently characterized (147) and has the unique feature of a tethered ligand. After thrombin binds the receptor through a hirudinlike anion-binding exosite, it cleaves the receptor to show a new receptor's amino acid terminus, which functions as the tethered ligand to activate the receptor. The molecule of thrombin thus remains free to activate other receptor sites and propagate the thrombotic process (148). This receptor has been cloned (149). A polyclonal antibody was raised against the peptide derived from the thrombin-binding exosite region of the cloned human thrombin receptor (150). This antibody serves as a selective inhibitor of the thrombin receptor.

CONCLUSION

1. Despite interdigitation of residues critical to its opposing biologic functions, the pro- and anticoagulant properties of

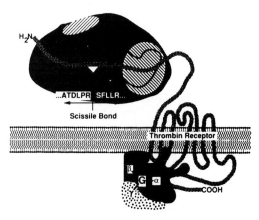

FIG. 9-5. Mechanism of thrombin receptor activation. Cleavage by thrombin of the Arg^{41}-Ser^{12} scissile bond in the native thrombin receptor shows the new amino terminal Ser-Phe-Leu-Leu-Arg ... sequence of the receptor, which serves as a tethered agonist ligand that directly activates the thrombin receptor, resulting in postreceptor signaling via specific G proteins. (From Ogletree, ref. 146, with permission.)

thrombin have been related to fast and slow allosteric forms of the enzyme, respectively, corresponding to distinct conformational states of the protein. None of the site-directed thrombin inhibitors blocks the procoagulant function only.

2. Advantages of all site-directed thrombin inhibitors over heparin are (a) selectivity and rapidity for interacting with functional domains of thrombin; (b) ability to inhibit both clot-bound thrombin and thrombin in the fluid phase; (c) independence of plasma proteins for their action; (d) absence of neutralization by natural anticoagulants, plasma proteins, endothelium and platelet factor 4; (e) predictable pharmacokinetic and pharmacodynamic profile; and (f) absence of immunologic reactions. For none of the specific site-directed thrombin inhibitors is an antidote available, and it has proven difficult to synthetize orally available specific thrombin inhibitors.

3. Desirudin at the low doses used in large-scale clinical trials in patients with acute myocardial infarction treated with al-

teplase or SK appears to be at least as effective as unfractionated heparin in terms of therapeutic benefit. Its therapeutic window in this setting is narrow because significantly more moderate bleeding occurs during i.v. desirudin than during unfractionated heparin administration.

4. In patients with unstable angina, low- and medium-high doses of desirudin resulted in a trend toward lower event rates at 7 days compared with unfractionated heparin at the cost of significantly more minor bleeding.

5. All trials to date have studied relatively short-term (3 to 5 days) desirudin administration. The potential benefits (or lack thereof) of longer-term administration of desirudin in unstable coronary syndromes and PTCA remain unknown.

6. In the prevention of postoperative deep venous thrombosis after orthopedic surgery, desirudin is significantly more effective than unfractionated heparin and low molecular-weight heparin without increase in bleeding risk.

7. There is a large clinical experience with bivalirudin in the treatment of unstable angina and as adjunctive therapy with thrombolytic drugs for acute myocardial infarction. Bivalirudin appears to be as effective as unfractionated heparin in the prevention of acute complications of PTCA in patients with unstable angina, but is significantly more effective than heparin in the cohort of patients with postinfarction angina. This advantage is associated with a 60% reduction of major bleeding complications. However, there was no significant benefit on event-free survival at 7 months in the subgroup.

8. Argatroban is more effective than heparin in animal models of thrombosis, but it is not demonstrated whether this is the case in patients. A drawback of the reversible thrombin inhibitor argatroban is that an infusion of short treatment may induce a thrombotic rebound phenomenon after cessation of infusion in clinical conditions in which the tendency toward thrombosis persists for days.

9. The safety and efficacy of hirunorm, efegatran, and napsagatran remain to be established through ongoing clinical trials. The clinical experience with inogatran has engendered dismay because no superiority over unfractionated heparin could be demonstrated in a large trial in patients with unstable angina or non–Q-wave infarction.

10. Several of the direct thrombin inhibitors also exhibit non–thrombin-mediated actions that are responsible for some of the additional pharmacologic effects that may also contribute to the antithrombotic/hemorrhagic balance. Direct thrombin inhibitors should be considered as a class of drugs, each compound having its own pharmacologic and therapeutic profile.

11. Direct thrombin inhibitors are easy to use, having a stable anticoagulant activity, lack of direct effects on platelet function, and uniformity of pharmacologic composition and activity, but no antidote is available.

REFERENCES

1. Dodt J, Machleidt W, Seemüller U, Maschler R, Fritz H. Isolation and characterization of hirudin isoinhibitors and sequence analysis of hirudin PA. *Biol Chem Hoppe Seyler* 1986;367:803–811.
2. Markwardt F. Development of hirudin as an antithrombotic agent. *Semin Thromb Hemost* 1989;15:269–282.
3. Stone SR, Hofsteenge J. Kinetics of the inhibition of thrombin by hirudin. *Biochemistry* 1986;25:4622–4628.
4. Rydel TJ, Ravichandran KG, Tulinsky A, et al. The structure of a complex of recombinant hirudin and human alpha-thrombin. *Science* 1990;249:277–280.
5. Märki WE, Wallis RB. The anticoagulant and antithrombotic properties of hirudin. *Thromb Haemost* 1990;64:344–348.
6. Pieters J, Lindhout T, Hemker HC. In situ-generated thrombin is the only enzyme that effectively activates factor VIII and factor V in thromboplastin-activated plasma. *Blood* 1989;74:1021–1024.
7. Fenton JW II, Villanueva GB, Ofosu FA, Maraganore JM. Thrombin inhibition by hirudin: how hirudin inhibits thrombin. *Haemostasis* 1991;21(suppl 1):27–31.
8. Hirsh J. Heparin. *N Engl J Med* 1991;324:1565–1574.
9. Zoldhelyi P, Chesebro JH, Owen WG. Hirudin as a molecular probe for thrombin in vitro and during systemic coagulation in the pig. *Proc Natl Acad Sci U S A* 1993;90:1819–1823.

10. Zoldhelyi P, Bichler J, Whyte G, et al. Persistent thrombin generation during specific thrombin inhibition with hirudin. *Circulation* 1994;90:2671–2678.

11. Zoldhelyi P, Bichler J, Owen WG, et al. Measurement of thrombin-hirudin complex documents persistent thrombin formation in patients with unstable angina during anticoagulation with recombinant hirudin [Abstract]. *Circulation* 1993;88(suppl I):319.

12. Garabedian HD, Gold HK, Newell JB, Collen D. Accelerated thrombin generation during anticoagulation in patients with unstable angina pectoris [Letter]. *Blood* 1994;83:1155.

13. Shionoya T. Studies in experimental extracorporeal thrombosis. Effects of certain anticoagulants (heparin and hirudin) on extracorporeal thrombosis and on the mechanism of thrombus formation. *J Exp Med* 1997;149:19–26.

14. Schmid JH, Jackson DP, Conley CL. Mechanism of action of thrombin on platelets. *J Clin Invest* 1962;41:543–553.

15. Hubbel JA, McIntire LV: Platelet active concentration profiles near growing thrombi. *Biophys J* 1986;50:937–945.

16. Heras M, Chesebro JH, Penny WJ, Bailey KR, Badimon L, Fuster V. Effects of thrombin inhibition on the development of acute platelet-thrombus deposition during angioplasty in pigs: heparin versus recombinant hirudin, a specific thrombin inhibitor. *Circulation* 1989;79:657–665.

17. Mruk JS, Zoldhelyi P, Chesebro JH, et al. Does antithrombotic therapy influence residual thrombus after thrombolysis of platelet-rich thrombus? Effects of recombinant hirudin, heparin, and aspirin. *Circulation* 1996;93:792–799.

18. Haskel EJ, Prager NA, Sobel BE, Abendschein DR. Relative efficacy of antithrombin compared with antiplatelet agents in accelerating coronary thrombolysis and prevention of reocclusion. *Circulation* 1991;83:1048–1056.

19. Kelly AB, Marzec UM, Krupski W, et al. Hirudin interruption of heparin-resistant arterial thrombus formation in baboons. *Blood* 1991;77:1006–1012.

20. Zoldhelyi P, Fuster V, Chesebro JH. Antithrombins as conjunctive therapy in arterial thrombolysis. *Coronary Artery Dis* 1992;3:1003–1009.

21. Inauen W, Baumgartner HR, Bombeli T, Haeberli A, Straub PW. Dose- and shear rate-dependent effects of heparin on thrombogenesis induced by rabbit aorta subendothelium exposed to flowing human blood. *Arteriosclerosis* 1990;10:607–615.

22. Heras M, Chesebro JH, Webster MWI, et al. Hirudin, heparin and placebo during deep arterial injury in the pig: the in vivo role of thrombin in platelet-mediated thrombosis. *Circulation* 1990;82:1476–1484.

23. Markwardt F, Kaiser B, Nowak G. Studies on antithrombotic effects of recombinant hirudin. *Thromb Res* 1989;54:377–388.

24. Verstraete M, Nurmohamed M, Kienast J, et al., on behalf of the European Hirudin in Thrombosis Group. Biologic effects of recombinant hirudin (CGP39393) in human volunteers. *J Am Coll Cardiol* 1993;22:1080–1088.

25. Marbet GA, Verstraete M, Kienast J, et al. Clinical pharmacology of intravenously administred recombinant desulfatohirudin (CGP39393) in healthy volunteers. *J Cardiovasc Pharmacol* 1993;22:364–372.

26. Zoldhelyi P, Webster MWI, Fuster V, et al. Recombinant desulfato hirudin in patients with chronic, stable coronary artery disease: safety, half-life, and effect on coagulation parameters. *Circulation* 1993;88:2015–2022.

27. Close P, Bichler J, Kerry R, et al., on behalf of the European Hirudin in Thrombosis Group (HIT group). Weak allergenicity of recombinant hirudin CGP 39393 in immunocompetent volunteers. *Coronary Artery Dis* 1994;5:943–949.

28. Markwardt F, Fink G, Kaiser B, et al. Pharmacological survery of recombinant hirudin. *Pharmazie* 1988;43:202–207.

29. van den Bos AA, Deckers JW, Heyndrickx GR, et al. Safety and efficacy of recombinant hirudin (CGP 39393) versus heparin in patients with stable angina undergoing coronary angioplasty. *Circulation* 1993;88:2058–2066.

30. Sarembock IJ, Gertz SD, Gimple LW, Owen RM, Powers ER, Roberts WC. Effectiveness of recombinant desulfatohirudin in reducing restenosis after balloon angioplasty of atherosclerotic femoral arteries in rabbits. *Circulation* 1991;84:232–243.

31. Serruys PW, Herrman JPR, Simon R, Rutsch W, Bode C, Laarman GJ, for the Helvetica Investigators. A comparison of hirudin with heparin in the prevention of restenosis after coronary angioplasty. *N Engl J Med* 1995;333:757–763.

32. Topol EJ, Fuster V, Harrington RA, Califf RM, Kleinmann NS, et al: Recombinant hirudin for unstable angina pectoris. *Circulation* 1994;89:1557–1566.

33. Organization to Assess Strategies for Ischemic Syndromes (OASIS) Investigators. Comparison of hirudin versus heparin and warfarin with control for unstable angina and non Q wave MI in a randomized controlled trial. *Circulation* 1995;92(suppl I):416.

34. Cannon CP, McCabe CH, Henry TD, et al., for the TIMI-5 Investigators. Hirudin reduces reocclusion compared to heparin following thrombolysis in acute myocardial infarction. Results of the TIMI-5 trial. *J Am Coll Cardiol* 1994;23:933–1003.

35. Lee LV, for the TIMI-6 Investigators. Initial experience with hirudin and streptokinase in acute myocardia infarction: results of the thrombolysis in myocardial infarction (TIMI) 6 trial. *Am J Cardiol* 1995;75:7–13.

36. Antman E for the TIMI-9A Investigators. Hirudin in myocardial infarction. Safety report from the thrombolysis and thrombin inhibition in myocardial infarction (TIMI) 9A trial. *Circulation* 1994;30:1624–1630.

37. The Global Use of Strategies to Open Occluded Coronary Arteries (GUSTO) IIa Investigators. Randomized trial of intravenous heparin versus recombinant-hirudin for acute coronary syndromes. *Circulation* 1994;90:1631–1637.

38. Neuhaus KL, von Essen R, Tebbe U, et al. Safety observations from the pilot study of the randomized r-hirudin for improvement of thrombolysis (HIT-III) study: a study of the Arbeitsgemeinschaft leiteder kardiologischer krankenhausärzte (ALK). *Circulation* 1994;90:1638–1642.

39. Zoldhelyi P, Janssens S, Lefevre G, Collen D, Van de Werf F, for the GUSTO-2 Investigators. Plasma hirudin and aPTT levels in acute patients of the GUSTO-2A compared with hirudin levels and aPTT in volunteers with stable coronary disease [Abstract]. *Eur J Cardiol* 1995;16(suppl):177.

40. The Global Use of Strategies to Open Occluded Coro-

nary Arteries (GUSTO) IIb Investigators. A comparison of recombinant hirudin with heparin for the treatment of acute coronary syndromes. *N Engl J Med* 1996;335:775–1782.

41. Antmann EM, for the TIMI-9B Investigatros. Hirudin in acute myocardial infarction. Thromobolyis and thrombin inhibition in myocardial infarction (TIMI) 9B trial. *Circulation* 1996;94:911–921.

42. Metz BK, White HD, Granger CB, et al., for the Global Use of Strategies to Open Occluded Coronary Arteries (GUSTO) IIb Investigators. Submitted for publication.

43. White HD. Clinical trials of direct thrombin inhibitors in acute ischaemic syndromes. *Thromb Haemost* 1997;78:364–366.

44. Zoldhelyi P, Janssens S, Lefèvre G, Collen D, Van de Werf F for the GUSTO-2A Investigators. Effects of heparin and hirudin (CGP 39393) on thrombin generation during thrombolysis for myocardial infarction [Abstract]. *Circulation* 1995;92(suppl I):740.

45. Rao AK, Sun L, Chesebro JH, et al. Distinct effects of recombinant desulfatohirudin (Revasc) and heparin on plasma levels of fibrinopeptide A and prothrombin fragment F1.2 in unstable angina—a multicenter trial. *Circulation* 1996;94:2389–2395.

46. Moliterno DJ, Califf RM, Aguirre FV, et al. Effect of platelet glycoprotein IIb/IIIa integrin blockade on activated clotting time during percutaneous transluminal coronary angioplasty or directional atherectomy (the EPIC trial). Evaluation of c7E3 Fab in the Prevention of Ischemic Complications trial. *Am J Cardiol* 1995; 75:559–562.

47. Andreotti F, Davies GH, Ujang SB, Sritara P. High-dose aspirin, thrombin, and coronary angioplasty [Letter]. *Lancet* 1993;341:1161.

48. Nicolini FA, Lee P, Rios G, Kottke-Marchant K, Topol EJ. Combination of platelet fibrinogen receptor antagonist and direct thrombin inhibitor at low doses markedly improves thrombolysis. *Circulation* 1994; 89:1802–1809.

49. Eriksson BI, Ekman S, Kälebo P, Zachrisson B, Bach D, Close P. Prevention of deep vein thrombosis after total hip replacement: direct thrombin inhibition with recombinant hirudin, CGP 39393. *Lancet* 1996;347: 632–633.

50. Schiele F, Vuillemot AR, Kramarz P, et al. A pilot study of subcutaneous recombinant hirudin (HBW 023) in the treatment of deep venous thrombosis. *Thromb Haemost* 1994;71:558–562.

51. Parent F, Bridey F, Dreyfus M, et al. Treatment of severe venous thrombo-embolism with intravenous hirudin, CGP 39393 (Revasc), compared to unfractionated heparin. *Circulation* 1994;90:I-569.

52. Schiele F, Vuillemot A, Kramarz P, et al. Use of recombinant hirudin as antithrombotic treatment in patients with heparin induced thrombocytopenia. *Am J Hematol* 1995;50:2025.

53. Ibbotson SH, Grant PJ, Kerry R, Findlay VS, Prentice CRM. The influence of 1-desamino-8-D-arginine vasopressin (DDAVP) in vivo on the anticoagulant effect of recombinant hirudin (CGP 39393) in vitro. *Thromb Haemost* 1991;65:64–66.

54. Butler KD, Dolan SL, Talbot MD, Wallis RB. Factor VIII and DDAVP reverse the effect of recombinant desulfatohirudin (CGP 39393) on bleeding in the rat. *Blood Coagulation Fibrinolysis* 1993;4:459–464.

55. Bove CM, Casey B, Marder VJ. DDAVP reduces

bleeding during continued hirudin administration in the rabbit. *Thromb Haemost* 1996;75:471–475.

56. Amin DM, Mant TGK, Walker SM, et al. Effect of a 15-minute infusion of DDAVP on the pharmacokinetics and pharmacodynamics of (TM)REVASC during a four-hour intravenous infusion in healthy male volunteers. *Thromb Haemost* 1997;77:127–132.

57. Cadroy Y, Maraganore JM, Hanson SR, Harker LA. Selective inhibition by a synthetic hirudin peptide of fibrin-dependent thrombosis in baboons. *Proc Natl Acad Sci U S A* 1991;88:1177–1181.

58. Jakubowski JA, Maraganore JM. Inhibition of coagulation and thrombin-induced platelet activation by a synthetic dodecapeptide modeled on the carboxy-terminus of hirudin. *Blood* 1990;75:399–406.

59. Couglin SR, Vu TH, Hung DT, Wheaton VI. Characterization of a functional thrombin receptor. *J Clin Invest* 1992;89:351–356.

60. Maraganore JM, Bourdon P, Jablonski J, Ramachandran KL, Fenton JW. Design and characterization of hirulogs: a novel class of bivalent peptide inhibitors of thrombin. *Biochem J* 1990;29:7095–7101.

61. Skrzypczak-Jankun E, Carperos VE, Ravichandran KG, Tulinsky A, Westbrook M, Maraganore JM. Structure of hirugen and hirulog 1 complexes of α-thrombin. *J Mol Biol* 1991;221:1379–1393.

62. Fox I, Dawson A, Loynds P, et al. Anticoagulant activity of hirulog, a direct inhibitor of thrombin. *Thromb Haemost* 1993;69:157–163.

63. Maraganore JM, Adelman BA. Hirulog: a direct thrombin inhibitor for management of acute coronary syndromes. *Coronary Artery Dis* 1996;7:438–448.

64. Qui X, Padmanabhan KP, Carperos VE, et al. Structure of the hirulog thrombin complex and nature of the 5′ subsides of substrates and inhibitors. *Biochem J* 1992;31:11689–11697.

65. Kelly A, Maraganore JM, Bourdon P, Hanson GR, Harker LA. Antithrombotic effects of synthetic peptides targeting different functional domains of thrombin. *Proc Natl Acad Sci U S A* 1992;89:6040–6044.

66. Klement P, Borm A, Hirsh J, Maraganore J, Wilson G, Weitz J. The effects of thrombin inhibitors on tissue plasminogen activator induced thrombolysis in a rat model. *Thromb Haemost* 1992;68:64–68.

67. Belmond BJ, Friederich PW, Levi M, Vlasuk GP, Büller HR, ten Cate JW. Comparison of sustained antithrombotic effects of inhibitors of thrombin and factor Xa in experimental thrombosis. *Circulation* 1996; 93:153–160.

68. Sarembock IJ, Gertz SD, Thome LM, et al. Effectiveness of hirulog in reducing restenosis after balloon angioplasty of atherosclerotic femoral arteries in rabbits. *J Vasc Res* 1996;33:308–314.

69. Cannon CP, Maraganore JM, Loscalzo JL, et al. Anticoagulant effects of hirulog, a novel thrombin inhibitor, in patients with coronary artery disease. *Am J Cardiol* 1993;71:778–782.

70. Lidon R-M, Théroux P, Juneau M, Adelman B, Maraganore J. Initial experience with a direct antithrombin, hirulog, in unstable angina. Anticoagulant, antithrombotic, and clinical effects. *Circulation* 1993; 1495–1501.

71. Fuchs J, Cannon CP, and the TIMI 7 Investigators. Hirulog in the treatment of unstable angina. Results of the Thrombin Inhibition in Myocardial Ischemia (TIMI) 7 Trial. *Circulation* 1995;92:727–733.

72. Lidon RM, Théroux P, Lespérance J, et al. A pilot, early angiographic patency study using a direct thrombin inhibitor as adjunctive therapy to streptokinase in acute myocardial infarction. *Circulation* 1994;89: 1567–1572.

73. Théroux P, Pérez-Villa F, Waters D, Lespérance J, Shabani F, Bonan R. Randomized double-blind comparison of two doses of hirulog with heparin as adjunctive therapy to streptokinase to promote early patency of the infarct-related artery in acute myocardial infarction. *Circulation* 1995;91:2132–2139.

74. Topol EJ, Bonan R, Jewitt D, et al. Use of a direct antithrombin, hirulog, in place of heparin during coronary angioplasty. *Circulation* 1993;87:1622–1629.

75. Bittl JA, Strony J, Brinker JA, et al., for the Hirulog Angioplasty Study Investigators.Treatment with bivalirudin (Hirulog) as compared with heparin during coronary angioplasty for unstable or postinfarction angina. *N Engl J Med* 1995;333:764–769.

76. Shah PB, Ahmed WH, Ganz P, Bittl JA. Hirulog compared with heparin during coronary angioplasty for thrombus-containing lesions [Abstract]. *Circulation* 1996;94(suppl I):197.

77. Ginsberg JS, Nurmohamed MT, Gent M, et al. Effects on thrombin generation of single injections of Hirulog™ in patients with calf vein thrombosis. *Thromb Haemost* 1994;72:523–525.

78. Ginsberg JS, Nurmohamed MT, Gent M, et al. Use of hirulog in the prevention of venous thrombosis after major hip or knee surgery. *Circulation* 1994;90: 2385–2389.

79. Badimon L, Badimon JJ. Interaction of platelet activation and coagulation. In: Fuster V, Ross R, Topol EJ (eds). *Atherosclerosis and Coronary Artery Disease, Vol. 1.* Philadelphia: Lippincott–Raven, 1996;639–656.

80. Weitz JJ. Biological rationale for the therapeutic role of specific antithrombins. *Coronary Arter Dis* 1996;7: 409–419.

81. Di Maio J, Gibbs B, Lefebvre J, Konishi Y, Munn D, Yi Yue S. Synthesis of a homologous series of ketomethylene arginyl pseudodipeptides and application to low molecular weight hirudin-like thrombin inhibitors. *J Med Chem* 1992;35:3331–3341.

82. Kline I, Hammond C, Boardon P, Maraganore JM. Hirulog peptides with scissile bond replacements resistant to thrombin cleavage. *Biochem Biophys Res Commun* 1991;177:1049–1055.

83. Cirillo R, Lippi A, Subissi A, Agnelli G, Criscuoli M. Experimental pharmacology of Hirunorm:a novel synthetic peptide thrombin inhibitor. *Thromb Haemost* 1996;76:384–392.

84. Lombardi A, Nastri F, Della-Morte R, et al. Rational design of true hirudin mimetics: synthesis and characterization of multisite-directed alpha-thrombin inhibitors. *J Med Chem* 1996;39:1008–2017.

85. Hijikata A, Okamoto S. A strategy for a rational approach to designing synthetic selective inhibitors. *Semin Thromb Hemost* 1992;18:135–149.

86. Kikumoto R, Tamao Y, Tezuka T, et al. Selective inhibition of thrombin by (2R,4R)-4-methyl-1-[N²-(3-methyl-1,2,3,4-tetrahydro-8-quinolinyl) sulfonyl]-arginyl]-2-piperidinecarboxylic acid. *Biochemistry* 1984;23:85–90.

87. Bush LR. Argatroban, at selective, potent thrombin inhibitor. *Cardiovasc Drug Rev* 1991;9:247–263.

88. Imura J, Stassen J-M, Collen D. Comparative antithrombotic effects of heparin, recombinant hirudin, and argatroban in a hamster femoral vein platelet-rich mural thrombus model. *J Pharmacol Exp Ther* 1992; 261:895–898.

89. Jang I, Gold HK, Ziskind AA, Leinbach RC, Fallon JT, Collen D. Prevention of platelet-rich arterial thrombosis by selective thrombin inhibition. *Circulation* 1990; 81:219–225.

90. Yasuda T, Gold HK, Yaoita H, et al. Comparative effects of aspirin, a synthetic thrombin inhibitor and a monoclonal antiplatelet glycoprotein IIb/IIIa antibody on coronary artery reperfusion, reocclusion and bleeding with recombinant tissue-type plasminogen activator in a canine preparation. *J Am Coll Cardiol* 1990; 16:714–722.

91. Fitzgerald DJ, FitzGerald GA. Role of thrombin and thromboxane A₂ in reocclusion following coronary thrombolysis with tissue-type plasminogen activator. *Proc Natl Acad Sci U S A* 1989;86:7585–7589.

92. Eidt JF, Allison P, Noble S, et al. Thrombin is an important mediator of platelet aggregation in stenosed canine coronary arteries with endothelial injury. *J Clin Invest* 1989;84:18–27.

93. Duval N, Lunven C, O'Brien DP, Grosset A, O'Connor SE, Berry CN. Antithrombotic actions of the thrombin inhibitor argatroban, in a canine model of coronary cyclic flow:comparison with heparin. *Br J Pharmacol* 1996;118:727–733.

94. Berry CH, Girard D, Lochot S, Lecoffre L. Antithrombotic actions of argatroban in rat models of venous, "mixed" and arterial thrombosis, and its effects on the tail transection bleeding time. *Br J Pharmacol* 1994; 113:1209–1214.

95. Berry CN, Girard D, Girardot C, Lochot S, Lunven C, Visconte C. Antithrombotic activity or argatroban in experimental thrombosis in the rabbit. *Semin Thromb Hemost* 1996;22:233–241.

96. Iida S, Komatsu T, Hirano T, et al. Pharmacokinetic studies of argipidine (MD-805) in dogs and rabbits. Blood or plasma level profile, metabolism, excretion and accumulation after single or consecutive intravenous administration of argipidine. *Oyo Yakuri (Pharmacometrics)* 1986;32:1171–1177.

97. Izawa O, Katsuki M, Komatsu T, et al. Pharmacokinetics studies of of argatroban (MD-805) in human volunteers of argatroban and its metabolites in plasma, urine and feces during and after drip intravenous infusion. *Jpn Pharm Ther* 1986;14:251–252.

98. Schwarz RP Jr, Becker JCP, Brooks RL, et al. State-of-the-Art Review. The preclinical and clinical pharmacology of Novastan (argatroban): a small-molecule, direct thrombin inhibitor. *Clin Appl Thromb Hemost* 1997;3:1–15.

99. Antman EM, for the TIMI 9A Investigators. Hirudin in acute myocardial infarction: safety report from the Thrombolysis and Thrombin Inhibition in Myocardial Infarction (TIMI) 9A trial. *Circulation* 1994;90: 1624–1630.

100. GUSTO IIa Investigators. Randomized trial of intravenous heparin versus recombinant hirudin for acute coronary syndromes. *Circulation* 1994;90:1631–1637.

101. Gold HK, Torres FW, Garabedian HD, et al. Evidence for a rebound coagulation phenomenon after cessation of a 4-hour infusion of a specific thrombin inhibitor in

patients with unstable angina pectoris. *J Am Coll Cardiol* 1993;21:1039–1047.

102. Willerson JT, Casscells W. Thrombin inhibitors in unstable angina:rebound or continuation of angina after argatroban withdrawal? *J Am Coll Cardiol* 1993;21:1048–1051.

103. Zoldhelyi P, Bichler J, Owen WG, et al. Persistent thrombin generation in humans during specific thrombin inhibition with hirudin. *Circulation* 1994;90:2671–2678.

104. Fitzgerald D, Murphy N. Argatroban: a synthetic thrombin inhibitor of low relative molecular mass. *Coronary Arter Dis* 1996;7:455–458.

105. Herrman PR, Suryapranata H, den Heijer P, Kutryk MJB, Gabriël L, Serruys PW. Argatroban during percutaneous transluminal angioplasty; results of a dose verification study. *J Thromb Thrombolysis* 1996;3:367–375.

106. Vermeer F, Vahanian A, Fels PW, Besse P, Radzik D, Simoons ML. Intravenous argatroban versus heparin as co-medication to alteplase in the treatment of acute myocardial infarction, preliminary results of the ARGAMI pilot trial [Abstract]. *J Am Coll Cardiol* 1997;29:185.

107. Bajusz S, Szell E, Badgy D, et al. Highly active and selective anticoagulants:D-Phe-Pro-Arg-H, a free tripeptide aldehyde prone to spontaneous inactivation, and its stable N-methyl derivative. *J Med Chem* 1990;33:1729–1735.

108. Williams JW, JF Morrison. The kinetics of reversible tight-binding inhibition. *Methods Enzymol* 1979;63:437–467.

109. Smith GF, Shuman RT, Craft TJ, et al. A family of arginal thrombin inhibitors related to efegatran. *Semin Thromb Hemost* 1996;22:173–183.

110. Kaiser B, Koza M, Walenga JM, Fareed J. Flow cytometric evaluation of the effect of various thrombin inhibitors on platelet activation in whole blood. *Thromb Res* 1996;82:257–263.

111. Callas DD, Hoppensteadt D, Fareed J. Comparative studies on the anticoagulant and protease generation inhibitory actions of newly developed site-directed thrombin inhibitory drugs. Efegatran, argatroban, hirulog, and hirudin. *Semin Thromb Hemost* 1995;21:177–183.

112. Jackson CV, Frank JD, Crowe VG, et al. Pharmacological assessment of the peptide thrombin inhibitor D-methyl-Phe-Pro-arginal (GYKI-14766) in a canine model of coronary thrombosis. *J Pharmacol Exp Ther* 1992;261:546–552.

113. Jackson CV, Wilson HC, Crowe VG, Shuman RT, Gesellchen PD. Reversible tripeptide thrombin inhibitors as adjunctive agents to coronary thrombolysis: a comparison to heparin in a canine model of coronary artery thrombosis. *J Cardiovasc Pharmacol* 1993;21:587–594.

114. Shetler TJ, Crowe VG, Bailey BD, Jackson CV. Antithrombotic assessment of the effects of combination therapy with the anticoagulants efegatran and heparin and the glycoprotein IIb–IIIa platelet receptor antagonist 7E3 in a canine model of coronary artery thrombosis. *Circulation* 1996;94:1719–1725.

115. Jackson CV, Sattewhite J, Roberts E. Preclinical and clinical pharmacology of efegatran (LY 294468): a novel antithrombin for the treatment of acute coronary syndromes. *Clin Appl Thromb Haemost* 1996;2:258–269.

116. Simoons M, Lenderink T, Scheffer M, et al. Efegatran, a new direct thrombin inhibitor: safety and dose response in patients with unstable angina [Abstract]. *Circulation* 1994;90:I-231.

117. Weaver WD, Fung A, Lorch G, et al. Efegatran and streptokinase vs t-PA and heparin for treatment of acute MI [Abstract]. *Circulation* 1996;94:430.

118. Ohman EM, Slovak JP, Anderson RL, et al., and the PRIME Group. Potent inhibition of thrombin with efegatran in combination with t-PA in acute myocardial infarction: results of a multicenter randomized dose ranging trial [Abstract]. *Circulation* 1996;94:430.

119. Hilpert K, Ackermann J, Banner DW, et al. Design and synthesis of potent and highly selective thrombin inhibitors. *J Med Chem* 1994;37:3889–3901.

120. Carteaux JP, Gast A, Tschopp TB, Roux S. The activated clotting time (ACT) as an appropriate test to compare heparin and direct thrombin inhibitors such as hirudin or Ro 46-6240 in experimental arterial thrombosis. *Circulation* 1995;91:1568–1574.

121. Tschopp TB, Ackermann J, Gast A, et al. Napsagatran, thrombin inhibitor, RO 46-6240. *Drugs Future* 1995;20:476–479.

122. Gast A, Tschopp TB, Schmid G, Hilpert K, Ackermann J. Inhibition of clot-bound and free (fluid-phase) thrombin by a novel synthetic thrombin inhibitor (Ro 46-6240), recombinant hirudin and heparin in human plasma. *Blood Coag Fibrinolysis* 1994;5:879–887.

123. Kirchhofer D, Tschopp TB, Hadváry P, Baumgartner HR. Endothelial cells stimulated with tumor necrosis factor-α express varying amounts of tissue factor resulting in inhomogenous fibrin deposition in a native blood flow system—effects of thrombin inhibitors. *J Clin Invest* 1994;93:2073–2083.

124. Gast A, Tschopp TB, Baumgartner HR. Thrombin plays a key role in late platelet thrombus growth and/or stability. Effect of a specific thrombin inhibitor on thrombogenesis induced by aortic subendothelium exposed to flowing rabbit blood. *Arterioscler Thromb* 1994;14:1466–1474.

125. Teger-Nilsson AC, Eriksson U, Gustafsson D, Bylund R, Fager G, Held P. Phase I studies on inogatran, a new selective thrombin inhibitor [Abstract]. *J Am Coll Cardiol* 1995;23:117–118.

126. Gustafsson D, Elg M, Lenfors S, Borjesson I, Teger-Nilsson AC. Effects of inogatran: a new low-molecular-weight thrombin inhibitor, in rat models of venous and arterial thrombosis, thrombolysis and bleeding time. *Blood Coag Fibrinolysis* 1996;7:69–79.

127. Chen LY, Nichols WW, Mattsson C, et al. Aspirin does not potentiate effect of suboptimal dose of the thrombin inhibitor inogatran during coronary thrombolysis. *Cardiovasc Res* 1995;30:866–874.

128. Andersen K, Delborg M, Emanuelson H, Grip L, Swedberg K. Thrombin inhibition with inogatran for unstable angina pectoris:evidence for reactivivated ischaemia after cessation of short-term treatment. *Coronary Arter Dis* 1996;7:673–681.

129. Grip L, Wallentin L, Dellborg M, et al. A low molecular weight, specific thrombin inhibitor inogatran, versus heparin, in unstable coronary artery disease [Abstract]. *Circulation* 1996;94(suppl I):430.

130. Harker LA, Hanson SR, Kelly AB. Antithrombotic

benefits and hemorrhagic risks of direct thrombin inhibitors. *Thromb Haemost* 1995;74:464–472.

131. Weitz JI. Biological rationale for the therapeutic role of specific thrombin inhibitors. *Coronary Arter Dis* 1996;7:409–419.

132. Philippides GJ, Loscalzo J. Potential advantages of direct-acting thrombin inhibitors. *Coronary Arter Dis* 1996;7:497–507.

133. Hauptmann J, Marckwardt F. Pharmacologic aspects of the development of selective thrombin inhibitors as anticoagulants. *Semin Thromb Hemost* 1992;18: 200–217.

134. Knabb RM, Kettner CA, Timmermans PB, Reilly TM. In vivo characterization of a new synthetic thrombin inhibitor. *Thromb Haemost* 1992;67:56–59.

135. Rote WR, Dempsey EM, Oldeschielte GL, et al. Evaluation of a novel orally active direct inhibitor of thrombin in animal models of thrombosis [Abstract]. *Circulation* 1994;90:344.

136. Cousins GR, Friedrichs GS, Sudo Y, et al. Orally effective CVS-1123 prevents coronary artery thrombosis in the conscious dog. *Circulation* 1996;94: 1705–1712.

137. Knapp A, Degenhardt T, Dodt J. Hirudisins; hirudin-derived thrombin inhibitors with disintegrin activity. *J Biol Chem* 1992;267:24230–24234.

138. Hung DT, Vu TK, Wheaton VI, et al. "Mirror image" antagonism of thrombin-induced platelet activation based on thrombin receptor structure. *J Clin Invest* 1992;89:444–450.

139. Bode C, Hudelmayer M, Mehwald P, et al. Fibrin-targeted recombinant hirudin inhibits fibrin depostion on experimental clots more efficiently than recombinant hirudin. *Circulation* 1994;90:1956–1963.

140. Bode C, Hanson SR, Schmedtje JF Jr, et al. Antithrombotic potency of hirudin is increased in nonhuman primates by fibrin targeting. *Circulation* 1997; 95:800–804.

141. Bock LC, Griffin LC, Latham JA, Vermaas EH, Toole JJ. Selection of a single-stranded DNA molecules that bind and inhibit human thrombin. *Nature* 1992;355: 564–566.

142. Griffin LC, Tidmarsh GF, Bock LC, Toole JJ, Leung LL. In vivo anticoagulant properties of a novel nucleotide-fased thrombin inhibitor and demonstration of regional anticoagulation in extracorporeal circuits. *Blood* 1993;81:3271–3276.

143. Li WX, Kaplan AV, Grant GW, Toole JJ, Leung LLK. A novel nucleotide-based thrombin inhibitor inhibits clot-bound thrombin and reduces arterial platelet thrombin formation. *Blood* 1994;83:677–682.

144. Vlasuk G, Vallar PL, Weinhouse MI, et al. A novel inhibitor of thrombin containing multiple recognition sequences linked by α-keto amide transition state. *Circulation* 1994;90:1–348.

145. Lewis SD, Ng AS, Lyle EA, et al. Inhibition of thrombin by peptides containing lysyl-α-keto carbonyl derivatives. *Thromb Haemost* 1995;74:1107–1112.

146. Ogletree ML. Thrombin receptor-mediated signaling in endothelial cells. In: Vane JR, Born GVR, Welzel D (eds). *The Endothelial Cells in Health and Disease.* Stuttgart: Schattauer Verlag, 1995;85–96.

147. Vu T-KN, Hung DT, Weaton VI Coughlin SR. Molecular cloning of a functional thrombin receptor reveals a novel proteolytic mechanism of receptor activation. *Cell* 1991;64:1057–1068.

148. Coughlin SR, Vu T-KH, Ilung DT, Wheaton VI. Characterization of a functional thrombin receptor, issues and opportunities. *J Clin Invest* 1992;89:351–355.

149. Nystedt S. Emilsson K, Wahlestedt C, Sundelin J. Molecular cloning of a potential proteinase activated receptor. *Proc Natl Acad Sci U S A* 1994;91:9208–9212.

150. Cook, Sitko GR, Bednar B, et al. An antibody against the exosite of the cloned thrombin receptor inhibits experimental arterial thrombosis in the African green monkey. *Circulation* 1995;91:2961–2971.

Cardiovascular Thrombosis: Thrombocardiology and Thromboneurology, Second Edition, edited by M. Verstraete, V. Fuster, and E. J. Topol, Lippincott–Raven Publishers, Philadelphia © 1998.

10

Specific Factor Xa Inhibitors

Meyer M. Samama, *Jeanine M. Walenga, †Brigitte Kaiser, and ‡Jawed Fareed

Service d'Hématologie Biologique, Hotel Dieu University Hospital, 75004 Paris, France;
**Cardiovascular Institute, Loyola University Medical Center, Maywood, Illinois 60153;*
†Center for Vascular Biology and Medicine, Friedrich Schiller University Jena,
D-99089 Erfurt , Germany; and ‡Department of Pathology and Pharmacology,
Loyola University Medical Center, Maywood, Illinois 60153

Today factor Xa targeting is one of the major focuses of drug development. The factor Xa inhibitor strategy was actually derived, in part, from heparin. The low molecular weight (LMW) heparins have higher anti-Xa activity than antithrombin (AT) activity, whereas heparin has equal factor Xa and thrombin inhibitory activities. An indirect evidence of the validity of the hypothesis that factor Xa inhibition is important for the control of thrombogenesis is given by the clinical antithrombotic efficacy of LMW heparins, which contain a large proportion of molecules with high anti–factor Xa activity (1). Pharmacologic development has now separated these two properties so that solely anti–factor Xa or AT agents are available.

The first development of factor Xa inhibitors was met with less interest than thrombin inhibitors. These early inhibitors had low affinity to factor Xa, low selectivity, and low potency (2,3). Because of the increase in enzymatic activity of the coagulation cascade once the prothrombinase complex is formed, a potent factor Xa inhibitor is required to have an extremely high affinity for the enzyme. The first factor Xa inhibitors did not fulfill this requirement.

Potent factor Xa inhibitors have several potential advantages. Factor Xa is in the common pathway of both the intrinsic and extrinsic systems, playing a central role in the coagulation pathway, so it is a logical focus of drug development for the control of thrombosis. Factor Xa is formed at an earlier stage than thrombin, and the procoagulant effect of factor Xa is strongly amplified by the prothrombinase complex. Factor Xa has no known activity other than as a procoagulant, as opposed to thrombin, which has multiple activation roles at various plasmatic and cellular levels (platelets, endothelial cells, smooth muscle cells, other cells), not the least of which is activation of the protein C inhibitor pathway. Inhibition of protein C by a thrombin inhibitor would lead to a reduced formation of activated protein C, an important natural anticoagulant.

Because factor Xa has relatively slow activation kinetics, as opposed to thrombin, opposing its function should result in easier management of the balance between the therapeutic and bleeding effects of a drug. From recent clinical trials, specific thrombin inhibitors have shown to have a relatively narrow safety/efficacy margin that could lead to an overdose of the therapeutic dose with a resultant bleeding complication (4,5). Because of their different mechanism of action, factor Xa inhibitors are expected to have a better efficacy/safety profile than thrombin inhibitors.

CLASSIFICATION

Factor Xa inhibitors are structurally diverse, ranging from peptides to proteins to heparin saccharidic sequences (6,7). They can be either naturally derived, recombinant, or synthetic in origin. Molecular size differs between the inhibitors, as does specificity and kinetics of factor Xa inhibition. The targeted binding site on factor Xa can differ between the inhibitors; they can be direct binding to factor Xa or indirect via a cofactor such as AT III. Binding to the enzyme can be either reversible or irreversible. The protein inhibitors are limited in the degree of activity they produce. Two possible reasons for this limitation are (a) size that limits access of the inhibitor to factor Xa bound within clots, and (b) when thrombin is bound to fibrin, the heparin binding site on thrombin is inaccessible for heparin. Other mechanisms may exist. Furthermore, protein inhibitors tend to be immunogenic, can carry viral or animal contaminants, and can become limited in supply.

Because of the structural differences, the primary mechanism of action (i.e., direct or indirect acting on factor Xa as well as other attributes) differs with the various agents. The factor Xa inhibitors that are in development are shown in Table 10-1. Only a few of these agents have moved out of the experimental and into the clinical realm.

MECHANISMS OF ACTION

Coagulation

The inhibition of factor Xa has multiple consequences for the plasmatic coagulation system (Fig. 10-1) as well as for cellular reactions that result in an effective anticoagulation and the prevention of thrombotic processes. Based on the amplification mechanisms in the coagulation cascade and the important role of the prothrombinase complex, highly effective

TABLE 10-1. *Factor Xa inhibitors*

Agent	Chemical nature	Source	Developmental status
Direct Inhibitors			
Yagin	Medicinal leech protein (85 amino acids)	Animal derived	Terminated
Antistasin	Mexican leech protein (119 amino acids)	Recombinant	Terminated
TAP	Tick protein (60 amino acids)	Recombinant	Preclinical
NAP-5	Hookworm protein	Recombinant	Preclinical
TFPI	Human protein	Recombinant	Preclinical
DX-9065a	Propanoic acid derivative	Synthetic	Phase II clinical trials
SEL 2711	Pentapeptide produced by combinatorial chemistry	Synthetic	Preclinical
YM-60828			Preclinical
Indirect inhibitors			
Heparin pentasaccharide	Oligosaccharide; requires binding to AT III	Synthetic	Phase II clinical trial

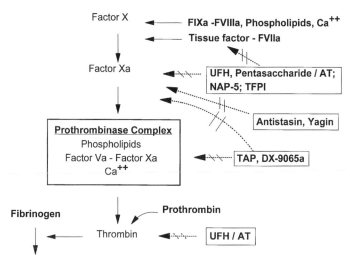

FIG. 10-1. Schematic representation of the coagulation cascade and the sites of action of factor Xa inhibitors. UFH, unfractionated heparin; AT, antithrombin III; ----, inhibition.

and selective factor Xa inhibitors are expected to strongly inhibit the generation of thrombin. This is probably the most important mechanism of factor Xa inhibitors with regard to their antithrombotic effectiveness. By this action, thrombin mediated positive feedback reactions such as the activation of the cofactors V and VIII that amplify thrombin formation, and the effect of thrombin on platelets and other cellular elements are also altered.

Free Versus Bound Factor Xa

An important aspect of the mechanism of the antithrombotic effect of factor Xa inhibitors is their capacity to inhibit clot-bound factor Xa. Because of the small size (500 to 800 daltons) of some of these inhibitors, they are able to inhibit bound prothrombinase as well as free factor Xa. Tick anticoagulant peptide (TAP) is particularly capable of inhibiting bound factor Xa.

Remnants of intravascular thrombi, known to induce activation of the coagulation system, may play a role in rethrombosis and restenosis after coronary thrombolysis. Preexisting thrombin, which is bound to fibrin and re-exposed during thrombolysis, has been thought to be the primary mediator of thrombus-associated procoagulant activity; thus,

thrombin inhibitors such as hirudin may be useful agents to prevent the recurrence of thrombosis after thrombolysis (8). However, recent results indicate that other clotting factors such as factor Xa are also bound to whole blood clots. Therefore, activation of prothrombin by clot-associated factors Xa/Va can significantly contribute to the procoagulant activity of intravascular thrombi (9).

The activity of clot-bound factor Xa is resistant to inhibition by AT III and AT III–dependent inhibitors such as the heparin pentasaccharide (due to its size or other mechanisms) (9,10). On the other hand, the activation of prothrombin can be inhibited by direct acting factor Xa inhibitors such as TAP as well as by tissue factor pathway inhibitor (TFPI) (10,11).

Restenosis

The inhibition of the proliferation of vascular smooth muscle cells (VSMCs) also may be controlled by factor Xa. Migration and proliferation of VSMCs as a reaction to injury of the endothelium and the resulting formation of a neointima mainly contribute to the development of restenosis and atherosclerosis. Platelets, thrombin, and other components of the thrombotic process are important factors in neointimal formation (12–15).

The serine protease thrombin is known to exert, besides its action in the plasmatic coagulation system, several cellular effects via the reaction with its specific receptor. By this mechanism it activates platelets and acts as a strong mitogen for endothelial cells, VSMC, fibroblasts, and macrophages. In limited studies on mitogenesis in cultured rat VSMCs, it was shown that factor Xa is also a potent mitogen that stimulates DNA synthesis and cell growth in VSMCs (16,17).

Most probably factor Xa exerts its effect indirectly via the platelet-derived growth factor (PDGF) receptor tyrosine kinase pathway. Factor Xa stimulates VSMCs to release pre-existing PDGF, which then, through the receptor tyrosine kinase pathway, leads to the activation of mitogen-activated protein kinases (MAPK) which are well-characterized intracellular mediators of cell proliferation (16). This action of factor Xa on VSCM seems to be related to its serine protease activity because in the presence of specific factor Xa inhibitors such as antistasin and TAP the mitogenic effect of factor Xa is blocked (16,17).

VSMCs proliferation, which is mediated by factor Xa, also might play an important role in reocclusion and restenosis after angioplasty in vivo. Therefore, specific inhibition of factor Xa can be expected to limit intimal hyperplasia after damage of the vascular endothelium and, thus, to diminish the restenosis rate after successful angioplasty.

Under experimental conditions the specific factor Xa inhibitors antistasin and TAP have been shown to limit restenosis after balloon angioplasty (18,19). A 2-hour infusion of antistasin resulted in significantly less restenosis and less luminal narrowing by plaque measured 28 days after balloon angioplasty of atherosclerotic femoral arteries in rabbits compared with controls (18). In a porcine model of severe coronary artery injury, a short-term administration of TAP for 60 hours resulted in a long-term decrease in neointimal thickness measured 28 days after injury (19).

These results implicate specific factor Xa inhibitors as effective substances to reduce neointimal hyperplasia either by preventing the mitogenic effects of factor Xa and/or by inhibiting the generation of thrombin which by itself is also a potent mitogen.

DIRECT INHIBITORS

Antistasin

Antistasin, purified several years ago from the Mexican leech (*Haementeria officinalis*), has an apparent molecular weight of 17,000 daltons (20). Due to antibody formation, it has fallen out of developmental interest and is no longer being developed. It inhibits factor Xa by forming a stable enzyme–inhibitor complex (21). Antistasin was more effective at prolonging the prothrombin time (PT) than was hirudin, but only slightly less effective than hirudin at prolonging the activated partial thromboplastin time (APTT) (6).

Yagin

Yagin, an 85–amino acid peptide isolated from the medicinal leech (*Hirudo medicinalis*), has 50% homology with antistasin. It is a slow, tightly binding inhibitor of factor Xa, where the inhibition is a time-dependent reaction effected by the order of addition of components (22). Optimization of production methods is in progress.

Tick Anticoagulant Peptide (TAP)

TAP was originally isolated from the tick *Ornithodorus moubata*. It is now produced through recombinant technology. This 60–amino acid peptide (6,850 daltons) is a slow, tightly binding inhibitor of human factor Xa that inhibits the enzyme via a two-step mechanism. Initially it forms a relatively weak complex with factor Xa, followed by a more stable enzyme–inhibitor complex (23,24). TAP is characterized by a much higher affinity of the inhibitor to the enzyme when it is assembled in the prothrombinase complex with an appropriately lower inhibition constant (K_i value 0.006 nmol/L versus 0.18 nmol/L for free factor Xa) (25,26).

Like other naturally derived inhibitors, TAP effectively inhibits factor Xa and has shown antithrombotic effects in various thrombosis models. Using TAP as a very selective and highly effective factor Xa inhibitor, it was shown under experimental conditions that the inhibition of thrombin generation is an effective approach to affect processes of thrombosis and restenosis. TAP inhibited in vivo the formation of venous thrombosis (27–29) and prevented platelet and fibrin deposition as well as thrombus formation in arterial thrombosis and in arteriovenous shunts (29–31) as well as in ex vivo human non-anticoagulated blood (32). It also accelerated perfusion during thrombolysis and prevented acute reocclusion in canines (33–35).

TAP has a different anticoagulant profile as measured by the APTT (26,27). In comparison with antistasin, for example, both in vitro and ex vivo, TAP was found to be much less potent than antistasin in prolonging the APTT despite nearly equal antithrombotic efficacies in a rabbit model of venous thrombosis. This reflects kinetic differences in the rate of factor Xa inactivation between various inhibitors, i.e., TAP shows a time dependent inhibition requiring an incubation period of 50 to 60 minutes to achieve maximal inhibition (27). On the other hand, in the celite activated clotting time (ACT) assay, TAP showed the most potent anticoagulant activity in comparison with heparin and other factor Xa inhibitors (Fig. 10-2). These differences show that the antithrombotic efficacy of a given anticoagulant cannot always be predicted by clotting assay values.

Besides the antithrombotic effectiveness of TAP found in experimental venous and arterial thrombosis, this factor Xa inhibitor showed favorable actions against the restenosis processes. TAP reduced angiographic restenosis and caused less luminal cross-sectional narrowing by plaque after short-term administration to rabbits (18), led to a long-term decrease in neointimal thickness in damaged pig coronary arteries (12), and inhibited mitogenesis in cultured rat aortic smooth muscle cells (17).

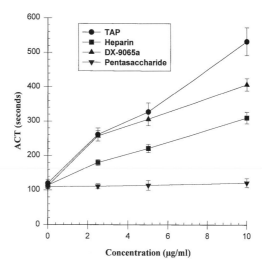

FIG. 10-2. In a comparative study the anticoagulant effects of TAP, DX-9065a, and heparin showed concentration-dependent effects in a celite-activated whole-blood clotting assay (ACT). At equigravimetric concentrations, TAP produced the strongest effect, followed by DX-9065a, and a weaker effect by heparin. Pentasaccharide, on the other hand, did not produce significant prolongation of the time to clot. These results demonstrate that in a test system where thrombin is generated by a strong activator, certain factor Xa inhibitors can produce a concentration-dependent anticoagulant effect whereas other factor Xa inhibitors do not have an effect, depending on their mechanism of action.

Factor Xa and the de novo activation of prothrombin may play an important role in the procoagulant activity of intravascular thrombi that may lead to reoccurrence of thrombosis after thrombolysis and to propagation of thrombi (9,36). The clot-associated factor Xa activity can be inhibited by TAP but not by AT III and AT III–dependent inhibitors (9,36).

NAP-5

NAP-5 is one of a family of anticoagulant proteins isolated from hookworm nematodes. It has a molecular weight of 8,700 daltons and inhibits factor Xa and the factor VII/TF complex after prior binding to factor Xa (37). It is in preclinical trials.

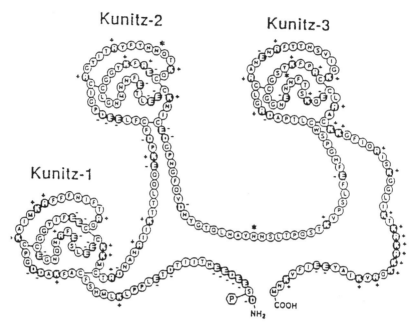

FIG. 10-3. Structure of tissue factor pathway inhibitor (TFPI), the endogenous inhibitor of the extrinsic coagulation pathway. (From Girard et al., ref. 90, with permission.)

Tissue Factor Pathway Inhibitor

TFPI is a human protein (43 kDa) (Fig. 10-3) identified over 40 years ago (38,39). TFPI is the endogenous inhibitor of the extrinsic coagulation pathway that, in addition to the inhibition of the factor VIIa/tissue factor complex in a final step, also binds to and inhibits factor Xa (9,36). Due to its mechanism of action, TFPI is an important regulator of coagulation. TFPI has been shown to inhibit venous thrombosis (40), rethrombosis after t-PA use (40), and platelet thrombosis after balloon injury to the vessel in experimental animals (41). Heparin and LMW heparins release endogenous TFPI upon administration; none of the factor Xa inhibitors tested to date are associated with the release of TFPI (11). A recombinant form is currently in preclinical trials. Defibrotide also releases TFPI (42).

DX-9065a

The Daiichi compound DX-9065a is a novel type of synthetic factor Xa inhibitor (Fig. 10-4 and Table 10-2). This nonpeptide, propanoic acid derivative, LMW compound (571 daltons) has been described as a potent, directly acting inhibitor of factor Xa. It inhibits factor Xa in a competitive manner with an inhibition constant in the nanomolar range (43,44). DX-9065a is also highly selective for factor Xa and shows limited oral absorption (44–47). It is in phase II clinical trials.

The factor Xa inhibitor DX-9065a is a promising antithrombotic agent. Effective antithrombotic activity was found in models of venous (Fig. 10-5) and arterial thrombosis (29,40,43,48,49), arteriovenous shunt thrombosis (29,43,50,51), acute disseminated intravascular coagulation (43,51–53) as well as hemodialysis in cynomolgus monkeys (54).

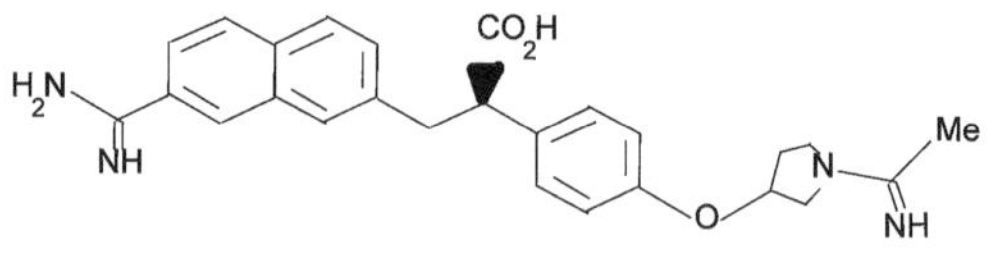

FIG. 10-4. Structure of DX-9065a the synthetic, nonpeptide factor Xa inhibitor. (From Dr. S. Kunitada, with permission.)

TABLE 10-2. *Characteristics of DX-9065a and the heparin pentasaccharide*

Pentasaccharide	DX-9065a
Synthetic	Synthetic
Oligosaccharide	Propanoic acid derivative
1,728 daltons	571 daltons
AT III–pentasaccharide complex binds factor Xa	Direct binding to factor Xa
Limited inhibition of clot-bound/prothrombinase-bound FXa	Inhibits clot-bound/prothrombinase-bound factor Xa
Prolongs the Heptest	Prolongs the APTT and PT
Does not prolong the APTT or PT	Does not prolong the Heptest
No platelet interactions in normal and HIT systems	No platelet interactions in normal and HIT systems
i.v. and s.c. half-life about 14 hr	i.v. half-life about 90 min
100% bioavailable s.c.	Orally bioavailable
Limited bleeding side effect	Limited bleeding side effect
Predictable dose response	Predictable dose response

HIT, heparin-induced thrombocytopenia.

Antithrombotic actions of DX-9065a were also demonstrated after oral administration of this agent (45,50–52). After an intravenous dose of 1 mg/kg, significant anticoagulant and anti–factor Xa activities could be measured in plasma up to 120 minutes in both rabbits and primates (Figs. 10-6 and 10-7).

DX-9065a in global clotting assays caused a significant dose-dependent prolongation of the APTT, the prothrombin time test (PT), and the ACT (Fig. 10-2) both in in vitro and ex vivo plasma (43,45,48,50–52). The PT assay was more sensitive to the anticoagulant effect of DX-9065a (Fig. 10-6). DX-9065a does not

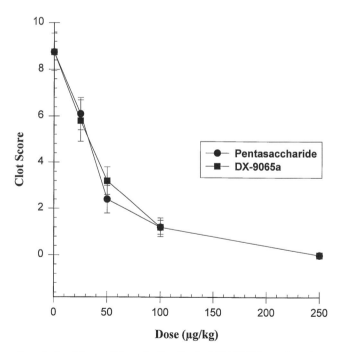

FIG. 10-5. Comparative study of the antithrombotic effect of DX-9065a and pentasaccharide in a modified Wessler rabbit stasis thrombosis model using FEIBA as a thrombogenic stimulus. At equigravimetric dosages, comparable antithrombotic activity was achieved with both agents. Thus direct and indirect acting factor Xa inhibitors are capable of producing inhibition of induced venous thrombosis.

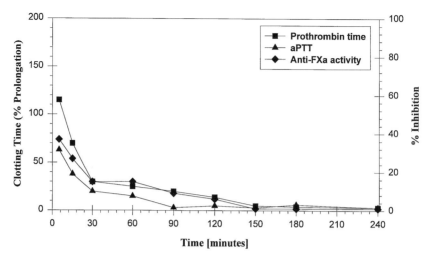

FIG. 10-6. Anticoagulant and anti-factor Xa activities of DX-9065a after administration of a 1 mg/kg intravenous dosage to rabbits (n = 5).

have any effect on preformed thrombin; however, the inactivation of factor Xa by DX-9065a can prevent the further generation of thrombin with resulting inhibition of thrombin-mediated feedback reactions. The formation of thrombin via the intrinsic pathway was more effected than the extrinsic thrombin

generation (43). The inhibition of thrombin generation was found in ex vivo samples after intravenous injection of DX-9065a into rabbits (43).

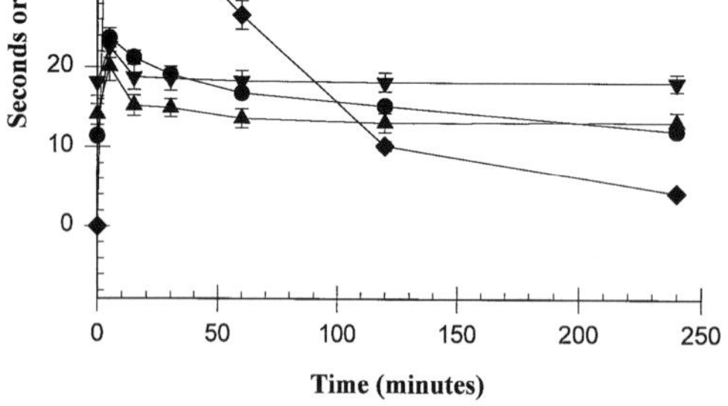

For unknown reasons the anticoagulant action of DX-9065a is species dependent, showing much less activity in rat, dog, and mouse plasma than in human and common squirrel monkey plasma (48,55).

Pharmacokinetic studies on DX-9065a showed a biologic half-life of about 6 minutes for the α phase and 99 minutes for the β phase when given intravenously (50). Oral administration produced peak plasma concentrations at 30 minutes, and plasma levels as well as anticoagulant effects gradually declined over about 6 to 8 hours (45,50). The bioavailability after oral administration was estimated to be approximately 5% to 12% (50).

DX-9065a does not compromise the hemostatic reaction of platelets. It does not affect platelet aggregation (45) and does not produce a positive platelet aggregation effect in a heparin-induced thrombocytopenia positive system in vitro (J. Fareed, unpublished data). As a competitive inhibitor of factor Xa, it does not completely suppress the production of thrombin. Small amounts of thrombin generated despite factor Xa inhibition can initiate primary hemostasis by forming platelet he-

FIG. 10-7. Anticoagulant and anti–factor Xa activities of DX-9065a after administration of a 1-mg/kg intravenous dose to nonhuman primates (*Macaca mulatta*) (n = 4).

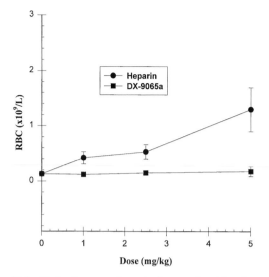

FIG. 10-8. Comparative studies on the bleeding effect of heparin and DX-9065a. The relative hemorrhagic effects of DX-9065a and heparin in a rabbit ear bleeding model show a markedly weaker effect of the factor Xa inhibitor in comparison with heparin. Even at a supratherapeutic dose of 5 mg/kg, the bleeding effect of DX-9065a was insignificant. Heparin, on the other hand, produced a dose-dependent effect. Thus, DX-9065a and most likely other factor Xa inhibitors have a wider therapeutic index than heparin, rendering them safer antithrombotic agents.

mostatic plugs. However, this small amount of thrombin would be insufficient to catalyze the conversion of fibrinogen to fibrin.

DX-9065a has nearly no effect in a rabbit ear bleeding model at doses higher than those shown to be effective for antithrombotic protection (Fig. 10-8). DX-9065a has been shown to have a favorable safety index regarding bleeding complications in animals (43,45,51).

Selectide Series

The Selectide (SEL) (Selectide Corp., Tucson, AZ) series of agents are pentapeptides produced by combinatorial chemistry (56). They are in the preclinical phase of development.

YM-60828

YM-60828 is an orally active agent in preclinical development. In animal models it has been shown to be effective against carotid arterial thrombosis and as an adjunct to thrombolysis after oral administration (57).

Summary

1. Numerous direct factor Xa inhibitors are under development as antithrombotic agents. These agents bind factor Xa and do not require any plasma cofactors. They can also inhibit clot-bound factor Xa.
2. TAP, a recombinant derived agent, is a selective and potent factor Xa inhibitor that has shown promise in experimental models of thrombosis. It is also being studied as an inhibitor of restenosis after angioplasty.
3. TFPI, a recombinant derived agent, is a natural human plasma-based anticoagulant. It is in human clinical trials.
4. DX-9065a is a synthetic factor Xa inhibitor with potent activity. It does not show bleeding effects in experimental models at antithrombotic dosages. It is in human clinical trials.

INDIRECT INHIBITORS

Heparin Pentasaccharide

The only available indirect factor Xa inhibitor is the heparin pentasaccharide. This agent produces its antithrombotic effect via high-affinity binding to AT III. It is the smallest heparin-based molecule (molecular weight 1,728 daltons) that retains antithrombotic activity, being composed of five saccharide units, two of the regular region of heparin and three of the irregular region (Fig. 10-9) (58). Pentasaccharide was developed in 1983 as proof of the hypotheses that a five-member heparin chain was the most minimum saccharide sequence for antithrombotic activity and that sole factor Xa inhibition was indeed antithrombotic (59–61). It was shown in experimental models that inhibition of factor Xa controls excessive thrombin generation, produces antithrombotic effect and has less bleeding risk than heparin (62–64).

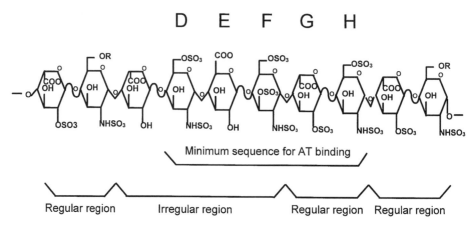

FIG. 10-9. Structure of the synthetic heparin pentasaccharide. (From Walenga et al., ref. 58, with permission.)

The heparin pentasaccharide is produced synthetically in a cooperative effort by Sanofi and Organon. Once the chemical synthesis process was established (60,61), other related agents that were structural modifications of the first pentasaccharide were synthetically produced. Of all materials synthesized, it was determined that the binding to AT III was most critical for expression of antithrombotic activity (65–68). These agents have stronger anti–factor Xa potencies and longer half-lives than the first synthetic pentasaccharide (65,68–70). Pentasaccharide is in phase II clinical trials for prophylaxis against venous thrombosis after hip and knee replacement; none of the modified agents are in clinical trial yet.

Because of its small size, it possesses anti–factor Xa activity with no inhibitory actions against thrombin or other serine proteases. The pentasaccharide–AT III complex has a potency of about 700 anti–factor Xa IU/mg in human plasma and 360 anti–factor Xa IU/mg in rabbit plasma (67). An equivalent amount of AT III is required for complete expression of the anti–factor Xa activity of pentasaccharide (71). Recently Lormeau et al. showed that pentasaccharide inhibits the coagulant activity of the factor VIIa-tissue factor complex (72). The antithrombotic activity was found to be related to the inhibition of

thrombin generation shown in in vitro and ex vivo settings, but the maximal inhibition was less than that for heparin (63,73–75). The same result was obtained after administration of pentasaccharide to humans (76). Thrombin generation inhibition after extrinsic pathway activation was stronger than the inhibition after intrinsic pathway activation.

The APTT was minimally affected (about 100 seconds at a very high dose) by pentasaccharide, and the PT and ACT (Fig. 10-2) were not affected at all (48,58). No platelet interactions have been observed for pentasaccharide in agonist-induced systems for aggregation or in heparin-induced thrombocytopenia test systems (77).

Pentasaccharide has shown dose-dependent antithrombotic activity in several animal models of thrombosis (Fig. 10-5), the degree of antithrombotic activity being dependent on the thrombogenic stimulus for venous thrombosis (40,62,64,78). Pentasaccharide was also effective against arterial thrombosis in a rat arteriovenous shunt model (64,79,80), in a modified arteriovenous shunt model in baboons (81), and in a laser-induced rat model (58,80). This agent also has been shown to facilitate fibrinolysis induced by tissue plasminogen activator in rabbits (82).

Pharmacokinetic studies show a prolonged half-life in both intravenous (approximately 4 hours) and subcutaneous (approximately 18 hours) dosing regimens (64,70,83). Subcutaneous bioavailability was near 100% (84). Human pharmacokinetics showed a similar half-life at about 13.5 hours and a linear correlation with dose (85). The majority of pentasaccharide was eliminated through the kidneys. In elderly subjects the half-life was prolonged to 14.5 hours, and plasma clearance was decreased (85). Bleeding studies in rats suggested very minor bleeding at dosages 100-fold higher than required for complete protection against induced thrombosis (58,64).

Clinical trials are in progress for the prophylaxis of venous thrombosis in orthopedic surgical patients. A brief study on the successful use of pentasaccharide with percutaneous transluminal coronary angioplasty has recently been reported (86). Pentasaccharide is more attractive than LMW heparins because it is a well-defined synthetic drug with a long half-life and 100% subcutaneous bioavailability. It does not appear to be related to the heparin-induced thrombocytopenic response and therefore may be used as a substitute antithrombotic agent in patients with heparin-induced thrombocytopenia (87). It appears to have minimal bleeding risks.

Summary

1. The heparin pentasaccharide is the only well-developed indirect factor Xa inhibitor. Its structure is based on heparin and it requires AT III to express activity. It is a well-defined synthetic agent.
2. Pentasaccharide has a long half-life (intravenous or subcutaneous). It has been shown to be antithrombotic in experimental models with no bleeding side effect.
3. Clinical trials of pentasaccharide as prophylaxis against thrombosis after hip and knee replacement surgery are nearing completion. If successful, the hypothesis that factor Xa inhibition is an effective means to produce antithrombotic activity will be validated.

CONCLUSION

Factor Xa plays a pivotal role in the coagulation process, being the common point between the extrinsic and intrinsic pathways. Although thrombin is an important enzyme, its generation is dependent on factor Xa. Thus, to control the activity of activated factor X would be to control excessive thrombin generation. With less thrombin, the rate of fibrin formation is slowed. A regulated control of the activation of the coagulation cascade would be achieved. With factor Xa inhibitors, bleeding risk would be minimal because some thrombin generation/clot formation is still possible under treatment because thrombin generation is not completely blocked.

The factor Xa inhibitors presently under clinical development are a diverse class of new antithrombotic agents with direct and indirect mechanisms of inhibition. The pentasaccharide represents a synthetic oligosaccharide that requires the endogenous cofactor AT III for its activity. TAP is a LMW peptide with direct inhibitory activity, whereas DX-9065a is a synthetic organic compound of lower molecular weight and direct inhibitory actions. DX-9065a is less specific than TAP. TFPI is also a promising agent.

Despite differences in their mechanisms of action and in vitro activities, pentasaccharide, DX-9065a, and TAP have been shown to be effective antithrombotic agents in experimental models of venous thrombosis, coronary artery occlusion, arterial thrombolysis and acute reocclusion, restenosis after angioplasty, dialysis, and disseminated intravascular coagulation (DIC). Preliminary results from human trials in orthopedic surgical patients are encouraging. Both TAP and DX-9065a produce measurable in vitro anticoagulant effects. In contrast, pentasaccharide does not produce an anticoagulant effect by the typical clot-based assays. Thus, with factor Xa inhibitors there is not necessarily a correlation between current laboratory assays and antithrombotic efficacy as there is with heparin.

Factor Xa inhibitors vary in their efficacy to inhibit factor Xa depending on molecular size, access to clot-bound factor Xa, access to prothrombinase bound factor Xa, specificity, and kinetics of inhibition. DX-9065a with a relatively lower molecular weight may be more effective in the inhibition of clot-bound factor Xa than TAP or pentasaccharide.

Based on in vivo experimental studies, factor Xa inhibitors can potentially be used for certain clinical indications where heparin is used as an anticoagulant. Factor Xa inhibitors would likely be suitable agents for prophylaxis of thrombotic processes where a control of thrombin formation is needed, especially in less severe indications, such as prophylaxis of venous thrombosis. Moreover, because the bioavailability of DX-9065a and pentasaccharide after subcutaneous administration is almost 100%, these drugs would have more readily accepted administration regimens. However, the half-life of some agents is rather short and they also do not all release endogenous TFPI. So a direct comparison to heparin for dosages and clinical effects is probably not possible.

Because of their unique properties, factor Xa inhibitors also may prove to be better adjunct drugs than heparin and thrombin inhibitors for the new antiplatelet agents clopidogrel and the glycoprotein IIb/IIIa inhibitors. This opens developmental applications for factor Xa inhibitors in arterial thrombosis such as coronary thrombosis prevention, unstable angina, and ischemic and thrombotic stroke. As adjunct agents, these drugs also may be ideal for thrombolytic therapy in both cardiovascular and cerebrovascular indications. Although factor Xa inhibitors may be extremely useful in the management of deep vein thrombosis prophylaxis, they also can be used at higher doses as therapeutic agents. Because of their predictable pharmacokinetics and relatively fewer interactions with the blood/vasculature, they may be more selective and controllable than heparin and AT agents. However, as antithrombotic agents, factor Xa inhibitors are expected to be weaker than AT agents because they cannot inhibit generated thrombin. Thus, clinical trials are needed to validate the true potential of these agents.

Further studies are needed to determine the relative importance of inhibition of clot-associated factor Xa or thrombin in the progression of thrombosis. One study has suggested that the inhibition of factor Xa but not of thrombin results in sustained attenuation of thrombus-associated procoagulant activity (88). For effective suppression of the procoagulant activity of intravascular thrombi and the resulting continuation of thrombotic processes, it may be useful to combine the inhibition of factor Xa with the inhibition of thrombin. Factor Xa inhibitors are able to inhibit thrombin generation but they do not have the capacity to inhibit pre-existing thrombin. Thrombin inhibitors can inhibit pre-existing thrombin as well as clot-bound thrombin and can release thrombin upon clot lysis. Is there an optimal site in the coagulation cascade where inhibition would prevent the thrombotic process, in terms of both safety and efficacy? Does the site differ for different clinical conditions where different rates of thrombin generation occur and there are different characteristics of the clot? Due to the differences in the site and mechanism of action, the resulting antithrombotic effect of both factor Xa and thrombin inhibitors could provide therapeutic benefit in a range of clinical indications (6,7,89). Factor Xa inhibitors may be useful in monotherapeutic and polytherapeutic modalities; however, synergistic effects need to be addressed when combining drugs.

In contrast to specific inhibitors of thrombin, the factor Xa inhibitors are devoid of bleeding effects even at dosages much higher than supratherapeutic levels, which in the case of heparin are responsible for bleeding. Thus, a dissociation between the bleeding and antithrombotic responses is expected for both DX-9065a and pentasaccharide.

None of the factor Xa inhibitors produce significant inhibition against agonist-induced platelet activation processes, and platelets have not been shown to be compromised in experimental settings. It can therefore be projected that the safety/efficacy profile of factor Xa inhibitors may be better than heparin and

AT agents. Furthermore, factor Xa inhibitors are devoid of heparin-induced thrombocytopenia and immunogenic responses, making them potentially useful alternative antithrombotic agents in patients in whom heparin is contraindicated.

There are potential advantages for factor Xa inhibitors over thrombin inhibitors, particularly a higher safety margin in prophylactic regimens and less frequent dosing requirements. With the development of factor Xa inhibitors it needs to be assured that the maximum benefit of factor Xa inhibitors has been achieved, be it in prophylactic or therapeutic use (i.e., in the choice of the clinical pathology, dose of drug, dosing regimen, etc. when establishing clinical trials). It is likely that each drug will have a role in specific clinical indications and that one drug will not be optimal for all thrombotic situations. How and where they are used clinically, and how they will compete with LMW heparins and direct thrombin inhibitors remains to be determined.

The limited data available on factor Xa inhibitors is favorable and thus warrants additional investigations to demonstrate the relative inhibitory profile of these agents in thrombotic and cardiovascular indications. The future holds promise for finding effective factor Xa inhibitors and their challenge to the widely accepted thrombin hypothesis.

ACKNOWLEDGMENTS

We acknowledge the generous gifts of DX-9065a from Dr. S. Kunitada of Daiichi (Tokyo, Japan) and pentasaccharide from Dr. J.M. Herbert of Sanofi (Paris, France).

REFERENCES

1. Clagett GP, Anderson FA Jr, Heit J, Levine MN, Wheeler HB. Prevention of venous thromboembolism. *Chest* 1995;108(suppl):312–334.
2. Stürzebecher J, Stürzebecher U, Vieweg H, Wagner G, Hauptmann J, Markwardt F. Synthetic inhibitors of bovine factor Xa and thrombin. Comparison of their anticoagulant efficiency. *Thromb Res* 1989;54:245–252.
3. Hauptmann J, Kaiser B, Nowak G, Stürzebecher J, Markwardt F. Comparison of the anticoagulant and antithrombotic effects of synthetic thrombin and factor Xa inhibitors. *Thromb Haemost* 1990;63:220–223.
4. The Global Use of Strategies to Open Occluded Coronary Arteries (GUSTO) IIb Investigators. A comparison of recombinant hirudin with heparin for the treatment of acute coronary syndromes. *N Engl J Med* 1996;335:775–782.
5. Antman EM for the TIMI 9B Investigators. Hirudin in acute myocardial infarction. Thrombolysis and thrombin inhibition in myocardial infarction (TIMI) 9B trial. *Circulation* 1996;94:911–921.
6. Kaiser B, Hauptmann J. Factor Xa inhibitors as novel antithrombotic agents: facts and perspectives. *Cardiovasc Drug Rev* 1994;12:225–236.
7. Kaiser B. Factor Xa versus factor IIa inhibitors. *Clin Appl Thromb Hemost* 1997;3:16–24.
8. Weitz JI, Hudoba M, Massel D, Maraganore J, Hirsh J. Clot-bound thrombin is protected from inhibition by heparin-antithrombin III but is susceptible to inactivation by antithrombin III-independent inhibitors. *J Clin Invest* 1990;86:385–391.
9. Eisenberg PR, Siegel JE, Abendschein DR, Miletich JP. Importance of factor Xa in determining the procoagulant activity of whole-blood clots. *J Clin Invest* 1993;91:1877–1883.
10. Meddahi S, Bara L, Uzan A, Samama MM. Pharmacologic modulation of human clots associated thrombin and prothrombinase activities by a direct anti Xa drug, r-hirudin and low molecular weight heparin. *Haemostasis* 1996;26(suppl 3):578.
11. Hoppensteadt D. Doctoral thesis: Tissue factor pathway inhibitor as a modulator of post-surgical thrombogenesis. Experimental and clinical studies. University of London, London, UK, October 1996.
12. Schwartz RS, Holmes Jr DR, Topol EJ. The restenosis paradigm revisited: an alternative proposal for cellular mechanisms. *J Am Coll Cardiol* 1992;20:1284–1293.
13. Kanthou C, Benzakour O. Cellular effects of thrombin and their signaling pathways. *Cell Pharmacol* 1995;2:293–302.
14. Benzakour O, Kanthou C. Cellular and molecular events in atherogenesis: basis for pharmacological and gene therapy approaches to restenosis. *Cell Pharmacol* 1996;3:7–22.
15. McNamara CA, Sarembock IJ, Bachhuber BG, et al. Thrombin and vascular smooth muscle cell proliferation: implications for atherosclerosis and restenosis. *Semin Thromb Hemost* 1996;22:139–144.
16. Ko FN, Yang YC, Huang SC, Ou JT. Coagulation factor Xa stimulates platelet-derived growth factor release and mitogenesis in cultured vascular smooth muscle cells of rat. *J Clin Invest* 1996;98:1493–1501.
17. Gasic GP, Arenas CP, Gasic TB, Gasic GJ. Coagulation factors X, Xa, and protein S as potent mitogens of cultured aortic smooth muscle cells. *Proc Natl Acad Sci U S A* 1992;89:2317–2320.
18. Ragosta M, Gimple LW, Gertz D, et al. Specific factor Xa inhibition reduces restenosis after balloon angioplasty of atherosclerotic femoral arteries in rabbits. *Circulation* 1994;89:1262–1271.
19. Schwartz RS, Holder DJ, Holmes DR Jr, et al. Neointimal thickening after severe coronary artery injury is limited by short-term administration of a factor Xa inhibitor. Results in a porcine model. *Circulation* 1996;93:1542–1548.

20. Tuszynski GP, Gasic TB, Gasic GJ. Isolation and characterization of antistasin. *J Biol Chem* 1987;262: 9718–9723.

21. Dunwiddie CT, Thornberry NA, Bull HG, et al. Antistasin, a leech-derived inhibitor of factor Xa. Kinetic analysis of enzyme inhibition and identification of the reactive site. *J Biol Chem* 1989;264:16694–16699.

22. Rigbi M, Jackson CM, Atamna H, et al. FXa inhibitor from the saliva of the leech *Hirudo medicinalis*. *Thromb Haemost* 1995;73:1306.

23. Jordan SP, Mao SS, Lewis SD, Shafer JA. Reaction pathway for inhibition of blood coagulation factor Xa by tick anticoagulant peptide. *Biochemistry* 1992;31: 5374–5380.

24. Jordan SP, Waxman L, Smith DE, Vlasuk GP. Tick anticoagulant peptide: kinetic analysis of the recombinant inhibitor with blood coagulation factor Xa. *Biochemistry* 1990;29:11095–11100.

25. Krishnaswamy S, Vlasuk GP, Bergum PW. Assembly of the prothrombinase complex enhances the inhibition of bovine factor Xa by tick anticoagulant peptide. *Biochemistry* 1994;33:7897–7907.

26. Vlasuk GP. Structural and functional characterization of tick anticoagulant peptide (TAP): a potent and selective inhibitor of blood coagulation factor Xa. *Thromb Haemost* 1993;70:212–216.

27. Vlasuk GP, Ramjit D, Fujita T, et al. Comparison of the in vivo anticoagulant properties of standard heparin and the highly selective factor Xa inhibitors antistasin and tick anticoagulant peptide (TAP) in a rabbit model of venous thrombosis. *Thromb Haemost* 1991;65: 257–262.

28. Fioravanti C, Burkholder D, Francis B, Siegl PKS, Gibson RE. Antithrombotic activity of recombinant tick anticoagulant peptide and heparin in a rabbit model of venous thrombosis. *Thromb Res* 1993;71:317–324.

29. Wong PC, Crain EJ Jr, Nguan O, Watson CA, Racanelli A. Antithrombotic actions of selective inhibitors of blood coagulation factor Xa in rat models of thrombosis. *Thromb Res* 1996;83:117–126.

30. Lynch JJ, Sitko GR, Lehman ED, Vlasuk GP. Primary prevention of coronary arterial thrombosis with the factor Xa inhibitor rTAP in a canine electrolytic injury model. *Thromb Haemost* 1995;74:640–645.

31. Schaffer LW, Davidson JT, Vlasuk GP, Siegl PKS. Antithrombotic efficacy of recombinant tick anticoagulant peptide. A potent inhibitor of coagulation factor Xa in a primate model of arterial thrombosis. *Circulation* 1991;84:1741–1748.

32. Ørvim U, Barstad RM, Vlasuk GP, Sakariassen KS. Effect of selective factor Xa inhibition on arterial thrombus formation triggered by tissue factor/factor VIIa or collagen in an ex vivo model of shear-dependent human thrombogenesis. *Arterioscler Thromb Vasc Biol* 1995; 15:2188–2194.

33. Mellott MJ, Stranieri MT, Sitko GR, Stabilito II, Lynch JJ, Vlasuk GP. Enhancement of recombinant tissue plasminogen activator-induced reperfusion by recombinant tick anticoagulant peptide, a selective factor Xa inhibitor, in a canine model of femoral arterial thrombolysis. *Fibrinolysis* 1993;7:195–202.

34. Sitko GR, Ramjit DR, Stabilito II, Lehmann D, Lynch JJ, Vlasuk GP. Conjunctive enhancement of enzymatic thrombolysis and prevention of thrombotic reocclusion with the selective factor Xa inhibitor tick anticoagulant

peptide. Comparison to hirudin and heparin in a canine model of acute coronary artery thrombosis. *Circulation* 1992;85:805–815.

35. Lifkovits J, Malycky JL, Rao JS, et al. Selective inhibition of factor Xa is more efficient than factor VIIa-tissue factor complex blockade at facilitating coronary thrombolysis in the canine model. *J Am Coll Cardiol* 1996;28:1858–1865.

36. Prager NA, Abendschein DR, McKenzie CR, Eisenberg PR. Role of thrombin compared with factor Xa in the procoagulant activity of whole blood clots. *Circulation* 1995;92:962–967.

37. Vlasuk GP, Bergum PW, Brunck TK, et al. Anticoagulant repertoire of hematophagous nematodes. *Thromb Haemost* 1995;73:1305.

38. Broze Jr GJ. Tissue factor pathway inhibitor. *Thromb Haemost* 1995;74:90–93.

39. Jort PFH. Intermediate reactions in the coagulation of blood with tissue thromboplastin. *Scand J Lab Invest* 1957;9(suppl 27):81–183.

40. Kaiser B, Jeske W, Hoppensteadt D, Walenga JM, Fareed J. Anticoagulant and antithrombotic effects of the synthetic heparin pentasaccharide and the direct factor Xa inhibitor DX-9065a after i.v. administration in rabbits. *Blood* 1996;88(suppl 1):67b.

41. Wang Z, Hebert D, Kaplan AV, Creasy A, Galluppi GR. Persistent inhibition to 12 hours of mural platelet thrombosis after a single local infusion of tissue factor pathway inhibitor at the site of angioplasty. *Circulation* 1996;94:I-268.

42. Fareed J, Callas D, Hoppensteadt D, Walenga J. Modulation of endothelium by heparin and related polyelectrolytes. In: Vane JR, Born GVR, Welzel D (eds). *The Endothelial Cell in Health and Disease.* Stuttgart: FK Schattauer Verlagsgesellschaft, 1995;165–182.

43. Herbert JM, Bernat A, Dol F, Hérault JP, Crepon B, Lormeau JC. DX 9065A, a novel, synthetic, selective and orally active inhibitor of factor Xa: in vitro and in vivo studies. *J Pharmacol Exp Ther* 1996;276: 1030–1038.

44. Nagahara T, Katakura S, Yokoyama Y, et al. Design, synthesis and biological activities of orally active coagulation factor Xa inhibitors. *Eur J Med Chem* 1995; 30(suppl):140–143.

45. Hara T, Yokoyama A, Ishihara H, Yokoyama Y, Nagahara T, Iwamoto M. DX-9065a, a new synthetic, potent anticoagulant and selective inhibitor for factor Xa. *Thromb Haemost* 1994;1:314–319.

46. Katakura S, Nagahara T, Hara T, Iwamoto M. A novel factor Xa inhibitor: structure-activity relationships and selectivity between factor Xa and thrombin. *Biochem Biophys Res Commun* 1993;197:965–972.

47. Katakura S, Nagahara T, Hara T, Kunitada S, Iwamoto M. Molecular model of an interaction between factor Xa and DX-9065a, a novel factor Xa inhibitor: contribution of the acetimidoylpyrrolidine moiety of the inhibitor to potency and selectivity for serine proteases. *Eur J Med Chem* 1995;30:387–394.

48. Fareed D, Wyma D, Ahmad S, Iqbal O, Kutinada S. Anticoagulant and antithrombotic effects of a synthetic factor Xa inhibitor (DX-9065a) [Abstract]. *Thromb Haemost* 1997 (in press).

49. Yamashita T, Tsuji T, Matsuoka A, Giddings JC, Yamamoto J. The antithrombotic effect of synthetic low molecular weight human factor Xa inhibitor, DX-

9065a, on He-Ne laser-induced thrombosis in rat mesenteric vessels. *Thromb Res* 1997;85:45–51.

50. Yokoyama T, Kelly AB, Marzec UM, Hanson SR, Kunitada S, Harker LA. Antithrombotic effects of orally active synthetic antagonists of activated factor X in non-human primates. *Circulation* 1995;92:485–491.

51. Hara T, Yokoyama A, Tanabe K, Ishihara H, Iwamoto M. DX-9065a, an orally active, specific inhibitor of factor Xa, inhibits thrombosis without affecting bleeding time in rats. *Thromb Haemost* 1995;74:635–639.

52. Yamazaki M, Asakura H, Aoshima K, et al. Effects of DX-9065a, an orally active, newly synthesized and specific inhibitor of factor Xa, against experimental disseminated intravascular coagulation in rats. *Thromb Haemost* 1994;72:393–396.

53. Yamazaki M, Asakura H, Saito M, Aoshima K, Morishita E, Matsuda T. Effects of DX-9065a, an orally active, newly synthesized and specific inhibitor of factor Xa against experimental disseminated intravascular coagulation in rats. *Thromb Haemost* 1995;73:1312.

54. Hara T, Morishima Y, Kunitada S. Selective factor Xa inhibitor, DX-9065a; suppressed hypercoagulable state during haemodialysis in cynomolgus monkeys. *Thromb Haemost* 1995;73:1311.

55. Hara T, Yokoyama A, Morishima Y, Kunitada S. Species differences in anticoagulant and anti-Xa activity of DX-9065a, a highly selective factor Xa inhibitor. *Thromb Res* 1995;80:99–104.

56. Ostrem JA, Stringer S, Al-Obeidi F, et al. Characterization of an orally available and highly specific synthetic factor Xa inhibitor. *Thromb Haemost* 1995;73:1306.

57. Kawasaki T, Sato K, Taniuchi Y, et al. Comparative studies of an orally-active factor Xa inhibitor, YM-60828, with various antithrombotic agents in a rat model of arterial thrombosis [Abstract]. *Thromb Haemost* 1997 (in press).

58. Walenga JM, Jeske WP, Bara L, Samama MM, Fareed J. State-of-the-art article. Biochemical and pharmacologic rationale for the development of a heparin pentasaccharide. *Thromb Res* 1997;86(1):1–36.

59. Choay J, Petitou M, Lormeau JC, Sinay P, Casu B, Gatti G. Structure-activity relationship in heparin: a synthetic pentasaccharide with high affinity for antithrombin III and eliciting high anti-factor Xa activity. *Biochem Biophys Acta* 1983;116:492–499.

60. Sinay P, Jaquinet JE, Petitou M, et al. Total synthesis of a heparin pentasaccharide fragment having high affinity for antithrombin III. *Carbohydr Res* 1984;132:C5–C9.

61. Petitou M, Duchaussoy P, Lederman I, et al. Synthesis of heparin fragments. A chemical synthesis of the pentasaccharide 0-(2-deoxy-2-sulfamido-6-O-sulfo-alpha-D-glucopyranosyl)-1→4)-0-(beta-D-glucopyranosyluronic acid)-(1→4)-0-(2-deoxy-2-sulfamido-3, 6-di-0-sulfo-alpha-D-glucopyranosyl)-(1→4)-0-(2-O-sulfo-alpha-L-idopyranosyluronic acid)-(1→4)-2-deoxy-2-sulfamido-6-O-sulfo-D-glucopyranose decasodium salt, a heparin fragment having high affinity for antithrombin III. *Carbohydr Res* 1986;147:221–236.

62. Walenga JM, Petitou M, Lormeau JC, Samama M, Fareed J, Choay J. Antithrombotic activity of a synthetic heparin pentasaccharide in a rabbit stasis thrombosis model using different thrombogenic challenges. *Thromb Res* 1987;46:187–198.

63. Walenga JM, Bara L, Petitou M, Samama M, Fareed J, Choay J. The inhibition of the generation of thrombin and the antithrombotic effect of a pentasaccharide with sole anti-factor Xa activity. *Thromb Res* 1988;51:23–33.

64. Hobbelen PMJ, van Dinther TG, Vogel GMT, van Boeckel CAA, Moelker HCT, Meuleman DG. Pharmacological profile of the chemically synthesized antithrombin III binding fragment of heparin (pentasaccharide). *Thromb Haemost* 1990;63:265–70.

65. Petitou M, van Boeckel CAA. Chemical synthesis of heparin fragments and analogues. *Prog Chem Org Nat Prod* 1992;60:143–210.

66. Van Boeckel CAA, Beetz T, Vos JN, et al. Synthesis of a pentasaccharide corresponding to the antithrombin III binding fragment of heparin. *J Carbohydr Chem* 1985;4:293–321.

67. Petitou M, Lormeau JC, Choay J. A new synthetic pentasaccharide with increased anti-factor Xa activity: possible role for anionic clusters in the interaction of heparin and antithrombin III. *Semin Thromb Res* 1993; 19(suppl 2):143–146.

68. Visser A, Buiting MT, van Dinther TG, van Boeckel CAA, Grootenhuis PG, Meuleman DG. The AT-III binding affinities of a series of synthetic pentasaccharide analogues. *Thromb Haemost* 1991;65:1296.

69. Meuleman DG, Hobbelen PMJ, van Dinther TG, Vogel GMT, van Boeckel CAA, Moelker HCT. Antifactor Xa activity and antithrombotic activity in rats of structural analogues of the minimal antithrombin III binding sequence: discovery of compounds with a longer duration of action than of the natural pentasaccharide. *Semin Thromb Hemost* 1991;17(suppl 1):112–117.

70. van Amsterdam RGM, Vogel GMT, Visser A, Kop WJ, Buiting MT, Meuleman DG. Synthetic analogues of the antithrombin III-binding pentasaccharide sequence of heparin. Prediction of in vivo residence times. *Arterioscler Thromb Vasc Biol* 1995;15:495–503.

71. Walenga JM, Bara L, Hoppensteadt D, Choay J, Fareed J, Samama M. AT III as a rate limiting factor for the measurement of pentasaccharide in laboratory assays. *Thromb Haemost* 1991;65:1314.

72. Lormeau JC, Hérault JP, Herbert JM. Antithrombin mediated inhibition of factor VIIa-tissue factor complex by the synthetic pentasaccharide representing the heparin binding site to AT. *Thromb Haemost* 1996;76:5–8.

73. Dol F, Gaich C, Petitou M, et al. The antithrombotic activity of synthetic pentasaccharides and fraxiparine is closely correlated with their respective ability to alter thromboplastin-triggered thrombin generation ex vivo. *Thromb Haemost* 1993;69:655.

74. Béguin S, Choay J, Hemker HC. The action of a synthetic pentasaccharide on thrombin generation in whole plasma. *Thromb Haemost* 1989;61:397–401.

75. Lormeau JC, Hérault JP. Comparative inhibition of extrinsic and intrinsic thrombin generation by standard heparin, a low molecular weight heparin, and a synthetic AT-III binding pentasaccharide. *Thromb Haemost* 1993;69:152–156.

76. Lormeau JC, Hérault JP. The effect of the synthetic pentasaccharide SR 90107/ORG 31540 on thrombin generation ex vivo is uniquely due to AT-mediated neutralization of factor Xa. *Thromb Haemost* 1995;74:1474–1477.

77. Walenga JM, Koza MJ, Lewis BE, Pifarré R. Relative heparin-induced thrombocytopenic potential of low molecular weight heparins and new antithrombotic agents. *Clin Appl Thromb Hemost* 1996;2(suppl 1): 21–27.

78. Amar J, Caranobe P, Sie P, Boneu B. Antithrombotic potencies of heparins in relation to their antifactor Xa and antithrombin activities: an experimental study in two models of thrombosis in the rabbit. *Br J Haematol* 1990;76:94–100.

79. Vogel GMT, van Amsterdam RGM, Kop WJ, Meuleman DG. Pentasaccharide and Orgaran arrest, whereas heparin delays thrombus formation in a rat arteriovenous shunt. *Thromb Haemost* 1993;69:29–34.

80. Weichert W, Breddin HK. Effect of low molecular weight heparins on laser-induced thrombus formation in rat mesenteric vessels. *Haemostasis* 1988;18(suppl 3):55–63.

81. Hérault JP, Pflieger AM, Savi P, et al. Comparative effects of two factor Xa inhibitors on prothrombinase assembled in different environments. *Haemostasis* 1996; 26:S3.

82. Bernat A, Hoffmann P, Sainte-Marie M, Herbert JM. The synthetic pentasaccharide SR 90107A/Org 31540 enhances tissue-type plasminogen activator-induced thrombolysis in rabbits. *Fibrinolysis* 1996;10:151–157.

83. Crépon B, Donat F, Bârzu T, Hérault JP. Pharmacokinetic (PK) parameters of AT binding pentasaccharides in three animal species: predictive value for humans. *Thromb Haemost* 1993;69:654.

84. Walenga JM, Fareed J. Preliminary biochemical and pharmacologic studies on a chemically synthesized pentasaccharide. *Semin Thromb Hemost* 1985;11:89–99.

85. Boneu B, Necciari J, Cariou R, et al. Pharmacokinetics and tolerance of the natural pentasaccharide (SR90107/ ORG31540) with high affinity to antithrombin III in man. *Thromb Haemost* 1995;74:1468–1473.

86. Schiele FJ, Vuillemenot AR, Meneveau NF, et al. Initial experience of a sulphated pentasaccharide, a pure factor Xa inhibitor, in coronary angioplasty. *Circulation* 1996; 94:I–742.

87. Elalamy I, Lecrubier C, Potevin F, et al. Absence of in vitro cross-reaction of pentasaccharide with the plasma heparin dependent factor of twenty-five patients with heparin associated thrombocytopenia. *Thromb Haemost* 1995;74:1384–1385.

88. McKenzie CR, Abendschein DR, Eisenberg PR. Sustained inhibition of whole-blood clot procoagulant activity by inhibition of thrombus-associated factor Xa. *Arterioscler Thromb Vasc Biol* 1996;16:1285–1291.

89. Fareed J, Callas DD, Hoppensteadt D, Jeske W, Walenga JM. Recent developments in antithrombotic agents. *Exp Opin Invest Drugs* 1995;4:389–412.

90. Girard TJ, Warren LA, Novotny WF. Functional significance of the Kunitz-type inhibitory domains of lipoprotein-associated coagulation inhibitor. *Nature* 1986;338: 518–519.

*Cardiovascular Thrombosis: Thrombocardiology
and Thromboneurology, Second Edition,*
edited by M. Verstraete, V. Fuster, and E. J. Topol,
Lippincott–Raven Publishers, Philadelphia © 1998.

11

Unfractionated and Low Molecular Weight Heparin

Jack Hirsh and *Christopher B. Granger

*Hamilton Civic Hospitals Research Centre, Hamilton, Ontario L8V 1C3, Canada; and
*Departments of Medicine and Cardiology, Duke University Medical Center,
Durham, North Carolina 27705*

UNFRACTIONATED HEPARIN

Mechanism of Action

Unfractionated heparin is a glycosaminoglycan (GAG) composed of chains of alternating residues of D-glucosamine and a uronic acid (1). Its major anticoagulant effect is accounted for by a unique pentasaccharide with a high-affinity binding sequence to antithrombin (AT), which is present in only one third of unfractionated heparin molecules (8–11). Heparin binds to AT (2–11) and produces a conformational change in AT (12–14) that markedly accelerates its ability to inactivate the coagulation enzymes thrombin (factor IIa), factor Xa, and factor IXa (3). After AT binds to form an irreversible complex with these coagulation enzymes, heparin dissociates from the complex and can be reutilized. Of the coagulation enzymes inactivated by the heparin–AT complex, thrombin is the most sensitive to inhibition (3,15–19).

Heparin catalyzes the inactivation of thrombin by AT by acting as a template to which both the enzyme and inhibitor bind to form a ternary complex (3,11,20,21). In contrast, the inactivation of factor Xa by AT–heparin complex does not require ternary complex formation and is achieved by binding of the enzyme to AT (1,3,6,7). Unfractionated heparin molecules that contain fewer than 18 saccharides are unable to bind thrombin and AT simultaneously and, therefore, are unable to accelerate the inactivation of thrombin by AT, but retain their ability to catalyze the inhibition of factor Xa by AT (21–23). Heparin also catalyzes the inactivation of thrombin by a second plasma cofactor, heparin cofactor II (HCII) (24). This second anticoagulant effect of unfractionated heparin is specific for thrombin, does not require the unique AT-binding pentasaccharide, and requires much higher doses of heparin (25–28) than those required to catalyze the activity of AT.

Unfractionated heparin is heterogeneous with respect to molecular size, anticoagulant activity, and pharmacokinetic properties. The molecular weight of unfractionated heparin ranges from 5,000 to 30,000 daltons with a mean molecular weight of 15,000 daltons (approximately 50 monosaccharide chains) (29–31). The anticoagulant activity of unfractionated heparin is heterogeneous because (a) only one third of the unfractionated heparin molecules administered to patients have anticoagulant activity; (b) the anticoagulant profile of unfractionated heparin is influenced by the chain length of the molecules; and (c) the clearance of unfractionated heparin is influenced by its molecular size, with the higher molecular weight species being cleared from the circulation more rapidly than the lower molecular weight species.

Administration, Pharmacokinetics, and Pharmacodynamics

Heparin must be given by injection; the two preferred routes are intravenous and subcutaneous. The efficacy and safety of unfractionated heparin administered by either the continuous intravenous method or by the subcutaneous route are comparable provided that the dosages used are adequate (32–34). When administered subcutaneously in high doses, the bioavailability of unfractionated heparin is reduced by about 10% (compared with heparin administered by continuous intravenous infusion), and its anticoagulant effect is delayed for 1 to 2 hours.

Unfractionated heparin binds to a number of plasma proteins, which contributes to its reduced plasma recovery (bioavailability) at low concentrations, to the variability of the anticoagulant response to fixed doses of heparin in patients with thromboembolic disorders (35), and to the laboratory phenomenon of heparin resistance (36). Binding of heparin to von Willebrand factor (VWF) results in the inhibition of VWF-dependent platelet function (37).

Heparin also binds to macrophages and endothelial cells (38). Unfractionated heparin is cleared through a combination of a rapid saturable and a much slower first-order mechanism of clearance (39–41). The saturable phase of heparin clearance is thought to be due to heparin binding to receptors on endothelial cells (42,43) and macrophages (44), where it is internalized, depolymerized, and metabolized into smaller and less sulfated forms (45,46). Clearance through the slower nonsaturable mechanism is partly renal. At therapeutic doses, a considerable proportion of the administered unfractionated heparin is cleared through the rapid saturable, dose-dependent mechanism of clearance. The apparent biologic half-life of unfractionated heparin increases from approximately 30 minutes with an intravenous bolus of 25 U/kg, to 60 minutes with an intravenous bolus of 100 IU/kg, to 150 minutes with an intravenous bolus of 400 U/kg (39–41).

LABORATORY MONITORING AND DOSE-RESPONSE RELATIONSHIPS OF HEPARIN

The anticoagulant effect of unfractionated heparin is usually monitored by the activated partial thromboplastin time (APTT). When unfractionated heparin is administered in fixed doses, the anticoagulant response to heparin varies among sick patients, including those with acute venous thromboembolism (47) and those with myocardial ischemia (48–51). This variability is caused by differences between patients in their plasma concentrations of heparin-neutralizing plasma proteins. In addition, elevated levels of factor VIII can occur in sick patients as part of the acute phase reaction response and result in a dissociation between the heparin levels and APTT. In such patients, the APTT response is reduced in relation to heparin levels (52).

The recommended therapeutic range for the APTT for the treatment of patients with venous thrombosis was originally based on a study performed in rabbits (53). This study demonstrated that thrombus extension is prevented by a heparin dose that prolongs the APTT above a ratio of 1.5, corresponding to a heparin level by protamine titration of 0.2 IU/ml; this is equivalent to an anti–factor Xa level of 0.3 IU/ml. Unfortunately, the different commercial APTT reagents vary in their responsiveness to heparin (54). For most currently used APTT reagents, a therapeutic effect is not achieved with an APTT ratio of 1.5 (measured by dividing the observed APTT by the mean of the laboratory control APTT) (54). For this reason, it is inappropriate to use the same APTT ratio for all reagents. Rather, the therapeutic range for each APTT reagent should be calibrated to be equivalent to a heparin level of 0.2 to 0.4 IU/ml by protamine titration or to an anti–factor Xa level of about 0.3 to 0.7 U/ml.

The APTT is sensitive over a heparin range of 0.1 to 1.0 IU/ml. It is therefore unsuitable for monitoring heparin dosage in high-risk angioplasty patients and those having cardiac bypass surgery because they may require heparin levels of greater than 1 U/ml. For both of these procedures, heparin monitoring is usually performed by the activated clotting time (ACT) because this test shows a graded response to heparin concentrations in the range of 1 to 5 IU/ml.

Relationship Between Anticoagulant Effect and Antithrombotic Efficacy and Safety

Treatment of Venous Thromboembolism

There is very good evidence that the efficacy of heparin is dependent on using an adequate starting dose of heparin and on using a maintenance dose that produces an adequate anticoagulant effect measured either by an APTT or a heparin level.

The clinical evidence supporting the use of a therapeutic range for the APTT is based on subgroup analysis of two prospective studies and from one randomized trial (55–57).

The first study reported by Basu and associates in 1972 (56) evaluating the relationship between the APTT and clinical efficacy was a prospective cohort study of 162 patients with venous thrombosis. Five of the 162 patients developed recurrent venous thromboembolism during their hospital stay, and all five had an APTT below 50 seconds (approximately 1.3 times control) for three or more consecutive days before recurrence. In contrast, there were no recurrences in patients whose APTT did not fall below 50 seconds for two consecutive days.

The second study reported by Hull and associates in 1986 (55) was a double-blind randomized trial in which patients were allocated to receive heparin administered either by continuous intravenous infusion or twice daily subcutaneous injection. A post hoc analysis showed that a higher proportion of patients had an APTT below the therapeutic range at 24 hours in the group randomized to receive heparin by subcutaneous injection than by continuous intravenous infusion (36 of 57 or 67% compared with 17 of 58 or 23%, respectively). There were 11 recurrences in the group receiving subcutaneous heparin after 3 months of follow-up, and 10 of the 11 patients had an APTT result below the therapeutic range in the first 24 hours of treatment. There were three recurrences in the continuous intravenous group after 3 months of follow-up, and all three patients had an APTT below the therapeutic range in the first 24 hours, and in two of these three the APTT remained below the therapeutic range for an additional 48 hours.

In the third study (57) patients with venous thromboembolism were randomly allocated to receive one of two continuous intravenous heparin regimens: either a dose of 5,000 IU as a bolus and 1,000 IU/hr by continuous infusion, or a weight-adjusted regimen consisting of an 80 IU/kg bolus followed by an infusion at 18 IU/kg/hr (equivalent to a 5,600 bolus and 12,600 IU/hr in a 70-kg person). Monitoring was performed by nomogram. Patients randomized to the weight-adjusted nomogram achieved an APTT in the therapeutic range more rapidly and with greater fequency than did those in the fixed-dose group. There was a significant relationship between achieving an APTT in the therapeutic range and subsequent recurrent venous thromboembolism.

Analysis of contemporary studies indicates that heparin administered by continuous infusion is very effective when initiated as a bolus dose of 5,000 IU followed by a continuous infusion of about 32,000 IU/24 hours with daily APTT monitoring.

Data on the relationship between excessive prolongation of APTT levels and bleeding complications are less conclusive. Some studies have suggested a relationship, whereas others have not (32). There is evidence, however, that bleeding is related to heparin dose (58,59), which is in turn related to the APTT, so it is likely that a relationship exists. However, there is even stronger evidence that patient-related factors, such as recent surgery, generalized hemostatic abnormalities, and local lesions (such as peptic ulcers or neoplasm) are important determinants of the risk of hemorrhagic complications.

Heparin Dose-Adjustment Nomograms

A number of methods for standardizing the management of intravenous heparin therapy have been developed to optimize dosage adjustment, including nomograms (47,57,60–62) and computer algorithms (63,64). Although initially developed for use in the treatment of venous thromboembolism, nomograms also have been used to manage heparin in conjunction with thrombolytic therapy for myocardial infarction (62,65). Recently, the weight-adjusted nomogram has been incorporated into the AHCPR (Agency for Health Care Policy and Research) guideline for treatment of unstable angina (66).

Because there are differences in heparin sensitivity of various partial thromboplastin reagents, it is important to determine the appropriate therapeutic range for the local laboratory reagent and adapt the recommended dosage adjustments of the nomogram to correspond to a therapeutic range equivalent to a heparin level of 0.2 to 0.4 IU/ml by protamine titration or 0.3 to 0.7 U/ml by anti–factor Xa heparin levels.

If the subcutaneous route is selected to treat patients with venous thromboembolism, a high initial dose should be used (35,000 IU/24 hours in two divided doses) to overcome the reduced bioavailability of subcutaneous injection (33). If a very rapid effect is required, the subcutaneous injection should be preceded by an intravenous bolus of 5,000 IU. Monitoring is performed 6 hours after injection with the aim of maintaining the APTT in the therapeutic range at this time (55).

Prevention of Venous Thromboembolism

A less intense anticoagulant effect is required to prevent venous thrombosis with heparin than to treat established thrombosis. Low-dose heparin, 5,000 IU subcutaneously twice or three times daily, is highly effective in preventing venous thrombosis in moderate-risk patients and is administered without laboratory monitoring. However, in very high risk patients such as those having hip surgery, the incidence of thrombosis is approximately 25% and of proximal vein thrombosis 10% to 12%, despite low-dose heparin prophylaxis (67–70). The results of three studies have demonstrated that the efficacy of low-dose heparin is improved without compromising safety by adjusting the dose to achieve a minimal heparin effect (71–73). The adjusted dose regimen has limitations for routine use because it requires careful monitoring and the use of a responsive APTT system.

Acute Coronary Syndromes

Unstable Angina

Aspirin reduces the risk of acute myocardial infarction and cardiac death in patients with unstable angina (74–77). Four recent randomized trials (76–79) have demonstrated that heparin is effective in reducing myocardial infarction during the period of heparin administration. There was also a general trend toward reduction in death. One trial (78) directly compared heparin (5,000-U bolus followed by 1,000 IU/hr and then titrated to 1.5 to 2.5 times control) versus aspirin 325 mg/day in a double-blind randomized trial of 484 patients with unstable angina. During the 5-day study drug period, myocardial infarction was significantly less common in the heparin group (0.8% versus 3.7%, $p = 0.035$).

However, because aspirin is universally recommended, the most important question concerning heparin is whether it provides incremental benefit. Six studies including a total of 1,353 patients (76,77,79–82) summarized in a meta-analysis (83) have randomized patients to aspirin versus aspirin plus heparin. The odds of death or myocardial infarction during the drug administration period for heparin plus aspirin was 0.67:1, with a 10.4% incidence with aspirin alone versus 7.9% with aspirin plus heparin ($p = 0.06$). These findings support the recommendation in the AHCPR guideline for treatment of unstable angina (84) that intravenous heparin and aspirin be standard treatment during the acute phase of unstable angina.

Although heparin is beneficial during the acute phase, whether heparin results in a sustained benefit is less clear. In studies that have evaluated longer term follow-up (77,79–82, 85), although there is a trend toward less death and myocardial infarction with heparin, the confidence intervals are wide and the results are inconclusive. Overall, ranging from in-hospital to 3 months follow-up, 68 of 684 patients (9.4%) treated with heparin and aspirin versus 73 of 635 patients (11.5%) treated with aspirin alone died or had myocardial infarction (odds ratio 0.80, $p = 0.20$). If there is a loss of early benefit, it could be explained in part by reactivation of thrombosis upon discontinuing intravenous heparin (83,85,86). The clinical reactivation of thrombosis is accompanied by hematologic evidence of a transient increase in both prothrombin fragment 1.2 as a measure of thrombin generation and fibrinopeptide A as a measure of thrombin activity (87).

The randomized trials demonstrating an early benefit with heparin added to aspirin used an APTT range of 1.5 to two times normal and treated for between 2 and 7 days (76,77,79–82). An observational analysis of the relationship between APTT and outcome from the TIMI IIIB trial found no fewer ischemic events with APTTs above the 1.5 to two times normal range (88).

Acute Myocardial Infarction

Without Thrombolytic Therapy. Heparin has been reported to reduce reinfarction and death in two open randomized trials that compared heparin with an untreated control group (89,90). Neither of these studies evaluated the added benefit or risks of adding heparin to aspirin; therefore, their results may not be relevant to the current practice.

The effect of heparin on the incidence of mural thrombosis has been evaluated in two randomized trials (49,90) that compared heparin in a fixed dose of 12,500 IU subcutaneously 12 hours with either an untreated control (90) or low-dose heparin (5,000 IU subcutaneously over 12 hours) (49). In these studies, moderate-dose heparin (12,500 IU subcutaneously over 12 hours) reduced the incidence of mural thrombosis detected by 2-D-echocardiography by 72% and 58%, respectively ($p < 0.05$ for each study).

High-dose intravenous heparin as a bolus, without thrombolytic therapy, has been studied as a method to improve early coronary artery patency in patients who are candidates for acute reperfusion therapy (within 6 hours of symptom onset and with ST-segment elevation). A pilot study of 50 patients treated with 300 IU/kg intravenous heparin bolus found a TIMI 2 or 3 patency rate of 56% at angiography 90 minutes later (91). This has led to a larger randomized trial, which is underway.

Adjuctive Treatment to Thrombolytic Therapy

Patency Studies

The effectiveness of heparin in preventing early coronary artery reocclusion after successful thrombolysis has been evaluated in a number of studies. In one study, a single intravenous bolus of 10,000 IU did not influence coronary artery patency at 90 minutes (92). In the four other studies using tissue plasminogen activator (t-PA), heparin was administered as a bolus of 5,000 IU intravenously followed by 1,000 IU/hr as a continuous infusion either during or at the end of the t-PA infusion. The dose of heparin was adjusted to maintain the APTT at 1.5 to 2.0 times control. In the Heparin-Aspirin Reperfusion Trial of 205 patients, the comparative group received 80 mg of acetylsalicylic acid (ASA)/day (93). Coronary artery patency at 18 hours was 82% in the heparin group and 52% in the aspirin group (p < 0.0002). In the trial reported by Bleich and associates of 83 patients, the comparative group received no treatment (94). Patency at 2 days was 71% in the heparin group and 44% in the control group (p < 0.023). In the European Coorperative Study Group-6 (ECSG-6) Trial, all 687 patients received aspirin and were randomized to heparin or no heparin. Patency at a mean of 81 hours was 80% in the heparin group and 75% in the comparative group (p < 0.01) (52). In the Australian National Heart Study Trial, all 202 patients received heparin for 24 hours (95). They were then randomized to either continuous intravenous heparin or to a combination of aspirin (300 mg) and dipyridamole (300 mg) daily. Patency at 1 week was 80% in both groups. The results of these studies suggest that heparin in a dose of 5,000 IU by intravenous bolus and 1,000 IU/hr by continuous infusion increases patency during the first few days after coronary thrombolysis with t-PA, probably by preventing rethrombosis. Moreover, higher levels of anticoagulation as measured by APTT were associated with higher levels of patency (96), with 90% TIMI 2 or 3 flow with APTTs of at least two times control, compared with 72% for lower APTTs (97).

Two other studies have evaluated the effect of adding heparin to aspirin given in adequate doses. The OSIRIS investigators treated 128 patients with streptokinase (SK) and aspirin and randomized the patients to either an intravenous bolus of heparin or no heparin, and reported no difference in coronary patency at 24 hours (86% versus 87%) (98). The Duke University Clinical Cardiology Studies (DUCCS-1) investigators treated 250 patients with anisoylated plasminogen–streptokinase activator complex (APSAC) and aspirin and randomized the patients into heparin or no heparin and found no significant difference in coronary artery patency (80% in the heparin group versus 74% in the control group) (99).

Thus, there is evidence that coronary patency with t-PA is improved by using full-dose intravenous heparin in therapeutic doses, but that heparin may not be important for sustained patency in patients who are treated with SK.

Studies Using Clinical Endpoints

The effectiveness of heparin in preventing reinfarction or death after thrombolytic therapy for acute myocardial infarction has been evaluated in a number of open randomized studies. In the ISIS-2 study (100), approximately half of the patients received intravenous heparin over 48 hours in a 2 × 2 factorial design that included SK and aspirin; heparin in this nonrandomized treatment comparison was associated with a small and nonsignificant decrease in recurrent infarction. In the Studio Sulla Calciparina Nell'Angina e Nella Trombosi Ventricolare

Nell'Infarto (SCATI) Study (90), in which the control group received no anticoagulant or aspirin treatment, mortality was reduced significantly in patients randomized to receive heparin (2,000-IU intravenous bolus followed by 12,500 IU subcutaneously 12 hours) after thrombolytic therapy for acute myocardial infarction.

In the Gruppo Italiano per lo Studio della Sopravvivenza nell'Infarto Miocardico (GISSI-2)/International Study (101,102), among the patients who received SK and heparin (90% of whom also received aspirin), the mortality rate was 7.9% (408 of 5,191), whereas it was 9.2% (479 of 5,205) in the group that received SK alone (p < 0.02). The mortality rate in the GISSI-2/International Study among the patients who received t-PA and heparin was 9.2% (476 of 5,170), whereas it was 8.7% (453 of 5,202) in those who received t-PA not followed by heparin (p = 0.393). After excluding the patients who died before heparin was started, the mortality rates were 5.9% (294 of 4,988) among those who received heparin and 5.9% (298 of 5,047) among those who did not (p = 0.984).

In the ISIS-3 study (103) the addition of heparin (12,500 IU subcutaneously over 12 hours starting 4 hours after commencing thrombolytic therapy) to aspirin and thrombolytic therapy produced a small excess of major noncerebral bleeds (1.0% compared with 0.8%, p < 0.01) and cerebral bleeds (0.56% to 0.40%, p < 0.05), as well as a nonsignificant reduction in reinfarction and death at 35 days. During the scheduled heparin treatment period, there was a modest reduction in both reinfarction in ISIS-3 (2.39% versus 2.81%, p < 0.01) as well as in mortality in GISSI-2 and ISIS-3 combined (6.8% versus 7.3%, p < 0.01).

Patients with evolving myocardial infarction in the Global Utilization of Streptokinase and Tissue Plasminogen Activator for Occluded Coronary Arteries (GUSTO) Study, which included a subgroup of about 20,000 patients, were randomized to receive SK and subcutaneous heparin or SK and intravenous heparin (65). The mortality rates were 7.2% and 7.4% in the subcutaneous and intravenous groups, respectively, whereas the rates of hemorrhagic stroke were 0.49% and 0.54%, respectively. The incidence of severe or life-threatening bleeding was 0.3% and 0.5%, respectively, and the incidence of moderate or severe bleeding was significantly lower in the subcutaneous versus the intravenous heparin group (11.8% versus 14.0%, p < 0.0001) (104). Thus, there was no advantage of using intravenous heparin in patients treated with SK.

In summary, the results of the GISSI-2 and the ISIS-3 studies show that the addition of heparin therapy to thrombolytic treatment increases the risk of bleeding (101,102): the reported incidence of minor bleeds was 594 of 6,195 (9.6%) among patients who received heparin and 328 of 6,206 (5.3%) among those who did not (relative risk 1.88, p < 0.001,) and that of major bleeds was 103 of 10,361 (1%) in the heparin group and 57 of 10,407 (0.5%) in the nonheparin group (relative risk 1.79, p < 0.01). In the ISIS-3 study (103), heparin produced a small but significant excess of major bleeding episodes and cerebral hemorrhages. As discussed above, the GUSTO study (65) showed no statistically significant difference in hemorrhagic strokes or severe extracranial bleeding between the intravenous and subcutaneous arms of the SK groups, although there was a significantly higher rate of moderate or severe bleeding in the intravenous heparin group.

One meta-analysis (105), which examined 26 randomized studies of heparin for acute myocardial infarction according to dose of heparin, use of aspirin, and use of oral anticoagulation, concluded that in the presence of aspirin and with thrombolysis, heparin has little additional effect on reducing mortality (five deaths fewer per thousand patients treated, p = 0.03) at the cost of three additional major bleeding episodes per thousand patients (p = 0.0001). However, there have been only three small randomized studies comparing intravenous heparin to no heparin with t-PA (106) with inadequate power to make a direct comparison based on clinical endpoints. Nevertheless, because the only trial to demonstrate that t-PA results in lower mortality than SK studied t-PA in an accelerated dose and with intravenous heparin, it seems prudent to include intravenous heparin as standard therapy with accelerated t-PA.

The APTT is used to monitor heparin treatment in patients with unstable angina or acute myocardial infarction. The guidelines for dosage adjustment are similar to those recommended for the treatment of venous thromboembolism, but the validity of a therapeutic range in patients with venous thromboembolism has never been evaluated in patients with unstable angina or acute myocardial infarction. In addition, recent studies in patients with acute myocardial infarction have highlighted the potential danger of heparin when used in conjunction with thrombolytic therapy. The first indication that the therapeutic window for heparin is narrower in patients with acute myocardial infarction who are treated with thrombolytic agents comes from a subgroup analysis of the GUSTO I study (65). The results of this study demonstrated that the risk of major bleeding, including intracranial bleeding, increased progressively as the APTT became prolonged above 75 seconds (86). Moreover, there was no lessening of risk of death or of reinfarction with higher APTTs. Consequently, it was suggested that care should be exercised to avoid exceeding the 75-second range when heparin is used in conjunction with thrombolytic therapy. This is consistent with the American College of Cardiology/American Heart Association practice guidelines for management of acute myocardial infarction, which recommend that intravenous heparin be used with t-PA, beginning with a weight-adjusted dose and using a nomogram to subsequently adjust the dose with a target APTT range of 50 to 75 seconds (107).

The results of the subgroup analysis of the GUSTO I study showing higher APTTs associated with worse outcomes are supported by the more recent findings in the GUSTO IIa and TIMI 9a studies (108,109). In both of these studies, there was an unacceptably high risk of major bleeding and intracranial bleed-

ing in patients receiving heparin. The dose of heparin used in these two studies was about 20% higher than in the GUSTO I study. In addition, the upper limit of the APTT range was less stringent in the GUSTO IIa and TIMI 9a studies than in the GUSTO I study. The dose of heparin was then reduced in the GUSTO IIb and TIMI 9b studies, and this modification was associated with a much lower incidence of intracranial bleeding (110).

Taken together, the results of these studies indicate that the risk-benefit ratio is narrow when heparin is used in conjunction with thrombolytic therapy. There is also evidence that the risk of bleeding is increased when full-dose heparin is used in combination with powerful antiplatelet agents such as platelet glycoprotein (GP)IIb-IIIa inhibitors (111).

Percutaneous Coronary Interventions

Coronary Angioplasty

Because coronary angioplasty involves severe plaque disruption with exposure of underlying thrombogenic surfaces, thrombin activation (112), and transient reduction in coronary blood flow, there is a sound rationale for antithrombotic therapy to reduce acute complications. Antiplatelet therapy has been found to be important in reducing early thrombotic complications. Pretreatment with aspirin decreases peri-procedural myocardial infarction by approximately 75% (113). Recently, three trials of over 1,000 patients each have demonstrated that the GPIIb/IIIa receptor antagonist abciximab reduces thrombotic complications of coronary angioplasty, including myocardial infarction, death, or urgent revascularization, by 34% to 68% (111,114,115).

In addition to antiplatelet therapy, since the beginning of coronary angioplasty, intravenous heparin in high doses has been used to prevent thrombosis related to both the coronary lesions being dilated as well as for the temporary placement of catheter equipment in the arterial system. The doses and plasma levels of heparin used during angioplasty, like those used for cardiopulmonary bypass, are above the level where the APTT-heparin response provides discriminative value; therefore, the ACT has become the standard measure. The two most common devices used to measure ACT—the Hemochron and the HemoTec—vary considerably, with the ACT from the Hemochron being approximately 50 seconds higher than the HemoTec with measurements in the 300-second range (116).

There are no randomized data addressing the optimal dose or degree of anticoagulation for routine coronary angioplasty. However, a series of retrospective studies have related the degree of anticoagulation during the coronary angioplasty procedure with subsequent thrombotic complications (117–119), all of which found a greater likelihood of complications with lower levels of anticoagulation. In one study (118), all patients received a 10,000-U bolus of intravenous heparin before the procedure followed by additional heparin according to the discretion of the responsible physician. Of a total of 1,469 patients undergoing angioplasty, 103 patients who died or had emergency bypass surgery were compared with 400 uncomplicated patients who had complete ACT data (measured by the HemoTec device) available. The ACT, both after the initial bolus and at the end of the procedure, was consistently an average of 60 to 80 seconds lower among patients with complications. Of patients with a final ACT of over 300 seconds, only 0.3% had complications. A second study (119) used a case-control design to evaluate the relationship of ACT (Hemochron) in 63 patients with abrupt closure, defined as angiographically documented vessel occlusion before hospital discharge, compared with 124 patients matched for other predictors of abrupt closure. The median ACT was 30 to 40 seconds lower among patients with abrupt closure, and there was a continuous relationship of lower ACT and higher risk of abrupt closure. In a multivariable logistic regression model, the risk of abrupt closure was approximately 10% with an initial ACT of 300 versus 5% with an ACT of 400 seconds. There was no significant relationship between initial ACT and bleeding risk. These

two studies have led to the recommendation that heparin be administered before angioplasty as an intravenous bolus of at least 10,000 IU, and that additional boluses be given to achieve and maintain an ACT of at least 300 (HemoTec) to 350 (Hemochron) seconds (120). Alternatively, the initial bolus may be given as a weight-adjusted 100-IU/kg dose, as has been adopted as the standard approach in some clinical trials (111,114).

It is now recommended that heparin need not be routinely administered after the angioplasty procedure, based on two small studies that randomized patients to 24 hours of continued intravenous heparin versus no additional heparin, with no difference in thrombotic complications (120–122). Moreover, early discontinuation of heparin with early femoral arterial sheath removal has been shown in a randomized study to result in a significant reduction in bleeding (123).

Although there was a substantial reduction of thrombotic events with abciximab in the Evaluation of 7E3 for the Prevention of Ischemic Complications (EPIC) trial, it was accompanied by a doubling of major bleeding complications. The trial used high-dose intravenous heparin for all patients, administered as a bolus of 10,000 to 20,000 IU, with additional heparin to maintain an ACT of 300 to 350 seconds, and continued for 12 hours to keep the APTT 1.5 to 2.5 times control. After adjusting for patient weight, the ACT was found to be prolonged by 35 seconds on average by abciximab (124). In attempts to retain the benefit seen in the EPIC trial while lowering bleeding risk, the EPILOG trial (114) tested abciximab with lower doses of heparin, using a bolus of 70 IU/kg and additional boluses to achieve and maintain an ACT of at least 200 seconds. Heparin was discontinued immediately after the procedure. The combination of abciximab and low-dose heparin was associated with at least as great a reduction in thrombotic events as was seen in the EPIC trial, with a much lower rate of major bleeding of 2.0%, and compared with 3.1% for standard-dose heparin alone. This lower dose heparin is recommended when abciximab is used during coronary angioplasty.

Coronary Stents

Because of concern about acute thrombosis during the early experience with coronary stent placement related to the exposed stent surface, intense antiplatelet and anticoagulant therapy had been the standard approach in the United States (125). The typical regimen included aspirin, dipyridamole, dextran, and high-dose heparin during and after the procedure until warfarin had become therapeutic. In 1995, however, an Italian group (126) reported a low incidence of thrombosis in a series of 359 patients with the use of ticlopidine without any procedural or postprocedural heparin anticoagulation. All patients included in the study underwent intravascular ultrasound to assure successful stent placement, which included high-pressure balloon inflation. Although the standard approach in the United States continues to be high-dose heparin during the stent deployment procedure, the use of routine postprocedural heparin and coumadin has been abandoned (125) after a randomized trial of 257 patients in which patients treated with postprocedural ticlopidine and aspirin without heparin had a 1.6% incidence of death, myocardial infarction, or repeat revascularization, compared with 6.2% for patients treated with postprocedural heparin and coumadin (127).

Cardiopulmonary Bypass

Heparin is used to prevent thrombosis in extracorporeal devices such as membrane oxygenators used in cardiac bypass surgery and to prevent coronary artery thrombosis and rethrombosis after coronary angioplasty and in patients with unstable angina or acute myocardial infarction. The very high doses of heparin required to prevent thrombosis in cardiac bypass circuits are monitored by the ACT, with the aim of maintaining the test result above 500 seconds.

Side Effects of Heparin

The most common side effect of heparin is hemorrhage. Other complications are thrombocytopenia with or without thrombosis (128,129), osteoporosis (130,131), skin necrosis (132), alopecia (133), hypersensitivity reactions (134), and hypoaldosteronism (135). Four variables have been reported to influence bleeding during heparin treatment: the dose of heparin, the patient's anticoagulant response, the method of heparin administration, and patient factors. There is indirect evidence that the frequency of bleeding is increased by heparin dose and anticoagulant effect (58,136). Studies comparing continuous intravenous heparin with subcutaneous heparin reported an average incidence of bleeding of 4.4% and 4.3%, respectively (odds ratio 1.0) (136). Other factors that predispose to anticoagulant-induced bleeding are serious concurrent illnesses (136,137) and chronic heavy alcohol consumption (138).

The concomitant use of aspirin has long been identified as a risk factor for heparin-induced bleeding (136,138,139). Aspirin increases operative and postoperative bleeding in patients who receive the very high doses of heparin required during open heart surgery (140). However, the risk of adding aspirin to a short course of regular therapeutic doses of heparin is likely to be much less and is acceptable in patients with ischemic heart disease. Renal failure and patient age and gender also have been implicated as risk factors for heparin-induced bleeding (136,141). The reported association with female gender has not been consistent among studies and remains in question.

Thrombocytopenia, a well-recognized complication of heparin therapy, has been reviewed recently (128,129). The reported incidence of heparin-associated thrombocytopenia varies widely. Thrombocytopenia is more common with heparin derived from bovine lung than from porcine gut (128). On pooled analysis of all prospective studies with porcine heparin, the mean incidence of thrombocytopenia is 2.4% for therapeutic heparin and 0.3% for prophylactic heparin. The incidence of arterial or venous thrombosis with heparin-associated thrombocytopenia is approximately 0.4% (129). Arterial thrombosis occurs as a consequence of platelet aggregation in vivo, but venous thrombosis could result from heparin resistance caused by the neutralizing effect of heparin-induced release of platelet factor 4. Thrombocytopenia usually begins between 3 and 15 days after starting heparin therapy (median 10 days) (129), but it has been reported within hours of commencing heparin in patients who have been previously exposed to heparin (129). The platelet count usually returns to baseline levels within 4 days of stopping heparin (129). Heparin-associated thrombocytopenia is thought to be caused by an immunoglobulin G (IgG)–heparin immune complex involving both the Fab and Fc portion of the IgG molecule (129). Although low molecular weight heparins can exhibit immunologic cross-reactivity with heparin (142), the heparinoid danaparoid sodium exhibits minimal cross-reactivity (143) and has been used successfully to manage a small number of patients with heparin-associated thrombocytopenia (143).

Pregnancy

Heparin is the anticoagulant of choice in pregnancy because it does not cross the placenta and its administration to the mother during pregnancy is not associated with untoward effects in the fetus or neonate. The drug should be given in therapeutic doses (approximately 15,000 IU subcutaneously over 12 hours) when used to treat pregnant patients with prosthetic heart valves or with venous thromboembolism. The use of heparin in doses of greater than 20,000 IU for more than 5 months is problematic because it can cause osteoporosis (130,131).

Limitations of Heparin

Heparin has biophysical and biologic limitations (32).

Pharmacokinetic Limitations

The pharmacokinetic limitations of heparin are caused by its nonspecific binding to pro-teins and cells (32). Because heparin is highly negatively charged, it binds in a pentasaccharide-independent fashion to a variety of plasma proteins (including histidine-rich glycoprotein, vitronectin, lipoproteins, fibronectin, and fibrinogen), as well as to proteins secreted by platelets (platelet factor 4) or endothelial cells (VWF) (32,38). Some of the heparin-binding plasma proteins are acute-phase reactants, the levels of which are elevated in sick patients (36). In addition, there is increased release of platelet factor 4 and VWF from platelets and endothelial cells during the clotting process. Although the affinity of heparin for many of heparin-binding proteins is much lower than its affinity for AT, the plasma concentration of many of these proteins is sufficiently high that they compete with AT for heparin binding.

The plasma levels of heparin-binding proteins are highly variable in patients with thromboembolic diseases (36). This variability likely reflects between-patient differences in the levels of inflammatory cytokines that stimulate the acute-phase response and thrombin that mediates release of VWF and platelet factor 4 from endothelial cells and platelets, respectively. The between-patient variability in the levels of heparin-binding proteins explains why the anticoagulant response to heparin is so unpredictable (36) and why some patients require extremely high doses of heparin to achieve a therapeutic anticoagulant response (52), so-called heparin resistance.

Biophysical Limitations

The biophysical limitations of heparin reflect the inability of the heparin–AT complex to inactivate thrombin bound to fibrin (144) and factor Xa bound to phospholipid surfaces within the prothrombinase complex (145). Thus, thrombin bound to fibrin retains its catalytic activity against macromolecular substrates, such as fibrinogen, factors V and VIII, and platelets and is protected from inactivation by AT even in the presence of heparin (144). The inability of AT to inactivate fibrin-bound thrombin may result from conformational changes in the active site of thrombin that occur when the enzyme binds to fibrin. The marked resistance of fibrin-bound thrombin to the heparin–AT complex occurs because the heparin binding site on thrombin (so-called exosite 2) is masked when thrombin binds to fibrin. The explanation for the protection of factor Xa from inactivation by heparin–AT is less well understood, but may reflect similar mechanisms. The inability of heparin to inactivate surface-bound thrombin and factor Xa may explain why heparin is of only limited efficacy in cardiopulmonary bypass surgery, unstable angina, high-risk coronary angioplasty, and coronary thrombolysis.

Biologic Limitations

The biologic limitations of heparin reflect its propensity to bind to platelets and to activate them (146). Platelet activation can contribute to bleeding because degranulated platelets have impaired hemostatic function. In addition, platelet factor 4 released from activated platelets can complex with heparin, thereby triggering the formation of the antibodies that cause heparin-induced thrombocytopenia (HIT) (147).

Low molecular weight heparins overcome the pharmacokinetic and biologic limitations of unfractionated heparin and share the same biophysical limitations. The biophysical limitations of both low molecular weight heparins and unfractionated heparins have provided an important rationale for the development of new antithrombotics.

LOW MOLECULAR WEIGHT HEPARINS

Low molecular weight heparins are a new class of anticoagulants which are replacing unfractionated heparin for many indications in Europe and are being used for more limited indications in North America.

Low molecular weight heparins are derived from unfractionated heparin by either chemical or enzymatic depolymerization to yield fragments that are approximately one third the size of heparin. Like heparin, they are heterogeneous with respect to molecular size and anticoagulant activity. Low molecular weight heparins have a mean molecular weight of 4,000 to 5,000 daltons with a molecular weight distribution of 1,000 to 10,000 daltons. Depolymerization of heparin into lower molecular weight fragments results in three main changes in the properties of heparin. Thus, the resultant low molecular weight heparins have (a) a change in their anticoagulant profile with a progressive loss of their ability to catalyze thrombin inhibition (11,21,29, 148); (b) reduced protein binding with an improvement in their pharmacokinetic properties (29,38,149–153); and (c) reduced interaction with platelets (146), which could be responsible for the reduced microvascular bleeding in experimental animal models and lower incidence of HIT (154). Two other glycosaminoglycans also have been developed for clinical use. These are dermatan sulfate and the heparinoid danaparoid sodium, which is a mixture of heparin sulfate (the major component making up 80% of the mixture) and smaller amounts of dermatan sulfate and chondroitin sulfates.

It should be noted that commercially available low molecular weight heparins are prepared using different methods of depolymerization; therefore, they are not necessarily clinically interchangeable.

Anticoagulant Effects of Low Molecular Weight Heparins

Like unfractionated heparin, low molecular weight heparins produce their major anticoagulant effect by binding to AT via a unique pentasaccharide sequence (6,7), which is present on less than one third of low molecular weight heparin molecules. Because a minimum chain length of 18 saccharides (including the pentasaccharide sequence) is required for ternary complex formation, only the 25% to 50% of low molecular weight heparin species that are above this critical chain length in the different commercial low molecular weight heparin preparations are able to inactivate thrombin. In contrast, all of the low molecular weight heparin fragments that contain the high-affinity pentasaccharide catalyzes the inactivation of factor Xa. Virtually all unfractionated heparin molecules contain at least 18 saccharide units (155,156). Therefore, in contrast to unfractionated heparin, which has a ratio of anti–factor Xa to anti–factor IIa activity of approximately 1:1, the various commercial low molecular weight heparins have anti–factor Xa to anti–factor IIa ratios that vary between 4:1 and 2:1, depending on their molecular size distribution.

Pharmacokinetics of Low Molecular Weight Heparins

The plasma recoveries and pharmacokinetics of heparin and low molecular weight heparins differ because of differences in their relative binding properties to plasma proteins and cells. Most heparin-binding proteins do not bind to or neutralize low molecular weight heparins (29,38,149–151,153). The absence of protein binding of low molecular weight heparins contributes to their excellent bioavailability at low doses (157) and to their more predictable anticoagulant response when administered in fixed doses (158). Low molecular weight heparin preparations also have a lower affinity than heparin for VWF (38), a property that could contribute to the observation that low molecular weight heparins produce less experimental bleeding than heparin for equivalent anticoagulant effects (159–165). Unlike heparin, low molecular weight heparins do not bind to endothelial cells in culture (39,166,167), a property that could be responsible for their longer plasma half-life (which is approximately two- to fourfold longer than that of heparin) (168–174). Low molecular weight heparins are cleared principally by the renal route, and their biologic half-life is increased in patients with renal failure (168,175,176).

Antithrombotic and Hemorrhagic Effects of Low Molecular Weight Heparins, Heparinoids, and Unfractionated Heparin in Experimental Models in Animals

The antithrombotic effects and hemorrhagic effects of heparin have been compared with low molecular weight heparins with the heparinoid danaparoid sodium and with dermatan sulfate in a variety of experimental animal models (159–165,177–181). In these models of thrombosis, temporary venous stasis is produced by ligating an appropriate vein, and blood coagulation is stimulated by injecting either serum, factor Xa, thrombin, or tissue factor (165,180,181). When compared on a gravimetric basis, low molecular weight heparins are slightly less effective than heparin as antithrombotic agents but produce much less bleeding than heparin in models measuring blood loss from a standardized injury (160–163,165,178,179).

These differences in the relative antithrombotic to hemorrhagic effects of these polysaccharides could be due in part to their different effects on platelet function (38,182,183) and vascular permeability (184).

Arterial Thrombosis

Low molecular weight heparins have been evaluated in a canine model of coronary artery thrombosis (185). Low molecular weight heparin in a dose of 2.5 mg/kg subcutaneously was as effective as unfractionated heparin in a dose of 10 mg/kg subcutaneously (185). A second study compared the relative efficacy and safety of a very low molecular weight heparin (CY222) with unfractionated heparin in an exteriorized femoral arteriovenous shunt in baboons (186). Skin bleeding times also were measured. In this platelet-dependent model, low molecular weight heparin demonstrated a more favorable antithrombotic to bleeding ratio than did unfractionated heparin.

Clinical Experience with Low Molecular Weight Heparin Preparations

Low molecular weight heparins have been evaluated in a large number of randomized clinical trials and have been shown to be safe and effective anticoagulants for the prevention and treatment of venous thrombosis. More recently, low molecular weight heparin preparations have been evaluated in patients with unstable angina (187,188) and with stroke (189), postfemoropopliteal arterial surgery (190), and for the prevention of restenosis after angioplasty (191).

The largest experience with low molecular weight heparin has been obtained in the prevention of venous thrombosis in high-risk patients. Experience with low molecular weight heparins for the treatment of venous thrombosis is growing, whereas studies evaluating low molecular weight heparins in arterial thrombosis are in their early stages.

Although the low molecular weight heparins in clinical use have many similarities, they also differ from one another in molecular weight distribution profiles, in their relative specific activities (anti-Xa to anti-IIa activities), in their rates of plasma clearance, and in their recommended dosage regimens and in experimental microvascular bleeding (Table 11-1). Therefore, it cannot be assumed that results obtained for a specific indication using one low molecular weight heparin would also be obtained with another low molecular weight heparin.

Prevention of Venous Thrombosis

The results of studies evaluating low molecular weight heparins for the prevention of venous thrombosis have been reviewed elsewhere (192).

For general surgical patients, low molecular weight heparins administered once daily by subcutaneous injection have been shown to reduce cardiovascular mortality when compared with placebo and to be approximately 30% more effective than unfractionated heparin 5,000 IU (administered by subcutaneous injection twice or three times daily) in preventing venous thrombosis without any difference in bleeding (192).

When compared with a control group, low molecular weight heparins have been shown to reduce the incidence of thrombosis in patients having major knee or hip surgery by about 70% without increasing the risk of bleeding (193–195). When compared directly with other forms of prophylaxis in orthopedic

patients, low molecular weight heparins are significantly more effective than heparin 5,000 IU subcutaneously administered twice or three times daily (196–198), significantly more effective than oral anticoagulants (199–201), significantly more effective than dextran (202,203), significantly more effective than aspirin (204), and significantly more effective than adjusted-dose heparin in preventing proximal vein thrombosis (205).

Low molecular weight heparins are very effective in preventing venous thrombosis in patients with thrombotic stroke (206,207) and in other high-risk medical patients (208), producing a relative risk reduction in venous thrombosis of between 60% and 90%. This beneficial effect occurred without an increase in clinically important bleeding. Low molecular weight heparins also have been shown to be significantly more effective than unfractionated heparin in preventing venous thrombosis in patients with paralytic stoke and in patients with spinal cord injury. Thus, in both studies comparing low molecular weight heparins with heparin, patients randomized to receive low molecular weight heparin showed a greater than 70% risk reduction in thrombosis, a statistically significant difference (209,210).

TREATMENT OF VENOUS THROMBOSIS

Treatment of Established Thrombosis

There is growing experience with the use of low molecular weight heparins for the treatment of venous thrombosis. Low molecular weight heparin has been compared with heparin in the treatment of venous thrombosis (Table 11-2). In the major studies, low molecular weight heparin was administered by subcutaneous injection (usually twice daily) and heparin was administered by continous intravenous infusion with APTT monitoring.

Eight trials (211–218) compared the effects of heparin and low molecular weight heparin by measuring the change in thrombus size after 5 to 10 days of treatment observed in a pretreatment and posttreatment venogram.

TABLE 11-1. *The anticoagulant profiles, molecular weights, plasma half-lives, and recommended doses of commercial low molecular weight heparins*

Agent	Anti-Xa to anti-IIa ratio	Molecular weight (range) [saccharide units]	Plasma half-life (min)	Recommended dose (converted into international anti-Xa units)		
				General surgery	Orthopedic surgery	Treatment
Enoxaparin sodium (Lovenox/Clexane) (Rhone-Poulenc Rorer)	2.7:1	4,500 (3,000–8,000) [10–27]	129–180	2,000 U s.c.	4,000 U s.c. daily or 3,000 U s.c. BID	7,000 U s.c. BID[a]
Dalteparin (Fragmin) (Kabi)	2.0:1	5,000 (2,000–9,000) [7–30]	119–139	2,500 U s.c.	2,500 U s.c. BID or 5,000 U s.c. daily	8,400 U s.c. BID[a]
Nadroparine calcium (Fraxiparin) (Sanofi)	3.2:1	4,500 (2,000–8,000) [7–27]	132–162	7,500 U/IC s.c. daily		31,500 U/IC daily[a]
	3.2:1	4,500 (2,000–8,000) [7–27]	132–162	7,500 U/IC s.c. daily		31,500 U/IC daily[a]
Innohep (Tinzaparin) (Leo Laboratories)	1.9:1	4,500 (3,000–6,000) [10–20]	111	3,500 U s.c. daily	50 U/kg s.c. daily	12,250 daily[a]
Ardeparin (Normoflo) (Wyeth-Ayerst)	2.0:1	6,000	200		50 U/kg s.c. BID	
Danaparoid sodium[b] (Orgaran) (NV Organon)	20:1	6,500 (2,000–15,000) [7–50]	1,100		750 U s.c. BID	1,250 U s.c. BID

[a]Weight-adjusted dose; stated dose for 70 kg patient.
[b]Danaparoid sodium (Orgaran) is a heparinoid.
U/IC, Institute Choay Units; 3 ICU, 1 International Unit.

TABLE 11-2. *Comparison of low molecular weight heparin with heparin (LMWH) in the treatment of venous thrombosis*

Study	LMWH	Route	Heparin	Repeat venography	Follow-up for recurrence
Bratt et al. (213)	Dalteparin (Fragmin)	i.v.	i.v.	Yes	No
Holm et al. (211)	Dalteparin (Fragmin)	s.c.	s.c.	Yes	No
Faivre et al. (212)	CY 222	s.c.	s.c.	Yes	No
Bratt et al. (214)	Dalteparin (Fragmin)	s.c.	i.v.	Yes	No[a]
Duroux and Beclere (215)	Nadroparine calcium (Fraxiparin)	s.c.	i.v.	Yes	No[a]
Prandoni et al. (217)	Nadroparine calcium (Fraxiparin)	s.c.	i.v.	Yes	Yes
Hull et al. (220)	Innohep (Tinzaparin)	s.c.	i.v.	No	Yes
Simonneau (216)	Enoxaparin sodium (Lovenox/Clexane)	s.c.	i.v.	Yes	Yes

[a]Not prospectively conducted at the study center.

The results of a pooled analysis of these studies show that there is a significant reduction of thrombus size in patients treated with low molecular weight heparin (p < 0.001) (Table 11-3). Thus, a reduction in thrombus size was observed in 64% of patients treated with a low molecular weight heparin and in 50% of patients treated with heparin, whereas an increase in thrombus size was observed in 6% of patients treated with low molecular weight heparin and 12% of patients treated with heparin (219).

A meta-analysis of randomized trials comparing low molecular weight heparin and heparin has been performed (219). The incidence of major bleeding was 3.2% (21 of 656) in the patients randomized to receive heparin and 0.9% (six of 652) in the patients randomized to receive a low molecular weight heparin for a risk reduction of 68% (p < 0.005). The incidence of recurrent venous throm-

boembolism in the pooled analysis of four studies was 7.0% (31 of 443) in the patients randomized to receive heparin and 2.7% (12 of 439) in those randomized to receive a low molecular weight heparin (p < 0.001).

The pooled mortality rate at long-term follow-up was 4.3% (19 of 439 patients) in the low molecular weight heparin group and 8.1% (36 of 443 patients) in the heparin group, a risk reduction of 48% in favor of low molecular weight heparin (p < 0.03) (Table 11-4).

Two relatively large studies used the clinically relevant endpoints of confirmed symptomatic recurrent thromboembolism as outcome measures. In the open randomized trial reported by Prandoni and associates (217), 170 patients with venographically confirmed proximal deep vein thrombosis were allocated to receive a low molecular weight heparin (nadroparin calcium, using a weight adjusted

TABLE 11-3. *Pooled analysis of studies comparing low molecular weight heparin and heparin for the treatment of venous thrombosis by comparison of posttreatment with pretreatment venography*

	Low molecular weight heparin[a]	Heparin[a]	p
Reduction	64%	50%	
Increase	6%	12%	<0.001

[a]Change in thrombus size.

Data from the following studies was pooled and analyzed: Holm et al., ref. 211; Faivre et al., ref. 212; Bratt et al., refs. 213 and 214; Duroux and Beclerc, ref. 215; Simonneau, ref. 216; Prandoni et al., ref. 217; and Albada et al., ref. 218.

TABLE 11-4. *Pooled analysis of studies comparing low molecular weight heparin and heparin for the treatment of venous thrombosis*

Event	Low molecular weight heparin	Heparin	Relative risk	p
Recurrent venous thromboembolism (four studies)	12/439 (2.7%)	31/443 (7. 0%)	61%	<0.005
Major bleeding (nine studies)	6/652 (0.9%)	21/656 (3.2%)	68%	<0.005
Mortality (four studies)	19/439 (4.3%)	36/443 (8.1%)	48%	<0.03

Data from Lensing et al., ref. 219.

regimen) or unfractionated heparin administered by continuous intravenous infusion adjusted to maintain the APTT at 1.5 to 2 times control (Table 11-5). At 10 days, four of 85 patients (4.7%) receiving heparin developed recurrence compared with one of 85 (1.2%) receiving low molecular weight heparin (p = 0.1). At 6 months, 11 of 85 (12.9%) developed recurrent thromboembolism compared with six of 85 low molecular weight heparin patients (7.1%) (p = 0.2). Bleeding occurred in 10.6% of the heparin patients compared with 3.5% of the low molecular weight heparin patients (p = 0.1). The mortality rate at 6 months was 12 of 85 patients (14.1%) in the heparin group and six of 85 (7.1%) in the low molecular weight heparin group, a nonsignificant difference. Most deaths were cancer related.

The second study reported by Hull and associates (220) was a double-blind trial performed in patients with proximal vein thrombosis (Table 11-6). A fixed dose of low molecular weight heparin (175 anti–factor Xa units/kg of body weight) of Tinzaparin (Leo, Denmark) given subcutaneously once daily was compared with adjusted-dose intravenous heparin given by continuous infusion. The patients in the intravenous heparin group received an initial intravenous bolus dose of 5,000 IU of heparin, followed by a continuous intravenous infusion of heparin. Objective tests were used to document clinical outcomes.

Six of 213 patients who received low molecular weight heparin (2.8%) and 15 of 219 patients who received intravenous heparin (6.9%) had new episodes of venous thromboembolism (p = 0.07). Major bleeding associated with initial therapy occurred in one patient receiving low molecular weight heparin (0.5%) and in 11 patients receiving intravenous heparin (5.0%), a reduction in risk of 91% (p = 0.006). Minor hemorrhagic compli-

TABLE 11-5. *Low molecular weight heparin treatment studies*

Endpoints	10 days	6 months
Recurrent venous thromboembolism		
Low molecular weight heparin	1/85	6/85
Heparin	4/85	12/85
Bleeding (major)		
Low molecular weight heparin	1/85	—
Heparin	3/85	—
Bleeding (minor)		
Low molecular weight heparin	3/85	—
Heparin	6/85	—
Mortality		
Low molecular weight heparin	—	6/85
Heparin	—	12/85

Data from the study of Prandoni et al., ref. 217, which was a comparison of subcutaneous low molecular weight heparin (nadroparine calcium [Fraxiparin]) and continuous heparin in the treatment of venous thrombosis.

TABLE 11-6. *Low molecular weight heparin treatment studies*

Endpoints	10 days	3 months
Recurrent venous thromboembolism		
Low molecular weight heparin	—	6/213
Heparin	—	15/213
Bleeding (major)		
Low molecular weight heparin	1/213	—
Heparin	10/213	—
Bleeding (minor)		
Low molecular weight heparin	6/213	—
Heparin	6/213	—
Mortality		
Low molecular weight heparin	—	9/213
Heparin	—	21/213

Data from the study of Hull et al., ref. 220, which was a comparison of subcutaneous low molecular weight heparin (Innohep [Tinzaparin]) and continuous intravenous heparin in the treatment of venous thrombosis.

cations occurred during or immediately after the initial therapy in five patients receiving low molecular weight heparin (2.4%) and in four patients receiving intravenous heparin (1.8%).

Ten patients assigned to receive low molecular weight heparin (4.7%) and 21 patients assigned to receive intravenous heparin (9.6%) died during the 3 months of follow-up (p = 0.062; reduction in risk, 51%).

The results of these studies suggest that in patients with proximal vein thrombosis, low molecular weight heparins administered in either a fixed or weight adjusted dose subcutaneously are more effective and produce less bleeding than conventional APTT-adjusted heparin administered by continuous infusion.

Since the publication of the pooled analysis, two large randomized trials have been completed (221,222) with a novel design which takes advantage of the more pre-dictable anticoagulant response of low molecular weight heparin. In both of these studies, low molecular weight heparin was administered subcutaneously on an outpatient basis and compared with the standard approach of heparin administered by continuous intravenous infusion in hospital. In the study reported by Levine and associates (221), eligible patients with proximal vein thrombosis were randomly assigned to intravenous heparin in hospital or a strategy of low molecular weight heparin (enoxaparin sodium) 1 mg/kg subcutaneously twice daily administered primarily at home. The design allowed outpatients to go home immediately on low molecular weight heparin and hospitalized patients to be discharged from hospital early on low molecular weight heparin. Thirteen (5.3%) of 247 low molecular weight heparin patients developed recurrent thromboembolism compared with 17 (6.7%) of 253 pa-

TABLE 11-7. *Incidence of recurrent thromboembolism*

	Treatment Group	
	LMWH enoxaparin sodium (Lovenox/Clexane) (n = 247)	Standard heparin (n = 253)
Total	13 (5.3%)	17 (6.7%)
DVT	11	15
PE	1	2[a]
DVT and PE	1	0

[a]Fatal pulmonary emboli.
LMWH, low molecular weight heparin.
Data from Levine et al., ref. 221.

TABLE 11-8. *Recurrent venous thromboembolism, major bleeding, and death in the study patients*

	Standard heparin (N = 198)	Low molecular weight heparin calcium nadroparine (Fraxiparin) (N = 202)
Recurrent venous thromboembolism	17 (8.6%)	14 (6.9%)
Major bleeding	4 (2.0%)	1 (0.5%)
Death	16 (8.1%)	14 (6.9%)

Adapted from Koopman et al., ref. 222.

tients in the heparin group (p = 0.57). Five low molecular weight heparin patients developed major bleeding compared with three heparin patients (Table 11-7). After randomization, the mean number of days in hospital for the low molecular weight heparin group was 1.1 days compared with 6.5 days for the heparin group. In the second study reported by Koopman and associates, patients with deep venous thrombosis were randomly assigned to intravenous heparin in hospital (5,000 IU as a bolus followed by 1,250 IU/hr with APTT monitoring) or low molecular weight heparin nadroparine calcium twice daily subcutaneously using a weight-adjusted dosage regimen. Patients weighing less than 50 kg received a daily dose of 8,200 anti-Xa units, those weighing between 50 and 70 kg received 12,300 anti-Xa units, and those weighing over 70 kg received 18,400 anti-Xa units (222). The design allowed outpatients to go home immediately on low molecular weight heparin and hospitalized patients to be discharged from hospital early on low molecular weight heparin. Fourteen (6.9%) of 202 low molecular weight heparin patients developed recurrent thromboembolism compared with 17 (8.6%) of 198 patients in the heparin group (p > 0.5). One low molecular

weight heparin patient developed major bleeding compared with four heparin patients (Table 11-8).

Thus, low molecular weight heparin administered on an out-of-hospital basis in eligible patients with deep venous thrombosis is as effective and safe as intravenous heparin administered in hospital. This approach has the potential to change our current approach to the treatment of venous thrombosis, thereby resulting in increased patient convenience and a marked reduction of health-care costs.

Low molecular weight heparin enoxaparin sodium also has been compared with warfarin in the longer term treatment of venous thrombosis. Pini and associates (223) treated 187 patients with deep vein thrombosis with heparin in-hospital for 10 days and then randomized the patients to receive low molecular weight heparin 4,000 anti-Xa units (40 mg) daily or warfarin to maintain the International Normalized Ratio (INR) at 2.0 to 3.5 for 3 months. The results are summarized in Table 11-9. There was no difference in the incidence of recurrent thrombosis between the two groups, but patients allocated to receive low molecular weight heparin had a significantly lower incidence of bleeding.

TABLE 11-9. *Low molecular weight heparin versus warfarin in the treatment of deep vein thrombosis*

	Enoxaparin sodium (Lovenox/Clexane) 40 mg s.c. daily (93)	Warfarin (94)
Recurrent DVT	6%	4%
Bleeding	4%	13%, p = 0.04

N = 187 patients. Treated with heparin in hospital for 10 days, then randomized to 3 months of enoxaparin or warfarin.
Data from Pini et al., ref. 223.

TABLE 11-10. *Low molecular weight heparin (nadroparine calcium [Fraxiparin]) in acute ischemic stroke*

Outcome	High dose (N =102)	Low dose (N = 101)	Placebo (N = 105)
Died	13	17	20
Dependent incomplete recovery	32	36	48
All poor outcomes	45 (45%)	53 (52%)	68 (65%)

Mortality and dependent incomplete recovery at 6 months; p = 0.005.
Data from Kay et al., ref. 189.

Low Molecular Weight Heparin in the Treatment of Acute Ischemic Stroke

Currently, there is no proven established treatment for patients with acute ischemic stroke. Early studies with heparin were either inconclusive or failed to show benefit. Recently, Kay and associates (189) performed a double-blind trial evaluating low molecular weight heparin dadroparine calcium in 312 patients with acute ischemic stroke (Table 11-10). Two dosage regimens (high dose and low dose) were compared with placebo. The high dose group received 4,100 anti–factor Xa units subcutaneously twice daily and the low dose group 4,100 anti–factor Xa units subcutaneously daily. The low molecular weight heparin regimens or placebo were administered within 48 hours of development of ischemic stroke and continued for 10 days. The primary outcome measure (death or permanent disability at 6 months) occurred in 45% of patients in the high-dose group, 52% in the low-dose group, and 65% in the placebo group. There was a significant dose-dependent effect among the three study groups in favor of low molecular weight heparin (p = 0.005). These results are promising but need to be reproduced in larger studies before the true role of low molecular weight heparin can be established in the treatment of acute ischemic stroke (189).

Low Molecular Weight Heparin in Unstable Angina

The combination of heparin and aspirin is the treatment of choice in patients with unstable angina. A small open trial comparing low molecular weight heparin and aspirin with heparin and aspirin or aspirin alone in unstable angina reported that low molecular weight heparin reduced the risk of acute myocardial infarction (82) (Table 11-11). This promising report was followed by two large studies of unstable angina. The first study (187) compared the low molecular weight heparin dalteparin (Fragmin, Pharmacia, Dublin, OH), 120 U/kg twice daily, with placebo followed by 7,500 anti-Xa units of dalteparin or placebo once daily for 35 to 45 days; all patients received aspirin. In the double-blind placebo-controlled trial (187), low molecular weight heparin was shown to reduce the risk of death or myocardial infarction by more than 60% at 6 days (Table 11-12). Thus, of the 741 patients allocated to receive low molecular weight heparin, 13 (1.8%) died or developed myocardial infarction, compared with

TABLE 11-11. *Low molecular weight heparin (LMWH) or aspirin in unstable angina*

	ASA (n = 73)	ASA + HEP (n = 70)	ASA + LMWH (n = 68)
Myocardial infarction	7 (9.6%)	4 (5. 7%)	0 (0.0%)
Recurrent angina	27 (37.0%)	31 (44.3%)	14 (20.6%)
Urgent revascularization	9 (12.3%)	7 (10.0%)	1 (1.5%)
Major bleed	0 (0.0%)	2 (2.9%)	0 (0. 0%)

Data from Gurfinkel et al., ref. 82.

TABLE 11-12. *Low molecular weight heparin in unstable angina*

	Dalteparin (Fragmin) (n = 741)	Placebo (n = 758)	p
Death or MI	13 (1.8%)	36 (4.7%)	0.001
AMI	10 (1.4%)	33 (4.4%)	0.001
Death	7 (0.9%)	8 (1.1%)	—

Data from the FRIC Study Group, ref. 187.

TABLE 11-14. *Low molecular weight heparin (LMWH) versus ASA + dipyridamole on graft patency*

	Femoropopliteal bypass grafts		
Graft	LMWH	ASA/DIP	
Survival	(94)	(106)	p = 0.031
1 year	78%	64%	

Values in parentheses, number of patients treated. Data from Edmondson et al., ref. 190.

36 of 758 patients (4.7%) who recieved placebo. In the second study (188) the low molecular weight heparin dalteparin, 120 anti-Xa units/kg twice daily, was compared with heparin (5,000-U bolus and 1,000 IU/kg by continuous infusion). The results summarized in Table 11-13 indicate that the treatment regimens were equivalent in efficacy and safety. At 6 days, 98 of 751 patients (13.0%) treated with low molecular weight heparin developed the composite outcome of death, myocardial infarction, recurrent angina, or revascularization, compared with 91 of 731 patients (12.5%) who were treated with heparin.

A larger randomized trial of low molecular weight heparin in unstable angina, the ESSENCE trial (224), included 3,171 patients with unstable angina or non–Q-wave myocardial infarct randomized in a double-blind fashion to enoxaparin 1 mg/kg every 12 hours subcutaneously versus unfractionated intravenous heparin for 2 to 8 days. There was a significant reduction in the primary endpoint of death, myocardial infarct, or recurrent angina at 14 days with enoxaparin: 19.8% in

the heparin group, 16.5% in the enoxaparin group, for a 17% relative risk reduction (p = 0.019). The TIMI 11B trial is testing a longer duration of treatment with enoxaparin versus unfractionated intravenous heparin.

Graft Patency after Femoropopliteal Bypass

Edmondson and associates (190) compared the relative efficacy and safety of low molecular weight heparin and the combination of aspirin and dipyridamole in patients undergoing femoropopliteal bypass grafting for peripheral vascular disease. Graft survival at 1 year was 78% in the low molecular weight heparin group and 64% in the aspirin and dipyridamole group (p = 0.031) (Table 11-14). These promising findings need to be confirmed in future studies.

SIDE EFFECTS OF LOW MOLECULAR WEIGHT HEPARIN PREPARATIONS

Risk of Thrombocytopenia

There is evidence from a large randomized trial of approximately 400 patients that the incidence of heparin-associated IgG and of thrombocytopenia are less in patients treated with prophylactic doses of low molecular weight heparin than those treated with low dose heparin (157).

However, there are reports that the administration of low molecular weight heparins can be associated with the development of thrombocytopenia both in previously unexposed individuals (225) and in those with a

TABLE 11-13. *Low molecular weight heparin in unstable angina*

	Dalteparin (Fragmin) (n = 751)	Heparin (n = 731)	p
Death, MI, recurrence	70 (9.3%)	57 (7.8%)	0.42
Revascularization	39 (5.2%)	42 (5.8%)	0.48
Composite	98 (13.0%)	91 (12.5%)	0.99

MI, myocardial infarction.
Data from the FRISC Study Group, ref. 188.

TABLE 11-15. *Incidence of cross-reactivity with heparin-induced antibody*

Heparin	100%
Dalteparin (Fragmin)	88%
Nadroparine calcium (Fraxiparin)	79%
Enoxaparin sodium (Lovenox/Clexane)	78%
Danaparoid sodium (Orgaran)	12%

Data from Chong et al., ref. 143.

history of HIT (225). There is also evidence that low molecular weight heparin preparations cross-react with plasma from patients with recent HIT (Table 11-15) (143,154). In contrast to the low molecular weight heparins, the heparinoid danaparoid sodium, which is said to be free of contaminating heparin, has minimal cross-reactivity in in vitro assays for HIT (143) and has been used successfully in patients with a history of HIT (143). Thus, low molecular weight heparins are associated with a lower risk of thrombocytopenia than heparin but often produce a positive in vitro test for HIT in patients with a history of HIT and may produce thrombocytopenia in these patients. The heparinoid danaparoid sodium has a lower frequency of cross-reactivity than low molecular weight heparins and has been used successfully in a fairly large number of patients with previous HIT (226).

Risk of Osteoporosis

The long-term use of heparin can be complicated with osteoporosis (131). Recent evidence suggests that the risk of osteoporosis is likely to be lower with low molecular weight heparin than with heparin. Results of studies comparing the effects of low molecular weight heparin with heparin in a fetal rat calvarium model suggest that the risk of bone loss is less when the calvarium is exposed to low molecular weight heparin (227). In this model, the effect of heparin fractions on bone loss was molecular size dependent, being minimal at a molecular weight of 3,000 and 5,000, and apparent at a molecular weight of 9,000.

Initial case reports of successful use of low molecular weight heparin in patients whose

treatment with heparin was complicated with symptomatic osteoporosis (228) has been supported by the results of a randomized study (229). Patients with venous thrombosis were randomly allocated to receive out-of-hospital low molecular weight heparin (dalteparin) or heparin; both treatments administered by subcutaneous injection for 3 to 6 months. In this small study, six of 34 patients treated with heparin and one of 39 patients who received low molecular weight heparin developed a fracture. Therefore, although the results are promising, the information is limited and additional appropriately designed studies are required before it can be concluded that this troublesome side effect of heparin can be avoided by using low molecular weight heparins.

Neutralization with Protamine Sulfate

The anticoagulant and hemorrhagic effects of heparin are neutralized by an equimolar concentration of protamine sulfate. Equimolar concentrations of protamine sulfate neutralize the anti–factor IIa activity but result in only partial neutralization of the anti–factor Xa of low molecular weight heparins (230–233), probably because protamine sulfate does not bind to the very low molecular weight components. Despite the failure of protamine sulfate to neutralize all of the anti–factor Xa activity of low molecular weight heparin, studies in experimental animal models indicate that increased microvascular bleeding produced by very high concentrations of low molecular weight heparins is neutralized by protamine sulfate (230) (Fig. 11-1). Whether protamine sulfate will neutralize clinically important bleeding is uncertain.

Use of Low Molecular Weight Heparin in Pregnancy

Heparin is the anticoagulant of choice in pregnancy because it does not cross the placenta and therefore does not affect fetal coagulation (234). Studies in humans indicate that low molecular weight heparins also do not

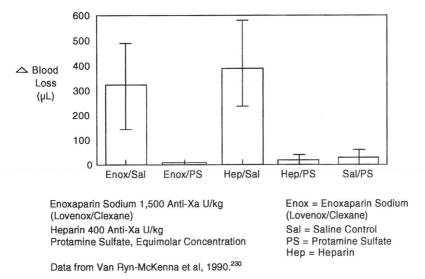

Enoxaparin Sodium 1,500 Anti-Xa U/kg
(Lovenox/Clexane)
Heparin 400 Anti-Xa U/kg
Protamine Sulfate, Equimolar Concentration

Enox = Enoxaparin Sodium
(Lovenox/Clexane)
Sal = Saline Control
PS = Protamine Sulfate
Hep = Heparin

Data from Van Ryn-McKenna et al, 1990.[230]

FIG. 11-1. Neutralizing effect of protamine sulfate on experimental blood loss induced by high doses of heparin on the low molecular weight heparin, enoxaparin sodium (lovenox/clexane).

cross the placental barrier (235–237) and descriptive studies suggest they are safe and effective (228). However, further studies are required to establish the safety of low molecular weight heparin during pregnancy.

CONCLUSION

Heparin is a heterogenous mixture of sulfated polysaccharide chains. Its mean molecular weight is 15,000 daltons with a range of 3,000 to 30,000 daltons. The anticoagulant effect of heparin is mediated through a unique pentasaccharide that is present on about one third of the heparin molecules. The anticoagulantly active heparin molecules catalyze the inactivation of thrombin and factor Xa by AT.

Heparin is an effective antithrombotic agent for the treatment of prevention of venous thromboembolism. When used in combination with aspirin it is effective in the short-term treatment of unstable angina, but whether these benefits are sustained is uncertain.

The value of heparin in patients with acute myocardial infarction is uncertain. It appears to be effective when used alone, but has not been evaluated adequately in combination

with aspirin. Heparin is not beneficial when used with SK, and its value when combined with t-PA has not been adequately evaluated using clinical endpoints.

High-dose heparin is used routinely in patients undergoing coronary angioplasty, but the optimal regimen is uncertain. There is evidence from retrospective studies that acute complications of coronary angioplasty are increased with lower levels of anticoagulation.

The major complication of heparin is bleeding. This is particularly problematic when heparin is used in combination with thrombolytic therapy or platelet GPIIb/IIIa inhibitors and when invasive procedures are used. In these circumstances it has been recommended that the dose of heparin should be reduced, although there is uncertainty as to whether these lower doses are of benefit.

Low molecular weight heparins are derived from unfractionated heparin by depolymerization. They are about one third the molecular weight of heparin and like heparin are heterogeneous in molecular size. Only about 20% of low molecular weight heparin molecules are anticoagulantly active. Low molecular weight heparins have the following advantages over unfractionated heparin: they have a more predictable dose response, better bioavailability when administered subcutaneously, longer plasma half-life, lower risk of HIT, and possibly a lower risk of osteoporosis.

Low molecular weight heparins have been shown to be more effective and as safe as heparin for the prevention of venous thrombosis after major orthopedic surgery. Low molecular weight heparins are also as effective and safe as heparin for the treatment of venous thrombosis, but unlike heparin they can be administered subcutaneously without laboratory monitoring, a characteristic that allows low molecular weight heparins to be administered outside the hospital setting. Low molecular weight heparins also have been compared with heparin in two large studies in patients with unstable angina. In one, the low molecular weight heparin was shown to be significantly more effective and in the other as effective as heparin.

Future studies are required to determine whether heparin has a role in acute myocardial infarction, particularly with thrombolytic therapy and antiplatelet agents, and whether low molecular weight heparins are more effective than heparin in acute myocardial ischemic syndromes.

REFERENCES

1. Choay J, Petitou M. The chemistry of heparin: a way to understand its mode of action. *Med J Aust* 1986; 144(HS):7–10.
2. Rosenberg RD, Lam L. Correlation between structure and function of heparin. *Proc Natl Acad Sci U S A* 1979;76:1218–1222.
3. Rosenberg RD. The heparin-antithrombin system: a natural anticoagulant mechanism. In: Colman RW, Hirsh J, Marder VJ, Salzman EW (eds). *Hemostasis and Thrombosis: Basic Principles and Clinical Practice.* 2nd ed. Philadelphia, PA: Lippincott, 1987; 1373–1392.
4. Lindahl U, Backstrom G, Hook M, Thunberg L, Fransson L-A, Linker A. Structure of the antithrombin-binding site of heparin. *Proc Natl Acad Sci U S A* 1979;76: 3198–3202.
5. Hook M, Bjork I, Hopwood J, Lindahl U. Anticoagulant activity of heparin: separation of high activity and low-activity heparin species by affinity chromatography on immobilized antithrombin. *FEBS Lett* 1976;66: 90–93.
6. Casu B, Oreste P, Torri G, et al. The structure of heparin oligosaccharide fragments with high anti-(factor

Xa) activity containing the minimal antithrombin-binding sequence. *Biochem J* 1981;197:599–609.
7. Choay J, Petitou M, Lormeau JC, Sinay P, Casu BJ, Gatti G. Structure-activity relationship in heparin: a synthetic pentasaccharide with high affinity for antithrombin and eliciting high anti-factor Xa activity. *Biochem Biophys Res Commun* 1983;116:492–499.
8. Lindahl U, Thunberg L, Backstrom G, Riesenfel J, Nordling K, Bjork I. Extension and structural variability of the antithrombin-binding sequence in heparin. *J Biol Chem* 1984;259:12368–12376.
9. Atha DH, Lormeau JC, Petitou M, Rosenberg RD, Choay J. Contribution of 3-0-and 6-0-sulfated blycosamine residues in the heparin-induced conformational change in antithrombin. *Biochemistry* 1987;26: 6454–6461.
10. Oosta GM, Gardner WT, Beeler DL, Rosenberg RD. Multiple functional domains of the heparin molecule. *Proc Natl Acad Sci U S A* 1981;78:829–833.
11. Rosenberg RD, Jordon RE, Favreau LV, et al. High active heparin species with multiple binding sites for antithrombin. *Biochem Biophys Res Commun* 1979;86: 1319–1324.
12. Nordenman B, Bjork I. Binding of low affinity and high affinity heparin to antithrombin. Ultraviolet difference spectroscopy and circular dichroism studies. *Biochemistry* 1978;17:3339–3344.
13. Olson ST, Srinivasan KR, Bjork I, et al. Binding of high affinity heparin to antithrombin: stopped flow kinetic studies of the binding interaction. *J Biol Chem* 1981;256:11073–11079.
14. Villanueva GB, Danishefsky I. Evidence for a heparin-induced conformational change on antithrombin. *Biochem Biophys Res Commun* 1977;74:803–809.
15. Ofosu FA, Modi GJ, Hirsh J, Buchanan M, Blajchman MA. Mechanisms for inhibition of the generation of thrombin activity by sulfated polysaccharides. *Ann NY Acad Sci* 1986;485:41–55.
16. Ofosu FA, Esmon CT, Blajchman MA, et al. Unfractionated heparin inhibits thrombin-catalyzed amplification reactions of coagulation more efficiently than those catalyzed by factor Xa. *Biochem J* 1989;257: 143–150.
17. Beguin S, Mardiguian J, Lindhout T, Hemker HC. The mode of action of low molecular weight heparin preparation (PK 10169) and two of its major components on thrombin generation in plasma. *Thromb Haemost* 1989;61:30–34
18. Hemker HC. The mode of action of heparin in plasma. In: Verstraete M, Vermylen J, Lijnen HR, Arnout J (eds). *XIth Congress on Thrombosis and Haemostasis.* Brussels, Leuven: Leuven University Press, 1987; 17–36.
19. Beguin S, Lindhout T, Hemker HC. The mode of action of heparin in plasma. *Thromb Haemost* 1989;60: 457–462.
20. Olson ST, Shore JD. Demonstration of a two-step reaction mechanism for inhibition of α-thrombin by antithrombin and identification of the step affected by heparin. *J Biol Chem* 1982;257:14891–14895.
21. Danielsson A, Raub E, Lindahl U, Bjork I. Role of ternary complexes in which heparin binds both antithromin and proteinase, in the acceleration of the reactions between antithrombin and thrombin or factor Xa. *J Biol Chem* 1986;261:15467–15473.

22. Jordan RE, Oosta GM, Gardner WT, Rosenberg RD. The kinetics of hemostatic enzyme-antithrombin interactions in the presence of low molecular weight heparin. *J Biol Chem* 1980;255:10081–10090.

23. Lane DA, Denton J, Flynn AM, Thunberg L, Lindahl U. Anticoagulant activities of heparin oligosaccharides and their neuralization by platelet factor 4. *Biochem J* 1984;218:725–732.

24. Tollefsen DM, Majerus DW, Blank MK. Heparin cofactor II. Purification and properties of thrombin in human plasma. *J Biol Chem* 1982;257:2162–2169.

25. Maimone MM, Tollefsen DM. Activation of heparin cofactor II by heparin oligosaccharides. *Biochem Biophys Res Commun* 1988;152:1056–1061.

26. Hurst RE, Poon MC, Griffith MJ. Structure-activity relationships of heparin. Independence of heparin charge density and antithrombin binding domains in thrombin inhibition by antithrombin and heparin cofactor II. *J Clin Invest* 1983;72:1042–1045.

27. Petitou M, Lormeau JC, Perly B, et al. Is there a unique sequence in heparin for interaction with heparin cofactor II? Structural and biological studies of heparin-derived oligosaccharides. *J Biol Chem* 1988;263:8685–8690.

28. Sie P, Petitou M, Lormeau JC, Dupouy D, Boneu B, Choay J. Studies on the structural requirements of heparin for the catalysis of thrombin inhibition by heparin cofactor II. *Biochem Biophys Acta* 1988;966:188–195.

29. Andersson L-O, Barrowcliffe TW, Holmer E, Johnson EA, Soderstrom G. Molecular weight dependency of the heparin potentiated inhibition of thrombin and activated factor X. Effect of heparin neutralization in plasma. *Thromb Res* 1979;15:531–541.

30. Harenberg J. Pharmacology of low molecular weight heparins. *Semin Thromb Hemost* 1990;16:12–18.

31. Johnson EA, Mulloy B. The molecular weight range of commercial heparin preparations. *Carbohydr Res* 1976;51:119–127.

32. Hirsh J. Heparin. *N Engl J Med* 1991;324:1565–1574.

33. Pini M, Pattachini C, Quintavalla R, et al. Subcutaneous vs. intravenous heparin in the treatment of deep venous thrombosis—a randomized clinical trial. *Thromb Haemost* 1990;64:222–226.

34. Hommes DW, Bura A, Mazzolai L, Buller HR, ten Cate JW. Subcutaneous heparin compared with continuous intravenous heparin administration in the initial treatment of deep vein thrombosis. A meta-analysis. *Ann Intern Med* 1992;116:279–284.

35. Hirsh J, van Aken WG, Gallus AS, Dollery CT, Cade JF, Yung WG. Heparin kinetics in venous thrombosis and pulmonary embolism. *Circulation* 1976;53:691–695.

36. Young E, Prins MH, Levine MN, Hirsh J. Heparin binding to plasma proteins, an important mechanism for heparin resistance. *Thromb Haemost* 1992;67:639–643.

37. Sobel M, McNeill PM, Carlson PL, et al. Heparin inhibition of von Willebrand factor-dependent platelet function in vitro and in vivo. *J Clin Invest* 1991;87:1787–1793.

38. Barzu T, Molho P, Tobelem G, Petitou M, Caen J. Binding and endocytosis of heparin by human endothelial cells in culture. *Biochem Biophys Acta* 1985;845:196–203.

39. de Swart CAM, Nijmeyer B, Roelofs JMM, Sixma JJ. Kinetics of intravenously administered heparin in normal humans. *Blood* 1982;60:1251–1258.

40. Olsson P, Lagergren H, Ek S. The elimination from plasma of intravenous heparin. An experimental study on dogs and humans. *Acta Med Scand* 1963;173:619–630.

41. Bjornsson TO, Wolfram BS, Kitchell BB. Heparin kinetics determined by three assay methods. *Clin Pharmacol Ther* 1982;31:104–113.

42. Glimelius B, Busch C, Hook M. Binding of heparin on the surface of cultured human endothelial cells. *Thromb Res* 1978;12:773–782.

43. Mahadoo J, Hiebert L, Jaques LB. Vascular sequestration of heparin. *Thromb Res* 1977;12:79–90.

44. Friedman Y, Arsenis C. Studies on the heparin sulphamidase activity from rat spleen. Intracellular distribution and characterization of the enzyme. *Biochem J* 1974;139:699–708.

45. Dawes J, Pepper DS. Catabolism of low-dose heparin in man. *Thromb Res* 1979;14:845–860.

46. McAllister BM, Demis DJ. Heparin metabolism: isolation and characterization of uroheparin. *Nature* 1966;212:293–294.

47. Cruickshank MK, Levine MN, Hirsh J, Roberts RS. A unfractionated heparin nomogram for the management of heparin therapy. *Arch Intern Med* 1991;151:333–337.

48. Turpie AGG, Robinson JG, Doyle DJ, et al. Comparison of high-dose with low-dose subcutaneous heparin to prevent left ventricular mural thrombosis in patients with acute transmural anterior myocardial infarction. *N Engl J Med* 1989;320:352–357.

49. Camilleri JF, Bonnet JL, Bouvier JL, et al. Thrombolyse intraveineuse dans l'infarctus du myocarde. Influence de la qualite de l'antiocoagulation sur le taux de recidives precoces d'angor ou d'infarctus. *Arch Mal Coeur* 1988;81:1037–1041.

50. Kaplan K, Davison R, Parker M, Mayberry B, Feiereisel P, Salinger M. Role of heparin after intravenous thrombolytic therapy for acute myocardial infarction. *Am J Cardiol* 1987;59:241–244.

51. de Bono DP, Simoons ML, Arnold AER, et al. Effect of early intravenous heparin on coronary patency, infarct size, and bleeding complications after alteplase thrombolysis: results of a randomised double blind European Cooperative Study Group Trial. *Br Heart J* 1992;67:122–128.

52. Levine M, Hirsh J, Gent M, et al. A randomized trial comparing activated thromboplastin time with heparin assay in patients with acute venous thromboembolism requiring large daily doses of heparin. *Arch Intern Med* 1994;154:49–56.

53. Chiu HM, Hirsh J, Yung WL, Rogoeczi E, Gent M. Relationship between anticoagulant and antithrombotic effects of heparin. *Blood* 1977;49:171–184.

54. Brill-Edwards P, Ginsberg JS, Johnston M, Hirsh J. Establishing a therapeutic range for heparin therapy. *Ann Intern Med* 1993;119:104–109.

55. Hull RD, Raskob GE, Hirsh J, et al. Continuous intravenous heparin compared with intermittent subcutaneous heparin in the initial treatment of proximal-vein thrombosis. *N Engl J Med* 1986;315:1109–1114.

56. Basu D, Gallus A, Hirsh J, Cade J. A prospective study of value of monitoring heparin treatment with the acti-

vated partial thromboplastin time. *N Engl J Med* 1972;287:324–327.

57. Raschke RA, Reilly BM, Guidry JR, Fontane JR, Srinivas S. The weight-based heparin dosing nomogram compared with a "standard care" nomogram. *Ann Intern Med* 1993;119:874–881.

58. Morabia A. Heparin doses and major bleedings. *Lancet* 1986;1:1278–1279.

59. Reilly B, Raschke R, Srinivas S, Nieman T. Intravenous heparin dosing: patterns and variations in internist's practices. *J Gen Intern Med* 1993;8:536–542.

60. Hull RD, Raskob GE, Rosenbloom D, et al. Optimal therapeutic level of heparin therapy in patients with venous thrombosis. *Arch Intern Med* 1992;152: 1589–1595.

61. Elliot GC, Hiltunen SJ, Suchyta M, et al. Physician-guided treatment compared with a heparin protocol for deep vein thrombosis. *Arch Intern Med* 1994;154: 999–1004.

62. Flaker GC, Bartolozzi J, Davis V, et al. Use of a standardized heparin nomogram to achieve therapeutic anticoagulation after thrombolytic therapy in myocardial infarction. *Arch Intern Med* 1994;154:1492–1496.

63. Mungall DR, Anbe D, Forrester PL, et al. A prospective randomized comparison of the accuracy of computer-assisted versus GUSTO nomogram-directed heparin therapy. *Clin Pharmacol Ther* 1994;55:591–596.

64. Kershaw B, White RH, Mungall DM, van Houten J, Brettfeld S. Computer-assisted dosing of heparin. *Arch Intern Med* 1994;154:1005–1011.

65. The GUSTO investigators. An international randomized trial comparing four thrombolytic strategies for acute myocardial infarction. *N Engl J Med* 1993;329: 673–682.

66. Braunwald E, Mark DB, Jones RH, et al. U.S. Department of Health and Human Services, Clinical Practice Guidelines. Unstable angina: diagnosis and management. AHCPR Publication No. 94-0602:63–64.

67. Venous Thrombosis Clinical Study Group. Small doses of subcutaneous sodium heparin in the prevention of deep vein thrombosis after elective hip operations. *Br J Surg* 1975;62:348–350.

68. Gallus AS, Hirsh J, Tuttle RJ, et al. Small subcutaneous doses of heparin in prevention of venous thrombosis. *N Engl J Med* 1973;288:545–551.

69. Sagar S, Nairn D, Stamatakis JD, et al. Efficacy of low-dose heparin in prevention of extensive deep-vein thrombosis in patients undergoing total-hip replacement. *Br J Surg* 1972;59:223–226.

70. Moskovitz PA, Ellenberg SS, Feffer HL, et al. Low-dose heparin for prevention of venous thromboembolism in total hip arthroplasty and surgical repair of hip fractures. *J Bone Joint Surg [Am]* 1978;60: 1065–1070.

71. Poller L, Taberner DA, Sandilands DG, Galasko CSB. An evaluation of APTT monitoring of low-dose heparin dosage in hip surgery. *Thromb Haemost* 1982; 47:50–53.

72. Leyvraz PF, Richard J, Bachmann F. Adjusted versus fixed dose subcutaneous heparin in the prevention of deep-vein thrombosis after total hip replacement. *N Engl J Med* 1983;309:954–958.

73. Taberner DA, Poller L, Thomson JM, Lemon G, Weighill FJ. Randomized study of adjusted versus fixed low dose heparin prophylaxis of deep vein thrombosis in hip surgery. *Br J Surg* 1989;76: 933–935.

74. Lewis HD, Davis JW, Archibald DG, et al. Protective effects of aspirin against acute myocardial infarction and death in men with unstable angina. Results of a Veterans Administration Cooperative Study. *N Engl J Med* 1983;309:396–403.

75. Cairns JA, Gent M, Singer J, et al. Aspirin, sulfinpyrazone, or both, in unstable angina: results of a Canadian multicenter clinical trial. *N Engl J Med* 1985;313: 1369–1375.

76. Theroux P, Ouimet H, McCans J, et al. Aspirin, heparin, or both to treat acute unstable angina. *N Engl J Med* 1988;319:1105–1111.

77. The RISC Group. Risk of myocardial infarction and death during treatment with low-dose aspirin and intravenous heparin in men with unstable coronary artery disease. *Lancet* 1990;336:827–830.

78. Theroux P, Waters D, Qiu S, McCans J, de Guise P, Juneau M. Aspirin versus heparin to prevent myocardial infarction during the acute phase of unstable angina. *Circulation* 1993;88:2045–2048.

79. Cohen M, Adams PC, Parry G, and the Antithrombotic Therapy in Acute Coronary Syndromes Research Group. Combination antithrombotic therapy in unstable rest angina and non–Q-wave infarction in nonprior aspirin users. *Circulation* 1994;89:81–88.

80. Cohen M, Adams PC, Hawkins L, Bach M, Fuster V. Usefulness of antithrombotic therapy in resting angina pectoris or non–Q-wave myocardial infarction in preventing death and myocardial infarction (a pilot study from the Antithrombotic Therapy in Acute Coronary Syndromes Study Group). *Am J Cardiol* 1990;66: 1287–1292.

81. Holdright D, Patel D, Cunningham D, et al. Comparison of the effect of heparin and aspirin versus aspirin alone on transient myocardial ischemia and in-hospital prognosis in patients with unstable angina. *J Am Coll Cardiol* 1994;24:39–45.

82. Gurfinkel EP, Manos EJ, Mejail RI, et al. Low molecular weight heparin versus regular heparin or aspirin in the treatment of unstable angina and silent ischemia. *J Am Coll Cardiol* 1995;26:313–318.

83. Oler A, Whooley MA, Oler J, Grady D. Adding heparin to aspirin reduces the incidence of myocardial infarction and death in patients with unstable angina. A meta-analysis. *JAMA* 1996;276:811–815.

84. Braunwald E, Mark DB, Jones RH, et al. *Unstable Angina: Diagnosis and Management.* Clinical practice guideline number X. AHCPR Publication No. 94-0682. Rockville, MD: Agency for Health Care Policy and Research and the National Heart, Lung, and Blood Institute, Public Health Service, U.S. Department of Health and Human Services. March 1994.

85. Theroux P, Waters D, Lam J, Juneau M, McCans J. Reactivation of unstable angina after the discontinuation of heparin. *N Engl J Med* 1992;327:141–145.

86. Granger C, Hirsh J, Califf RM, et al. Activated partial thromboplastin time and outcome after thrombolytic therapy for acute myocardial infarction. Results from the GUSTO-1 Trial. *Circulation* 1996;93:870–878.

87. Granger CB, Miller JM, Bovill EG, et al. Rebound increase in thrombin generation and activity after cessation of intravenous heparin in patients with acute coronary syndromes. *Circulation* 1995;91:1929–1935.

88. Becker RC, Cannon CP, Tracy RP, et al. Relation between systemic anticoagulation as determined by activated partial thromboplastin time and heparin measurements and in-hospital clinical events in unstable angina and non-Q wave myocardial infarction. Thrombolysis in Myocardial Ischemia III B Investigators. *Am Heart J* 1996;131:421–433.

89. Serneri GGN, Rovelli F, Gensini GF, Pirelli S, Carnovali M, Fotini A. Effectiveness of low-dose heparin in prevention of myocardial reinfarction. *Lancet* 1987;1:937–942.

90. The SCATI (Studio sulla Calciparina nell'Angina e nella Thrombosi Ventricolare nell'Infarto) Group. Randomised controlled trial of subcutaneous calcium-heparin in acute myocardial infarction. *Lancet* 1989;2: 182–186.

91. Verheugt FWA, Marsh RC, Been G, Bronzwaer JGF, Zijlstra F. Megadose bolus heparin as reperfusion therapy for acute myocardial infarction: results of the HEAP pilot study. *J Am Coll Cardiol* 1996;27(suppl A):11.

92. Topol EJ, George BS, Kereiakes DJ, et al., and the TAMI Study Group. A randomized controlled trial of intravenous tissue plasminogen activator and early intravenous heparin in acute myocardial infarction. *Circulation* 1989;79:281–286.

93. Hsia J, Hamilton WP, Kleiman N, Roberts R, Chaitman BR, Ross AM, for the Heparin-Aspirin Reperfusion Trial (HART) Investigators. A comparison between heparin and low-dose aspirin as adjunctive therapy with tissue plasminogen activator for acute myocardial infarction. *N Engl J Med* 1990;323:1433–1437.

94. Bleich SD, Nichols TC, Schumacher RR, et al. Effect of heparin on coronary arterial patency after thrombolysis with tissue plasminogen activator in acute myocardial infarction. *Am J Cardiol* 1990;66:1412–1417.

95. The Australian National Heart Study Trial. A randomized comparison of oral aspirin/dipyridamole versus intravenous heparin after rtPA for acute myocardial infarction [Abstract]. *Circulation* 1989;80(suppl II):114.

96. Hsia J, Kleiman NS, Aguirre FV, Chaitman BR, Roberts R, Ross AM. Heparin-induced prolongation of partial thromboplastin time after thrombolysis: relation to coronary artery patency. *J Am Coll Cardiol* 1992;20:31–35.

97. Arnout J, Simoons M, de Bono D, Rapold HJ, Collen D, Verstraete M. Correlation between level of heparinization and patency of the infarct-related coronary artery after treatment of acute myocardial infarction with alteplase (rt-PA). *J Am Coll Cardiol* 1992;20: 513–519.

98. Col J, Decoster O, Hanique G, et al. Infusion of heparin conjunct to streptokinase accelerates reperfusion of acute myocardial infarction: results of a double blind randomized study (OSIRIS) [Abstract]. *Circulation* 1992;(suppl):I-259.

99. O'Connor C, for the DUCCS Study Group. Duke University Clinical Cardiology Studies (DUCCS-1). Presented at the American Heart Association, Anaheim, California, 1992.

100. ISIS-2 (Second International Study of Infarct Survival) Collaborative Group. Randomized trial of intravenous streptokinase, oral aspirin, both, or neither among 17,187 cases of suspected acute myocardial infarction: ISIS-2. *Lancet* 1988;2:349–360.

101. Gruppo Italiano per lo studio della sopravvivenza nel-

l'infarto miocardico. GISSI-2: a factorial randomized trial of alteplase versus streptokinase and heparin versus no heparin among 12,490 patients with acute myocardial infarction. *Lancet* 1990;336:65–71.

102. The International Study Group. In-hospital mortality and clinical course of 20,891 patients with suspected acute myocardial infarction randomised between alteplase and streptokinase with or without heparin. *Lancet* 1990;336:71–75.

103. ISIS-3 Study Group. A randomised comparison of streptokinase vs tissue plasminogen activator vs anistreplase and of aspirin plus heparin vs aspirin alone among 41,299 cases of suspected acute myocardial infarction. *Lancet* 1992;339:753–770.

104. Berkowitz SD, Granger CB, Pieper KS, et al., for the Global Utilization of Streptokinase and Tissue Plasminogen Activator for Occluded Coronary Arteries (GUSTO) I Investigators. Incidence and predictors of bleeding following contemporary thrombolytic therapy for myocardial infarction. *Circulation* 1997;95: 2508–2516.

105. Collins R, MacMahon S, Flather M, et al. Clinical effects of anticoagulant therapy in suspected acute myocardial infarction: systematic overview of randomised trials. *Br Med J* 1996;313:652–659.

106. Mahaffey KW, Granger CB, O Connor CM, et al. Overview of randomized trials of intravenous heparin in patients with acute myocardial infarction treated with thrombolytic therapy. *Am J Cardiol* 1996;77: 551–556.

107. Ryan TJ, Anderson JL, Antman EM, et al. ACC/AHA Guidelines for the management of patients with acute myocardial infarction a report of the American College of Cardiology/American Heart Association Task Force on practice guidelines (Committee on Management of Acute Myocardial Infarction). *J Am Coll Cardiol* 1996;28:1328–1419.

108. GUSTO IIa Investigators. Global use of strategies to open coronary arteries (GUSTO) IIa investigators. Randomized trial of intravenous heparin versus recombinant hirudin for acute coronary syndromes. *Circulation* 1994;90:1631–1637.

109. Antman EM for the TIMI 9A Investigators. Hirudin in acute myocardial infarction. Safety report from the thrombolysis and thrombin inhibition in myocardial infarction (TIMI) 9A trial. *Circulation* 1994;90: 1624–1630.

110. Antman EM, Braunwald E. Trials and tribulations of thrombin inhibition. *Eur Heart J* 1996;17:971–973.

111. EPIC Investigators. Use of a monoclonal antibody directed against the platelet glycoprotein IIb/IIIa receptor in high-risk coronary angioplasty. *N Engl J Med* 1994;330:956–961.

112. Manolis AS, Melita-Manolis H, Stefanadis C, Toutouzas P. Plasma level changes of fibrinopeptide A after uncomplicated coronary angioplasty. *Clin Cardiol* 1993;16:548–552.

113. Schwartz L, Bourassa MG, Lesperance J, et al. Aspirin and dipyridamole in the prevention of restenosis after percutaneous transluminal coronary angioplasty. *N Engl J Med* 1988;318:1714–1719.

114. EPILOG Investigators. Platelet glycoprotein IIb/IIIa receptor blockade and low-dose heparin during percutaneous coronary revascularization. *N Engl J Med* 1997;336:1689–1696.

115. Van de Werf F. More evidence for a beneficial effect of platelet glycoprotein IIb/IIIa-blockade during coronary interventions. Latest results from the EPILOG and CAPTURE trials. *Eur Heart J* 1996;17:325–326.

116. Ferguson JJ. All ACTs are not created equal [Editorial]. *Tex Heart Inst J* 1992;19:1–3.

117. McGarry TF Jr, Gottlieb RS, Morganroth J, et al. The relationship of anticoagulation level and complications after successful percutaneous transluminal coronary angioplasty. *Am Heart J* 1992;23:1445–1451.

118. Ferguson JJ, Dougherty KG, Gaos CM, Bush HS, Marsh KC, Leachman DR. Relation between procedural activated coagulation time and outcome after percutaneous transluminal coronary angioplasty. *J Am Coll Caridol* 1994;23:1061–1065.

119. Narins CR, Hillegass WB Jr, Nelson CL, et al. Relation between activated clotting time during angioplasty and abrupt closure. *Circulation* 1996;93:667–671.

120. Popma JJ, Coller BS, Ohamn EM, et al. Antithrombotic therapy in patients undergoing coronary angioplasty. *Chest* 1995;108(suppl):486–501.

121. Ellis SG, Roubin GS, Wilentz J, Douglas JS Jr, King SB 3d. Effect of 18- to 24-hour heparin administration for prevention of restenosis after uncomplicated coronary angioplasty. *Am Heart J* 1989;117:777–782.

122. Friedman HZ, Cragg DR, Glazier SM, et al. Randomized prospective evaluation of prolonged versus abbreviated intravenous heparin therapy after coronary angioplasty. *J Am Coll Cardiol* 1994;24:1214–1219.

123. Lincoff AM, Tcheng JE, Califf RM, et al., for the PROLOG Investigators. A multicenter, randomized, double-blind pilot trial of standard versus low dose weight-adjusted heparin in patients treated with the platelet GP IIb/IIIa receptor antibody fragment c7E3 Fab (abciximab) during percutaneous coronary revascularization. *J Am Coll Cardiol* 1997;79(3):286–291.

124. Moliterno DJ, Califf RM, Aguirre FV, et al. Effect of platelet glycoprotein IIb/IIIa integrin blockade on activated clotting time during percutaneous transluminal coronary angioplasty or directional atherectomy (the EPIC trial). Evaluation of c7E3 Fab in the Prevention of Ischemic Complications trial. *Am J Cardiol* 1995; 75:559–562.

125. Pepine CJ, Holmes DR Jr. Coronary artery stents. American College of Cardiology. *J Am Coll Cardiol* 1996;28:782–794.

126. Columbo A, Hall P, Nakamura S, et al. Intracoronary stenting withoug anticoagulation accomplished with intravascular ultrasound guidance. *Circulation* 1995; 91:1676–1688.

127. Schomig A, Neumann FJ, Kastrati A, et al. A randomized comparison of antiplatelet and anticoagulant therapy after the placement of coronary-artery stents. *N Engl J Med* 1996;334:1084–1089.

128. King DJ, Kelton JG. Heparin-associated thrombocytopenia. *Ann Intern Med* 1984;100:535–540.

129. Warkentin TE, Kelton JG. Heparin-induced thrombocytopenia. In: Creger WP (ed). *Annual Review in Medicine.* Volume 40. California: Annual Review Medicine, 1989;31–44.

130. Ginsberg JS, Hirsh J. Use of anticoagulants during pregnancy. *Chest* 1989;95(suppl):156–160.

131. Ginsberg JS, Kowalchuk G, Hirsh J, et al. Heparin effect on bone density. *Thromb Haemost* 1990;64:286–289.

132. White RW, John RS, Richard EN. Thrombotic complications of heparin therapy including six cases of heparin-induced skin necrosis. *Ann Surg* 1979;190: 595–608.

133. Jacques LB. Heparins—anionic polyelectrolyte drugs. *Pharmacol Rev* 1980;31:99–106.

134. Curry N, Bandana EJ, Pirofsky B. Heparin sensitivity: report of a case. *Arch Intern Med* 1973;132: 744–745.

135. O'Kelly R, Magee F, McKenna J. Routine heparin therapy inhibits adrenal aldosterone production. *J Clin Endocrinol Metab* 1983;56:108–112.

136. Levine MN, Hirsh J, Kelton JG. Heparin-induced bleeding. In: Lane DA, Lindahl U (eds). *Heparin: Chemical and Biological Properties. Clinical Applications.* London, England: Edward Arnold, 1989;517–532.

137. Landefeld S, Cook F, Flatley M, Weisberg M, Goldman L. Identification and preliminary validation of predictors of major bleeding in hospitalized patients starting anticoagulant therapy. *Am J Med* 1987;82: 703–713.

138. Walker AM, Jick H. Predictors of bleeding during heparin therapy. *JAMA* 1980;244:1209–1212.

139. Yett HS, Skillman JJ, Salzman EW. The hazards of heparin plus aspirin. *N Engl J Med* 1978;244: 1209–1212.

140. Sethi GK, Copeland JG, Goldman S, Moritz T, Zadina K, Henderson WG. Implications of preoperative administration of aspirin in patients undergoing coronary artery bypass grafting. *J Am Coll Cardiol* 1990;15: 15–20.

141. Jick H, Sloan D, Borda IT, Chapiro S. Efficacy and toxicity of heparin in relation to age and sex. *N Engl J Med* 1968;279:284–286.

142. Leroy J, Leclerc MH, Delahousse B, et al. Treatment of heparin-associated thrombocytopenia and thrombosis with low molecular weight heparin (CY 216). *Semin Thromb Haemost* 1985;11:326–329.

143. Chong BH, Ismail F, Cade J, Gallus AS, Gordon S, Chesterman CN. Heparin-induced thrombocytopenia: studies with a low molecular weight heparinoid, ORG 10172. *Blood* 1989;73:1592–1596.

144. Weitz JI, Hudoba M, Massel D, Maraganore J, Hirsh J. Clot-bound thrombin is protected from inhibition by heparin-antithrombin but is susceptible to inactivation by antithrombin III-independent inhibitors. *J Clin Invest* 1990;86:385–391.

145. Marciniak E. Factor X_a inactivation by antithrombin. 3. Evidence for biological stabilization of factor X_a by factor V-phospholipid complex. *Br J Haematol* 1973; 24:391–400.

146. Salzman EW, Rosenberg RD, Smith MH, Lindon JN, Favreau L. Effect of heparin and heparin fractions on platelet aggregation. *J Clin Invest* 1980;65:64–73.

147. Kelton JG, Smith JW, Warkentin TE, Hayward CPM, Denomme GA, Horsewood P. Immunoglobulin G from patients with heparin-induced thrombocytopenia binds to a complex of heparin and platelet factor 4. *Blood* 1994;83:3232–3239.

148. Jordan RE, Favreau LV, Braswell EH, Rosenberg RD. Heparin with two binding sites for antithrombin or platelet factor 4. *J Biol Chem* 1982;257:400–406.

149. Lane DA, Pejler G, Flynn AM, Thompson EA, Lindahl U. Neutralization of heparin-related saccharides by histidine-rich glycoprotein and platelet factor 4. *J Biol Chem* 1986;261:3980–3986.

150. Preissner KT, Muller-Berghaus G. Neutralization and binding of heparin by S-protein/vitronectin in the inhibition of factor Xa by antithrombin. *J Biol Chem* 1987;262:12247–12253.

151. Dawes J, Pavuk N. Sequestration of therapeutic glycosaminoglycans by plasma fibronectin [Abstract]. *Thromb Haemost* 1991;65:829.

152. Young E, Wells P, Holloway S, Weitz J, Hirsh J. Exvivo and in-vitro evidence that low molecular weight heparins exhibit less binding to plasma proteins than unfractionated heparin. *Thromb Haemost* 1994;71: 300–304.

153. Lane DA. Heparin binding and neutralizing protein. In: Lane DA, Lindahl U (eds). *Heparin, Chemical and Biological Properties, Clinical Applications.* London: Edward Arnold, 1989;363–374

154. Warkentin TE, Levine MN, Hirsh J, Horsewood P, Roberts RS, Gent M. Heparin-induced thrombocytopenia in patients treated with low-molecular-weight heparin or unfractionated heparin. *N Engl J Med* 1995;332:1330–1335.

155. Holmer E, Kurachi K, Soderstrom G. The molecular-weight dependence of the rate-enhancing effect of heparin on the inhibition of thrombin, factor Xa, factor IXa, factor XIa, factor XIIa and kallikrein by antithrombin. *Biochem J* 1981;193:395–400.

156. Holmer E, Soderberg K, Bergqvist D, Lindahl U. Heparin and its low molecular weight derivatives: anticoagulant and antithrombotic properties. *Haemostasis* 1986;16(suppl 2):1–7.

157. Bara L, Billaud E, Gramond G, Kher A, Samama M. Comparative pharmacokinetics of low molecular weight heparin (PK 10169) and unfractionated heparin after intravneous and subcutaneous administration. *Thromb Res* 1985;39:631–636.

158. Handeland GF, Abildgaard GF, Holm HA, Arnesen K-E. Dose adjusted heparin treatment of deep venous thrombosis: a comparison of unfractionated and low molecular weight heparin. *Eur J Clin Pharmacol* 1990;39:107–112.

159. Andriuolli G, Mastucchi R, Barnti M, Sarret M. Comparison of the antithrombotic and hemorrhagic effects of heparin and a new low molecular weight heparin in the rat. *Haemostasis* 1985;15:324–330.

160. Bergqvist D, Nilsson B, Hedner U, Pederson PC, Ostergaard PB. The effects of heparin fragments of different molecular weight in experimental thrombosis and haemostasis. *Thromb Res* 1985;38:589–601.

161. Cade JF, Buchanan MR, Boneu B, Ockelford P, Carter CJ, Cerskus ALH. A comparison of the antithrombotic and haemorrhagic effects of low molecular weight heparin fractions: The influence of the method of preparation. *Thromb Res* 1984;35:613–625.

162. Carter CJ, Kelton JG, Hirsh J, Cerskus A, Santos AV, Gent M. The relationship between the hemorrhagic and antithrombotic properties of low molecular weight heparins and heparin. *Blood* 1982;59:1239–1245.

163. Esquivel CO, Bergqvist D, Bjork C-G, Nilsson B. Comparison between commerical heparin, low-molecular weight heparin and pentosan polysulphate on haemostasis and platelets in vivo. *Thromb Res* 1982; 28:389–399.

164. Holmer E, Matsson C, Nilsson S. Anticoagulant and antithrombotic effects of low molecular weight heparin fragments in rabbits. *Thromb Res* 1982;25:475–485.

165. Ockelford PA, Carter CJ, Mitchell L, Hirsh J. Discordance between the anti-Xa activity and antithrombotic activity of an ultra-low molecular weight heparin fraction. *Thromb Res* 1982;28:401–409.

166. Barzu T, Molho P, Tobelem G, Petitou M, Caen JP. Binding of heparin and low molecular weight heparin fragments to human vascular endothelial cells in culture. *Nouv Rev Fr Haematol* 1984;26:243–247.

167. Barzu T, Van Rijn JLMC, Petitou M, Tobelem G, Caen JP. Heparin degradation in the endothelial cells. *Thromb Res* 1987;47:601–609.

168. Boneu B, Caranobe C, Cadroy Y, et al. Pharmacokinetic studies of standard unfractionated heparin, and low molecular weight heparins in the rabbit. *Semin Thromb Hemost* 1988;14:18–27.

169. Bradbrook ID, Magnani HN, Moelker HC, et al. ORG 10172: a low molecular weight heparinoid anticoagulant with a long half life in man. *Br J Clin Pharmacol* 1987;23:667–675.

170. Bratt G, Tornebohm E, Widlund L, Lockner D. Low molecular weight heparin (KABI 2165, FRAGMIN): pharmacokinetics after intravenous and subcutaneous administration in human volunteers. *Thromb Res* 1986;42:613–620.

171. Briant L, Caranobe C, Saivin S, Byrou B, Houin G, Boneu B. Unfractionated heparin and CY216. Pharmacokinetics and bioavailabilities of the anti-factor Xa and IIa. Effects of intravenous and subcutaneous injection in rabbits. *Thromb Haemost* 1989;61:348–353.

172. Frydman A, Bara L, Leroux Y, Woler M, Chauliac F, Samama M. The antithrombotic activity and pharmacokinetics of Enoxaparin, a low molecular weight heparin, in man given single subcutaneous doses of 20 up to 80 mg. *J Clin Pharmacol* 1988;28:608–618.

173. Matzsch T, Bergqvist D, Hedner U, Ostergaard P. Effect of an enzymatically depolymerized heparin as compared with conventional heparin in healthy volunteers. *Thromb Haemost* 1987;57:97–101.

174. Stiekema JC, Wijnand HP, Van Dinther TG, et al. Safety and pharmacokinetics of the low molecular weight heparinoid ORG 10172 administered to healthy elderly volunteers. *Br J Clin Pharmacol* 1989;27:39–48.

175. Caranobe C, Barret A, Gabaig AM, Dupouy D, Sie P, Boneu B. Disappearance of circulating anti-Xa activity after intravenous injection of unfractionated heparin and of low molecular weight heparin (CY216) in normal and nephrectomized rabbits. *Thromb Res* 1985;40:129–133.

176. Palm M, Mattsson CH. Pharmacokinetics of heparin and low molecular weight heparin fragment (Fragmin) in rabbits with impaired renal or metabolic clearance. *Thromb Haemost* 1987;58:932–935.

177. Boneu B, Buchanan MR, Cade JF, van Ryn J, Fernandez FF, Ofosu FAH. Effects of heparin, its low molecular weight fractions and other glycosaminoglycans on thrombus growth in vivo. *Thromb Res* 1985;40:81–89.

178. Henny CP, ten Cate H, ten Cate JW, et al. A randomized blind study comparing standard heparin and a new low molecular weight heparinoid in cardiopulmonary bypass surgery in dogs. *J Lab Clin Med* 1985;106:187–196.

179. Hobbelen PM, Vogel GM, Meuleman DG. Time courses of the antithrombotic effects, bleeding enhancing effects and interactions with factors Xa and thrombin after administration of low molecular weight he-

parinoid ORG 10172 or heparin to rats. *Thromb Res* 1987;48:549–558.

180. Van Ryn-McKenna J, Gray E, Weber E, et al. Effects of sulphated polysaccharides on inhibition of thrombus formation initiated by different stimuli. *Thromb Haemost* 1989;61:7–9.

181. Van Ryn-McKenna J, Ofosu FA, Hirsh J, Buchanan MR. Antithrombotic and bleeding effects of glycosaminoglycans with different degrees of sulfation. *Br J Haematol* 1989;71:265–269.

182. Fabris F, Fussi F, Casonato A, et al. Normal and low molecular weight heparins: interaction with human platelets. *Eur J Clin Invest* 1983;13:135–139.

183. Fernandez F, Nguyen P, Van Ryn J, Ofosu FA, Hirsh J, Buchanan MR. Hemorrhagic doses of heparin and other glycosaminoglycans induce a platelet defect. *Thromb Res* 1986;43:491–495.

184. Blajchman MA, Young E, Ofosu FA. Effects of unfractionated heparin, dermatan sulfate and low molecular weight on vessel wall permeability in rabbits. *Ann NY Acad Sci* 1989;556:245–254.

185. Mestre M, Clairefond P, Mardiguian J, Trillou M, Le Fur G, Uzan A. Comparative effects of heparin and PK 10169, a low molecular weight fraction, in a canine model of arterial thrombosis. *Thromb Res* 1985;38:389–399.

186. Cadroy Y, Harker LA, Hanson SR. Inhibition of platelet-dependent thrombosis by low molecular weight heparin (CY 222): comparison with standard heparin. *J Lab Clin Med* 1989;114:349–357.

187. Klein W, Buchwald A, Hillis SE, et al. Comparison of low molecular weight heparin with unfractionated heparin acutely and with placebo for 6 weeks in the management of unstable coronary artery disease—the Fragmin is unstable coronary artery disease study (FRIC). *Circulation* 1997;96:61–68.

188. FRISC Study Group. Low-molecular-weight heparin during instability in coronary artery disease. Fragmin during instability in Coronary Artery Disease (FRISC) study group. *Lancet* 1996;347:561–568.

189. Kay R, Sing Wong K, Yu YK, et al. Low molecular weight heparin for the treatment of acute ischemic stroke. *N Engl J Med* 1995;333:1588–1593.

190. Edmondson RA, Cohen AT, Das SK, et al. Low molecular weight heparin versus asprin and dipyridamole after femoropopliteal bypass grafting. *Lancet* 1994;344:914.

191. Cairns JA, Gill J, Morton B, et al., and the EMPAR Collaborators. Fish oils and low molecular weight heparin for the reduction of restenosis following percutaneous transluminal coronary angioplasty (PTCA). *Circulation* 1996;94:1553–1560.

192. Hirsh J, Levine MN. Low molecular weight heparin. *Blood* 1992;79:1–17.

193. Turpie AGG, Levine MN, Hirsh J, et al. A randomized controlled trial of a low molecular weight heparin (enoxaparin) to prevent deep vein thrombosis in patients undergoing elective hip surgery. *N Engl J Med* 1986;315:925–929.

194. Leclerc JR, Geerts WH, Desjardins L, et al. Prevention of deep vein thrombosis after major knee surgery. A randomized double-blind trial comparing a low molecular weight heparin fragment (enoxaparin) to placebo. *Thromb Haemost* 1992;67:417–423.

195. Hoek JA, Nurmohamed MT, Hamelynck KJ, et al. Prevention of deep vein thrombosis following total hip replacement by low molecular weight heparinoid. *Thromb Haemost* 1992;67:28–32.

196. Planes A, Vochelle N, Mazas F, et al. Prevention of postoperative venous thrombosis: a randomized trial comparing unfractionated heparin with low molecular weight heparin in patients undergoing total hip replacement. *Thromb Haemost* 1988;60:407–410.

197. Estoppey D, Hochreiter J, Breyer HG, et al. ORG 10172 (Lomoparin) versus heparin-DHE in prevention of thromboembolism in total hip replacement—a multicentre trial [Abstract]. *Thromb Haemost* 1989; 62(suppl):356.

198. Eriksson BI, Kalebo P, Anthmyr BA, Wadenvik H, Tengborn L, Risberg B. Prevention of deep vein thrombosis and pulmonary embolism after total hip replacement. *J Bone Joint Surg [Am]* 1991;73:484–493.

199. Hull R, Raskob G, Pineo G, et al. A comparison of subcutaneous low-molecular-weight heparin with sodium for prophylaxis against deep-vein thrombosis after hip or knee implantation. *N Engl J Med* 1993; 329:1370–1376.

200. RD Heparin Arthroplasty Group. RD Heparin compared with warfarin for prevention of venous thromboembolic disease following total hip or knee arthroplasty. *J Bone Joint Surg [Am]* 1994;76:1174–1185.

201. Leclerc JR, Geerts WH, Desjardins L, et al. Prevention of venous thromboembolism (VTE) after knee arthroplasty—a randomized double-blind trial, comparing enoxaparin to warfarin sodium [Abstract]. *Hemostasis* 1994;24(suppl 1):232.

202. Bergqvist D, Kettunen K, Fredin H, et al. Thromboprophylaxis in hip fracture patients—a prospective randomized comparative study between ORG 10172 and dextran. *Surgery* 1991;109:617–622.

203. Borris LC, Hauch O, Jorgensen LN, the Danish Enoxaparin Study Group. Low-molecular-weight heparin (enoxaparin) vs dextran 70. The prevention of postoperative deep vein thrombosis after total hip placement. *Arch Intern Med* 1991;151:1621–1624.

204. Gent M, Hirsh J, Ginsberg JS, et al. Low-molecular-weight heparinoid orgaran is more effective than aspirin in the prevention of venous thromboembolism after surgery of hip fracture. *Circulation* 1996;93:80–84.

205. Leyvraz PF, Bachmann F, Bohnet J, et al. Thromboembolic prophylaxis in total hip replacement: a comparison between the low molecular weight heparinoid lomoparan and heparin-dihydroergotamine. *Br J Surg* 1992;79:911–914.

206. Turpie AGG, Levine MN, Hirsh J, et al. A double-blind randomized trial of ORG 10172 low molecular weight heparinoid in the prevention of deep vein thrombosis in thrombotic stroke. *Lancet* 1987;1:523–526.

207. Prins MH, den Ottolander GJH, Gelsema R, van Woerkon TCM. Deep vein thrombosis prophylaxis with a low molecular weight heparin (Kabi 2165) in stroke patients [Abstract 418]. *Thromb Haemost* 1987;58(suppl 1):117.

208. Dahan R, Houlbert D, Caulin C, et al. Prevention of deep vein thrombosis in elderly medical patients by a low molecular weight heparin: a randomized double-blind trial. *Haemostasis* 1986;16:159–164.

209. Green D, Lee MY, Lim AC, et al. Prevention of thromboembolism after spinal cord injury using low molecular weight heparin. *Ann Intern Med* 1990;113:571–574.

210. Turpie AGG, Gent M, Cote R, et al. A low-molecular-weight heparinoid compared with unfractionated heparin in the prevention of deep vein thrombosis in patients with acute ischemic stroke. *Ann Intern Med* 1992;117:353–357.

211. Holm HA, Ly B, Handeland GF, et al. Subcutaneous heparin treatment of deep vein thrombosis: a comparison of unfractionated and low molecular weight heparin. *Haemostasis* 1986;16(suppl 2):30–37.

212. Faivre R, Neuhart E, Kieffer Y, et al. Subcutaneous administration of a low molecular weight heparin CY222 compared with subcutaneous administration of standard heparin in patients with acute deep vein thrombosis. *Thromb Haemost* 1987;58(suppl):430.

213. Bratt G, Tornebohm E, Granqvist S, Aberg W, Lockner D. A comparison between low molecular weight heparin Kabi 2165 and standard heparin in the intravenous treatment of deep vein thrombosis. *Thromb Haemost* 1985;85:813–817.

214. Bratt G, Aberg W, Johansson M, Tornebohm E, Granqvist S, Lockner D. Two daily subcutaneous injections of fragmin as compared with intravenous standard heparin in the treatment of deep venous thrombosis. *Thromb Haemost* 1990;64:506–510.

215. Duroux P, Beclere A. A randomized trial of subcutaneous low molecular weight heparin (CY216) compared with intravenous unfractionated heparin in the treatment of deep vein thrombosis. *Thromb Haemost* 1991;65:251–256.

216. Simonneau G. Subcutaneous fixed dose of enoxaparin versus intravenous adjusted dose of unfractionated heparin in the treatment of deep venous thrombosis. *Thromb Haemost* 1991;65(suppl):754.

217. Prandoni P, Lensing AWA, Buller HR, et al. Comparison of subcutaneous low-molecular-weight heparin with intravenous standard heparin in proximal deep-vein thrombosis. *Lancet* 1992;339:441–445.

218. Albada J, Nieuwenhuis HK, Sixma JJ. Treatment of acute venous thromboembolism with low molecular weight heparin. *Circulation* 1989;80:935–940.

219. Lensing AWA, Prins MH, Davidson BL, Hirsh J. Treatment of deep venous thrombosis with low-molecular-weight heparins. A meta-analysis. *Arch Intern Med* 1995;155:601–607.

220. Hull RD, Raskob GE, Pineo GF, et al. Subcutaneous low-molecular weight heparin compared with continuous intravenous heparin in the treatment of proximal-vein thrombosis. *N Engl J Med* 1992;326:975–982.

221. Levine M, Gent M, Hirsh J, et al. A comparison of low molecular weight heparin administered primarily at home with unfractionated heparin administered in the hospital for proximal deep vein thrombosis. *N Engl J Med* 1996;334:677–681.

222. Koopman MMW, Prandoni P, Piovella F, et al. Treatment of venous thrombosis with intravenous unfractionated heparin administered in the hospital as compared with subcutaneous low-molecular-weight heparin administered at home. *N Engl J Med* 1996;334:682–687.

223. Pini M, Alello S, Manotti C, et al. Low molecular weight heparin versus warfarin in the prevention of recurrences after deep vein thrombosis. *Thromb Haemost* 1994;72:191–197.

224. Cohen M, Demers C, Gurfinkel E, Fromell F, Langer A, Turpie AGG, ESSENCE Group. Primary end point analysis from the ESSENCE Trial: enoxaparin vs unfractionated heparin in unstable angina and non–Q wave infarction. *Circulation* 1996;94(suppl I):554.

225. Vitoux JF, Mathieu JF, Roncato M, et al. Heparin associated thrombocytopenia: treatment with low molecular weight heparin. *Thromb Haemost* 1986;55:37.

226. Magnani H. Heparin-induced thrombocytopenia (HIT): an overview of 230 patients treated with Organan (Org 10172). *Thromb Haemost* 1993;70:554–561.

227. Shaughnessy SG, Young E, Deschamps P, Hirsh J. The effects of low molecular weight and standard heparin on calcium loss from fetal rat calvaria. *Blood* 1995;86:1368–1373.

228. Melissari E, Parker CJ, Wilson NV, et al. Use of low molecular weight heparin in pregnancy. *Thromb Haemost* 1992;68:652–656.

229. Monreal M, Lafoz E, Olive A, del Rio L, Vedia C. Comparison of subcutaneous unfractionated heparin with a low molecular weight heparin (fragmin) in patients with venous thromboembolism and contraindications to coumarin. *Thromb Haemost* 1994;71:7–11.

230. Van Ryn-McKenna J, Cai L, Ofosu FA, Hirsh J, Buchanan MR. Neutralization of enoxaparine induced bleeding by protamine sulfate. *Thromb Haemost* 1990;63:271–274.

231. Massonet-Castel S, Pelissier E, Bara L, et al. Partial reversal of low molecular weight heparin (PK 10169) anti Xa activity by protamine sulfate: in vitro and in vivo study during cardiac surgery with extracorporeal circulation. *Haemostasis* 1986;16:139–146.

232. Harenberg J, Wurzner B, Zimmermann R, Schettler G. Bioavailability and antagonization of the low molecular weight heparin CY 216 in man. *Thromb Res* 1986;44:549–554.

233. Racanelli A, Fareed J, Walenga JM, et al. Biochemical and pharmacologic studies on the protamine interactions with heparin, its fractions and fragments. *Semin Thromb Hemost* 1985;11:176–189.

234. Ginsberg JS, Hirsh J, Levine MN, Burrows R. Risk to the fetus of anticoagulant therapy during pregnancy. *Thromb Haemost* 1989;61:197–203.

235. Forestier F, Daffos F, Capella-Pavlovsky M. Low molecular weight heparin (PK 10169) does not cross the placenta during the second trimester of pregnancy: study by direct fetal blood sampling under ultrasound. *Thromb Res* 1984;34:557–560.

236. Forestier F, Daffos F, Rainaut M, Toulemonde F. Low molecular weight heparin (CY 216) does not cross the placenta during the third trimester of pregnancy. *Thromb Haemost* 1987;57:234.

237. Omri A, Delaloye JF, Andersen H, Bachmann F. Low molecular weight heparin NOVO (LHN-1) does not cross the placenta during the second trimester of pregnancy. *Thromb Haemost* 1989;61:55–56.

*Cardiovascular Thrombosis: Thrombocardiology
and Thromboneurology, Second Edition,*
edited by M. Verstraete, V. Fuster, and E. J. Topol,
Lippincott–Raven Publishers, Philadelphia © 1998.

12

Heparinoids

Walter Ageno and Alexander G. G. Turpie

*Department of Medicine, McMaster University,
Hamilton, Ontario L8L 2X2, Canada*

DANAPAROID

Chemistry

Danaparoid (Lomoparan, Orgaran, ORG 10172) is a low molecular weight heparinoid with antithrombotic activity similar to that of heparins. It is a mixture of glycosaminoglycans derived from porcine intestinal mucosa with an average molecular weight of approximately 6,000 daltons and it consists mainly of heparan sulphate (84%), a small quantity of dermatan sulphate (12%), and a little chondroitin-4- and chondroitin-6-sulphate (4%) (Table 12-1). The glycosaminoglycans in danaparoid are composed of repeating dimer units consisting of uronic acid, glucosamine and galactosamine in varying degrees of sulphation and acetylation (1). Compared with heparin, danaparoid has a lower degree of sulphation and a lower charge density, which is assumed to be relevant for its pharmacologic profile (2). Both factors play an important role in the binding to plasma proteins and blood platelets and, thus, in its pharmacologic properties. The difference in chemical composition is reflected by the structural dissimilarity of the major repeating units of the polysaccharide chains: the major repeating unit of

heparan sulphate, the principal component of danaparoid, contains mostly glucuronic acid, whereas iduronic acid 2-sulphate predominates in heparin and low molecular weight heparins (LMWH) (3). Danaparoid contains mostly N-acetyl-glucosamine, whereas heparin and LMWH contain mainly glucosamine-N-sulphate; moreover, neither heparin nor LMWH contain galactosamine (4).

Anticoagulant Profile of Danaparoid

Danaparoid exerts its anticoagulant effect by catalyzing serine protease inhibitors (serpins), which are the endogenous inhibitors of activated coagulation factors. Its individual components have different affinities for serpins: a heparan sulphate fraction with high affinity for antithrombin III (AT III) acts via selective inhibition of factor Xa; the heparan sulphate fraction with low affinity for AT III lacks effects on coagulation factors Xa and IIa, but contributes significantly to the antithrombotic activity, most likely by an endothelial cellular mechanism; dermatan sulphate contributes to the antithrombotic activity of danaparoid by its catalyzing effect on thrombin inactivation via heparin cofactor

TABLE 12-1. *Characteristics of danaparoid*

Constituents	
Heparan sulphate	84%
Dermatan sulphate	12%
Chondroitin sulphate	4%
Specific anti-Xa activity	14 U/mg
Specific anti-IIa activity	<0.5 U/mg
Mean molecular weight	6,000 daltons

II (HC II) (5). Danaparoid exerts a stronger catalytic effect on the inactivation of factor Xa than on the inactivation of thrombin, with an antifactor Xa/antithrombin ratio of greater than 28 (6). On a weight basis, the potency of danaparoid with respect to factor Xa inactivation is approximately 10% of that of heparin and less than 1% with respect to thrombin inactivation (1). Nonanticoagulant plasma proteins such as histidine-rich glycoprotein, vitronectin, and platelet factor 4 may interact with unfractionated heparin in plasma to modulate its anticoagulant activity, whereas histidine-rich glycoprotein is the only plasma protein likely to affect the efficacy of danaparoid by direct competition with AT III. Nevertheless danaparoid appears to be more resistant to its neutralization than unfractionated heparin (7).

Effect on Experimental Models

Danaparoid exerts antithrombotic effects in a variety of experimental thrombosis models. In the stasis models, experimental thrombosis is produced by a combination of venous stasis and a hypercoagulable state (6). Such models result in the generation of a thrombus consisting almost exclusively of red cells enmeshed in fibrin. Vogel et al. (8) have compared the antithrombotic effects of danaparoid with those of heparin in a rat venous stasis model and found that danaparoid, heparin, and LMWH had similar antithrombotic activity with identical dose-response curves. Boneu et al. (9) demonstrated that danaparoid was superior to both heparin and LMWH in inhibiting the extension of established venous thrombi in rabbits. This effect may partly explain the high efficacy of danaparoid in conditions in which the thrombogenic stimulus precedes the initial dose, such as fractured hip surgery (6). Meuleman et al. (10) found that danaparoid in an arteriovenous shunt model in rats inhibited thrombus formation in a dose-dependent manner and displayed an antithrombotic activity that was on a basis of anti-Xa activity comparable to that of commercial unfractionated heparin (10). The thrombi formed in this model consisted of a blood platelet core surrounded by a fibrin-rich clotlike extension, induced by contact of the circulating blood with a nonhematocompatible surface in the shunt. Commercial heparin reduced the blood platelet and the fibrin content in these thrombi, whereas danaparoid primarily reduced the fibrin content, leaving the blood platelet deposition undisturbed even at much higher doses. Using a similar model, Vogel et al. (11) compared heparin and danaparoid by measuring thrombus weight, the number of platelets adhered to the thrombus, and thrombus-induced thrombin generation. At a dose of 80 anti-Xa U/kg intravenously (i.v.) both compounds inhibited thrombus growth after 15 minutes by 30% and inhibited a systemic decrease of 27% of platelet numbers in the placebo group by 63%. After 45 minutes, thrombi that had formed in the presence of danaparoid, but not in the presence of heparin, became less thrombogenic or nonthrombogenic as reflected by inhibition of the local deposition of platelets and of ex vivo thrombus-induced thrombin generation. The suppression of the local thrombin generation potency is correlated more with thrombus growth than systemic anticoagulant activity. According to Vogel, this suppression is likely to be due to the anti-Xa activity. Moreover, the loss of activity of heparin during the development of the thrombus can be explained by local neutralization by platelet factor 4 (PF 4) released by activated platelets. PF 4 does not reduce the activity of danaparoid because only mainly large molecules are affected. Using an in vitro thrombosis model, which contains exclusively human materials, Lozano et al. (12) found a more potent antithrombotic effect with danaparoid than with two different

LMWH. They suggested that this may be due to the presence of dermatan sulphate, because dermatan sulphate–heparin cofactor II complexes are able to inhibit thrombin adsorbed to fibrin, whereas antithrombin III–heparin complexes cannot accomplish this.

Danaparoid was also compared with both heparin and LMWH in a number of animal bleeding models. Using the rabbit ear bleeding model, Cade et al. (13) demonstrated that danaparoid caused significantly less bleeding than either heparin or LMWH at equivalent antithrombotic doses. After i.v. administration of 3,200 anti-Xa U/kg of danaparoid, approximately a two-fold increase in blood loss over placebo control was seen, whereas 400 anti-Xa U/kg of heparin gave a tenfold increase in blood loss over control. Using a modification of the rabbit ear bleeding model, Nurmohamed et al. (5) showed that danaparoid, given i.v. at dosages of up to five times those used to obtain effective antithrombotic activity, has only minor effect on blood loss. Using experimental bleeding models in rats, Meuleman et al. (10) demonstrated that after i.v. equipotent antithrombotic doses, danaparoid had less hemorrhagic activity than did commercial heparin. Meuleman demonstrated that to achieve a twofold increase in blood loss compared with placebo, a fourfold higher i.v. dose of danaparoid than of heparin was needed.

The improved benefit to risk ratio of danaparoid may be due to the difference in anticoagulant profile because danaparoid inhibits thrombin generation linearly over a much broader concentration range than heparin and LMWH. It is also probably due to the lack of effect on normal blood platelet function.

Effect on Platelets

It has been demonstrated that heparin impairs the formation of primary hemostatic plugs in rats and human volunteers and retards the degranulation process. Danaparoid has minimal effects on physiologic platelet function, and it does not affect degranulation. Meuleman et al. (14) investigated the effects

of danaparoid and heparin in the rat arteriovenous shunt model. At effective antithrombotic doses, heparin inhibited blood platelet deposition, but danaparoid had only a marginal effect. This minimal effect on hemostatic plug formation is probably due to its lower direct anti-IIa activity compared with heparin. In healthy volunteers, bleeding time was significantly prolonged 10 minutes after i.v. injection of heparin, but not after danaparoid administration (15). Both platelet aggregation and thromboxane A2 release, in response to several agonists or even in the absence of any aggregating agent, were enhanced after heparin but not after danaparoid administration. Lozano et al. (12) studied the effect of danaparoid on platelet adhesion in an in vitro model and found high platelet adhesion apparently not due to a direct effect on platelet adhesion, but to a lower microaggregate formation as compared with heparin. Nurmohamed et al. (5) tested the activity of danaparoid in the heparin-induced platelet activation (HIPA) and heparin-induced thrombocytopenia screening (HIT) systems. The HIPA system tests platelet aggregation/agglutination in the presence of an antithrombotic agent. The HIT system tests platelet aggregation/agglutination in the presence of HIT-positive (heparin) serum and an antithrombotic agent. Danaparoid produced relatively weak effects in the two test systems in comparison with heparin. Heparin also may cause HIT, which occasionally results in severe or life-threatening paradoxic thromboembolic complications. Danaparoid has been reported to be relatively safe in such patients because its cross-reactivity rate with heparin-dependent antibodies is about 12% in contrast to a rate of 88% observed with LMWH (16).

Toxicology

Toxicity of danaparoid has been studied on both rats and dogs and has been shown to be low (14). In rats, the lethal dose$_{50}$ (LD$_{50}$) after a single subcutaneous (s.c.) injection is approximately 15,200 anti-Xa U/kg, and in dogs, i.v. doses up to 28,000 anti-Xa U/kg are well tolerated without significant adverse effects. Danaparoid administered to both rats and dogs i.v. for 6 months or s.c. for 6 weeks at doses of 1,600 anti-Xa U/kg/day has also shown to be nontoxic. Administration of danaparoid to pregnant female rabbits does not exacerbate postimplantation fetal loss or produce teratogenicity. The treatment with danaparoid of sexually mature female rats did not affect fertility, gestation, or fetal growth in utero. Thus, danaparoid appears to be free of any embryotoxic or teratogenic effects in experimental animals (14).

Pharmacokinetic Profile

Because of its compositional heterogeneity, there are no simple assay methods to directly measure danaparoid in plasma. Standard coagulation tests, such as activated partial thromboplastin time (APTT), prothrombin time (PT), and thrombin time (TT), are of little value because, at therapeutic dosages, danaparoid has only a minimal effect on these tests. The pharmacokinetics of danaparoid have thus been studied by monitoring the kinetics of its biologic activities by measurement of plasma anti-Xa activity, plasma anti-IIa activity, or thrombin generation inhibition (TGI) (17).

Absorption

The absorption phase of plasma anti-Xa activity in humans after s.c. injection of danaparoid is relatively rapid (absorption half-life 2 to 3 hours). Peak plasma anti-Xa levels occur within approximately 4 to 5 hours (Table 12-2), and maximum thrombin generation inhibition activity is reached 2 to 3 hours after injection (18). Much less pronounced differences between peak and trough concentrations are observed after s.c. administration compared with i.v. administration. This is considered advantageous because high peak levels immediately after administration might be associated with an increased bleeding risk. After both i.v. or s.c. administration, danaparoid shows linear kinetics, which contrasts

TABLE 12-2. *Pharmacokinetic parameters of danaparoid*

Anti-Xa activity	
Peak plasma levels	4–5 hr
Elimination half-life	25 hr
Volume of distribution	9 L
Anti-IIa activity	
Peak plasma levels	2–3 hr
Elimination half-life	4 hr
Volume of distribution	9 L
IIa generation inhibition	
Peak plasma levels	2–3 hr
Elimination half-life	7 hr
Volume of distribution	17 L

with the nonlinear pharmacokinetics of heparin (19). This property of danaparoid offers more predictable plasma levels in clinical practice.

Bioavailability

In humans, the bioavailability of danaparoid after s.c. administration is almost 100%, in striking contrast with unfractionated heparin, which has a bioavailability of only 20% to 30% after s.c. injection, with considerable intraindividual and interindividual variation (20,21). In addition, in contrast with heparin, heparin neutralizing factor does not neutralize danaparoid. The result of a complete bioavailability is a lower variability in the plasma levels after s.c. administration, thus suggesting that danaparoid may have a clinical advantage over heparin.

Distribution

Danaparoid has a total distribution volume of its anti-Xa activity of approximately 9 L (20).

Elimination

The kidney has a predominant role in clearing danaparoid from the circulation, accounting for at least 40% to 50% of the total plasma clearance of its anti-Xa activity (19). The importance of renal excretion has been confirmed in renal failure patients on long-term hemodialysis in whom accumulation of danaparoid has been reported. Consequently, danaparoid is contraindicated in patients with severely impaired renal function. In animal studies, it has been clearly demonstrated that the liver is not involved in the metabolism of the fraction of danaparoid displaying anti-Xa activity. Also, in humans, the disposition of danaparoid appears to be relatively insensitive to changes in hepatic function (22). The elimination half-life of anti-Xa activity is approximately 25 hours, and the elimination half-life of anti-IIa activity is approximately 4 hours. The thrombin generation-inhibiting activity is eliminated with a half-life of approximately 7 hours (18) (Table 12-2). Although these data suggest that once-daily dosing with danaparoid may be sufficient, clinical experience has shown that twice-daily dosing is optimal for danaparoid. Pharmacokinetically, this can be correlated with the relatively rapid elimination of some of the components of danaparoid. Because the antithrombotic effect of danaparoid is the result of a complex interaction between its various components, they all need to be present in sufficient concentration.

Drug Interactions

No significant interactions have been observed when danaparoid was administered in association with other drugs. Interaction studies included drugs selected on the basis of their effects on hemostasis (i.e., acetylsalicilic acid, acenocumarol, ticarcillin, cloxacillin) (23–25) or their frequency of use (i.e. digoxin, chlortalidone) (26,27).

Antidote

Danaparoid has minimal bleeding-enhancing effects when it is used in the prophylaxis of DVT at a dosage of 750 anti-Xa units twice daily, thus bleeding problems have not been encountered. In surgery, severe bleeding is commonly associated with conditions related to the intervention rather than with danaparoid. The potential of protamine chloride on the effects of danaparoid has been tested in

healthy volunteers (28), and no neutralizing effects on the anti-Xa activity were seen, whereas a partial neutralizing effect on the anti-IIa and on the thrombin generation-inhibiting activity was observed. Also, no effects were seen on the prothrombin time, the APTT, and the bleeding time. Because protamine chloride itself can provoke serious adverse reactions, its use cannot be recommended. Therefore, in the rare event of unexpected severe bleeding, there is currently no specific fully active antidote to danaparoid.

Clinical Evaluation of Danaparoid

The safety and efficacy of danaparoid have been studied for the prophylaxis of deep vein thrombosis (DVT) in a number of large-scale trials in patients at high risk for venous thromboembolism (VTE) and bleeding.

Venous Thromboembolism Prophylaxis in Orthopedic Surgery

DVT and fatal pulmonary embolism (PE) are a common complication in major orthopedic surgery, with an incidence of DVT between 45% and 70% in the absence of prophylaxis, and an incidence of fatal PE of approximately 1% to 3% (29). Fracture of the hip is one of the highest risk settings for the development of DVT and PE. The high-risk period for developing venous thrombosis begins with the initial trauma itself, and subsequently the trauma caused by the surgical procedure increases the overall risk. DVT can occur to approximately 50% of hip fracture patients undergoing surgery without appropriate prophylaxis. The high incidence of fatal PE poses a special problem: in the absence of prophylaxis, fatal PE occurs in 5.9% to 7.5% of these patients (30).

Danaparoid has been investigated for the prevention of DVT and PE in four studies in fractured hip surgery (Table 12-3). In all studies it was given s.c. twice daily at a dose of 750 anti-Xa units. The first study was reported by Bergqvist et al. (31). Danaparoid

TABLE 12-3. *Randomized trials of danaparoid in preventing DVT following fractured hip surgery*

	Total DVT	Proximal DVT
Bergqvist et al. (1991)		
Danaparoid	13.1%	4.7%
Dextran	34.8%	8.7%
Gerhardt et al. (1991)		
Danaparoid	7.0%	2.3%
Warfarin	21.0%	5.4%
Roise et al. (1993)		
Danaparoid	5.7%	3.8%
Fragmin	8.8%	5.3%
Clexane	15.4%	3.8%
	Total VTE	Proximal DVT/PE
Gent et al. (1996)		
Danaparoid	27.8%	6.8%
Aspirin	44.3%	14.3%

was compared with dextran in a randomized assessor-blind study. Study drugs were started preoperatively immediately after admission, and danaparoid prophylaxis was continued until day 10 to 12. DVT was diagnosed by bilateral venography performed in all patients at the end of the study period or earlier if detected by fibrinogen leg scanning. DVT occurred in 14 (13.1%) of 107 patients receiving danaparoid compared with 40 (34.8%) of 115 patients given dextran (p < 0.001). Proximal DVT occurred in 4.7% of the patients on danaparoid and in 8.7% of the patients on dextran. PE occurred in 3.1% and 0% in the dextran and danaparoid groups, respectively. The frequency of postoperative transfusions was significantly greater (p < 0.01) in the dextran group, and no other differences were found in the various bleeding parameters. The second study, reported by Gerhart et al., compared danaparoid with warfarin (32). Both drugs were begun preoperatively after admission. One group received danaparoid until the ninth postoperative day, plus warfarin added to the regimen on the seventh postoperative day and continued until discharge. The other group received only warfarin for 14 days. DVT was assessed by fibrinogen leg scanning and impedance plethysmography and confirmed whenever possible by ultrasound or

venogram. DVT was reduced from 21% in the warfarin alone group to 7% in the danaparoid plus warfarin group (p < 0.001). Proximal vein thrombosis was reduced from 5.4% in the warfarin group to 2.3% in the danaparoid group; 6% of patients in this latter group suffered major bleeding episodes, 3.8% in the warfarin group. There was no difference in intraoperative blood loss or transfusion requirements between the two treatment groups.

The third study was performed by Gent et al. and compared danaparoid with aspirin (33). Both regimens were started 12 to 24 hours after surgery and continued for 14 days. All patients had postoperative fibrinogen leg scanning and impedance plethysmography, plus venography if one or both tests were positive. Otherwise, venography was performed at day 14. VTE was reduced from 44.3% in the aspirin group to 27.8% in the danaparoid group (p = 0.028). Proximal DVT or PE occurred in 6.8% of the patients in the danaparoid group and 14.3% in the aspirin group (p = 0.137). Hemorrhagic complications occurred in 1.6% of the danaparoid group and in 6.4% in the aspirin group. In a pilot study, Roise et al. (34) compared danaparoid with two LMWH, dalteparin (5,000 IU once daily) and enoxaparin (40 mg once daily). All treatments started preoperatively and continued for 10 days. Bilateral venography was performed on all patients at study exit. DVT was detected in 15.4% of patients in the enoxaparin group, 8.8% of patients from the dalteparin group and 5.7% of patients from the danaparoid group. No difference within the three groups was found for proximal DVT and no PEs were detected.

Total hip replacement surgery is associated with a high incidence of thromboembolic complications. In the absence of prophylaxis there is a 40% to 60% incidence of calf vein thrombosis, a 20% incidence of proximal vein thrombosis, and a 1% to 5% incidence of fatal PE (35). This high incidence of proximal vein thrombosis is thought to result from the intraoperative manipulation of the leg, which causes local vessel wall damage and stasis (36). Three studies evaluated the efficacy and safety of danaparoid for the prevention of VTE in such patients (Table 12-4). Hoek et al. (37) randomized 196 patients to receive either 750 anti-Xa units of danaparoid s.c. twice daily or placebo. Treatment was started 15 to 45 minutes before anesthesia and continued until the tenth postoperative day. All patients underwent bilateral venography around day 10. Incidence of DVT was reduced from 56.6% in the placebo group to 15.5% in the danaparoid-treated patients (p < 0.0001); proximal DVT was reduced from 25.3% to 8.2% in the danaparoid group (p < 0.005). No major bleeding complications were reported, but 6.2% of the patients in the danaparoid group developed wound hematomas, although they were minor and none required surgical intervention. Leyvraz et al. (38) compared danaparoid (750 anti-Xa units s.c. twice daily) to unfractionated heparin (5,000 units s.c. twice daily) plus dihydroergotamine (DHE; 0.5 mg twice daily) in 284 patients. The initial dose was administered 2 hours before surgery and treatment was continued until the tenth postoperative day. Bilateral venography was performed on all patients around day 10. DVT occurred in 17% of the patients in the danaparoid group and in 32% of the patients receiving heparin–DHE (p < 0.007). The frequency of proximal DVT was 4.8% in the danaparoid group and 6.5% in the heparin-DHE group. Major bleeding occurred in one patient from each group. Danaparoid (750 anti-Xa units) and heparin (5,000 IU), both administered s.c. twice daily, were compared by Agnelli et al. (39) in the prevention

of DVT in 174 patients undergoing elective hip replacement. Treatment was started 2 hours before surgery and continued for approximately 10 days. Bilateral venography was performed on all patients around day 10. DVT was diagnosed in 36.3% of patients treated with heparin, and in 20.9% of patients in the danaparoid group (p = 0.038). Proximal DVT was observed in 17% of the patients in the heparin group and in 8% of the patients treated with danaparoid (p = 0.12). However, there was no significant difference in the bleeding parameters between the two groups.

Abdominothoracic Surgery for Cancer

Patients who undergo surgery for malignant disease are at high risk for VTE. Danaparoid given in a dose of 750 anti-Xa units twice daily s.c. was shown to be as effective as 5,000 units of unfractionated heparin given three times daily s.c. in the prevention of DVT in a prospective, single-blind, randomized study of 121 patients undergoing surgery for gastrointestinal tract cancer reported by Blum et al. (40). DVT was detected in 11% of the patients in the danaparoid group and in 10% of the patients treated with heparin, and no significant differences in bleeding complications were reported. Gallus et al. (41) randomized 490 patients undergoing elective surgery for malignant abdominal or thoracic disease to receive either heparin (5,000 U) or danaparoid (750 anti-Xa units) s.c. twice daily. Treatment was started 1 to 2 hours before surgery and was continued for 6 days. The incidence of DVT was 14.9% in the former group and 10.4% in the latter, a trend that was not statistically significant (p > 0.1). There was no difference in bleeding complications between the two study groups.

Ischemic Stroke Patients

VTE is a common complication in patients with acute ischemic stroke. Without prophylaxis, DVT occurs in 60% to 70% of patients with dense hemiplegia and 1% to 2% suffer fatal PE (42). Three studies evaluated the ef-

TABLE 12-4. *Randomized trials of danaparoid in preventing DVT following elective hip surgery*

	Total DVT	Proximal DVT
Hoek et al. (1992)		
Danaparoid	15.5%	8.2%
Placebo	56.6%	25.3%
Leyvraz et al. (1992)		
Danaparoid	17.0%	4.8%
Heparin/DHE	32.0%	6.5%
Agnelli et al. (1995)		
Danaparoid	20.9%	8.0%
Heparin	36.3%	17.0%

ficacy and safety of danaparoid in preventing VTE in patients with acute nonhemorrhagic stroke (Table 12-5). In the two studies performed by Turpie et al. (43,44), danaparoid was given in doses of 750 anti-Xa units twice daily s.c. (43,44). The first study (43), with a group of 75 patients, was placebo controlled, and DVT was detected by fibrinogen leg scanning and impedance plethysmography, followed by venography when either test was positive. Prophylaxis was started within 7 days of onset of stroke, and a loading dose of 1,000 anti-Xa units given i.v. preceded the s.c. administration. Treatment was continued for 14 days. In this study the incidence of DVT was reduced from 28% of the patients in the placebo group to 4% of patients in the danaparoid group (p < 0.005). Proximal DVT occurred, respectively, in 16% and 0%. One major and one minor hemorrhage occurred in the danaparoid group and in the placebo-treated patients, respectively. In the second study (44), danaparoid was compared with unfractionated heparin (5,000 U s.c. twice daily), and DVT was detected by fibrinogen leg scanning and confirmed by ascending venography. Eighty-seven patients with marked lower limb paralysis secondary to stroke were randomized and treated for up to 14 days. DVT occurred in 31% in the heparin-treated group and 8.9% in the danaparoid group (p = 0.014), and the corresponding rates of proximal DVT were 11.9% and 4.4%, respectively (p = 0.255). There was no significant difference in the frequency of bleeding complications in the two groups. A third study was performed

by Dumas et al. (45) in 175 patients with limb paresis after acute ischemic stroke. Danaparoid given s.c. once daily at a dose of 1,250 anti-Xa units was compared to standard heparin (5,000 IU s.c. twice daily) in preventing DVT. Prophylaxis started within 72 hours of the onset of stroke and continued for approximately 9 days. Patients underwent daily fibrinogen leg scanning, which when positive was followed by venography. DVT was diagnosed in 14.6% of the patients in the danaparoid group and in 19.8% of the patients treated with heparin (p = 0.392). PE was diagnosed in one patient in each group. One major hemorrhage occurred in each group.

Treatment of Deep Vein Thrombosis

De Valk et al. (46) compared two s.c. doses of danaparoid with continuous i.v. administration of unfractionated heparin in the treatment of VTE on 209 patients. Low-dose danaparoid was given in an i.v. loading dose of 1,250 U followed by 1,250 U administered s.c. twice daily. High-dose danaparoid was given in an i.v. loading dose of 2,000 U followed by 2,000 U administered s.c. twice daily. A significant reduction in recurrence or extension of VTE was seen in patients receiving high-dose danaparoid (13%) compared with patients receiving heparin (28%), whereas occurrence of major and minor bleeding was similar in the three groups.

Treatment of Ischemic Stroke

Among the several therapies tested for the treatment of acute ischemic stroke, danaparoid has been evaluated in two pilot studies, and a large trial is currently underway in the United States. The two pilot studies performed were a phase I study, testing five escalating doses of danaparoid, and a phase II study, providing information about its safety and possible efficacy (47,48). In the first study with 26 patients, infusion rates were adjusted to achieve five target anti-Xa levels from 0.2 to 1.0 anti-Xa U/ml for 7 days. After the loading dose, plasma anti-Xa levels

TABLE 12-5. *Randomized trials of danaparoid in preventing DVT in ischemic stroke patients*

	Total DVT	Proximal DVT
Turpie et al. (1987)		
Danaparoid	4.0%	0%
Placebo	28.0%	16.0%
Turpie et al. (1992)		
Danaparoid	8.9%	4.4%
Heparin	31.0%	11.9%
Dumas et al. (1994)		
Danaparoid	14.6%	5.6%
Heparin	19.8%	9.3%

reached target levels, but after starting the maintenance infusion, levels decreased to a nadir at 6 hours. Thereafter, the levels of inhibition gradually increased over the next 4 days to reattain postloading dose levels. Thus, danaparoid administered i.v. demonstrated a multicompartmental kinetic profile. The second study in 57 patients was designed to achieve steady-state plasma anti-Xa activity of 0.8 U/ml from the beginning of the 7-day treatment period. This study confirmed that the treatment regimen could achieve the desired levels, and although patients still required dosage adjustments, the decline of anti-Xa levels after bolus administration was avoided, and the mean daily levels of anti-Xa activity remained relatively constant in a range of 0.5 to 0.8 U/ml. Four patients had minor bleeding episodes that did not require stopping of the infusion. Severe bleeding episodes that required discontinuation of the study drug developed in three patients. Three months after the stroke, 37 patients (65%) had a favorable outcome. The randomized, double-blind, placebo-controlled trial of Org 10172 in Acute Stroke Treatment (TOAST) is now involving 20 major medical centers in the United States and it is designed to enroll 1,300 patients in order to detect a 20% improvement in stroke outcome.

Danaparoid in Heparin-Induced Thrombocytopenia

HIT is a well-recognized complication of heparin therapy. It is an immune disorder mediated by an immunoglobulin G (IgG) heparin-dependent antibody, with an incidence of approximately 1% to 3% (49). Recent studies suggest that 30% to 90% of patients with HIT develop paradoxic thrombosis. The definitive treatment of HIT remains controversial. Heparin should be stopped even if the patients have a recent thrombosis requiring continuing anticoagulant therapy (50). Anticoagulation with vitamin K antagonists may be inadequate due to the delayed action of warfarin. Moreover, several HIT patients were observed with venous limb gangrene while on warfarin, prob-

ably for a variant of the warfarin-induced skin necrosis syndrome. LMWH have shown to be highly cross-reactive (80% to 90%) with HIT-IgG (49). Because danaparoid structure is devoid of any heparin component, danaparoid has been proposed as a useful antithrombotic agent in HIT patients. Several observations have been reported on danaparoid cross-reactivity with IgG and on its safety and efficacy in such patients. Chong et al. (50) reported 57 patients with suspected HIT treated with danaparoid for arterial or venous thrombosis, prophylaxis for VTE, hemodialysis, and anticoagulation for vascular surgery or plasmapheresis. All but one patient had resolution of thrombocytopenia, and five major bleeds and two deaths likely to be related to HIT were observed. An overview of 230 patients with HIT treated with danaparoid was performed by Magnani (51). A 92.8% success rate was reported, and the mortality rate in such patients was reduced from 30% to 5.1%, whereas 3% of danaparoid-related deaths due to bleeding, thrombosis, and septic shock were observed. Ortel et al. (52) treated six HIT patients with danaparoid who required primary treatment for specific medical problems (n = 4 patients) or anticoagulation during a surgical procedure (n = 2 patients). Neither exacerbation of thrombocytopenia nor thromboembolic complications were reported. Three patients had sustained hemorrhagic complications. Danaparoid was used to treat or to prevent thrombosis in 10 HIT patients, three of whom had presented 4 to 6 years earlier, in a study by Tardy-Poncet et al (53). One patient did not recover completely from thrombocytopenia, one had recurrent HIT, and one experienced minor bleeding. Vun et al. (54) compared three LMWH (dalteparin, enoxaparin, nadroparin) and danaparoid in their cross-reactivity rates with the HIT antibody and found a 7% reactivity rate for danaparoid and 89%, 83%, and 86% reactivity rates, respectively, for dalteparin, enoxaparin, and nadroparin.

Danaparoid also has been used in the prevention of recurrent VTE in a patient with hereditary antithrombin III deficiency who developed HIT and disseminated intravascular coagulation after heparin administration in the first weeks of pregnancy (55). After warfarin therapy from the 14th week, danaparoid was started at the 36th week of gestation and continued to the fourth day postpartum, when warfarin was restarted. No hemostatic abnormalities or symptoms of thromboembolic complications were encountered while on danaparoid treatment.

Additional Clinical Applications

Several case reports and small uncontrolled studies provide data on the application of danaparoid in a variety of thrombotic disorders.

Danaparoid has been shown to be safe and effective in hemodialysis patients, although with some limitations. Henny et al. (56) used danaparoid during 55 hemodialysis sessions in 12 patients with acute renal failure and at high risk for bleeding. No fibrin depositions were noted on the dialysis membranes and no hemorrhagic complications occurred. Frei et al. (21) compared danaparoid with heparin in 14 patients with chronic renal failure. No significant difference was found in blood loss or dialyzer blood retention, but the mean half-life of anti-Xa activity of danaparoid was almost double the value found in healthy volunteers. This is indeed an important limit to the use of heparinoids in patients with renal failure.

Ten Cate et al. (57) assessed s.c. danaparoid in patients undergoing transurethral resection of the prostate (TURP) and found dose-dependent postoperative bleeding. In a placebo-controlled study on 48 patients, Gallus et al. (58) measured the effects of danaparoid in prophylactic doses on blood loss after TURP. There was no increased perioperative blood loss, but danaparoid caused more urinary bleeding after surgery than did placebo.

Ten Cate et al. (59) gave i.v. danaparoid to four patients with intracerebral hematoma and DVT and one patient with a large hemorrhagic infarct and a left ventricular thrombus. One patient died as a result of status epilecticus and had an unexplained decrease in hemoglobin level. The other four patients had resolution of their thrombi without bleeding complications.

Four patients with acute promyelocytic leukemia and clinical and laboratory manifestations of disseminated intravascular coagulation were treated by Nieuwenhuis and Sixma during induction chemotherapy with danaparoid (60). Bleeding symptoms ceased and fibrinogen levels improved in the first week in all patients, and two patients developed bleeding due to primary fibrinolysis in the second week.

DERMATAN SULPHATE

Dermatan sulphate is a natural glycosaminoglycan that catalyzes thrombin inhibition by heparin cofactor II. Whereas antithrombin inactivates thrombin and activated factors X and IX, heparin cofactor II exclusively inhibits thrombin, thus exerting a selective antithrombin activity and a reduced influence on conventional coagulation tests (61). In vitro studies found dermatan sulphate being a more potent inhibitor of thrombin bound to fibrin than heparins. Experimental studies on animals showed the effectiveness of dermatan sulphate in preventing thrombosis and inhibiting further growth of an existing thrombus. Moreover, bleeding complications were found to be remarkably low (62,63).

Van Ryn-McKenna et al. (64) studied the use of dermatan sulphate after thrombolysis in a rabbit model of arterial thrombosis. Several clinical studies suggested that the patency rate achieved with thrombolytic therapy is greater in those patients who receive tissue plasminogen activator (t-PA) plus heparin than in those patients who receive t-PA alone. Heparin acceleration of thrombin inhibition by antithrombin prevents thrombus growth, allowing for more rapid thrombolysis by t-PA. Because dermatan sulphate has been shown to prevent fibrin accretion and subsequent thrombus growth more effectively than heparin, the Canadian group compared heparin with dermatan sulphate after t-PA–induced fibrinolysis. They concluded that both drugs enhanced t-PA–induced thrombolysis, but heparin also enhanced bleeding, whereas dermatan sulphate did not.

The first clinical trial aimed to assess the efficacy and safety of dermatan sulphate in the prevention of DVT in hip fracture was performed by Agnelli et al. (65). Two dosage regimens were evaluated in two consecutive study phases, the treatment was started within 48 hours from the trauma and continued for 14 days for patients not undergoing surgery or until the tenth postoperative day. At an intramuscular dosage of 100 mg twice daily, the incidence of DVT was not reduced from that on placebo and no bleeding was detected. At an intramuscular dosage of 300 mg twice daily, the incidence of DVT was reduced from 64% in the placebo group to 38% in the dermatan sulphate group (p = 0.01), with a reduction in proximal DVT from 42% to 20%. No significant differences were found in hemorrhagic complications between the two groups. Two years later, Imbimbo et al. (66) studied the relationship between pharmacokinetics and antithrombotic efficacy of intramuscular dermatan sulphate in patients with hip fracture. The clinical efficacy of the drug was found to be dependent on the plasma concentration of dermatan sulphate and it was concluded that plasma levels greater than 9 µg/ml are advisable to optimize efficacy in hip fracture patients.

Prandoni et al. (67) compared dermatan sulphate (100 mg intramuscularly once daily) with unfractionated heparin (5,000 U s.c. three times daily) in the prevention of DVT after elective major surgical operations. Both treatments were initiated before intervention and continued until discharge. The incidence of DVT was not statistically different between the two groups, whereas the incidence of clinically overt hemorrhage was 5.7% with dermatan sulphate and 17.6% with unfractionated heparin (p < 0.01). A dose-finding trial with dermatan sulphate in the prophylaxis of DVT in elective hip surgery was performed by Cohen et al. (68). Three dosage regimens were studied: 200 mg once daily, 200 mg twice daily, and 300 mg twice daily, all administered from the second preoperative day until the tenth postoperative day. The incidence of DVT was, respectively, 53% and 51% with the lower dosages and 34% with 300 mg twice daily. Excessive bleeding requiring treatment withdrawal occurred in only one patient in the 200 mg twice-daily regimen. The incidence of bleeding episodes was similar in the three groups.

Lane et al. (69) reported a series of dose-finding studies on the use of dermatan sulphate as an anticoagulant in patients on maintenance hemodialysis. Three studies were performed at the Charing Cross Hospital in London on patients on 5 to 6 hours of dialysis. With a dosing regimen of 5 mg/kg in bolus followed by 1 mg/kg/hr of infusion over 5 hours, a trouble-free dialysis of the same duration as with standard heparin dosage was obtained.

Three more studies were conducted at the Academic Medical Center in Amsterdam. Out of different bolus injection doses (2.0, 2.5, 3.0, 4.5, and 6.0 mg/kg), a bolus injection of 6.0 mg/kg of dermatan sulphate allowed a successful completion of all dialyses without significant difference in clot formation in the extracorporeal circuit as compared with heparin and without any serious bleeding event.

Dermatan sulphate also has been evaluated to prevent cardiopulmonary bypass (CPB) pump occlusion during cardiac surgery. Brister et al. (70) compared it with heparin in pigs and found that a successful CPB could be achieved with lower doses of dermatan sulphate than heparin, thus resulting in less bleeding events.

CONCLUSION

Danaparoid is a low molecular weight heparinoid composed of a mixture of glycosaminoglycans with different affinities for serine protease inhibitors. Its main fraction, heparan sulphate, selectively inhibits factor Xa, thus giving danaparoid an overall anti–factor Xa/anti–factor IIa ratio of more than 28. With respect to unfractionated heparin, danaparoid has a much higher bioavailability and a longer half-life. Danaparoid has minimal inhibitory activity on platelet function, moreover, it has low cross-reactivity against the platelet-activating antibody responsible for the heparin-induced thrombocytopenia. Because of that, danaparoid is currently considered one of the anticoagulants of choice for patients with HIT. The recommended therapy protocol consists of an i.v. loading dose of 2,250 U bolus, followed by an infusion of 400 U/hr for 4 hours, followed by 300 U/hr for 4 hours, then a maintenance dosage of 150 to 200 U/hr, with subsequent dose adjustments made according to the anti-Xa levels (target range 0.5 to 0.8 anti-Xa U/ml), if available. Danaparoid is also recommended in the prevention of DVT in patients with previous HIT. The dosage is always 750 antifactor Xa IU twice daily administered s.c. Clinical trials have shown that danaparoid has the potential to be used as a first-choice drug in the prophylaxis and treatment of VTE, in hemodialysis patients, and in the treatment of acute ischemic stroke.

Dermatan sulphate, a heparinoid that inhibits thrombin by selectively interacting with heparin cofactor II, is not approved currently for clinical use. Additional randomized clinical trials are needed to evaluate dermatan sulphate, but because it is more potent than heparins in inhibiting thrombin bound to fibrin (and thus prevents fibrin accretion and thrombus growth), it is a very promising drug, particularly in situations such as prophylaxis in hip fracture surgery, where the initial trauma can determine an early development of DVT.

From a clinical point of view it is important that neither of these heparinoids can be monitored by routine coagulation tests, and that no specific antidote is available for danaparoid and dermatan sulphate.

REFERENCES

1. Meuleman DG. Synopsis of the anticoagulant and antithrombotic profile of the low molecular weight heparinoid ORG 10172 in experimental models. *Semin Thromb Haemost* 1989;15:370–371.
2. Casu B. Structural features of chondroitin sulphates, dermatan sulphate and heparan sulphate. *Semin Thromb Haemost* 1991;17(suppl 1):9–14.
3. van Dedem G, de Leeuw den Bouter H, Damm J, Overklift G. The nature of the glucosaminoglycan in Orgaran (ORG 10172) [Abstract]. *Thromb Haemost* 1993;69:652.
4. Gordon DL, Linhardt R, Adams HP. Low-molecular-weight heparins and heparinoids and their use in acute or progressing ischaemic stroke. *Clin Neuropharmacol* 1990;13:522–543.
5. Nurmohamed MT, Fareed J, Hoppensteadt D, Walenga JM, ten Cate JW. Pharmacological and clinical studies with Lomoparan, a low molecular weight glycosaminoglycan. *Semin Thromb Haemost* 1991;17(suppl 2): 205–213.
6. Meuleman DG. Orgaran (Org 10172): Its pharmacological prophile in experimental models. *Haemostasis* 1992;22:58–65.
7. Zammit A, Dawes J. Low-affinity material does not contribute to the antithrombotic activity of Orgaran (Org 10172) in human plasma. *Thromb Haemost* 1994;71:759–767.
8. Vogel GMT, Meuleman DG, Bourgondien F, Hobbelen PMJ. Comparison of two experimental thrombosis models in rats. *Thromb Res* 1989;54:399–410.
9. Boneu B, Buchanan MR, Cade JF, et al. Effects of heparin, its low molecular weight fractions and other glycosaminoglycans on thrombus growth in vivo. *Thromb Res* 1985;40:81–89.
10. Meuleman DG, Hobbelen PMJ, van Dedem G, Moelker HCT. A novel antithrombotic heparinoid (ORG 10172) devoid of bleeding enhancing capacity: A survey of its pharmacological properties in experimental animal models. *Thromb Res* 1982;27:353–363.
11. Vogel GMT, van Amsterdam RGM, Kop WJ, Meuleman DG. Pentasaccharide and Orgaran arrest, whereas heparin delays thrombus formation in a rat arteriovenous shunt. *Thromb Res* 1993;69:29–34.
12. Lozano M, Bos A, de Groot PG, et al. Suitability of low-molecular weight heparin(oid)s and a pentasaccharide for an in vitro human thrombosis model. *Arterioscler Thromb* 1994;14:1215–1222.
13. Cade JF, Buchanan MR, Boneu B, et al. A comparison of the antithrombotic and haemorrhagic effects of low molecular weight heparin fractions: the influence of the method of preparation. *Thromb Res* 1984;35: 613–625.
14. Meuleman DG, van Dinther T, Hobbelen PMJ, et al. Effects of the low molecular weight heparinoid Org 10172 in experimental thrombosis and bleeding models: comparison with heparin. *Thromb Haemorragic Disord* 1990;2:25–29.
15. Mikhailidis DP, Fonseca VA, Barradas MA, Jeremy JY, Dandona P. Platelet activation following intravenous injection of a conventional heparin: absence of effect with a low molecular weight heparinoid (ORG 10172). *Br J Clin Pharmacol* 1987;24:415–424.
16. Borris LC, Lassen MR. A comparative review of the adverse effect profiles of heparins and heparinoids. *Drug Safety* 1995;12:26–31.
17. Dawes J, Prowse DV, Pepper DS. The measurement of heparin and other therapeutic sulphated polysaccharides in plasma, serum and urine. *Thromb Haemost* 1985;54: 630–634.
18. Danhof M, de Boer A, Magnani HN, Stiekema JCJ. Pharmacokinetic considerations on Orgaran (ORG 10172) therapy. *Haemostasis* 1992;22:73–84.
19. Bradbrook ID, Magnani HN, Moelker CT, et al. ORG 10172: a low molecular weight heparinoid anticoagu-

lant with a long half-life in man. *Br J Clin Pharmacol* 1987;23:667–675.

20. Stiekema JCJ, Wijnand HP, van Dinther TG, et al. Safety and pharmacokinetics of the low molecular weight heparinoid ORG 10172 administered to healthy elderly volunteers. *Br J Pharmacol* 1989;27:39–48.

21. Frei U, Wilks MF, Boehmer S, et al. Gastrointestinal blood loss in hemodialysis patients during use of a low molecular weight heparinoid. *Nephrol Dial Transplant* 1988;3:435–439.

22. De Boer A, Stiekema JCJ, Danhof M, Breimer DD. The influence of Org 10172, a low molecular weight heparinoid, on oxidative drug metabolizing enzyme activity and vice versa in healthy male volunteers. *Br J Clin Pharmacol* 1991;32:23–29.

23. De Boer A, Danhof M, Cohen AF, Magnani HN, Breimer DD. Interaction study between Org 10172 (Lomoparan) a low molecular weight heparinoid and acetylsalicilic acid in healthy male volunteers. *Thromb Haemost* 1991;66:202–209.

24. Stiekema JCJ, De Boer A, Danhof M, et al. An interaction study of the new low molecular weight heparinoid Lomoparan and Acenocoumarol in healthy volunteers. *Haemostasis* 1990;20:136–146.

25. De Boer A, Stiekema JCJ, Danhof M, et al. Interaction studies of a low molecular weight heparinoid (Org 10172) with cloxacillin and ticarcillin in healthy male volunteers. *Antimicrob Agents Chemoter* 1991;35:2110–2115.

26. De Boer A, Stiekema JCJ, Danhof M, Breimer DD. An interaction study of Org 10172 (Lomoparan) and digoxin in six healthy male volunteers. *Eur J Clin Pharmacol* 1991;41:245–250.

27. De Boer A, Stiekema JCJ, Danhof M, Breimer DD. The influence of chlortalidone on the pharmacokinetics and pharmacodynamics of Org 10172 (Lomoparan) on low molecular weight heparinoid in healthy volunteers. *J Clin Pharmacol* 1991;31:611–617.

28. Stiekema JCJ, Wijnand HP, Ten Cate H, et al. Partial in vivo neutralisation of plasma anticoagulant effects of Lomoparan (Org 10172) by protamine chloride. *Thromb Res* 1991;63:157–167.

29. The Office of Medical Application of Research, National Institutes of Health. Prevention of venous thrombosis and pulmonary embolism; consensus conference. *JAMA* 1986;256:744–749.

30. Bergqvist D. *Postoperative Thromboembolism: Frequency, Etiology, Prophylaxis.* Berlin: Springer-Verlag, 1983.

31. Bergqvist D, Kettunen K, Fredin H, et al. Thromboprophylaxis in patients with hip fractures: a prospective, randomized, comparative study between ORG 10172 and dextran 70. *Surgery* 1991;109:617–622.

32. Gerhart TN, Yett HS, Robertson LK, Lee MA, Smith M, Salzman EW. Low-molecular-weight heparinoid compared with warfarin for prophylaxis of deep vein thrombosis in patients who are operated on for fracture of the hip. *J Bone Joint Surg* 1991;73:494–502.

33. Gent M, Hirsh J, Ginsberg JS, et al. Low-molecular-weight heparinoid Organan is more effective than aspirin in the prevention of venous thromboembolism after surgery for hip fracture. *Circulation* 1996;93:80–84.

34. Roise O, Nurmohamed M, Reijnders P, et al. A multicenter, randomised, assessor-blind, pilot study comparing the efficacy in the prophylaxis of DVT and the safety of Orgaran (Org 10172), Fragmin, Clexane/Lovenox in patients undergoing surgery for a fractured hip [Abstract]. *Thromb Haemost* 1993;69:620.

35. Turpie AGG. Thromboprophylaxis in orthopaedic surgery. *Orthop Int* 1993;1:396–401.

36. Stamatakis JD, Kakkar VV, Sagar S, Lawrence D, Nairn D, Bentley PG. Femoral vein thrombosis and total hip replacement. *Br Med J* 1977;2:223–225.

37. Hoek JA, Nurmohamed MT, Hamelynk KJ, et al. Prevention of deep vein thrombosis following total hip replacement by low molecular weight heparinoid. *Thromb Haemost* 1992;67:28–32.

38. Leyvraz P, Bachmann F, Bohnet J, et al. Thromboembolic prophylaxis in total hip replacement: a comparison between the low molecular weight heparinoid Lomoparan and heparin dihydroergotamine. *Br J Surg* 1992;79:911–914.

39. Agnelli G, Damiani M, Veschi F, et al. A double blind randomized trial on Orgaran versus unfractionated heparin in the prevention of deep vein thrombosis after elective hip replacement [Abstract]. *Thromb Haemost* 1995;73:1103.

40. Blum A, Desruennes E, Elias A, Lagrange G, Loriferne JF. DVT prophylaxis in surgery for digestive tract cancer comparing the LMW heparinoid ORG 10172 (Lomoparan) with calcium heparin [Abstract]. *Thromb Haemost* 1989;62:126.

41. Gallus A, Cade J, Ockelford P, et al. Orgaran (Org 10172) or heparin for preventing venous thrombosis after elective surgery for malignant disease? A double-blind, randomised, multicenter comparison. *Thromb Haemost* 1993;70:562–567.

42. Warlow C, Ogston D, Douglas AS. Venous thrombosis following strokes. *Lancet* 1972;1:1305–1306.

43. Turpie AGG, Levine MN, Hirsh J, et al. Double-blind randomised trial of ORG 10172 low molecular weight heparinoid in prevention of deep vein thrombosis in thrombotic stroke. *Lancet* 1987;1:523–526.

44. Turpie AGG, Gent M, Cote R, et al. A low-molecular-weight heparinoid compared with unfractionated heparin in the prevention of deep vein thrombosis in patients with acute ischemic stroke. *Ann Intern Med* 1992;117:353–357.

45. Dumas R, Woitinas F, Kutnowsky M, et al. A multicenter, double-blind, randomized study to compare the safety and efficacy of once-daily ORG 10172 and twice-daily low-dose heparin in preventing deep vein thrombosis in patients with acute ischemic stroke. *Age Ageing* 1994;23:512–516.

46. de Valk HW, Banga JD, Wester JWJ, et al. Comparing subcutaneous Danaparoid with intravenous unfractionated heparin for the treatment of venous thromboembolism. *Ann Intern Med* 1995;123:1–9.

47. Biller J, Massey EW, Marler JR, et al. A dose escalation study of ORG 10172 (low molecular weight heparinoid) in stroke. *Neurology* 1989;39:262–265.

48. Massey EW, Biller J, Davis JN, et al. Large-dose infusions of heparinoid ORG 10172 in ischemic stroke. *Stroke* 1990;21:1289–1292.

49. Warkentin TE, Levine MN, Hirsh J, et al. Heparin-induced thrombocytopenia in patients treated with low-molecular-weight heparin or unfractionated heparin. *N Engl J Med* 1995;332:1330–1335.

50. Chong BH, Magnani HN. Organan in heparin-induced thrombocytopenia. *Haemostasis* 1992;22:85–91.

51. Magnani HN. Heparin-induced thrombocytopenia (HIT): an overview of 230 patients treated with Orgaran (Org 10172). *Thromb Haemost* 1993;70:554–561.
52. Ortel TL, Gockerman JP, Califf RM, et al. Parenteral anticoagulation with the heparinoid Lomoparan (Org 10172) in patients with heparin induced thrombocytopenia and thrombosis. *Thromb Haemost* 1992;67:292–296.
53. Tardy-Poncet B, Reynaud J, Tardy B, et al. Efficacy and safety of Orgaran anticoagulation in patients with heparin induced thrombocytopenia [Abstract]. *Thromb Haemost* 1995;73:1323.
54. Vun CM, Evans S, Chong BH. Cross-reactivity study of low molecular weight heparins and heparinoid in heparin-induced thrombocytopenia. *Thromb Res* 1996;81:525–532.
55. Henny CP, ten Cate H, ten Cate JW, Prummel MF, Peters M, Buller HR. Thrombosis Prophylaxis in an AT III deficient pregnant woman: application of a low-molecular weight heparinoid. *Thromb Haemost* 1986;55:301.
56. Henny CP, ten Cate H, ten Cate JW, et al. Use of a new heparinoid as anticoagulant during acute haemodialysis of patients with bleeding complications. *Lancet* 1983;1:890–893.
57. ten Cate H, Henny CP, ten Cate JW, Buller HR, Dabhoiwala NF. Randomized, double-blind, placebo controlled safety study of a low molecular weight heparinoid in patients undergoing transurethral resection of the prostate. *Thromb Haemost* 1987;57:92–96.
58. Gallus A, Murphy W, Nacey J, et al. The influence of ORG 10172, an antithrombotic heparinoid, on urinary blood loss after transurethral prostatectomy. *Thromb Res* 1989;56:229–238.
59. ten Cate H, Henny CP, Buller HR, ten Cate JW, Magnani HN. Use of a heparinoid in patients with haemorragic stroke and thromboembolic disease. *Ann Neurol* 1984;15:268–270.
60. Nieuwenhuis HK, Sixma JJ. Treatment of disseminated intravascular coagulation in acute promyelocytic leukemia with low molecular weight heparinoid Org 10172. *Cancer* 1986;58:761–764.
61. Tollefsen DM, Petska CA, Monafo WJ. Activation of heparin cofactor II by dermatan sulfate. *J Biol Chem* 1983;258:6713–6716.
62. Merton RE, Thomas DP. Experimental studies on the relative efficacy of dermatan sulphate and heparin as antithrombotic agents. *Thromb Haemost* 1987;58:839–842.
63. Van Ryn-McKenna J, Gray E, Weber E, Ofosu FA, Buchanan MR. Effects of sulphated polysaccharides on inhibition of thrombus formation initiated by different stimuli. *Thromb Haemost* 1989;61:7–9.
64. Van Ryn-McKenna J, Ofosu FA, Buchanan MR. The effects of heparin and dermatan sulphate on t-PA-induced thrombolysis and blood loss in rabbits. *Fibrinolysis* 1993;7:75–81.
65. Agnelli G, Cosmi B, Di Filippo P, et al. A randomised, double-blind, placebo-controlled trial of dermatan sulphate for prevention of deep vein thrombosis in hip fracture. *Thromb Haemost* 1992;67:203–208.
66. Imbimbo BP, Sie' P, Agnelli G, et al. Intramuscular dermatan sulfate MF701 in patients with hip fracture: relationship between pharmacokinetics and antithrombotic efficacy. *Thromb Haemost* 1994;71:553–557.
67. Prandoni P, Meduri F, Cuppini S, et al. Dermatan sulphate: a safe approach to prevention of postoperative deep vein thrombosis. *Br J Surg* 1992;79:505–509.
68. Cohen AT, Phillips MJ, Edmonson RA, Melissari E, Vaidyanathan I, Kakkar VV. Dermatan sulphate for prophylaxis of deep vein thrombosis in elective hip surgery: a dose finding trial [Abstract]. *Thromb Haemost* 1983;69:621.
69. Lane DA, Ryan K, Ireland H, et al. Dermatan sulphate in haemodialysis. *Lancet* 1992;339:334–335.
70. Brister SJ, Ofosu FA, Heigenhauser GJF, Gianese F, Buchanan MR. Is heparin the ideal anticoagulant for cardiopulmonary bypass? Dermatan sulphate may be an alternate choice. *Thromb Haemost* 1994;71:468–473.

Cardiovascular Thrombosis: Thrombocardiology and Thromboneurology, Second Edition,
edited by M. Verstraete, V. Fuster, and E. J. Topol,
Lippincott–Raven Publishers, Philadelphia © 1998.

13

Dextran

David Bergqvist

Department of Surgery, University Hospital, S-75185 Uppsala, Sweden

BACKGROUND

The polysaccharide dextran was first described in the 1870s as a by-product of beet sugar refining. Its use as a plasma substitute was first conceived during World War II by Ingelman and Grönwall in Sweden (1,2). Two findings secured dextran's place in the history of medicine: it failed to provoke immunologic response on infusion into animals and was completely metabolized by the body. Dextran had advantages over blood and plasma: it eliminated the risk of transfusion-transmitted infections, was stable, required no cross-matching, and was cheaper.

The first clinical studies on dextran as a volume expander were performed between 1944 and 1946 (3), and in 1947 dextran was launched as a 6% solution. Around 1953, dextran production was improved, whereby average molecular weight was lowered and the molecular weight distribution narrowed. This product was designated "dextran 70" (average molecular weight 70,000 daltons). In the beginning of the 1960s, dextran 40 was introduced (average molecular weight 40,000 daltons), and because of flow-promoting properties, it was used in ischemic conditions and arterial surgery (4–6).

The antithrombotic effect of dextran was first demonstrated experimentally in rabbits by Borgström et al. (7) and in patients by Koekenberg (8).

GENERAL ASPECTS

Dextran is formed by the enzyme dextran sucrase when the bacterium *Leuconostoc mesenteroides* B 512 acts on saccharose. It is a neutral, high molecular weight polymer composed of glucose molecules bound to each other by α-1-6-glucosidic bonds, forming a chain, side chains being formed via one to three glucose bonds. A higher degree of branching induces more adverse effects. Clinically useful dextrans form only about 1% of the molecular weight spectrum of raw dextran, which is hydrolyzed to produce fractions of desired molecular weight (Medisan AB, Sweden).

Excretion rate via the kidneys is molecular weight dependent, molecules below 40,000 to 50,000 daltons being rapidly excreted (9). Approximately 50% of dextran 40 is excreted renally in 2 to 3 hours compared with 24 hours for dextran 70.

Dextran is temporarily taken up by various organs. Dextran not excreted via the kidneys is degraded to carbon dioxide and water by dextranase in the reticuloendothelial system.

MECHANISMS OF ACTION

Colloid Osmotic (Oncotic) Effect

The water-binding capacity is 20 to 25 ml water/g dextran, compared with 18 ml/g for albumin. The water not available in the circulatory system is absorbed from the extracellular space. An approximately 2.5% solution of dextran 40 and 3.5% solution of dextran 70 is nearly iso-oncotic with blood in vitro. In vivo, however, allowance should be made for rapid extravascular loss of small molecules through the glomerular and capillary membranes. In hypovolemic individuals and those with a lowered colloid osmotic pressure, the volume-expanding effect is more prolonged. The volume effect of dextran exceeds that of hydroxyethyl starch (10).

Effect on Erythrocyte Aggregation

Dextran below 60,000 in molecular weight has a cellular disaggregating effect ascribed to an increase in the electronegativity of the cells (10). Above 60,000 molecular weight in vitro (80,000 in vivo), dextran induces a progressive increase in red cell aggregation (11). As a consequence, peripheral resistance is increased, and nutritive flow is impaired with the development of hypoxia (12–15).

Coating of the Vessel Wall Endothelium

Coating of the endothelium and blood cells with a thin dextran film (16) changes the electrical potential (17) and may be of importance for the thromboprophylactic mechanism.

Influence on the Hemostatic System

Infusion of dextran in doses up to 1.5 g/kg body weight does not affect the number of platelets (18), but the platelet adhesiveness decreases with a maximum 2 to 6 hours after the infusion, i.e., when the dextran concentration in serum is decreasing (19–21). Dextran infusion prevents platelet adherence to various artificial surfaces during extracorporeal circulation (22), grafting (23), and stenting (24). Platelet aggregation in vitro induced by several stimuli is inhibited by dextran, as is adenosine diphosphate–induced platelet aggregation in vivo (25).

With the exception of factor VIII, the different coagulation factors are not influenced by dextran more than what could be explained by the hemodilution (26,27). Factor VIII has been suggested to decrease more (28), which has been considered due to von Willebrand factor (VIII R:Ag) as the coagulation activity (VIII:C) remains unchanged (29). However, this specific effect on VIIIR:Ag has recently been challenged (30,31).

In vitro, dextran accelerates fibrinogen coagulation on addition of thrombin (fibrinoplastic effect) (32), and the fibrin network is coarser (33,34). Clots formed in vitro in the presence of dextran are more easily lysed by plasmin than control clots (34). Dextran is capable of reducing the fibrinolysis-inhibitive activity (α_2-antiplasmin) in serum, and postoperative t-PA levels are increased in dextran-treated patients (35). As an overall effect, the activation rate of plasminogen is enhanced (36). The increase in ongoing coagulation reflected by fibrinopeptide A and decrease in fibrinolysis (plasminogen activator) associated with monocyte dysfunction after trauma is also counteracted by dextran (37).

The plasmin-induced lysis of thrombi formed ex vivo increases with blood from dextran-treated patients, reaching a maximum 2 to 4 hours after dextran infusion, whereas dextran added in vitro does not alter lysability (38). Concurrently with increased lysability, the structure of the thrombi is altered. The platelets become more evenly distributed throughout the thrombus instead of being localized to its head, giving more fragile thrombi. The weight of the thrombi is significantly less, this effect being dose dependent (39). Volume expansion with albumin does not affect the thrombi.

The formation of experimental venous thrombi in vivo is also counteracted by dextran with increased thrombus fragility and lysability (40,41).

In 1954 it was noted that dextran could prolong the bleeding time in patients (42,43), the maximal influence occurring some hours after the dextran infusion.

Both molecular weight and the dose of dextran are decisive for the effect on initial hemostasis (44,45). The more frequent reports of bleeding complications in the early history of dextran appears to be related to the presence of a greater proportion of large molecules in early clinical dextran than today.

Influence on Hemodynamics

The effect on hemodynamics is due to a combination of the following factors:

1. Interaction with cell surfaces, reducing or preventing red blood cell aggregation, platelet adhesiveness, leukocyte plugging (46).
2. Hemodilution with decreased viscosity (47).
3. Passive dilatation of microvessels due to the colloid osmotic effect (48).

There is an increased resting arterial volume blood flow and increased arterial and venous cross-sectional area after dextran infusion to patients (49). Increased arterial circulation and microcirculatory flow velocity also have been demonstrated experimentally (50–52).

PREVENTION OF DEEP VEIN THROMBOSIS

Comparison with Untreated Controls

In the first clinical study, Koekenberg (8) randomly replaced intraoperative blood loss with either bank blood or dextran. The frequency of clinical deep vein thrombosis (DVT) decreased from 21% to 4% in the dextran group. In a double-blind study, Jansen (53) confirmed the reduction in frequency of clinically diagnosed thrombi.

There are seven open randomized studies in orthopedic surgery between dextran and no prophylaxis with phlebographic diagnosis of DVT (54–60). Bilateral phlebography was not performed in all studies, which tends to underestimate the DVT frequency. In all studies, dextran was the better alternative. The mean frequency of DVT was reduced from 48.4% to 17.5% (124 of 256 to 42 of 240; p < 0.01).

In 15 open randomized studies the diagnosis was based on the fibrinogen uptake test (FUT) (61–75). Two dealt with hip surgery (64,67), for which the FUT test is not optimal (76), but the studies were randomized. The beneficial effect of dextran was not as obvious as when phlebography was used, but overall there was a reduction in the frequency of DVT (26.1% to 19.8%; 218 of 835 to 173 of 872; p < 0.05). In most studies, dextran 70 was used, but no data indicate dextran 40 to be inferior in this respect. In a meta-analysis, Clagett and Reisch (77) found that dextran produced a moderate but significant reduction in frequency of postoperative DVT diagnosed by the FUT (from 24.2% to 15.6%).

Comparison with Other Prophylactic Methods

In Tables 13-1 to 13-3, randomized studies comparing dextran with anticoagulants are shown. In the investigations in Table 13-1, phlebography was used for diagnosis, all in hip surgery patients. In Table 13-2, the FUT was used, positive tests being confirmed with phlebography, as well as in hip surgery pa-

TABLE 13-1. *Deep vein thrombosis confirmed by phlebography in orthopedic studies where dextran is compared with anticoagulant prophylaxis[a]*

| Ref. | Dextran | | Anticoagulation | | Type of surgery | Type of anticoagulation |
	No. of patients	No. of DVT	No. of patients	No. of DVT		
Andersen et al. (55)	29	5	36	7	HF	Heparin DHE, TED in all
Bergquist et al. (78)	75	25	63	19	HF	Dicoumarol
Bergqvist et al. (79)	138	43	139	14	HF	Danaparoid
Bronge et al. (80)	74	31	61	21	THR	Dicoumarol
Danish Enoxaparin Study (81)	111	24	108	7	THR	Enoxaparin
Francis et al. (82)[b]	51	12	52	2	THR	Heparin + AT III
Francis et al. (83)[b]	43	19	57	11	THR	Warfarin
Francis et al. (84)[b]	38	31	39	14	TKR	Heparin + AT III
Fredin et al. (85)	58	27	58	29	THR	Heparin DHE
Fredin et al. (86)	46	25	50	21	THR	Heparin DHE
Fredin et al. (87)	114	49	93	41	THR	Heparin DHE
Harris et al. (88)[b]	61	14	55	10	THR	Warfarin
Myhre and Holen (59)	55	11	50	9	HF	Warfarin
Heparin	474	192 (40.5%)	467	128 (27.4%)		
Oral anticoagulant	308	100 (32.5%)	286	70 (24.5%)		
Total	893	316	861	205		
Overall frequency (%)		35.3		23.8		$p < 0.01$

DHE, dihydroergotamine; TED, thromboembolic deterrent stocking; LMWH, low molecular weight heparin; AT III, antithrombin III; HF, hip fracture; THR, total hip replacemement; TKR, total knee replacement.
[a]Phlebography was used for diagnosis. Overall frequency (%) is provided in parentheses.
[b]Dextran 40.

tients. In Table 13-3, only FUT was used, most studies being nonorthopedic. All studies in the tables are randomized and all are open. It is difficult to blind the dextran infusion versus the subcutaneous (s.c.) injectons of the comparative substances. The predominant finding in all types of surgery is that anticoagulants (oral anticoagulants, low-dose heparin, or low molecular weight heparins) are more effective than dextran. In the study by Lambie et al. (100), the frequency of DVT is significantly higher in the warfarin group, but warfarin was not started until 36 hours postoperatively. At least in comparison with oral

TABLE 13-2. *Deep vein thrombosis in hip surgery studies where dextran is compared with anticoagulant prophylaxis[a]*

| Ref. | Dextran | | Anticoagulation | | Type of surgery | Type of anticoagulation |
	No. of patients	No. of DVT	No. of patients	No. of DVT		
Eriksson et al. (89)	49	22	49	10	THR	Dalteparin
Fredin et al. (90)	41	8	27	6	HF	PZ 68
Myrvold et al. (91)	55	20	39	16	HF	Heparin
Mätzsch et al. (92)	49	18	47	9	THR	Tinzaparin
Mätzsch et al. (93)	123	36	120	22	THR	Tinzaparin
Total	317	104	282	63		
Overall frequency (%)		32.8		22.3		$p < 0.05$

PZ 68, sodium pentosan polysulphate.
[a]The fibrinogen uptake test was used for surveillance with phlebographic verification.

TABLE 13-3. *Deep vein thrombosis as detected with fibrinogen uptake test in studies where dextran is compared with anticoagulant prophylaxis, except Lindström (electric stimulation)*[a]

Ref.	Dextran		Anticoagulation		Type of surgery	Type of anticoagulation
	No. of patients	No. of DVT	No. of patients	No. of DVT		
Barber et al. (94)	51	26	58	34	THR	Warfarin
Bergqvist and Dahlgren (95)	43	19	32	16	HF	Dicoumarol
Bergqvist et al. (64)	27	13	28	18	HF	Heparin
Bergqvist et al. (64)	70	40	72	35	THR	Heparin
Bergqvist and Hallböök (63)	52	15	46	6	General	Heparin
Bergqvist et al. (96)	56	39	59	10	THR	Heparin DHE
Bergqvist et al. (96)	29	21	25	20	HF	Heparin DHE
Bergqvist and Ljugnér (97)	52	10	34	1	General	PZ 68
Davidson et al. (98)	30	3	30	4	Gynecology	Warfarin
Gruber et al. (68)[b]	37	9	33	3	General	Heparin
Hedlund (69)	37	10	38	13	Urology	Heparin
Hohl et al. (99)	117	17	115	2	Gynecology	Heparin
Lambie et al. (100)	40	4	40	12	Gynecology	Warfarin
Lindström et al. (73)	35	7	37	5	General	Electric stimulation
McCarthy et al. (101)	61	11	64	7	Gynecology	Heparin
Rosell Pradas and Vara-Thorbeck (102)[b]	56	6	57	5	General	Heparin
Ruckley (74)	130	33	128	15	General	Heparin
Total heparin (nonorthopedic)	542	111	515	52		
Overall frequency (%)		20.5		10.1		p < 0.01

[a]The fibrinogen uptake test was used for diagnosis.
[b]Dextran 40.

anticoagulants given before operation, the risk for hemorrhage is less for dextran (103).

Combination Prophylaxis

Considering that thrombogenesis is a multifactorial process, combination prophylaxis seems reasonable.

The concomitant combination of dextran and oral anticoagulants increases bleeding problems and is therefore not recommended. The concomitant combination of dextran and low-dose heparin or low molecular weight heparin fragments is insufficiently documented. Experimentally, however, clinical doses of dextran potentiated the thromboprophylactic effect of s.c. low molecular weight heparin (104) without increasing bleeding (105). In the clinical setting, Rutherford et al. (106) found that a standard dextran dose combined with 100 IU/kg intravenous (i.v.) unfractionated heparin provided protection against early graft failure without bleedings.

Dextran combined with mechanical methods shows an additive thromboprophylactic effect and is therefore of potential clinical interest, especially with graded compression stockings (107–111) without increasing the bleeding risk.

The combination of acetylsalicylic acid (ASA) and dextran 40 may lead to postoperative bleeding problems (112).

PREVENTION OF PULMONARY EMBOLISM

In a double-blind trial, Kline et al. (113) noted a significant reduction in the number of fatal pulmonary emboli (FPE) after administration of dextran 70 at surgery. In the control group, 14 FPEs occurred among 435 patients, and in the dextran group four occurred in 396 patients (p < 0.05).

The study by Ljungström (114) is in part historical, but its strength lies in the total coverage within one hospital and the fact that the four periods with and without dextran alternated in 2-year sequences. The frequency of FPE during nondextran periods was 0.69% (35 of 5,094) and during dextran periods 0.20% (10 of 4,881), a significant reduction.

In Table 13-4, the available dextran studies (n = 29) are pooled to compare the rates of FPE, between dextran and no antithrombotic prophylaxis. A reduction from 1.5% to 0.3% with dextran is seen. In a meta-analysis, Clagett and Reisch (77) arrived at the same conclusion. The frequency in the control group was 1.5% and in the dextran group 0.27%.

In Table 13-5 dextran is compared with anticoagulants. Although there are several types of anticoagulants, this group appears as effective as dextran in preventing FPE. This is in keeping with a randomized study from Tubingen (127), where dextran 60 (2,945 patients) was compared with heparin and oral anticoagulants (3,014 patients). The incidence of FPE was 0.36% in the anticoagulant group and 0.30% in the dextran group. Hemorrhagic complications were noted in 1.1% of the anticoagulant group and in 0.6% of the subjects treated with dextran (p < 0.05).

Based on these open but randomized trials, dextran appears to be as effective as anticoagulant prophylaxis in preventing FPE. Apart from the specific effects of dextran, hemodilution in itself also may contribute to the protection achieved (128).

IMPROVEMENT OF ARTERIAL CIRCULATION DURING ISCHEMIA

Most experimental work conducted to date has been of acute character with virtually no

TABLE 13-4. *Data on fatal pulmonary embolism (FPE) and total mortality in studies on dextran versus control*

Ref.	Dextran			Control		
	No. of patients	No. of deaths	No. of FPE	No. of patients	No. of deaths	No. of FPE
Ahlberg et al. (54)	39	6	0	45	14	2
Atik et al. (115)	49	7	1	77	14	8
Becker and Schampi (61)	42	1	0	35	1	0
Bergman et al. (62)	30	0	0	30	0	0
Bergqvist et al. (64)	27	2	0	26	3	0
Bergqvist et al. (64)	70	1	0	71	2	2
Bergqvist and Hallböök (63)	52	2	0	51	7	0
Brisman et al. (116)	89	8	0	90	5	0
Carter and Eban (66)	106	0	0	101	0	0
Edwards et al. (117)	31	3	2	31	7	6
Elsner-Mackey et al. (118)	391	0	0	427	0	0
Evarts and Feil (56)[a]	50	0	0	50	0	0
Gruber et al. (68)[a]	37	4	1	38	6	2
Hedlund (69)	37	0	0	40	0	0
von Hospenthal et al. (70)	39	0	0	47	0	0
Hurson et al. (119)	55	1	0	51	0	0
Hutter et al. (71)[a]	92	0	0	100	0	0
Huttunen et al. (72)	150	4	1	75	0	0
Huttunen et al. (120)	100	1	1	100	6	4
Jansen (53)	304	13	1	301	19	4
Johnsson et al. (58)	27	0	0	25	0	0
Kline et al. (113)	396	27	1	435	35	7
Myhre and Holen (59)	55	3	0	55	6	2
Nillius et al. (60)	38	0	0	29	1	1
Rothermel et al. (121)[a]	60	1	1	60	1	0
Ruckley (74)	130	0	0	128	1	1
Stadil (122)	424	21	1	397	22	5
Stephenson et al. (75)	34	0	0	46	0	0
Welin-Berger et al. (123)	20	0	0	20	0	0
Total	2,964	107	10	2,981	148	44
Overall frequency (%)		3.6	0.34		5.0	1.5	p < 0.01

[a]Dextran 40.

TABLE 13-5. *Data on fatal pulmonary embolism and total mortality in studies on dextran versus anticoagulation*

	Dextran			Anticoagulation			
Ref.	No. of patients	No. of deaths	No. of FPE	No. of patients	No. of deaths	No of FPE	Type of anticoagulation
Barber et al. (94)	51	1	1	58	0	0	Warfarin
Bergquist et al. (78)	75	9	0	63	12	1	Dicoumarol
Bergqvist et al. (64)	27	2	0	28	4	1	Heparin
Bergqvist et al. (64)	70	1	0	72	0	0	Heparin
Bergqvist and Hallböök (63)	52	2	0	46	2	0	Heparin
Bergqvist et al. (96)	56	0	0	59	0	0	Heparin DHE
Bergqvist et al. (96)	29	1	0	25	3	1	Heparin DHE
Bergqvist and Ljungnér (97)	52	1	0	34	0	0	PZ 68
Bergqvist et al. (79)	138	8	3	139	9	0	Org 10172
Danish Enoxaparin Study (81)	111	0	0	108	1	0	Enoxaparin
Eriksson et al. (89)	49	0	0	49	0	0	Dalteparin
Francis et al. (82)[a]	51	0	0	52	0	0	Heparin + AT III
Francis et al. (83)[a]	43	0	0	57	0	0	Warfarin
Francis et al. (84)[a]	38	0	0	39	2	1	Heparin + AT II
Fredin et al. (90)	41	4	0	27	0	0	PZ 68
Fredin et al. (85)	58	0	0	58	2	0	Heparin DHE
Fredin et al. (86)	46	0	0	50	0	0	Heparin DHE
Fredin et al. (87)	114	0	0	93	0	0	Heparin DHE
Gruber et al. (68)[a]	37	4	1	33	2	1	Heparin
Gruber et al. (124)	2,159	38	5	2,193	37	3	Heparin
Gruber (125)	3,715	27	9	3,698	28	6	Heparin DHE
Harris et al. (126)[a]	113	0	0	114	1	0	Warfarin
Harris et al. (88)[a]	61	0	0	55	0	0	Warfarin
Hedlund (69)	37	0	0	38	0	0	Heparin
Hohl et al. (99)	117	0	0	115	0	0	Heparin
Lambie et al. (100)	40	0	0	40	0	0	Warfarin
McCarthy et al. (101)	68	0	0	64	0	0	Heparin
Myhre and Holen (59)	55	3	0	50	4	1	Warfarin
Myrvold et al. (91)	55	2	2	39	2	2	Heparin
Mätzsch et al. (92)	49	0	0	47	0	0	Tinzaparin
Mätzsch et al. (93)	123	1	0	120	1	0	Tinzaparin
Rosell-Pradas and Vara-Thorbeck (102)[a]	56	0	0	40	0	0	Heparin
Ruckley (74)	130	0	0	128	0	0	Heparin
Welin-Berger et al. (123)	20	0	0	20	0	0	Heparin
Heparin, LMWH	7,498	91	20	7,414	93	15	
Oral anticoagulant	438	13	1	437	17	2	
Total	7,936	104	21	7,851	110	17	
Overall frequency (%)		1.3	0.26		1.4	0.22	p = NS

[a]Dextran 40.

documentation from chronic studies. Moreover, experimental models simulating chronic extremity ischemia in humans do not exist.

Several studies demonstrate increased blood flow with dextran, both in healthy persons and in patients with occlusive lower extremity disease (129–131).

There are no controlled studies on the effect of dextran in relieving rest pain or delaying amputation in patients with critical ischemia. However, there are clinical reports claiming at least relief of pain (132–134).

Clinical data are few but indicate a flow-promoting effect of dextran in patients with acute and possibly also in chronic ischemia. Long-term flow measurements, however, are lacking. Although some evidence suggests that hemodilution with dextran improves critical parameters in claudication, threatening gangrene and wound healing (135–138), further work to objectively establish these observations in well-controlled studies is required.

The incidence of thromboembolic complications after angiography seems to be reduced by dextran 40 and 70 (139,140).

PROPHYLAXIS AGAINST EARLY GRAFT FAILURE

Several experimental studies have documented the beneficial effect of dextran during the immediate postoperative course. Thus, dextran increases graft patency (23,141–143), prevents thrombus formation (144–146), inhibits platelet deposition and distal embolization (147), prevents microvascular thrombosis (148–150), and increases patency in anastomoses (151,152) and in synthetic grafts in the venous circulation (153). The combination of low molecular weight heparin and dextran may have a potentiating effect (154), especially when arterial flow is restricted.

Data from controlled clinical studies on the effect of dextran on complications after arterial reconstructive surgery are few. Investigators who have used dextran routinely in uncontrolled series of different vascular reconstructions are satisfied (155,156).

Waibel (157) studied postoperative occlusion within 3 days of arterial reconstruction. One group was randomized to dextran 40 peroperatively and postoperatively for 4 days, the other to peroral anticoagulants started postoperatively. The three first postoperative days were uninfluenced by the anticoagulation therapy, and the group served as a control. Dextran had a significant effect in preventing early occlusion in patients undergoing iliaco-femoro-popliteal reconstructions compared to aorto-iliac reconstructions, and the effect was seen in patients with impaired outflow.

In a controlled study by Sawyer et al. (158) on complications after peripheral vascular surgery, one group received no pharmacologic treatment and one group got a combination of dextran 40 and heparin. The frequency of total as well as thrombotic complications was significantly reduced in the treated group. The results are not presented in suffi-

TABLE 13-6. *Occlusion rate of femorodistal bypass versus postoperative interval*

Interval	Dextran 40	Control
1 day	0/95 (0%)	10/100 (10%)
1 week	6/95 (6%)	22/100 (22%)
1 month	15/95 (16%)	22/100 (22%)

From Rutherford et al., ref. 106.

cient detail to evaluate different types of complications. The conclusions can only be drawn for the combined treatment.

In another randomized trial in difficult femorodistal reconstructions, dextran 40 for 3 days provided significantly better patency both at 1 week and 1 month postoperatively than one single dose of heparin during cross-clamping (Table 13-6) (106). This finding has been verified in a recent randomized study with dextran 70 (159). However, dextran 70 seems to have more problems with heart failure than dextran 40.

DOSAGE AND TIMING ASPECTS

There are considerable variations in dosage and dose interval in the various studies, but there does not appear to be a clear correlation between dose and effect.

In clinical praxis it is reasonable to recommend infusion of dextran 500 ml intraoperatively (over 1 to 2 hours) and 500 ml after operation, i.e., a total 1,000 ml during the day of surgery (over 6 to 8 hours). In hip surgery, it has been suggested that additional infusions (500 ml per day over 4 hours), for instance on days 3 and 5, would be of prophylactic value (56,160), especially if the patients were not mobilized. Concerning timing, the most important infusion seems to be the intraoperative one.

Recently, 3% dextran 60 has been introduced as a plasma substitute in blood component therapy and for volume expansion (161–163). There is no evidence to suggest any clinical difference between dextran 60 and 70, and 3% colloid seems optimal for perioperative volume treatment (164). In doses up to 1.5 g/kg body weight, 3% dextran 60/70 does not significantly interfere with hemostatic factors in patients undergoing orthopedic surgery (165). Three percent dextran 60 is more effective than Ringer's lactate in maintaining hemodynamic stability and carries a lower risk of cardiac overloading than does 6% dextran. A quantity of 1,000 ml of the 3% solution gives the same amount of dextran as 500 ml of the 6% solution; thus, there is no reason to expect any difference in thromboprophylactic effect.

In patients with critical ischemia not undergoing surgery, 500 ml of dextran 40 every second day for 1 week may be tried.

SIDE EFFECTS

Cardiac Overload

Because dextran is a volume expander, particularly when given rapidly, there is a small risk of cardiac overload, but this can usually be avoided by slow infusion (50 to 100 ml/hr). Rutherford et al. (106) found no increase in cardiac complications in a series where dextran 40 (18% versus 5% in the control group) was compared with heparin in connection with femorodistal arterial surgery, despite the high frequency of ischemic heart disease in this predominantly elderly patient population.

Hemorrhagic Complications

Dextran doses of 1 to 1.5 g/kg body weight and lower do not impair hemostasis.

In most studies on dextran, no increased blood loss has been reported. In trials where the exact blood loss has been reported, it has not been increased (63,64,107,124). In a multicenter study comparing dextran 70 with low-dose heparin for a week, there was no difference in the blood loss during operation, but more blood was transfused to dextran-treated patients (124). This phenomenon has been noted in other studies. It might be that the lowered hematocrit in dextran hemodiluted patients triggers the need for blood transfusion. If the hemodilution effect of dextran is exploited optimally, however, it would be possible to save donor blood.

Heparin and dextran act at different levels of the hemostatic mechanism. A combination should therefore be advantageous from a thromboprophylactic point of view, but for the same reason, surgery may raise the risk for bleeding (166). In an experimental study on hemostatic plug formation, the combination did not impair hemostasis compared with either substance alone (105), but combining dextran and heparin in the clinical setting has yielded mixed results concerning bleeding complications (106,166–168). Enoxaparin and dextran in combination slightly increased the need for transfusion in elective hip surgery compared with enoxaparin alone (169), but dalteparin and dextran did not increase blood loss in patients undergoing transurethral prostatectomy (170).

An increased diffuse oozing has been reported in association with dextran, but this is difficult to assess objectively and is probably related to the improved capillary perfusion. In patients with hemostatic defects, dextran should be administered with caution.

Anaphylactoid Reactions

Like other colloids, dextran may rarely elicit anaphylactoid reactions. Hypersensitivity to dextran has been known since the mid-1960s (171,172). Although crudely fractionated high molecular weight dextrans (more than 80,000 daltons) can induce antibody formation, modern clinical fractions are not considered immunogenic. However, they may cross-react with preformed circulating antibodies to related polyglucans in dental plaques or in the capsules of bacteria (173).

The symptomatology of dextran reaction can be classified as follows:

I. Skin symptoms and/or slight fever.
II. Measurable, but not life-threatening, cardiovascular reaction (hypotension, tachycardia); respiratory disturbances; nausea, vomiting.
III. Severe hypotension ($\geq$40 to 60 mmHg); life-threatening bronchospasm.
IV. Cardiac and/or respiratory arrest.
V. Death.

Specific immune complexes are probably involved in the serious reactions (174). There is a reaction between dextran-reactive immunoglobulin G antibodies and dextran, causing large immune complexes to form (175). The complement system, platelets, leukocytes, and the coagulation cascade are activated, and vasoactive substances are released (172,176,177). Metabolic acidosis is always present in severe cases (178). Circulation is not normalized until the acidosis has been corrected.

The incidence per infused unit of dextran varies between 0.008% and 0.23% (124, 179–181).

Using low molecular weight dextran (dextran 1, molecular weight 1,000 daltons), the binding sites on the antibody are blocked, and aggregate formation is prevented (hapten inhibition). The hapten inhibition principle is effective in clinical practice, reducing the frequency of severe anaphylactoid reactions by at least 35-fold. In Sweden the incidence of grade III to V reactions (per patient) diminished from one in 2,000 in 1975 to 1979 to 1 in 70,000 in 1983 to 1992 (173).

In practice, 20 ml of dextran 1 is given i.v. immediately before the first infusion of dextran 40 or 70. Renewed injection of dextran 1 is recommended when the interval between dextran infusions exceeds 48 hours.

Should a serious reaction occur despite hapten preinfusion, the dextran infusion should be stopped immediately. Theophylline or β_2-agonists and adrenaline have been recommended in cases of bronchospasm. The metabolic acidosis must be corrected. Large doses of corticosteroids and crystalloid infusions seem beneficial.

Renal Dysfunction

Because the dextran solutions are hyperoncotic, concurrent crystalloid fluid administration is required, especially in dehydrated patients (182). Renal dysfunction may occur when large quantities of dextran are administered to dehydrated patients or to patients with underlying renal disease. This applies primar- ily to dextran 40, which, in the form of Rheomacrodex (Medisan Pharmaceuticals, Parsippany, NY), is a 10% solution. Some findings suggest the risk of renal failure being higher if the arterial circulation is diminished (183). Large quantities of dextran 40 induce a pronounced, but reversible, morphologic vacuolization (osmotic nephrosis) of the cytoplasm of proximal tubular cells, but their function is not influenced (184).

CONCLUSION

In addition to its plasma volume-expanding effect, dextran has specific properties that make it useful in indications associated with a high risk of thromboembolism and impaired circulation.

In comparison with no prophylaxis, dextran gives a significant but moderate reduction in postoperative DVT, particularly in orthopedic and trauma surgery. It reduces postoperative fatal pulmonary embolism to the same extent as heparin prophylaxis. It improves arterial circulation in situations of acute ischemia and improves early patency after femorodistal reconstructions.

Further studies are warranted to establish:

1. The efficacy and safety of dextran in combination with other prophylactic methods.
2. Whether dextran reduces the frequency of microembolic complications, e.g., in carotid artery surgery.
3. Optimal administration such as dose, dose intervals, duration, and time for first infusion.
4. Whether it is possible to relieve pain, increase wound healing rate, and reduce the risk for amputation in patients with critical limb ischemia.
5. The exact role in reconstructive arterial surgery.

ACKNOWLEDGMENTS

This work was supported by the Swedish Medical Research Council (Grant 00759) and the Swedish Heart and Lung Foundation.

REFERENCES

1. Grönwall A, Ingelman B. Untersuchungen über Dextran und sein Verhalten bei parenteraler Zufuhr. *Acta Physiol Scand* 1944;7:97–107.
2. Grönwall A, Ingelman B. Dextran as a substitute for plasma. *Nature* 1945;155:45.
3. Bohmansson G. Dextran as substitute for plasma. *North Med Assoc* 1947;23:126–131.
4. Gelin L-E, Ingelman B. Rheomacrodex—a new dextran solution for rheological treatment of impaired capillary flow. *Acta Chir Scand* 1961;122:294–302.
5. Bergentz SE, Eiken O, Gelin LE. Rheomacrodex in vascular surgery. *J Cardiovasc Res* 1963;4:388–392.
6. Bergqvist D, Bergentz S-E. The role of dextran in severe ischemic extremity disease and arterial reconstructive surgery. A review. *VASA* 1983;12:213–218.
7. Borgström S, Gelin L-E, Zederfeldt B. The formation of vein thrombi following tissue injury. *Acta Chir Scand* 1959;247(suppl):1–37.
8. Koekenberg LJL. Experimental use of macrodex as a prophylaxis against postoperative thromboembolism. *Exp Med Amst* 1961;40:123–130.
9. Wallenius G. Renal clearance of dextran as a measure of glomerular permeability. *Acta Soc Med Ups* 1954;4(suppl):1–91.
10. Hiippala S. Teppo A-M. Perioperative volume effect of HES 120/0.7 compared with dextran 70 and Ringer acetate. *Ann Chir Gynaecol* 1996;85:333–339.
11. Thorsén G, Hint H. Aggregation, sedimentation and intravascular sludging of erythrocytes. An experimental study. *Acta Chir Scand* 1950;154(suppl):1–51.
12. Gelin L-E. Studies in anemia of injury. *Acta Chir Scand* 1956;210(suppl):1–130.
13. Zederfeldt B. Studies on wound healing and trauma. *Acta Chir Scand* 1957;224(suppl):1–85.
14. Gelin L-E. Zederfeldt B. Low molecular weight dextran as a therapeutic agent against capillary stagnation. *Bibl Anat* 1960;1:265–273.
15. Gelin L-E, Shoemaker WC. Hepatic blood flow and microcirculatory alterations induced by dextran of high and low viscosity. *Surgery* 1961;49:713–718.
16. Ponder E, Ponder RV. Haematology, age and molecular weight of dextrans, their coating effects, and their interaction with serum albumin. *Nature* 1961;190:277–278.
17. Ross S, Ebert R. Microelectrophoresis of blood platelets and the effect of dextran. *J Clin Invest* 1959;38:155–160.
18. Gelin L-E, Korsan-Bengtsen K, Ygge J, Zederfeldt B. Influence of low viscous dextran on the hemostatic mechanism. *Acta Chir Scand* 1961;12:324–328.
19. Bennett PN, Dhall DP, McKenzie FN, Matheson NA. Effects of dextran infusion n the adhesiveness of human blood-platelets. *Lancet* 1966;2:1001–1003.
20. Bygdeman S, Eliasson R, Gullbring B. Effect of dextran infusion on the adenosine diphosphate induced adhesiveness and the spreading capacity of human blood platelets. *Thromb Haemost* 1966;15:451–456.
21. Dhall DP, Bennett PN, Matheson NA. Effect of dextran on platelet behaviour after abdominal operations. *Acta Chir Scand* 1967;387(suppl):75–59.
22. Watson W, Chang T. Platelet-surface interaction: effects of dextran 70 on platelet retention in extracorporeal surfaces. *Biomater Med Devices Art Organs* 1975;3:489–502.
23. Shoenfeld NA, Eldrup-Jorgensen J, Conolly R, et al. The effect of low molecular weight dextran on platelet deposition onto prosthetic materials. *J Vasc Surg* 1987;5:76–82.
24. Palmaz JC, Garcia O, Kopp DT, et al. Balloon expandable intra-arterial stents: effect of antithrombotic medication on thrombus formation. In: Zeitler E, Seyferth W (eds). *Pros and Cons in PTA and Auxilliary Methods*. Berlin: Springer Verlag, 1989;170–178.
25. Arfors K-E, Hint HC, Dhall DP, Matheson NA. Counteraction of platelet activity at sites of laser-induced endothelial trauma. *Br Med J* 1968;4:430–431.
26. Jacobsen U. Studies on the effect of dextran on the coagulation of blood. *Diss Med Karolinska Inst* 1957, Stockholm.
27. Nilsson IM, Eiken O. Further studies on the effect of dextran of various molecular weight on the coagulation mechanism. *Thromb Haemost* 1964;11:40–40.
28. Cronberg S, Robertson B, Nilsson IM, Niléhn J-E. Suppressive effect of dextran on platelet adhesiveness. *Thromb Haemost* 1966:16:384–394.
29. Kladetzky RG, Popov-Cenic S, Müller N, Hack G, Lang U. The effect of dextan 70 on the intra- and postoperative behaviour of haemostasis. *Bibl Anat* 1977;16:463–465.
30. Lethagen S, Rugarn P, Åberg M, Nilsson IM. Effects of desmopressin acetate (DDAVP) and dextranon hemostatic and thromboprophylactic mechanisms. *Acta Chir Scand* 1990:156:597–602.
31. Flordal PA, Svensson J, Ljungström K-G. Effects of desmopressin and dextran on coagulation and fibrinolysis in healthy volunteers. *Thromb Res* 1991;62:335–364.
32. Laurell AB. Influence of dextran on the conversion of fibrinogen to fibrin. *Scand J Clin Lab Invest* 1951;3:262–266.
33. Dugdale M, Nofzinger JD, Murphey F. Some effects of low molecular weight dextran on coagulation. *Thromb Haemost* 1966;15:118–130.
34. Tangen O, Wik KO, Almqvist IAM, Arfors K-E, Hint HC. Effects of dextran on the structure and plasmin induced lysis of human fibrin. *Thromb Res* 1972;1:487–492.
35. Eriksson M, Saldeen T. Effect of dextran on plasma tissue plasminogen activator (t-PA) and plasminogen activator inhibitor-1 (PAI-1) during surgery. *Acta Anaesthesiol Scand* 1995;39:163–166.
36. Carlin G, Karlström G, Modig J, Saldeen T. Effect of dextran on fibrinolysis inhibition activity in the blood after major surgery. *Acta Anaesth Scand* 180;24:375–378.
37. Miller CL, Lim RC. Dextran as a modulator of immune and coagulation activities in trauma patients. *J Surg Res* 1985;39:183–191.
38. Åberg M, Bergentz S-E, Hedner U. The effect of dextran on the lysability of ex vivo thrombi. *Acta Chir Scand* 1975;181:342–345.
39. Esquivel C, Bergqvist D, Björck C, Nilsson B, Bergentz S-E. Effect of volume expanders on the lysability of ex vivo thrombi in the rabbit. *Acta Chir Scand* 1982;148:359–362.
40. Ah-See A-K, Arfors K-E, Bergqvist D, Tangen O. Effect of dextran on experimental venous thrombosis in rabbits. *Thromb Haemost* 1974;32:284–291.
41. Bergqvist D, Björck C-G, Esquivel C, Nilsson B. Ef-

fect of platelet inhibition on experimental venous thrombosis in rabbit. *Acta Chir Scand* 1985;151: 429–431.

42. Carbone JV, Furth FW, Scott R, Crosby WH. A haemostatic defect associated with dextran infusion. *Proc Soc Exp Biol Med* 1954;85:101–103.

43. Bronwell W, Artz C, Sako Y. Evaluation of blood loss from a standarized wound after dextran. *Surg Forum* 1954;5:809–814.

44. Arfors K-E, Bergqvist D. Microvascular haemostatic plug formation in rabbit mesentery. Effect of blood flow velocity, thrombocytopenia and dextran treatment. *Bibl Haemotol* 1975;41:84–97.

45. Bergqvist D. The influence of plasma volume expanders on initial haemostasis in the rabbit mesentery. *Acta Anaesthesiol Scand* 1985;29:607–609.

46. Arfors K-E, Buckley PB. Pharmacological characteristics of artificial colloids. In: Haljamae H (ed). *Plasma Volume Support. Bailliere's Clinical Anaesthesiology* 1997;11:15–48.

47. Barker JH, Hammersen F, Galla TJ, et al. Direct monitoring of capillary perfusion following normovolemic hemodilution in an experimental skin-flap model. *Plast Reconstr Surg* 1990;86:946–954.

48. Hint H. Pharmacology of dextran and the physiological background for the clinical use of Rheomacrodex and Macrodex. *Acta Anaesthesiol Belg* 1968;2:119–138.

49. Lindblad B, Bergqvist D, Efsing HO, Hallböök T, Lindell S-E. Changes in peripheral haemodynamics induced by dextran 70, dihydroergotamine and their combination. A study using ultrasonic serial phlebography, plethysmography and isotope clearance techniques. *VASA* 1984;13:165–170.

50. Lindblad B, Bergqvist D. Central hemodynamic effects of dextran 70, dihydroergotamine and their combination. A study in dogs. *Acta Chir Scand* 1983;149: 459–465.

51. Lindblad B, Jensen N, Dougan P, Bergqvist D. Does dextran reduce early graft thrombogenicity? An experimental investigation on patency and platelet deposition on prosthetic graft materials in sheep. *Eur J Vasc Surg* 1990;4:341–344.

52. Frost-Arner L, Åberg M, Brueciner UG, Wieslander JB, Messmer K. Effects of normovolemic hemodilution on blood flow in the rabbit ear. *Microsurgery* 1990:11:19–24.

53. Jansen H. Postoperative thromboembolism and its prevention with 500 ml dextran given during operation. With a special study of the venous flow pattern in the lower extremities. *Acta Chir Scand* 1972;427(suppl): 1–73.

54. Ahlberg Å, Nylander G, Robertson B, Cronberg S, Nilsson IM. Dextran in prophylaxis of thrombosis in fractures of the hip. *Acta Chir Scand* 1968;387(suppl): 83–85.

55. Andersen P, Kjaersgaard E, Beyer-Holdersen R, Frederiksen E. DHEH and Dextran 70 in thromboprophylaxis after hip fracture. *Acta Orthop Scand* 1986;57: 469.

56. Evarts C, Feil E. Prevention of thromboembolic disease after elective surgery in the hip. *J Bone Joint Surg* 1971;53:1271–1280.

57. Harper DR, Dhall DP, Woodruff WH. Prophylaxis in iliofemoral venous thrombosis. The major amputee as a clinical research model. *Br J Surg* 1973;60:831.

58. Johnson SR, Bygdeman S, Eliasson R. Effect of dextran on postoperative thrombosis. *Acta Chir Scand* 1968;387(suppl):80–82.

59. Myhre H, Holen A. Thrombosis prophylaxis. Dextran or sodium warfarin? A controlled clinical study [in Norwegian]. *Nord Med* 1969;82:1534–1537.

60. Nillius SA, Ahlberg Å, Arborelius M Jr, Rosberg B. Preoperative normovolemic naemodilution with dextran 70 as a thromboembolic prophylaxis in total hip replacement. *Int Orthop* 1979;3:197–202.

61. Becker J, Schampi B. The incidence of postoperative venous thrombosis of the legs. A comparative study on the prophylactic effect of dextran 70 and electrical calf-muscle stimulation. *Acta Chir Scand* 1973;139: 357–367.

62. Bergman B, Bergqvist D, Dahlgren D. The incidence of venous thrombosis in the lower limbs following elective gall-bladder surgery. A study with the ^{125}I-fibrinogen test. *Ups J Med Sci* 1975;80:40–45.

63. Bergqvist D, Hallböök T. Prophylaxis of postoperative venous thrombosis in a controlled trial comparing dextran 70 and low-dose heparin. A study with ^{125}I-fibrinogen test. *World J Surg* 1980;4:239–243.

64. Bergqvist D, Efsing HO, Hallböök T, Hedlund T. Thromboembolism after elective and posttraumatic hip surgery—a controlled prophylactic trial with dextan and low-dose heparin. *Acta Chir Scand* 1979;145: 213–218.

65. Bowman HW. Clinical evaluation of dextran as a plasma volume expander. *JAMA* 1953;153:24–26.

66. Carter AE, Eban R. The prevention of postoperative deep venous thrombosis with dextran 70. *Br J Surg* 1973;60:681–683.

67. Daniel WJ, Moore AR, Flanc C. Prophylaxis of deep vein thrombosis (DVT) with dextran 70 in patients with a fractured neck of the femur. *Aust NZ J Surg* 1972;41:289.

68. Gruber UF, Rem J, Altofer R, et al. Efficacy of dextran 40 or heparin in the prevention of deep vein thrombosis after major surgery. *Eur Surg Res* 1973;5:15–16.

69. Hedlund PO. Postoperative venous thrombosis in benign prostatic disease. A study of 316 patients with the ^{125}I-fibrinogen uptake test. *Scand J Urol Nephrol* 1975;27(suppl):1–100.

70. von Hospenthal J, Frey C, Rutishauser G, Gruber UF. Thromboseprophylaxe bei transurethraler Prostataresektionen. *Urologe* 1977:16:88–92.

71. Hutter O, Duckert F, Fridrich R, Gruber UF. Dextran 40 zur Prophylaxe tiefer Venenthrombosen in der Chirurgie. *Dtsch Med Wochenschr* 1976;101:1834–1837.

72. Huttunen H, Mattila MAK, Alhava EM, Kettunen K, Karjalainen P, Huttunen K. Preoperative infusion of dextran 70 and dextran 40 in the prevention of postoperative deep venous thrombosis as confirmed by the ^{125}I-labelled fibrinogen uptake method. *Ann Chir Gynecol Fenn* 1977;66:79–81.

73. Lindström B, Holmdahl D, Jonsson O, et al. Prediction and prophylaxis of postoperative thromboembolism— a comparative calf muscle stimulation with groups of impulses and dextran 40. *Br J Surg* 1982;69:633–637.

74. Ruckley CV. A multi-unit controlled trial of heparin and dextran in the prevention of venous thromboembolic disease. In: Kakkar VV, Thomas DP (eds). *Heparin, Chemistry and Clinical Usage.* London: Academic, 1976;325–335.

75. Stephenson CBS, Wallace JG, Vaughan JV. Dextran 70 in the preventin of postoperative deep-vein thrombosis with observations on pulmonary embolism. Report on a pilot study. *NZ Med J* 1973;77:302–305.

76. Faun P, Suomalainen O, Bergqvist D, et al. The use of fibrinogen uptake test in screening for deep vein thrombosis in patients with hip fracture. *Thromb Res* 1990;60:185–190.

77. Clagett GP, Reisch JS. Prevention of venous thromboembolism in general surgical patients. *Ann Surg* 1988;208:227–240.

78. Bergquist E, Bergqvist D, Bronge A, Dahlgren S, Lindquist B. An evaluation of early thrombosis prophylaxis following fracture of the femoral neck. A comparison between dextran and dicoumarol. *Acta Chir Scand* 1972;138:689–693.

79. Bergqvist D, Kettunen K, Fredin H, et al. Thromboprophylaxis in hip fracture patients—a prospective randomized comparative study between Org 10172 and dextran 70. *Surgery* 1991;109:617–622.

80. Bronge A, Dahlgren S, Lindquist B. Prophylaxis against thrombosis in femoral neck fractures—a comparison between dextran 70 and dicoumarol. *Acta Chir Scand* 1971;137:29–35.

81. The Danish Enoxaparin Study Group. Low-molecular-weight heparin (Enoxaparin) versus dextran 70. The prevention of postoperative deep vein thrombosis after total hip replacement. *Arch Intern Med* 1991;151:1621–1624.

82. Francis CW, Pellegrini VD, Marder VJ, Harris CM, Totterman S, Gabriel KR. Prevention of venous thrombosis after total hip arthroplasty. *J Bone Joint Surg [Am]* 1989;71:327–335.

83. Francis C, Marder V, Evarts M, Yaukoolbodi S. Two-step warfarin therapy. Prevention of postoperative venous thrombosis without excessive bleeding. *JAMA* 1983;249:374–378.

84. Francis C, Pellegrini V, Stulberg B, Millar M, Totterman S, Marder V. Prevention of venous thrombosis after total knee arthroplasty. Comparison of antithrombin III and low dose heparin with dextran. *J Bone Joint Surg [Am]* 1990;72:976–982.

85. Fredin H, Gustafson C, Rosberg B. Hypotensive anesthesia, thromboprophylaxis and postoperative thromboembolism in total hip arthroplasty. *Acta Anaesthesiol Scand* 1984;28:503–507.

86. Fredin HO, Rosberg B, Arborelius M, Nylander G. On thromboembolism after total hip replacement in epidural analgesia: a controlled study of dextran 70 and low-dose heparin combined with dihydroergotamine. *Br J Surg* 1984;71:58–60.

87. Fredin H, Nilsson B, Rosberg B, Tengborn L. Pre- and postoperative levels of antithrombin III with special reference to thromboembolism after total hip replacment. *Thromb Haemost* 1983;49:158–161.

88. Harris WH, Salzman EH, Athanasoulis C. Comparison of warfarin. Low-molecular-weight dextran, aspirin and subcutaneous heparin in prevention of venous thromboembolism following total hip replacement. *J Bone Joint Surg* 1974;56:1552–1562.

89. Eriksson BI, Zacharisson BE, Teger-Nilsson AC, Risberg B. Thrombosis prophylaxis with low molecular weight heparin in total hip replacement. *Br J Surg* 1988;75:1053–1057.

90. Fredin HO, Nillius SA, Bergqvist D. Prophylaxis of deep vein thrombosis in patients with fracture of the femoral neck. *Acta Orthop Scand* 1982;53:413–417.

91. Myrvold HE, Persson J-E, Svensson B, Wallensten S, Vikterlöf KJ. Prevention of thrombo-embolism with dextran 70 and heparin in patients with femoral neck fractures. *Acta Chir Scand* 1973;139:609–616.

92. Mätzsch T, Bergqvist D, Fredin H, Hedner U. Low molecular weight heparin compared with dextran as prophylaxis against thrombosis after total hip replacement. *Acta Chir Scand* 1990;156:445–450.

93. Mätzsch T, Bergqvist D, Fredin H, Hedner U, Lindhagen A, Nistor L. Comparison of the thromboprophylactic effect of low molecular weight heparin versus dextran in total hip replacement. *Thromb Haemorrh Disord* 1991;3:25–29.

94. Barber HM, Feil EJ, Galasko GA. A comparative study of dextran 70, warfarin and low-dose heparin for the prophylaxis of thromboembolism following total hip replacement. *Postgrad Med J* 1977;53:130–133.

95. Bergqvist D, Dahlgren S. Leg vein thrombosis diagnosed by ^{125}I-fibrinogen test in patients with fracture of the hip: a study of early prophylaxis with dicoumarol or dextran 70. *VASA* 1973;2:121–126.

96. Bergqvist D, Elfsing HO, Hallböök T, Lindblad B. Prevention of postoperative thromboembolic complications. A prospective comparison between dextran 70, dihydroergotamine heparin and a sulfated polysaccharide. *Acta Chir Scand* 1980;146:559–568.

97. Bergqvist D, Ljungnér H. A comparative study of dextran 70 and a sulphated poly-saccharide in the prevention of postoperative thromboembolic complications in patients undergoing abdominal surgery. *Br J Surg* 1981;68:449–451.

98. Davidson AI, Brunt ME, Matheson NA. A further trial comparing dextan 70 with warfarin in the prophylaxis of postoperative venous thrombosis. *Br J Surg* 1972;59:314.

99. Hohl MK, Lüsher KP, Tichy J, et al. Prevention of postoperative thromboembolism by dextran 70 or low-dose heparin. *Obstet Gynecol* 180;55:497–500.

100. Lambie JM, Barber DC, Dhall DP, Matheson NA. Dextran 70 in prohylaxis of postoperative venous thrombosis. A controlled trial. *Br Med J* 1970;2:144–145.

101. McCarthy TG, McQueen J, Johnston FD, Weston J, Campbell S. A comparison of low-dose subcutaneous heparin and intravenous dextran 70 in the prophylaxis of deep venous thrombosis after gynaecological surgery. *J Obstet Gynaecol* 1974;81:486–491.

102. Rosell Pradas J, Vara-Thorbeck R. Dextran versus heparin subcutána en la profilaxis de la trombosis venosa profunda (T.V.P) postcirugría biliar. *Rev Esp Enf Ap Dig* 1988;74:521–524.

103. Bergqvist D. *Postoperative Thromboembolism. Frequency, Etiology, Prophylaxis.* Berlin: Springer Verlag, 1983.

104. Matthiasson S, Lindblad B, Holst J, Bergqvist D. Effect of low molecular weight heparin, dextran and their combination on experimental venous thrombosis in rabbits. In: Raymond-Martimbeau P, Prescott R, Zummo M (eds). *Phlebologie 92*. Paris: John Libbey Eurotext, 1992;451–453.

105. Holst J, Lindblad B, Mätzsch T, Bergqvist D. Effect on primary haemostasis of prophylactic regimens of low molecular weight heparin, unfractionated heparin,

dextran and their combinations. An experimental dou-
ble-dummy study. *Thromb Res* 1992;65:651–656.

106. Rutherford R, Jones D, Bergentz S-E, et al. The efficacy of dextran 40 in preventing early postoperative
thrombosis following difficult lower extremity bypass. *J Vasc Surg* 1984;1:765–773.

107. Smith RC, Elton RA, Orr JD, et al. Dextran and intermittent pneumatic compression in prevention of postoperative deep vein thrombosis. *Br Med J* 1978;1:
952–954.

108. Bergqvist D, Lindblad B. The thromboprophylactic effect of graded elastic compression stockings in combination with dextran 70. *Arch Surg* 1984;119:
1329–1331.

109. Harris WH, Athanasoulis CA, Waltman AC, Salzman
EW. Prophylaxis of deep-vein thrombosis after total
hip replacement. *J Bone Joint Surg [Am]* 1985;67:
57–62.

110. Boström S, Holmgren E, Jonsson O, et al. Postoperative thromboembolism in neurosurgery. A study on the
prophylactic effect of calf muscle stimulation plus
dextran compared to low-dose heparin. *Acta Neurochir*
1986;80:83–89.

111. Fredin H, Bergqvist D, Cederholm C, Lindblad B, Ny-
man U. Thromboprophylaxis in hip arthroplasty. Dextran with graded compression or preoperative dextran
compared in 150 patients. *Acta Orthop Scand*
1989;60:678–681.

112. Pini M, Spadini E, Caluccio L, et al. Dextran/aspirin
versus heparin/dihydroergotamine in preventing
thrombosis after hip fractures. *J Bone Joint Surg [Br]*
1985;67:305–309.

113. Kline A, Hughes LE, Campbell H, Williams A, Zlos-
nick J, Leach KG. Dextran 70 in prohylaxis of thromboembolic disease after surgery: a clinically oriented
randomized double-blind trial. *Br Med J* 1975;2:
109–112.

114. Ljungström KG. Dextran prophylaxis of fatal pulmonary embolism. *World J Surg* 1983;7:767–772.

115. Atik M, Harkness JW, Wichman H. Prevention of fatal
pulmonary embolism. *Surg Gynecol Obstet* 1970;130:
403–413.

116. Brisman R, Parks LC, Haller A. Dextran prohylaxis in
surgery. *Ann Surg* 1971;137–141.

117. Edwards DH, Steel WM, Bentley G. Prophylaxis with
dextran 70 against thrombosis in patients with fractures of the upper end of the femur. *Injury* 1975;6:
250–253.

118. Elsner-Mackey P, Ledermair O, Schastok H, Vinazzer
H. Zur Wirkung von Macrodex auf die postoperative
Thromboembolie-Frequenz. *Wien Med Wochenschr*
1969;119:149–153.

119. Hurson B, Ennis JT, Corrigan TP, Macauley P. Dextran
prophylaxis in total hip replacement: a scintigraphic
evaluation of the incidence of deep vein thrombosis
and pulmonary embolus. *Ir J Med Sci* 1979;148:
140–144.

120. Huttunen H, Mattila MAK, Hakelehto J, Kettunen K,
Rehnberg V, Babinski M. Single infusion of dextran 70
in the prophylaxis of postoperative deep venous thrombosis. *Ann Chir Gynecol Fenn* 1971;60:119–122.

121. Rothermel JE, Wessinger JB, Stinchfield FE. Dextran
40 and thromboembolism in total hip replacement
surgery. *Arch Surg* 1973;106:135–137.

122. Stadil F. Prevention of postoperative vein thrombosis

with dextran 70 [in Danish]. *Ugeskr Laeg* 1970;132:
1817–1820.

123. Welin-Berger T, Bygdeman S, Mebius C. Deep vein
thrombosis following hip surgery. Relation to activated
factor C inhibitor activity: effect of heparin and dextran. *Acta Orthop Scand* 1982;53:937–945.

124. Gruber UF, Saldeen T, Brokop T, et al. Incidences of
fatal postoperative pulmonary embolism with dextran
70 and low-dose heparin. An internatinal multicentre
study. *Br Med J* 1980;280:69–72.

125. Gruber UF, Allemann U, Wettler H. Erster direkter Vergleich der allergischen Nebemvirkungen des Dextrans
mit ohne Hapten. *Schweiz Med Wochenschr* 1982;112:
605–612.

126. Harris WH, Salzman EW, DeSanctis RW, Coutts RD.
Prevention of venous thromboembolism following total hip replacement. Warfarin vs dextran 40. *JAMA*
1972;220:1319–1322.

127. Lüders H, Konold P, Otten GL, Koslowski L. Postoperative Thromboseprophylaxe. Randomisierte, pros-
pektive Untersuchung zum Vergleich einer Throm-
boemboliprophylaxe mit Antikoagulantien (Heparin-
Marcumar) und Dextran 60 (Macrodex). *Chirurgie*
1973;4:563–569.

128. Bombardini T. Borghi B, Montebuganoli M, Picano E,
Caroli GC. Effect of normovolemic hemodilution on
fatal postoperative pulmonary embolism in major
elective orthopaedic surgery. A retrospective analysis
of 4653 patients. *Vasc Surg* 1996;30:125–144.

129. Gottstein U. Sedmeyer I, Schöttler M, Gülk V. Der Ef-
fekt von niedermolekularem Dextran auf die Durch-
blutung von Gesunden und von Kranken mit peripheren arteriellen Zirkulationsstörungen. *Deutsch Med
Wochenschr* 1970;95:1955.

130. Humphreys WV, Walker A, Charlesworth C. The effect
of an infusion of low molecular weight dextran on peripheral resistance in patients with arteriosclerosis. *Br
J Surg* 1976;63:691.

131. Bollinger A, Simon HJ, Köhler R, Lüthy E. Wirkung
von niedermolekylarem Dextran auf Blutviskosität
und Extremitätendurchblutung. *Z Kreislaufforsch*
1968;57:456–465.

132. Bergan JJ, Trippel OH, Kaupp A, Kukral JC, Nowlin
WF. Low molecular weight dextran in treatment of severe ischemia. *Arch Surg* 1965;91:338.

133. Powley P. Rheomacrodex in peripheral ischemia.
Lancet 1953;1:1189.

134. Skalkeas G, Balas P, Katsogianis A, Bakoulas G, Kara-
gianokas R. A new approach to the treatment of ischemic conditions of the extremities; continuous intraarterial infusion therapy. *Angiology* 1969;20:144.

135. Ernst E, Kollar L, Matrai A. A double-blind trial of
dextran-haemodilution vs placebo in claudicants. *J Intern Med* 1990;227:19–24.

136. Stoltz JF, Cheraud C, Voisin Ph, Burdin D, Streiff F,
Laxenaire MC. Association albumine diluée-dextran
40 dans le traitment de lártériopathie des membres in-
férieurs par hémodilution normovolémique. *J Mal
Vasc* 1986;11:344–350.

137. von Stoltz J, Bartel M. Einfluss einer adjuvanten Infu-
sionstherapie von niedermolekularen Dextranen (Infu-
koll M-40) und deproteinsiertem Hämoderivat
(Actovegin) bei chronisch arteriellen Durchblutungs-
störungen im Stadium IV nach Fontaine. *Zentralbl
Chir* 1988;112:1044–105.

138. Rieger H, Köhler M, Schoop W, Schmid-Schöönbein H, Roth FJ, Leyhe A. Hemodilution (HD) in patients with ischemic skin ulcers. *Klin Wochenschr* 1979;57: 1153–1161.

139. Jacobsson B. Effect of pretreatment with dextran 70 on platelet adhesiveness and thromboembolic complications following percutaneous arterial catheterization. *Acta Radiol* 1969;8:289.

140. Langsjoen P, Best EB. Studies in the prevention of complications of angiography. *AJR* 1969;106:425.

141. Davidson SF, Brantley SK, Das SK. Comparison of single-dose antithrombotic agents in the prevention of microvascular thrombosis. *J Hand Surg [Am]* 1991; 16:585–589.

142. Frost-Arner L, Bergqvist D. Effect of isovolemic hemodilution with dextran and albumin on thrombus formation in artificial vessel grafts inserted into the abdominal aorta of the rabbit. *Microsurgery* 1995;16: 357–361.

143. Lindblad B, Jensen N, Dougan P, Bergqvist D. Does dextran 40 reduce early graft thrombogenicity? An experimental investigation on patency and platelet deposition on prosthetic graft materials in sheep. *Eur J Vasc Surg* 1990;4:341–344.

144. Winfrey EW, Foster J. Low molecular weight dextran in small artery surgery. *Arch Surg* 1964;88:78.

145. Mason RG, Wolf RH, Zucker WH, Shinoda BA, Mohammed SF. Effects of antithrombotic agents evaluated in a nonhuman primate vascular shunt model. *Am J Pathol* 1976;83:557.

146. Pasternak R, Baugham K, Fallon J, Block P. Scanning electron microscopy after coronary transluminal angioplasty of normal canine arteries. *Am J Cardiol* 1980;45:591.

147. Christenson JT, Al-Huneidi W, Abu Saleh R. Distal embolisation from the surface of PTFE grafts in vivo and the effect of low molecular weight dextran. *Eur J Vasc Surg* 1988;2:121–125.

148. Rothkopf DM. Chu B, Bern S, May JW. The effect of dextran on microvascular thrombosis in an experimental rabbit model. *Plast Reconstr Surg* 1993;92:511–515.

149. Zhang B, Wieslander JB. Dextran's antithrombotic properties in small arteries are not altered by low-molecular-weight heparin or the fibrinolytic inhibitor tranexamic acid: an experimental study. *Microsurgery* 1993;14:289–295.

150. Wolfort, SF, Angel MF, Knight KR, Amiss LR, Morgan RF. The beneficial effect of dextran on anastomotic patency and flap survival in a strongly thrombogenic model. *J Reconstr Microsurg* 1992;8:375–378.

151. Sasamoto Y. Experimental studies on continuous local infusion of anticoagulants for reconstruction of small arteries. *J Kumamoto Med Soc* 1970;44:839.

152. Dagher F, Slim M, Abraham E, Meneshian G. Effect of dextrans on small arterial anastomosis. *Arch Surg* 1972;103:581.

153. Shoenfeld NA, Yeager A, Conolly R, et al. A new primate model for the study of intravenous thrombotic potential and its modification. *J Vasc Surg* 1988;8: 49–54.

154. Matthiasson SE, Bergqvist D, Lundell A, Lindblad B. Effect of dextran and enoxaparin on early ePTFE graft thrombogenicity in sheep. *Eur J Vasc Endovasc Surg* 1995;9:284–292.

155. Bergentz S-E, Gelin L-E, Rudenstam C-M, Zederfeldt B. The viscosity of whole blood in trauma. *Acta Chir Scand* 1963;126:289.

156. Thomas J, Silva J. Dextran 40 in the treatment of peripheral vascular disease. *Arch Surg* 1973;106:138.

157. Waibel P. Antikoagulation in der Gefässchirurgie. *VASA* 1976;5:107.

158. Sawyer PN, Stillman RM, Faller J, Sophie Z, Stanczewski B, Solimon F. Dextran-heparin antithrombotic therapy following vascular reconstruction. *Surg Rounds* 1979;Nov:37–45.

159. Logason K, Bergqvist D on behalf of Swedvasc. The effect of low molecular weight heparin in early graft patency—a randomized comparison with dextran. *Eur J Surg* (in press).

160. McManus F. The incidence of deep venous thrombosis after total hip replacement using dextran 70 prophylaxis—a venographic study. *Ir J Med Sci* 1976;145: 201–206.

161. Schött U, Sjöstrand U, Thorén T, Berséus O. Three per cent dextran-60 as a plasma substitute in blood component therapy. I. An alternative in surgical blood loss replacement. *Acta Anaesthesiol Scand* 1985;29:767–774.

162. Schött U, Thorén T, Sjöstrand U, Berséus O, Söderholm B. Three per cent dextran-60 as a plasma substitute in blood component therapy. II. Comparative studies on pre- and postoperative blood volume. *Acta Anaesthesiol Scand* 1985;29:775–781.

163. Schött U, Lindbom L-O, Sjöstrand U. Hemodynamic effects of colloid concentration in experimental hemorrhage: a compariosn of Ringer's acetate, 3% dextran-60 and 6% dextran-70. *Crit Care Med* 1988;16:346–352.

164. Dawidson IJ, Willms C, Sandor ZF, Coorpender LL, Reisch JS, Fry WJ. Ringer's lactate with or without 3% dextran-60 as volume expanders during abdominal aortic surgery. *Crit Care Med* 1991;19:36–42.

165. Bergman A, Andreen M, Blombäck M. Plasma substitution with 3% dextran-60 in orthopaedic surgery: influence on plasma colloid osmotic pressure, coagulation parameters, immunoglobulins and other plasma constituents. *Acta Anaesthesiol Scand* 1990;34:21–29.

166. Schöndorf T, Weber U. Heparin prophylaxis combined with DHE or dextran in hip operations. *Thromb Haemost* 1979;42:249–263.

167. Korttila K, Layritsalo K, Särmo A, Goridn A, Sundberg S. Suitability of plasma expanders in patients receiving low-dose heparin for prevention of venous thrombosis after surgery. *Acta Anaesthesiol Scand* 1983;27:104–107.

168. Morrison ND, Stephenson CBS, Maclean D, Stanhope JM. Deep vein thrombosis after femoropopliteal bypass grafting with observations on the incidence of complications following the use of dextran 70. *NZ Med J* 1976;84:233–236.

169. Lisander B, Jacobsson S-A, Ivarsson I, Vegfors M, Engdahl O. Giving both enoxaparin and dextran increases the need for transfusion in revision hip arthroplasty. *Eur J Surg* 1996;162;861–866.

170. Hjerrberg H, Olsson J, Ekström T, et al. Combining dalteparin and dextran does not increase the blood loss in transurethral resection of the prostate. *Acta Anaesthesiol Scand* 1995;105(suppl)39:159.

171. Bauer Å, Östling G. Dextran-induced anaphylactoid reactions in connection with surgery. *Acta Anaesth Scand* 1970;38(suppl):182–185.

172. Hedin H. Dextran-induced anaphylactoid reactions in

man. Immunological in vitro and in vivo studies. *Acta Univ Ups Abst Diss Fac Med* 432:1–43.

173. Ljungström K-G. Safety of dextran in relation to other colloids—ten years experience with hapten inhibition. *Infusionsther Transfusionsmed* 1993;20:206–210.

174. Smedgård G. Anaphylactic shock. Pathophysiology of aggregate and cytotropic anaphylaxis in the monkey. *Acta Univ Ups Diss Fac Sci* 1980;548:1–44.

175. Kraft D, Hedin H, Richter W, Scheiner O, Rumpold H, Devey ME. Immunoglobulin class and subclass distribution of dextran-reactive antibodies in human reactors and non reactors to clinical dextran. *Allergy* 1982;37: 481–489.

176. Hedin H, Smedegård G. Complement profiles in monkeys subjected to aggreparticulate polysaccharides. *Int Arch Allergy Appl Immunol* 1979;60:286–294.

177. Hedin H, Richter W. Pathomechanisms of dextran-induced anaphylactoid/anaphylactic reactions in vein. *Int Arch Allerg Appl Immunol* 1982;62:122–126.

178. Ljungström K-G, Renck H. Metabolic acidosis in dextran-induced anaphylactic reactions. *Acta Anaesthesiol Scand* 1987;31:157–160.

179. Paull J. A prospective study of dextran-induced anaphylactoid reactions in 5745 patients. *Anaesth Intens Care* 1987;15:163–167.

180. Ring J, Messmer K. Anaphylaktoide Reaktionen nach Infusion kolloidaler Volumenersatzmittel. *Internist Prax* 1976;16:579–588.

181. Furhoff A-K. Anaphylactoid reaction to dextran—a report of 133 cases. *Acta Anesthesiol Scand* 1977;21: 161–167.

182. Gelin L-E. Use and misuse of Rheomacrodex [in Swedish]. *Svensk Läkartidn* 1966;63:1377–1380.

183. Mailloux L, Swarz CD, Capizzi R, et al. Acute renal failure after administration of low-molecular-weight dextran. *N Engl J Med* 1976;21:1113–1118.

184. Engberg A, Ericsson JLE. Effects of dextran 40 on proximal renal tubule. Electron microscopic and cytochemical studies in the mouse. *Acta Chir Scand* 1969;135:263–274.

Cardiovascular Thrombosis: Thrombocardiology and Thromboneurology, Second Edition,
edited by M. Verstraete, V. Fuster, and E. J. Topol,
Lippincott–Raven Publishers, Philadelphia © 1998.

14

Other Antithrombotics

Marc Verstraete

The Center for Molecular and Vascular Biology, University of Leuven, B-3000 Leuven, Belgium

The previous six chapters describe the advantages but also the limitations of different classes of antithrombotic drugs. Substantial research is focusing on other compounds with antithrombotic properties, which are briefly discussed here.

THROMBOMODULIN

Thrombomodulin is an endothelial cell surface protein that forms a reversible 1:1 stoichiometric complex with thrombin. After formation of this complex, thrombin no longer has procoagulant activity but does acquire the potential to activate protein C 1000-fold compared to free thrombin (1–3). The term *thrombomodulin* is appropriate because this protein changes the substrate specificity of thrombin, apparently by an allosteric mechanism. Activated protein C, in the presence of protein S, inactivates blood coagulation factors Va and VIIIa (4,5). Thus, by accelerating the activation of protein C, thrombomodulin plays an important role as endogenous regulator of coagulation at the surface of the vascular wall.

Furthermore, thrombomodulin inhibits the proteolytic action of thrombin on macromolecular substrates, and because thrombomodulin contains a galactosaminoglycan, it accelerates the inactivation of thrombin by antithrombin III.

The thrombin–thrombomodulin complex is also involved in the regulation of fibrinolysis as it activates another macromolecular substrate, termed Thrombin Activatable Fibrinolysis Inhibitor (TAFI), by cleavage of a single proteolytic cleavage (6,7). The enzyme, TAFIa, is a carboxypeptidase with specificity for carboxy terminal arginine and lysine residues (8) and is a potent inhibitor of fibrinolysis (6,9,10). This suppression of fibrinolysis is most likely obtained by downregulation of the cofactor function of partially degraded fibrin (removing plasminogen binding sites). The existence of TAFI explains the apparent profibrinolytic effect of activated protein C.

The lethal effect of deletion of thrombomodulin gene in the mouse was demonstrated (11). Thrombomodulin mutation cosegregates with thromboembolic disease (12).

Thrombomodulin is an integral membrane glycoprotein containing 575 amino acids and 5 domains. it is present on the vascular surface of endothelial cells of arteries, veins, capillaries, and lymphatic vessels (Fig. 14-1). Thrombomodulin purified from human urine has a potent antithrombotic effect in the rat disseminated intravascular coagulation model (13). The human thrombomodulin cDNA has been isolated (4) and expressed in Chinese hamster ovary (CHO) cells (14). This soluble human thrombomodulin contains only the domains 1, 2, and 3 (amino acids 1–491) but not the transmembrane module and cytoplasmic tail of native single-chain thrombomodulin.

Recombinant human soluble thrombomodulin is effective in the rat model of arteriovenous shunt thrombosis (15) and in disseminated intravascular coagulation models in mice and rats, also when the levels of antithrombin III are reduced. The presence of chondroitin sulfate on recombinant human soluble thrombomodulin results in a higher affinity for thrombin, a greater ability to inhibit thrombin-induced fibrin formation and

platelet activation, and is associated with antithrombin III–dependent inactivation of thrombin (16,17). Administration of thrombomodulin prolongs the thrombin time (TT), prothrombin time (PT), and activated partial thromboplastin time (APTT). Recombinant human thrombomodulin may be a means to generate endogenous activated protein C.

The parenteral administration of soluble recombinant thrombomodulin has been associated with antithrombotic effects without bleeding in cancer patients (18).

PROTEIN C

Activated protein C is a natural coagulation inhibitor that plays a key role in the regulation of blood coagulation by selectively degrading coagulation cofactors Va and VIIIa and thereby inhibits thrombus generation (19). Thus, activated protein C stops the positive feedback actions of thrombin on the coagulation cascade (thrombin activates factors VIII and V), thereby limiting the coagulation process and thrombus propagation (Fig. 14-2).

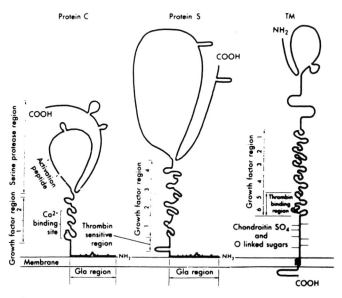

FIG. 14-1. Schematic representation of protein C, protein S, and thrombomodulin (TM). The Gla residues (γ-carboxyglutamic acid) are indicated as small Y-shaped symbols on protein C and protein S. These residues are required for biological activity and depend on vitamin K for their biosynthesis. (From Esmon CT, ref. 3, and Esmon ML, ref. 107, with permission.)

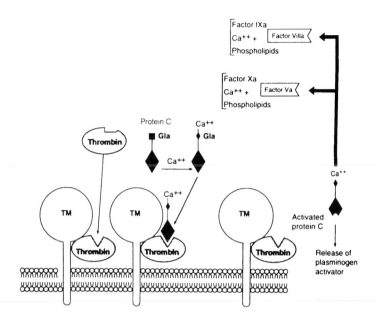

FIG. 14-2. Thrombin forms a complex with the endothelium-bound protein thrombomodulin (TM). This complex activates circulating protein C, which inhibits factor Va and VIIIa and releases tissue plasminogen activator from the endothelial cells. Binding of activated protein C to phospholipids is facilitated by protein S. Gla, γ-carboxyglutamic acid.

Protein C is one of the vitamin K–dependent plasma proteins; it is activated on the surface of intact endothelial cells by thrombin bound to thrombomodulin. The anticoagulant effect of activated protein C is enhanced by protein S, which is another vitamin K–dependent plasma protein (20). It has been reported that protein S increases the affinity of activated protein C for thrombogenic phospholipids approximately 10-fold and that protein S abrogates the protective effect of factor Xa against activated protein C–mediated degradation of factor Va in the prothrombinase complex.

An endothelial cell protein C receptor has been identified (21). It is a transmembrane protein that is expressed at high levels only on a subset of endothelial cells. These receptors augment protein C activation. Binding to the receptor is Ca^{2+}-dependent and is mediated in part by the Gla domain of the protein.

Human plasma contains 4 mg/L of protein C. The protein can be purified from plasma or obtained by recombinant technology (22). Because of its endogenous origin and specificity

of action, activated protein C is a potentially attractive antithrombotic agent. Earlier studies have shown that activated protein C inhibits disseminated intravascular coagulation in rabbits (23) and blocks the lethal effects of *Escherichia coli* infusion in baboons (24). Moreover, human activated protein C has been shown to reduce jugular vein thrombus formation in dogs, to delay the time to occlusion in anodal current-induced rat aorta thrombosis (25), and to reduce intermittent platelet thrombus formation in rat microvessels (26). Human activated protein C inhibits thrombus formation on thrombogenic grafts interposed in arteriovenous shunts in baboons, when infused into the shunt just proximal to the thrombogenic site (27).

Using a bovine protein C preparation in a microarterial thrombosis model in the rabbit, antithrombotic efficacy was demonstrated but was associated with significant bleeding (28).

Thrombin mutants with selectivity for endogenous protein C have been developed (29, 30). Activated protein C administration does not impair hemostasis (31), which supports the proposal to either use protein C or increase its plasmatic level by administering thrombin mutants without affecting the fibrinogen conversion.

DEFIBROTIDE

Defibrotide is the sodium salt of a single-strand polydeoxyribonucleotide (aptamers) of a well-defined base sequence and composition that binds to thrombin. The compound has a mean molecular weight of 15 to 30 kDa with a defined ratio of purine to pyrimidine bases of >0.85. It is prepared by controlled depolymerization of deoxyribonucleic acid (DNA) obtained from porcine organs.

In most studies, particularly those using a three- to fourfold higher dose than that recommended for patients, defibrotide stimulates PGI_2 and PGE_2 production without change in thromboxane A_2 levels and is associated with reduced leukotriene B4 levels (32). The drug also stimulates the fibrinolytic system, as shown by a decrease of the euglobulin lysis time and dilute clot lysis time. Furthermore, the lysis area of euglobulin on standard fibrin plates increases (33,34). There are conflicting observations regarding the effect of defibrotide on activity in blood of tissue-type plasminogen activator (t-PA), plasminogen activator inhibitor type 1 (PAI-1), and α_2-antiplasmin (35).

Defibrotide appears to be largely devoid of anticoagulant properties as determined by a lack of clinically significant effects on coagulation parameters, including APTT and the prothrombin time. The drug appears to have no effect on von Willebrand factor, factor VIII, factor Xa, and prekallikrein, whereas its effect on antithrombin III, fibrinogen, and protein C requires further confirmation.

Defibrotide has been reported to have little effect on platelet numbers, but may inhibit platelet function, possibly by stimulating the formation of PGI_2 and blocking calcium ions' entry into cells by interfering with the adenosine receptor (36). It has recently been shown that defibrotide stimulates expression of

thrombomodulin in cultured human umbilical vein endothelial cells (37).

Investigation of the pharmacokinetic behavior of defibrotide is difficult because the drug is degraded in the body to a number of products and the identity of the active derivative(s) in humans is unclear. To date, the majority of pharmacokinetic data have been determined by following the fate of the carbohydrate moiety of the drug 6-deoxyribose. Elimination of defibrotide in humans follows different kinetic models depending on the dose, with a one-compartment model being the most appropriate following administration of low doses, and a two-compartment model better suited following high doses. The elimination half-life is short and increases with dose, with values of between 9.8 and 27.1 minutes after intravenous doses of 0.5 to 16 mg/kg or a single intravenous injection of 200 mg. The elimination half-life appears to be independent of the route of administration, with similar values being obtained after oral and intravenous administration.

An antithrombotic action of defibrotide has been demonstrated in a number of animal models of venous thrombosis, in which the drug

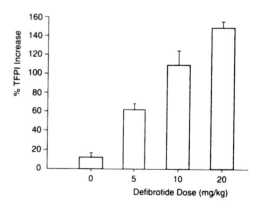

FIG. 14-3. Effect of oral administration of defibrotide on plasma tissue factor pathway inhibitor (TFPI) levels in normal healthy volunteers. Defibrotide was administered at 5, 10, and 20 mg/kg dosages to groups of healthy individuals ($n = 10$). Blood samples were drawn 4 hours after the administration of defibrotide. (From Fareed et al., ref. 108, with permission.)

was able to attenuate the formation of collagen-, activated prothrombin complex–, thrombin-, and mechanically induced venous thrombosis, and to reduce the size and alter the composition of the thrombi that are formed (38). Furthermore defibrotide has a protective effect in animal models on myocardial, liver, and kidney ischemia (39). When healthy volunteers were treated with oral dosages of 5, 10, and 20 mg/kg defibrotide, a dose-dependent increase in the release of the tissue factor pathway inhibitor (TFPI) was observed (Fig. 14-3). This suggest that, similar to heparin, defibrotide is capable of releasing TFPI.

Defibrotide has been demonstrated to be more effective than placebo for the prevention of postoperative deep vein thrombosis but does not appear to be superior to subcutaneous unfractionated heparin (35,40).

TISSUE FACTOR PATHWAY INHIBITOR

Coagulation at a site of injury is initiated by exposure of blood to cell surface tissue factor and formation of the tissue factor– factor VIIa complex. The latter then activates both factors IX and X, leading to thrombin generation and fibrin formation. Tissue factor pathway inhibitor (TFPI) plays a primary role in regulating tissue factor–induced coagulation. Human plasma contains a tissue factor pathway inhibitor, formerly termed anticonvertin (41), external pathway inhibitor (42), or lipoprotein-associated coagulation inhibitor (LACI) (43).

Tissue factor (TF) is an integral membrane protein of the vascular endothelium, primarily synthesized by the endothelium, that functions as an essential cofactor for the proteolytic activity of factor VII toward its substrates, factors IX and X (44,45).

This endogenous protease inhibitor of 42,000 Da is a 276-amino acid polypeptide consisting of three Kunitz-type serine protease inhibitor domains (Fig. 14-4). The majority (85%) of human TFPI remains associated with apolipoprotein AII, possibly via a mixed disulfide linkage. TFPI interacts with the target proteins of factors VIIa and Xa in a

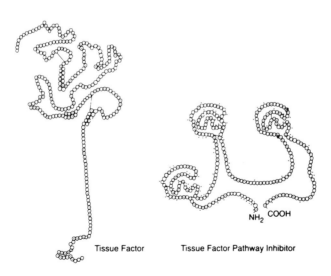

Tissue Factor   Tissue Factor Pathway Inhibitor

FIG. 14-4. A comparison of the primary structure of tissue factor (TF) with tissue factor pathway inhibitor (TFPI). TF is a transmembrane protein with both plasmatic and TF activating properties. TFPI is capable of selectively inhibiting TF and its mediated responses. Thus, in addition to controlling coagulation activation, this inhibition is also involved in the control of inflammatory responses. (From Fareed et al., ref. 108, with permission.)

two-step fashion. In the first step, which is independent of calcium, TFPI binds to factor
Xa by the second Kunitz domain, presumably
through an active arginyl site (Fig. 14-5). This
reaction does not involve the Gla residues on
factor Xa. The bimolecule then induces a
feedback inhibition of tissue factor– factor
VIIa complex, thereby inhibiting the extrinsic
pathway of coagulation. In this second step,
the binding occurs through the first Kunitz
domain. This reaction requires calcium and
the Gla residues on factor Xa are essential
(43). The function of the third Kunitz-like domain is unknown but a segment of it, including the C-terminal tail, may be involved in
binding to cell surface glycosaminoglycans
(46). TFPI may also inhibit factor VIIa–tissue
factor complexes in the absence of factor Xa
(47). This may be an additional mechanism of
action when recombinant TFPI is considered
for use as a therapeutic agent (48). Thus TFPI

inhibits factor Xa directly, whereas inhibition
of factor VIIa requires the simultaneous presence of factor Xa to form a quaternary complex TFPI–factor Xa and VIIa–tissue factor.

There is accumulating evidence that the tissue factor–induced coagulation system is involved in arterial thrombosis and atherogenesis. Atherosclerotic plaques contain tissue
factor–synthesizing cells, and plaque rupture
leads to exposure of tissue factor activity to
the circulating blood (49–54). Elevated TFPI
activity has been demonstrated in patients
with myocardial infarction (54), even at a
young age (56), suggesting that TFPI level
adapts to changes in the activity of factor VII.

Recombinant TFPI is available either at
full length (prepared from Chinese hamster
ovary cells) (44) or in a truncated form
(TFPI$_{1-161}$) lacking the basic C-terminal region and the third Kunitz domain and is produced in yeast cells (57). The two forms of

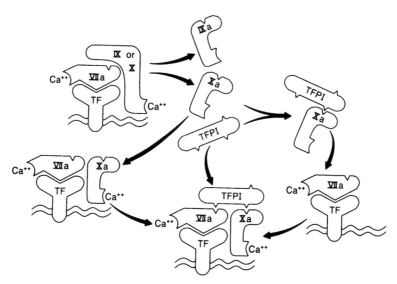

FIG. 14-5. Proposed mechanism for the inhibition of factor Xa and the factor VIIa–tissue factor complex by tissue factor plasminogen inhibitor (TFPI). The indentations represent the active site of fac-
tor VIIa and factor Xa; the protrusions represent the three Kunitz-type domains of TFPI. In the factor
Xa–TFPI complex, the active site of factor Xa is bound to the second Kunitz domain of TFPI. In the
final quaternary factor Xa–TFPI–factor VIIa/tissue factor complex, factor Xa is bound at its active site
to the second Kunitz domain of TFPI and factor VIIa is bound at its active site to the first Kunitz domain of TFPI. Two potential pathways for the formation of the final quaternary inhibitory complex are
depicted: on the left, TFPI binds to a preformed factor Xa–factor VIIa/tissue complex; on the right,
TFPI binds to factor Xa and the factor Xa–TFPI complex then binds to factor VIIa/tissue factor. (From
Broze, ref. 109, with permission.)

rTFPI have different pharmacokinetic and activity profiles. Full-length rTFPI binds to factor Xa at a much faster rate; it also binds to endothelial glycosaminoglycans in microvessels in contrast to the two-domain rTFPI (58). Full-length rTFPI is also cleared more rapidly from circulation. The truncated form of TFPI, in contrast to full-length TFPI, does not bind to heparin but has dose-related antithrombotic activity in experimental venous thrombosis in rabbits induced by a combination of endothelium destruction and restricted blood flow (59). Although $TFPI_{1-161}$ displayed a dose-dependent increase in activity in the anti-factor Xa, APTT, and PT assays, APTT and PT were, for the same antithrombotic effect, much less prolonged compared with low molecular weight heparin. TFPI has no direct effect on thrombin and does not prolong the clotting time in the anti-factor IIa assay, even at high dose. No bleeding was observed in rabbits or rats receiving 10 mg/kg $TFPI_{1-161}$/day, an antithrombotic dose as effective as 60 anti-factor Xa IU/kg of tinzaparin sodium (60). Full-length recombinant TFPI expressed in *E. coli* (61,62) appears to be a much more potent antithrombotic. It completely prevented arterial reocclusion after vessel wall injury that yielded platelet-rich thrombi (63,64) and reduced coagulopathic and lethal effects in the baboon gram-negative model of septic shock (65). The same compound administered for 3 days in a rabbit atherosclerosis injury model reduced angiographic restenosis and decreased neointimal hyperplasia compared with controls (66). This indicates the importance of early inhibitors of the extrinsic pathway in response to arterial injury. Brief inhibition of the coagulation system by administration of TFPI sustains patency of arteries recanalized by pharmacologic fibrinolysis in the dog without markedly perturbing the coagulation system (67).

The hookworm, *Ancylostoma caninum,* produces TFPI which has been characterized and cloned. This small recombinant protein (9500 Da), administered subcutaneously or intravenously, reduces in a dose-dependent manner coronary and carotid artery occlusions in rat and pig models and in a chronic model of deep venous thrombosis in rats (68). A nematode low molecular weight protein has similar properties.

Administration of recombinant TFPI may become an interesting antithrombotic drug targeted to exposed subendothelium. Full-length rTFPI is presently being used in clinical trials in patients with sepsis and in those with microvascular surgery (7).

INACTIVATED TISSUE FACTOR

Tissue factor has a dominant role in the thrombus formation in arterial wall damage or ruptured atherosclerotic plaques. One may use inactivated factor VIIa (factor VIIai) as a competitive inhibitor of tissue factor–dependent activation of factor X.

Vascular thrombosis at sites of carotid endarterectomy in baboons was prevented by bolus intravenous administration of 1 mg/kg factor VIIai (31,66,69,70). In these experiments hemostasis was not compromised and the bleeding time remained normal. Monoclonal antibodies against tissue factor or against factor VII can also be considered. Synthetic peptides based on nematode-derived peptide antagonists of FVIIa/FVII have also been investigated (68,71).

BLOCKERS OF THE THROMBIN RECEPTOR FUNCTION

There are two thrombin receptors on the platelet membrane that undergo activation by thrombin-mediated cleavage of the terminal peptides yielding neoamino terminal peptide sequences that activate the receptors as tethered ligands (72). Protease-activated receptors 1 and 3 (PAR-1, PAR-3) are reactivated by thrombin and PAR-2 by trypsin (73). Monoclonal antibodies against human PAR-1 and PAR-3 raised in rabbits were tested in nonhuman primates and found to be antithrombotic (74). This approach is attractive as it produces dose-dependent interruption of platelet thrombosis while sparing cleavage of fibrinogen for the formation of hemostatic plugs (70).

HUMAN PLASMA–DERIVED AND RECOMBINANT ANTITHROMBIN III

The natural plasma protein antithrombin III is a relatively poor inhibitor of thrombin, but its inhibitory effect is increased 10,000-fold in the presence of heparin. In vivo the interaction between antithrombin and heparin probably takes place at the endothelial cell surface where the protein binds to the heparin-like glycosaminoglycan, heparan sulfate. It has been shown that for tight binding of heparin to antithrombin III a particular pentasaccharide sequence must be present (75). This pentasaccharide brings about a change in conformation in antithrombin, which involves an arginine residue that is sufficient for near-maximal acceleration of the inhibition of factor Xa (76). In contrast, much longer heparin species are required for significant acceleration of the rate of inhibition of thrombin by antithrombin III because this reaction appears to be accelerated principally by simultaneous binding of both thrombin and antithrombin III to the same heparin molecule, increasing the inhibition rate of thrombin by antithrombin III encounter frequency (77).

Concentrates of human plasma–derived antithrombin III are available. As with all plasma products, the potential for viral infection must be weighed against the therapeutic benefits and alternatives. The concentrates contain some nonfunctioning, cross-reacting material and so the effect of therapy should be monitored by functional rather than antigenic antithrombin assays (77). The biological half-life of antithrombin from concentrates ranges from a mean of 61 hours (78) to 92 hours (79). The half-life is not affected by the presence of coumarins (74) but is shortened by heparin (80) and in the postoperative period (77).

Because of the moderate survival time of antithrombin III in the circulation, alternate-day substitution is usually sufficient, although activity should be monitored regularly; it seems reasonable to maintain activity above 80% of the normal blood level during the treatment period.

In septicemia, where there is widespread endothelial damage, the action of antithrombin III may be impaired. In addition, under conditions of a fulminant inflammatory response, as occurs during *E. coli* sepsis, the expression of heparin-like receptors on the vascular endothelium may be downregulated in the same manner as the thrombomodulin and protein S receptors. This may in part explain why high concentrations of antithrombin III are necessary to prevent shock in animal models of sepsis (81,82). Theoretically, combined antithrombin and heparin therapy should be more effective than antithrombin alone in the management of shock, but unfortunately this form of treatment did not improve the outcome in shocked patients and was associated with an increased risk of bleeding.

In humans, two randomized trials compared antithrombin III with a synthetic protease inhibitor (83) or antithrombin III with heparin (84). Both studies documented a significant attenuation of disseminated intravascular coagulation (DIC) after antithrombin III treatment, but neither included a placebo control group. A placebo-controlled, double-blind trial in patients with septic shock and DIC treatment with a plasma concentrate of antithrombin III achieved significantly earlier correction of DIC but failed to decrease mortality in a significant manner (85).

Compared with heparin alone, adjunctive intracoronary therapy with a plasma antithrombin III concentrate does not appear to have any beneficial effect on procedural outcome as well as type and frequency of acute complications during percutaneous coronary angioplasty (PTCA), even in subgroups of patients with a high risk for thrombotic complications (86). Thus, a local deficiency of antithrombin III does not seem to play a major role for the failure of heparin to abolish thrombotic complications during PTCA. It should be noted that antithrombin III in combination with heparin inhibits coronary restenosis in atherosclerotic swine subjected to balloon overstretch (87). A similar study has not been conducted in patients. In a critical authoritative review of the clinical use of antithrombin III concentrates it was concluded that antithrombin III is only beneficial in a few clinical situations in patients with hereditary antithrombin III deficiency (such as delivery, acute thromboembolic complications, and postoperative prophylaxis). In acquired antithrombin III deficiency, there is no proven indication for the use of antithrombin III concentrates (88).

Different recombinant antithrombin III molecules are now available. Numerous problems had to be solved due to the failure to obtain satisfactory expression of functional or reactivatable antithrombin III from *E. coli* (89). Even expression in yeast gave only poor levels of active antithrombin (90). The majority of reports on active wild-type and variant antithrombin III have thus involved mammalian cell or baculovirus expression. In addition to the greater time involved in obtaining protein from such a system compared to *E. coli,* there is the further problem of heterogeneous glycosylation, which would be absent in bacterial expression. Differences in glycosylation of antithrombin have been shown to affect the affinity of the antithrombin for heparin (91–93). No randomized controlled trials with recombinant antithrombin III were published.

INHIBITORS OF FACTOR VIII

A synthetic 12-amino-acid peptide corresponding to a light-chain residue of factor VIII inhibits cleavage by thrombin of the heavy chain required for the activation of the procoagulant activity of factor VIII and also of the light chain required to dissociate factor VIII from von Willebrand factor. Tyrosine sulfation of the peptide potentiates its recognition by factor VIII (94).

Several other glycosaminoglycans (such as suleparoide, hemoclar, arteparon) and dermatan sulfates (such as heparin sulfate) are being developed, but clinical experience with these as antithrombotic drugs is limited. The same holds true for synthetic hypersulfated bis-lactobionic acid amide (aprosulfate).

NAROPARCIL

It is known that the majority of mammalian tissues produce chondroitin sulfate and heparin sulfate glycosaminoglycan chains when provided with exogenous β-D-xylasides. This is considered to be achieved by competition between the exogenous β-D-xylaside and the xylosylated serines on the core proteins of the endogenous proteoglycans undergoing biosynthesis (95). Naroparcil is a β-D-xylaside (4-[4-cyanobenzoyl]-phenyl)-1.5-dithio-β-D-xylopyranoside (96,97).

Naroparcil reduced thrombus weight in a Wessler stasis model of jugular vein thrombosis in rabbits in a dose-related manner giving an ED_{50} of 21.9 mg/kg and 36.0 mg/kg after intravenous and oral administration, respectively (97). Venous antithrombotic activity was maximal 2 to 3 hours after intravenous administration and 4 to 8 hours after oral administration. This suggests that naroparcil is not acting directly and that further metabolism is required, even after intravenous administration; this hypothesis is in line with the absence of any in vitro anticoagulant effect of the compound.

The antithrombotic effect of naroparcil occurs without increases in either APTT or thrombin time and without detectable antifactor Xa or antithrombin activity, although a dose-dependent reduction in thrombin generation (only 50% when the antithrombotic effect was maximal) and an increase in plasma dermatan sulfate–like material was observed. At antithrombotic doses no significant effect of naroparcil on bleeding time was noted.

These interesting findings of naroparcil on a venous thrombosis model in the rabbit have to be confirmed in venous and arterial thrombosis models in other animals. It is interesting that the bioavailability following oral administration of naroparcil in rabbits is high.

COAGULATION INHIBITORS DERIVED FROM APROTININ

Recently, a series of potential coagulation inhibitors derived from the bovine pancreatic trypsin inhibitor aprotinin was described.

These aprotinin-derived analogues showed significantly increased inhibition activity toward factor X, factor VIIa–tissue factor complex, factor XIa, and plasma kallikrein (98). In flow chamber experiments with human blood, these compounds significantly inhibited fibrin formation and platelet deposition on extracellular matrix from phorbol ester stimulated human endothelial cells under both high- and low-shear stress and in the presence of low molecular weight heparin (99).

Platelet-dependent thrombus deposition was quantified by dedicated image analysis after transillumination of the hamster femoral vein to which a standardized vascular trauma was applied. All tested aprotinin-derived agents, except for aprotinin, induced a dose-dependent decrease of thrombus formation and concomitant prolongation of the APTT with a complete inhibition of thrombus formation at two- to threefold prolongation of the APTT (100).

These results are to be confirmed in other animal species and the safety profile is to be established before these compounds can be considered as potential candidates for antithrombotic therapy.

INHIBITORS OF FACTOR XIII

In blood, factor XIII is present in two forms. Plasma factor XIII is produced in the liver and consists of a heterotetramer with two catalytic A subunits and two noncatalytic B units (A_2B_2) (101). Platelet factor XIII consists of only two A subunits (102). Both plasma and platelet forms of factor XIIIa contribute to fibrin cross- linking and to fibrin α_2-antiplasmin ligation in plasma (103). Factor XIIIa also cross-links other plasma proteins to fibrin, such as α_2-antiplasmin (103) and fibronectin (104); cross-linked fibrin is largely resistant to thrombolytics. This accounts for the interest in finding agents that inhibit the activation of factor XIII or impede its action. Monoclonal antibodies inhibit both plasma and platelet factor XIII (101,104) and a thiadiazole inhibitor (L-722,151) was used in vivo as an antithrombotic agent in thrombolysis experiments (105,106).

CONCLUSION: THE IDEAL ANTITHROMBOTIC DRUG

It is obvious that commercial antithrombotic drugs currently available for clinical use all have serious drawbacks. Moreover, the assays applied to monitor unfractionated heparin (APTT) and vitamin K antagonist (PT) also have serious shortcomings.

The combination of very-low-dose oral anticoagulants (targeted INR-2) with a potent antiaggregation may be a welcome way out in the prevention of thromboembolic complications in patients at low or medium-high thrombotic risk. Future drugs or drug combinations will all have to be tailored in accordance with the pathogenesis of the thrombus (venous versus arterial thrombus, thrombus induced by mechanical trauma as in PTCA, thrombus on foreign surfaces as on stents, platelet-rich versus platelet-poor thrombus). Local delivery of antithrombotic drugs or targeting to the thrombus may increase the local concentration where most needed and allow lower systemic levels, thereby reducing the bleeding risk. With recombinant technology human natural anticoagulants can be obtained in liberal quantities (antithrombin III, thrombomodulin, protein C, TFPI) and allows the creation of mutants and hybrids.

Table 14-1 summarizes what the ideal anticoagulant should be. It is hoped that the properties of one of the numerous antithrombotic drugs in development would correspond to this hematologist's dream of obtaining an antithrombotic drug without anticoagulant prop-

TABLE 14-1. *Ideal antithrombotic agent*

Oral as well as parenteral effectiveness
Rapid onset of action, <1 hour
Rapid cessation of effect by nontoxic antidote
Satisfactory therapeutic index, absence of side effects
No cumulative action or toxicity from long-term use
Predictable quantitative relation between dose and anticoagulant action
Antithrombotic effect not requiring laboratory monitoring
No or limited interaction with commonly used drugs
Large benefit-to-risk ratio
Inexpensive

erties. In the meantime the unabated search for the Holy Grail continues.

REFERENCES

1. Esmon NL, Owen WG, Esmon CT. Isolation of a membrane-bound cofactor for thrombin-catalyzed activation of protein C. *J Biol Chem* 1982;257:859–864.
2. Esmon NL, Carroll RC, Esmon CT. Thrombomodulin blocks the ability of thrombin to activate platelets. *J Biol Chem* 1983;258:12238–12242.
3. Esmon CT. The roles of protein C and thrombomodulin in the regulation of blood coagulation. *J Biol Chem* 1989;264:4743–4746.
4. Marlar RA, Kleiss AJ, Griffin JH. Mechanism of action of human activated protein C, a thrombin-dependent anticoagulant enzyme. *Blood* 1982;59:1067–1072.
5. Suzuki K, Kusumoto H, Deyashiki Y, et al. Structure and expression of human thrombomodulin, a thrombin receptor on endothelium acting as a cofactor for protein C activation. *EMBO J* 1987;6:1891–1897.
6. Bajzar L, Manuel R, Nesheim ME. Purification and characterization of TAFI, a thrombin activatable fibrinolysis inhibitor. *J Biol Chem* 1995;270:14477–14484.
7. Bajaj MS, Bajar SP. Tissue factor pathway inhibitor: potential therapeutic applications. *Thromb Haemost* 1997;78:471–477.
8. Eaton DL, Malloy BE, Tasai SP, Henzel W, Drayna D. Isolation, molecular cloning, and partial characterization of a novel carboxypeptidase B from human plasma. *J Biol Chem* 1991;269:21833–21838.
9. Bajzar L, Morser J, Nesheim M. TAFI, or plasma procarboxypeptidase B, couples the coagulation and fibrinolytic cascades through the thrombin-thrombomodulin complex. *J Biol Chem* 1996;271:16603–16608.
10. Nesheim M, Wang W, Boffa M, Nagashima M, Morser J, Bajzar L. Thrombin, thrombomodulin and TAFI in the molecular link between coagulation and fibrinolysis. *Thromb Haemost* 1997;78:386–391.
11. Healy AM, Rayburn HB, Rosenberg RD, Weiler H. Absence of the blood clotting regulator thrombomodulin causes embryonic lethality in mice before development of a functional cardiovascular system. *Proc Natl Acad Sci USA* 1995;92:850–854.
12. Ohlin AK, Norlund L, Marlar RA. Thrombomodulin gene variations and thromboembolic disease. *Thromb Haemost* 1997;78:396–400.
13. Takahashi Y, Hosaka Y, Nina H, et al. Soluble thrombomodulin purified from human urine exhibits a potent anticoagulant effect in vitro and in vivo. *Thromb Haemost* 1995;73:805–811.
14. Gomi K, Zushi M, Honda G, et al. Antithrombotic effect of recombinant human thrombomodulin on thrombin-induced thromboembolism in mice. *Blood* 1990;75:1396–1399.
15. Ono M, Nawa K, Marumoto Y. Antithrombotic effects of recombinant human soluble thrombomodulin in a rat model of vascular shunt thrombosis. *Thromb Haemost* 1994;72:421–425.
16. Nawa K, Sakano K, Fujiwara H, et al. Presence and function of chondrotin-4-sulfate on recombinant human soluble thrombomodulin. *Biochem Biophys Res Commun* 1990;171:729–737.

17. Nawa K, Ono M, Uchiyama T, Sugiyama N, Marumoto Y. Recombinant human thrombomodulin as a proteoglycan. *Trends Glycosc Glycotech* 1994;6:111–120.
18. Maruyama I, Saito H, Matsuda T, Aoki N. Antithrombotic effect of recombinant soluble human thrombomodulin on disseminated intravascular coagulation [Abstract]. *Zimmerman Conf Proc* 1996;I:82.
19. Dahlbäck B, Stenflo J. A natural anticoagulant pathway. Biochemistry and physiology of proteins C, S, C4b-binding protein and thrombomodulin. In: Bloom AL, Forbes CD, Thomas DP, Tuddenham EGD (eds). *Haemostasis and Thrombosis* (3rd ed). London: Churchill Livingstone, 1994;671–698.
20. Dahlbäck B. Protein S and C4b-binding protein. Components involved in the regulation of the protein C anticoagulant system. *Thromb Haemost* 1991;66:49–61.
21. Esmon CT, Ding W, Yasuhiro K, et al. The protein C pathway. *Thromb Haemost* 1997;78:70–74.
22. Grinnell BW, Berg DT, Walls J, Yan SB. Trans-activated expression of fully γ-carboxylated recombinant human protein C, an antithrombotic factor. *Biotechnology* 1987;5:1189–1992.
23. Emekli NB, Ulutin ON. The protective effect of autoprothrombin II-anticoagulant on experimental DIC formed animals. *Haematologica* 1980;65:655–651.
24. Taylor FB Jr, Chang A, Esmon CT, D'Angelo A, Vigano-D'Angelo S, Blick KE. Protein C prevents the coagulopathic and lethal effects of *Escherichia coli* infusion in the baboon. *J Clin Invest* 1987;79:918–925.
25. Smirnov MD, Pyzh MV, Borovikov DV, et al. Low doses of activated protein C delay arterial thrombosis in rats. *Thromb Res* 1990;57:645–650.
26. Araki H, Nishi K, Ishihara N, Okajima K. Inhibitory effects of activated protein C and heparin on thrombotic arterial occlusion in rat mesenteric arteries. *Thromb Res* 1991;652:209–216.
27. Gruber A, Hanson SR, Kelly AB, et al. Inhibition of thrombus formation by activatd protein C in a primate model of arterial thrombosis. *Circulation* 1990;82:578–585.
28. Arnljots B, Bergqvist D, Dahlbÿ84ck B. Inhibition of microarterial thrombosis by activated protein C in a rabbit model. *Thromb Haemostas* 1994;72:415–420.
29. Wu QY, Sheehan JP, Tsiang M, Lentz SR, Birktoft JJ, Sadler JE. Single amino acid substitutions dissociate fibrinogen-clotting and thrombomodulin-binding activities of human thrombin. *Proc Natl Acad Sci USA* 1991;88:6775–6779.
30. Gibbs CS, Coutre SE, Tsiang M, et al. Conversion of thrombin into an anticoagulant by protein engineering. *Nature* 1995;378:413–416.
31. Harker LA, Hanson SR, Kelly AB. Antithrombotic benefits and hemorrhagic risks of direct thrombin antagonists. *Thromb Haemost* 1995;74:464–472.
32. Biagi G, Legnani C, Rodorigo G, Coccheri S. Modulation of arachidonic metabolite generation in human blood by oral defibrotide. *Arzneim Forsch/Drug Res* 1991;41:511–514.
33. Coccheri S, De Rosa V, Dettori AG, et al. Effect on fibrinolysis of a new antithrombotic agent: fraction P (Defibrotide): a multicentre trial. *Int J Clin Pharmacol Res* 1982;3:227–245.

34. Coccheri S, Biagi G, Legnani C, Bianchini B, Grauso F. Acute effects of defibrotide, an experimental antithrombotic agent on fibrinolysis and blood prostanoids in man. *Eur J Clin Pharmacol* 1988;35:151–156.

35. Palmer KJ, Goa KL. Defibrotide. A review of its pharmacodynamic and pharmacokinetic properties, and therapeutic use in vascular disorders. *Drugs* 1993;45:259–294.

36. Pasini FL, Frigerio C, Capecchi PL, et al. Modulation of venous endothelial activity and transcellular calcium transport by defibrotide: the adenosine hypothesis. *Semin Thromb Hemost* 1996;22(suppl 1):15–20.

37. Zhou Q, Chu X, Ruan C. Defibrotide stimulates expression of thrombomodulin in human endothelial cells. *Thromb Haemost* 1994;71:507–510.

38. Fareed J, Walenga JM, Cornelli U. Antithrombotic drugs in pelvic surgery. *Semin Thromb Hemost* 1989;15:230–232.

39. Coccheri S, Nazzari M. Defibotide as a possible antiischemic drug. *Semin Thromb Hemost* 1996;22(suppl 1):9–14.

40. Coccheri S, Biagi G. Defibrotide. *Cardiovasc Drug Dev* 1991;9:172–196.

41. Hjort PF. Intermediate reactions in the coagulation inhibitor of blood with tissue thromboplastin. *Scand J Clin Lab Invest* 1957;9:1–173.

42. Rao LVM, Rapaport SI. Studies on the mechanism inhibiting the initiation of the extrinsic pathway of coagulation. *Blood* 1987;69:645–651.

43. Broze GJ Jr, Warren LA, Novotny WF, Higuchi DA, Girard TJ, Miletich JP. The lipoprotein-associated coagulation inhibitor that inhibits factor VII–tissue factor complex also inhibits Xa: insight into its possible mechanism of action. *Blood* 1988;71:335–343.

44. Silverberg SA, Nemerson Y, Zur M. Kinetics of the activation of bovine coagulation factor X by components of the extrinsic pathway. *J Biol Chem* 1977;252:8481–8488.

45. Zur M, Nemerson Y. Kinetics of factor IX activation via the extrinsic pathway. *J Biol Chem* 1980;255:5703–5707.

46. Enjyoji K, Miyata K, Kamikubo Y, Kato H. Effect of heparin on the inhibition of factor Xa by tissue factor pathway inhibitor: a segment, zGly212-Phe243, of the third Kunitz domain is a heparin binding site. *Biochemistry* 1995;34:5725–5735.

47. Callande NS, Rao LVM, Nordfang O, Sandset PM, Warn-Cramer B, Rapaport SI. Mechanisms of binding of recombinant extrinsic pathway inhibitor (rEPI) to cultured cell surfaces. *J Biol Chem* 1992;267:876–882.

48. Sandset M, Bendz B. Tissue factor pathway inhibitor: clinical deficiency states. *Thromb Haemost* 1997;78:467–470.

49. Wilcox JN, Smith KM, Schwartz SM, Gordon D. Localization of tissue factor in the normal vessel wall and in the atherosclerotic plaque. *Proc Natl Acad Sci USA* 1989;86:2839–2843.

50. Moreno PR, Bernardi VH, Lopez-Cuellar J, et al. Macrophages, smooth muscle cells, and tissue factor in unstable angina. Implications for cell-mediated thrombogenicity in acute coronary syndromes. *Circulation* 1996;94:3090–3097.

51. Toschi V, Gallo R, Lettino M, et al. Tissue factor modulates the thrombogenicity of human atherosclerotic plaques. *Circulation* 1997;85:594–599.

52. Fuster V, Fallon JT, Nemerson Y. Coronary thrombosis. *Lancet* 1996;348(suppl 1):s7–s10.

53. Fuster V, Fallon JT, Badimon JJ, Nemerson Y. The unstable atherosclerotic plaque: clinical significance and therapeutic intervention. *Thromb Haemost* 1997;78:247–255.

54. Semeraro N, Colucci M. Tissue factor in health and disease. *Thromb Haemost* 1997;78:759–764.

55. Sandset PM, Sirnes PA, Abildgaard U. Factor VII and extrinsic pathway inhibitor in acute coronary disease. *Br J Haematol* 1989;72:391–396.

56. Moor E, Hamsten A, Karpe F, Båvenholm P, Blombäck M, Silveiro A. Relationship of tissue factor pathway inhibitor activity to plasma lipoproteins and myocardial infarction at a young age. *Thromb Haemotas* 1994;71:707–712.

57. Petersen JGL, Meyn G, Rasmussen JS, et al. Characterization of human tissue factor pathway inhibitor variants expressed in Saccharomyces cerevisae. *J Biol Chem* 1993;268:13344–13351.

58. Nordfang O, Bjorn SE, Valantin S, et al. The C-terminus of tissue factor pathway inhibitor is essential to its anticoagulant activity. *Biochemistry* 1991;30:10371–10376.

59. Holst J, Lindblad B, Bergqvist D, et al. Antithrombotic effect of recombinant truncated tissue factor pathway inhibitor (TFPI$_{1-161}$) in experimental venous thrombosis—a comparison with low molecular weight heparin. *Thromb Haemost* 1994;71:214–219.

60. Holst J, Lindblad B, Matthiasson SE, et al. Experimental haemorrhagic effect of two-domain non-glycosylated tissue factor pathway inhibitor compared to low molecular weight heparin. *Thromb Haemost* 1996;75:586–589.

61. Wun TC, Kretzmar KK, Girard TJ, Miletich JP, Broze GJ Jr. Cloning and characterization of a cDNA coding for the lipoprotein associated coagulation inhibitor shows that its consists of three tandem Kunitz-type inhibitory domains. *J Biol Chem* 1988;263:6001–6004.

62. Diaz-Collier JA, Palmier MO, Kretzmer KK, et al. Refold and characterization of recombinant tissue factor pathway inhibitor expressed in *Escherichia coli*. *Thromb Haemost* 1994;71:339–346.

63. Haskel EJ, Torr SR, Day KC, et al. Prevention of arterial reocclusion after thrombolysis with recombinant lipoprotein-associated coagulation inhibitor. *Circulation* 1991;84:821–827.

64. Rote WE, Oldeschulte GL, Dempsey EM, Vlasuk GP. Evaluation of a novel small protein inhibitor of the blood coagulation factor VIIa/tissue factor complex in animal models of arterial and venous thrombosis [Abstract]. *Circulation* 1996;94:695.

65. Can C, Bild GS, Chang AC, et al. Recombinant *E. coli*- derived tissue factor pathway inhibitor reduce coagulopathic and lethal effects in the baboon gram-negative model of septic shock. *Circ Res* 1994;44:126–137.

66. Jang Y, Guzman LA, Lincoff AM, et al. Influence of blockade of specific levels of the coagulation pathway cascade on restenosis in a rabbit atherosclerotic femoral artery injury model. *Circulation* 1995;92:3041–3050.

67. Abendschein DR, Meng YY, Torr-Brown S, Sobel BE.

Maintenance of coronary patency after fibrinolysis with tissue factor pathway inhibitor. *Circulation* 1995; 92:944–949.

68. Rote WE, Oldeschulte GL, Dempsey EM, Vlasuk GP. Evaluation of a novel small protein inhibitor of the blood coagulation factor VIIa/tissue factor complex in animal models of arterial and venous thrombosis [Abstract]. *Circulation* 1996;94(suppl I):I-596.

69. Harker LA, Maraganore JM, Hirsh J. Novel antithrombotic agents. In: Colman RW, Hirsh J, Marder VJ, Salzman EW (eds). *Hemostasis and Thrombosis: Basic Principles and Clinical Practice* (3rd ed). Philadelphia: Lippincott–Raven, 1994;1638–1660.

70. Harker LA, Hanson SR, Kelly AB. Antithrombotic strategies targeting thrombin activates; thrombin receptors and thrombin generation. *Thromb Haemost* 1997;78:736–741.

71. Maki SL, Ruf W, Huang S, Kelly C, Vlasuk GP. Nematode anticoagulant protein C2 (C2): a potent inhibitor of factor VIIa/tissue factor complex (FVIIa/TF) requires an exosite on factor Xa (Fxa) that overlaps a factor Va (Fva) binding site [Abstract]. *Circulation* 1996;94(suppl I):I-694.

72. Coufgkub SR, Vu T-KH, Hung DT, Wheaton VI. Characterization of a functional thrombin receptor. Issues and opportunities. *J Clin Invest* 1992;89:351–355.

73. Ishihara H, Connolly AJ, Zeng D, et al. Protease-activated receptor 3 is a second thrombin receptor in humans. *Nature* 1997;386:502–506.

74. Cook JJ, Sitko GR, Bednar B, et al. An antibody against the exosite of the cloned thrombin receptor inhibits experimental arterial thrombosis in the African green monkey. *Circulation* 1995;91:2961–2971.

75. Choay J, Petitou M, Lormeau JC, Sinay P, Casu B, Gatti G. Structure–activity relationships in heparin: a synthetic pentasaccharide with high affinity for antithrombin III and eliciting high anti-factor Xa activity. *Biochem Biophys Res Commun* 1983;116:492–499.

76. Olson ST, Björk I, Sheffer R, Craig PA, Shore JD, Choay J. Role of the antithrombin-binding pentasaccharide in heparin acceleration of antithrombin-proteinase reactions. Resolution of the antithrombin conformational change contribution to heparin rate enhancement. *J Biol Chem* 1992;267:12528–12538.

77. Mannucci PM, Boyer C, Wolf M, Tripodi A, Larrieu MJ. Treatment of congential antithrombin III deficiency with concentrates. *Br J Haematol* 1982;50:531–535.

78. Menache D, O'Malley P, Schorr JB, Wagner B, Williams C, and the Cooperative Study Group. Evaluation of the safety, recovery, half-life, and clinical efficacy of antithrombin III (human) in patients with hereditary antithrombin III deficiency. *Blood* 1990;75:33–39.

79. Schwartz RS, Bauer KA, Rosenberg RD, Kavanaugh EJ, Davies DC, Bogdanoff DA. Clinical experience with antithrombin III concentrate in treatment of congential and acquired deficiency of antithrombin. The Antithrombin III Study Group. *Am J Med* 1989;87 (suppl 3B):53S–60S.

80. Knot EA, de Jong E, ten Cate JW, Gie LK, van Royen EA. Antithrombin III biodistribution in healthy volunteers. *Thromb Haemost* 1987;58:1008–1011.

81. Büller HR, ten Cate JW. Acquired antithrombin III deficiency: laboratory diagnosis, incidence, clinical im-

plications, and treatment with antithrombin III concentrate. *Am J Med* 1989;87(suppl 3B):44S–48S.

82. Vinazzer HA. Antithrombin III in shock and disseminated intravascular coagulation. *Clin Appl Thromb/Hemost* 1995;1:62–65.

83. Maki M, Terao T, Ikenoue T, et al. Clinical evaluation of antithrombin III concentrate (BI 6.013) for disseminated intravascular coagulation in obstetrics. *Gynecol Obstet Invest* 1987;23:230–240.

84. Blauhut B, Kramar H, Vinazzer H, Bergmann H. Substitution of antithrombin III in shock and DIC: a randomized study. *Thromb Res* 1985;39:81–89.

85. Fourrier F, Huart J-J, Runge I, Caron C, Goudemand J, Chopin C. Results of a double-blind, placebo-controlled trial of antithrombin III concentrates in septic shock with DIC. In: Müller-Berghaus G, Madlener K, Blombäck M, ten Cate JW (eds). *DIC: Pathogenesis, Diagnosis and Therapy of Disseminated Intravascular Fibrin Formation.* Amsterdam: Excerpta Medica, 1993;221–226.

86. Schächinger V, Allert M, Kasper W, Just H, Vach W, Zeiher AM. Adjunctive intracoronary infusion of antithrombin III during percutaneous transluminal coronary angioplasty. Results of a prospective, randomized trial. *Circulation* 1994;90:2258–2266.

87. Nadier Ali M, Mazur W, Kleiman NS, et al. Inhibition of coronary restenosis by antithrombin III in atherosclerotic swine. *Coron Art Dis* 1996;7:851–861.

88. Lechner K, Kyrle PA. Antithrombin III concentrates. Are they clinically useful? *Thromb Haemost* 1995;73:340–348.

89. Bock SC, Wion KL, Vehar GA, Lawn RM. Cloning and expression of the cDNA for human antithrombin III. *Nucl Acids Res* 1982;10:8113–8125.

90. Bröker M, Ragg H, Karges HE. Expression of human antithrombin III in Saccharomyces cerevisiae and Saccharomyces pombe. *Biochem Biophys Res Commun* 1987;908:203–213.

91. Björk I, Ylinenjärvi K, Olson ST, Hermentin P, Conradt HS, Zettlmeissl G. Decreased affinity of recombinant antithrombin for heparin due to increased glycosylation. *Biochem J* 1992;286:793–800.

92. Fan B, Crews BC, Turko IV, Choay J, Zettlemeissl G, Gettins P. Hererogeneity of recombinant human antithrombin III expressed in baby hamster kidney cells. Effect of glycosylation differences on heparin binding and structure. *J Biol Chem* 1993;268:17588–17596.

93. Zettlmeissl G, Conad HS, Nimtz M, Karges HE. Characterization of recombinant human antithrombin III synthesized in Chinese hamster ovary cells. *J Biol Chem* 1989;264:21153–21159.

94. Maraganore JR, Healy JF, Parker ET, Lollar P. Inhibition of thrombin activation of factor VIII by a synthetic peptide corresponding to residues 1675–1686 in factor VIII [Abstract]. *Circulation* 1992;86:413.

95. Cöster J, Harnnäs J, Malmström A. Biosynthesis of dermatan sulfate proteoglycans. The effect of β-D-xylaside addition in the polymer-modification process in fibroblast cultures. *Biochem J* 1994;276:533–539.

96. Bellamy F, Horton D, Millet J, Picard F, Samreth G, Chazan FB. Glycosylated derivatives of benzophenone benzhydrol.N.benzhydril as potential venous antithrombotic agents. *J Med Clin* 1993;36:898–903.

97. Millet J, Theveneaux J, Brown ML. The venous antithrombotic profile of naroparcil in the rabbit. *Thromb Haemost* 1994;72:874–879.

98. Stanssens P, De Maeyer M, Lambeir AM, et al. Design of inhibitors of serine protease. Use of site selective and random mutagenesis to define the pharmacophore and conformational selectivity of Künitz inhibitors towards factor Xa and VIIa. Submitted.

99. Stassen JM, Lambeir DM, Matthyssens G, et al. Characterisation of a novel series of aprotinin-derived anticoagulants. I. In vitro and pharmacological properties. *Thromb Haemost* 1995;74:646–654.

100. Stassen JM, Lambeir AM, Vreys I, et al. Characterisation of a novel series of aprotinin-derived anticoagulants. II. Comparative antithrombotic effects on primary thrombus formation in vivo. *Thromb Haemost* 1995;74:655–659.

101. Schwartz ML, Pizzo SV, Hill RL, McKee PA. Human factor XIII from plasma and platelets: molecular weights, subunit structure, proteolytic activation and crosslinking of fibrinogen and fibrin. *J Biol Chem* 1973;248:1395–1407.

102. Reed G, Lukacova D. Generation and mechanism of action of a potent inhibitor of factor XIII function. *Thromb Haemost* 1995;74:680–685.

103. Pisano JJ, Bronzert TJ, Peyton MP, Finlayson JS. e-(g-Glutamyl) lysine cross-links: determination in fibrin from normal and factor XIII–deficient individuals. *Ann NY Acad Sci* 1972;202:98–113.

104. Tamaki T, Aoki N. Cross-linking of ($_2$-plasmin inhibitor and fibronectin to fibrin by fibrin-stabilizing factor. *Biochim Biophys Acta* 1981;661:280–286.

105. Shebuski RJ, Sitko GR, Claremon DA, Baldwin JJ, Remy DC, Stern AM. Inhibition of factor XIIIa in a canine model of coronary thrombosis: effect on reperfusion and acute reocclusion after recombinant tissue-type plasminogen activator. *Blood* 1990;75:1455–1459.

106. Parameswaran KN, Velasco PT, Wilson J, Lorand L. Labeling of e-lysine crosslinking sites in proteins with peptide substrates of factor XIIIa and transglutaminase. *Proc Natl Acad Sci USA* 1990;87:8472–8475.

107. Esmon ML. The roles of protein C and thrombomodulin in the regulation of blood coagulation. *J Biol Chem* 1989;264:4743–4746.

108. Fareed J, Callas D, Hoppensteadt D, Walenga J. Modulation of endothelium by heparin and related polyelectrolytes. In: Vane JR, Born GVR, Welzel D (eds). *Endothelial Cell in Health and Disease.* Stuttgart, Germany: Schattauer 1995;165–182.

109. Broze GJ. The tissue factor pathway of coagulation: factor VII, tissue factor, and tissue factor pathway inhibitor. In: Bloom AL, Forbes KD, Thomas DP, Tuddenham EGD (eds). *Haemostasis and Thrombosis.* Edinburgh: Churchill Livingstone, 1994;349–377.

*Cardiovascular Thrombosis: Thrombocardiology
and Thromboneurology, Second Edition,*
edited by M. Verstraete, V. Fuster, and E. J. Topol,
Lippincott–Raven Publishers, Philadelphia © 1998.

15

Stable Prostacyclin Analogues

Jill J. F. Belch and Margaret McLaren

*Department of Medicine, Ninewells Hospital and
Ninewells Medical School, Dundee DD1 9SY, United Kingdom*

Prostaglandin (PG) research has provided one of the most rapidly growing areas in cardiovascular medicine. It had its beginning with the detection of PG activity in the early 1930s, which was rapidly followed by the isolation and determination of PG structures coupled with the discovery that PGs are synthesized from essential fatty acids in nearly all animal cells. In 1971 it was shown conclusively that aspirin and aspirin-like drugs acted through the prevention of biosynthesis of the PGs. In 1976, Moncada and Vane (1) established that the blood vessel wall manufactures an unstable PG, initially called PGX and later renamed prostacyclin (PGI_2). This discovery of PGI_2 was followed by massive research into its formation, activity, and potential uses in pharmacotherapy. Given the

ubiquitous nature of the PGs and their potent and far-reaching effects on many biological systems, it is not surprising that many diverse clinical indications have been evaluated. This is particularly true in the field of cardiovascular disease where prostacyclins have potent vasodilator and antiplatelet effects (2) (Fig. 15-1).

However, PGI_2 is chemically unstable and rapidly metabolized within the body to its essentially inert metabolite 6-κ-$PGF_1\alpha$(3). The former property meant that cold storage of the crystalline sodium salt was required. Thereafter it was required to be dissolved in a glycine buffer with pH 10.5. Accidental infusion into the tissues produced chemical trauma and this, compounded with its short half life meant that an intensive search for

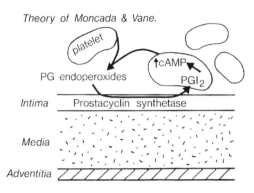

FIG. 15-1. Theory of Moncada and Vane. In the intact vessel PGI$_2$ production by the endothelium prevents platelet aggregation. When the vessel is breached, thromboxane A$_2$ (TXA$_2$) is produced ensuring platelet plugging over the area. Intact endothelium downstream prevents extension of the platelet plug via further PGI$_2$ production.

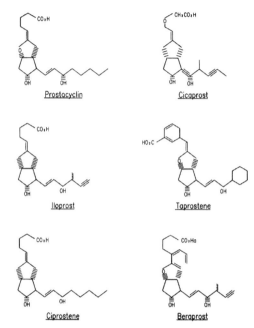

FIG. 15-2. Chemical structures of prostacyclin and its analogues.

chemically and metabolically stable PGI2 analogues was undertaken. As there was already evidence of some potential clinical indications for PGI$_2$ therapy (4–6), these analogues also had to have the same biological profiles and potency. The first analogue to meet these criteria was the modified carbacyclin derivative iloprost (7,8). In the last 15 years, iloprost has been studied intensively and has entered clinical practice as a therapy for peripheral arterial obstructive disease (PAOD). As this compound has been the best studied of the prostacyclin analogues, it will be the most fully reviewed later. Other PGI$_2$ analogues have been developed including cicaprost (9,10), which is metabolically stable and is excreted unchanged. Ataprost (11,12) and the less potent ciprostene (13,14), as well as the interphenylene analogues naxaprostene (15,16) and taprostene (17,18), are potent antiplatelet agents with less vasodilator activity. The orally active racemic compound beraprost (19,20) is used in Japan and is currently undergoing clinical trials in other indications. Figure 15-2 shows the chemical structure of these compounds and their relationship to PGI$_2$.

ILOPROST

Iloprost is the most extensively and best studied PGI$_2$ analogue. Much is now known about its pharmacokinetics and therapeutic use in cardiovascular disease, particularly in peripheral vascular disease such as PAOD and Raynaud's phenomenon (RP).

Pharmacology

The main pharmacologic actions of iloprost are the same as those of prostacyclin. Iloprost occupies the PGI$_2$ membrane receptor and its actions are similarly mediated via an increase in intracellular cyclic AMP. Iloprost inhibits, in a dose-dependent fashion, all phases of platelet activation. This includes shape change, adhesion, and aggregation. It does not inhibit platelet-agglutinating agents such as ristocetin. Both iloprost and prostacyclin are equiefficient in inhibiting ADP-induced platelet aggregation in humans (21). Iloprost is a vasodilator of arterial and venous vessels of all sizes. There are reports of some differences between these two actions of iloprost such that it may be a more potent antiplatelet agent with less profound vasodilator activity than native prostacyclin; however, in vitro platelet effects are similar (22).

Microvascular and Hemorheologic Features of Cardiovascular Disease

The role of platelets in the formation of arterial thrombosis has been well described (23,24). If platelets are activated either as a primary event or secondarily by ulcerated atherosclerotic plaques or in poststenotic vortices in the proximal arteries, the organ can be perfused with a high proportion of activated cells. When platelets are activated, they release vasoconstrictor substances such as thromboxane A_2 (TXA$_2$) and serotonin (5-HT). Aggregates are formed that may aggravate the disease by further decreasing blood flow. Platelet aggregation is increased in PAOD (23) and in coronary artery disease (24) and circulating platelet aggregates have been detected in critical limb ischemia (CLI) (23). An excess of TXA$_2$ relative to vasodilator PG production has been suggested in animal studies as the cause of CLI (25). Furthermore, increased levels of its stable metabolite TXB$_2$ are found in vascular disease (26) and rise further after exercise suggesting increased platelet–vessel wall interaction (26). Serotonin, weaker in effect than TXA$_2$, also induces platelet aggregation and vasoconstriction, and studies suggest that atherosclerosis potentiates the vasoconstrictor response to serotonin (27). Patients with arterial disease have lower intraplatelet serotonin and higher plasma levels than controls, consistent with increased release through activation (28). Other platelet release products are also elevated in vascular disease and parallel the well- documented increased rate of platelet aggregation (23).

The part played by red blood cells (RBCs) has also been studied. Its diameter of approximately 7 μm is greater than that of some of the capillaries so flow in the microcirculation may be critically dependent on RBC deformability. In the ischemic organ RBC aggregation is further increased under the low flow, low shear, and reduced temperature conditions (29). RBC aggregation is known to be promoted by plasma fibrinogen, the levels of which are known to be increased in vascular disease (29). Furthermore, an increased RBC number is inversely correlated with arterial graft survival (30,31) and the degree of susceptibility of the red cells to auto-oxidation correlates with clinical measures of blood flow (32). These findings lead to the suggestion that decreased whole blood flow filterability in vascular disease was secondary to RBC rigidity; however, newer tests involving removal of the white blood cells (WBCs) combined with measurement of WBC deformability suggest that the predominant influence may be increased rigidity to the activated WBC (33). Indeed, the total WBC count is a predictor of future vascular events (34). Thus, it has become apparent that there is an important role for the WBC in maintaining flow in blood vessels. Polymorphonuclear leukocytes (PMNs) are about 2,000 times less deformable than erythrocytes (35). When they become activated, they project pseudopods and their cytoplasmic stiffness increases further. Adhesion to the endothelium can occlude the vessel and adhesion to other cells including other WBCs can lead to the formation of microaggregates (36). Once the WBC has become fixed in the microcirculation it can deliver a variety of further insults to the vessel lining including the release of free radicals (FRs). Radical scavengers are decreased in vascular disease and there is an increase in the products of FR activity (37), which is further augmented by exercise (38), or immediately after ischemia/reperfusion such as occurs during the process of angioplasty (39). These adverse effects can be reversed by surgical vascularization (40).

It is not just the cellular components of the blood that are important in vascular disease but also the plasma constituents. Several epidemiologic studies have confirmed that fibrinogen is an important independent predictor of cardiovascular events (31) and the mechanisms whereby increased fibrinogen may promote cardiovascular disease include increased plasma viscosity, fibrin formation, platelet aggregation, and infiltration of the vessel wall. Increased fibrinogen may also be of prognostic value in that it may affect the long-term patency vein grafts (31). Fibrin deposition, however, is not only dependent on fibrinogen level but is modulated by the activation and inhibition of fibrinolysis. Fibrinolysis is largely controlled by the endothelium through its ability to produce tissue plasminogen activator (t-PA) and plasminogen activator inhibitor (PAI). Patients with vascular disease with impaired fibrinolysis are in a state that may favor atherogenesis, arterial thrombosis, and microemboli formation (41). Endothelial damage is probably relevant in the pathogenesis of vascular disease. There is a spectrum of endothelial injury ranging from subtle alterations in cell surface constituents through the new injury where individual cells become detached and are rapidly replaced by neighboring cells, with loss of endothelial cover. Any of these forms of endothelial injury may promote release of the blood clotting factor, factor VIII, and von Willebrand factor antigen (vWF). Patients with vascular disease have increased plasma levels of vWF (42), which not only marks vascular damage but in itself can propagate the disease by participation in the coagulation cascade and by promoting platelet aggregation. Other endothelial constituents such as endothelium-derived relaxing factor, now known to be nitric oxide (NO), and endothelin are also known to be abnormal in patients with vascular disease (43,44). As can be seen from the above, there are a number of microvascular abnormalities occurring in patients with vascular disease. These abnormalities are not only present in patients with established disease but also in patients with risk factors for them (45), thus suggesting some role in the pathogenesis of the disease. How then may the prostacyclin analogues be of use in such diseases?

Iloprost as a Treatment for Cardiovascular Disease: Theoretical Considerations

The impaired endothelial function, activated WBCs and platelets, plus rigid red cells will contribute to impaired flow in the microcirculation in patients with vascular diseases and the correction by iloprost could produce clinical improvement. Iloprost is a potent antiplatelet and vasodilator agent (3) but it also has other effects. Di Perri et al. (46) described a statistically significant decrease in whole blood viscosity associated with the increased RBC filterability during iloprost therapy. A similar effect was seen on WBCs where a decrease in WBC aggregation was detected with iloprost (47). Adhesion of activated PMNs to human umbilical vein endothelium was significantly decreased by iloprost (48), and at increased concentrations iloprost inhibited neutrophil chemotaxis and slightly inhibited oxygen free radical production (49). The infusion of iloprost in patients with vascular disease has also been shown to enhance blood fibrinolytic activity (50). A decrease in euglobulin clot lysis time was consistently seen in subjects treated with a single infusion. Bertele et al. confirmed this above work indicating that iloprost can significantly increase fibrinolytic activity (51). Interestingly, in this population where fibrinolytic activity was decreased prior to treatment, iloprost restores normal fibrinolytic response. Interestingly, this change was detectable at 6 days but not the first day of treatment. It has been hypothesized that iloprost can stimulate the release of t-PA from blood vessel walls (50), but the lack of a consistent and significant rise in plasma t-PA during therapy suggested an additional mechanism, perhaps the release of t-PA inhibitor from platelets, may be involved (51). All of the above, in particular the WBC free radical scavenging effects combined with the enhanced ability for endothelial repair following iloprost treatment, probably contribute to so-called "cytoprotective" effect (52,53). Clinically, this has been demonstrated as an ability of iloprost to improve tissue resistance to ischemia (54). The above effects appear to be a drug class effect with many of these potentially beneficial effects occurring either in prostacyclin (55) or the other stable analogues (56,57).

Clinical Pharmacology

Administration of iloprost to humans has most frequently been by venous infusion. Oral preparation is also available (58). During infusions of iloprost there is clinical evidence of vasodilatation as shown by skin flushing and vascular headache. Alteration in pulse rate and in systemic blood pressure is not seen in healthy subjects receiving an iloprost dose that is sufficient to inhibit platelet activity consistently (59). An increase in heart rate is frequently noted in arteriopathic patients and in these subjects significant decrease in systolic and diastolic pressure can also incur (60). At our usual therapeutic dose of 2 ng per kg per minute, the heart rate is increased by about 10% with a fall in blood pressure of about 5% to 10% (61). There is an increase in cardiac output and microcirculatory blood flow, with a decrease in total peripheral resistance and in pulmonary vascular resistance. Iloprost increases cardiac output in cardiac index in a dose-dependent manner. No tachyphylaxis of the hemodynamic changes have been reported following infusion times to 72 hours. Interestingly, this is in contrast to the antiplatelet effects where some tachyphylaxis has been seen and has thus led to the current intermittent regime of administration. The platelet inhibitory action of the drug is also dose-dependent. The threshold for this effect is 0.5 to 1.0 ng per kg per minute.

Iloprost is metabolized by β oxidation of the upper side chain to give dinor- and tetra-noriloprost. The metabolites have no pharmacologic activity. Excretion is via urine (68%) and feces (12%). There is no evidence of enterohepatic circulation of active drug.

Therapeutic Use

Indications

A number of clinical indications have been suggested for the use of iloprost. These are listed in Table 15-1. A product license for iloprost has been granted by approximately 20 countries worldwide for the following indications:

1. Peripheral occlusive arterial disease especially with rest pain and/or ischemic ulceration (Figs. 15-3 and 15-4).

TABLE 15-1. *Clinical indications for iloprost therapy*

Proven indications
Critical limb ischemia
Thromboangiitis obliterans
Raynaud's phenomenon
Potential indications
Pulmonary hypertension
Cardiopulmonary bypass
Hemodialysis
Thrombotic stroke
Transplantation
No benefit
Intermittent claudication
Angina
Acute myocardial infarction
Scientific studies completed
Critical limb ischemia
Thromboangiitis obliterans
Raynaud's phenomenon
Scientific studies either small or currently underway
Pulmonary hypertension
Cardiopulmonary bypass
Hemodialysis
Stroke
Transplant
Scientific studies suggest no benefit
Intermittent claudication
Angina/myocardial infarction

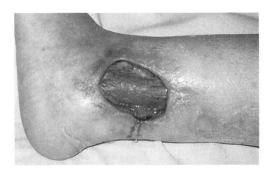

FIG. 15-3. Ischemic ulceration in critical limb ischemia.

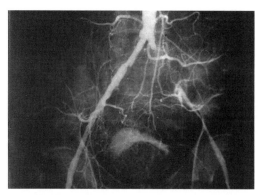

FIG. 15-4. Angiogram of occluded vessel causing severe claudication.

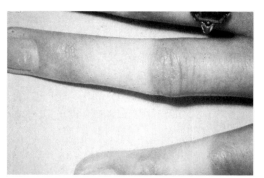

FIG. 15-6. Raynaud's phenomenon.

2. Thromboangiitis obliterans (Buerger's disease) (Fig. 15-5).
3. Raynaud's phenomenon (Fig. 15-6).

The oral formulation of the drug is currently under investigation for these indications (62). A further anticipated indication is in the field of pulmonary hypertension and this area is currently under investigation (63). In this later indication, other formulations are also being evaluated (64).

Contraindications

Usual contraindications apply. These include pregnancy and lactation and conditions where the effect on platelets increases the risk of hemorrhage, e.g., active peptic ulceration, trauma, or intracranial hemorrhage.

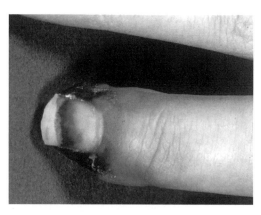

FIG. 15-5. Thromboangiitis obliterans.

Mode of Use

The recommended intravenous dose rate is between 0.5 and 2 ng per kg per minute, ideally for 6 hours per day. The duration of treatment varies depending on the indication, e.g., for ischemic leg ulcer rest pain 28 days is recommended, whereas for Raynaud's phenomenon 5 days is usually adequate. Dose titration is to be recommended in each individual treated. The most unpleasant adverse effects, which are related to its vasodilatory properties, can then be avoided and the maximum tolerated dose given.

Scientific Evidence in Support of Iloprost Usage

Peripheral Arterial Occlusive Disease

Intermittent Claudication

Efficacy studies using iloprost in peripheral arterial occlusive disease presenting as intermittent claudication have consistently shown platelet aggregation to be inhibited in the blood of these patients during iloprost infusions (65). However, no clinically significant improvement in walking distance has been demonstrated when compared to placebo (66–68).

Critical Limb Ischemia

In patients with severe limb ischemia, rest pain or ischemic ulceration can develop. Several major international placebo-controlled studies have reported that between 14 and 28 days of intermittent treatment with iloprost produced significant healing of lesions and relief of rest pain (69–74). In six published multicentered trials (69–76), 740 patients were studied in a prospective, placebo-controlled, and double-blind fashion. Three of the trials had a formal follow-up in terms of major amputation and death for a total of 6 months. All of the studies evaluated relief of rest pain and degree of ulcer healing at the end of follow-up. Using an intention-to-treat diagnosis in five of the six studies, more patients showed evidence of ulcer healing in the iloprost group and in three studies the difference was statistically significant. More patients were completely free of rest pain at the end of treatment in the iloprost group when compared to those receiving placebo. In one study, this difference was statistically significant. Iloprost was equally effective in diabetics and nondiabetic patients (73,74). Where amputation and death were recorded at 6 months in three studies, the decrease in the rates of major amputation and death in the actively treated group was between 14% and 19%. A published meta-analysis of six of the studies (69–74) showed that iloprost had a significant beneficial effect by increasing the probability of being alive with both legs intact at the 6-month follow-up (p < 0.05) (76). In this meta analysis, the prostaglandin also had a significant beneficial effect on ulcer healing and pain relief (p < 0.05).

Thromboangiitis Obliterans

In the study by Fissenger and Schafer, 133 patients were enrolled with half given 100 mg of aspirin per day and the other half iloprost in the standard regimen of six hourly infusions per day up to a maximum dose of 2 ng per kg per minute for 28 days (77). At the end of the treatment period there appeared to be significantly enhanced healing in the iloprost-treated group. This was associated with increased pain relief and these two effects were maintained 5 months following therapy. At this study endpoint, 88% of the patients who received iloprost reported themselves to be improved compared to 21% of those treated with aspirin. There is no difference in amputation requirements between the two treatment legs. In general, the amputation rate was low.

Raynaud's Phenomenon

Iloprost was initially studied in Raynaud's phenomenon (RP) in an open study of 13 patients with RP secondary to systemic sclerosis (SSc) (78). Two nanograms per kilogram per minute of iloprost was given intravenously for 8 hours per day for 3 days. Analysis of the diary cards was not possible due to poor completion of the cards. However, in 19 of 26 patients, digital ulcers healed over 10 weeks and 9 of 13 patients reported subjective improvement. The peripheral vascular resistance also fell after treatment and this was maintained for up to 6 weeks. Subsequently, two prospective placebo-controlled double-blind studies were reported (79,80). Unfortunately, the study designs were crossover. Where a drug is capable of producing a variable long-term effect, some hangover of this effect into the next treatment phase can occur and attenuate the response and cloud the evaluation of such crossover studies. This was demonstrated in these two studies. Nevertheless, they both showed a significant decrease in duration of severity of the Raynaud's attacks over the study period of 6 weeks. In these trials and in two prospective parallel group studies (81,82), iloprost did appear to be effective in curtailing the symptomatology of Raynaud's phenomenon. Vasodilatation produced the majority of side effects and a further study comparing dosage regimes of 2 ng per kg per minute and 0.5 ng per kg per minute was completed to see if the lower dose could be effective without producing the same degree of vasodilatation (83). In this study both appeared to be equally effective in decreasing the frequency, duration, and severity of the spasm attacks in the 55 patients studied. Ulcer healing occurred in 44% of patients receiving the standard dose and 39% of patients receiving the low dose, i.e., to a similar degree. As one might have expected, the lower dose was associated with fewer side effects and was much better tolerated.

The current gold standard treatment for RP is calcium channel blockage using nifedipine. There have been two studies comparing iloprost to nifedipine (84,85). In the published study (84), 23 patients were enrolled and given either iloprost in the standard regime or nifedipine 30 to 60 mg per day. Both treatments effectively reduced the vasospastic attacks; however, nifedipine was less effective in digital ulcer healing and appeared to produce more side effects.

Despite its equitable potency with nifedipine, as shown above, and despite its apparent efficacy, iloprost remains a second-choice treatment because its mode of administration, intravenously, poses logistical problems.

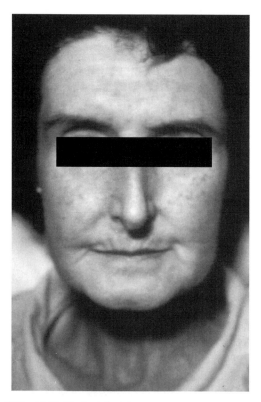

FIG. 15-7. Typical facial appearance of patient with systemic sclerosis.

Orally administered iloprost is now being evaluated and early pilot work has been published (62) (Fig. 15-7).

Pulmonary Hypertension

Prostacyclin has been evaluated in pulmonary hypertension and it now has a license for this indication in some countries. This has lead to studies of iloprost in this same indication. Similar acute effects on hemodynamics within the lung have been demonstrated using iloprost (86,87) This drug has also been used successfully over the longer term to treat patients with this condition secondary to their connective tissue disease (63) where the work is ongoing in this area.

Others

Angina and Myocardial Infarction

Ischemic heart disease is the most common manifestation of cardiovascular disease with its clinical presentations of angina pectoris (AP) and acute myocardial infarction (MI). It has been suggested that prostacyclin and its analogues may be used in such conditions and possible mechanisms of action of these compounds in angina and MI include vasodilatation, antiplatelet activity, and the effects on neutrophils. Prostacyclin and its analogues have been studied in several in vivo models of acute (MI) and in different species. A major difference between the models was whether the drug was administered prior to or after coronary vessel occlusion. Administration of prostacyclin prior to the occlusion uses information about mechanisms involved in the development of MI but infusion of the PG after the event is therapeutically more relevant. In an open-chest pig model, the time required to elicit an electrically induced coronary thrombosis was prolonged by iloprost (88). In another study, infusion of iloprost starting 30 minutes before ligation of the coronary artery in an open-chest dog did not improve collateral blood flow to the ischemic region but improved functional recovery during reperfusion

(89). Similar results were seen in pigs (99,91). If iloprost was given after coronary ligation, a favorable effect on infarct size, with a reduction in the necrotic zone by about 50%, was reported in some species (92) and not in others (93). Both prostacyclin and iloprost have been studied in patients with stable coronary disease manifested by angina. Both treatments lowered the systemic blood pressure and provoked chest pain and ECG changes in some of the patients studied (94,95). Myocardial blood flow was increased by both treatments. Similar findings were reported by the same group in a separate study (96) and by others (97). Iloprost has been studied with respect to its effect during physical exercise in patients with stable coronary disease. Once again, similar results were obtained for both prostacyclin and iloprost in that patients developed chest pain and ST segment depression on the electrocardiogram (ECG) (98). Thus, in patients with stable coronary disease, both prostacyclin and iloprost when infused in doses sufficient to lower coronary vascular resistance may produce myocardial ischemia and cause the symptom of chest pain to develop. This probably is a consequence of coronary steal caused by their potent vasodilator activity.

There are no data available on the use of iloprost in unstable angina. However, prostacyclin has been studied (99) and was not found to be effective. The results in variant angina (Prinzmetal's angina) demonstrated no effect of iloprost and the total number of episodes of ST segment elevation. Indeed the infusion increased the number of symptomatic episodes and consumption of glyceryl trinitrate in the subjects (100). Work with prostacyclin in acute MI failed to show any benefit in three different randomized studies (101–103).

Adjunctive Therapy

Prostacyclin and/or its analogues have been evaluated as adjunctive therapies in patients with both angina and MI. Iloprost combined with t-PA therapy in a closed-chest canine model of thrombosis has been studied. Iloprost was found to increase the time to reperfusion by 50% in comparison with control (104). This possibly unexpected result could be explained by an increase in plasma clearance of t-PA in the presence of the PG. Unfavorable results were also reported in patients with MI given t-PA with or without iloprost (105). Reocclusion at 1 week was not affected by iloprost. Ejection fraction increased after 1 week in patients in the placebo group compared to those receiving iloprost.

Thus initial experiments on animals or small open uncontrolled clinical trials tended to present positive findings of prostacyclin or iloprost in these conditions. However, these findings could not be confirmed in human studies when the studies had sufficient power and were double-blind and placebo-controlled. With the currently available information, it does not appear that iloprost is useful as an adjunct to thrombolytic therapy in patients with MI.

Stroke Disease

In patients with stroke an antiplatelet vasodilator agent with cytoprotective effects to protect against reperfusion injury might be expected to be of benefit. In cerebrally ischemic rats, an iloprost infusion reduced cerebral edema, diminished accumulation of calcium in the brain, and improved the healing capacity of the injured animals (106). Only a few trials in humans evaluating prostacyclin-type drugs have been published, however (107). This early open study lead to the completion of a controlled randomized trial. Disappointingly, however, a significant alleviation of neurologic deficit which occurred early after treatment with prostacyclin was not sustained at the 2-week follow-up period (108). Other studies of prostacyclin failed to show a benefit in this group of patients (109,110). Again, there does not appear to be any competitive studies of iloprost in the published literature but it may be that results would be similar to those seen with prostacyclin.

Extracorporeal Circulation

Extracorporeal circuits are frequently used in clinical medicine. Hemodialysis for patients with chronic renal failure is one such frequent use of extracorporeal circuits. When blood is exposed to an artificial surface there is a potential for activation of blood coagulation to occur triggered through platelet aggregation. An antiplatelet agent might be expected to be of use. Indeed prostacyclin has a license for use in some countries for this indication (111,112). Studies comparing prostacyclin and iloprost have been undertaken (113) and results from the two treatments seem similar.

Prostacyclin has been studied in cardiopulmonary bypass and benefits were confirmed in two placebo-controlled trials (114,115). Iloprost was given to dogs during cardiopulmonary bypass and this resulted in less platelet consumption and myocardial platelet deposition (116). Clearly in these indications a prostacyclin analogue such as iloprost offers some advantages over prostacyclin in terms of chemical stability. However, there are few studies using PGI_2 and much work in this area must still be completed.

Organ Transplant

Organ viability following cold ischemia is of crucial importance in the procedure of transplantation. A number of noxious insults are involved in organ damage including ischemia/reperfusion injury. Prostacyclin has been used as an addition to organ preservation fluids. Iloprost improves pulmonary function after lung transplantation (117,118). Studies in this area are small and must be regarded as pilots. Further work in this area is required.

Conclusion

A number of indications have been evaluated as potential clinical areas for iloprost use. Its potent vasodilatory effect and subsequent coronary steal has made evaluation in myocardial disease disappointing. Its potential as a treatment for peripheral vascular diseases, however, has been better realized and its licensing for use in critical limb ischemia, thromboangiitis obliterans, and Raynaud's phenomenon in a number of countries worldwide has allowed this compound to enter into the therapeutic armamentarium against peripheral vascular disease.

CICAPROST

Pharmacology

There is only about 20% bioavailability on oral application of iloprost but modification of the lower side chain has resulted in the biologically more potent cicaprost (10). Cicaprost is metabolically stable and is excreted unchanged in urine and feces (119).

Therapeutic Use

In vitro animal studies have shown cicaprost to inhibit platelet aggregation (120). In a study of its effects on platelet aggregation and other indices of cell function and fibrinolysis in patients with RP secondary to SSc, cicaprost, in doses up to 5 g tid failed to modify the blood coagulation elements but did produce potent vasodilatation (56).

Conclusion

Cicaprost is less likely to be a clinically important drug in the treatment of vascular disease than it is for patients receiving cancer surgery or as a preventative against the spread of cancers (121,122).

CIPROSTENE

Pharmacology

Ciprostene is also a carbocyclin analogue of prostacyclin and is more stable than the native prostacyclin. It has antiplatelet vasodilator effects and may also suppress endothelial tissue factor expression indirectly by inhibiting the amplification produced by monocyte-derived cytokines (123).

Therapeutic Use

Ciprostene has been studied in a number of clinical areas. These include patients with PAOD and critical limb ischemia, intermittent claudication, and those undergoing therapeutic transluminal coronary angioplasty.

Intermittent Claudication

Wolf et al. (124) evaluated 10 patients with claudication given ciprostene through a portable infusion pump. Ciprostene was infused over 8 hours on 1 day per week for 4 consecutive weeks. Patients successfully maintained the pump strapped to their waists. The drug delivery was accurate as planned. Headache, flushing, and infusion site irritation were the most commonly reported side effects. Blood pressure remained unchanged. Disappointingly, the relative claudication times on the treadmill remained unchanged. However, absolute claudication times increased ($p < 0.05$) but only by about 3 minutes.

Severe Limb Ischemia

A single randomized double-blind study has investigated the effects of ciprostene in patients with ischemic ulcers (57). A total of 211 patients received either ciprostene (120 nm per kg per minute) or placebo in 8 hourly infusions for 7 days. Disappointingly, there was poor compliance with only 45% of the patients receiving ciprostene and 55% of the placebo patients completing the trial. The reduction of ulcer size by at least 50% occurred more frequently in the ciprostene treated group at month 4 ($p = 0.005$). Interestingly, there was a similar decrease in patients' perception of pain severity in both the ciprostene and placebo groups. The drug was reasonably well tolerated with vasodilatory side effects occurring. The therapeutic benefit was limited to a partial reduction in ulcer size.

Transluminal Coronary Angioplasty

Ciprostene was studied for its potential beneficial effects on restenosis in patients with coronary artery disease undergoing percutaneous transluminal coronary angioplasty (PTCA) (125). In a double-blind randomized placebo-controlled trial 32 patients were enrolled. The infusion of the medication was begun before the introduction of the balloon catheter into the coronary artery and continued for 36 hours thereafter. There was a further tailing-off period when the drug dosage was gradually decreased until 48 hours. The coronary artery stenosis at 6 months in the ciprostene group was significantly less than the pre-PTCA value when compared to placebo ($p < 0.05$). When patients were characterized according to their clinical status, these differences were accounted for by the patients with unstable angina receiving ciprostene. Thus it was concluded that ciprostene appeared to reduce restenosis 6 months after coronary angioplasty in patients with unstable angina. The infusion rate of 40 ng per kg per minute followed by 120 ng per kg per minute was well tolerated although the incidence of catheter-associated bleeding was increased.

Others

There have been few studies on ciprostene in humans in other indications. Animal work looking at skin flap survival is of interest, however. In this study administration of ciprostene and indomethacin either alone or together partially reversed the pathophysiologic mechanisms that caused necrosis of random skin flap distal end (126). A potential property of ciprostene—that of cytoprotection—may also be of use in future clinical indications such as organ transplant (127).

In the study by Demke et al., whereby ciprostene was given in PTCA (128), an additional benefit of ciprostene was seen over and above that of protection against restenosis. In this study the ciprostene-treated patients had significantly fewer major clinical events (MI, death, repeat PTCA or coronary artery bypass graft surgery to the study vessel) than did placebo-treated patients. Ciprostene-treated patients also had a significantly greater improvement in the New York Heart Association Angina Classification than did placebo-treated patients.

Conclusion

In conclusion, there are tantalizing data regarding ciprostene's efficacy already published in the literature. However, these studies have not been supported by further substantive studies. Such supportive data are required to more fully assess the potential for ciprostene to act as an effective vascular medication.

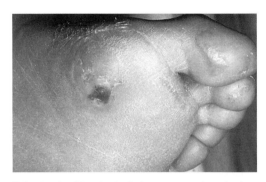

FIG. 15-8. Classical diabetes-associated plantar ulceration in a patient in the taprostene critical limb ischemia study.

TAPROSTENE

Pharmacology

Taprostene sodium is a stable prostacyclin analogue with less inhibitory effect on platelet aggregation than the natural prostacyclin (129). However, taprostene sodium is also less hypotensive than its natural counterpart. It was hypothesized, therefore, that taprostene could still inhibit platelet aggregation without producing vasodilator side effects. Additional actions that caused it to be considered as a therapy for vascular disease were platelet disaggregation (130), inhibition of neutrophil–endothelial interactions (131), and scavenging of the hydroxy free radical (132).

Therapeutic Use

Taprostene has been evaluated in critical limb ischemia (Fig. 15-8) in patients with coronary vascular disease and in association with thrombolytic therapy.

Critical Limb Ischemia

The European PARTNER studies (peripheral artery disease response to taprostene with newly established response definitions) evaluated the clinical safety and efficacy of taprostene in the treatment of peripheral arterial disease of Fontaine stages III and IV in a randomized double-blind placebo-controlled grouping of multicenter trials (133). Over 300 patients were enrolled into these studies of critical limb ischemia where patients received 200 to 600 µg of taprostene over 2×2 hours per day or placebo. Randomization was on a 2:1 patient basis in most cases. One study was controlled by PGE_1. At least 30 infusions were administered to all the patients and the endpoints were amputation rate at 12 months and total mortality. Disappointingly, the individual studies failed to show a significant beneficial effect of the infusions (134). Taprostene was well tolerated in the treated group.

Coronary Vascular Disease

Taprostene has been investigated in an open preliminary study and then in a double-blind crossover study versus placebo investigating its influence on ischemic ST segment depression during exercise stress testing of patients with angiographically proven coronary heart disease and stable angina (135). Taprostene was well tolerated and blood pressure and the ECG parameters did not change. The double-blind study showed no variation in the extent of ischemic ST segment depression when compared to placebo. This indicated that taprostene while not being an effective treatment for myocardial ischemia was unlikely to produce the increase in angina symptoms seen with prostacyclin and other analogues.

Adjunctive Therapy

It was considered that taprostene might be a useful adjuvant to thrombolytic agents when given to patients with acute MI. In a placebo-controlled dose rising study, taprostene or placebo was intravenously infused in 80 patients treated with the thrombolytic agent saruplase (rscu-PA) for acute MI. Disappointingly, taprostene did not affect 90-minute patency. However, there was a trend to better persistence of patency after rescue PTCA had been undertaken (136).

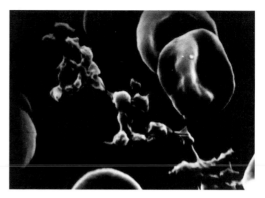

FIG. 15-9. Platelet aggregates in blood of patient with vascular disease.

Extracorporeal Circulation

When administered at a dosage of 25 to 35 ng per kg per minute to chronic renal failure patients undergoing hemodialysis with heparin for 5 hours, inhibition of platelet aggregation ex vivo was noted (137). Although marked heparin-sparing was achieved, dialysis with taprostene alone resulted in thrombus formation and premature termination of the procedure. Also the therapeutic ratio of this analogue appeared to be small, as the 35 ng per kg per minute infusion resulted in nausea and headache in all subjects. This is in contrast to the peripheral and coronary artery studies where the drug appeared to be very well tolerated.

Conclusion

The studies with taprostene have been well conducted. It is therefore disappointing that such poor clinical results were achieved. It may be that drug dosage was not sufficiently high and it might be worth pursuing studies of this compound at a higher dose levels in the future.

BERAPROST

Pharmacology

Beraprost sodium is another stable analogue of prostacyclin that has potent vasodilator and antiplatelet effects (Fig. 15-9) (138). Additional properties which might contribute to its usefulness as a therapeutic agent for vascular disease include beneficial effects on RBC deformability (139) and positive ionotropic and chronotropic effects on animal myocardium (140).

Therapeutic Use

Beraprost is still at the fairly early stages of its clinical trial program but studies have already been completed in intermittent claudication, stroke and autonomic nerve dysfunctioning patients with diabetes. Pulmonary hypertension is also being investigated.

Intermittent Claudication

The efficacy and safety of three doses of beraprost sodium has been compared to placebo in patients with intermittent claudication (141). One hundred sixty-four patients were randomized to receive either placebo, 20 g, 40 g, or 60 g of beraprost sodium three times a day administered orally in a double-blind fashion over 12 weeks. Exercise treadmill tests were performed. At week 10 all groups showed an increase in pain-free walking distance but this distance was greatest in the groups receiving the 60 and 120 g per day of beraprost (p = 0.055). At week 12 a similar pattern was observed and the difference was then statistically significant between the groups (p = 0.023). The compound was reasonably well tolerated but the question remains as to why the highest dose used (180 g per day) showed a lower efficacy than the two middle doses. Nevertheless, this initial study suggested that beraprost was a promising drug for consideration in a further study of intermittent claudication. Objective measures of blood flow in the lower limb also showed an improvement during test dosing with beraprost in two patients with non-insulin-dependent diabetes mellitus and arterial disease (142).

Stroke Disease

Beraprost was administered in a dose of 1 g per kg per minute to dogs with cerebral ischemia. Residual blood flow in the ischemic medulla oblongata was not improved. However, the decrease in baroreceptor reflex sensitivity was abolished. The authors conclude that the beneficial action of beraprost in this brain ischemia was exerted through "cytoprotection" (143). The effect of beraprost in stroke disease in humans has yet to be evaluated.

Raynaud's Phenomenon

A controlled multicenter double-blind trial of beraprost in primary Raynaud's phenomenon has been reported (144). The aim was to compare the efficacy and tolerance of beraprost to placebo. One hundred and twenty-five patients with disabling primary Raynaud's disease participated in this 8-week study, which was conducted during the winter months. The number of vasospastic attacks decreased significantly in both groups (confidence intervals of improvement were 35% to 53% in the beraprost group and 25% to 49% in the placebo group) but did not differ significantly between the two groups. Similar results were found for the severity of the vasospastic attacks and overall disability reported by the patients. Thus, disappointingly, beraprost did not appear to produce more benefit than placebo in this study.

Pulmonary Hypertension

The short-term hemodynamic effects of beraprost have been investigated in both pri-
mary and secondary pulmonary hypertension (145). In this pilot study beraprost did appear to be reasonably effective as a pulmonary vasodilator agent. This supported the early promising animal work (146).

Others

Very little other human work has been reported but beraprost does appear to improve autonomic nerve dysfunction in patients with diabetes in a small pilot study (147). Another small study evaluated beraprost as a treatment for levido vasculitis in four patients. Clinical improvement was seen but it should be stressed that neither of these two studies was placebo-controlled (148). Animal work suggests that this compound should be evaluated in skin flap viability (149) and possibly other areas requiring cytoprotection (150).

Conclusion

Beraprost is a fairly recently developed prostacyclin analogue. Conclusions regarding its clinical efficacy cannot yet be made as the studies are in the early stages with most reports relating to uncontrolled studies containing small numbers of patients. The only study of major size, that of the patients with Raynaud's phenomenon (144), proved negative, thus stressing the importance of properly designed and powered studies in this field.

CONCLUSION

The enthusiasm and excitement that gripped the scientific world after discovery of prostacyclin and its analogues has not been fully sustained. The hopes for this new therapeutic agent have not been fully realized, although the area of peripheral arterial disease seems to be the most promising field. Some of the earliest discovered compounds have been particularly well studied. These include prostacyclin itself and iloprost. Other compounds have not yet been fully evaluated and no conclusions can be drawn about their therapeutic effectiveness at this stage. It should be remembered that it is not just prostacyclin and its analogues that might have potential benefits in the area of vascular disease but also some of the PGE chemicals. This is particularly so in critical limb ischemia (151) with analogues of PGE_1 (152).

REFERENCES

1. Moncada S, Gryglewski RJ, Bunting S, Vane JR. An enzyme isolated from arteries transforms prostaglandin endoperoxides to an unstable substance that inhibits platelet aggregation. *Nature* 1971;231: 663–665.

2. Szczeklik A, Skawinski A, Gluszko P, Nizankowski R, Szczeklik, RJ Gryglewski. Successful therapy of advanced arteriosclerosis obliterans with prostacyclin. *Lancet* 1979;1:1111–1114.

3. Hanss JG, Taylor GW. Metabolism and toxicology of the prostaglandins. In: Vane J, O'Grady J (eds). *Therapeutic Applications of Prostaglandins.* 1993;37–48.

4. Belch JJF, McArdle B, Pollock JG, Forbes CD, et al. Epoprostenol (prostacyclin) and severe arterial disease. A double-blind trial. *Lancet* 1983;1:315–317.

5. Belch JJF, Newman P, Drury JK, et al. Intermittent prostacyclin infusions in patients with Raynaud's syndrome: a double blind trial. *Lancet* 1983;1:313–315.

6. Virgolini I, Fitscha P, Linet OI, O'Grady J, Sinzinger H. A double blind placebo controlled trial of intravenous prostacyclin (PGI_2) in 108 patients with ischaemic peripheral vascular disease. *Prostaglandins* 1990;39:657–664.

7. Stock G. Iloprost: a stable analog of prostacyclin. In: Rubanyi GM, Vanhoutte OD (eds). *Endothelium-derived relaxing factors. Proceedings of the First International Symposium on Endothelium-Derived Vasoactive Factors.* Philadelphia:Philadelphia Press, 1989;260–264.

8. Belch JJF, Greer IA, McLaren M, et al. The effects of intravenous infusion of ZK36374, a synthetic prostacyclin derivative, on normal volunteers. *Prostaglandins* 1984; 28:67–78.

9. *Drugs of the Future.* New York: Raven Press, 1986;11: 913–917.

10. Skuballa W, Schillinger E, Stuerzebecher CS, Vorbrueggen H. Synthesis of a new chemically and metabolocally stable prostacyclin analogue with high and long-lasting oral activity. *J Med Chem* 1986;29: 313–315.

11. Sodeoka M, Ogawa Y, Kirio Y, Shibasaki M. Stereocontrolled synthesis of exocyclin olefins using arene tricarbonyl chromin complex-catalyzed hydrogenation. I. Efficient synthesis of carbacyclin and its analogs. *Chem Pharm Bull* 1991;39:309–322.

12. Fujitani B, Wakitani K. Studies on antiplatelet effects of OP-41483, a prostaglandin I_2 analog, in experimental animals. I. Effect on platelet function and thrombosis. *Pharmacology* 1990;52:123–130.

13. Linet OI, Luderer JR, Froeschke M, Welch S, Metxler CM, Eckert SM. Ciprostene in patients with peripheral vascular disease (PVD). An open-label, tolerance trial. *Prostaglandins Leukot Essent Fatty Acids* 1988;34:9–14.

14. O'Grady J, Hedges A, Whittle BJR, et al. A chemically stable analog, 9β-methylcarbarbacyclin, with similar effects to epoprostenol (prostacyclin, PGI_2) in man. *Br J Clin Pharmacol* 1984;18:921–33.

15. *Drugs of the Future.* New York:Raven Press, 1990;15: 233–236.

16. Flohe L, Boehlke H, Frankus E, et al. Designing prostacyclin analogs. *Arznei Forsch/Drug Res* 1983; 33:1240–1248.

17. Michael G, Seipp U. In vitro studies with the stabilized epoprostenol analog taprostene. Effect on platelets and erythrocytes. *Arzneim Forsch/Drug Res* 1990;40: 817–822.

18. Michael G, Seipp U. In vivo studies with the stabilized epoprostenol analog taprostene. Effects on platelet functions and blood clotting. *Arzneim Forsch/Drug Res* 1990;40:932–914.

19. Murata T, Sakaya S, Hoshino T, Umetsu T, Hiranto T, Mishio S. General pharmacology of beraprost sodium, 1st communication: effect on the central nervous system. *Arzneim Forsch/Drug Res* 1989;29(II):860–866.

20. Murata T, Murai T, Kanai T, et al. General pharmacology of beraprost sodium, 2nd communication: effect on the autonomic cardiocvascular and gastro-intestinal systems,and other effects. *Arzneim Forsch/Drug Res* 1989;29(II):867–76.

21. Schillinger E, Losert WF. Identification of PGI_2 receptors, and CAMP levels in platelets and femoral arteries. *Acta Therapeutica* 1980;6(suppl):37.

22. Schror K, Ohlendorf R, Darius H. Beneficial effects of a new carbacyclin derivative, ZK 36 374 in acute myocardial ischaemia. *J Pharmacol Exp Ther* 1981;219: 243–249.

23. Galt SW, McDaniel MD, Ault KA, Mitchell J, Cronenwett JL. Flow cytometric assessment of platelet function in patients with peripheral arterial occlusive disease. *J Vasc Surg* 1991;14:749–755.

24. Zahavi J, Zahavi M. Enhanced platelet release reaction shortened platelet survival time and increased platelet aggregation and plasma thromboxane B_2 in chronic obstructive arterial disease. *Thromb Haemost* 1985;53: 105–109.

25. Feng LJ, Berger BE, Lysz TW, Shaw WW. Vasoactive prostaglandins in the impending no-reflow state: evidence for a primary disturbance in microvascular tone. *Plast Reconstr Surg* 1988;81:755–767.

26. Wennmalm A, Edlund A, Sevastik B, FitzGerald GA. Excretion of thromboxane A2 and prostacyclin metabolites during treadmill exercise in patients with intermittent claudication. *Clin Physiol* 1988;8:243–253.

27. Heistad DD, Harrison DG, Armstrong ML. Serotonin and experimental vascular disease. *Int J Cardiol* 1987; 14:205–212.

28. Barradas MA, Gill DS, Fonseca VA, Mikhailidis DP, Dandona O. Intra-platelet serotonin in patients with diabetes mellitus and peripheral vascular disease. *Eur J Clin Invest* 1988;18:399–404.

29. Lowe GDO. Pathophysiology of critical limb ischaemia. In: Dormandy J, Stock G. *Critical Leg Ischaemia: Its Pathophysiology and Management.* Heidelberg: Springer, 1990:17–40.

30. Wiseman S, Kenchington G, Dain R, et al. Influence of smoking and plasma factors on patency of femoropopliteal vein grafts. *Br Med J* 1989;299: 643–646.

31. Bouhoutsos J, Morris T, Chavatzas D, Martin P. The influence of haemoglobin and platelet levels on the results of arterial surgery. *Br J Surg* 1974;61:984–986.

32. Dormandy JA, Hoare E, Colley J, Arrowsmith DE, Dormandy TL. Clinical haemodynamic, rheological,

and biochemical findings in 126 patients with intermittent claudication. *Br Med J* 1973; December: 576–581.

33. Ciuffetti G, Mercuri M, Mannarino E, Robinson MK, Lennie SE, Lowe G. Peripheral vascular disease. Rheologic variables during controlled ischemia. *Circulation* 1989;80:348–352.

34. Belch JJF. Chapter 47. White cells, free radicals and scavengers. In: Bloom AL, Forbes CD, Thomas DP, Tuddenham EGD (eds). *Haemostasis and Thrombosis* (3rd ed). Edinburgh: Churchill Livingstone, 1994: 1089–1106.

35. Belch JJF. The role of the white blood cell in arterial disease. *Blood Coag Fibrin* 1990;1:183–192.

36. Belch JJF. The white blood cells as a risk factor for thrombotic vascular disease. *Vasc Med Rev* 1990; 1:203–213.

37. Belch JJF, Chopra M, Hutchison S, et al. Free radical pathology in chronic arterial disease. *Free Rad Biol Med* 1989;6:375–378.

38. Shearman CP, Gosling P, Gwynn BR, Simms MH. Systemic effects associated with intermittent claudication. A model to study biochemical aspects of vascular disease? *Eur J Vasc Surg* 1988;2:401–404.

39. Lau CS, Scott N, Brown JE, Shaw W, Belch JJF. Increased activity of oxygen free radicals during reperfusion in patients undergoing percutaneous peripheral artery balloon angioplasty. *Int Angiol* 1991;10: 244–246.

40. Hickey NC, Gosling P, Baar S, Shearman C. Effects of surgery on the systemic inflammatory response to intermittent claudication. *Br J Surg* 1990;77:1121–1124.

41. D'Angelo Y, Villa S, Mysllvvlec M, Donati MB, De Gaetano G. Defective fibrinolytic and prostacyclin like activity in human atheromatous plaques. *Thromb Haemost* 1978;39:535–536.

42. Belch JJF, Zoma A, Richards I, Forbes CD, Sturrock RD. Vascular damage and factor VIII related antigen in the rheumatic disease. *Rheumatol Int* 1987;7:107–111.

43. Ludmet PL, Selwyn AP, Wayne RR, Mudge GH, Alexander RW, Ganz P. Impaired endothelial-dependent coronary dilation in patients with coronary artery disease. *J Am Coll Cardiol* 1986;7:2091.

44. McMurray JJ, Ray SG, Ibrahin A, Dargie HV, Morton JJ. Plasma endothelin in chronic heart failure. *Circulation* 1992;85:1374–1379.

45. Bridges AB, Hill A, Belch JJF. Cigarette smoking increases white blood cell aggregation in whole blood. *J R Soc Med* 1993;86:139–140.

46. Di Perri T, Laghi Pasini F, Acciavatti A, Pieragalli D, Domini L, et al. Haemodynamics, rheology and mechanism of action of iloprost in man. *Clin Hemorr* 1990;10:171–183.

47. Belch JJF, Ansell D, Saniabadi A, Forbes CD, Sturrock RD. Transdermally applied iloprost (ZK36-374) decreases whole blood platelet aggregation in normal volunteers. *Prog Clin Biol Res* 1987;242:413–417.

48. Riva CM, Morganroth ML, Marks RM, et al. Iloprost inhibits activated human neutrophil (PMN) adherence to endothelial cells via increased cyclic AMP. *Clin Res* 1989;37:949A.

49. Nicolini FA, Metha P, Lawson D, Mehta JL. Reduction in human neutrophil chemotaxis by the rostacyclin analogue iloprost. *Thromb Res* 1990;59:669–674.

50. Musial J, Wilczynska M, Sladek K, et al. Fibrinolytic activity of prostacyclin and iloprost in patients with peripheral arterial disease. *Prostaglandins* 1986;31: 61–70.

51. Bertele V, Mussoni L, de Rosso G, et al. Defective fibrinolytic response in atherosclerotic patients—effect of iloprost and its possible mechanism of action. *Thromb Haemost* 1988;60:141–144.

52. Sinzinger H, O'Grady J, Cromwell M, Hofer R. Epoprostenol (prostacyclin) decreases platelet deposition on vascular prosthetic grafts. *Lancet* 1983;1: 1275–1276.

53. Thiemermann C, Steinhagen-Thiessen E, Schror K. Inhibition of oxygen centred free radical formation by the stable prostacyclin mimetic iloprost (ZK36 374) in acute myocardial ischaemia. *J Cardiovasc Pharmacol* 1984;6:365–366.

54. Andreozzi GM, Pino LD, Pira ML, Butto G, Martini R, Signorelli S. Iloprost stable analogue of prostacyclin is able to improve the tissue resistance to ischaemia. *Int Angiol* 1994;68–69.

55. Belch JJF, Lowe GDO, Drummond MM, Forbes CD, Prentice CRM. Prostacyclin reduces red cell deformability. *Thromb Haemost* 1981;45;189.

56. Lau CS, McLaren M, Saniabadi A, Scott N, Belch JJF. The pharmacological effects of cicaprost, an oral prostacyclin analogue, in patients with Raynaud's syndrome secondary to systemic sclerosis—a preliminary study. *Clin Exp Rheumatol* 1991;9:271–273.

57. The Ciprostene Study Group. The effect of ciprostene in patients with peripheral vascular disease (PVD) characterized by ischemic ulcers. *J Clin Pharmacol* 1991;31:81–87.

58. Belch JJF, Capell HA, Cooke ED, et al. Oral iloprost as a treatment for Raynaud's Syndrome: a double blind multicentre placebo controlled study. *Ann Rheum Dis* 1995;54:197–200.

59. Yardumian DA, Mackie IJ, Brennan EC, Bull H, Machin SJ. Platelet function studies during and after infusions of ZK36 375, a stable prostacyclin analogue to healthy volunteers. *Haemostasis* 1986;16:20–26.

60. Ylitalo P, Kaukinen S, Nurmi A, Pessi T, Kraus T, Vapaatalo H. Pharmacological effects of iloprost, ZK36 374, a stable prostacyclin analogue in man. *Biomed Biochim Acta* 1984;43:S399–S402.

61. Schillinger E, Krain T, Lehman M, Stock G. Iloprost. In: Scriabine A (ed). *New Cardiovascular Drugs*. New York: Raven, 1986;209–301.

62. McHugh NJ, Csuka M, Watson H, et al. Infusion of iloprost, a prostacyclin analogue, for the treatment of Raynaud's phenomenon in systemic sclerosis. *Ann Rheum Dis* 1988:47:43–47.

63. De la Mata J, Gomez Sanchez MA, Aranzana M, Gomez Reino JJ. Long term iloprost infusion therapy for severe pulmonory hypertension in patients with connective tissue diseases. *Arthritis Rheum* 1994; 37:1528–1533.

64. Olschewski H, Walmrath D, Schermuly R, Ghofrani A, Grimminger F, Seeger W. Aerosolized prostacyclin and iloprost in severe pulmonary hypertension. *Ann Intern Med* 1996;124:820–824.

65. Fitscha P, Tiso B, Sinzinger H. Iloprost in peripheral vascular disease: platelet function and clinical outcome. In: Sinzinger H, Schror K (eds). *Progress in Clinical and Biological Research* (vol 242). New York: Liss, 1987;463–468.

66. Hay CR, Waller PC, Carter C, et al. Lack of effect of 24 hour infusion of iloprost in intermittent claudication. *Thromb Res* 1987;46:317–324.

67. Sinzinger H, Fitscha P, Popovic R, Krias T. Clinical and platelet effects of ZK36 374 (iloprost) a stable prostacyclin analogue in peripheral vascular disease. *Thromb Haemost* 1985;54:294.

68. Wilkinson D, Vowden P, McNulty T, Parkin A, Kester RC. A placebo-controlled trial using iloprost in intermittent claudication. *J Cardiovasc Surg* 1988;29:72.

69. Diehm C, Abrio O, Baitsch G, et al. Iloprost, a stable prostacyclin derivative in the treatment of stage iv arterial disease. A placebo controlled multicentre trial (Ger). *Ideutsche Medizinische Wochenschrift* 1989; 114:783–788.

70. Brock F, Abri O, Baitsch G, et al. Iloprost in der Behandlung ischamischer Gwebslasionen bei Diabetikern Schweiz. *Med Wochenschrift* 1990;120: 1477–1482.

71. Norgren L, Alwmark A, Angqvist B, et al. A stable prostacyclin analogue (iloprost) in the treatment of ischaemic ulcers of the lower limb. *Eur J Vasc Surg* 1990;4:463–467.

72. Balzer K, Bechara G, Bisler H, et al. Placebo controlled double blind multicentre study in the efficacy of iloprost in the treatment of ischaemic rest pain in patients with peripheral arterial circulatory disease. *Vasa* 1987;20(suppl):379–381.

73. Bliss B, Wilkins D, Campbell WB, et al. Treatment of limb threatening ischaemia with intravenous iloprost. A randomised double blind placebo controlled study. *Eur J Vasc Surg* 1991;5:511–516.

74. Guilmot JL, Diot E. Treatment of lower limb ischaemia due to atherosclerosis in diabetic and non-diabetic patients with iloprost. A stable analogue of prostacyclin: results of the French multicentre trial. *Drug Invest* 1991;3:351–359.

75. Balzer K, Bechara G, Bisler H, et al. Reduction of ischaemic rest pain in advanced peripheral arterial occlusive disease. A double blind placebo controlled trial with iloprost. *Int Angiol* 1991;10:229–232.

76. Loosemore TM, Chalmers TC, Dormandy JA. A meta-analysis of randomized placebo control trials in Fontaine stages III and IV peripheral occlusive arterial disease. *Int Angiol* 1994;13:133–142.

77. Fissenger JN, Schafer M. A randomised double blind study comparing iloprost and aspirin in the treatment of critical ischaemia due to thromboangitis obliterans. *Lancet* 1990;335:555–557.

78. Rademaker M, Thomas RHM, Provost G, et al. Prolonged increase in digital blood flow following iloprost infusion in patients with systemic sclerosis. *Postgrad Med J* 1987;63:617–620.

79. Yardumian DA, Isenberg DA, Rustin M, et al. Successful treatment of Raynaud's syndrome with iloprost, a chemically stable prostacyclin analogue. *Br J Rheum* 1988;27:220–226.

80. McHugh NJ, Csuka M, Watson H, Belcher G, Amadi A, Ring FEJ. Infusion of iloprost, a prostacyclin analogue for treatment of Raynaud's phenomenon in systemic sclerosis. *Ann Rheum Dis* 1988;47:43–47.

81. Wigley F, Seibold J, Wise R, et al. Intravenous iloprost treatment of Raynaud's phenomenon and ischaemic ulcers to systemic sclerosis. *J Rheumatol* 1992;19: 1407–1414.

82. Wigley F, Wise R, Seibold J, et al. Intravenous iloprost infusion in patients with Raynaud's phenomenon secondary to systemic sclerosis. *Ann Intern Med* 1994; 120:199–206.

83. Torley HI, Madhok R, Capell HA, et al. A double blind, randomised, multicentre comparison of two doses of intravenous iloprost in the treatment of Raynaud's phenomenon secondary to connective tissue diseases. *Ann Rheum Dis* 1991;50:800–804.

84. Rademaker M, Cooke ED, Almond NE, et al. Comparison of intravenous infusions of iloprost and oral nifedipine in treatment of Raynaud's phenomenon in patients with systemic sclerosis. A double blind randomised study. *Br Med J* 1989;298:561–564.

85. Mascagni B, Sardina M, Alvino S, Berruti V, Bazzi S, Scorza R. Effects of iloprost in comparison to nifedipine in patients with Raynaud's phenomenon secondary to progressive systemic sclerosis. *Int Angiol* 1994; 13(suppl 1):81–82.

86. Scott JP. Higenbottam TW, Wallwork J. The acute effect of the synthetic prostocyclin analogue iloprost in primary pulmonary hypertension. *Br J Pharmacol* 1990;6:231–234.

87. Butt AY, Dinh-Xuar AT, Tako M. et al. Treatment of pulmonary hypertension with prostacyclin analogue iloprost. *J Am Coll Cardiol* 1994;375A.

88. Holmes DR Jr, Vlietstra RE. Percutaneous transluminal coronary angioplasty. Current status and future trends. *Mayo Clin Porc* 1986;61:865–876.

89. Holmes DR Jr, Vliestra RE. Angioplasty in total coronary arterial occlusion. *Herz* 1985;10:292–297.

90. Holmes DR Jr, Smith HC, Vlietstra RE, et al. Percutaneous transluminal coronary angioplasty, alone or in combination with streptokinase therapy, during acute myocardial infarction. *Mayo Clin Proc* 1985;60: 449–456.

91. Papapierto SE, MacLean WAH, Stanley AWH Jr, et al. Percutaneous transluminal coronary angioplasty after intracoronary streptokinase in evolving acute myocardial infarction. *Am J Cardiol* 1985;55:48–53.

92. Leimgruber PP, Roubin GS, Hollman J, et al. Restenosis after successful coronary angioplasty in patients with single vessel disease. *Circulation* 1986;73: 710–717.

93. Ernst SMPG, van der Feltz TA, Bal ET, el al. Long term angiographic follow up, cardiac events, and survival in patients undergoing percutaneous transluminal coronary angioplasty. *Br Heart J* 1987;57:220–225.

94. Holmes Dr Jr, Vlietstra RE, Reeder Gs, et al. Balloon angioplasty for total coronary occlusion not associated with evolving myocardial infarction. *J Am Coll Cardiol* 1986;7:211A.

95. Wexman MP, Murphy MC, Fishman-Rosen J, et al. Factors predicting recurrence in patients who have had angioplasty (PTCA) of totally occluded vessels. *J Am Coll Cardiol* 1986;7:20A.

96. Mata LA, Bosch X, David PR, et al. Clinical and angiographic assessment 6 months after double vessel percutaneous coronary angioplasty. *J Am Coll Cardiol* 1985;6:1239–1244.

97. DiSciascio G, Cowley MJ, Vetrovec GW. Angiographic patterns of restenosis after angioplasty to multiple coronary arteries. *Am J Cardiol* 1986;58: 922–925.

98. Hollman J, Galan K, Franci I, et al. Recurrent stenosis

after coronary angioplasty. *J Am Coll Cardiol* 1986; 7:20A.

99. Uebis R, von Essen R, vom Dahl J, et al. Recurrence rate after PTCA in relationship to the initial length of coronary artery narrowing. *J Am Coll Cardiol* 1986; 7:62A.

100. Hirshfeld JW Jr, Goldberg S, MacDonald R, et al. Lesion and procedure-related variables predictive of restenosis after PTCA—a report from the M-HEART study. *Circulation* 1987;76:IV-215.

101. White CW, Chaitman B, Laser TA, et al. Antiplatelet agents are effective in reducing the immediate complications of PTCA. Results from the Ticlopidine Multicenter Trial. *Circulation* 1987;76:IV-400.

102. Barnathan ES, Schwartz JS, Taylor L, et al. Aspirin and dipyridamole in the prevention of acute coronary thrombosis complicating coronary angioplasty. *Circulation* 1987;76:125–34.

103. Hartxler GO, Rutherford BD, McConahay DR, et al. High dose steroids for prevention of recurrent restenosis post OTCA. A randomized trial. *J Am Coll Cardiol* 1987;9:185A.

104. Pepine CJ, Hill JA, Lambert CR. Therapeutic cardiac catherization. Part 2. *Mod Concepts Cardiovasc Dis* 1990;59:61–66.

105. Jaffe E, Physiologic functions of normal endothelial cells. *Ann NY Acad Sci* 1985;454:279.

106. Borzeix MG, Cahn R, Cahn J. Effects of new chemically and metabolically stable prostacyclin analogues (iloprost and ZK 96480) on early consequences of a transient cerebral oligaemia in the rat. *Prostaglandins* 1988;35:653–664.

107. Gryglewski RJ, Nowak S, Kostka-Trabka E, et al. Treatment of ischaemic stroke with prostacyclin. *Stroke* 1983;14:197–202.

108. Huczynski J, Kosta-Trabka E, Sotowska W, et al. Double-blind controlled trial of the therapeutic effects of prostacyclin in patients with completed ischaemic stroke. *Stroke* 1985;16:810–814.

109. Martin JF, Hamdy N, Nicholl J, et al. Double-blind controlled trial of prostacyclin in cerebral infarction. *Stroke* 1985;16:386–390.

110. Hsu CY, Faught RE Jr, Furlan AJ, et al. Intravenous prostacyclin in acute nonhemorrhagic stroke: a placebo controlled double-blind trial. *Stroke* 1987; 18:352–358.

111. Woods HF, Ash G, Weston MJ, Bunting S, Moncada S, Vane JR. Prostacyclin can replace heparin in haemodialysis in dogs. *Lancet* 1978;2:1075–1077.

112. Turney JH, Williams LC, Fewell MR, Parsons V, Weston MJ. Platelet protection and heparin sparing with prostacyclin during regular dialysis therapy. *Lancet* 1980;2:219–222.

113. Dibble JB, Kalra PA, Orchard MA, Turney JH, Davies JA. Prostacyclin and iloprost do not affect action of standard dose heparin on haemostatic function during haemodialysis. *Thromb Res* 1988;29:385–392.

114. Longmore DB, Hoyle PM, Gregory A, et al. Prostacyclin administration during cardiopulmonary bypass in man. *Lancet* 1981;1:800–804.

115. Walker ID, Davidson JF, Faichney A, Wheatley DJ, Davidson KG. A double-blind study of prostacyclin in cardiopulmonary bypass surgery. *Br J Haematol* 1981; 49:415–423.

116. Cottrell ED, Kappa JR, Stenach N, et al. Temporary inhibition of platelet function with iloprost (ZK36374) preserves canine platelets during extracorporeal membrane oxygenation. *J Thorac Cardiovasc Surg* 1988;96:535–541.

117. Klepetko W, Muller M, Khurl-Brady G. Beneficial effect of iloprost on early pulmonary function after lung preservation with modified Euro-Collins solution. *Thorac Cardiovasc Surg* 1989;37:174–178.

118. Sanchez-Urdazpal L, Gores G, Ferguson D, Krom R. Improved liver preservation with addition of iloprost to Euro-Collins and University of Wisconsin storage solutions. *Transplantation* 1991;52:1105–1107.

119. Hildebrand M, Staks T, Schuett A, Matthes H. Pharmacokinetics of ^{3}H-cicaprost in healthy volunteers. *Prostaglandins* 1989;37:259–273.

120. Sturzebecher CST, Loge O, Schroder G, Muller B, Witt W. Cardiovascular and antithrombotic effects of XK 96480, an oral metabolically stable carbacyclin derivative with oral activity. In: Sinzinger H, Schror K (eds). *Progress in Clinical and Biological Research.* New York: Liss, 1987;425–431.

121. Schirner M, Schneider MR. Cicaprost inhibits metastases of animal tumors. *Prostaglandins* 1991;42: 451–461.

122. Ostrom RS, Ehlert FJ. M2 Muscarinic receptor inhibition of agonist-induced cyclic adenosine monophosphate accumulation and relaxation in the guinea pig ileum. *J Pharmacol Exp Ther* 1997;280:189–199.

123. Crutchley DJ, Conanan LB, Toledo AW, Solomon DE, Que BG. Effects of prostacyclin analogues on human endothelial cell tissue factor expression. *Arterioscler Thromb* 1993;13:1082–1089.

124. Wolf DL, Metzler CM, Froeschke MO, Luderer JR. Continuous intravenous dosing with ciprostene using a portable pump in ambulatory patients. *J Clin Pharmacol* 1993;33:150–153.

125. Darius H, Nixdorff U, Zander J, Rupprecht HJ, Erbel R, Meyer J. Effects of ciprostene on restenosis rate during therapeutic transluminal coronary angioplasty. *Agents Actions* 1992;379(suppl):305–311.

126. Salerno GM, McBride DM, Bleicher JN, Watson P, Stromberrg BV. Ciprostene and indomethacin partially reverse the mechanisms of distal necrosis in the rat random skin flap. *Ann Plast Surg* 1992;28:526–533.

127. Kmiec Z. Prostaglandin cytoprotection of galactosamine-incubated hepatocytes isolated from young and old rats. *Ann NY Acad Sci* 1994;717:216–225.

128. Demke DM, for the Ciprostene Study Group. Double-blind, placebo-controlled efficacy study of ciprostene (U-61, 431F) in percutaneous transluminal coronary angioplasty (PTCA). *Br J Haematol* 1990;76:20.

129. Lefer AM, Darius H. Taprostene (CG-4203). *Cardiovasc Drug Rev* 1989;7:39–50.

130. McLaren M, Bancroft A, Belch JJF. Effects of prostacyclin analogue taprostene on platelet aggregation and intracellular calcium release. *Thromb Haemost* 1993; 69:674 (Abs).

131. Lefer AM, Murohara T, Buerke M. Effects of taprostene on neutrophil-endothelial interactions in isolated coronary arteries. *Meth Find Exp Clin Pharmacol* 1994;16:623–631.

132. Arroyo CM, Wade JV, Ichimori K, Nakazawa H. The scavenging of hydroxyl radical (.OH) by a prostacyclin analogue, taprostene. *Chem Biol Interact* 1994;91:29–38.

133. Belch JJF, Diehm C, Sohngen M, Sohngen W. Critical Limb Ischaemia: a case against Consensus II. *Int Angiol* 1995;14:353–356.

134. Belch JJF. Taprostene versus placebo as a treatment of patients with Critical Limb Ischaemia: the Scottish-Finish-Swedish PARTNER Study [Abstract]. *Int Angiol* 1994;13:6.

135. Hopf R, Schofl E, Frings M, Sohngen W. Effect of the prostacyclin analog taprostene on ischemic ST-segment depression in the stress ECG of coronary patients. *Z Kardiol* 1994;83:258–263.

136. Bar FW, Meyer J, Michels R, et al. The effect of taprostene in patients with acute myocardial infarction treated with thrombolytic therapy: results of the START study. Saruplase Taprostene Acute Reocclusion Trial. *Eur Heart J* 1993;14:1118–1126.

137. Maurin N, Ballmann M. Prevention of coagulation during hemodialysis by a combination of the stable prostacyclin analogue CG4203 and low-dose heparin. *Clin Nephrol* 1988;30:35–41.

138. Nony P, Ffrench P, Girard P, et al. Platelet-aggregation inhibition and hemodynamic effects of beraprost sodium, a new oral prostacyclin derivative: a study in healthy male subjects. *Can J Physiol Pharmacol* 1996; 74:887–893.

139. Hayashi J, Ishida N, Sato H, Hata Y, Saito T. Effect of beraprost, a stable prostacyclin analogue, on red blood cell deformability impairment in the presence of hypercholesterolemia in rabbits. *J Cardiovasc Pharmacol* 1996;27:527–531.

140. Ueno Y, Okazaki S, Isogaya M, et al. Positive inotropic and chronotropic effects of beraprost sodium, a stable analogue of prostacyclin in isolated guinea pig myocardium. *Gen Pharmacol* 1996;27:101–103.

141. Lievre M, Azoulay S, Lion L, Morand S, Girre JP, Boissel JP. A dose effect study of beraprost sodium in intermittent claudication. *J Cardiovasc Pharmacol* 1996;27:788–793.

142. Okuda Y, Sone H, Mizutani S, et al. Acute effect of beraprost sodium on lower limb circulation in patients with non-insulin-dependent diabetes mellitus-evaluation by colour Doppler ultrasonography and laser cutaneous blood flowmetry. *Prostaglandins* 1996;52: 375–384.

143. Kurihara J, Sahara T, Kato H. Protective effect of beraprost sodium, a new chemically stable prostacyclin analogue, against deterioration of baroreceptor reflex following transient global cerebral ischaemia in dogs. *Br J Pharmacol* 1990;99:91–96.

144. Vayssairat M. Controlled multicenter double blind trial of an oral analog of prostacyclin in the treatment of primary Raynaud's phenomenon. French Microcirculation Society Multicentre Group for the Study of Vascular Acrosyndromes. *J Rheumatol* 1996;23:1917–1920.

145. Saji T, Ozawa Y, Ishikita T, Matsuura H, Matsuo N. Short-term hemodynamic effect of a new oral PG12 analogue, beraprost, in primary and secondary pulmonary hypertension. *Am J Cardiol* 1996;78:244–247.

146. Miyata M, Ueno Y, Sekine H. Protective effect of beraprost sodium, a stable prostacyclin analogue in development of monocrotaline-induced pulmonary hypertension. *J Cardiovasc Pharmacol* 1996;27:20–26.

147. Noda K, Umeda F, Nawata H. Effect of beraprost sodium on response to tests of autonomic control of heart rate in patients with diabetes mellitus. *Diabetes Res Clin Pract* 1996;31:119–124.

148. Tsutsui K, Shirasaki F, Takata M, Takenhara K. Successful treatment of livedo vasculitis with beraprost sodium: a possible mechanism of thrombomodulin upregulation. *Dermatology* 1996;192:120–124.

149. Alexandrou K, Hata Y, Matsuka K, Matsuda H. Effect of beraprost sodium (Procylin), a stable prostaglandin 12 analogue, on a dorsal skin flap model in rats. *Scand J Plast Reconstr Surg Hand Surg* 1996;30:17–22.

150. Battal MN, Hata Y, Matsuka K, et al. Reduction of progressive burn injury by a stable prostaglandin 12 analogue, beraprost sodium (Procylin): an experimental study in rats. *Burns* 1996;22:531–538.

151. Belch JJF, Shaw B, Sturrock RD, Madhok R, Leiberman P, Forbes CD. Double-blind trial of CL115, 347: a transdermally absorbed prostaglandin E$_2$ analogue in treatment of Raynaud's phenomenon. *Lancet* 1985; 1:1180–1183.

152. Belch JJF, Bell PRF, Creissen D, et al. Randomized, double-blind, placebo-controlled study evaluating the efficacy and safety of AS-013, a Prostaglandin E$_1$ prodrug in patients with intermittent claudication. *Circulation* 1997;95:2298–2302.

*Cardiovascular Thrombosis: Thrombocardiology
and Thromboneurology, Second Edition,*
edited by M. Verstraete, V. Fuster, and E. J. Topol,
Lippincott–Raven Publishers, Philadelphia © 1998.

16

Vitamin K Antagonists

Eliot C. Williams and *John W. Suttie

*Department of Medicine, University of Wisconsin Hospital and Clinics, Madison, Wisconsin 53792;
and *Department of Biochemistry, University of Wisconsin, Madison, Wisconsin 53706*

The involvement of vitamin K in the procoagulant phase of hemostasis was apparent from the earliest studies of this essential dietary factor. In the late 1920s, Henrik Dam (1), working at the University of Copenhagen, designed a series of experiments to demonstrate the dietary essentialness of cholesterol. During the studies, he noted a hemorrhagic condition in chicks fed lipid-free diets. It was soon demonstrated that the addition of alfalfa meal or a lipid extract of alfalfa would prevent this condition, and continued study of this response led to the isolation, characterization, and synthesis of the active compound 2-Me-3-phytyl-1,4-naphthoquinone (phylloquinone) in the early 1930s. In Saint Louis, Missouri, Edward Doisy and his collaborators subsequently demonstrated (2) that in addition to phylloquinone in green plants, vitamin K activity was present in many bacteria as a series

of menaquinones, 2-Me-1,4-naphthoquinones substituted at the 3 position with an unsaturated polyisoprenoid chain (Fig. 16-1). In 1941, Dam and Doisy were awarded the Nobel Prize for their discovery of this fat-soluble vitamin.

At about the same time that vitamin K was discovered, Link discovered a naturally occurring antagonist of the vitamin (3). A hemorrhagic disease of cattle was prevalent in the American upper midwest and western Canada in the 1920s, and the cause of the disease was traced to the consumption of improperly cured sweet clover hay. Animals with "sweet clover disease" could be aided by transfusion with whole blood from healthy animals, and by the early 1930s it was established that the cause of the prolonged clotting times was a decrease in the prothrombin activity of blood (4). A number of investigators attempted to

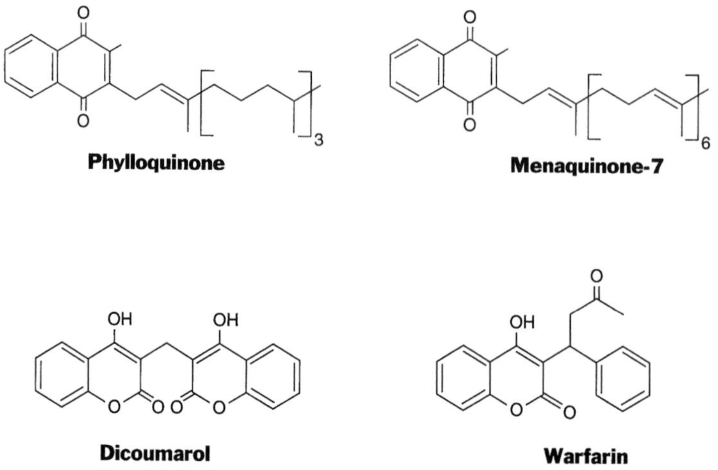

FIG. 16-1. Structures of compounds with vitamin K activity and vitamin K antagonists. Phylloquinone is the form of the vitamin found in green plants, and menaquinone-7 (MK-7) is an example of a series of unsaturated polyisoprenoid derivatives of 2-Me-1,4-naphthoquinones produced by anaerobic bacteria. Dicoumarol was the vitamin K antagonist isolated as a naturally occurring hemorrhagic agent, whereas warfarin is the 4-hydroxycoumarin anticoagulant most commonly used in North America.

isolate the compound in spoiled sweet clover which was responsible for this disease, but it was first isolated and characterized as 3-3′-methylbis-4-(hydroxycoumarin) by Link's group at the University of Wisconsin (4) and called dicumarol (Fig. 16-1).

BIOCHEMICAL ROLE OF VITAMIN K

The biochemical basis for antagonism of vitamin K action by the 4-hydroxycoumarins cannot be understood without reference to the metabolic role of vitamin K in clotting factor biosynthesis. The classical vitamin K–dependent plasma clotting factors, prothrombin, factor VII, factor IX, and factor X, were known to have many similar properties, including a Ca^{2+}-dependent interaction with negatively charged phospholipids. The basis for this interaction was clarified in the mid-1970s when Stenflo (5) and Nelsestuen (6) demonstrated that prothrombin contained a number of residues of a previously unidentified amino acid, γ-carboxyglutamic acid (Gla). This amino acid was missing or was present in decreased amounts in prothrombin isolated from patients or cattle treated with warfarin or other coumarin deriv-

atives. Vitamin K–dependent proteins present in plasma following warfarin treatment did not exhibit their normal Ca^{2+}-dependent phospholipid binding and lacked biological activity. Antagonism of the formation of Gla residues by warfarin was therefore identified as the basis for its anticoagulant action.

A rat liver microsomal activity that would fix $^{14}CO_2$ into glutamyl residues of endogenous precursor proteins to form ^{14}C-γ-carboxyglutamyl residues in the presence of vitamin K was described (7) soon after the presence of Gla residues in prothrombin was reported. This activity (Fig. 16-2) was soon shown to require O_2, the reduced form of vitamin K (vitamin KH_2) and CO_2. Early studies of the molecular action of vitamin K demonstrated that the vitamin was a cofactor utilized to labilize the hydrogen on the γ position of the glutamyl residue to allow CO_2 attack at this position. The mechanism of the carboxylation reaction (8) is now known to be coupled to the vitamin K epoxidase activity, which converts vitamin KH_2 to the 2,3-epoxide of the vitamin and is catalyzed by the same protein. The available data are consistent with the general reaction mechanism shown in Fig. 16-3.

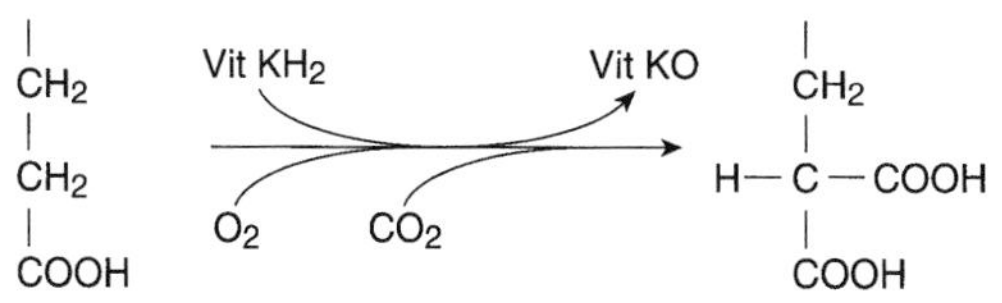

FIG. 16-2. The vitamin K–dependent carboxylase. The hepatic enzyme catalyzes the carboxylation of specific Glu residues in the "Gla" domain of prothrombin, factors VII, IX, and X, and
proteins C and S to Gla residues. The enzyme
requires O_2, and in the reaction the reduced form
of vitamin K (KH_2) is converted to the 2,3-epox-
ide of the vitamin (KO).

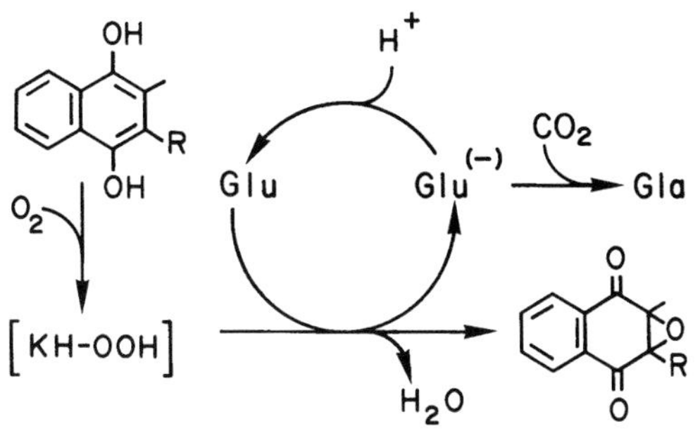

FIG. 16-3. Generalized mechanism of action of
the vitamin K–dependent carboxylase/epoxi-
dase system. The available data strongly support the vitamin K–dependent formation of a carbanion on the position of the Glu residue
followed by carboxylation in a step not involving
the vitamin. The chemical nature of the oxygenated intermediate (KH-OOH) has not been
definitely established, and the detailed mechanism by which hydrogen abstraction is linked to
epoxide formation cannot be determined from
the available data.

Details of the bioorganic mechanism by
which an oxygenated form of vitamin K
could be used to drive the carboxylation reaction is are speculative. Most investigators
have suggested that hydrogen removal from
the glutamyl residue occurs as the abstraction of a proton to leave a formal carbanion.
The enzyme has been demonstrated to catalyze a vitamin KH_2 and oxygen-dependent
exchange of ^3H from ^3H_2O into the γ position
of a substrate Glu residue, and this exchange
is decreased at HCO_3^- concentrations (9).
This suggests that the active intermediate
can partition between accepting CO_2 or a
proton. An understanding of the hydrogen
abstraction mechanism and proof of this hypothesis will, however, require a much
clearer understanding of the nature of the
presumed oxygenated intermediate and of
the mechanism by which hydrogen abstraction is coupled to epoxide formation. A recent chemical model (10) has suggested a
possible mechanism involving oxygen attack
leading to a dioxetane ring, which can generate a strongly basic alkoxide intermediate.
Direct biochemical evidence that demonstrates the presence of these intermediates is
lacking, but a great many indirect data are
consistent with this mechanism.

The vitamin K–dependent carboxylase has
now been purified (11), cloned, and expressed
(12) in various cell lines; and details of the association of this protein to the endoplasmic
reticulum and to its multiple substrates are being elucidated.

METABOLIC ACTION OF THE
4-HYDROXYCOUMARIN
ANTICOAGULANTS

As soon as the vitamin K–dependent carboxylase was discovered, it was revealed that
this enzyme was not particularly sensitive to
inhibition by these drugs. It was also shown
that the agonist/antagonist relationship seen
between vitamin K and warfarin in animal
studies did not hold in vitro and that inhibition of the carboxylase enzyme by warfarin
could not be reversed by high concentrations
of vitamin. The nature of the inhibition of
clotting factor synthesis by warfarin was only
apparent when the hepatic metabolism of vitamin K was better understood.

The coproduct of microsomal Gla formation is vitamin K epoxide, and microsomes
contain an efficient mechanism for recycling
this metabolite to the active substrate form of
the vitamin, vitamin KH_2. The microsomal-
associated activities that have been identified
as being involved in these metabolic inter-
conversions of the liver vitamin K pool are
shown in Fig. 16-4, and include a vitamin K
epoxide reductase and two or more vitamin K

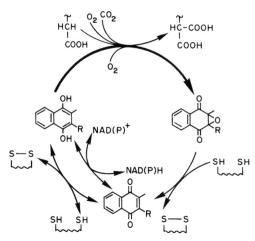

FIG. 16-4. Vitamin K metabolism in hepatic microsomes. In addition to the carboxylase/epoxidase system, liver microsomes contain a dithiol-linked vitamin K epoxide reductase and a dithiol-linked vitamin K quinone reductase. It is likely that these two dithiol-linked reductase activities, which are strongly inhibited by the 4-hydroxycoumarin anticoagulants, are catalyzed by the same enzyme or share a common subunit. The NAD(P)H linked quinone reductase activity may be catalyzed by more than one enzyme.

quinone reductases. The microsomal epoxide reductase requires a dithiol rather than a reduced pyridine nucleotide coenzyme for activity, and dithiothreitol is commonly used as a reductant in vitro. The physiologically relevant reductase for this enzyme system has not yet been identified with certainty. Elucidation of the mechanism of action of warfarin began with the demonstration that the 2,3-epoxide of vitamin K was a normal metabolite in rat liver and that the ratio of vitamin K epoxide to vitamin K was increased by warfarin administration (13,14). Inhibition of vitamin K epoxide reduction by warfarin increases the fraction of the vitamin present as the epoxide and decreases the amount of the enzymatically active reduced form to the extent that the action of the carboxylase is limited.

Acceptance of this theory was aided by observations utilizing a strain of wild rats resistant to the action of the common 4-hydroxycoumarin anticoagulants. It was demonstrated

that the vitamin K epoxide reductase preparation obtained from livers of the warfarin-resistant rats was relatively insensitive to inhibition by warfarin (15,16). These preparations were, however, strongly inhibited by a second 4-hydroxycoumarin, difenacoum, which had been developed as an effective rodenticide for control of the warfarin-resistant rat population. These data provided the final proof that the inhibition of epoxide reductase by warfarin was related to its anticoagulant action. The dithiol-dependent vitamin K quinone reductase (Fig. 16-4) has also been shown (17) to be warfarin-sensitive, and this activity, like that of the epoxide reductase, is less sensitive to warfarin when assayed in tissues of the warfarin-resistant rat (18,19). It is therefore likely that the effects of the 4-hydroxycoumarin anticoagulants involve not only the reduction of vitamin K epoxide to the quinone, but also the reduction of the quinone to the hydroquinone. The NADH-dependent quinone reductases are less sensitive to warfarin inhibition and constitute a pathway for vitamin K quinone reduction in the anticoagulant-treated animal. The presence of this pathway explains the ability of administered vitamin K to counteract the hemorrhagic condition resulting from a massive dose of warfarin (20).

The alteration of these two enzyme activities by what has been assumed to be a single mutation responsible for the development of warfarin resistance in the wild rat population raises some interesting questions in terms of the structural relationship of the proteins involved. However, many data support the theory that the same enzyme catalyzes both activities (21). Whether or not the two microsomal dithiol-dependent activities, vitamin K epoxide reductase and vitamin K quinone reductase, are catalyzed by the same or two active sites on the protein has been undecided because of difficulty in purifying this enzyme. A recent report (22) indicates that this has been accomplished, and the availability of this preparation will also help in clarifying the detailed mechanism of inhibition.

CONSEQUENCE OF WARFARIN ADMINISTRATION

The pharmacologic effect of warfarin administration is a decreased ability of the liver to effectively carry out the posttranslational conversion of glutamyl to γ-carboxyglutamyl residues during the intracellular processing of vitamin K–dependent proteins. In the human and cow, but not in the rat (23), this results in the secretion to the plasma of vitamin K–dependent proteins lacking all or a portion of the normal complement of Gla residues. The under-γ-carboxylated form of prothrombin has been most extensively studied, and this pool of prothrombin has sometimes been called "abnormal prothrombin," or PIVKA-II (Protein Induced by Vitamin K Absence, or Antagonism-II) where the II specifically identifies the protein as factor II, or prothrombin (24).

It is possible to fractionate the plasma abnormal prothrombin pool into fractions that contain from one to seven moles of Gla per mole of prothrombin (25). The rate of activation of these proteins to thrombin is dependent on the number of Gla residues in the molecule and is greatly decreased by the loss of as few as three Gla residues per mole. This response has been shown to be related to an increase in the apparent K_m for the binding of prothrombin to the rest of the "prothrombinase" complex and is a function of the Ca^{2+} and phospholipid binding properties of these proteins (26). The structure of the Gla domain of the vitamin K–dependent proteins has been determined (27), and the critical importance of some of the Gla residues to this structure can be seen. Studies of protein C mutants lacking specific Gla residues have confirmed the importance of specific sites (28). The relationship between the concentration of various partially γ-carboxylated proteins and alterations in the assays used to monitor warfarin therapy are not clear. However, it appears that failure of some under-γ-carboxylated species to bind to the protein–phospholipid complexes that are involved in the thrombotic cascade is important and that in some cases binding of nonfunctional but partially carboxylated species may prevent the binding of functional proteins to the activation complexes (29).

CLINICALLY USEFUL COUMARIN DERIVATIVES

Several coumarin derivatives have been developed for clinical use as oral anticoagulants. Of these, racemic warfarin has the most favorable pharmacologic profile and is essentially the only coumarin derivative prescribed in the United States. Acenocoumarol, phenprocoumon, and ticlomarol are widely used in Europe. Indanedione derivatives, including phenindione, diphenadione, and anisindione, are also prescribed in some parts of the world, although these drugs, particularly phenindione, produce more toxicity than warfarin and other coumarin derivatives. This chapter discusses the pharmacology and clinical use of warfarin, although most of the principles discussed are also applicable to other coumarin derivatives.

SOURCES OF VARIABILITY IN THE ANTICOAGULANT EFFECT OF WARFARIN

The magnitude of the anticoagulant effect produced by a given dose of warfarin varies by as much as 20-fold between individuals and may vary by several fold in an individual patient over time. Several factors, including warfarin's absorption and metabolism, the amount of vitamin K available to the liver, the synthetic capacity of the liver, and the rates of turnover of the vitamin K–dependent clotting factors, contribute to this variability. Differences in warfarin metabolism and vitamin K availability in particular are probably the most important factors that determine warfarin's anticoagulant effect. Determinants of warfarin's anticoagulant effect are summarized in Table 16-1.

Warfarin is efficiently absorbed from the small intestine, and malabsorption is rarely a cause of warfarin resistance, even in patients who have had most of their small bowel re-

TABLE 16-1. *Factors that modify the effect of coumarin derivatives*

Mechanism	Example	Expected effect on anticoagulant action
Reduced vitamin K intake	Reduced oral intake	Increased
Increased vitamin K intake	Vitamin supplementation; oral or parenteral hyperalimentation (100,101); consumption of foods with high vitamin K intake (102,103)	Decreased
Reduced vitamin K absorption	Biliary tract obstruction; fat malabsorption (34)	Increased
Reduced vitamin K production in gut	Antibiotics	Increased, particularly if reduced oral vitamin K intake
Binding of warfarin in gut	Cholestyramine	Decreased
Displacement of warfarin from plasma albumin	Aspirin, anionic drugs	Minimal (increased clearance balances increased free warfarin)
Induction of hepatic P450, increased warfarin metabolism	Many drugs, alcohol (chronic use)	Decreased
Stereoselective inhibition of R-warfarin clearance	Several drugs	Increased
Stereoselective inhibition of S-warfarin clearance	Cimetidine, omeprazole	Increased
Non-stereo-selective inhibition of warfarin clearance	Amiodarone	Increased
Interference with vitamin K cycle by warfarin-like effect	Second- and third-generation cephalosporins	Increased
Unknown (reduced affinity of warfarin receptor?)	Hereditary resistance to warfarin	Decreased (marked)
Reduced hepatic synthesis of coagulation proteins	Liver disease; alcohol (acute intoxication)	Increased
Increased catabolism of coagulation proteins or vitamin K (?)	Hypermetabolic states (hyperthyroidism) (36)	Increased
Decreased catabolism of coagulation proteins or vitamin K (?)	Hypometabolic states (hypothyroidism) (104)	Decreased
Coexisting hemostatic defect	Concomitant administration of anticoagulant/antiplatelet drugs (105)	Increased

moved (30). An exception to this rule occurs in patients taking cholestyramine, which binds warfarin in the gut and inhibits its absorption. Warfarin is highly protein-bound, mainly to serum albumin. Drugs that displace it from albumin increase its bioavailability, but this effect is balanced by an increase in warfarin metabolism and so has little influence on its anticoagulant effect (31). Warfarin is metabolized by the cytochrome P450 system in the liver, and so its effect is modified by drugs that inhibit or stimulate this system. Drug effects on warfarin anticoagulant activity are summarized in Table 16-2. Alcohol may either promote warfarin's effect by inhibiting hepatic synthesis of coagulation proteins or (when consumed chronically) inhibit warfarin's effect by stimulating its metabolism. However, consumption of moderate amounts of alcohol has little impact on warfarin's anticoagulant effect unless there is concomitant liver disease (32,33).

Changes in vitamin K intake have a major influence on warfarin's anticoagulant effect. Diminished vitamin K absorption due to fat malabsorption (34) or dietary deficiency amplifies the effect of warfarin, whereas increased vitamin K intake has the opposite effect. Alteration in menaquinone (vitamin K_2) production by enteric bacteria (as a consequence of antibiotic use, for example) does not seem to play a major role in determining warfarin's effect unless there is a concomitant lack of dietary vitamin K (35). Consumption of foods with high vitamin K con-

TABLE 16-2. *Warfarin–drug interactions (30,33,48,55)*

Drugs that may potentiate warfarin

Alcohol (with coexistent liver disease)
Allopurinol
Amiodarone
Aminoglycoside antibiotics
Ampicillin
Anabolic steroids
Aspirin (high doses)
Azathioprine
Cephalosporin antibiotics
Clofibrate
Chloral hydrate
Chloramphenicol
Chlorpromazine
Chlorpropamide and other oral hypoglycemics
Cimetidine
Ciprofloxacin and other fluoroquinolones
Disulfiram
Erythromycin
Ethacrynic acid
Fluconazole
Glucagon
Heparin
Indomethacin
Influenza vaccines
Isoniazide
Ketoconazole
Metronidazole and related antifungals
Methotrexate
Monoamine oxidase inhibitors
Omeprazole
Penicillin (high doses)
Phenylbutazone
Phenytoin
Piroxicam
Propafenone
Propranolol
Quinidine
Ranitidine
Simvastatin
Sulfinpyrazone
Tamoxifen
Thyroxine
Trimethoprim-sulfisoxazole

Drugs that may counteract warfarin

Barbiturates
Carbamazepine
Chlordiazepoxide
Cholestyramine
Griseofulvin
Diuretics
Dicloxacillin
Lipid emulsion (intravenous)
Nafcillin
Rifampin
Sucralfate
Sulfinpyrazone (with prolonged treatment)
Vitamin K (vitamin supplements, enteral feeds, avocado and other vitamin K–rich foods)

Drugs in boldface are those for which interactions are considered definite, highly probable, or probable (33).

tent (e.g., a diet rich in leafy green vegetables) tends to counteract the effect of warfarin, as does administration of an oral or parenteral nutritional supplement containing vitamin K.

If the synthesis of clotting factors by the liver is diminished by liver disease the anticoagulant effect of warfarin is magnified. Conditions that result in accelerated turnover of vitamin K–dependent clotting factors (e.g., hyperthyroidism) also enhance warfarin's effect (36). The bleeding risk caused by warfarin-induced clotting deficiency is increased if there is an additional hemostatic defect, such as that caused by another anticoagulant (e.g., heparin) or an antiplatelet drug such as aspirin, ticlopidine, or clopidogrel.

Hereditary warfarin resistance is a rare condition in which very high doses (5 to 20 times normal) and plasma levels of warfarin are required to achieve an anticoagulant effect. This condition seems to be inherited in a dominant fashion. Its biochemical basis is unknown but has been postulated to be due to a reduced affinity of the vitamin K epoxide reductase. It can be distinguished from warfarin resistance due to noncompliance or malabsorption by the finding of a disparity between warfarin plasma level and its anticoagulant effect (37–39).

Patients taking warfarin should be counseled to consult their physician or pharmacist before taking any new medication or radically changing their diet. They should not attempt to restrict vitamin K intake in the mistaken belief that this will enhance the effectiveness of warfarin but should be made aware of the vitamin K content of various foods so that they maintain a reasonably constant intake of the vitamin.

Sensitivity to warfarin is greater in older patients for unknown reasons (40,41). Because older patients are also more likely to have other conditions that predispose to bleeding and because the morbidity associated with bleeding may be greater in older patients, particular care must be exercised when initiating warfarin therapy in this population and a relatively low starting dose is appropriate.

RELATIONSHIP BETWEEN THE CLINICAL ANTICOAGULANT EFFECT OF WARFARIN AND CLOTTING FACTOR LEVELS

Warfarin administration causes plasma levels of four procoagulants—factors II (prothrombin), VII, IX, and X—and two anticoagulants—proteins C and S—to decline. In animals, protection against thrombosis by warfarin correlates best with decreased concentrations of factors II and X (42). In plasma from warfarin-treated patients, in vitro thrombin generation shows a linear relationship to the factor II concentration but is unaffected by decreases in concentrations of factors X, IX, and VII until levels of these factors fall below 30%, 20%, and 5% of normal, respectively (43). Studies in human patients suggest that the clinical effects of warfarin correlate better with the plasma factor II concentration than with more global indicators of procoagulant levels such as the prothrombin time (44–46).

INITIATION OF WARFARIN THERAPY

The goal of warfarin treatment is gradual reduction of the plasma levels of the vitamin K–dependent procoagulant proteins, typically to steady state levels 20% to 30% of normal. As noted above, reductions in the plasma levels of factors II and X make the greatest contributions to the clinical anticoagulant effect of warfarin. Because these factors normally have plasma half-lives of 1–2 days, it will usually take at least 4 to 5 days to achieve the desired reductions in their plasma levels. In contrast, factor VII, which is less important in terms of the clinical anticoagulant activity of warfarin but makes an important contribution to the effect of warfarin on the prothrombin time, and protein C, which is a major physiologic anticoagulant, both have plasma half-lives of 12 hours or less. The practice of initiating warfarin therapy with a high loading dose may therefore be counterproductive, prolonging the prothrombin time and diminishing plasma anti-

coagulant activity more than it reduces physiologically important procoagulant protein levels. A randomized trial comparing 5- and 10-mg loading doses of warfarin found that factor VII and protein C levels did indeed drop faster in the group receiving 10 mg of warfarin, whereas there was no difference between the two groups in the rate at which plasma levels of factor II dropped. Excessive anticoagulation requiring vitamin K administration was more likely in patients receiving a 10-mg loading dose (47).

Warfarin therapy should therefore usually be initiated with a dose equal to the estimated maintenance dose. The mean dose needed to maintain an International Normalized Ratio (INR; see below) of 2 to 3 in a large group of anticoagulated patients was found to be approximately 5 mg per day (48), so this is a reasonable starting dose in the absence of any factors known to increase or decrease susceptibility to warfarin (Table 16-1).

In patients receiving heparin, an overlap period of at least 4 to 5 days during which both drugs are given is necessary to ensure that adequate reductions in factor II and X levels have been achieved. Prolongation of the prothrombin time or INR early in the course of warfarin therapy is not a reliable indication that an anticoagulant effect exists because it is likely to be due mainly to decreased plasma factor VII activity (47,49,50).

MONITORING WARFARIN THERAPY

The prothrombin time (PT) is the method most often used to monitor the anticoagulant effect of warfarin. Warfarin-induced depression of plasma levels of factors II, VII, and X causes prolongation of the PT. Immediately after beginning warfarin therapy or increasing the dose of warfarin, prolongation of the PT is primarily due to a decline in factor VII activity because of that factor's short plasma half-life (49,50). The PT does not accurately reflect the antithrombotic effect of warfarin until plasma concentrations of factors II and X approach their new steady state levels, about 4 to 5 days later.

The PT is the clotting time of a mixture of citrate-anticoagulated plasma, calcium, and thromboplastin; thromboplastin is a mixture of phospholipid and tissue factor or tissue factor–containing tissue extract. Commercial thromboplastin reagents vary widely in their compositions and functional characteristics. Some contain extracts of animal tissue (e.g., rabbit brain), some are derived from human tissue (e.g., placenta), and some contain recombinant human tissue factor. Some reagents are much more sensitive than others to the effects of depressed levels of various clotting factors (51). Therefore, plasma from a warfarin-treated patient may yield very different PTs when tested with different thromboplastins. These differences in prothrombin time values may result in variability in the dosing of warfarin (52). To overcome this problem a calibration system was devised. The International Normalized Ratio (INR) is a standardized method for reporting prothrombin time results that is designed to minimize this variability (53).

The International Sensitivity Index (ISI) is a variable that allows interconversion of PT ratios (patient PT/mean normal PT) obtained with different thromboplastins (54). The ISI is derived by comparing PT ratios obtained with a particular thromboplastin to those obtained with a reference standard. The INR is a function of the PT ratio and the ISI, according to the following formula:

$$(PT\ ratio)^{ISI} = INR$$

The ISI is affected by the composition of the thromboplastin and, to a lesser extent, by the method and instrumentation used to measure the PT. The ISI varies from approximately 1.0 to 3.0 or higher. It would be more accurately termed an "insensitivity index" because a higher ISI indicates lower sensitivity to changes in clotting factor concentrations. Because the ISI magnifies any errors or variability in the PT measurement, the precision of the INR is also inversely proportional to the ISI (53,55). It is important to realize that INR values obtained from a given plasma sample using different thromboplastins sometimes differ significantly (56,57) (Fig. 16-5). Imprecision and variability in the INR can be minimized by using more sensitive thromboplastins (i.e., those with relatively low ISI values) and by using an ISI value specific to both the thromboplastin and the instrument used to perform the PT (58).

Alternatives to the PT may be useful for monitoring warfarin therapy in some circumstances. For example, the PT does not accurately reflect the effect of warfarin in the pres-

PATIENT #	REAGENT E (ISI 2.98) INR	REAGENT B (ISI 0.96) INR
1	3.4	2.7
2	2.8	2.5
3	3.5	2.3
4	2.6	2
5	2.2	1.2
6	2.3	2.4
7	1.9	1.7
8	3	2.8
9	2.2	2.7
10	4	4

FIG. 16-5. International Normalized Ratio (INR) values obtained by testing identical plasma samples from ten randomly selected patients on stable warfarin therapy, using two thromboplastin reagents with different International Sensitivity Index (ISI) values. Reagent E is derived from rabbit brain and reagent B contains recombinant human tissue factor. (Data courtesy of Sue Hoffman, M.T., A.S.C.P.)

ence of an interfering substance such as a lupus anticoagulant (59), an antibody to bovine thrombin (60), or a high concentration of heparin. The antithrombotic effect of warfarin is most closely related to the degree to which it depresses the plasma factor II (prothrombin) level (42,43). Two randomized trials have shown that in warfarin-treated patients monitoring therapy by measurement of the plasma native (fully γ-carboxylated) prothrombin antigen leads to more accurate prediction of clinical outcome and a lower complication rate than does monitoring the PT (45,46). The native prothrombin antigen assay is not widely available, however. As an alternative, a more readily available test such as measurement of plasma prothrombin activity by a standard one-stage assay may be useful in selected problem cases. A prothrombin activity in the range of 20% to 25% of normal represents a level of anticoagulation considered adequate for the secondary prevention of venous thromboembolism.

Warfarin exerts an anticoagulant effect even at low doses that have little effect on the PT (61,62). Such very-low-intensity or "minidose" warfarin therapy reduces intravascular thrombin formation (as shown by a reduction in the plasma level of the prothrombin activation peptide fragment 1.2) in patients with thrombotic disorders (61,63). Administration of 1 mg per day warfarin to a group of normal subjects did not cause a significant change in the PT, factor VII activity, factor II activity, or F1.2 level but did cause significant increases in plasma levels of undercarboxylated prothrombin and osteocalcin, particularly in older subjects (64). Minidose warfarin has had mixed success as a thromboprophylactic agent in clinical trials. It has been effective in reducing the incidence of central venous catheter-associated thrombosis (65) and the incidence of deep venous thrombosis in patients undergoing major gynecologic surgery (66), but ineffective in high-risk patients such as those undergoing joint replacement (67,68). While the precise role of very-low-intensity warfarin therapy in the management of thrombotic disorders remains

to be determined, it seems possible that such a role does exist. Whether the F1.2 assay or another sensitive indicator of coagulation system activation will be clinically useful for monitoring very-low-intensity warfarin therapy is a subject that deserves additional study.

COMPLICATIONS OF WARFARIN THERAPY AND THEIR MANAGEMENT

Bleeding

Bleeding is the most common complication of anticoagulant therapy. In patients taking warfarin the bleeding risk is directly related to the INR (69,70) (Fig. 16-6). Most bleeding episodes that occur in the presence of a therapeutic INR (< 4.0) are associated with an anatomic lesion (peptic ulcer, gastrointestinal neoplasm, etc.) (71,72). Other important risk factors for bleeding are concomitant aspirin (or other antiplatelet drug, e.g., ticlopidine) use, the presence of comorbid disease (particularly if there is an associated hemostatic defect such as in liver or kidney failure), and a history of prior bleeding (particularly gastrointestinal bleeding) or stroke (70,73–75). Older patients are at increased risk of bleeding. Most of this increase can be attributed to the higher prevalence of other risk factors for

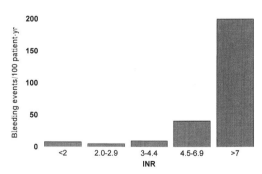

FIG. 16-6. Risk of bleeding according to level of anticoagulation (expressed as the International Normalized Ratio or INR) in a prospective study of 2,745 patients taking warfarin or acenocoumarol who were treated in 1 of 34 anticoagulation clinics. (From Palareti et al., ref. 70, with permission.)

bleeding in older people; old age *per se* does not seem to increase bleeding risk (76,77).

Reversal of Warfarin Anticoagulation

It usually takes 4 to 5 days for the INR of a stably anticoagulated patient to drop from within the therapeutic range (2.0 to 3.0) to < 1.2 if warfarin is withheld (78). If more rapid reversal is necessary, vitamin K should be administered; this often results in correction of the INR within 12 to 24 hours. If the effect of warfarin must be reversed as quickly as possible, as in the case of life-threatening bleeding (e.g., intracranial bleeding or major gastrointestinal hemorrhage), fresh frozen plasma or prothrombin complex concentrate should be infused in addition to vitamin K (79). It should be kept in mind that if high doses of vitamin K are administered, reestablishment of adequate levels of anticoagulation with a vitamin K antagonist may take days to weeks longer than usual. Recommendations for reversal of warfarin anticoagulation are shown in Table 16-3.

There is evidence that a rebound phenomenon, with a transient increase in thrombin generation, occurs when warfarin therapy is abruptly discontinued (80–82). The increase in thrombin formation can be detected by sensitive measurements such as the plasma F1.2 peptide or fibrinopeptide level; its magnitude is usually small and it lasts a few days to a week after withdrawal of oral anticoagulation. The clinical significance of this phenomenon is unclear and probably minimal in most cases.

Skin Necrosis

Skin necrosis is a rare complication of warfarin therapy (83). It typically begins within a few days of initiation of warfarin therapy and most commonly involves the skin over the thigh, abdominal wall, female breast, and penis (84). The lesions initially may resemble ecchymoses but quickly develop hemorrhagic bullae and other evidence of necrosis (85) (Fig. 16-7). Skin grafting or amputation is often necessary. There is usually evidence of microvascular injury, with fibrin deposition in the venules and small veins, in the skin and subcutaneous tissue; the pathologic findings are similar to those found in infants with homozygous protein C deficiency. Affected patients usually have an underlying defect in the protein C anticoagulant pathway, most commonly inherited partial protein C deficiency (83,86,87). Warfarin administration causes a rapid decline in plasma protein C activity (due to that protein's short half-life), leading to transient imbalance between plasma procoagulant and anticoagulant activity (49,50). This imbalance is particularly severe in individuals with underlying protein C deficiency,

TABLE 16-3. *Reversal of warfarin anticoagulation*

INR	Action
< 6.0, no bleeding	Withhold warfarin until INR therapeutic, restart at lower dose
< 6.0, rapid reversal desired for elective surgery, etc.	Vitamin K, 1–2 mg s.c.
6.0–10.0, or if patient has significant bleeding	Vitamin K, 1–2 mg s.c. (give additional 0.5–1.0 mg if INR still supratherapeutic at 24 hr)
10.0–20.0	Vitamin K, 3 mg s.c. or slow IV infusion, recheck INR q 6 hr and repeat dose as needed
>20.0	Vitamin K, 10 mg s.c. or slow IV infusion; repeat q 6–12 hr as needed. Consider giving fresh frozen plasma or, if patient is bleeding, prothrombin complex concentrate.

Adapted from Hirsh et al., ref. 79, with permission.
Note: In the presence of potentially life-threatening bleeding (e.g., major gastrointestinal bleeding or intracranial bleeding), fresh frozen plasma or prothrombin complex concentrate should be administered in addition to vitamin K.
INR, International Normalized Ratio.

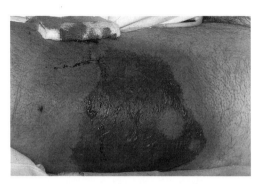

FIG. 16-7. Warfarin-induced skin necrosis. The patient developed painful ecchymoses on the thigh and abdomen on the twelfth day of warfarin therapy for deep venous thrombosis. He was subsequently found to have heterozygous protein C deficiency and heterozygous activated protein C deficiency. (Description adapted from Conlan et al., ref. 85, with permission.)

which probably accounts for the preponderance of such patients among those with skin necrosis. There are reports of defibrination (88) and hemorrhagic infarction of the adrenal glands (85) following initiation of warfarin therapy in protein C–deficient patients; these complications probably have a similar pathophysiologic basis.

Warfarin-induced skin necrosis is usually treated by discontinuation of warfarin and administration of vitamin K and/or fresh frozen plasma. Protein C concentrate should in theory be an effective treatment, but clinical experience with this treatment is limited (89). Heparin administration may be beneficial, although skin necrosis often occurs despite concurrent heparin therapy. A history of warfarin-induced skin necrosis is not an absolute contraindication to further warfarin administration; patients with such a history have been successfully anticoagulated by initiating therapy with a very low dose of warfarin and increasing the dose in small increments until the desired level of anticoagulation (INR level) was achieved (85). Concomitant administration of protein C concentrate until a stable anticoagulant effect is achieved may also be of benefit (89). Avoidance of high loading doses

of warfarin should help prevent this rare complication of warfarin therapy.

Cholesterol Embolism

Warfarin may inhibit thrombus formation on a ruptured atheromatous arterial plaque, thereby allowing the contents of the plaque to embolize. Cholesterol embolism can cause gangrene of fingers or toes, livedo reticularis, renal failure, intestinal infarction, and a variety of other ischemic complications (90–92). Blood eosinophilia and complement consumption may occur, and some cases closely resemble inflammatory vasculitis. Discontinuation of anticoagulant therapy may help some patients, but reported mortality rates are high (60% to 80%) (92).

Use in Cancer

Patients with cancer may have an anomalous response to warfarin. Administration of warfarin causes a significant increase in fibrin degradation product levels (in the absence of disseminated intravascular coagulation or clinically evident thrombosis) in patients with carcinoma (93). Some patients with cancer and thrombosis (Trousseau's syndrome) treated with warfarin develop recurrent superficial or deep venous thrombosis, skin necrosis (94), and, in extreme cases, severe defibrination and widespread arterial and venous thrombosis resembling purpura fulminans (95). Such patients require long-term anticoagulation with heparin or heparin derivatives.

Use in Pregnancy

Warfarin and its congeners are teratogenic. Administration of coumarin derivatives during the first trimester of pregnancy causes a characteristic embryopathy consisting of nasal hypoplasia and epiphyseal stippling, whereas fetuses exposed to warfarin during the second and third trimester have developed central nervous system and eye disorders (96). Therefore, whenever possible administration of coumarin derivatives should be avoided during pregnancy; heparin and its derivatives (low molecular weight heparins or heparinoids) are preferred alternatives.

Other Complications

An association has been reported between long-term warfarin use and decreased bone mineral density (97); however, this association has not been substantiated in other studies. At present there is very little evidence that long-term warfarin use results in clinically significant bone disease. Rare complications of chronic warfarin administration include alopecia (98) and ectopic calcification of the tracheobronchial tree (99).

CONCLUSION

Vitamin K is required as a substrate for a liver microsomal enzyme that carboxylates specific glutamyl residues in a limited number of proteins to γ-carboxyglutamyl residues. These proteins include prothrombin, factors VII, IX, and X, and proteins C and S. Without this posttranslational modification, the proteins lack biological activity. The coproduct of this carboxylation reaction is an epoxide of the vitamin which is normally recycled to the active form of the vitamin by a microsomal vitamin K epoxide reductase. Warfarin and other 4-hydroxycoumarins block this reaction, and the induced vitamin K deficiency results in decreased activity of these proteins and a prolonged prothrombin time.

The anticoagulant effect of warfarin varies among individuals and over time in a given individual due to differences in drug absorption and metabolism, interactions with other drugs, and varying availability of vitamin K. Warfarin therapy must therefore be monitored carefully. The prothrombin time is the most clinically useful method for monitoring warfarin therapy and is most accurate when performed with a sensitive thromboplastin reagent and expressed as the International Normalized Ratio (INR). Warfarin therapy

should be initiated at a dose no greater than the estimated maintenance dose for that patient; use of a higher loading dose is not recommended. When converting a patient from heparin to warfarin anticoagulation, the two drugs should overlap for at least 4 to 5 days to ensure that an adequate anticoagulant effect has been attained.

Bleeding is the major risk of warfarin therapy and is directly related to the INR. In the absence of an anatomic lesion, serious bleeding is unusual unless the INR is well above 4.0. Most cases of warfarin overdose can safely be managed by withholding warfarin until the INR falls within the desired range. Patients with severe warfarin overdose and/or major bleeding should be given vitamin K and/or fresh frozen plasma. Skin necrosis is a rare, but potentially serious, complication of warfarin therapy that occurs primarily in individuals with protein C deficiency.

REFERENCES

1. Dam H. Vitamin K, its chemistry and physiology. *Adv Enzymol* 1942;2:285–324.
2. Doisy EA, Binkley SB, Thayer SA. Vitamin K. *Chem Rev* 1941;28:477–517.
3. Link KP. The discovery of dicumarol and its sequels. *Circulation* 1997;19:97–107.
4. Owen CA, Bowie EWJ. The history of the development of oral anticoagulant drugs. In: Poller L, Hirsch J (eds). *Oral Anticoagulants.* London: Arnold, 1996;1–8.
5. Stenflo J, Ferlund P, Egan W, Roepstorff P. Vitamin K dependent modifications of glutamic acid residues in prothrombin. *Proc Natl Acad Sci USA* 1974;71:2730–2733.
6. Nelsestuen GL, Zytkovicz TH, Howard JB. The mode of action of vitamin K. Identification of gamma-carboxyglutamic acid as a component of prothrombin. *J Biol Chem* 1974;249:6347–6350.
7. Esmon CT, Sadowski JA, Suttie JW. A new carboxylation reaction. The vitamin K–dependent incorporation of H-14-CO_3^- into prothrombin. *J Biol Chem* 1975; 250:4744–4748.
8. Suttie JW. Synthesis of vitamin K–dependent proteins. *FASEB J* 1993;7:445–452.
9. McTigue JJ, Suttie JW. vitamin K–dependent carboxylase. Demonstration of a vitamin K- and O_2-dependent exchange of 3H from $3H_2O$ into glutamic acid residues. *J Biol Chem* 1983;258:12129–12131.
10. Dowd P, Ham SW, Naganathan S, Hershline R. The mechanism of action of vitamin K. *Annu Rev Nutr* 1995;15:419–440.
11. Wu SM, Morris DP, Stafford DW. Identification and purification to near homogeneity of the vitamin K–dependent carboxylase. *Proc Natl Acad Sci USA* 1991; 88:2236–2240.

12. Wu SM, Cheung WF, Frazier D, Stafford DW. Cloning and expression of the cDNA for human gamma-glutamyl carboxylase. *Science* 1991;254:1634–1636.
13. Bell RG, Matschiner JT. Warfarin and the inhibition of vitamin K activity by an oxide metabolite. *Nature* 1972;237:32–33.
14. Matschiner JT, Bell RG, Amelotti JM, Knauer TE. Isolation and characterization of a new metabolite of phylloquinone in the rat. *Biochim Biophys Acta* 1970; 201:309–315.
15. Zimmermann A, Matschiner JT. Biochemical basis of hereditary resistance to warfarin in the rat. *Biochem Pharmacol* 1974;23:1033–1040.
16. Whitlon DS, Sadowski JA, Suttie JW. Mechanism of coumarin action: significance of vitamin K epoxide reductase inhibition. *Biochemistry* 1978;17:1371–1377.
17. Fasco MJ, Principe LM. R- and S-Warfarin inhibition of vitamin K and vitamin K 2,3-epoxide reductase activities in the rat. *J Biol Chem* 1982;257:4894–4901.
18. Fasco MJ, Hildebrandt EF, Suttie JW. Evidence that warfarin anticoagulant action involves two distinct reductase activities. *J Biol Chem* 1982;257:11210–11212.
19. Hildebrandt EF, Suttie JW. Mechanism of coumarin action: sensitivity of vitamin K metabolizing enzymes of normal and warfarin-resistant rat liver. *Biochemistry* 1982;21:2406–2411.
20. Wallin R, Patrick SD, Martin LF. Vitamin K1 reduction in human liver. Location of the coumarin-drug-insensitive enzyme. *Biochem J* 1989;260:879–884.
21. Gardill SL, Suttie JW. Vitamin K epoxide and quinone reductase activities. Evidence for reduction by a common enzyme. *Biochem Pharmacol* 1990;40:1055–1061.
22. Wallin R, Guenthner TM. Purification of warfarin sensitive vitamin K epoxide reductase. *Meth Enzymol* 1997;282:395–408.
23. Shah DV, Swanson JC, Suttie JW. Abnormal prothrombin in the vitamin K-deficient rat. *Thromb Res* 1984; 35:451–458.
24. Hemker HC, Veltkamp JJ, Loeliger EA. Kinetic aspects of the interaction of blood clotting enzymes. 3. Demonstration of an inhibitor of prothrombin conversion in vitamin K deficiency. *Thrombosis et Diathesis Haemorrhagica* 1968;19:346–363.
25. Malhotra OP. Dicoumarol-induced prothrombins. *Ann NY Acad Sci* 1981;370:426–437.
26. Malhotra OP, Nesheim ME, Mann KG. The kinetics of activation of normal and gamma-carboxyglutamic acid-deficient prothrombins. *J Biol Chem* 1985;260: 279–287.
27. Soriano-Garcia M, Padmanabhan K, de Vos AM, Tulinsky A. The Ca^{2-} ion and membrane binding structure of the Gla domain of Ca-prothrombin fragment 1. *Biochemistry* 1992;31:2554–2566.
28. Zhang L, Castellino FJ. The contributions of individual gamma-carboxyglutamic acid residues in the calcium-dependent binding of recombinant human protein C to acidic phospholipid vesicles. *J Biol Chem* 1993;268: 12040–12045.
29. Sadowski JA, Booth SL, Mann KG, Malhotra OP, Bovill EG. Structure and mechanism of activation of vitamin K antagonists. In: Poller L, Hirsch, J (eds). *Oral Anticoagulants.* London, Arnold; 1996:9–29.
30. Owens JP, Mirtallo JM, Murphy CC. Oral anticoagulation in patients with short-bowel syndrome. *DICP* 1990;24:585–589.
31. Yacobi A, Udall JA, Levy G. Intrasubject variation of warfarin binding to protein in serum of patients with cardiovascular disease. *Clin Pharmacol Ther* 1976;20: 300–303.
32. Sellers EM, Holloway MR. Drug kinetics and alcohol ingestion. *Clin Pharmacokinet* 1978;3:440–452.
33. Wells PS, Holbrook AM, Crowther NR, Hirsh J. Interactions of warfarin with drugs and food. *Ann Intern Med* 1994;121:676–683.
34. Talstad I, Gamst ON. Warfarin resistance due to malabsorption. *J Intern Med* 1994;236:465–467.
35. O'Reilly RA. Warfarin metabolism and drug-drug interactions. *Adv Exp Med Biol* 1987;214:205–212.
36. Kellett HA, Sawers JS, Boulton FE, Cholerton S, Park BK, Toft AD. Problems of anticoagulation with warfarin in hyperthyroidism. *Q J Med* 1986;58:43–51.
37. Alving BM, Strickler MP, Knight RD, Barr CF, Berenberg JL, Peck CC. Hereditary warfarin resistance. Investigation of a rare phenomenon. *Arch Intern Med* 1985;145:499–501.
38. Diab F, Feffer S. Hereditary warfarin resistance. *South Med J* 1994;87:407–409.
39. Hallak HO, Wedlund PJ, Modi MW, et aL. High clearance of (S)-warfarin in a warfarin-resistant subject. *Br J Clin Pharmacol* 1993;35:327–330.
40. Shepherd AM, Hewick DS, Moreland TA, Stevenson IH. Age as a determinant of sensitivity to warfarin. *Br J Clin Pharmacol* 1977;4:315–320.
41. Gurwitz JH, Avorn J, Ross-Degnan D, Choodnovskiy I, Ansell J. Aging and the anticoagulant response to warfarin therapy. *Ann Intern Med* 1992;116:901–904.
42. Zivelin A, Rao LV, Rapaport SI. Mechanism of the anticoagulant effect of warfarin as evaluated in rabbits by selective depression of individual procoagulant vitamin K–dependent clotting factors. *J Clin Invest* 1993; 92:2131–2140.
43. Xi M, Beguin S, Hemker HC. The relative importance of the factors II, VII, IX and X for the prothrombinase activity in plasma of orally anticoagulated patients. *Thromb Haemost* 1989;62:788–791.
44. Furie B, Liebman HA, Blanchard RA, Coleman MS, Kruger SF, Furie BC. Comparison of the native prothrombin antigen and the prothrombin time for monitoring oral anticoagulant therapy. *Blood* 1984;64: 445–451.
45. Furie B, Diuguid CF, Jacobs M, Diuguid DL, Furie BC. Randomized prospective trial comparing native prothrombin antigen with the prothrombin time for monitoring oral anticoagulant therapy. *Blood* 1990; 75:344–349.
46. Kornberg A, Francis CW, Pellegrini VD Jr, Gabriel KR, Marder VJ. Comparison of native prothrombin antigen with the prothrombin time for monitoring oral anticoagulant prophylaxis. *Circulation* 1993;88:454–460.
47. Harrison L, Johnston M, Massicotte MP, Crowther M, Moffat K, Hirsch J. Comparison of 5-mg and 10-mg loading doses in initiation of warfarin therapy. *Ann Intern Med* 1997;126:133–136.
48. James AH, Britt RP, Raskino CL, Thompson SG. Factors affecting the maintenance dose of warfarin. *J Clin Pathol* 1992;45:704–706.
49. Weiss P, Soff GA, Halkin H, Seligsohn U. Decline of proteins C and S and factors II, VII, IX and X during the initiation of warfarin therapy. *Thromb Res* 1987; 45:783–790.

50. Vigano S, Mannucci PM, Solinas S, Bottasso B, Mariani G. Decrease in protein C antigen and formation of an abnormal protein soon after starting oral anticoagulant therapy. Br J Haematol 1984;57:213–220.

51. Zucker S, Cathey MH, Sox PJ, Hall EC. Standardization of laboratory tests for controlling anticoagulent therapy. Am J Clin Pathol 1970;53:348–354.

52. Bussey HI, Force RW, Bianco TM, Leonard AD. Reliance on prothrombin time ratios causes significant errors in anticoagulation therapy. Arch Intern Med 1992;152:278–282.

53. Loeliger EA, van den Besselaar AM, Lewis SM. Reliability and clinical impact of the normalization of the prothrombin times in oral anticoagulant control. Thromb Haemost 1985;53:148–154.

54. Poller L. A simple nomogram for the derivation of international normalised ratios for the standardisation of prothrombin times. Thromb Haemost 1988;60:18–20.

55. Taberner DA, Poller L, Thomson JM, Darby KV. Effect of international sensitivity index (ISI) of thromboplastins on precision of international normalised ratios (INR). J Clin Pathol 1989;42:92–96.

56. Le DT, Weibert RT, Sevilla BK, Donnelly KJ, Rapaport SI. The international normalized ratio (INR) for monitoring warfarin therapy: reliability and relation to other monitoring methods. Ann Intern Med 1994; 120:552–558.

57. Ng VL, Levin J, Corash L, Gottfried EL. Failure of the International Normalized Ratio to generate consistent results within a local medical community. Am J Clin Pathol 1993;99:689–694.

58. Hirsh J, Poller L. The international normalized ratio. A guide to understanding and correcting its problems. Arch Intern Med 1994;154:282–288.

59. Rapaport SI, Le DT. Thrombosis in the antiphospholipid-antibody syndrome. N Engl J Med 1995;333:665.

60. Ortel TL, Charles LA, Keller FG, et al. Topical thrombin and acquired coagulation factor inhibitors: clinical spectrum and laboratory diagnosis. Am J Hematol 1994;45:128–135.

61. Bauer KA, Rosenberg RD. The pathophysiology of the prethrombotic state in humans: insights gained from studies using markers of hemostatic system activation. Blood 1987;70:343–350.

62. Holm J, Berntorp E, Carlsson R, Erhardt L. Low-dose warfarin decreases coagulability without affecting prothrombin complex activity. J Intern Med 1993;234: 303–308.

63. Millenson MM, Bauer KA, Kistler JP, Barzegar S, Tulin L, Rosenberg RD. Monitoring "mini-intensity" anticoagulation with warfarin: comparison of the prothrombin time using a sensitive thromboplastin with prothrombin fragment F1-2 levels. Blood 1992;79:2034–2038.

64. Bach AU, Anderson SA, Foley AL, Williams EC, Suttie JW. Assessment of vitamin K status in human subjects administered "minidose" warfarin 1-3. Am J Clin Nutr 1996;64:894–902.

65. Bern MM, Lokich JJ, Wallach SR, et al. Very low doses of warfarin can prevent thrombosis in central venous catheters. A randomized prospective trial. Ann Intern Med 1990;112:423–428.

66. Poller L, McKernan A, Thomson JM, Elstein M, Hirsch PJ, Jones JB. Fixed minidose warfarin: a new approach to prophylaxis against venous thrombosis after major surgery. Br Med J 1987;295:1309–1312.

67. Fordyce MFJ, Baker AS, Staddon GE. Efficacy of fixed minidose warfarin prophylaxis in total hip replacement. Br Med J 1991;303:219–220.

68. Dale C, Gallus A, Wycherley A, Langlois S, Howie D. Prevention of venous thrombosis with minidose warfarin after joint replacement. Br Med J 1991;303:224.

69. Levine MN, Raskob G, Landefeld S, Hirsh J. Hemorrhagic complications of anticoagulant treatment. Chest 1995;108:276S–290S.

70. Palareti G, Leali N, Coccheri S, et al. Bleeding complications of oral anticoagulant treatment: an inception-cohort, prospective collaborative study (ISCOAT). Italian Study on Complications of Oral Anticoagulant Therapy. Lancet 1996;348:423–428.

71. Landefeld CS, Rosenblatt MW, Goldman L. Bleeding in outpatients treated with warfarin: relation to the prothrombin time and important remediable lesions. Am J Med 1989;87:153–159.

72. Wilcox CM, Truss CD. Gastrointestinal bleeding in patients receiving long-term anticoagulant therapy. Am J Med 1988;84:683–690.

73. Landefeld CS, Goldman L. Major bleeding in outpatients treated with warfarin: incidence and prediction by factors known at the start of outpatient therapy. Am J Med 1989;87:144–152.

74. Gitter MJ, Jaeger TM, Petterson TM, Gersh BJ, Silverstein MD. Bleeding and thromboembolism during anticoagulant therapy: a population-based study in Rochester, Minnesota. Mayo Clin Proc 1995;70: 725–733.

75. Fihn SD, McDonell M, Martin D, et al. Risk factors for complications of chronic anticoagulation. A multicenter study. Warfarin Optimized Outpatient Follow-up Study Group. Ann Intern Med 1993;118:511–520.

76. Fihn SD, Callahan CM, Martin DC, McDonell MB, Henikoff JG, White RH. The risk for and severity of bleeding complications in elderly patients treated with warfarin. The National Consortium of Anticoagulation. Ann Intern Med 1996;124:970–979.

77. Gurwitz JH, Goldberg RJ, Holden A, Knapic N, Ansell J. Age-related risks of long-term oral anticoagulant therapy. Arch Intern Med 1988;148:1733–1736.

78. White RH, McKittrick T, Hutchinson R, Twitchell J. Temporary discontinuation of warfarin therapy: changes in the international normalized ratio. Ann Intern Med 1995;122:40–42.

79. Hirsh J, Dalen JE, Deykin D, Poller L, Bussey H. Oral anticoagulants. Mechanism of action, clinical effectiveness, and optimal therapeutic range. Chest 1995; 108:231S–246S.

80. Palareti G, Legnani C, Guazzaloca G, et al. Activation of blood coagulation after abrupt or stepwise withdrawal of oral anticoagulants—a prospective study. Thromb Haemost 1994;72:222–226.

81. Palareti G, Legnani C. Warfarin withdrawal. Pharmacokinetic-pharmacodynamic considerations. Clin Pharmacokinet 1996;30:300–313.

82. Genewein U, Haeberli A, Straub PW, Beer JH. Rebound after cessation of oral anticoagulant therapy: the biochemical evidence. Br J Haematol 1996;92:479–485.

83. Comp PC, Elrod JP, Karzenski S. Warfarin-induced skin necrosis. Semin Thromb Hemost 1990;16:293–298.

84. Green D. Warfarin. N Engl J Med 1984;311:1578–1579.

85. Conlan MG, Bridges A, Williams E, Marlar R. Familial type II protein C deficiency associated with war-

farin-induced skin necrosis and bilateral adrenal hemorrhage. *Am J Hematol* 1988;29:226–229.

86. Craig A, Taberner DA, Fisher AH, Foster DN, Mitra J.
    Type I protein S deficiency and skin necrosis. *Postgrad
    Med J* 1990;66:389–391.

87. Makris M, Bardhan G, Preston FE. Warfarin induced
    skin necrosis associated with activated protein C resis-
    tance. *Thromb Haemost* 1996;75:523–524.

88. Francis RB, McGehee WG. Defibrination during war-
    farin therapy in a man with protein C deficiency.
    Thromb Haemost 1985;53:249–251.

89. Schramm W, Spannagl M, Bauer KA, et al. Treatment
    of coumarin-induced skin necrosis with a monoclonal
    antibody purified protein C concentrate. *Arch Derma-
    tol* 1993;129:753–756.

90. Hyman BT, Landas SK, Ashman RF, Schelper RL,
    Robinson RA. Warfarin-related purple toes syndrome
    and cholesterol microembolization. *Am J Med* 1987;
    82:1233–1237.

91. Dahlberg PJ, Frecentese DF, Cogbill TH. Cholesterol
    embolism: experience with 22 histologically proven
    cases. *Surgery* 1989;105:737–746.

92. Rhodes JM. Cholesterol crystal embolism: an impor-
    tant "new" diagnosis for the general physician. *Lancet*
    1996;347:1641.

93. Edwards RL, Rickles FR, Moritz TE, et al. Abnormal-
    ities of blood coagulation tests in patients with cancer.
    Am J Clin Pathol 1987;88:596–602.

94. Stone MS, Rosen T. Acral purpura: an unusual sign of
    coumarin necrosis. *J Am Acad Dermatol* 1986;14:
    797–802.

95. Bell WR, Starksen NF, Tong S, Porterfield JK.
    Trousseau's syndrome. Devastating coagulopathy in
    the absence of heparin. *Am J Med* 1985;79:423–430.

96. Shaul WL, Hall JG. Multiple congenital anomalies as-
    sociated with oral anticoagulants. *Am J Obstet Gy-
    necol* 1977;127:191–198.

97. Fiore CE, Tamburino C, Foti R, Grimaldi D. Reduced
    axial bone mineral content in patients taking an oral
    anticoagulant. *South Med J* 1990;83:538–542.

98. Umlas J, Harken DE. Warfarin-induced alopecia. *Cutis*
    1988;42:63–64.

99. Taybi H, Capitanio MA. Tracheobronchial calcifica-
    tion: an observation in three children after mitral valve
    replacement and warfarin sodium therapy. *Radiology*
    1990;176:728–730.

100. Martin JE, Lutomski DM. Warfarin resistance and en-
     teral feedings. *J Parent Ent Nutr* 1989;13:206–208.

101. Lutomski DM, Palascak JE, Bower RH. Warfarin re-
     sistance associated with intravenous lipid administra-
     tion. *J Parent Ent Nutr* 1987;11:316–318.

102. Kempin SJ. Warfarin resistance caused by broccoli. *N
     Engl J Med* 1983;308:1229–1230.

103. Blickstein D, Shaklai M, Inbal A. Warfarin antagonism
     by avocado. *Lancet* 1991;337:914–915.

104. Stephens MA, Self TH, Lancaster D, Nash T. Hy-
     pothyroidism: effect on warfarin anticoagulation.
     South Med J 1989;82:1585–1586.

105. Meade TW, Roderick PJ, Brennan PJ, Wilkes HC,
     Kelleher CC. Extra-cranial bleeding and other symp-
     toms due to low dose aspirin and low intensity oral an-
     ticoagulation. *Thromb Haemost* 1992;68:1–6.

Cardiovascular Thrombosis: Thrombocardiology and Thromboneurology, Second Edition,
edited by M. Verstraete, V. Fuster, and E. J. Topol,
Lippincott–Raven Publishers, Philadelphia © 1998.

17

Thrombolytic Agents

Roger H. Lijnen, Désiré Collen, and Marc Verstraete

The Center for Molecular and Vascular Biology,
University of Leuven, B-3000 Leuven, Belgium

Cardiovascular diseases, comprising acute myocardial infarction, stroke, and venous thromboembolism, have as their immediate underlying cause thrombosis of critically situated blood vessels with loss of blood flow to vital organs. One approach to the treatment of thrombosis consists of infusing thrombolytic agents to dissolve the blood clot and to restore tissue perfusion and oxygenation. Thrombolytic agents are plasminogen activators which activate the blood fibrinolytic system by activation of the proenzyme, plasminogen, to the active enzyme plasmin. Plasmin in turn digests fibrin to soluble degradation products. Inhibition of the fibrinolytic system occurs both at the level of the plasminogen activators, by plasminogen activator inhibitors (PAI-1 and PAI-2), and at the level of plasmin, mainly by α_2-antiplasmin. Currently, five thrombolytic agents are available for clinical use: streptokinase, anisoylated plasminogen streptokinase activator complex (APSAC), two-chain urokinase-type plasminogen activator (tcu-PA), single-chain u-PA (scu-PA, prourokinase), and tissue-type plasminogen activator (t-PA).

Streptokinase, APSAC, and tcu-PA induce extensive systemic plasmin generation; α_2-antiplasmin inhibits circulating plasmin but may become exhausted during thrombolytic therapy because its plasma concentration is only about half that of plasminogen. As a result, plasmin, which has a broad substrate specificity, will degrade several plasma proteins, such as fibrinogen, coagulation factors V, VIII, and XII, and von Willebrand factor. These thrombolytic agents are therefore considered to be non-fibrin-specific. In contrast, the physiologic plasminogen activators, t-PA and scu-PA, are more fibrin-specific because they activate plasminogen preferentially at the fibrin surface and less in the circulation. Plasmin, associated with the fibrin surface, is protected from rapid inhibition by α_2-antiplasmin because its lysine binding sites are not available and may thus efficiently degrade the fibrin of a thrombus (1,2). The molecular interactions determining the fibrin specificity of plasminogen activators are schematically illustrated in Fig. 17-1.

In patients with acute myocardial infarction, reduction of infarct size, preservation of

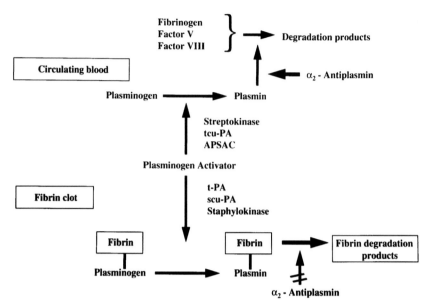

FIG. 17-1. Molecular interactions determining the fibrin specificity of thrombolytic agents. Non-fibrin-specific agents (streptokinase, tcu-PA, APSAC) extensively activate plasminogen in the circulating blood, whereas fibrin-specific agents (t-PA, scu-PA, staphylokinase) preferentially activate fibrin-associated plasminogen.

ventricular function, and reduction in mortality has been demonstrated with streptokinase, recombinant t-PA (rt-PA), and APSAC. The GUSTO (Global Utilization of Streptokinase and t-PA for Occluded Coronary Arteries) trial has conclusively established a correlation between early coronary patency and reduction in mortality (3).

Nevertheless, all available thrombolytic agents suffer from significant shortcomings, including large therapeutic doses, short plasma half-lives, limited efficacy and fibrin specificity, reocclusion, and bleeding complications (1,2,4). At best, a brisk coronary flow (TIMI 3 grade) within 90 min is obtained in approximately half of the myocardial infarction patients treated with thrombolytic drugs. To obtain this antegrade coronary flow requires an average of 45 minutes, and reocclusion occurs in roughly 10% of patients. In most trials the residual mortality in patients treated with thrombolytic drugs is not less than half of that without thrombolytic treatment. In the treatment of

myocardial infarction and ischemic stroke, a second limitation is the length of time to treatment; earlier and accelerated administration of thrombolytic drugs should be the first and immediately applicable goal. Rapid recanalization of an occluded artery may reflect not only the velocity of plasminogen activation in the thrombus, but also the ease with which the thrombolytic agent reaches and diffuses into the thrombus, and the speed with which the thrombolytic therapy can be initiated. These ideas have encouraged the development of "front-loaded" or "bolus" administration schedules. In the early years of thrombolytic therapy, a rapid countering of the thrombolytic effect was thought to be an advantage, in that thrombolysis could be interrupted rapidly if complications occurred. This has proved more difficult to achieve than anticipated because plasminogen activation may continue within a thrombus after systemic thrombolytic activity has returned to normal. Conversely, agents with rapid termination of action may be unsatisfactory because it might be difficult to ensure completion of clot lysis without the technical difficulties of a carefully controlled infusion. Another limitation is the lack of significant impact of aspirin and heparin on the speed of thrombolysis or resistance to lysis and, importantly, the fact that they do not consistently prevent reocclusion. Paradoxically, fibrinolytic drugs themselves can exert procoagulant effects through generation of plasmin, which may activate the coagulation system resulting in a retardation of apparent thrombolysis, failure of initial recanalization, and virtually instantaneous reocclusion. Thus, vigorous, concomitant anticoagulation is needed. Specific reduction of platelet aggregation is presently being explored with monoclonal antibodies or synthetic peptides against the platelet receptor GPIIb/IIIa. Another approach is the use of selective inhibitors of thrombin, of factor Xa, or of factor VIIa. Furthermore, it is possible that the desired profile for a thrombolytic agent to be used in patients with an acute coronary or carotid-vertebral occlusion, with its emphasis on speed, may not be optimal for agents to be used for other indications, such as venous occlusion.

Therefore the search continues for better thrombolytic agents or regimen. Recent approaches to improve the thrombolytic properties of plasminogen activators include the production of mutant plasminogen activators, of chimeric molecules comprising portions of different plasminogen activators, of antibody-targeted plasminogen activators using fibrin-specific or platelet-specific monoclonal antibodies, and of plasminogen activators from animal or bacterial sources (5–7). Some of these new thrombolytic agents have shown promise in animal models of venous or arterial thrombosis and in pilot clinical studies (7). In this chapter, we will focus on the biochemistry, mechanism of action, and pharmacodynamic properties of presently available thrombolytic agents and of some new and promising agents that are being developed for clinical use.

FIBRIN-SPECIFIC THROMBOLYTIC AGENTS

Wild-type Tissue-type Plasminogen Activator

Physicochemical Properties

The cDNA of t-PA has been cloned and the complete amino acid sequence has been determined (8). The human t-PA gene, localized on chromosome 8 (bands 8.p.12 → q.11.2) consists of 14 exons, and the intron–exon organization suggests that the assembly occurred according to the "exon shuffling" principle, whereby the distinct structural domains are encoded by a single exon or by adjacent exons (for references, cf. 9). The proximal promoter sequences in the human t-PA gene contain typical TATA and CAAT boxes, and potential recognition sequences for several transcription factors have been identified (10,11). Consensus sequences of a cAMP-responsive element and of an AP-2 binding site have been identified, which may have a cooperative effect on constitutive t-PA gene expression (12).

Human t-PA was first isolated as a single-chain serine proteinase of 70 kDa, consisting of 527 amino acids with Ser as the NH_2-terminal amino acid (8); it was subsequently shown that native t-PA contains an NH_2-terminal extension of three amino acids, but in general the initial numbering system has been maintained (Fig. 17-2). Limited plasmic hydrolysis of the Arg^{275}-Ile^{276} peptide bond converts t-PA to a two-chain molecule held together by one interchain disulfide bond. The t-PA molecule contains four domains: (a) an NH_2-terminal region of 47 residues (residues 4 to 50) (F domain), which is homologous with the finger domains mediating the fibrin affinity of fibronectin; (b) residues 50 to 87 (E domain), which are homologous with epidermal growth factor; (c) two regions comprising residues 87 to 176 and 176 to 262 (K_1 and K_2 domains), which share a high degree of homology with the five kringles of plasminogen; and (d) a serine proteinase domain

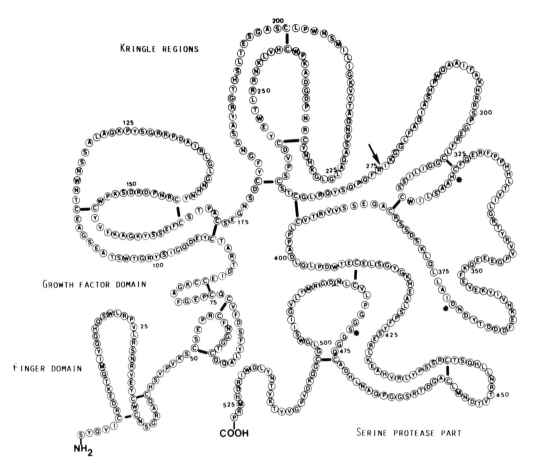

FIG. 17-2. Schematic representation of the primary structure of rt-PA. The amino acids are represented by their single- letter symbols and black bars indicate disulfide bonds. The active site residues are indicated with an asterisk. The arrow indicates the plasmin cleavage site for conversion of single-chain rt-PA to two-chain rt-PA. In reteplase (BM 06.022), the sequence comprising Val[4] through Glu[175] has been deleted. In TNK-rt-PA, Thr[103] is substituted by Asn, Asn[117] by Gln, and the sequence Lys[296]-His-Arg-Arg[299] is mutagenized to Ala-Ala-Ala-Ala.

(P, residues 276 to 527) with the active site residues His[322], Asp[371], and Ser[478]. There are three potential N-glycosylation sites, at Asn[117] (K₁), Asn[184] (K₂), and Asn[448] (P). t-PA preparations usually contain a mixture of variant I (with all three glycosylation sites) and variant II (lacking carbohydrate at Asn[184]) (8). The t-PA molecule is ellipsoidal and relatively compact (13), with the individual domains folded within the molecule yielding a globular structure, which is stabilized by strong interactions between the proteinase domain and the F and/or E domains (14,15). In contrast to the single-chain precursor form of most serine proteinases, single-chain t-PA is enzymatically active. On the basis of conformational similarities between single-chain and two-chain t-PA, it was postulated that the activity of single-chain t-PA would involve an equilibrium between an active and a zymogenic conformation, which would be shifted to the active conformation upon substrate binding (16). Amino acid Lys[156] appears to play a role in the enzymatic activity of single-chain t-PA by stabilizing the active conformation (17).

Inhibition of t-PA by its physiologic inhibitor PAI-1 involves formation of a 1:1 stoichiometric reversible complex, followed by covalent binding between the hydroxyl group of the active site Ser^{478} residue of t-PA and the carboxyl group of the P_1 residue at the reactive center (Arg^{346}) of the inhibitor. The reversible high-affinity second-site interaction occurs between a negatively charged sequence in PAI-1 (residues 350 to 355) and a positively charged region in t-PA (residues 296 to 304) (for references, cf. 9).

Mechanism of Action

As all known plasminogen activators, t-PA converts its substrate plasminogen to plasmin by cleavage of a single Arg^{561}-Val^{562} peptide bond. t-PA is a poor enzyme in the absence of fibrin, but the presence of fibrin strikingly enhances the activation rate of plasminogen. Optimal stimulation is only obtained after early plasmin cleavage in the COOH-terminal α chain and the NH_2-terminal β chain of fibrin, yielding fragment X polymer (18). Kinetic data (19) support a mechanism in which fibrin provides a surface to which t-PA and plasminogen adsorb in a sequential and ordered way yielding a cyclic ternary complex. Formation of this complex allows an enhanced affinity of t-PA for plasminogen, resulting in an up to three orders of magnitude higher catalytic efficiency for plasminogen activation. Plasmin formed on the fibrin surface has both its lysine binding sites and active site occupied and is thus only slowly inactivated by α_2-antiplasmin; in contrast, free plasmin, when formed, is very rapidly inhibited by α_2-antiplasmin (for references, cf. 9).

Pharmacokinetic Properties

rt-PA (predominantly two-chain material) is cleared from the circulation in a biphasic manner with an initial half-life of 6 minutes and a terminal half-life of 64 minutes in humans (20). The initial and terminal half-lives of single-chain rt-PA, following infusion of 8.3 µg per kg per minute over 30 minutes in healthy volunteers, were 3.3 and 26 minutes (21). In patients with acute myocardial infarction, clearance of single-chain rt-PA was found to be 30% to 40% more rapid than two-chain rt-PA (22). Clearance is the result of interaction with several receptor systems. Liver endothelial cells have a mannose receptor that recognizes the high-mannose-type carbohydrate side chain at Asn^{117} in the K_1 domain, whereas liver parenchymal cells contain a calcium-dependent receptor that interacts mainly with the growth factor domain of t-PA (23,24). In addition, the low-density lipoprotein receptor–related protein (LRP), expressed in high copy number on hepatocytes, binds free t-PA and complexes with PAI-1 (25,26).

Dosage

The recommended dose of recombinant t-PA (alteplase, Activase, Actilyse) for the treatment of acute myocardial infarction was 100 mg administered as 60 mg in the first hour (of which 6 to 10 mg is administered as a bolus over the first 1 to 2 minutes), 20 mg over the second hour, and 20 mg over the third hour. More recently, it was proposed to give the same total dose of 100 mg but "front-loaded," starting with a bolus of 15 mg followed by 50 mg in the next 30 minutes and the remaining 35 mg in the following hour (27). In the GUSTO trial, a dose of 15 mg intravenous bolus of alteplase followed by 0.75 mg per kg over 30 minutes (not to exceed 50 mg) and then 0.50 mg per kg over 60 minutes (not to exceed 35 mg) was utilized (3). In the COBALT trial, double-bolus administration of rt-PA (50 mg given 30 minutes apart) was evaluated in patients with myocardial infarction (28). Whichever regimen is used, it is important to coadminister intravenous heparin during and after alteplase treatment. For catheter-directed local thrombolysis with alteplase in patients with recent peripheral arterial occlusion, a dose of 0.05 to 0.10 mg per kg per hour over an 8-hour period is usually recommended.

Mutants and Variants of Tissue-type Plasminogen Activator

By deletion or substitution of functional domains, by site-specific point mutations, and/or by altering the carbohydrate composition, mutants of rt-PA have been produced with higher fibrin specificity, more zymogenicity, slower clearance from the circulation, and resistance to plasma proteinase inhibitors.

During thrombolytic therapy there is a vast excess of t-PA over PAI-1 in the circulation, but critical lysis occurs at the surface of an arterial thrombus where the local PAI-1 concentration can be very high (29). Therefore, mutants with resistance to PAI-1 may be useful to reduce reocclusion. In addition, mutants with prolonged half-life may allow efficient thrombolysis by bolus administration at a reduced dose. Several mutants and variants of t-PA are presently evaluated at the preclinical level in animal models of venous and arterial thrombosis and in pilot studies, mainly in patients with acute myocardial infarction. These agents include reteplase (Rapilysin or Ecokinase), TNK-rt-PA, and the vampire bat (*Desmodus rotundus*) salivary plasminogen activator.

Physicochemical Properties

Reteplase (BM 06.022) is a single-chain nonglycosylated deletion variant consisting only of the kringle 2 and the proteinase domain of human t-PA; it contains amino acids 1–3 and 176–527 of rt-PA (deletion of Val^4-Glu^{175}; cf. Fig. 17-2). The Arg^{275}-Ile^{276} plasmin cleave site is maintained (30).

In TNK-rt-PA, replacement of Asn^{117} with Gln (N117Q) deletes the glycosylation site in K_1 whereas substitution of Thr^{103} by Asn(T103N) reintroduces a glycosylation site in K_1, but at a different locus; these modifications substantially decrease the plasma clearance rate. In addition, the amino acids Lys^{296}-His^{297}-Arg^{298}-Arg^{299} were each replaced with Ala (cf. Fig. 17-2) (31).

Different molecular forms of the *Desmodus* salivary plasminogen activator (DSPA) have been purified, characterized, cloned, and expressed. Two high molecular weight forms, DSPAα₁ (43 kDa) and DSPAα₂ (39 kDa), exhibit about 85% homology to human t-PA, but contain neither a kringle 2 domain nor a plas-

min-sensitive cleavage site. DSPAβ lacks the finger domain and DSPAγ lacks the finger and epidermal growth factor domains (32–34).

Mechanism of Action

The active site in the proteinase domain of reteplase and of t-PA and their plasminogenolytic activity in the absence of a stimulator do not differ, but the plasminogenolytic activity of reteplase in the presence of CNBr fragments of fibrinogen as a stimulator was found to be fourfold lower as compared to t-PA, whereas the binding of reteplase to fibrin was fivefold lower (30,35). These differences might possibly be due to the missing finger domain in reteplase. It is known that fibrin binding is mediated through both the finger domain and the lysine binding site in the kringle 2 domain of t-PA. Reteplase and t-PA are inhibited by PAI-1 to a similar degree. The affinity of reteplase for binding to endothelial cells and monocytes is reduced as compared to t-PA, probably as a consequence of deletion of the finger and epidermal growth factor domains in reteplase which seem to be involved in the interaction with endothelial cell receptors (36).

TNK-rt-PA has a similar ability as wild-type rt-PA to bind to fibrin and to lyse fibrin clots in a plasma milieu (31). It has an enhanced fibrin specificity, resistance to inhibition by PAI-1, and slower plasma clearance (37).

DSPAα1 and DSPAα2 exhibit a specific activity in vitro that is equal to or higher than that of rt-PA, a relative PAI-1 resistance, and a greatly enhanced fibrin specificity with a strict requirement for polymeric fibrin as a cofactor (32,34).

Pharmacokinetic Properties

Pharmacokinetic analysis of plasma activity in the rabbit revealed a half-life of 18.9 ± 1.5 minutes for reteplase and 2.1 ± 0.1 minutes for alteplase, with a 4.3-fold slower plasma clearance for reteplase than for alteplase (38). In healthy human volunteers (39) and in patients with acute myocardial infarction (40), an initial half-life of 14 to 18 minutes was observed for reteplase.

TNK-rt-PA has a slower clearance and marked resistance to PAI-1. It was shown to have an increased thrombolytic potency on platelet-rich clots in rabbits, to conserve fibrinogen, and to be effective upon bolus administration at half the dose of rt-PA (31,41). Similar results were obtained in a combined arterial and venous thrombosis model in the dog (42) and in a rabbit carotid artery thrombosis model (43). In patients with acute myocardial infarction, TNK-rt-PA has a plasma clearance of 151 ± 55 ml per minute and a half-life of 17 ± 7 minute, as compared to 572 ± 132 ml per minute and 3.5 ± 1.4 minute for wild-type rt-PA (44).

In several animal models of thrombolysis, DSPAα1 has a 2.5 times higher potency and four- to eightfold slower clearance than t-PA (45–49). Recombinant DSPAα1 produced in mammalian cell culture may be suitable for bolus administration, whereby its long half-life and high specific activity may allow a reduction of the therapeutic dose (49).

Dosage

Different doses of reteplase in patients with acute myocardial infarction were evaluated in two open nonrandomized pilot trials (50,51). The randomized RAPID I trial showed that reteplase, when given as a double bolus of 10 plus 10 MU 30 minutes apart, achieves more rapid, complete, and sustained thrombolysis than standard dose alteplase (100 mg over 3 hours) (52). In the RAPID II trial, the same reteplase dose regimen appeared to achieve higher rates of early reperfusion than frontloaded alteplase (53). In the INJECT study, a double-blind randomized trial in patients with acute myocardial infarction, administration of two boluses of 10 MU reteplase given 30 min apart was compared with streptokinase (1.5 MU intravenously over 60 minutes) (54).

In the Thrombolysis in Myocardial Infarction (TIMI) 10A trial, a phase 1 dose-ranging

pilot study in patients with acute myocardial infarction, single-bolus TNK-rt-PA was administered over 5 to 10 seconds with doses ranging from 5 to 50 mg (44). The agent was fibrin-specific with initial patency and safety profile at 30- to 50-mg doses, which appeared encouraging.

Single-Chain Urokinase-type Plasminogen Activator

Physicochemical Properties

Urokinase (u-PA) was first found in urine at relatively high concentrations (200 to 300 ng/ml) and was later identified in human plasma at a level of about 3 to 5 ng/ml. u-PA is secreted as a single-chain molecule (scu-PA, pro-urokinase) that may be converted to a chain–chain form (tcu-PA). The cDNA has been cloned and expressed (55).

scu-PA is a serine proteinase of 411 amino acids in a single polypeptide chain, with active site triad His^{204}, Asp^{255}, and Ser^{356} (Fig. 17-3). The molecule contains an NH$_2$-terminal growth factor domain and one kringle structure homologous to the five kringles found in plasminogen and the two kringles in t-PA (51). u-PA contains only one N-glycosylation site (at Asn^{302}), and contains a fucosylated threonine residue at position 18. Conversion of scu-PA to tcu-PA occurs after proteolytic cleavage at position Lys^{158}-Ile^{159} by plasmin (56), but also by kallikrein (57), trypsin, cathepsin B, human T-cell–associated serine proteinase-1, and thermolysin. A fully active tcu-PA derivative is obtained after additional proteolysis by plasmin at position Lys^{135}-Lys^{136}. A low molecular weight form of scu-PA (32 kDa) can be obtained by selective cleavage at position Glu^{143}-Leu^{144} (58); this cleavage can be obtained with matrix metalloproteinase Pump-1 (59). In contrast, scu-PA is converted to an inactive two-chain molecule by thrombin after proteolytic cleavage at position Arg^{156}-Phe^{157} (57). This inactivation is strongly enhanced in the presence of thrombomodulin and is dependent on the 0-linked glucosaminoglycan of thrombomod-

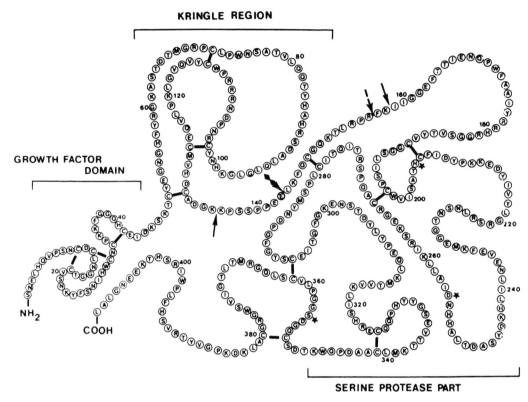

FIG. 17-3. Schematic representation of the primary structure of scu-PA. The amino acids are represented by their single letter symbols and black bars indicate disulfide bonds. The active site residues are indicated with an asterisk. The arrows indicate the plasmin cleavages sites for conversion of 54 kDa scu-PA to 54 kDa tcu-PA (Lys[158]-Ile[159]), and of 54 kDa tcu-PA to 33 kDa tcu-PA (Lys[135]-Lys[136]), the thrombin cleavage site (Arg[156]-Phe[157]) yielding inactive 54 kDa tcu-PA, and the conversion site to 32 kDa scu-PA (Glu[143]-Leu[144]).

ulin (60). The cofactor effect of thrombomodulin on the inactivation of scu-PA by thrombin could be demonstrated in a perfused rabbit heart model (61).

Mechanism of Action

u-PA is a serine proteinase with a high substrate specificity for plasminogen. In contrast to tcu-PA, scu-PA displays very low activity toward low molecular weight chromogenic substrates. Scu-PA appears to have some intrinsic plasminogen activating potential, which represents ≤ 0.5% of the catalytic efficiency of tcu-PA (62,63). However, other investigators have claimed that scu-PA has no measurable intrinsic amidolytic or plasmino-

gen activator activities (64). The occurrence of a transitional state of scu-PA with a higher catalytic efficiency for native plasminogen than tcu-PA has been postulated (65). Furthermore, it was reported that fibrin fragment E-2 selectively promotes the activation of plasminogen by scu-PA, mainly by enhancing the catalytic rate constant of the activation (66). Indeed scu-PA is not an efficient activator of plasminogen bound to internal lysine residues on intact fibrin, but it develops a higher activity toward plasminogen bound to newly generated COOH-terminal lysine residues on partially degraded fibrin (67). Subsequent studies confirmed that the fibrin specificity of scu-PA does not require its conversion to tcu-PA but appears to be mediated by enhanced binding of plasminogen to partially digested fibrin (68).

In plasma, in the absence of fibrin, scu-PA is stable and does not activate plasminogen; in the presence of a fibrin clot, scu-PA, but not tcu-PA, induces fibrin-specific clot lysis (62). scu-PA does not bind to a significant extent to fibrin, although in the presence of Zn^{2+} ions some binding has been reported (69). The intrinsic activity of scu-PA toward fibrin-bound plasminogen may contribute to its fibrin specificity. Furthermore, α_2-antiplasmin in plasma prevents conversion of scu-PA to tcu-PA outside the clot and thus preserves fibrin specificity (70).

Pharmacokinetic Properties

The turnover of different molecular forms of u-PA in blood of different animal species occurs with an initial half-life of approximately 3 to 7 minutes (62,71–74). Because similar turnover rates were observed for ^{125}I-labeled tracer, enzymatic activity, and antigen, this short half-life seems to be an inherent property of u-PA. The main mechanism of removal of u-PA from the blood appears to occur by hepatic clearance. Experimental hepatectomy in rabbits indeed markedly prolongs the initial half-life of scu-PA (from 3 minutes to 20 to 30 minutes) (71). scu-PA is taken up in the liver via a recognition site on parenchymal cells and is subsequently degraded in the lysosomes (75).

The rapid clearance of u-PA apparently is not mediated via carbohydrate receptors because very similar turnover characteristics are observed for both the scu-PA and tcu-PA forms of unglycosylated recombinant molecules are of glycosylated natural molecules. It does not occur via reaction with plasma proteinase inhibitors and subsequent rapid clearance of the complexes because active site blocked tcu-PA and scu-PA, which do not react with plasma protease inhibitors, have the same half-life as the active tcu-PA forms (71). In addition, the similar half-life observed for 32 kDa scu-PA indicates that clearance is not

mediated via the NH_2-terminal portion of the molecule (72).

Following intravenous infusion of natural or recombinant scu-PA in patients with acute myocardial infarction, a biphasic disappearance was observed with initial half-lives in plasma (postinfusion) of 4 minutes or 8 minutes, respectively (76,77). This short half-life suggests that the maintenance of a therapeutic level of the agent in plasma may require its continuous infusion.

Dosage

Saruplase is the generic name for full-length unglycosylated human recombinant scu-PA obtained from *Escherichia coli*. With a preparation containing 160,000 IU per mg, the dose used successfully in patients with acute myocardial infarction (PRIMI Study) was 20 mg given as a bolus and 60 mg over the next 60 minutes, immediately followed by an intravenous heparin infusion (20 IU per kg per hour) for 72 hours (78). In the LIMITS Study in patients with acute myocardial infarction, the same dose regimen of saruplase was used, but with a prethrombolytic heparin bolus of 5,000 IU and an intravenous heparin infusion for 5 days starting 30 minutes after completion of thrombolysis (79). A recombinant glycosylated form of prourokinase (A-74187) has been evaluated in patients with acute myocardial infarction using 60 or 80 mg monotherapy or 60 mg primed with a preceding bolus of 250,000 IU of recombinant tcu-PA, always combined with aspirin and intravenous heparin (80).

Staphylokinase

Physicochemical Properties

Staphylokinase, a plasminogen activator produced by certain strains of *Staphylococcus aureus* , was shown to have profibrinolytic properties more than four decades ago (81,82). Natural staphylokinase has been purified from *S. aureus* strains that were transformed with bacteriophages containing the staphylokinase gene or that had undergone lysogenic conversion to staphylokinase production (83,84). In addition, the staphylokinase gene has been cloned from the bacteriophages *sakøC* (85) and *sak*42D (86) as well as from the genomic DNA (*sak*STAR) of a lysogenic *S. aureus* strain (84).

The staphylokinase gene encodes a protein of 163 amino acids with amino acid 28 corresponding to the NH₂-terminal residue of the mature protein, which consists of 136 amino acids in a single polypeptide chain without disulfide bridges. The mature proteins SakSTAR, SakøC, and Sak42D differ in only three amino acids; amino acid 34 is Ser in SakSTAR but Gly in SakøC and Sak42D; amino acid 36 is Gly in SakSTAR and in SakøC, but Arg in Sak42D; and amino acid 43 is His in SakSTAR and in SakøC, but Arg in Sak42D (87–89). In purified preparations, different molecular forms of staphylokinase with slightly different molecular weight and isoelectric points have been observed; molecular forms have been characterized lacking the 6 or the 10 NH₂-terminal amino acid (84,88,89).

Mechanism of Action

Staphylokinase forms a 1:1 stoichiometric complex with plasmin(ogen) (90,91). It is not an enzyme, and generation of an active site in its equimolar complex with plasminogen requires conversion of plasminogen to plasmin. Thus, the plasmin–staphylokinase complex is the active enzyme (92,93). This is in contrast with streptokinase, which produces a complex with plasminogen that exposes the active site in the plasminogen moiety without proteolytic cleavage (94). Kinetic data suggest the following mechanism for plasminogen activation in a buffer milieu.

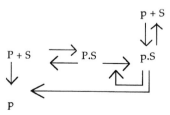

Plasmin (P) and staphylokinase (S) produce an inactive 1:1 stoichiometric complex (P–S), which does not activate plasminogen. The activation reaction appears to be initiated by trace amounts of plasmin (p), which generates active plasmin–staphylokinase complex (p–S) (93). In mixtures with excess plasminogen over staphylokinase, generated p–S converts excess plasminogen to plasmin. In addition, kinetic analysis has revealed that generated p–S converts P–S to p–S, thus representing a potential positive feedback mechanism (95). However, the main pathway for plasmin generation in the above scheme appears to be via activation of P by p–S formed by binding of S to p. This is supported by binding data obtained with fluorescently labeled staphylokinase, showing that it has a much higher affinity for plasmin than for native plasminogen (96).

In a buffer milieu, α₂-antiplasmin rapidly inhibits the p–S complex if the lysine binding sites in the plasmin moiety of the complex are available (92,97,98). Fibrin, but not fibrinogen, reduces the inhibition rate of the complex by α₂-antiplasmin by competing for interaction with the lysine binding site(s). By delaying inhibition of plasmin or p–S complex by α₂-antiplasmin, fibrin thus facilitates generation of active p–S complex (99). However, staphylokinase dissociates from the p–S complex following neutralization by α₂-antiplasmin and is recycled to other plasmin(ogen) molecules (100). Thus, extensive systemic plasminogen activation with staphylokinase would be expected in plasma, which is in contradiction with its observed fibrin specificity. This may be explained by the finding that in the absence of fibrin no significant amounts of p–S are generated because traces of plasmin are inhibited by α₂-antiplasmin. In the presence of fibrin, generation of the p–S complex is facilitated because traces of fibrin-bound plasmin are protected from α₂-antiplasmin and, furthermore, inhibition of p–S by α₂-antiplasmin at the clot surface is delayed more than 100-fold. Thus, generated p–S may efficiently convert P–S to p–S and excess P to p. Recycling of staphylokinase to fibrin-bound plasmin, after slow neutralization of the p–S complex, will result in more efficient generation of the complex. In addition, binding data obtained with fluorescently labeled staphylokinase indicate that it does not bind to a significant extent to plasminogen in circulating plasma, but binds with high affinity to plasmin and to plasminogen which is bound to partially degraded fibrin (96).

Recently, biochemical studies with highly purified recombinant staphylokinase, initial experiments in animal models of thrombosis, and pilot studies in patients with acute myocardial infarction or peripheral arterial occlusion have revealed that staphylokinase is an efficient and highly fibrin-specific plasminogen activator (101,102).

Pharmacodynamic Properties

In patients with acute myocardial infarction treated with an intravenous infusion of 10 mg staphylokinase (SakSTAR) over 30 minutes, the concentration of staphylokinase-related antigen in blood at the end of the infusion increased to between 0.9 and 1.7 µg/ml. The postinfusion disappearance of staphylokinase-related antigen from plasma occurred in a biphasic manner with a $t_{1/2\alpha}$ of 6.3 minutes and a $t_{1/2\beta}$ of 37 minutes, corresponding to a plasma clearance of 270 ml/min (103). In the STAR trial, SakSTAR antigen levels in 25 patients with acute myocardial infarction receiving 10 mg IV over 30 minutes were 0.56 ± 0.06 µg/ml at 25 minutes and 0.16 ± 0.04 µg/ml at 90 minutes, with corresponding levels of 1.9 ± 0.22 µg/ml and 0.42 ± 0.06 µg/ml in 23 patients receiving 20 mg SakSTAR over 30 minutes (104).

Unfortunately, the somewhat low-grade antigenicity of staphylokinase, as suggested by early dog and baboon experiments, is not extended to patients. The vast majority of patients with either myocardial infarction (103,104) or peripheral arterial occlusion (105) developed neutralizing antibodies to SakSTAR, albeit after a long lag phase of 7 to 12 days, that remained elevated well above pretreatment levels for several months after administration (106). However, the titers of preformed anti-SakSTAR antibodies in the general population appeared to be lower than those of antistreptokinase antibodies (107), and even systemic *S. aureus* infections failed to induce SakSTAR-neutralizing antibodies in most patients (105), possibly reflecting the low proportion of *S. aureus* strains that produce staphylokinase. The boost of neutralizing antibody titers upon infusion of SakSTAR, however, predicts therapeutic refractoriness on repeated administration. Therefore, the restriction to single use applies probably both to streptokinase and staphylokinase. The absence of cross-reactivity to streptokinase of antibodies elicited by SakSTAR, and vice versa, suggests that the consecutive use of both plasminogen activators may be feasible (107). Furthermore, variants of recombinant staphylokinase with reduced immunogenicity have been obtained by site-directed mutagenesis (108–112). Thus, substitution mutagenesis in recombinant staphylokinase (SakSTAR) of clusters of two or three charged amino acids with alanine identified two variants, SakSTAR.M38 (with K35, E38, K74, E75, and R77 substituted with A) and SakSTAR.M89 (with K74, E75, R77, E80, and D82 substituted with A) that had a markedly reduced expression of two of the three immunodominant epitopes of SakSTAR but also had an approximately 50% reduced specific activity. These mutants did not recognize approximately one third of the antibodies elicited in patients by treatment with wild-type SakSTAR, and elicited markedly less circulating neutralizing antibodies and significantly less resistance to thrombolysis in rabbits than wild-type SakSTAR. In patients with peripheral arterial occlusion given doses of 6.5 to 12 mg of compound, SakSTAR.M38 and SakSTAR.M89 induced significantly less neutralizing antibody and staphylokinase-specific IgG than wild-type SakSTAR (109).

In a subsequent study, the effect of the reversal of one or more of these substituted amino acids on the ratio of activity to antigenicity was evaluated (111). In pooled plasma from patients with peripheral arterial occlusion treated with wild-type SakSTAR, about 40% of the antibodies depended on K74 of epitope K74, E75, and R77 for binding, whereas epitopes K35, E38 and E80, and D82 had a negligible contribution toward antibody recognition. SakSTAR (K74), with a single substitution of Lys^{74} with Ala, had an intact specific activity but did not absorb 40% of the antibodies induced in patients by treatment with wild-type SakSTAR. The thrombolytic potency and antibody induction of SakSTAR (K74) and of SakSTAR (K74ER) with Lys^{74}, Glu^{75}, and Arg^{77} replaced by Ala were studied in more detail (112). Intra-arterial administration in patients with peripheral arterial occlusion of SakSTAR (K74) or SakSTAR (K74ER) induced significantly less circulating neutralizing antibody than SakSTAR. Overt neutralizing antibody induction (>10 µg compound neutralized/ml plasma) occurred in all 9 patients given wild-type SakSTAR, in 6 of the 11 SakSTAR (K74) patients, and in 2 of the 6 SakSTAR (K74ER) patients. Thus, SakSTAR (K74) and SakSTAR (K74ER) appear to have intact thrombolytic potencies but induce significantly less antibody formation in patients.

These variants provide proof of concept that reduction of the immunogenicity and immunoreactivity of recombinant staphylokinase by protein engineering may be feasible.

Dosage

In the first pilot recanalization studies, patients with acute myocardial infarction were given 10 mg IV SakSTAR, as a 1-mg bolus followed by infusion of 9 mg over 30 minutes (103). In the STAR trial, patients randomized to intravenous SakSTAR were given 10 mg over 30 minutes in the first half of the study and, following a prospectively planned interim analysis, 20 mg over 30 minutes in the second half, always with an initial 10% bolus (104). In a phased, angiographically controlled pilot study on bolus Sak42D infusion for coronary thrombolysis, 20 mg Sak42D was given over 5

minutes at study entry, with a second bolus of 10 mg over 5 minutes at 60 minutes if angiography showed TIMI perfusion grade 0, 1, or 2 (113). The encouraging experience obtained in this pilot study inspired a multicenter randomized trial in patients with evolving myocardial infarction, comparing accelerated rt-PA with a double bolus of 15 mg Sak42D given 30 minutes apart.

In a pilot study in patients with peripheral arterial occlusion, intra-arterial catheter-directed SakSTAR was given as a bolus of 1 mg, followed by a continuous infusion of 0.5 mg per hour, or as a 2-mg bolus followed by an infusion of 1 mg per hour, together with heparin. Complete recanalization was obtained in 83% of the patients after 7.0 ± 0.7 mg SakSTAR infused over 8.7 ± 1.0 hours (105).

NON-FIBRIN-SPECIFIC THROMBOLYTIC AGENTS

Two-Chain Urokinase-type Plasminogen Activator

Physicochemical Properties

Urokinase is a naturally occurring plasminogen activator excreted in human urine, from which it can be extracted; urokinase can also be isolated from tissue cultures of human embryonic kidney cells. It is a trypsin-like enzyme composed of two polypeptide chains (a light chain with 158 amino acids and a heavy chain with 253 amino acids). Urokinase occurs in two molecular forms designated S_1 (33 kDa, low molecular weight u-PA) and S_2 (54 kDa, high molecular weight u-PA), the former being a proteolytic degradation product of the latter generated by plasmin cleavage of the Lys^{135}-Lys^{136} peptide bond (114). The two-chain 54-kDa molecule is generated by proteolytic cleavage of the single-chain precursor scu-PA (cf. supra).

Mechanism of Action

tcu-PA activates plasminogen directly following Michaelis-Menten kinetics. The two-chain molecule has no specific affinity for fibrin and activates fibrin-bound and circulating plasminogen relatively indiscriminately. Extensive plasminogen activation and depletion of α_2-antiplasmin may occur following treatment with tcu-PA, leading to a systemic lytic state with low fibrinogen levels. The pharmacokinetic properties of tcu-PA are described in the section on scu-PA (cf. supra).

Dosage

As the level of inhibitors in plasma is relatively constant, a fixed dosage regimen can be used. In acute myocardial infarction, the dose of urokinase is either 2×10^6 units as a bolus or 3×10^6 units over 90 minutes (115). For over a decade, an initial intravenous dose of 4,000 units per kg body weight over 10 minutes followed by the same maintenance dose per kg hourly has been recommended for the treatment of acute major pulmonary embolism. At present, a bolus dose in the right atrium of 15,000 units per kg of body weight has been recommended in this indication; an intravenous infusion of 3×10^6 units of urokinase (1×10^6 units over 10 minutes and 2×10^6 units over the next 110 minutes) has also been tested.

Streptokinase

Physicochemical Properties

Streptokinase is a nonenzyme protein produced by several strains of hemolytic streptococci. It consists of a single polypeptide chain of 47 to 50 kDa and containing 414 amino acids (116). The region comprising amino acids 1 to 230 shows some homology with trypsin-like serine proteinases but lacks an active site serine residue.

Mechanism of Action

Streptokinase activates plasminogen indirectly, following a three-step mechanism (117). In the first step, streptokinase forms an equimolar complex with plasminogen, which undergoes a conformational change resulting in the exposure of an active site in the plas-minogen moiety (94,118). In the second step, this active site catalyzes the activation of plasminogen to plasmin. In a third step, plasminogen-streptokinase molecules are converted to plasmin–streptokinase complexes (119). The plasminogen activating potential of the plasminogen–streptokinase complex is two- to threefold higher than that of the plasmin–streptokinase complex (120). The activation of native plasminogen by the plasminogen–streptokinase complex is enhanced 6.5-fold in the presence of fibrin and 2-fold in the presence of fibrinogen (121).

The equimolar plasminogen–streptokinase complex converts rapidly to the plasmin–streptokinase complex by proteolytic cleavage of both the plasminogen and the streptokinase moieties. In plasminogen, the Arg^{561}-Val^{562} and the Lys^{77}-Lys^{78} peptide bonds are cleaved (122,123); four modified forms of streptokinase differing in molecular weight by 4 to 5 kDa have been observed depending on the species origin of the plasminogen (124). With human plasminogen, a major proteolytic derivative of 36 kDa is generated (125). The plasmin–streptokinase complex can also be formed by mixing plasmin and streptokinase; it is extremely rapidly formed and very stable (126). The active site residues in the plasmin–streptokinase complex are the same as those in the plasmin molecule. The main differences between the enzymatic properties of plasmin and the plasmin–streptokinase complex are found in their interaction with plasminogen and with α_2-antiplasmin. Plasmin, in contrast to its complex with streptokinase, is unable to activate plasminogen, and it is rapidly neutralized by α_2-antiplasmin, which does not inhibit the plasmin(ogen)–streptokinase complex. Because streptokinase generates free circulating plasmin, its use is associated with generation of a systemic lytic state.

Pharmacokinetic Properties

The elimination half-life of streptokinase in humans is approximately 20 minutes (initial half-life of 4 minutes and terminal half-life of 30 minutes) (127). The level of antistreptokinase antibodies from previous infections with β-hemolytic streptococci varies greatly among individuals. About 350,000 units of streptokinase is required to neutralize the circulating antibodies in 95% of a healthy population, with individual requirements ranging between 25,000 and 3×10^6 units (124). A few days after streptokinase administration, the antistreptokinase titer rises rapidly to 50 to 100 times the preinfusion value and remains high for at least 4 to 6 months, during which period renewed thrombolytic treatment with streptokinase or compounds containing streptokinase is impracticable because exceedingly high doses are required to overcome the antibodies.

Dosage

The initial dose of streptokinase must be adequate to neutralize the plasma levels of antistreptococcal antibodies: the streptokinase–antibody complex thus formed is rapidly cleared from the circulation. The initial dose for an individual patient can be determined either by the streptokinase resistance test or, more practically, a standard initial intravenous dose ranging from about 0.5 to 0.75 million units can be given over 10 to 30 minutes, followed by a continuous intravenous maintenance dose of 100,000 units hourly for 1 or more days. Such a fixed dosage regimen produces a satisfactory thrombolytic effect in most patients (128,129). Moreover, laboratory control is simplified and thrombolytic treatment can be started without delay. In the last 15 years, however, high-dose (1.5 million units), short-term (15 to 60 minutes infusion) streptokinase treatment has been routinely used in patients with acute myocardial infarction.

Anisoylated Plasminogen Streptokinase Activator Complex

Anisoylated plasminogen streptokinase activator complex (APSAC) was constructed with the intention of controlling the enzymatic activity of the plasmin(ogen)–streptokinase complex by a specific reversible chemical protection of its catalytic center. This approach should prevent premature neutralization of the agent in the bloodstream and enable its activation to proceed in a controlled and sustained manner (130).

Physicochemical Properties and Mechanism of Action

Anistreplase (APSAC, Eminase) is an equimolar noncovalent complex between human lysine-plasminogen and streptokinase (Fig. 17-4). The catalytic center is located at the COOH-terminal region of plasminogen,

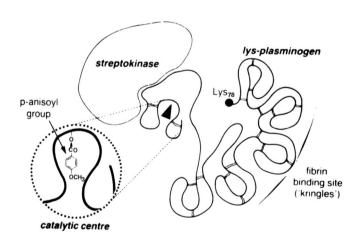

FIG. 17-4. Schematic representation of APSAC. (From Ferres et al., ref. 132, with permission.)

whereas the lysine binding sites are contained in the NH_2-terminal region of the molecule. Specific acylation of the catalytic center is achieved by the use of a reversible acylating agent, *p*-amidinophenyl-*p'*-anisate.HCl. The cationic amidino group is positioned to interact with the anionic carboxyl group of Asp^{735} within the catalytic center of plasminogen. The anisoyl head is located at a position near the Ser^{741} residue of the active center, so that the required acyl transfer can take place (130).

The reversible blocking of the catalytic site by acylation delays the formation of plasmin but has no influence on the lysine binding sites involved in binding of the complex to fibrin, although the affinity of plasminogen for fibrin is very weak. Deacylation starts immediately after dissolution of the lyophilized material and proceeds gradually after intravenous injection. Deacylation uncovers the catalytic center, which converts plasminogen to plasmin. This deacylation of the complex occurs both in the circulation and at the fibrin surface, and the fibrin specificity of thrombolysis by anistreplase is only marginal.

Pharmacokinetic Properties

Streptokinase slowly dissociates from the plasminogen-streptokinase complex with a rate constant of $<10^{-4}$ per second. In aqueous solution or in plasma, the deacylation (activation) rate constant of APSAC, however, is greater than 10^{-4} per second (131), and the activity of the complex is controlled by the deacylation rate rather than by dissociation. The deacylation half-life of anistreplase in human plasma was claimed to be 105 to 120 minutes (132), although it was previously reported to be 40 minutes in buffer (130). In healthy volunteers, an apparent clearance half-life of 70 minutes was found for anistreplase, as compared to 25 minutes for the plasminogen–streptokinase complex formed upon administration of streptokinase alone (127). In patients with acute myocardial infarction treated with anistreplase, half-lives of 90 to 112 minutes were reported for the plasma clearance of fibrinolytic activity (133).

Dosage

The recommended dose of anistreplase in acute myocardial infarction is 30 units (1 mg = 1 unit and 30 mg contains approximately 1.1 million units of streptokinase) to be given as a bolus injection. In aggregate, comparative studies indicate that the efficacy for coronary thrombolysis (angiographic patency) of anistreplase is comparable or somewhat higher than intravenous streptokinase but lower than intracoronary streptokinase (134).

In trials comparing anistreplase (30 units) versus intravenously infused streptokinase (1.5×10^6 U over 60 minutes), the same fall in fibrinogen concentrations and the same incidence of adverse events were noted (135). Because anistreplase contains streptokinase, it causes immunization. The antibody titer may increase up to 60-fold within 2 to 3 weeks and still be very high after 3 months (135,136).

CONCLUSION

Presently available (first-generation) thrombolytic agents include non-fibrin-specific plasminogen activators (streptokinase, tcu-PA, APSAC) and fibrin-specific agents (t-PA, scu-PA, staphylokinase). The clinical benefits of thrombolytic therapy in patients with acute myocardial infarction are well documented, and a close correlation between early coronary artery recanalization and clinical outcome is established. However, all available thrombolytic agents still have significant shortcomings, including the need for large therapeutic doses, limited fibrin specificity, and significant associated bleeding tendency and reocclusion. As a promising new development toward improvement of thrombolytic agents, mutants and variants of tissue-type plasminogen activator have been produced with reduced plasma clearance and lower reactivity with proteinase inhibitors and with maintained or enhanced plasminogen activator potency and/or fibrin specificity (e.g., reteplase, TNK-rt-PA, and the *Desmodus* salivary plasminogen activator). In addition, the bacterial plasminogen activator staphylokinase has shown promise for fibrin-specific thrombolysis, although neutralizing antibodies are elicited in most patients. The potential therapeutic benefit of these new second-generation agents over the presently available agents remains to be evaluated in large-scale randomized efficacy and safety studies in patients with thromboembolic disease.

REFERENCES

1. Collen D, Lijnen HR. Basic and clinical aspects of fibrinolysis and thrombolysis. *Blood* 1991;78:3114–3124.
2. Collen D, Lijnen HR. Molecular basis of fibrinolysis, as relevant for thrombolytic therapy. *Thromb Haemost* 1995;74:167–171.
3. The GUSTO Investigators. An international randomized trial comparing four thrombolytic strategies for acute myocardial infarction. *N Engl J Med* 1993;329: 673–682.
4. Collen D. Towards improved thrombolytic therapy. *Lancet* 1993;342:34–36.
5. Lijnen HR, Collen D. Strategies for the improvement of thrombolytic agents. *Thromb Haemost* 1991;66: 88–110.
6. Madison EL. Probing structure-function relationships of tissue-type plasminogen activator by site-specific mutagenesis. *Fibrinolysis* 1994;8(Suppl 1):221–236.
7. Verstraete M, Lijnen HR, Collen D. Thrombolytic agents in development. *Drugs* 1995;50:29–42.
8. Pennica D, Holmes WE, Kohr WJ, et al. Cloning and expression of human tissue-type plasminogen activator cDNA in *E. coli. Nature* 1983;301:214–221.
9. Lijnen HR, Collen D. Regulation of the fibrinolytic system. In: Agnelli G (ed). *Thrombolysis Yearbook 1995*. Amsterdam: Excerpta Medica, 1995;1–29.
10. Feng P, Ohlsson M, Ny T. The structure of the TATA-less rat tissue-type plasminogen activator gene. Species-specific sequences divergences in the promoter predict differences in regulation of gene expression. *J Biol Chem* 1990;265:2022–2027.
11. Kooistra T, Bosma PJ, Toet K, et al. Role of protein kinase C and cyclic adenosine monophosphate in the regulation of tissue-type plasminogen activator, plasminogen activator inhibitor-1, and platelet-derived growth factor mRNA levels in human endothelial cells. Possible involvement of proto-oncogenes c-jun and c-fos. *Arterioscl Thromb* 1991;11:1042–1052.
12. Medcalf RL, Ruegg M, Schleuning WD. A DNA motif related to the cAMP-responsive element and an exon-located activator protein-2 binding site in the human tissue-type plasminogen activator gene promoter cooperate in basal expression and convey activation by phorbol ester and cAMP. *J Biol Chem* 1990;265:14618–14626.
13. Margossian SS, Slayter HS, Kaczmarek E, McDonagh J. Physical characterization of recombinant tissue plasminogen activator. *Biochim Biophys Acta* 1993;1163: 250–256.
14. Novokhatny VV, Ingham KC, Medved LV. Domain structure and domain-domain interactions of recombinant tissue plasminogen activator. *J Biol Chem* 1991; 266:12994–13002.
15. Downing AK, Driscoll PC, Harvey TS, et al. Solution structure of the fibrin binding finger domain of tissue-type plasminogen activator determined by 1H nuclear magnetic resonance. *J Mol Biol* 1992;225:821–833.
16. Nienaber VL, Young SL, Birktoft JJ, Higgins DL, Berliner LJ. Conformational similarities between one-chain and two-chain tissue plasminogen activator (t-PA): implications to the activation mechanism on one-chain t-PA. *Biochemistry* 1992;31:3852–3861.
17. Tachias K, Madison EL. Converting tissue-type plasminogen activator into a zymogen. Important role of Lys[156]. *J Biol Chem* 1997;272:28–31.
18. Thorsen S. The mechanism of plasminogen activation and the variability of the fibrin effector during tissue-type plasminogen activator-mediated fibrinolysis. *Ann NY Acad Sci* 1992;667:52–63.
19. Hoylaerts M, Rijken DC, Lijnen HR, Collen D. Kinetics of the activation of plasminogen by human tissue plasminogen activator. Role of fibrin. *J Biol Chem* 1982;257:2912–2919.
20. Verstraete M, Bounameaux H, De Cock F, Van de Werf F, Collen D. Pharmacokinetics and systemic fibrinogenolytic effects of recombinant human tissue-type plasminogen activator (rt-PA) in man. *J Pharmacol Exp Ther* 1985;235:506–512.
21. Seifried E, Tanswell P, Rijken DC, et al. Pharmacokinetics of antigen and activity of recombinant tissue-type plasminogen activator after infusion in healthy volunteers. *Arzneim Forschung/Drug Res* 1988;38: 418–422.
22. Garabedian HD, Gold HK, Leinbach RC, et al. Comparative properties of two clinical preparations of recombinant human tissue-type plasminogen activator in patients with acute myocardial infarction. *J Am Coll Cardiol* 1987;9:599–607.
23. Otter M, Zockova P, Kuiper J, et al. Isolation and characterization of the mannose receptor from human liver potentially involved in the plasma clearance of tissue-type plasminogen activator. *Hepatology* 1992;16: 54–59.
24. Kuiper J, Van't Hof A, Otter M, Biessen EA, Rijken DC, van Berkel TJ. Interaction of mutants of tissue-type plasminogen activator with liver cells: effect of domain deletions. *Biochem J* 1996;313:775–780.
25. Orth K, Madison EL, Gething MJ, Sambrook JF, Herz J. Complexes of tissue-type plasminogen activator and its serpin inhibitor plasminogen-activator inhibitor type 1 are internalized by means of the low density lipoprotein receptor-related protein/alpha 2-macroglobulin receptor. *Proc Natl Acad Sci USA* 1992;89: 7422–7426.
26. Bu G, Williams S, Strickland DK, Schwartz AL. Low density lipoprotein receptor-related protein/alpha 2-macroglobulin receptor is an hepatic receptor for tissue-type plasminogen activator. *Proc Natl Acad Sci USA* 1992;89:7427–7431.
27. Neuhaus KL, Feuerer W, Jeep-Tebbe S, Niederer W, Vogt A, Tebbe U. Improved thrombolysis with a modified dose regimen of recombinant tissue-type plasminogen activator. *J Am Coll Cardiol* 1989;14:1566–1569.
28. Van de Werf F, on behalf of the COBALT Investigators. Randomized study of continuous infusion vs double bolus administration of alteplase (rt-PA): the COBALT trial [Abstract 511]. *Circulation* 1996;94 (suppl):I89.

29. Fay WP, Eitzman DT, Shapiro AD, Madison EL, Ginsburg D. Platelets inhibit fibrinolysis in vitro by both plasminogen activator inhibitor-1-dependent and -independent mechanisms. *Blood* 1994;83:351–361.

30. Kohnert U, Rudolph R, Verheijen JH, et al. Biochemical properties of the kringle 2 and protease domains are maintained in the refolded t-PA deletion variant BM 06.022. *Protein Engineer* 1992;5:93–100.

31. Keyt BA, Paoni NF, Refino CJ, et al. A faster-acting and more potent form of tissue plasminogen activator. *Proc Natl Acad Sci USA* 1994;91:3670–3674.

32. Gardell SJ, Hare TR, Bergum PW, Cuca GC, O'Neill-Palladino L, Zavodny SM. Vampire bat salivary plasminogen activator is quiescent in human plasma in the absence of fibrin unlike human tissue plasminogen activator. *Blood* 1990;76:2560–2564.

33. Kratzschmar J, Haendler B, Langer G, et al. The plasminogen activator family from the salivary gland of the vampire bat Desmodus rotundus: cloning and expression *Gene* 1991;105:229–237.

34. Bergum PW, Gardell SJ. Vampire bat salivary plasminogen activator exhibits a strict and fastidious requmirement for polymeric fibrin as its cofactor, unlike human tissue-type plasminogen activator. A kinetic analysis. *J Biol Chem* 1992;267:17726–17731.

35. Stürzebecher J, Neumann U, Kohnert U, Kresse GB, Fischer S. Mapping of the catalytic site of CHO-t-PA and the t-PA variant BM 06.022 by synthetic inhibitors and substrates. *Protein Sci* 1992;1:1007–1013.

36. Hajjar KA. The endothelial cell tissue plasminogen activator receptor. Specific interaction with plasminogen. *J Biol Chem* 1991;266:21962–21970.

37. Paoni NF, Keyt BA, Refino CJ, et al. A slow clearing, fibrin-specific, PAI-1 resistant variant of t-PA (T103N,KHRR296-299AAAA). *Thromb Haemost* 1993;70:307–312.

38. Martin U, Fischer S, Kohnert U, et al. Thrombolysis with an Escherichia coli-produced recombinant plasminogen activator (BM 06.022) in the rabbit model of jugular vein thrombosis. *Thromb Haemost* 1991;65:560–564.

39. Martin U, van Möllendorf E, Akpan W, Kientsch Engel R, Kaufmann B, Neugebauer G. Dose-ranging study of the novel recombinant plasminogen activator BM 06.022 in healthy volunteers. *Clin Pharmacol Ther* 1991;50:429–436.

40. Mülller M, Haerer W, Ellbrück D, et al. For the GRECO Study Group. Pharmacokinetics and effects on the hemostatic system of bolus application of a novel recombinant plasminogen activator in AMI patients [Abstract 63]. *Fibrinolysis* 1992;6(suppl 2):26.

41. Refino CJ, Paoni NF, Keyt BA, et al. A variant of t-PA (T103N, KHRR 296-299 AAAA) that, by bolus, has increased potency and decreased systemic activation of plasminogen. *Thromb Haemost* 1993;70:313–319.

42. Collen D, Stassen JM, Yasuda T, et al. Comparative thrombolytic properties of tissue-type plasminogen activator and of a plasminogen activator inhibitor-1-resistant glycosylation variant, in a combined arterial and venous thrombosis model in the dog. *Thromb Haemost* 1994;72:98–104.

43. Benedict CR, Refino CJ, Keyt BA, et al. New variant of tissue plasminogen activator (t-PA) with enhanced efficacy and lower incidence of bleeding compared with recombinant human t-PA. *Circulation* 1995;92:3032–3040.

44. Cannon CP, McCabe CH, Gibson CM, et al. TNK-tissue plasminogen activator in acute myocardial infarction: results of the Thrombolysis in Myocardial Infarction (TIMI) 10A dose-ranging trial. *Circulation* 1997;95:351–356.

45. Gardell SJ, Ramjit DR, Stabilito II, et al. Effective thrombolysis without marked plasminemia after bolus intravenous administration of vampire bat salivary plasminogen activator in rabbits. *Circulation* 1991;84:244–253.

46. Mellott MJ, Stabilito II, Holahan MA, et al. Vampire bat salivary plasminogen activator promotes rapid and sustained reperfusion without concomitant systemic plasminogen activation in a canine model of arterial thrombosis. *Arterioscl Thromb* 1992;12:212–221.

47. Mellott MJ, Ramjit DR, Stabilito II, et al. Vampire bat salivary plasminogen activator evokes minimal bleeding relative to tissue-type plasminogen activator as assessed by a rabbit criticle bleeding time model. *Thromb Haemost* 1995;73:478–483.

48. Witt W, Baldus B, Bringmann P, Cashion L, Donner P, Schleuning WD. Thrombolytic properties of Desmodus rotundus (vampire bat) salivary plasminogen activator in experimental pulmonary embolism in rats. *Blood* 1992;79:1213–1217.

49. Witt W, Maass B, Baldus B, Hildebrand M, Donner P, Schleuning WD. Coronary thrombolysis with Desmodus salivary plasminogen activator in dogs. Fast and persistent recanalization by intravenous bolus administration. *Circulation* 1994;90:421–426.

50. Neuhaus KL, von Essen R, Vogt A, et al. Dose finding with a novel recombinant plasminogen activator (BM 06.022) in patients with acute myocardial infarction: results of the German recombinant plasminogen activator study. *J Am Coll Cardiol* 1994;24:55–60.

51. Tebbe U, von Essen R, Smolarz A, et al. Open, noncontrolled dose-finding study with a novel recombinant plasminogen activator (BM 06.022) given as a double bolus in patients with acute myocardial infarction. *Am J Cardiol* 1993;72:518–524.

52. Smalling RW, Bode C, Kalbfleisch J, et al. More rapid, complete, and stable coronary thrombolysis with bolus administration of reteplase compared with alteplase infusion in acute myocardial infarction. RAPID Investigators. *Circulation* 1995;91:2725–2732.

53. Bode C, Smalling RW, Berg G, et al. Randomized comparison of coronary thrombolysis achieved with double-bolus reteplase (recombinant plasminogen activator) and front-loaded, accelerated alteplase (recombinant tissue plasminogen activator) in patients with acute myocardial infarction. *Circulation* 1996;94:891–898.

54. International Joint Efficacy Comparison of Thrombolytics. Randomised, double-blind comparison to reteplase double-bolus administration with streptokinase in acute myocardial infarction (INJECT): trial to investigate equivalence. *Lancet* 1995;346:329–336.

55. Holmes WE, Pennica D, Blaber M, et al. Cloning and expression of the gene for pro-urokinase in Escherichia coli. *Biotechnology* 1985;3:923–929.

56. Günzler WA, Steffens GJ, Ötting F, Kim SMA, Frankus E, Flohe L. The primary structure of high molecular mass urokinase from human urine. The

complete amino acid sequence of the A chain. *Hoppe-Seyler's Z Physiol Chem* 1982;363:1155–1165.

57. Ichinose A, Fujikawa K, Suyama T. The activation of pro-urokinase by plasma kallikrein and its inactivation by thrombin. *J Biol Chem* 1986;261:3486–3489.

58. Stump DC, Lijnen HR, Collen D. Purification and characterization of a novel low molecular weight form of single-chain urokinase-type plasminogen activator. *J Biol Chem* 1986;261:17120–17126.

59. Marcotte PA, Kozan IM, Dorwin SA, Ryan JM. The matrix metalloproteinase Pump-1 catalyzes formation of low molecular weight (pro)urokinase in cultures of normal human kidney cells. *J Biol Chem* 1992;267: 13803–13806.

60. de Munk GA, Parkinson JF, Groeneveld E, Bang NU, Rijken DC. Role of the glycosaminoglycan component of thrombomodulin in its acceleration of the inactivation of single-chain urokinase-type plasminogen activator by thrombin. *Biochem J* 1993;290:655–659.

61. Molinari A, Giorgetti C, Lansen J. Thrombomodulin is a cofactor for thrombin degradation of recombinant single-chain urokinase plasminogen activator "in vitro" and in a perfused rabbit heart model. *Thromb Haemost* 1992;67:226–232.

62. Gurewich V, Pannell R, Louie S, Kelley P, Suddith RL, Greenlee R. Effective and fibrin-specific clot lysis by a zymogen precursor form of urokinase (pro-urokinase). A study in vitro and in two animal species. *J Clin Invest* 1984;73:1731–1739.

63. Lijnen HR, Van Hoef B, Nelles L, Collen D. Plasminogen activation with single-chain urokinase-type plasminogen activator (scu-PA). Studies with active site mutagenized plasminogen (Ser^{740}→Ala) and plasmin resistant scu-PA (Lys^{158}→Glu). *J Biol Chem* 1990; 265:5232–5236.

64. Husain SS. Single-chain urokinase-type plasminogen activator does not possess measurable intrinsic amidolytic or plasminogen activator activities. *Biochemistry* 1991;30:5797–5805.

65. Liu J, Pannell R, Gurewich V. A transitional state of pro-urokinase that has a higher catalytic efficiency against Glu-plasminogen than urokinase. *J Biol Chem* 1992;267:15289–15292.

66. Liu J, Gurewich V. Fragment E-2 from fibrin substantially enhances pro-urokinase-induced Glu-plasminogen activation. A kinetic study using the plasmin-resistant mutant pro-urokinase Ala-158-rpro-UK. *Biochemistry* 1992;31:6311–6317.

67. Fleury V, Gurewich V, Anglés-Cano E. A study of the activation of fibrin-bound plasminogen by tissue-type plasminogen activator, single chain urokinase and sequential combinations of the activators. *Fibrinolysis* 1993;7:87–96.

68. Fleury V, Lijnen HR, Anglés-Cano E. Mechanism of the enhanced intrinsic activity of single-chain urokinase-type plasminogen activator during ongoing fibrinolysis. *J Biol Chem* 268:1993;18554–18559.

69. Husain SS. Fibrin affinity of urokinase-type plasminogen activator. Evidence that Zn^{2+} mediates strong and specific interaction of single-chain urokinase with fibrin. *J Biol Chem* 1993;268:8574–8579.

70. Declerck PJ, Lijnen HR, Verstreken M, Collen D. Role of α_2-antiplasmin in fibrin-specific clot lysis with single-chain urokinase-type plasminogen activator in human plasma. *Thromb Haemost* 1991;65:394–398.

71. Collen D, De Cock F, Lijnen HR. Biological and thrombolytic properties of proenzyme and active forms of human urokinase. II. Turnover of natural and recombinant urokinase in rabbits and squirrel monkeys. *Thromb Haemost* 1984;52:24–26.

72. Stump DC, Kieckens L, De Cock F, Collen D. Pharmacokinetics of single chain forms of urokinase-type plasminogen activator. *J Pharmacol Exp Ther* 1987; 242:245–250.

73. Collen D, Stump DC, Van de Werf F, Jang IK, Nobuhara M, Lijnen HR. Coronary thrombolysis in dogs with intravenously administered human pro-urokinase. *Circulation* 1985;72:384–388.

74. Flameng W, Vanhaecke J, Stump DC, et al. Coronary thrombolysis by intravenous infusion of recombinant single chain urokinase-type plasminogen activator or recombinant urokinase in baboons. *J Am Coll Cardiol* 1986;8:118–124.

75. Kuiper J, Rijken DC, de Munk GAW, van Berkel TJ. In vivo and in vitro interaction of high and low molecular weight single-chain urokinase-type plasminogen activator with rat liver cells. *J Biol Chem* 1992;267: 1589–1595.

76. Van de Werf F, Nobuhara M, Collen D. Coronary thrombolysis with human single chain urokinase-type plasminogen activator (scu-PA) in patients with acute myocardial infarction. *Ann Intern Med* 1986;104: 345–348.

77. Van de Werf F, Vanhaecke J, De Geest H, Verstraete M, Collen D. Coronary thrombolysis with recombinant single-chain urokinase-type plasminogen activator (rscu-PA) in patients with acute myocardial infarction. *Circulation* 1986;74:1066–1070.

78. PRIMI Trial Study Group. Randomised double-blind trial of recombinant pro-urokinase against streptokinase in acute myocardial infarction. *Lancet* 1989;1: 863–868.

79. Tebbe U, Windeler J, Boesl I, et al, behalf of the LIMITS Study Group. Thrombolysis with recombinant unglycosylated single-chain urokinase-type plasminogen activator (Saruplase) in acute myocardial infarction: influence on early patency rate (LIMITS Study). *J Am Coll Cardiol* 1995;26:365–373.

80. Weaver WD, Hartmann JR, Anderson JL, Reddy PS, Sobolski JC, Sasahara AA, for the Prourokinase Study Group. New recombinant glycosylated prourokinase for treatment of patients with acute myocardial infarction. *J Am Coll Cardiol* 1994;24:1242–1248.

81. Lack CH. Staphylokinase: an activator of plasma protease. *Nature* 1948;161:559–560.

82. Lewis JH, Ferguson JH. A proteolytic enzyme system of the blood. III. Activation of dog serum profibrinolysin by staphylokinase. *Am J Physiol* 1951;166: 594–603.

83. Winkler KC, DeWaart J, Grootsen C, Zegers BJM, Tellier NF, Vertegt CD. Lysogenic conversion of staphylococci to loss of beta-toxin. *J Gen Microbiol* 1965;39: 321–333.

84. Collen D, Silence K, Demarsin E, De Mol M, Lijnen HR. Isolation and characterization of natural and recombinant staphylokinase. *Fibrinolysis* 1992;6:203–213.

85. Sako T, Tsuchida N. Nucleotide sequence of the staphylokinase gene from Staphylococcus aureus. *Nucleic Acids Res* 1983;11:7679–7693.

86. Behnke D, Gerlach D. Cloning and expression in Es-

cherichia coli, Bacillus subtilis, and Streptococcus sanguis of a gene for staphylokinase—a bacterial plasminogen activator. *Mol Gen Genet* 1987;210:528–534.

87. Collen D, Zhao ZA, Holvoet P, Marynen P. Primary structure and gene structure of staphylokinase. *Fibrinolysis* 1992;6:226–231.

88. Sako T. Overproduction of staphylokinase in Escherichia coli and its characterization. *Eur J Biochem* 1985;149:557–563.

89. Gerlach D, Kraft R, Behnke D. Purification and characterization of the bacterial plasminogen activator staphylokinase secreted by a recombinant Bacillus subtilis. *Zentralbl Bakteriol Mikrobiol Hyg A* 1988;269:314–322.

90. Kowalska-Loth B, Zakrzewski K. The activation by staphylokinase of human plasminogen. *Acta Biochim Pol* 1975;22:327–339.

91. Lijnen HR, Van Hoef B, Collen D. Interaction of staphylokinase with different molecular forms of plasminogen. *Eur J Biochem* 1993;211:91–97.

92. Lijnen HR, Van Hoef B, De Cock F, et al. On the mechanism of fibrin-specific plasminogen activation by staphylokinase. *J Biol Chem* 1991;266:11826–11832.

93. Collen D, Schlott B, Engelborghs Y, et al. On the mechanism of the activation of human plasminogen by recombinant staphylokinase. *J Biol Chem* 1993;268:8284–8289.

94. Reddy KN, Markus G. Mechanism of activation of human plasminogen by streptokinase. Presence of active center in streptokinase-plasminogen complex. *J Biol Chem* 1972;247:1683–1691.

95. Silence K, Hartmann M, Guhrs KH, et al. Structure-function relationships in staphylokinase as revealed by "clustered charge to alanine" mutagenesis. *J Biol Chem* 1995;270:27192–27198.

96. Sakharov DV, Lijnen HR, Rijken DC. Interactions between staphylokinase, plasmin(ogen) and fibrin: staphylokinase discriminates between free plasminogen and plasminogen bound to partially degraded fibrin. *J Biol Chem* 1996;271:27912–27918.

97. Sakai M, Watanuki M, Matsuo O. Mechanism of fibrin-specific fibrinolysis by staphylokinase: participation of alpha 2-plasmin inhibitor. *Biochem Biophys Res Commun* 1989;162:830–837.

98. Lijnen HR, Van Hoef B, Matsuo O, Collen D. On the molecular interactions between plasminogen-staphylokinase, alpha 2-antiplasmin and fibrin. *Biochim Biophys Acta* 1992;1118:144–148.

99. Silence K, Collen D, Lijnen HR. Regulation by alpha 2-antiplasmin and fibrin of the activation of plasminogen with recombinant staphylokinase in plasma. *Blood* 1993;82:1175–1183.

100. Silence K, Collen D, Lijnen HR. Interaction between staphylokinase, plasmin(ogen), and alpha 2-antiplasmin. Recycling of staphylokinase after neutralization of the plasmin-staphylokinase complex by alpha 2-antiplasmin. *J Biol Chem* 1993;268:9811–9816.

101. Collen D, Lijnen HR. Staphylokinase, a fibrin-specific plasminogen activator with therapeutic potential? *Blood* 1994;84:680–686.

102. Lijnen HR, Collen D. Staphylokinase, a fibrin-specific bacterial plasminogen. *Fibrinolysis* 1996;10:119–126.

103. Collen D, Van de Werf F. Coronary thrombolysis with recombinant staphylokinase in patients with evolving myocardial infarction. *Circulation* 1993;87:1850–1853.

104. Vanderschueren S, Barrios L, Kerdsinchai P, et al. A randomized trial of recombinant staphylokinase versus alteplase for coronary artery patency in acute myocardial infarction. *Circulation* 1995;92:2044–2049.

105. Vanderschueren S, Stockx L, Wilms G, et al. Thrombolytic therapy of peripheral arterial occlusion with recombinant staphylokinase *Circulation* 1995;92:2050–2057.

106. Vanderschueren SMF, Stassen JM, Collen D. On the immunogenicity of recombinant staphylokinase in patients and in animal models. *Thromb Haemost* 1994;72:297–301.

107. Declerck PJ, Vanderschueren S, Billiet J, Moreau H, Collen D. Prevalence and induction of circulating antibodies against recombinant staphylokinase. *Thromb Haemost* 1994;71:129–133.

108. Collen D, Bernaerts R, Declerck P, et al. Recombinant staphylokinase variants with altered immunoreactivity. I. Construction and characterization. *Circulation* 1996;94:197–206.

109. Collen D, Moreau H, Stockx L, Vanderschueren S. Recombinant staphylokinase variants with altered immunoreactivity. II. Thrombolytic properties and antibody induction. *Circulation* 1996;94:207–216.

110. Vanderschueren S, Stassen JM, Collen D. Comparative antigenicity of recombinant staphylokinase (SakSTAR) and a selected mutant (SakSTAR.M38) in a baboon thrombolysis model. *J Cardiovasc Pharmacol* 1996;27:809–815.

111. Collen D, De Cock F, Demarsin E, et al. Recombinant staphylokinase variants with altered immunoreactivity. III. Species variability of antibody binding patterns. *Circulation* 1997;95:455–462.

112. Collen D, Stockx L, Lacroix H, Suy R, Vanderschueren S. Recombinant staphylokinase variants with altered immunoreactivity. IV. Identification of variants with reduced antibody induction but intact potency. *Circulation* 1997;95:463–472.

113. Vanderschueren S, Collen D, Van de Werf F. A pilot study on bolus administration of recombinant staphylokinase for coronary artery thrombolysis. *Thromb Haemost* 1996;76:541–544.

114. White WF, Barlow GH, Mozen MM. The isolation and characterization of plasminogen activators (urokinase) from human urine. *Biochemistry* 1966;5:2160–2169.

115. Mathey DG, Schofer J, Sheehan FH, Becher H, Tilsner V, Dodge HT. Intravenous urokinase in acute myocardial infarction. *Am J Cardiol* 1985;55:878–882.

116. Jackson KW, Tang J. Complete amino acid sequence of streptokinase and its homology with serine proteases. *Biochemistry* 1982;21:6620–6625.

117. Reddy KNN. Mechanism of activation of human plasminogen by streptokinase. In: Kline DL, Reddy KNN (eds). *Fibrinolysis*. Boca Raton: CRC Press, 1980; 71–94.

118. McClintock DK, Bell PH. The mechanism of activation of human plasminogen by streptokinase. *Biochem Biophys Res Commun* 1971;53:694–702.

119. Summaria L, Wohl RC, Boreisha JG, Robbins KC. A virgin enzyme derived from human plasminogen. Specific cleavage of the arginyl-560-valyl peptide bond in the diisoproxyphosphinyl virgin enzyme by plasminogen activators. *Biochemistry* 1982;21:2056–2059.

120. Markus G, DePasquale JL, Wissler FC. Quantitative determination of the binding of E-aminocaproic acid to native plasminogen. *J Biol Chem* 1978;253:727–732.

121. Camiolo SM, Markus G, Evers JL, Hobika GH. Augmentation of streptokinase activator activity by fibrinogen or fibrin. *Thromb Res* 1980;17:697–706.

122. McClintock DK, Englert ME, Dziobkowski C, Snedeker EH, Bell PH. Two distinct pathways of the streptokinase-mediated activation of highly purified human plasminogen. *Biochemistry* 1974;13:5334–5344.

123. Bajaj SP, Castellino FJ. Activation of human plasminogen by equimolar levels of streptokinase. *J Biol Chem* 1977;252:492–498.

124. Reddy KNN. Kinetics of active center formation in dog plasminogen by streptokinase and activity of a modified streptokinase. *J Biol Chem* 1976;251:6624–6629.

125. Siefring Jr GE, Castellino FJ. Interaction of streptokinase with plasminogen. Isolation and characterization of a streptokinase degradation product. *J Biol Chem* 1976;251:3913–3920.

126. Cederholm-Williams SA, De Cock F, Lijnen HR, Collen D. Kinetics of the reactions between streptokinase, plasmin and α_2-antiplasmin. *Eur J Biochem* 1979;100:125–132.

127. Staniforth DH, Smith RAG, Hibbs M. Streptokinase and anisoylated streptokinase plasminogen complex. Their action on haemostasis in human volunteers. *Eur J Clin Pharmacol* 1983;24:751–756.

128. Verstraete M, Vermylen J, Amery A, Vermylen C. Thrombolytic therapy with streptokinase using a standard dosage scheme. *Br Med J* 1966;5485:454–456.

129. Hirsh J, O'Sullivan EF, Martin M. Evaluation of a standard dosage schedule with streptokinase. *Blood* 1970;35:341–349.

130. Smith RAG, Dupe RJ, English PD, Green J. Fibrinolysis with acyl-enzymes: a new approach to thrombolytic therapy. *Nature* 1981;290:505–508.

131. Esmail AF, Dupe RJ, English PD, Smith RAG. Pharmacokinetic and pharmacodynamic comparisons of acylated streptokinase plasminogen complexes with different deacylation rate constants. *Haemostasis* 1984;14:84.

132. Ferres H, Hibbs M, Smith RAG. Deacylation studies in vitro on anisoylated plasminogen streptokinase activator complex. *Drugs* 1987;33(suppl 3):80–82.

133. Nunn B, Esmail A, Fears R, Ferres H, Strandring R. Pharmacokinetic properties of anisoylated plasminogen streptokinase activator complex and other thrombolytic agents in animals and in humans. *Drugs* 1987;33(suppl 3):88–92.

134. Verstraete M. Thrombolytic treatment in acute myocardial infarction. *Circulation* 1990;82(suppl 3):II96–II109.

135. Hoffmann JJML, Bonnier JJRM, de Swart JBRM, Cutsers P, Vijgen M. Systemic effects of anisoylated plasminogen streptokinase activator complex and streptokinase therapy in acute myocardial infarction. *Drugs* 1987;33(suppl 3):242–246.

136. Jalihal S, Morris GK. Antistreptokinase titers after intravenous streptokinase. *Lancet* 1990;335:184–185.

Cardiovascular Thrombosis: Thrombocardiology and Thromboneurology, Second Edition,
edited by M. Verstraete, V. Fuster, and E. J. Topol,
Lippincott–Raven Publishers, Philadelphia © 1998.

18

Agents Lowering Blood Viscosity, Including Defibrinogenating Agents

Gordon D. O. Lowe

Department of Medicine, Royal Infirmary, Glasgow G31 2ER, United Kingdom

There is increasing interest in study of the flow properties of blood (hemorheology) in relation to cardiovascular diseases (especially ischemia of the heart, brain, or lower limb; and venous thromboembolism) and in rheologic therapies (1–5). This chapter considers in turn:

The determinants of blood flow properties (e.g., blood viscosity);
The overt hyperviscosity states that arise in hematologic disorders, which occasionally cause thrombosis and ischemia, and which often indicate urgent rheologic treatments such as erythrapheresis, plasmapheresis, or leukapheresis;
The contributions of hemorheologic variables within their normal ranges to thrombosis and ischemia; and
Therapeutic agents that influence blood rheology and their current (or potential) uses in cardiovascular disease.

DETERMINANTS OF THE FLOW PROPERTIES OF BLOOD AND OVERT CLINICAL HYPERVISCOSITY STATES

Blood Viscosity

Clinical hemorheology research studies, performed in specialized rheologic laboratories, have used a range of methods to study the complex flow properties of blood (1–5).

Bulk whole-blood viscosity is the intrinsic resistance of blood to flow in wide vessels (arteries and veins): it can be measured either in simple capillary viscometers or in more complex rotational viscometers. Blood is a non-newtonian fluid, i.e., its apparent viscosity depends on the flow conditions of measurement, including the geometric constraints (vessel diameter) and the imposed shear stresses. Viscosity is defined as the ratio of shear stress to shear rate:

$$\text{Viscosity (mPa·s)} = \frac{\text{shear stress (mPa)}}{\text{shear rate (s}^{-1})}$$

The viscosity of water, plasma, and whole blood is temperature-dependent, with an increase in temperature decreasing viscosity. It is therefore customary to measure blood viscosity at normal body temperature (37°C).

When measured at 37°C in a capillary viscometer under high-shear conditions (shear rate >300 s^{-1}), when bulk blood viscosity achieves an asymptotic minimum value, mean blood viscosity in large random samples of the general population is about 3.5 mPa·s (SD = 0.5) in adult men, and 3.2 (SD = 0.5) in adult women (5). With decreasing shear rates of measurement, blood viscosity increases exponentially, due to both loss of shear-induced red cell deformation, and to increasing red cell aggregation under low-shear conditions. When measured in rotational viscometers, apparent blood viscosity (37°C) rises to about 18 mPa·s at a shear rate of 1 s^{-1}. Such low-shear conditions may arise in vivo in several circumstances (1–5):

At arterial bends and bifurcations (due to flow separation), which may be relevant to atherogenesis;

Distal to arterial stenoses (due to flow separation), which may be relevant to arterial thrombogenesis following plaque rupture;

In the ischemic microcirculation (distal to an atherothrombotic stenosis or occlusion), which may be relevant to the pathogenesis of both acute ischemia and chronic intermittent ischemia (stable angina or claudication);

In the deep leg veins of immobile persons (which may be relevant to venous thrombogenesis).

Although whole-blood viscosity is not measured in routine clinical hematology laboratories, such laboratories do routinely measure two of its major determinants: the cell volume fraction of blood (hematocrit), and a rheologic measure of acute or chronic phase reactant proteins such as fibrinogen [either plasma viscosity or erythrocyte sedimentation rate (ESR)].

Plasma viscosity has many advantages over the ESR (6) but paradoxically is less widely measured in routine hematology laboratories.

In the microcirculation, blood viscosity falls due to a dynamic reduction in hematocrit: this tends to minimize the effects of increasing hematocrit on ischemia. Plasma viscosity and the deformability of individual red cells are major hemorheologic determinants of microcirculatory blood flow. White cells have lower deformability than red cells and when activated adhere to microvascular walls, further reducing microcirculatory flow. Pathologic disturbance in red cell deformability (hemolytic disorders), white cell numbers and deformability (hyperleukocytic leukemias), or in platelet count causing platelet aggregation (thrombocythemias) are all factors that can disturb microcirculatory flow, resulting in ischemic syndromes (2–4). These hemorheologic disorders have little effect on bulk blood viscosity, measured in wide-bore viscometers; however, they markedly affect blood filterability through micropore filters with pore diameters of about 5 μm (Table 18-1). Like blood viscosity, blood filterability is not currently routinely performed in clinical hematology laboratories.

Hematocrit and Polycythemias

The sex difference in blood viscosity is largely due to the high hematocrit in men compared to women: 46% (SD = 3.5) versus 42% (SD = 3.5) using the microhematocrit method (5). In all patients with ischemia or thrombosis, a hematocrit should be performed routinely to exclude polycythemias (hematocrit over 53% in men and over 50% in women). Polycythemias are associated with increased risks of both venous and arterial thrombosis, and of ischemia. Possible mechanisms include not only hyperviscosity but also increased platelet adhesion to the vessel wall (due to mechanical displacement by red cells) and increased platelet activation (by both mechanical stresses imposed by red cells, as well as release of adenosine diphos-

TABLE 18-1. *Determinants of the flow properties (rheology) of blood, and of overt clinical hyperviscosity states*

Bulk blood viscosity (macrocirculation)		Hyperviscosity states
Hematocrit	Red cell count	Polycythemias
	Mean red cell volume (MCV)	
White cell count and volume		Hyperleukocytic leukemias
Plasma viscosity	Temperature	
	Fibrinogen, other acute phase proteins	
	Lipoproteins	
	Immunoglobulins	Myeloma, macroglobulinemias, polyclonal (e.g., rheumatoid arthritis, systemic lupus erythematosus)
Red cell deformation	Shear stress, hematocrit, plasma viscosity	
	MCV, shape	Hemolytic disorders, e.g.,
	Mean cell hemoglobin concentration (MCHC)	sickle cell anemia
Red cell aggregation	Shear stress, temperature, hematocrit	
	Fibrinogen, other acute phase proteins	
	Lipoproteins	
	Immunoglobulins	
Blood filterability (microcirculation)		
Hematocrit, plasma viscosity, red cell aggregation		
Red cell deformation		Hemolytic disorders
White cell deformation	Cell and nuclear geometry	Hyperleukocytic leukemias
	Activation	
Platelet aggregation, adhesion		Thrombocythemias

phate from red cells) (1–5). Hematologic advice should be sought for appropriate management. Absolute polycythemias (increased red cell mass) can be distinguished from relative polycythemias (decreased plasma volume or vascular compartment) by clinical assessment and blood volume studies.

Absolute polycythemias can be subclassified into primary proliferative polycythemia; idiopathic erythrocytosis; and secondary polycythemias due to hypoxic lung disease, cyanotic congenital heart disease, high altitude, and high oxygen affinity hemoglobins: their management has been reviewed (7). Treatment options to reduce risks of ischemia and thrombosis include venesection, isovolemic hemodilution, and erythrapheresis (Table 18-2).

Relative polycythemias may reflect primary contraction of the plasma volume, due to dehydration, capillary leak syndromes (e.g., burns), reduced oncotic pressure (hypoalbu-minemias), third-space syndrome (edema, ascites, effusions); or primary contraction of the vascular compartment, due to hypoxia, smoking, stress, hypertension, myocardial infarction, stroke, head injury, or pheochromocytoma (8). Management has been reviewed: it largely involves treatment of the underlying causes, but occasionally justifies regular venesection (8).

Plasma Viscosity, Red Cell Aggregation, and Plasma Hyperviscosity Syndromes

Unlike whole blood, plasma is a newtonian fluid whose viscosity is constant regardless of flow conditions. When measured at 37°C in capillary viscometers, plasma viscosity in large random samples of the general population is about 1.30 mPa.s (SD = 0.5) in adult men and women. The effect of individual plasma proteins on plasma viscosity increases with their concentration, molecular size, and

TABLE 18-2. *Therapeutic agents influencing blood viscosity or filterability*

Reduction in hematocrit	Venesection
	Isovolemic hemodilution, erythrapheresis
	Hypervolemic hemodilution
	Oral agents: vasodilators, antimalarials, cytotoxic agents
Reduction in plasma viscosity/ red cell aggregation	Plasmapheresis, plasma exchange, cytotoxics
	Lipoproteins: HELP, statins (LDL/cholesterol), fibrates (VLDL/triglyceride)
	Fibrinogen: thrombolytic agents, defibrinogenating enzymes (ancrod, batroxobin), fibrates (except gemfibrozil)
Increase in red cell deformability	Exchange transfusion
	Oral agents—see text
Increase in white cell deformability	Leukapheresis, cytotoxic agents, other oral agents (see text)
Reduction in platelet aggregation	Antiplatelet agents

asymmetry: thus, fibrinogen has a stronger effect than serum globulins (lipoproteins, immunoglobulins), which in turn have stronger effects than albumin. In acute and chronic diseases, the plasma protein pattern changes: there is an increase in fibrinogen and, later, in immunoglobulins, and a fall in albumin. Plasma viscosity therefore increases and is used clinically as a routine measure of acute and chronic phase proteins in disease (6).

These plasma protein changes in disease also increase red cell aggregation under low-shear conditions. The routine clinical red cell aggregation test of such plasma protein changes is the erythrocyte sedimentation rate (ESR) (6). Red cell aggregation also increases blood viscosity under low-shear conditions, as noted above.

Extreme elevations in plasma viscosity and ESR occur in paraproteinemias, causing the clinical plasma hyperviscosity syndrome (9). This can occur in myeloma (especially types IgG and IgA), in Waldenström's macroglobulinemia (IgM), or in rheumatic or autoimmune disease (due to increases in rheumatoid factors or polyclonal IgG polymers). Plasmapheresis or plasma exchange is effective in treatment, usually with concomitant cytotoxic drugs to inhibit proliferation of malignant clones producing the paraproteins (9).

Red Cell Deformability and Sickle Cell Disorders

Red cell deformability not only minimizes bulk blood viscosity, facilitating blood flow in the macrocirculation; it also permits rapid passage of individual red cells (whose resting diameter is 7 to 8 μm) through nutritive capillaries (whose diameter in human heart, brain, and skeletal muscle is 2 to 6 μm). Red cell deformation is promoted by increases in shear stress, hematocrit, and plasma viscosity; it therefore partially compensates for pathologic increases in hematocrit or plasma viscosity. Normal red cell deformability depends on mean red cell volume, normal shape, and mean cell hemoglobin concentration (MCHC), which determines internal cell viscosity. In hemolytic anemias, abnormalities in these variables decrease red cell deformability, contributing to hemolysis.

In the sickle cell disorders, more marked decreases in red cell deformability (especially under hypoxic conditions) contribute to microcirculatory occlusion and clinical vaso-occlusive crises (10). Treatment options for such crises include supportive care (analgesia, rehydration), transfusion or exchange transfusion (avoiding raising the hematocrit above 35% because higher hematocrits increase blood viscosity), and oral antisickling agents (10).

White Cell Deformability and Hyperleukocytic Leukemias

White cells are 700 times less numerous than red cells in venous blood samples but are 700 times more likely than red cells to plug micropore filters with pore diameters of about

5 μm in blood filtration tests. This ability of normal leukocytes to plug capillaries reflects their larger volume than red cells, and their nuclei and organelle-rich cytoplasm, which increase internal cell viscosity. In hyperleukocytic leukemias, high circulating concentrations (over 50×10^9/L) of immature, poorly deformable leukocytes can cause microcirculatory occlusion and the clinical hyperleukocytic syndrome (11). Treatment options include leukapheresis, cytotoxic drugs, and radiotherapy (11).

Thrombocythemia

The role of platelets in thrombosis has been considered in Chapter 2 and antiplatelet drugs in Chapter 8. Thrombocythemia can present with thrombotic or ischemic symptoms, due to occlusive platelet-rich thrombi in the macrocirculation and/or microcirculation (12). Antiplatelet agents such as aspirin may be beneficial in such patients (12).

CONTRIBUTION OF BLOOD RHEOLOGY TO THROMBOSIS AND ISCHEMIA IN THE ABSENCE OF OVERT HYPERVISCOSITY STATES

All patients with clinical symptoms of thrombosis or ischemia merit a routine clinical and laboratory screen to exclude overt hyperviscosity syndromes, due to the uncommon (but treatable) hematologic disorders reviewed in the previous section. A routine full blood count (which includes hematocrit, white cell count, and platelet count), plasma viscosity or ESR, and, if clinically suspected, tests for sickle cell diseases usually detect or exclude such disorders.

There is, however, increasing interest in the contributions of hemorheologic variables to thrombosis and ischemia, within their normal ranges, in the general population (2–5). Virchow's triad of factors predisposing to thrombosis includes local blood flow, which is influenced not only by cardiac output and local vascular geometry but also by the intrinsic flow resistance of blood (its viscosity). If extreme disturbances in blood flow properties can cause ischemia and thrombosis, even in the relative absence of cardiovascular disease (see previous section), it is quite possible that less extreme variations in blood rheology might also promote ischemia and thrombosis, especially in the presence of cardiovascular disease. As noted previously, the non-newtonian properties of blood can result in local increases in blood viscosity in areas of the vascular tree where atherogenesis, arterial thrombogenesis, ischemia, and venous thrombogenesis occur. At the microcirculatory level, there is increasing interest in the ability of leukocytes to block microvessels and to perpetuate ischemia under low-flow conditions (13).

Prospective epidemiologic studies (reviewed in 2–5) have shown that blood viscosity and its major determinants (hematocrit, plasma viscosity, red cell aggregation as measured by the ESR) as well as white cell count (13) are consistent predictors of both ischemic heart disease (IHD) and stroke. We have recently reported that whole blood viscosity was significantly associated with incident IHD and stroke in the Edinburgh Artery Study: a random population sample of 1,500 men and women aged 55 to 74 years (14); and with incident IHD in the West of Scotland Coronary Prevention Study of 6,595 men aged 45 to 64 years with moderate hypercholesterolemia (15). This association of whole blood viscosity with incident ischemic events was attributable equally to the association of hematocrit with IHD and stroke, which has been observed in other prospective studies (2–5,16–18); and to the association of plasma viscosity with incident ischemic events, which has also been observed in other prospective studies (19,20). These associations of blood viscosity, hematocrit, and plasma viscosity with incident ischemic events were partly due to their mutual associations with other cardiovascular risk factors such as cigarette smoking, blood pressure, and cholesterol; however, they remained statistically significant after multivariate analyses including these variables. Rheologic factors may therefore be mechanisms through which conventional risk factors promote CHD and stroke, possibly via influences on atherogenesis, thrombosis, and ischemia (5).

Approximately half of the association between plasma viscosity and incident CHD is attributable to fibrinogen (20), which is a strong determinant of plasma viscosity as well as risk of CHD and stroke (21; see also Chapter 5). Lipoproteins also contribute to the association of plasma viscosity and CHD (2–5,15). Fibrinogen is also associated with CHD risk independently of its effects on plasma viscosity (20), possibly due to its effects on atherogenesis and thrombogenesis (see also Chapter 5).

The potential importance of rheologic variables in acute coronary thrombosis is illustrated by their associations with adverse outcome in unstable angina (22,23). The potential importance of rheologic variables in chronic ischemia is illustrated by the association of plasma viscosity with intermittent claudication in the older population, even following statistical adjustment for the extent of stenoses/occlusions in arteries supplying the lower limb, as measured by the ankle-brachial systolic pressure index (ABPI) (24). There is also evidence for a role of rheologic variables in venous thromboembolism (25).

The results of these studies therefore suggest that rheologic therapies merit evaluation, not only in the overt hyperviscosity states due to uncommon hematologic disorders that were reviewed in the previous section, but also in the routine prevention and treatment of ischemic diseases as well as venous thrombosis.

THERAPEUTIC AGENTS INFLUENCING BLOOD RHEOLOGY IN CARDIOVASCULAR DISEASE

Table 18-2 summarizes therapeutic agents that influence blood rheology (blood viscosity or filterability) in cardiovascular disease. The four main approaches are reduction in hematocrit; reduction in plasma lipoproteins, which influence plasma viscosity and red cell aggregation; reduction in plasma fibrinogen, which

also influences plasma viscosity and red cell aggregation; and increase in red cell or white cell deformability (26).

Reduction in Hematocrit

While reduction in hematocrit is potentially beneficial in reducing blood viscosity, platelet activation, and cardiovascular risk, potentially adverse effects include reduced oxygen transport capacity, acute changes in blood volume, thrombocytosis and iron deficiency following venesection, and reactions to infused fluids (26). The management of polycythemias has been reviewed elsewhere (7,8). Possible approaches to hematocrit reduction are listed in Table 18-2.

Primary prevention in persons without evidence of cardiovascular disease and with moderately elevated hematocrit who are not overtly polycythemic is problematic. Hematocrits repeatedly above 0.50 are associated with a two- to fourfold increase in risk of CHD and stroke, partly associated with increased blood viscosity (2–5,14–18). Global assessment of cardiovascular risk should be followed by treatment of risk factors, especially cigarette smoking and hypertension. Reduction in cigarette smoking and treatment of hypertension (especially with vasodilator drugs) may be followed by a reduction in hematocrit. If not, antiplatelet prophylaxis (e.g., with aspirin) may be justified, in view of the increased risk of CHD and stroke, and of the results of primary prevention trials (27). Regular venesection is of unproven benefit: A randomized trial (28) was prematurely terminated due to poor recruitment (T. C. Pearson, personal communication). Regular blood donation is associated with decreased risk of CHD (29), and while this cannot be prescribed, it should not be advised against in persons with high-normal hematocrit who have no contraindications to blood donation.

Acute hematocrit reduction in acute ischemia is of unproven benefit. Hemodilution with dextran is ineffective in acute stroke (29); however, customized hemodilution with albumin, monitoring hematocrit and hemodynamics may be beneficial but requires monitoring in an intensive care unit (30). There are no randomized trials of hematocrit reduction in acute myocardial or peripheral ischemia.

Chronic Hematocrit Reduction in Chronic Intermittent Stable Ischemia (Stable Angina or Claudication)

Randomized trials of hemodilution have shown benefit in claudication (31); however, this treatment is tedious and an exercise program may be equally beneficial in reducing viscosity and increasing claudication distance (32,33). There are no reported randomized trials of hematocrit reduction in stable angina.

Secondary Prevention of Coronary Heart Disease and Stroke

Hematocrit reduction has not been evaluated in controlled trials. In persons with evidence of cardiovascular disease and high-normal hematocrit, it would seem reasonable to follow the management advice as for primary prevention (see above).

Other Conditions

Preoperative isovolemic hemodilution has an established place in elective major surgery; there is also evidence that it reduces the risk of deep vein thrombosis after elective hip replacement (34). Controlled trials have also reported benefit from this procedure in central retinal vein occlusion (35).

Reduction in Plasma Viscosity/ Red Cell Aggregation

Lipoproteins

Heparin-induced extracorporeal LDL precipitation (HELP) is highly effective in reducing plasma levels of LDL, as well as fibrinogen, hence reducing plasma and blood viscosity as well as cholesterol and triglyceride (36). It is expensive but may have a role in prevention of IHD in persons with severe hypercholesterolemia (36).

Statins (HMG CoA reductase inhibitors), including fluvastatin, pravastatin, and simvastatin, are also effective in lowering low-density lipoprotein (LDL) cholesterol and, to a lesser extent, in lowering very-low-density lipoprotein (VLDL) cholesterol and triglyceride and in raising high-density lipoprotein (HDL) cholesterol. Recent studies have shown that statins are effective in both primary and secondary prevention of IHD; this is only partly explained by reducing progression of atherosclerosis (37). The largest primary prevention trial was the West of Scotland Coronary Prevention Study, in which pravastatin (40 mg per day) reduced the relative risk of IHD death or nonfatal myocardial infarction by 31% (38). In this study, we observed that pravastatin significantly lowered plasma and blood viscosity after 1 year, by about one fourth of a standard deviation (15). This was largely attributable to reduction in LDL (by 25%) and partly to reduction in VLDL (by 10%): pravastatin had no significant effects on fibrinogen or hematocrit. The plasma viscosity reduction was consistent with decreases in hazard ratios for IHD of about 6% to 8% in the WOSCOPS Study (15,38) and in other prospective studies of plasma viscosity (14,19,20). It is therefore plausible that viscosity reduction may account for about one fourth of the risk reduction by pravastatin, whereas the remaining risk reduction may reflect other mechanisms including effects on coronary artery plaques, endothelial function, and thrombotic tendency (37).

Fibrates, which include bezafibrate, ciprofibrate, clofibrate, fenofibrate, and gemfibrozil, are less effective in lowering LDL cholesterol than statins. However, they are more effective in lowering VLDL cholesterol and triglyceride than statins; furthermore (with the exception of gemfibrozil, which appears to have no consistent effect), they lower plasma fibrinogen, on average by about 20% (39–42). In epidemiologic terms, these reductions in fibrinogen (14,15,19–21,43) and triglyceride (44) have significant potential to reduce risk of IHD, over and above any reduction in LDL by fibrates. In part, such reduction in risk could be mediated partly by reduced plasma and blood viscosity (14,15,19–21,39,45,46).

The WHO study of primary prevention with clofibrate (47,48) showed significant reductions in plasma fibrinogen (48) and myocardial infarction (47), but a significant increase in total mortality (48) that has never been explained. A recent study of bezafibrate in secondary prevention of IHD following myocardial infarction showed significant reductions both in recurrence and in angiographic progression of coronary atherosclerosis (49), similar to that observed in trials of statins. Ongoing, larger randomized trials of bezafibrate in secondary prevention following myocardial infarction (50) or peripheral arterial disease (41) will clarify both the role of fibrates in secondary prevention of cardiovascular events and the role of fibrinogen in the pathogenesis of such events (21). Peripheral arterial disease is a particularly attractive area for trials of fibrinogen reduction by fibrates because of the epidemiologic evidence that fibrinogen (and hence, plasma and blood viscosity) is strongly related to peripheral atherosclerosis (24,51), claudication in the presence of a standard degree of peripheral arterial stenosis, mortality, and occlusion of peripheral bypass arterial grafts (54,55). Reduction in fibrinogen and viscosity by fibrates might be beneficial for claudication (39,56) as well as for reduction in arterial events.

Reduction in restenosis after coronary or peripheral angioplasty by fibrates also merits investigation (57) because fibrinogen is a risk factor for restenosis (58,59).

Fibrinogen

Lifestyle changes that may lower fibrinogen include stopping smoking, exercise, moderate alcohol consumption, and possibly weight reduction (42). However, compliance with lifestyle advice is notoriously poor. Chronic reduction in plasma fibrinogen with *oral agents* is achieved most effectively by certain fibrates (see previous section). Other oral

drugs that lower plasma fibrinogen levels by at least 10% include anabolic steroids, whose use is limited by adverse effects including hyperlipidemia and myocardial infarction (60); and the platelet inhibitor ticlopidine (61). The latter will probably be replaced by its derivative, clopidogrel, which has fewer adverse effects (62) but does not lower fibrinogen levels (63). There is little evidence that other oral drugs lower fibrinogen (42).

Thrombolytic Agents

These have been reviewed in Chapter 17. In addition to their thrombolytic actions, these plasminogen activators generate plasmin, which digests not only fibrin but also plasma fibrinogen, lowering plasma viscosity, red cell aggregation, and blood viscosity (especially at low shear rates) (26,62–65). These rheologic effects may be relevant to maintenance of blood flow in ischemic tissues, reduction in infarct size, and clinical benefits (reduction in morbidity and mortality). Streptokinase and anistreplase have similar effects on plasma fibrinogen, rapidly reducing levels of clottable fibrinogen and increasing levels of terminal fibrin(ogen) degradation products (FDP) (62–64). Alteplase reduces fibrinogen to a lesser extent, generates earlier FDP of higher molecular weight, and hence has a lesser rheologic effect than streptokinase (64), although there is a lesser difference when alteplase is given as a bolus (66). This may partly explain why alteplase and streptokinase have similar clinical benefits in acute myocardial infarction, despite early coronary artery patency with alteplase (67).

Chronic low-dose intermittent *urokinase* (500,000 IU three times weekly for 3 to 12 weeks) lowers plasma fibrinogen by about 35%, plasma viscosity by 6%, and red cell aggregation by 20%; it has been reported to give symptomatic benefit in end-stage IHD (refractory angina pectoris) or peripheral arterial disease (critical limb ischemia) (68). Randomized trials are required to assess this approach to therapy.

Defibrinogenating Agents

Ancrod and *batroxobin* are thrombin-like enzymes purified from pit viper venoms (69,70). In contrast to thrombin, they release only fibrinopeptide A (not B) from fibrinogen, and do not activate coagulation factor XIII which cross-links fibrin. Thus following intravenous or subcutaneous injection in humans, soluble fibrin is formed that is rapidly cleared from the circulation (probably by the reticuloendothelial system, and the plasmin system because plasma plasminogen falls markedly). As a result, plasma fibrinogen falls rapidly and terminal plasma FDP increase markedly; these effects are similar to those of thrombolytic agents, but the risk of bleeding is less, presumably because of the lack of a direct fibrinolytic effect upon hemostatic plugs and the lack of effect on factors V and VIII.

Most clinical studies have been performed with ancrod. Following intravenous infusion of ancrod, plasma fibrinogen levels can be maintained at under 0.5 g/L by repeated intravenous injections once or twice daily. Such treatment provides effective anticoagulation, and is an effective alternative to conventional heparin infusions for treatment of deep vein thrombosis (71), e.g., in the presence of heparin-induced thrombocytopenia/thrombosis (72–74). Ancrod is available by compassionate release for this purpose in the United States (74). Subcutaneous injections maintain plasma fibrinogen levels at about 1 g/L when given daily; they are more convenient than intravenous therapy, have a lower risk of reactions, and appear to reduce plasma viscosity, blood viscosity, and red cell aggregation as effectively (70). Plasma viscosity falls by about 10% (to a value approaching serum viscosity), and high-shear blood viscosity falls to a similar extent (75–77). Red cell aggregation and hence low-shear blood viscosity fall to a greater extent (78). These rheologic effects may be relevant to both the antithrombotic effects of ancrod (71,76) and its potential benefits in ischemia (see below). After 4 to 6 weeks of therapy, ancrod and batroxobin are frequently inactivated by antibodies and fibrinogen levels return to normal; however, adverse clinical reactions due to these antibodies appear rare (70).

Randomized trials of ancrod have shown it to be effective in both prevention (76) and treatment (71) of deep vein thrombosis; however, in view of the widespread use of unfractionated (and, recently, of low molecular weight) heparins its use is currently reserved for uncommon situations such as heparin-induced thrombocytopenia/thrombosis (72–74). The author has occasionally used ancrod successfully in cases of progressive thrombosis despite conventional heparin/warfarin therapy in patients with malignant disease (in whom high levels of cancer procoagulants and fibrinogen, and low levels of protein C and S, may result in resistance to heparin and warfarin). There are also observational reports of ancrod in retinal vein thrombosis and in the prevention of thrombosis in venous grafts (70).

In peripheral arterial disease, there are observational reports of ancrod in severe intermittent claudication (78) or critical limb ischemia (71); however, three small randomized trials showed no benefit over placebo (77,79,80). In ischemic heart disease, only small observational studies in unstable angina have been reported (81,82). There are no reported studies in acute myocardial infarction; however, the possibility that ancrod might reduce the incidence of reinfarction by maintaining low plasma fibrinogen and viscosity levels following thrombolytic therapy merits future investigation.

In acute ischemic stroke, small trials of ancrod demonstrated its feasibility (83–85), apparent safety (lack of intracranial hemorrhage), and an indirect effect in promoting thrombolysis (85). A larger randomized trial in 132 patients with moderate to severe ischemic stroke, starting ancrod within 6 hours of stroke onset, showed that this treatment appeared safe and was associated with dose-dependent (plasma fibrinogen level) reductions in both cerebral infarct size and adverse clinical outcome (86). Two larger randomized trials (starting ancrod within 3 hours of stroke onset) are currently in progress in the United States and Europe to determine whether or not defibrinogenation results in clinical benefit. If it does, ancrod therapy may be competitive (at less hemorrhagic risk) in acute ischemic stroke with alteplase, which has recently been shown to improve clinical outcome when started within 3 hours of stroke onset, but at a cost of increased intracranial hemorrhage (87).

Agents Affecting Red or White Blood Cells

This is a controversial area in therapeutics. There is increasing evidence that red cell and white cell deformability have important influences on both blood filterability ex vivo and microcirculatory flow in vivo especially under ischemic conditions (88,89); and that they can be modified by stable prostacyclin analogues (see Chapter 15), antioxidants, and agents licensed for treatment of chronic peripheral and/or cerebral ischemia including cinnarizine, naftidrofuryl oxalate (90), and oxpentifylline (pentoxifylline) (91,92). Potentially, these agents may act by increasing oxygen delivery to ischemic tissues (93); hence they may be worthy of trial in patients whose daily activities are severely curtailed, especially by intermittent claudication (94, 95). Further advances in this area may result from epidemiologic studies relating objective measures of peripheral ischemia to markers of leukocyte activation such as plasma levels of neutrophil elastase (24); from improved methodology in evaluation of the rheologic effects of pharmacologic agents (96); and from improved methodology in trials in patients with peripheral arterial disease (97) or dementia (98).

CONCLUSION

Cardiologists should appreciate that ischemia and/or thrombosis may arise not only from arterial narrowing but from changes in the flow properties of the blood (hemorheology). While bulk blood viscosity (a global measure of its intrinsic resistance to flow in arteries and veins) and blood filterability (a global measure of its intrinsic resistance to flow in the nutritive microcirculation) are not currently measured in routine clinical laboratories, routine measurements of hematocrit, ESR or plasma viscosity, white cell count, and platelet count should be routinely scrutinized in patients with ischemia and/or thrombosis to detect *overt hyperviscosity syndromes* (99). Such syndromes are best managed in conjunction with hematologists.

Even in the absence of overt hyperviscosity states, cardiologists should recognize that there is increasing evidence from epidemiologic studies that variations in blood rheology in the normal range are associated with increased risk of not only ischemic heart disease, but also of stroke and peripheral vascular disease. Evaluation of hematocrit, white cell count, ESR or plasma viscosity, and fibrinogen may therefore merit equal consideration as conventional risk factors such as smoking, blood pressure, and serum lipids/lipoproteins. Indeed, part of the impact of conventional risk factors may be mediated through rheologic factors (e.g., smoking via fibrinogen, hematocrit, and viscosity; lipoproteins through direct effects on plasma and blood viscosity).

Hematocrits >0.50 are associated with increased risks of IHD and stroke. Reduction in smoking, treatment of hypertension (especially with vasodilator drugs), regular exercise and aspirin, and regular blood donation should be considered.

Lipoproteins and fibrinogen each increase plasma viscosity, red cell aggregation, and hence blood viscosity. Statins (LDL) and fibrates (VLDL, fibrinogen) may reduce cardiovascular risk partly by lowering plasma levels of proteins that have rheologic effects. Further trials are in progress to test this hypothesis.

Thrombolytic drugs may be beneficial in acute myocardial infarction partly through their rheologic effects (reduction in plasma fibrinogen and hence in plasma viscosity, red cell aggregation, and blood viscosity).

Defibrinogenation with ancrod (which has similar rheologic effects to thrombolytic drugs but less risk of bleeding) is currently under evaluation in acute ischemic stroke.

Oral agents that influence red or white blood cell deformability are currently under evaluation in chronic symptomatic peripheral or cerebral ischemia.

REFERENCES

1. Goldsmith HL, Turitto VT. Rheological aspects of thrombosis and haemostasis: basic principles and applications. *Thromb Haemost* 1986;55:415–435.
2. Chien S, Dormandy J, Ernst E, Matrai A (eds). *Clinical Hemorheology*. Dordrecht: Nijhoff, 1987.
3. Lowe GDO (ed). Blood rheology and hyperviscosity syndromes. *Baillière's Clin Haematol* 1987;1:597–861.
4. Lowe GDO (ed). *Clinical Blood Rheology*. Boca Raton: CRC Press, 1988.
5. Lowe GDO. Blood rheology, haemostasis and vascular disease. In: Bloom AL, Forbes CD, Thomas DP, Tuddenham EGD (eds). *Haemostasis and Thrombosis* (3rd ed). Edinburgh: Churchill Livingstone, 1994; 1169–1188.
6. Lowe GDO. Should plasma viscosity replace the ESR? *Br J Haematol* 1994;86:6–11.
7. Pearson TC. Rheology of the absolute polycythaemias. *Baillière's Clin Haematol* 1987;1:637–664.
8. Ishister JP. The contracted plasma volume syndromes (relative polycythaemias) and their haemorheological significance. *Baillière's Clin Haematol* 1987;1: 665–693.
9. Somer T. Rheology of paraproteinaemias and the plasma hyperviscosity syndrome. *Baillière's Clin Haematol* 1987;1:695–723.
10. Stuart J, Johnson CS. Rheology of the sickle cell disorders. *Baillière's Clin Haematol* 1987;1:747–775.
11. Lichtman MA, Heal J, Rowe JM. Hyperleukocytic leukemia: rheological and clinical features and management. *Baillière's Clin Haematol* 1987;1:725–746.
12. Wright SD, Tuddenham EGD. Myeloproliferative and metabolic causes. *Baillière's Clin Haematol* 1994;7: 591–635.
13. Ernst E, Hammerschmidt DE, Bagge U, Matrai A, Dormandy JA. Leukocytes and the risk of ischemic diseases. *JAMA* 1987;257:2318–2324.
14. Lowe GDO, Lee AJ, Rumley A, Price JF, Fowkes FGR. Blood viscosity and risk of cardiovascular events: the Edinburgh Artery Study. *Br J Haematol* 1997;96: 168–173.
15. Rumley A, Lowe GDO, Norrie J, Ford I, Shepherd J, Cobbe SM, for the West of Scotland Coronary Prevention Study Group. Blood rheology and outcome in the West of Scotland Coronary Prevention Study: is the benefit of lipoprotein reduction partly due to lower viscosity? *Br J Haematol* 1997;97(suppl 1):78.
16. Gagnon DR, Zhang TJ, Brand FN, Kannel WB. Hematocrit and the risk of cardiovascular disease—the Framingham Study: a 34 year follow-up. *Am Heart J* 1994; 127:674–682.
17. Wannamethee G, Shaper AG, Whincup PH. Ischaemic heart disease: association with haematocrit in the British Regional Heart Study. *J Epidemiol Commun Hlth* 1994;48:112–118.
18. Wannamethee G, Perry IJ, Shaper AG. Haematocrit, hypertension and risk of stroke. *J Intern Med* 1994;235: 163–168.
19. Yarnell JWG, Baker IA, Sweetnam PM, et al. Fibrinogen, viscosity and white blood cell count are major risk factors for ischemic heart disease: the Caerphilly and Speedwell Collaborative Heart Disease Studies. *Circulation* 1991;83:836–844.
20. Sweetnam PM, Thomas HF, Yarnell JWG, Beswick AD, Baker ID, Elwood PC. Fibrinogen, viscosity and the 10-year incidence of ischaemic heart disease. The Caerphilly and Speedwell Studies. *Europ Heart J* 1996; 17:1814–1820.
21. Lowe GDO, Fowkes FGR, Koenig W, Mannucci PM (eds). Fibrinogen and cardiovascular disease. *Eur Heart J* 1995;16(suppl A):1–63.
22. Fuchs J, Pinhas A, Davidson E, Rotenberg Z, Agmon J, Weinburger I. Plasma viscosity, fibrinogen and haematocrit in the course of unstable angina. *Eur Heart J* 1990;11:1029–1032.
23. Newmann F-J, Katus HA, Hoberg E, et al. Increased plasma viscosity and erythrocyte aggregation: indicators of an unfavourable clinical outcome in patients with unstable angina pectoris. *Br Heart J* 1991;66:425–430.
24. Lowe GDO, Fowkes FGR, Dawes J, Donnan PT, Lennie SE, Housley E. Blood viscosity, fibrinogen and activation of coagulation and leukocytes in peripheral arterial disease and the normal population in the Edinburgh Artery Study. *Circulation* 1993;87:1915–1920.
25. Lowe GDO. Blood rheology and venous thrombosis. *Clin Hemorheol* 1984;4:571–588.
26. Lowe GDO. Rheological therapy. In: Lowe GDO (ed). *Clinical Blood Rheology*. Boca Raton: CRC Press, 1988;vol II:1–22.
27. Patrono C. Aspirin as an antiplatelet drug. *N Engl J Med* 1994;330:1287–1294.
28. Tuomainen TP, Salonen R, Nyyssönen K, Salonen JT. Cohort study of relation between donating blood and risk of myocardial infarction in 2682 men in Eastern Finland. *Br Med J* 1997;314:793–794.
29. Adams HP Jr, Brott TG, Crowell RM, et al. Guidelines for the management of patients with acute ischemic stroke. *Stroke* 1994;25:1901–1914.
30. Goslinga H, Eijzenbach VJ, Heuvelmans JHA, et al. Custom-tailored hemodilution with albumin and crystalloids in acute ischemic stroke. *Stroke* 1992;23:181–188.
31. Ernst E, Matrai A, Kollar L. Placebo-controlled, double-blind study of haemodilution in peripheral arterial disease. *Lancet* 1987;1:1449–1451.
32. Ernst E, Matrai A. Intermittent claudication, exercise and blood rheology. *Circulation* 1987;76:1110–1114.
33. Gardner AW, Poehlman ET. Exercise rehabilitation programs for the treatment of claudication pain. *JAMA* 1995;274:975–980.
34. Vara-Thorbeck R, Rosell J. Invited commentary. *World J Surg* 1988;12:353–355.
35. Hansen LL, Danisevskis P, Arutz HR, Hovener G, Widerholt M. A randomised prospective study on treatment of central retinal vein occlusion in isovolaemic haemodilution and photocoagulation. *Br J Ophthalmol* 1985;65:108–114.

36. Seidel D. The HELP system: mode of action and clinical utility. In: Koenig W, Hombach V, Bond MG, Kramsch DM (eds). *Progression and Regression of Atherosclerosis*. Vienna: Blackwell Wissenschaft, 1995; 319–327.

37. Vaughan CJ, Murphy MB, Buckley BM. Statins do more than just lower cholesterol. *Lancet* 1996;348: 1079–1082.

38. Shepherd J, Cobbe SM, Ford I, et al. Prevention of coronary heart disease with pravastatin in men with hypercholesterolemia. *N Engl J Med* 1995;333:1301–1307.

39. Dormandy JA, Gutteridge JMC, Hoare E, Dormandy TL. Effect of clofibrate on blood viscosity in intermittent claudication. *Br Med J* 1974;iv:259–262.

40. Branchi A, Rovellini A, Sommariva D, et al. Effect of three fibrate derivatives and two HMG-CoA reductase inhibitors on plasma fibrinogen level in patients with primary hypercholesterolaemia. *Thromb Haemost* 1993;70: 241–243.

41. Meade TW. Fibrinogen and ischaemic heart disease. *Eur Heart J* 1995;16(suppl A):31–35.

42. Ernst E, Resch KL. Therapeutic interventions to lower plasma fibrinogen concentrations. *Eur Heart J* 1995; 16(suppl A):47–53.

43. Ernst E, Resch KL. Fibrinogen as a cardiovascular risk factor: a meta-analysis and review of the literature. *Ann Intern Med* 1993;118:956–963.

44. Hokanson JE, Austin MA. Plasma triglyceride level is a risk factor for cardiovascular disease independent of high-density lipoprotein cholesterol level: a meta-analysis of population-based prospective studies. *J Cardiovasc Risk* 1996;3:213–219.

45. Caimi G, Francavilla G, Romano A, Catania A, Santonocito G, Sarno A. Blood rheology changes during bezafibrate treatment. *Br J Clin Pract* 1988;42: 456–458.

46. Bo M, Bonino F, Neirotti M, et al. Hemorheologic and coagulative pattern in hypercholesterolemic subjects treated with lipid lowering drugs. *Angiology* 1991;42: 106–113.

47. Oliver MF, Heady JA, Morris JN, Cooper J. A co-operative trial in the primary prevention of ischaemic heart disease using clofibrate. *Br Heart J* 1978;40:1069–1118.

48. Green KG, Heady A, Oliver MF. Blood pressure, cigarette smoking and heart attack in the WHO co-operative trial of clofibrate. *Int J Epidemiol* 1989;18:355–360.

49. Ericsson CG, Hamsten A, Nilsson J, et al. Angiographic assessment of effects of bezafibrate in progression of coronary artery disease in young male postinfarction patients. *Lancet* 1996;347:849–853.

50. Goldbourt U, Behar S, Reicher-Reiss H, et al. Rationale and design of a secondary prevention trial of increasing serum high-density lipoprotein cholesterol and reducing triglycerides in patients with clinically manifest atherosclerotic heart disease (the Bezafibrate Infarction Prevention Trial). *Am J Cardiol* 1993;71:909–914.

51. Fowkes FGR, Pell JP, Donnan PT, et al. Sex differences in susceptibility to etiologic factors for peripheral atherosclerosis: importance of blood viscosity and plasma fibrinogen. *Arterioscler Thromb* 1994;14:865–865.

52. Banerjee AK, Pearson J, Gilliland EL, et al. A six year prospective study of fibrinogen and other risk factors associated with mortality in stable caludicants. *Thromb Haemost* 1992;68:261–263.

53. Fowkes FGR, Lowe GDO, Housley E, et al. Cross-linked fibrin degradation products, risk of coronary heart disease, and progression of peripheral arterial disease. *Lancet* 1993;342:84–86.

54. Wiseman S, Kenchington G, Dain R, et al. Influence of smoking and plasma factors on patency of femoropopliteal vein grafts. *Br Med J* 1989;299:643–646.

55. Woodburn KR, Rumley A, Lowe GDO, et al. Clinical, biochemical and rheological factors affecting the outcome of infra-inguinal bypass grafting. *J Vasc Surg* 1996;24:639–646.

56. Postlethwaite JC, Dormandy JA. Results of ankle systolic pressure measurements in patients with intermittent claudication being treated with clofibrate. *Ann Surg* 1975; 181:799–802.

57. Specht-Leible N, Schlierg G, Lang PD, et al. Fibrinogen and bezafibrate—a pilot study in patients following percutaneous transluminal coronary angioplasty (PTCA). *Clin Hemorheol* 1993;13:679–685.

58. Montalescot G, Ankri A, Vicart E, et al. Fibrinogen after coronary angioplasty as a risk factor for restenosis. *Circulation* 1995;92:31–38.

59. Stein D, Schaebel FC, Heins M, et al. Lipoprotein (a) and fibrinogen in restenosis after percutaneous transluminal coronary angioplasty. *Clin Hemorheol* 1995;15: 737–747.

60. Lowe GDO, Small M. Stimulation of endogenous fibrinolysis. In: Kluft C, ed. *Tissue-type Plasminogen Activator (t-PA): Physiological and Clinical Aspects*. Boca Raton: CRC Press, 1988;129–169.

61. Boisseau MR, Mazoyer E, Ripoll L, Drouet L. Does ticlopidine treatment lower plasma fibrinogen? A review of the literature. *Clin Hemorheol* 1994;14: 171–180.

62. Bruhn HD. Rheological consequences of fibrinolysis and of anticoagulation. *Clin Hemorheol* 1984;4:29–34.

63. Moriarty AJ, Highes R, Nelson SD, et al. Streptokinase and reduced plasma viscosity: a second benefit. *Eur J Haematol* 41:25–36.

64. Douglas JT, Hillis WS, Dunn FG, et al. Coagulation, fibrinolysis and viscosity during thrombolytic therapy of acute myocardial infarction with recombinant tissue plasminogen activator (rt-PA), APSAC and streptokinase. *Fibrinolysis* 1988;2(suppl 1):85.

65. Douglas JT, Hogg KJ, Gemmill JD, et al. Relationship of coronary artery patency to plasma fibrinogen, viscosity and plasmin activity following thrombolytic therapy with streptokinase or anistreplase in acute myocardial infarction. *Fibrinolysis* 1990;4(suppl 3):134.

66. Douglas JT, Gemmill JD, Hogg KJ, et al. Haemostatic and haemorheological changes and coronary reperfusion following bolus injection of rt-PA in acute myocardial infarction. *Fibrinolysis* 1990;4(suppl 3):68.

67. Collins R, Peto R, Baigent C, Sleight P. Aspirin, heparin and fibrinolytic therapy in suspected acute myocardial infarction. *N Engl J Med* 1997;336:847–860.

68. Leschke M, Schoebel FC, Straker BE. Low-dose intermittent urokinase therapy in chronic symptomatic end-stage arterial disease—clinical relevance for patients with coronary artery disease or peripheral arterial occlusive disease. *Clin Hemorheol Microcirc* 1997;17:59–66.

69. Stocker K. Defibrination with thrombin-like snake venom enzymes. In: Markwardt F (ed). *Fibrinolytics and Anti-fibrinolytics*. Berlin: Springer, 1978;481–484.

70. Lowe GDO. Defibrination, blood flow and blood rheology. *Clin Hemorheol* 1984;4:15–28.

71. Davies JA, Merrick MV, Sharp AA, Holt JM. Controlled trial of ancrod and heparin in treatment of deep vein thrombosis of lower limb. *Lancet* 1972;1:113–115.

72. Demers C, Ginsberg JS, Brill-Edward P, et al. Rapid anticoagulation using ancrod for heparin-induced thrombocytopenia. *Blood* 1991;78:2194–2197.

73. Souter RL, Ginsberg JS. Uses of heparin. Ancrod for heparin-induced thrombocytopenia. *Br Med J* 1993;306:1410.

74. George JN. Heparin-induced thrombocytopenia. In: Hull R, Pineo GF (eds). *Disorders of Thrombosis*. Philadelphia: Saunders, 1996;359–373.

75. Ehrly AM. Influence of Arwin on the flow properties of blood. *Biorheology* 1973;10:453–456.

76. Lowe GDO, Campbell AF, Meek DR, Forbes CD, Prentice CRM, Cummings SW. Subcutaneous ancrod in prevention of deep vein thrombosis after operation for fractured neck of femur. *Lancet* 1978;2:698–700.

77. Lowe GDO, Dunlop D, Lawson DH, et al. Double-blind controlled trial of ancrod in the relief of ischaemic rest pain of the leg. *Angiology* 1982;33:46–50.

78. Dormandy JA, Coyle KB, Reid HL. Treatment of severe intermittent claudication by controlled defibrination. *Lancet* 1977;1:625–626.

79. Martin M, Hirdes E, Auel H. Defibrinogenation treatment in patients suffering from severe intermittent claudication—a controlled study. *Thromb Res* 1976;9:47–57.

80. Tønnessen KH, Sager P, Gormsen J. Treatment of severe foot ischaemia by defibrination with ancrod: a randomised blind study. *Scand J Clin Lab Invest* 1978;38:431–435.

81. Leube G, Sondern W. Klinische Anwendung von Arwin bei Schwerer Angina pectoris. *Folia Angiol* 1975;23:411–414.

82. von Spottl F, Pimmingstorfer E, Fraschaker J. Therapeutic defibrination by Arwin in unstable angina pectoris combined with hyperfibrinogenaemia. *Wein Klin Wochenschr* 1978;22:792–796.

83. Hossmann V, Heiss W-D, Bewermeyer H, et al. Controlled trial of ancrod in ischemic stroke. *Arch Neurol* 1983;40:803–808.

84. Olinger CP, Brott TG, Barson WG, et al. Use of ancrod in acute or progressing ischemic cerebral infarction. *Ann Emerg Med* 1988;17:1208–1209.

85. Pollak VE, Glas-Greenwalt P, Olinger CP, et al. Ancrod causes rapid thrombolysis in patients with acute stroke. *Am J Med Sci* 1990;299:319–325.

86. Ancrod Stroke Study Investigators. Ancrod for the treatment of acute ischemic brain infarction. *Stroke* 1994;25:1755–1759.

87. The National Institute of Neurological Disorders and Stroke rtPA Stroke Study Group. Tissue plasminogen activator for acute ischemic stroke. *N Engl J Med* 1995;333:1588–1593.

88. Ciuffetti G, Mercuri M, Mannarino E, Robinson MK, Lennie SE, Lowe GDO. Peripheral vascular disease: rheologic variables during controlled ischemia. *Circulation* 1989;80:348–352.

89. Ciuffetti G, Balendra R, Lennie SE, Anderson J, Lowe GDO. Impaired filterability of white cells in acute cerebral infarction. *Br Med J* 1989;298:930–931.

90. Lehert P, Riphagen FE, Gaward S. The effect of naftidrofuryl on intermittent claudication: a meta-analysis. *J Cardiovasc Pharmacol* 1990;16(suppl 3):S81–S86.

91. Porter JM, Cutler BS, Lee BY, et al. Pentoxyfylline efficiency in the treatment of intermittent claudication: multicenter controlled double-blind trial with objective assessment. *Am Heart J* 1982;104:66–72.

92. Lindgarde F, Jelnes R, Bjorkman H, et al. Conservative drug treatment in patients with moderately severe chronic occlusive peripheral arterial disease. *Circulation* 1989;80:1549–1556.

93. Lowe GDO. Drugs that modify red blood cell characteristics. In: Fleming JS (ed). *Drugs and the Delivery of Oxygen to Tissue*. Boca Raton: CRC Press, 1990;253–264.

94. Lowe GDO. Conservative management of chronic occlusive arterial disease. In: Galland RB, Clyne CAC (eds). *Clinical Problems in Vascular Surgery*. London: Arnold, 1994;41–48.

95. Coffman JD. Intermittent claudication. In: Tooke JE, Lowe GDO (eds). *A Textbook of Vascular Medicine*. London: Arnold, 1996;207–220.

96. Nash GB. Measurements of blood rheology for the evaluation of pharmacological agents. In: Nimmo WS, Tucker GT (eds). *Clinical Measurement in Drug Evaluation*. Chichester: Wiley, 1995;99–119.

97. Demol P, Weihrauch TR. What are the valid measurements of drug efficacy in paitents with intermittent claudication? In: Nimmo WS, Tucker GT (eds). *Clinical Measurement in Drug Evaluation*. Chichester: Wiley, 1995;151–171.

98. Whalley LJ, Gerhard SJ. What to measure in dementia. In: Nimmo WS, Tucker GT (eds). *Clinical Measurement in Drug Evaluation*. Chichester: Wiley, 1995;23–43.

99. Frewin R, Henson A, Provan D. Haematological emergencies: hyperviscosity syndrome. *Br Med J* 1997;314:1333–1336.

*Cardiovascular Thrombosis: Thrombocardiology
and Thromboneurology, Second Edition,*
edited by M. Verstraete, V. Fuster, and E. J. Topol,
Lippincott–Raven Publishers, Philadelphia © 1998.

19

Mechanical Thrombectomy Approaches

Alexios P. Dimas and *Patrick L. Whitlow

*Hygeia Hospital, Athens, Greece; and
Department of Cardiology, The Cleveland Clinic Foundation, Cleveland, Ohio 44195

THE PROBLEM

The increased incidence and ominous consequences of complications arising when performing interventions in thrombus-containing lesions have been well recognized (1–6). Acute closure, myocardial infarction, and distal embolization are clearly increased with intervention in this setting. This issue of high risk is exemplified in the prototypical thrombus-laden lesion of a degenerated saphenous vein graft where the incidence of distal embolization has been found to be as high as 17.2% (7–11). The reported rates of distal embolization are certainly underestimating the scope of the problem because angiography is somewhat insensitive in detecting it (5,12). Graft age (7,13,14), extent of disease (13,15), and plaque burden indices (15) have been implemented as predictors of embolic events.

The Coronary Angioplasty Versus Excisional Atherectomy Trial (CAVEAT-II) investigators, besides identifying the use of the directional atherectomy catheter (a bulky device when compared to an angioplasty balloon) and the presence of thrombus as predictors of

distal embolization, have elucidated the acute and midterm (12-month) sequelae of such an event (16). Patients with distal embolization had a higher incidence of death (7% versus 1%) and myocardial infarction (68% versus 17%) than patients without embolization. At 12 months, distal embolization was associated with an increased incidence of myocardial infarction (odds ratio: 4.39) and composite endpoint for adverse outcome (odds ratio: 3.5) (Fig. 19-1A, B).

MECHANICAL THROMBECTOMY DEVICES

A host of devices aiming at mechanical removal or dissipation of thrombus have been proposed and applied in clinical practice or are currently under evaluation. The number of devices underscores both the difficulties encountered in combating intravascular thrombus and the intense effort to circumvent the problem. This chapter will focus on devices with coronary application; however, all currently available devices for intravascular thrombus removal will be included.

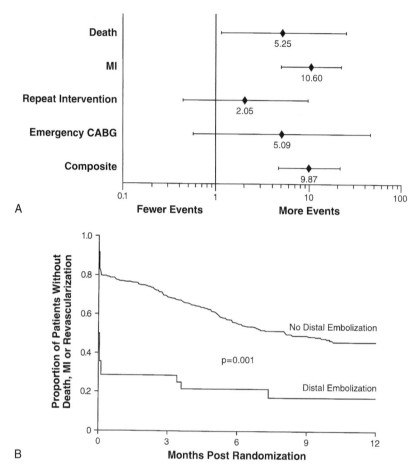

FIG. 19-1. A: Odds ratios and 95% confidence intervals for in-hospital outcomes after distal embolization in CAVEAT-II. MI indicates myocardial infarction; CABG, coronary artery bypass graft; and Composite, composite endpoint including death, MI, repeat intervention, or emergency CABG. **B:** Kaplan-Meier plots for freedom from the composite clinical endpoint of death, MI, repeat intervention, or CABG for patients (Pts) with and without distal embolization. (From Lefkovits et al., ref. 16, with permission.)

Transluminal Extraction Endarterectomy Catheter

Device Description (17-19)

The transluminal extraction endarterectomy catheter (TEC, InterVentional Technologies, San Diego, California) device is an over-the-wire, motor-driven, rotating torque tube with a cutter on the end designed to excise and extract atherosclerotic plaque and thrombus. Plaque is excised by two stainless steel blades arranged in a conical configuration at-

tached to the distal end of the hollow torque tube, and suction is applied via an external vacuum bottle (Fig. 19-2). These cutters are available in 5.0 to 7.5 French (Fr) sizes for coronary and 5.0-Fr to 15.0-Fr sizes for peripheral application.

The catheter drive unit houses a motor and trigger and has sites for attachment of a remote battery source and a vacuum bottle for retrieval of excised material. The trigger simultaneously activates cutting blade rotation (750 rpm) and suction. An operator-con-

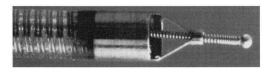

FIG. 19-2. Tip of the Transluminal Extraction-Endarterectomy Catheter (TEC) with the torque tube and the conical cutter head over a 0.014-in. TEC guidewire. (From Sketch et al., ref. 18, with permission.)

trolled sliding lever on top of the catheter drive unit initiates advancement and retraction of the cutter over a unique 0.014-in. guidewire. This wire with a rigid, extra support style shaft contains a radiopaque floppy tip with a terminal 0.021-in. ball to prevent wire tip entrapment in the rotating blades.

The procedure is performed using a percutaneous transfemoral approach following customary percutaneous transluminal coronary angioplasty (PTCA) premedication. A 10-Fr arterial sheath is placed allowing the introduction of a 10-Fr guiding catheter over a 0.063-in. wire or a 0.035-in. wire/catheter introducer to minimize trauma to the aortoiliac wall. After removal of the wire and/or introducer system and engagement of the target vessel, the 0.014-in. TEC wire is positioned across the lesion. The cutter is then advanced over the wire to the proximal end of the lesion with the advancer in the proximal, retracted position. Intracoronary nitroglycerin is administered prior to cutter activation to limit coronary spasm. Warmed (37°C) lactated Ringer's or saline solution is infused under pressure into the guiding catheter to create a dilute particulate slurry to facilitate aspiration of the excised material. The cutter is advanced and retracted slowly across the lesion to remove atherosclerotic material and thrombus.

Clinical Application

There have been three relatively large series pertaining to the specific use of TEC in the presence of intraluminal thrombus.

In a multicenter prospective nonrandomized trial (17) of 650 vein graft lesions in 538 patients (13.8% presenting with acute myocardial infarction), 183 lesions contained intraluminal thrombus. In the thrombus containing subgroup, a 90% angiographic success rate was achieved. Unfortunately, there is no separation of the complications noted according to the presence or absence of thrombus. Angiographically apparent distal embolization was 3.7% per lesion or 4.3% per patient for the entire cohort, and the major complication rate (death, myocardial infarction, coronary artery bypass graft) was 4.3% (3.4% in nonacute myocardial infarction patients). Although these rates compare favorably with the major complication rate of 14.9% reported by Platko et al. (7) for a similar group of patients undergoing balloon angioplasty, there are obvious limitations in such a comparison.

In a single-center experience (20), a 75% angiographic success rate was noted in 59 thrombus-containing lesions (group I) compared to 89% in 124 lesions without angiographic evidence of thrombus (group II). The clinical success rates were 69% and 88%, respectively. The composite endpoint of death, coronary bypass grafting, and Q-wave myocardial infarction occurred in 13.3% of group I versus 2.4% of group II patients (p < 0.001). With regard to angiographic complications, there was no difference between group I and group II in abrupt closure (5% versus 3%) or distal embolization (8% versus 6%), whereas the incidence of no reflow was significantly higher in group I (19 versus 5%, p < 0.05). In 74% of group I lesions, there was no angiographic evidence of thrombus following TEC application. Insensitive as the angiographic assessment of thrombus is, a similar rate (75%) of thrombus removal with TEC was found in a small series of 14 patients with unstable angina or acute myocardial infarction utilizing angioscopy (12)

The TEC or PTCA in Thrombus (TOPIT) study is attempting to determine whether extraction atherectomy prior to conventional PTCA is advantageous to patients presenting with acute ischemic syndromes. The primary endpoint is event-free survival at 6 months. An interim report of the first 153 patients ran-

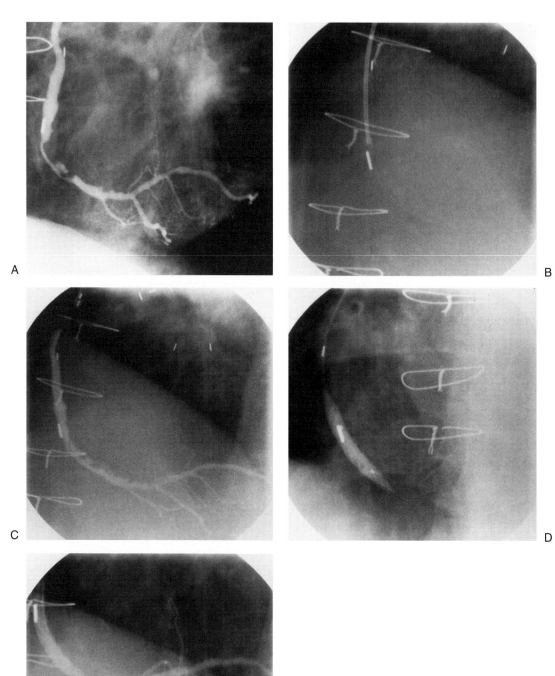

FIG. 19-3. A: A complex thrombotic vein graft lesion is visualized in this saphenous vein graft to the right coronary artery. **B:** Sequential 2.1-mm and 2.5-mm TEC devices are passed through the lesion. **C:** Angiography post TEC shows improvement in the stenosis and resolution of intravascular haziness. **D:** A 5-mm Palmaz stent is balloon expanded in the lesion. **E:** Postprocedure angiography documents resolution of the lesion without distal embolization.

domized (28.7% presenting with acute myocardial infarction, 12.5% with thrombolytic failure, 27.9% with postmyocardial infarction, and 30.9% with unstable angina) revealed a trend toward worse outcome in PTCA compared to the TEC group. Patients with unstable and postmyocardial infarction angina treated with PTCA had a higher incidence of five times normal postprocedure creatine kinase release, 7.1% for TEC versus 31.3% for PTCA (p = 0.045) (21).

In summary, TEC likely modestly decreases the risk of distal embolization and non-Q-wave infarction in thrombus-containing lesions. In combination with stenting to maximize lumen diameter and optimize flow dynamics, its benefit may be further enhanced and favorably influence complication profile and long-term results. However, any theoretical synergistic effect remains to be proven in a prospective, core laboratory–controlled, randomized study. A typical case of a saphenous vein graft with a thrombotic lesion treated with TEC and stenting is shown in Fig. 19-3.

Ultrasound Thrombolysis

Device Description (22)

The ultrasound thrombolysis device (Angiosonics, Wayne, NJ) is a 140-cm-long solid aluminum alloy probe ensheathed in a plastic catheter and connected to a piezoelectric transducer at its proximal end. Ultrasonic energy (45 kHz) is transmitted from the transducer as longitudinal vibrations of the probe that impart energy to the arterial segment. The last 18 cm of the device is a three-wire flexible segment with a 1.6-mm tip designed to optimize the thrombolytic effect of ultrasound. The three-wire tip design permits the use of proximal catheter solid metal for optimal ultrasound transmission while still achieving distal flexibility. The device fits into a 10-F angioplasty guide catheter and accepts a 0.014-in. guidewire through a coaxial central lumen in a monorail fashion. Power output and frequency at the handpiece (18 W)

is controlled by an integrated computer designed to ensure constant power output at the distal tip (10 longitudinal displacements) under the variable loading conditions encountered during the procedure.

Procedure Performance

The usual percutaneous interventional procedural protocol is followed. Patients are pretreated with aspirin and intravenous heparin to maintain an activated clotting time (ACT) >300 throughout the procedure. A 10-Fr guiding catheter is positioned as described for TEC atherectomy. A 0.014-in. typical angioplasty exchange length wire is positioned beyond the lesion. Optimal technique requires positioning of the ultrasound probe over the guidewire, 1 to 2 mm past the proximal end of the occlusion. During sonication, the probe is either left stationary or moved slowly back and forth with a small amplitude (approx. 3 mm). Sonication is carried out at 60-second intervals up to a total period of ≤3 minutes. Sonication is typically followed by PTCA and/or stenting.

Clinical Application

The safety and efficacy of percutaneous coronary ultrasound thrombolysis (CUT) has been tested in the Analysis of Coronary Ultrasound Thrombolysis Endpoints in Acute Myocardial Infarction (ACUTE) trial (22,23). The primary endpoint of the trial was normalization of perfusion (TIMI grade 3 flow) induced by coronary ultrasound thrombolysis. Secondary endpoints included vessel patency (TIMI grade flow ≥3) at 10 minutes and at 12–24 hours. Clinical events in the cardiac catheterization laboratory and during hospitalization were also tabulated.

Twenty-four clinically and angiographically eligible patients with evidence of acute anterior myocardial infarction and TIMI grade 0 to 1 flow in the left anterior descending artery were treated with the device. Following failure of CUT in the first patient, the technique was modified and remained unchanged for the re-

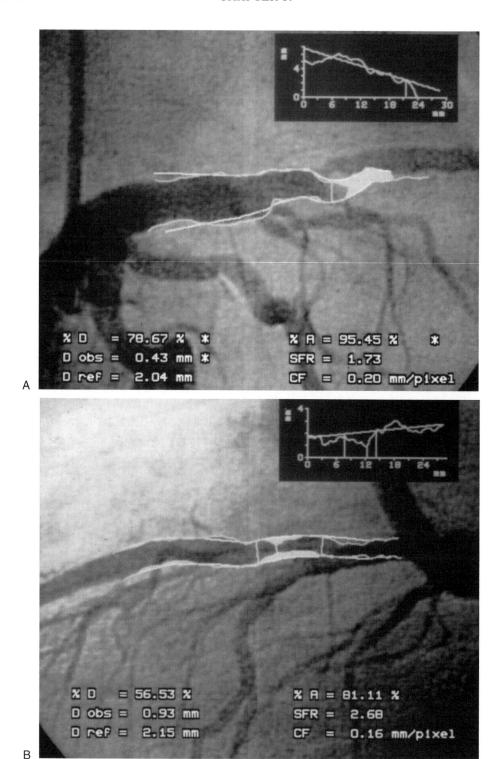

FIG. 19-4. A typical case of ultrasound thrombolysis. **A:** Total occlusion of the middle left anterior descending artery in a patient presenting with acute anterior myocardial infarction. **B:** Reestablishment of flow after 2 minutes of sonication.

mainder of the study. In the subsequent 23 patients, sonication achieved arterial patency in 22 (96%) with TIMI 3 flow in 83%, and post-ultrasound minimal lumen diameter (MLD) of 1.5 ± 0.8 mm with a residual stenosis of 48 ± 24%. There were no cases of dissection, perforation, embolization, side-branch occlusion, spasm, or no reflow. Adjunct PTCA resulted in final MLD of 2.4 ± 0.6 mm and residual stenosis of 20 ± 12%. A typical case is illustrated in Fig. 19-4. In-hospital reinfarction occurred in two patients (9%). Both were retreated with PTCA. There were no deaths, bleeding, or need for vascular repair. Eleven of the first 15 patients (feasibility phase of the study) experienced idioventricular rhythm at reperfusion. For the same feasibility subgroup patients at 6-month follow-up, there were no deaths, although myocardial infarction occurred in one patient associated with a new culprit lesion. Target lesion revascularization was required in four patients (27%).

Data from upcoming multicenter studies are needed to accurately determine the role of CUT across the spectrum of acute ischemic syndromes and in vein graft disease. A smaller size device compatible with a 7 Fr guiding catheter is planned and is expected to contribute to wider application of the technique in the future.

The Possis AngioJet (Possis Medical, Minneapolis, Minnesota)

Device Description (24)

The AngioJet is a three-component system consisting of an external and portable drive unit, a disposable connection tubing and pump set, and a disposable LF140 catheter. The catheter is introduced over a typical angioplasty guidewire. Thrombectomy is accomplished by the introduction of a pressurized high-velocity saline stream through

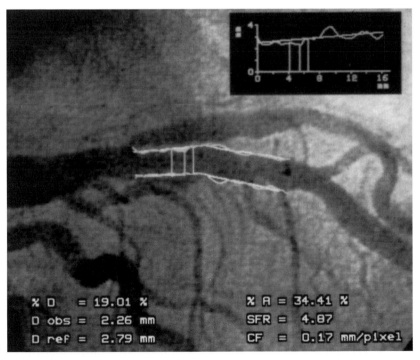

FIG. 19-4 *Continued.* **C:** Final result after low-pressure balloon angioplasty. (Courtesy of Uri Rosenschein, M.D., Tel Aviv, Israel.)

directed orifices in the catheter distal tip, so that thrombus is entrained by the low pressure created by the high-velocity saline, dissipated, and evacuated through the catheter and associated tubing. The external high-pressure pulsatile pump generates the flow necessary for the dissociation and evacuation of thrombus through connection tubing into an effluent bag.

AngioJet LF140 Catheter

The single use AngioJet LF140 catheter (Fig. 19-5) consists of a connection manifold, catheter body, and distal tip. The catheter's stainless steel tip components are 5 Fr in diameter, whereas the shaft diameter tapers to 3.5 Fr immediately proximal to the tip components. The manifold contains connections for the high-pressure saline input supply and effluent removal lines, and a hemostasis valve for sealing around the 0.014- to 0.018-in.-diameter guidewire. A stainless steel hypodermic tube traverses the catheter carrying high-

pressure saline to the distal tip. This hypodermic tube occupies one lumen of a dual lumen plastic tube. The other, larger lumen is used for the evacuation effluent and for passage of the guidewire. This lumen may also be used for hand injection of contrast when the pump is not activated.

The catheter tip is a stainless steel subassembly through which the stainless steel hypodermic tube extends and terminates in a loop. The loop contains six proximally directed jet orifices which deliver high-velocity saline back up the exhaust lumen. Openings in the catheter tip proximal to the jets transmit a Bernoulli effect–induced vacuum that sucks in thrombus, which is then dissipated by the saline jets and driven down the exhaust lumen of the catheter.

AngioJet Pump Set

The single-use pump set consists of a high-pressure saline supply line, a high-pressure pulsatile pump, an effluent evacuation line,

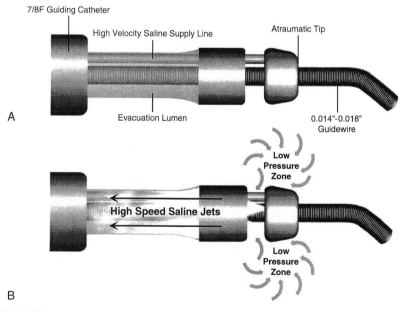

FIG. 19-5. A: LF140 catheter with atraumatic tip, high- pressure line, and exhaust lumen. **B:** Activated saline jets and a low- pressure zone that is created. The thrombus is drawn around the catheter tip for evacuation. (Courtesy of Possis Medical, Minneapolis, Minnesota.)

and an effluent collection bag. The pulsatile pump is a stainless steel assembly capable of functioning over a range of approximately 0 to 15,000 psi; however the drive unit controls the pump operation in the range of 8,000 to 13,000 psi.

AngioJet Drive Unit

This component generates the force to operate the pump set and catheter. The power for driving the high-pressure pump is generated by means of an electronically controlled, motor-driven mechanism. A peristaltic pump is located on the drive unit to control the rate of removal of thrombotic debris containing effluent. The drive unit is built into a mobile cart containing all mechanical and electronic components needed for operating the unit with the exception of the system-activating foot switch.

Description of the AngioJet Procedure

Patients are pretreated with aspirin and calcium channel blocker as for most standard percutaneous procedures. An 8-Fr guiding catheter is placed and positioned per usual technique. Heparin should be administered to maintain the ACT at ≥ 300 seconds. An exchange length 0.014- to 0.018-in. PTCA guidewire is positioned distal to the treatment site.

Because preliminary experience with the AngioJet procedure during the VeGAS 1 (see below) trial documented occasional bradycardia similar to that observed with rotational atherectomy, particularly when treating the right coronary circulation, it is recommended that a temporary pacing electrode be placed prior to the procedure.

The AngioJet catheter is advanced to the site of thrombus over a guidewire. A foot pedal control switch activates the high-pressure saline jets. Thrombectomy may be achieved by either distal-to-proximal or proximal-to-distal catheter movement. Several passes may be required to complete thrombectomy. Cineangiography should be obtained before and after

each AngioJet pass until visible thrombus is removed. This is usually accomplished in one to two passes. Adjunctive PTCA and/or stenting is generally required to optimize lumen dimensions (Fig. 19-6).

Clinical Application

The device has been tested in humans in the phase 1 trial *Vein Graft AngioJet Study* (VeGAS 1) (25). In this study, 90 consecutive patients with angiographic evidence of thrombus in either native coronary arteries ($n = 35$) or saphenous vein grafts ($n = 52$), presenting with unstable angina (68%) or acute myocardial infarction, (32%) were treated with rheolytic thrombectomy. In 7% of the enrolled patients, cardiogenic shock complicated the acute myocardial infarction.

AngioJet treatment alone reduced the thrombus area from 79 mm^2 to 21 mm^2 with the mean diameter stenosis improving from $77 \pm 21\%$ to $48 \pm 25\%$. Definitive adjunctive treatment was required in 97% of patients (stenting in 73%). Major complications occurred in 5 patients (3 deaths, 1 coronary artery bypass graft before discharge, and 1 Q-wave myocardial infarction). Angiographic complications included transient no reflow in 8 patients (11%) and abrupt closure in 3 patients (4%). Transient heart block requiring temporary pacing occurred in 20%. The overall procedural success was 87.7%, and the clinical success was 80%.

The European experience with the AngioJet (26) encompasses 35 patients (9 with saphenous vein graft thrombus). AngioJet success was achieved in 80%, whereas the procedural success was 86%. There were no deaths. Of note, temporary pacing was required in 63%.

Based on the encouraging phase 1 and European multicenter results, the multicenter VeGAS 2 trial was planned and has been underway since September 1996 (24). In this two-arm randomized equivalency clinical trial, 500 patients with angiographic evidence of thrombus without acute myocardial infarction within 3 days will be randomized at ap-

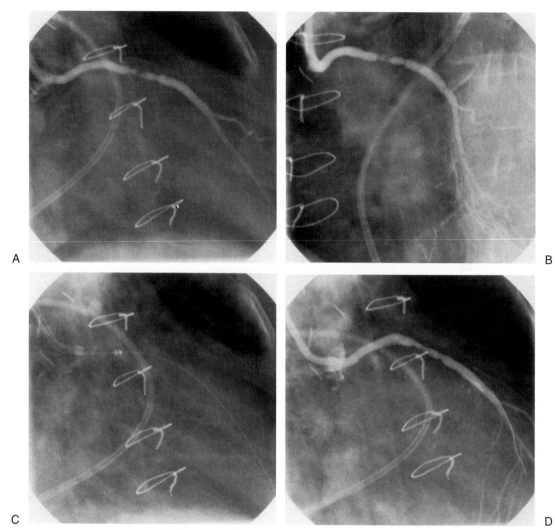

FIG. 19-6. AngioJet application in a thrombus-laden saphenous vein graft. **A:** Thrombotic lesion in a saphenous vein graft to the left anterior descending artery in the right anterior oblique view. **B:** Left anterior oblique view of the vein graft before treatment with the AngioJet. **C:** AngioJet just proximal to the lesion. **D:** Right anterior oblique view after AngioJet treatment.

proximately 20 American and Canadian centers to receive either AngioJet and definitive treatment or intracoronary urokinase and definitive treatment. All angiograms will be analyzed by a core angiographic laboratory.

The primary endpoint of the trial is successful acute clinical outcome defined as >20% improvement in MLD, final diameter stenosis <50%, and TIMI grade 3 flow, in the absence of death, stroke, Q- or non-Q-wave myocardial infarction, recurrent thrombotic vessel closure, emergent bypass surgery, or repeat target site revascularization within 30 days of the index procedure.

A series of secondary endpoints will also be assessed, including non-Q-wave myocardial infarction (with detailed stratification of creatine kinase-myocardial band [CK-MB] release), percutaneous access complications, hemolysis, hemorrhagic events, various an-

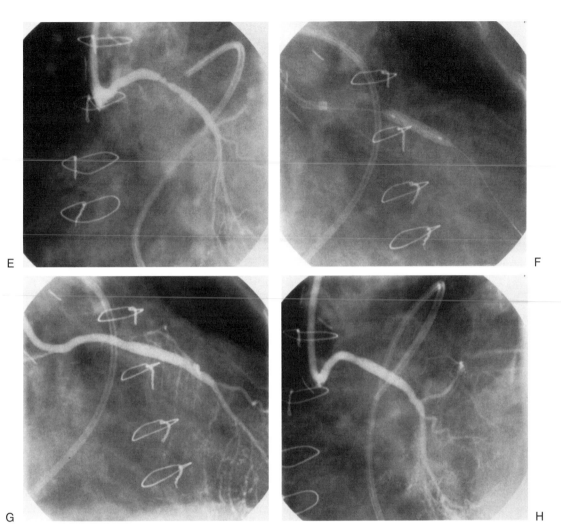

FIG. 19-6. *(Continued).* **E:** Left anterior oblique view post AngioJet treatment. **F:** Stent placement. **G:** Final result following stenting in the right anterior oblique view. **H:** Final result following stenting in the left anterior oblique view.

giographic outcomes, as well as 1-year target vessel success.

Extracardiac applications of rheolytic thrombectomy have been approved by the Food and Drug Administration and include thrombosed hemodialysis access sites where success rates of up to 100% have been reported (27). Peripheral arterial and venous occlusions and pulmonary embolism have also been successfully treated with the AngioJet.

Hydrolyser

Device Description (28)

The Hydrolyser (Cordis Europa, Roden, The Netherlands) is a double-lumen, over-the-wire, 7-Fr catheter consisting of a small (0.6 mm diameter) injection and a large (1 mm diameter) exhaust lumen with a sidehole located near the distal tip (Fig. 19-7). The catheter, which accommodates a 0.025-in.

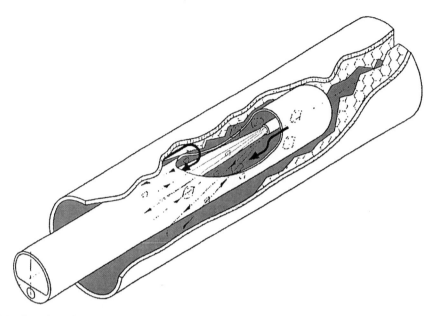

FIG. 19-7. Drawing of the tip of the Hydrolyser. The small lumen is the injection, and the larger is the outflow lumen. Injection of saline solution causes a Venturi effect at the nozzle at the tip of the catheter. (From Reeker et al., ref. 29, with permission.)

guidewire through the exhaust lumen, is made of nylon and has limited flexibility. The small injection lumen is connected to a standard contrast power injector that is filled with saline. At the tip of the catheter is a nozzle where the small injection lumen makes a U turn so as to direct the saline jet (infused at 3 ml per second at 750 psi) into the larger lumen. A negative pressure is thereby generated around the nozzle sidehole and suction is created. The thrombus sucked in by the negative pressure created by the high-velocity saline jet is fragmented on entry into the sidehole and is then removed as a mixture of thrombotic material and saline through the large exhaust lumen.

Clinical Application

Current indications include fresh or soft thrombotic occlusions up to 2 weeks old in vessels of 5 to 10 mm in diameter. This obviously limits the use of the device to large vessels. The two main areas of application to date are arterial thrombosis below the inguinal lig-

ament and thromboses of hemodialysis fistulas. Additional indications encompass pulmonary embolism and suprainguinal arterial thrombosis.

In a series of 28 patients (29) with arterial thrombosis below the inguinal ligament (11 native vessels and 17 grafts), successful thrombosuction (removal of more than 90% of angiographically assessed thrombus) was achieved in 23 (82%) patients (73% in native arteries, 88% in synthetic or composite grafts). Clinical success (defined as restoration of antegrade flow to the foot, with or without additional local therapy and resolution of symptoms related to the thrombotic occlusion by the time of hospital discharge) was 61% (73% for native vessels, 53% in grafts). The 30-day clinical success rate was 50% (73% and 35%, respectively). Amputation could not be avoided in three patients (11%).

Distal and proximal displacement of thrombotic material was observed only in grafts (7 patients) and led to modification of technique with subsequent elimination of this embolization problem. Overall 42% of patients required additional lysis as a result of either inability to access vessels smaller than 5 mm with the current design of the device or of distal thrombus displacement.

The first experience with recently (6 to 48 hours) thrombosed hemodialysis shunts included a series of 14 patients with 16 shunt thromboses (30). Successful thrombectomy was performed in 15 shunts. Early rethrombosis within 24 hours occurred in 5 shunts. At 6 months, cumulative patency was 41%.

In a clinical trial aimed at determining the safety and efficacy of the Hydrolyser in acutely thrombosed hemodialysis arteriovenous fistulas (n = 20) and prosthetic implant grafts (n = 17), the success rate with adjunctive use of balloon angioplasty in 95% and 80% of the cases was high (80% and 100%, respectively) (31). Patency at 1 month was 58% and 53%, respectively.

Finally, there have been reports of successful device use in arterial occlusions above the inguinal ligament, in pulmonary embolism, and in large venous (subclavian, iliac, caval, arm) thromboses (32). There has also been one report of Hydrolyser use in saphenous vein grafts with thrombus (33). Percutaneous thrombectomy was performed in seven patients with mean graft diameter of 3.9 mm and mean thrombus length of 15 mm. Successful thrombus removal was achieved in all cases; adjunctive balloon angioplasty was performed in six. No distal embolization was observed.

This preliminary experience outlines the potential of the Hydrolyser for coronary applications provided that smaller devices also become available.

The Clot Buster Amplatz Thrombectomy Device

Device Description and Procedural Technique (34)

The Clot Buster Amplatz Thrombectomy Device (ATD, MicroVena Corporation, White Bear Lake, Minnesota) is a mechanical thrombectomy catheter that performs percutaneous thrombus maceration (Fig. 19-8). The ATD is powered by compressed air. A drive shaft, extending the length of the polyurethane catheter, rotates an encapsulated impeller housed at the distal end of the device (Fig. 19- 9). At speeds exceeding 100,000 rpm, this miniature impeller creates a recirculating vortex that homogenizes the thrombus. There is a side port that allows for high-pressure infusion of saline and/or contrast media for cooling of the system and graft visualization. No guidewire lumen is available.

The device comes in 8-Fr size and two different lengths (50 and 120 cm). It is placed through a sheath or a guide catheter and positioned proximal to the thrombus. Upon activation and while the ATD is simultaneously flushed with saline, the device is advanced toward the thrombus under fluoroscopic guidance. As the thrombus is drawn into the distal hub, the ATD recirculates and macerates the thrombus creating a particulate slurry consisting of very small particles (95% <13 μm).

A device for coronary application is also in evolution.

Clinical Application

The device has thus far been applied in thrombosed dialysis grafts, pulmonary embolism, arterial and central venous thrombosis.

In a company-sponsored study, a total of 72 thrombosed dialysis grafts were treated with an acute procedure success rate (>90% of thrombus removed) of 92.5%, acute functional procedure success rate of 91.7%, and a 30-day postprocedure graft patency rate of 62.2% (incomplete follow-up). The study included a surgical thrombectomy arm consisting of 45 grafts for which the acute success rate was 95.5%, the acute functional success rate was 77.4%, and 30-day patency rate was 62.3%. Similar results were reported in a smaller randomized series of ATD (n = 19) or surgically (n = 18) treated grafts (35). Technical success rates were 89% and 83% with secondary 30-day patency of 68% and 77%, respectively. With the ATD increased, plasma free hemoglo-

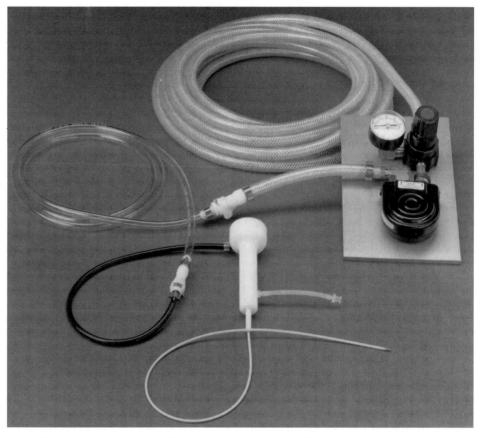

FIG. 19-8. The Clot Buster Amplatz Thrombectomy Device (ATD). (Courtesy of MicroVena Corporation, White Bear Lake, Minnesota.)

bin levels were noted in 63% of the cases, with normalization in 88% within 24 hours.

In five patients with massive pulmonary embolism, the device achieved marked perfusion improvement in one and moderate improvement in three patients (36).

The device has been successfully used in a variety of acute or subacute arterial occlusions (37,38) and central venous thromboses (39).

The hemolytic effect of the device lasts <24 hours and appears to be innocuous clinically (40). Nonetheless, since plasma free hemoglobin promotes intranephronal cast formation and may precipitate acute renal failure, the activation time probably should be restricted to <5 minutes when the device is used in patients with borderline renal function.

Arrow Trerotola Device

Device Description—Technique (41)

The Arrow-Trerotola Percutaneous Thrombolytic Device (PTD) (Arrow International, Reading, Pennsylvania) consists of a low-speed (3,000 rpm) nitinol fragmentation cage attached to a drive cable. The cage and drive cable are housed in a 5-Fr catheter that constrains the self-expanding cage in the closed position. In the open position, the cage expands to 9 mm (Fig. 19-10). Rotation of the open cage at the optimal clot fragmentation speed of 3,000 rpm is accomplished by a separate hand-held rotator unit. The device is designed for use in thrombosed synthetic grafts.

The PTD, which is not an over-the-wire device, is introduced into the clotted graft from

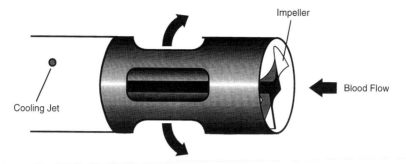

FIG. 19-9. Schematic drawing of the distal tip of the ATD. A recessed impeller is driven by a drive shaft at high speed in a 5-mm metal capsule, creating a recirculating vortex. The thrombus is homogenized and expelled through the side ports. (From Uflacker, et al., ref. 34, with permission.)

the arterial side through a 5-Fr sheath and advanced beyond the clot. There the cage is deployed by retracting the 5-Fr catheter. A second 5-Fr sheath is placed retrograde from the venous side of the graft. The rotator unit is activated and the cage is pulled slowly through the clot resulting in maceration and stripping of the clot from the graft wall. The vast majority of the particles created are smaller than 1 mm and are flushed out through the venous sheath.

Experimental Data

Concern has been raised regarding the potential for pulmonary embolism with percutaneous thrombolytic devices and also with pulse- spray pharmacomechanical thrombolysis (PSPMT). In an experimental study utilizing a dog dialysis-graft model, 10 of 11 perfusion lung scans were positive after PSPMT versus 2 of 11 after the Arrow device (p < 0.001) (41). In the same animal model, 38

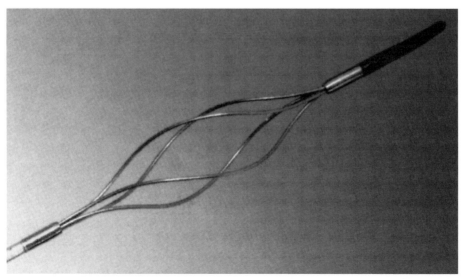

FIG. 19-10. The Arrow Percutaneous Thrombolytic Device fragmentation basket in the open position (FDA market clearance is pending). (Courtesy of Arrow International, Reading, Pennsylvania.)

procedures were performed with a 100% success rate (42). A single arterial embolus occurred.

Clinical Application

There are obvious limitations in extrapolating animal data to humans. A multicenter trial comparing PTD and PSPMT has been underway, and 113 patients out of a target of 122 have been enrolled (43). Preliminary data indicate no difference in success (97%) between groups, whereas procedure times were shorter with the Trerotola device (76 versus 94 minutes). Long-term patency is also similar.

Shredding Embolectomy Thrombectomy

The Shredding Embolectomy Thrombectomy (SET) (Convergenza, San Diego, California) is expected to enter clinical trials in thrombosed dialysis grafts in the near future. The device, available in 5 to 10 Fr and 0.018-in.-guidewire compatible, is driven either by an external drive or an angiographic injector, and achieves thrombolysis via a Venturi effect. No published data are available regarding this device.

CONCLUSION: THROMBECTOMY VERSUS THROMBUS MODULATION— A CASE FOR PHARMACOMECHANICAL SYNERGISM

In a complex biological phenomenon such as intravascular thrombus, mechanical devices constitute a conceptually simplistic approach that should not be anticipated to provide the sole solution, no matter how intelligently designed and effective at dissipating formed thrombus. Mechanical restoration of flow will also have to be paired with additional adjunctive mechanical approaches to minimize obstruction and normalize flow in the majority of cases. Likewise, antiplatelet and/or anticoagulant therapy will still be necessary to successfully treat the prothrombotic intravascular lesion. Perhaps the need for

thrombolytic agents may be minimized as effective mechanical devices are developed, but a complex approach with both mechanical and pharmacologic agents will still be required.

An optimal strategy will only emerge from the future evolution of mechanical devices and thrombopharmacology, proven by the results of randomized trials. Thoughtful and careful study will finally determine the appropriate use of these devices and their most efficacious utilization in thrombus management. The future seems bright despite the fact that much work is needed.

REFERENCES

1. Mabin TA, Holmes DR Jr, Smith HC, et al. Intracoronary thrombus: role in coronary occlusion complicating percutaneous transluminal coronary angioplasty. *J Am Coll Cardiol* 1985;5:198–202.
2. Ellis SG, Roubin GS, King SB III, et al. Angiographic clinical predictors of acute closure after native vessel coronary angioplasty. *Circulation* 1988;77:372–379.
3. Deligonul U, Gabliani GI, Caralis DG, Kern MJ, Vandormael MG. Percutaneous transluminal coronary angioplasty in patients with intracoronary thrombus. *Am J Cardiol* 1988;62:474–476.
4. Arora R, Platko W, Bhadwar K, Simpfendorfer C. Role of intracoronary thrombus in acute complications during percutaneous transluminal coronary angioplasty. *Cathet Cardiovasc Diag* 1989;16:226–229.
5. White CJ, Ramee SR, Collins TJ, et al. Coronary thrombi increase PTCA risk. Angioscopy as a clinical tool. *Circulation* 1996;93:253–258.
6. Hartmann JR, McKeever LS, O Neill WW, et al. Recanalization of chronically occluded aortocoronary saphenous vein bypass grafts with long-term, low dose direct infusion of urokinase (ROBUST): a serial trial. *J Am Coll Cardiol* 1996;27:60–66.
7. Platko WP, Hollman J, Whitlow PL, Franco I. Percutaneous transluminal coronary angioplasty of saphenous vein graft stenosis: long-term follow-up. *J Am Coll Cardiol* 1989;14:1645–1650.
8. Cowley MJ, Whitlow PL, Baim DS, Hinohara T, Hall K, Simpson JB. Directional coronary atherectomy of saphenous vein graft narrowings: investigational experience. *Am J Cardiol* 1993;72:30E–34E.
9. Popma JJ, Leon MB, Mintz GS, Kent KM, Satler LF, Garland TJ, Pichard AD. Results of coronary angioplasty using the transluminal extraction catheter. *Am J Cardiol* 1992;70:1526–1532.
10. Safian RD, Grines CL, May MA, et al. Clinical and angiographic results of transluminal extraction coronary atherectomy in saphenous vein bypass grafts. *Circulation* 1994;89:302–312.
11. Hong MK, Popma JJ, Pichard AD, et al. Clinical significance of distal embolization after transluminal extraction atherectomy in diffusely diseased saphenous vein grafts. *Am Heart J* 1994;127:1496–1503.

12. Annex BH, Larkin TJ, O Neill WW, Safian RD. Evaluation of thrombus removal by transluminal extraction coronary atherectomy by percutaneous coronary angioscopy. *Am J Cardiol* 1994;74:606–609.

13. Cote G, Myler RK, Stertzer SH, et al. Percutaneous transluminal angioplasty of stenotic coronary artery bypass grafts; 5 years' experience. *J Am Coll Cardiol* 1987;9:8–17.

14. De Feyter PJ, van Suylen RJ, de Jaegere PPT, Topol EJ, Serruys PW. Balloon angioplasty for the treatment of lesions in saphenous vein bypass grafts. *J Am Coll Cardiol* 1993;21:1539–1549.

15. Liu MW, Douglas JS, Lembo NJ, King SB. Angiographic predictors of a rise in serum creatine kinase (distal embolization) after balloon angioplasty of saphenous vein coronary artery bypass grafts. *Am J Cardiol* 1993;72:514–517.

16. Lefkovits J, Holmes DR, Califf RM, et al., for the CAVEAT-II Investigators. Predictors and sequelae of distal embolization during saphenous vein graft intervention from the CAVEAT-II trial. *Circulation* 1995;92:734–740.

17. Sketch MH, Labinaz M, Stack RS. Extraction atherectomy. In: Topol EJ (ed). *Textbook of Interventional Cardiology* (2nd ed). Philadelphia: Saunders, 1994;668–672.

18. Sketch MH Jr, Phillips HR, Lee M-M, Stack RS. Coronary transluminal extraction-endarterectomy. *J Invas Cardiol* 1991;3:13–18.

19. Meany TB, Leon MB, Kramer BL, et al. Transluminal extraction catheter for the treatment of diseased saphenous vein grafts: a multicenter experience. *Cathet Cardiovasc Diagn* 1995;34:112–120.

20. Dooris M, Hoffman M, Glazier S, et al. Comparative results of transluminal extraction coronary atherectomy in saphenous vein graft lesions with and without thrombus. *J Am Coll Cardiol* 1995;25:1700–1705.

21. O'Neill WW. Mechanical alternatives to thrombolytics and PTCA in acute ischemic syndrome. *J Invas Cardiol* 1996;8(suppl C):28C–33C.

22. Rosenschein U, Roth A, Rasin T, Basan S, Laniado S, Miller HI. Analysis of coronary ultrasound thrombolysis endpoints in acute myocardial infarction (ACUTE Trial): results of the feasibility phase. *Circulation* 1997; 95:1411–1416.

23. Rosenschein U. Ultrasound thrombolysis in acute myocardial infarction [Abstract]. *J Invas Cardiol* 1997; 9(suppl C):17C.

24. Vein Graft AngioJet Study (VeGAS 2) Investigational Plan and Manual of Operations, 1996. Possis Medical, Inc., Minneapolis, Minn.

25. Ramee SR, Schatz RA, Carrozza JP, et al. Results of the VeGAS I pilot study of the Possis Coronary AngioJet Thrombectomy Catheter [Abstract]. *Circulation* 1996; 94(suppl I):I–619.

26. Hamburger JN, de Feyter PJ, di Mario C, et al. Preliminary experience with the coronary angiojet rheolytic thrombectomy catheter: a preamble to the Euro-ARTS study [Abstract suppl]. *Eur Heart J* 1996;17:181.

27. Ramee SR, Collins TJ, Karsan A, Escobar A, White CJ. Percutaneous recanalization of thrombosed hemodialysis access sites using rheolytic thrombectomy: acute results [Abstract]. *Circulation* 1994;90(Pt 2):I–10.

28. Reeker JA, Kromhout JG, van der Waal K. Catheter for percutaneous thrombectomy. First clinical experience. *Radiology* 1993;188:871–874.

29. Reeker JA, Kromhout JG, Spithoven HG, et al. Arterial thrombosis below the inguinal ligament: percutaneous treatment with a thrombosuction catheter. *Radiology* 1996;198:49–53.

30. Vorwerk D, Sohn M, Schurmann K, Hoogeveen Y, Gladziwa U, Gunther RW. Hydrodynamic thrombectomy of hemodialysis fistulas: first clinical results. *J Vasc Interv Radiol* 1994;5:813–821.

31. Unpublished Cordis Corporation sponsored study on the Hydrolyser (Cordis Europa, Roden, The Netherlands).

32. Vorwerk D, Gunther RW, Wendt G, Nuerburg J, Schurmann K. Iliocaval stenosis and iliac venous thrombosis in retroperitoneal fibrosis: percutaneous treatment by use of hydrodynamic thrombectomy and stenting. *Cardiovasc Interv Radiol* 1995;19:40–42.

33. Fajadet J, Bar O, Jordan C, et al. Human percutaneous thrombectomy using the new Hydrolyser catheter: preliminary results in saphenous vein grafts [Abstract]. *J Am Coll Cardiol* 1994;220A.

34. Uflacker R, Rajagopalan PR, Vujic J, Stutley J. Treatment of thrombosed dialysis access grafts: randomized trial of surgical thrombectomy with the Amplatz device. *J Vasc Interv Radiol* 1996;7:185–192.

35. Company-sponsored study in accordance with investigational device exemption, reported in instructions-for-use booklet. MicroVena Corporation, White Bear Lake, Minnesota.

36. Uflacker R, Strange C, Vujic J. Massive pulmonary embolism: preliminary results of treatment with the Amplatz Thrombectomy Device. *J Vasc Interv Radiol* 1996; 7:519–528.

37. Uflacker R, Vujic J. Feasibility study of the Amplatz Thrombectomy Device in acute and subacute thrombosis. *SCVIR Meet Abstr* 1996;7:112.

38. Rilinger N, Gorich J, Scharrer-Pamler R, Sokiranski R, Vogel T, Brambs H. Amplatz Thrombectomy Device in the treatment of acute lower limb occlusion, preliminary experience with 40 patients. *SCVIR Meet Abstr* 1996;7: 244.

39. Edwards RD, Rowlands PC, Meany J. Central venous thrombosis: treatment with the Amplatz Thrombectomy Device. *SCVIR Meet Abstr* 1995;6:1.

40. Nazarian GK, Qian Z, Coleman CC, Rengel G, Castaneda-Zuniga GK, Amplatz K. Hemolytic effect of the Amplatz Thrombectomy Device. *J Vasc Interv Radiol* 1994;5:155–160.

41. Trerotola SO, Johnson MS, Schauwecker DS, et al. Pulmonary emboli from pulse spray and mechanical thrombolysis: evaluation with an animal dialysis-graft model. *Radiology* 1996;200:169–176.

42. Trerotola SO, Davidson DD, Filo RS, Dreesen RG, Forney M. Preclinical in vivo testing of a rotational mechanical thrombolytic device. *J Vasc Interv Radiol* 1996;7:717–723.

43. Trerotola SO. Overview of mechanical thrombolysis of hemodialysis grafts. *Proceedings of the Ninth Annual Interventional Symposium on Vascular Diagnosis and Intervention.* January 1997:325–330.

Cardiovascular Thrombosis: Thrombocardiology
and Thromboneurology, Second Edition,
edited by M. Verstraete, V. Fuster, and E. J. Topol,
Lippincott–Raven Publishers, Philadelphia © 1998.

20

The Technical Aspects of Antithrombotic Approaches in Vascular Surgery

Michael D. Malone, Anthony J. Comerota, and Paul L. Cisek

Department of Surgery, Temple University Hospital, Philadelphia, Pennsylvania 19140

Prebypass Evaluation   353
**Choice and Preparation of the Vascular
    Conduit   355**
**Adjunctive Measures to Prolong Patency of
    Infrainguinal Grafts   356**
  Distal Arteriovenous Fistula   356
  Anastomotic Vein Cuff or Vein Patch   356
  Prevention of Clamp Injury   356
**Intraoperative Evaluation of Vascular
    Reconstruction   357**

Hand-held Continuous Wave Doppler   357
Duplex Imaging   357
Angioscopy   358
Intraoperative Completion
    Arteriography   358
**Patching Following Carotid
    Endarterectomy   358**
Advances in Venous Thrombectomy   359
Conclusion   360

Although the title of this chapter suggests the use of pharmacologic intervention to extend the functional life of vascular reconstructive procedures, it will instead address some of the many technical aspects of vascular reconstruction designed to reduce short- and long-term thrombotic complications. Pharmacologic manipulation before, during, and after revascularization procedures are increasingly important, and routinely used. These adjuncts are covered in depth in Chapter 38 and it would be difficult to add to the expertise expressed there.

Despite the major advances in our understanding and use of antithrombotics and anticoagulants, the best pharmacologic manipulation will fail in the presence of a technically disadvantaged vascular reconstruction. Vascular surgeons have developed techniques and established principles that have improved short- and long-term outcome of revascular-

ization procedures. Although nonsurgeons traditionally have little interest in the technical aspects of operative procedures, it is appropriate for nonsurgeons to appreciate the basics of good operative care. Because proper technique will offer pharmacologic manipulation the best chance of long-term success, it is increasingly important for nonsurgeons to understand the basic principles of revascularization procedures. This chapter reviews many of the techniques that are applied to infrainguinal, carotid, and venous reconstructive procedures.

PREBYPASS EVALUATION

The best outcome of any revascularization procedure begins with a proper prebypass evaluation. Such an evaluation must include a complete anatomic and physiologic assessment of the patient, identifying the disease causing the patient's problem, which will then lay the foundation for the appropriate vascular reconstruction.

In most instances it is inappropriate to base a vascular reconstruction solely on arteriographic (or other anatomically based imaging modality) studies. Obtaining a complete physiologic assessment ensures the hemodynamic significance of the pathology in question, offers objective documentation, and provides a basis for the evaluation of success of the revascularization procedure as well as the basis for long-term follow-up.

Proper physiologic assessment depends on the portion of the vascular tree being evaluated. When one considers lower extremity revascularization, segmental Doppler pressures (including toe pressures) and pulse wave recordings are the mainstay to evaluate lower extremity occlusive disease. Arterial duplex imaging is becoming popular; however, it rarely provides information that allows the clinician to quantify the degree of ischemia but rather offers an opportunity to directly interrogate a segment of the arterial tree and the magnitude of disease in that arterial segment. Treadmill exercise testing is important when evaluating the functional significance of arterial occlusive disease causing intermittent claudication.

Carotid duplex imaging and transcranial Doppler are important in the evaluation of patients with cerebrovascular disease and are the mainstays of clinical decision making. The functional significance of renal artery stenoses can be assessed with duplex imaging, nuclear medicine scans using angiotensin enzyme inhibitors, and renal vein renin levels. Mesenteric vascular stenoses can be functionally assessed with arterial duplex imaging in the fasting and postprandial states. Venous evaluations are best performed with duplex imaging in the supine and upright position as well as the use of air plethysmography. Both the anatomy and physiology of the venous system are evaluated, and the contribution of obstruction as well as valvular incompetence of both the superficial and deep venous systems can be assessed.

Complete imaging of that portion of the vascular tree in question is a necessity to ensure proper selection of inflow and outflow vessels. Contrast two-plane arteriography is the standard for evaluation of patients with arterial occlusive disease. However, it is an "anatomic" evaluation and cannot be used to assess the hemodynamics of a given lesion. Proximal lesions in the aortoiliac segments can be assessed hemodynamically by measuring pressure gradients across the lesion. If prebypass pressure gradients are not performed, or if normal and a lesion remains suspicious, recording distal pressures after pharmacologically reducing the peripheral vascular resistance will "stress" the stenosis in question and assess whether the lesion might become hemodynamically significant with exercise or following a more distal bypass.

Intra-arterial pressure measurements remain the standard for evaluation of the hemodynamic significance of aortoiliac occlusive disease (1). Resting segmental pressure measurements alone are incomplete because subcritical stenoses at rest may become hemodynamically important during exercise as a result of induced lower extremity vasodilatation with the resultant drop in peripheral vascular resistance. This follows the equation $P = Q \times R$, where P = pressure, Q = flow, and R = resistance. In the presence of an arterial stenosis, maximal blood flow is fixed. If the peripheral resistance drops and the flow is "fixed," the pressure recorded distally will necessarily drop. Measurement of the intra-arterial pressure in the common femoral artery during lower extremity vasodilatation improves the hemodynamic evaluation of suspected proximal lesions. If a significant pressure gradient is detected following intra-arterial infusion of a peripheral vasodilator such as papaverine, correction of the proximal stenosis prior to infrainguinal revascularization will provide maximal inflow to the leg and optimize success of the bypass (2–4).

Reduction in outflow resistance may serve to unmask a potential hemodynamically significant stenosis. An induced pressure gradient of 15% or more is considered hemodynamically significant, and most proximal occlusive lesions should be corrected prior to infrainguinal reconstruction, assuming that correction of the proximal disease would not add significant risk of major morbidity or mortality.

Magnetic resonance arteriography is becoming increasingly popular to assess the arterial tree. While it is often assumed to be an anatomic study, the image is based on the sum of moving blood cells in the artery. Turbulence can portray an area of stenosis more severe than it is anatomically, and it often shows a segmental occlusion when only a stenosis is present.

CHOICE AND PREPARATION OF THE VASCULAR CONDUIT

Appropriate selection and preparation of the vascular conduit is reasonably simple today. For large central vascular reconstructions of the aorta, prosthetic grafts are the mainstay. Most are constructed from Dacron or polytetrafluoroethylene (PTFE). Dacron grafts are either knitted or woven. It is our opinion that Dacron grafts placed in a central location (chest or abdomen) should be of the woven variety. The advantage of knitted grafts is that they handle well. The handling characteristics of woven Dacron grafts have improved to be comparable to knitted grafts. Knitted grafts are disadvantaged by their propensity for dilatation over time, the need for preclotting or application of a protein sealant to reduce intraoperative bleeding, and the risk of future trans-graft bleeding should the patient require thrombolytic therapy for myocardial infarction, stroke, or arterial graft occlusion. Because these patients have considerable risk for additional arterial thrombotic occlusion, and because the likelihood of receiving therapeutic thrombolysis is increasing, it seems appropriate to avoid potential future hemorrhagic complications.

In patients undergoing infrainguinal revascularization, the best choice of a conduit is autogenous vein. Autogenous vein has superior long-term patency for infrainguinal reconstruction. In these authors' opinion, based on personal experience and all of the available data, it is inappropriate to use prosthetic grafts in an infrainguinal location if autogenous vein is available (saphenous or other location). The argument that the saphenous vein should be "saved" for a future bypass procedure (coronary or peripheral) has no merit because patients who have a successful initial bypass do not require subsequent ipsilateral bypass and only 5% of these patients will require future coronary revascularization. With the increasing popularity of the internal mammary arteries and radial arteries for coronary revascularization, patients having coronary artery bypass have more options for autogenous revascularization than patients with extremity occlusive disease. It is our belief that the arterial revascularization should use the best conduit available to ensure the best patency rates.

If the ipsilateral saphenous vein is a good conduit, free of varicosities or sclerosis and 4 mm or more in diameter, it probably does not make much difference whether the graft is constructed as an in situ, reversed, or excised non-reversed. If a major size discrepancy exists between the proximal and distal saphenous vein or if the distal vein tapers to <4 mm, there is merit in constructing an in situ or an excised non-reversed graft to take advantage of an improved size match at both anastomoses and avoid narrowing the proximal anastomosis. During preparation of an autogenous graft it is important for the venous endothelium to remain in contact with blood. Therefore, heparinized blood is used for graft preparation in preference to saline.

If ipsilateral greater saphenous vein is not available or is found to be inadequate, other options for autogenous tissue are residual segments of previously harvested ipsilateral greater saphenous vein, contralateral greater saphenous vein, lesser saphenous veins, and upper extremity veins. The superficial femoral-proximal popliteal venous segment can also be used. Preoperative venous duplex imaging has been helpful to evaluate potential sources of autogenous vein. In the absence of good lower extremity saphenous vein and if the arm veins are small, a radial artery to cephalic vein fistula can be constructed to allow an arm vein to develop into a reasonable conduit. This technique can be used if the patient's ischemia permits a 2- to 4-week delay in their revascularization procedure.

ADJUNCTIVE MEASURES TO PROLONG PATENCY OF INFRAINGUINAL GRAFTS

Distal Arteriovenous Fistula

The addition of a femoral arteriovenous fistula produced higher flow rates and increased the patency rates of a Dacron iliac interposition grafts in the animal model (5). The first clinical use of arteriovenous fistula was by Blaidsell (6,7). Ibrahim et al. (8) and Dardik et al. (9) have described the use of arteriovenous fistula constructed as part of the distal anastomosis. In a high-risk group of patients with multiple failed reconstructions, they achieved a 1-year patency rate of 39% and a limb salvage rate of 52%. In a study by Paty et al. (10), femoral-tibial bypass graft reconstructions were performed with PTFE followed by the construction of an arteriovenous fistula 5 to 15 cm below the distal anastomosis in the same artery to the adjacent vein. In that study they achieved a 1-year patency rate of 67% with a 75% limb salvage rate.

An arteriovenous fistula reduces outflow resistance thereby increasing flow through the graft and the intervening artery and often through the distal artery. This produces a greater graft flow velocity, which may overcome the "thrombotic threshold velocity" of the prosthetic material and increase the patency of the distal graft (11,12). Usually these grafts are prosthetic. Evaluated prospectively, infrapopliteal bypasses were found to have a 12% primary patency rate at 4 years. The poor results of prosthetic materials is based on three main factors. First, synthetic material has an inherent thrombogenecity higher than that of endothelialized autogenous vein. Sec-

ond, this increased thrombogenic state predisposes to neointimal hyperplasia at a rate higher than that of autogenous material. Finally, in the distal bypass grafts there is an inherent low flow volume and velocity which contributes to early thrombosis (13,14).

Anastomotic Vein Cuff or Vein Patch

One of the factors attributed to the poor results of infrapopliteal reconstruction with prosthetic grafts is a graft artery compliance mismatch at the distal anastomosis (15). Several techniques have been designed in which a segment of vein is placed between the PTFE graft and the native artery to overcome the compliance mismatch. The rationale for the addition of a vein cuff or patch to the distal anastomosis is to prevent anastomotic narrowing caused by intimal hyperplasia by widening the anastomosis with autogenous tissue (16). Anastomotic hyperplasia is thought to be responsible for approximately 25% of graft failures that occur more than a month after insertion and is second only to progression of distal disease (17,18).

The use of a vein cuff or patch with prosthetic femorodistal bypass grafts in patients without adequate vein has had favorable results. Taylor et al. (17) reports 5-year patency rates of 71% for popliteal and 54 % for infrapopliteal grafts. Raptis and Miller (19) also demonstrated improved patency with prosthetic femoral-distal popliteal bypasses in which vein cuffs were used compared to grafts without a cuff (57% versus 28%).

Prevention of Clamp Injury

Seemingly small alterations in vascular technique can have a significant effect on immediate and long-term success. Despite an open lumen, the distal target vessel frequently has plaque and calcium in its wall. Circumferential dissection and the application of vascular clamps tight enough to achieve a hemostatic seal may crush the plaque/calcium producing a permanent deformity, compromising the lumen. The direct vessel wall injury is known to promote degenerative changes in the intima and media of the vessel leading to accelerated atherosclerosis and neointimal hyperplasia (20). DePalma et al. (21) found that endothelial damage coupled with hyperlipidemia resulted in accelerated atherosclerotic lesions in a canine model. Slayback et al. (22) found that prior heparinization did not prevent platelet and thrombus formation at the site of intimal damage from clamp injury. Plaque fracture, dissection and thrombosis have all been reported as complications of vascular clamps (23).

Application of vascular clamps to distal vessels can be avoided by the use of a pneumatic tourniquet to the thigh or upper calf. This is often an effective substitute for vascular clamps when performing popliteal and tibial artery anastomoses (22,24). Insertion of an intraluminal vascular occluder through the arteriotomy provides additional hemostasis in calcified vessels and can improve exposure of the arterial wall during construction of the anastomosis (24).

INTRAOPERATIVE EVALUATION OF VASCULAR RECONSTRUCTION

Technical precision during vascular reconstructive procedures cannot be overemphasized. Once the appropriate procedure and conduit have been identified, it is the surgeon's responsibility to ensure that the reconstructive procedure is free of any technical flaw which might threaten its outcome. After the vascular reconstruction is completed, it should be evaluated prior to wound closure for any potentially correctable defect (which include arterial clamp injury, intimal flap, anastomotic stenosis, luminal thrombus, retained valve, etc.).

The appropriate method of intraoperative evaluation will vary with the type of reconstructive procedure performed. Available methods include hand-held continuous wave Doppler, duplex ultrasound, angioscopy, intraluminal vascular ultrasound, and completion arteriography.

Hand-held Continuous Wave Doppler

This is the easiest, most inexpensive, and least time-consuming method of assessing vascular reconstruction. It should be part of every revascularization procedure, and the results can be compared to the prebypass status. The surgeon can evaluate whether the expected hemodynamics (velocity profile) are observed, i.e., pandiastolic flow in the carotid, renal, mesenteric system and the ischemic lower extremity (if the distal anastomosis is beyond disease). While this technique is somewhat subjective, the surgeon with experience using the Doppler becomes proficient in predicting whether a technical defect is present.

For lower extremity revascularization, the hand-held Doppler can quickly identify retained valve cusps, arteriovenous fistulae, and anastomotic stenoses. This should be the minimal method of evaluating any completed reconstructive procedure.

Duplex Imaging

Duplex imaging provides a B-mode image plus a velocity profile of blood flow. Many units offer color-coded velocity profiles of the vessel lumen. Some believe that duplex imaging is better than arteriography because the entire graft and both anastomoses can be visualized in multiple views, both in longitudinal and transverse planes.

Bandyk has found that a low peak systolic velocity <45 cm/second would predict failure of the in situ saphenous vein graft. Also the definition of a hemodynamically significant stenosis, >50% diameter reduction, has been defined based on parameters such as increased peak systolic velocity of >150 cm/sec (25–28). The application of intraoperative duplex scanning allows for optimization of early graft patency and provides cost-effective care by minimizing the number of early graft revision procedures (29). Yu et al. found that intraoperative duplex imaging was less expensive, less invasive, quicker, and equally accurate in comparison to arteriography when used as an adjunct to assess surgical results of arterial reconstructions (30).

There are two main problems associated with operative duplex imaging. The first is the lack of direct experience of most surgeons. The second problem is the lack of available equipment for intraoperative use. Once the problems of duplex imaging are overcome, it can become a valuable technique that poses no risk to the patient and can be effectively and expediently used in experienced hands.

Angioscopy

Improvement in fiberoptics, cameras, and projection capability have expanded the role of angioscopy in vascular diseases. It now permits the vascular surgeon to evaluate the intraluminal condition in real time before leaving the operating room (31). Its use as an adjunct to infrainguinal reconstruction allows for thorough prebypass evaluation of the venous conduit, examining for segments of adherent thrombus, segmental fibrosis, or luminal recanalization (31–36). The surgeon has the opportunity to assess the adequacy of vein valve lysis for in situ or excised nonreversed bypasses, and to examine for potential vein wall injury (34,38–41).

Angioscopy permits full inspection of arteries or grafts following thrombectomy and to assess for residual thrombus and anastomotic stenoses. It can be used to evaluate arterial runoff vessels distal to the bypass graft for atherosclerotic disease. Baxter et al. (41) compared completion arteriography with angioscopy and found angioscopy to be more sensitive than arteriography in identifying potential defects. Gilbertson et al. (35) compared duplex imaging, arteriography, and angioscopy in patients undergoing infrainguinal reconstruction. They found that angioscopy correctly identified all residual vein valve cusps compared to only 22% by arteriography and 11% by duplex imaging. Additionally, they reported a false-positive rate of anastomotic stenoses to be 20% for arteriography, 10% for duplex scanning, while angioscopy failed to demonstrate a lesion which did not exist. Harward et al. (31) found better early

patency in infrainguinal bypass grafts evaluated with arteriography and angioscopy than arteriography alone.

Complications of angioscopy are endothelial damage, vessel wall injury leading to intimal flaps, and fluid overload.

Intraoperative Completion Arteriography

Contrast arteriography has been the standard method of evaluating technical adequacy of the completed bypass. Generally, the lumen of the bypass graft, distal anastomosis, and recipient vessels are imaged. Unfortunately, many areas of the vascular tree are not accessible to good completion arteriography. In addition to detecting abnormalities within the graft or the anastomosis, the completion arteriogram can image the downstream arterial bed to evaluate "runoff" following revascularization. In a study by Liebman et al (42), intraoperative completion arteriography was found to detect a correctable abnormality in 5% of femoropopliteal and femorotibial bypass grafts.

Early graft failure may occur as a result of inadequate runoff despite a well-placed graft and a precise anastomosis. Information about the runoff may be important in the surgeons' decision about subsequent care. With badly diseased runoff, it is unlikely that technical modifications of an occluded but well-constructed bypass can offer improved patency; therefore, repeated operations would be ill advised.

An inherent weakness of intraoperative arteriography is that there are areas of the vascular tree that are inaccessible to visualization, such as the proximal anastomosis. Also, the single plane of visualization may miss some defects. Air bubbles introduced during the arteriogram can cause false positive results, and the risk of renal toxicity in patients with compromised renal function is always a concern.

PATCHING FOLLOWING CAROTID ENDARTERECTOMY

Carotid endarterectomy is the most commonly performed vascular procedure. It has been shown to significantly reduce subsequent stroke and can be performed with a low operative morbidity and mortality. Patching of the arteriotomy is increasingly popular because it is associated with reduction in operative neurologic deficits and recurrent stenoses. Primary closure of the longitudinal arteriotomy narrows the lumen, at least slightly. If the carotid artery is large, such luminal restriction is negligible. However, with a smaller carotid, primary closure can cause substantial relative reduction in diameter. Closing the arteriotomy with a patch prevents luminal compromise and allows some degree of "forgiveness" with the development of subsequent neointimal fibroplasia (43–47).

Accepted indications for carotid patching include (a) a small internal carotid artery with a diameter <5 mm, (b) a long arteriotomy that extends >3 cm beyond the origin of the internal carotid artery, and (c) a looped or kinked internal carotid artery requiring resection, or (d) a spiraled or crooked arteriotomy (48).

Studies comparing patch closure with primary closure have demonstrated a reduction in subsequent recurrent stenosis in patched carotids. Lord et al. (49) found that carotid arteries undergoing primary closure had more than a sixfold risk of developing recurrent stenosis than those with patch closure (21% versus 3.5%; p < 0.05). Eikelboom et al. (50) demonstrated that most recurrent stenoses occurred in the first 6 months following endarterectomy and the rate of recurrent carotid stenosis is reduced by patch closure.

There does not appear to be an appreciable difference in type of patch used, Dacron, PTFE, or autogenous vein. In our practice, essentially all of the women and approximately 85% of the men undergo patch closure of their carotid endarterectomy.

ADVANCES IN VENOUS THROMBECTOMY

Iliofemoral deep vein thrombosis represents the most extreme form of acute deep venous thrombosis (DVT). These patients suffer the most severe acute symptoms of pain, swelling, and discoloration but also have the most serious long-term sequelae (51). Because of the acute and chronic morbidity of iliofemoral DVT, we believe that the thrombus in the iliofemoral venous system should be eliminated. The two most effective techniques of eliminating the iliofemoral clot are catheter-directed thrombolysis and venous thrombectomy. If patients have a contraindication to thrombolytic therapy, venous thrombectomy is recommended. Although regarded for many years as an ineffective operation, venous thrombectomy has evolved into a highly effective treatment option.

The operative technique of venous thrombectomy has improved significantly since the early reports, when the procedure was usually a blind thrombectomy associated with high operative morbidity and failure. The principles of successful venous thrombectomy are listed in Table 20-1. All patients require preoperative contralateral iliocaval phlebography to evaluate the status of the contralateral iliofemoral venous segment and vena cava. Surgeons should be prepared to use fluoroscopy to assess adequacy of thrombus removal and examine the iliac veins for a stenotic proximal lesion, which might have contributed to the acute iliofemoral venous thrombosis.

Through an inguinal incision, exposure of the common femoral vein, saphenofemoral junction, superficial femoral vein, and profunda femoris vein is performed. Either a transverse or a longitudinal venotomy can be used, depending on location and access to the profunda venous system and location of the thrombus.

The leg is elevated and exsanguinated with a rubber bandage to expel clot from below. In patients with extensive infrainguinal DVT, occasionally a cut down to the posterior tibial vein in the lower leg is performed and a no. 3 Fogarty catheter advanced proximally and brought out through the common femoral venotomy. A no. 4 Fogarty catheter is secured and guided distally into the lower leg to perform a mechanical thrombectomy. A larger bore infusion catheter is then placed into the posterior tibial vein and large volumes of heparinized saline flushed through the lower leg,

TABLE 20-1. *Principles of venous thrombectomy*

1. Define full extent of thrombosis (contralateral iliofemoral phlebography is essential).
2. Obtain blood specimens for complete hypercoagulable evaluation (before anticoagulation).
3. Fully anticoagulate with heparin and continue throughout procedure and postoperatively.
4. Prepare operating room for fluoroscopy and radiography.
5. Make inguinal incision to expose and control common femoral, saphenous, superficial femoral, and profunda femoris veins.
6. Perform right retroperitoneal caval control and caval venotomy for removal of caval thrombus.
7. Exsanguinate leg with rubber bandage and expel clot from below.
8. Pass venous thrombectomy catheter part way into iliac vein for several passes before advancing into vena cava.
9. If caval filter is in place, use fluoroscopy for thrombectomy with contrast to fill balloon.
10. In selected patients with severe infrainguinal thrombosis, cut down to posterior tibial vein and advance no. 3 Fogarty catheter to femoral venotomy. Attach and guide no. 4 Fogarty catheter retrograde in leg to allow balloon catheter thrombectomy in selected (especially patients with thrombosed profunda in or inadequate drainage from profunda) and repeat as needed. Flush leg with high- volume/pressure heparin-saline solution. Infuse urokinase, 500,000 U, before ligating posterior tibial vein. (Consider leaving catheter in posterior tibial vein for heparin infusion.)
11. After completing thrombectomy, evaluate iliofemoral system with completion phlebogram/fluoroscopy.
12. Correct underlying vein stenosis (if present) with angioplasty/stent. If unsuccessful, perform a cross-pubic venous bypass with 10-mm externally supported polytetrafluoroethylene (PTFE) graft plus arteriovenous fistula.
13. Construct 4-mm arteriovenous fistula with saphenous vein (or large proximal branch of saphenous vein) end to side to superficial femoral artery.
14. Slip piece of PTFE graft, 5 to 6 mm in diameter, around saphenous vein before arteriovenous fistula, and leave small loop of 0-prolene with clip in subcutaneous wound (in case of arteriovenous fistula becomes necessary).
15. Measure femoral vein pressure before and after arteriovenous fistula is open. If pressure increases, band arteriovenous fistula to decrease flow and normalize pressure. If pressure increases with arteriovenous fistula, look for proximal iliac vein stenosis or large arteriovenous anastomosis.
16. Continue full anticoagulation postoperatively.
17. Apply external pneumatic compression garment postoperatively.

while aspiration of the drainage from the femoral venotomy takes place. It is surprising how much additional acute thrombus can be flushed from the leg with this maneuver. A solution of urokinase (250,000 to 500,000 U) is infused and the posterior tibial vein ligated. A venous thrombectomy catheter (no. 8 or 10) is initially passed part way into the iliac vein, progressively removing segments of thrombus, and subsequently advanced into the vena cava. After completing the thrombectomy, the iliofemoral system is evaluated with completion phlebography/fluoroscopy. If an underlying iliac vein stenosis is present, angioplasty and/or stent placement can be performed. A 3.5- to 4-mm arteriovenous fistula is constructed, sewing the end of the transected saphenous vein (or a large proximal branch) to the side of the superficial femoral artery. Because the diameter of the A-V fistulas small the venous pressure is not increased,

however, the velocity of venous return is accelerated.

Venous thrombectomy with an arteriovenous fistula has been compared to standard anticoagulation in a prospective manner and found to be superior in terms of maintaining patency of the iliofemoral venous system as well as clinical outcome (52). Contemporary venous thrombectomy is now combined with catheter-directed thrombolysis as a unified approach to patients with iliofemoral DVT (51).

CONCLUSION

In this chapter we reviewed the various technical aspects of vascular reconstruction designed to reduce short- and long-term thrombotic complications. The value of a preoperative evaluation inclusive of a complete anatomic and physiologic examination of the patient cannot be over emphasized. Selecting the appropriate revascularization procedure and conduit should follow. Improving the results of infrapopliteal reconstruction with prosthetic grafts by adding a vein cuff or arteriovenous fistula appear to improve patency rates in patients with no available autogenous conduit. In addition to technical precision, the role of intraoperative evaluation and postoperative surveillance of the vascular reconstruction is important to preserve immediate satisfactory and long-term results. The role of venous thrombectomy as an adjunct to catheter-directed thrombolysis in patients with iliofemoral DVT was also reviewed in this chapter, since it is a vascular reconstructive procedure.

The problem of neointimal fibroplasia following reconstructive procedures continues. Unfortunately, there is no definitive intervention or prophylaxis as yet which can be recommended to avoid this common problem of vessel wall injury.

RERERENCES

1. Flannigan DP, Ryan TJ, Williams LR, et al. Aortofemoral or femoropopliteal revascularization? A prospective evaluation of the papaverine test. *J Vasc Surg* 1984;1;1215–223.
2. Berguer R, Hwang NHC. Critical arterial stenosis. A theoretical and experimental solution. *Ann Surg* 1973; 178:39–50.
3. Flanigan DP, Tullis JP, Streeter VL, et al. Multiple Subcritical Arterial Stenoses. Effect on post stenotic pressure and flow. *Ann Surg* 1977;186:663–668.
4. Flanigan DP, Williams LR, Schwartz JA, et al. Hemodynamic evaluation of the aorto-iliac system based on pharmacologic vasodilatation. *Surgery* 1983;93: 709–714.
5. Dean RE, Read RC. The influence of increased blood flow on thrombosis in prosthetic grafts. *Surgery* 1964; 55:581–585.
6. Blaidsell FW, Lim RC, Hall AD, et al. Reconstruction of small arteries. *Arch Surg* 1966;92:206–211.
7. Blaidsell FW, Lim RC, Hall AD, et al. Revascularization of severely ischemic extremities with an arteriovenous fistula. *Am J Surg* 1966;112:166–173.
8. Ibrahim IM, Sussman B, Dardik H, et al. Adjunctive arteriovenous fistula with tibial and peroneal reconstruction for limb salvage. *Am J Surg* 1980;140:46–51.
9. Dardik H, Sussman B, Ibrahim IM, et al. Distal arteriovenous fistula as an adjunct to maintaining arterial and graft patency for limb salvage. *Surgery* 1983;94: 478–486.
10. Paty PS, Shah DM, Saifi J, et al. Remote distal arteriovenous fistula to improve infrapopliteal bypass patency. *J Vasc Surg* 1990; 11:171–178.
11. Strandness DE, Sumner DS. *Hemodynamics for Surgeons.* New York: Grune & Stratton, 1975;346–349.
12. Sauvage LE, Berger KE, Mansfield PB, et al. Future directions in the development of arterial prostheses for small and medium caliber arteries. *Surg Clin North Am* 1974;54:213–218.
13. Rutherford RB, Jones DN, Bergentz SE, et al. Factors affecting infrainguinal bypass. *J Vasc Surg* 1988;8: 236–246.
14. Ascer E, Collier P, Gupta SK, et al. Reoperation for polytetrafluoroethylene bypass failure; the importance of distal outflow site and operating technique in determining outcome. *J Vasc Surg* 1987;5:298–310.
15. Karacaagil S, Narbani A, Almgren B, et al. Modified vein cuff technique for distal polytetrafluoroethylene graft anastomosis; how we do it. *Eur J Surg* 1995;161: 47–48.
16. Parsons RE, Suggs WD, Veith FJ, et al. Polytetrafluoroethylene bypasses to infrapopliteal arteries without cuffs or patches: a better option than amputation in patients without autologous vein. *J Vasc Surg* 1996;23: 347–356.
17. Taylor RS, Loh A, McFarland RJ, et al. Improved technique for polytetrafluoroethylene bypass grafting: long term results using anastomotic vein patching. *Br J Surg* 1992;79:348–354.
18. Taylor RS, McFarland RJ, Cox MI. An investigation into the causes of failure of PTFE grafts. *Eur J Vasc Surg* 1987;1:335–343.
19. Raptis S, Miller J. Influence of a vein cuff on polytetrafluoroethylene grafts for primary femoropopliuteal bypass. *Br J Surg* 1995;82:487–491.
20. Bernhard VM, Boren CH, Towne JB, et al. Pneumatic tourniquet as a substitute for vascular clamps in distal bypass surgery. *Surgery* 1980;87:709–713.
21. DePalma RG, Chidi CC, Sternfeld WC, et al. Pathogenesis and prevention of trauma provoked atheromas. *Surgery* 1977;82:429–437.
22. Slayback JB, Bowen WW, Hinshaw DB. Intimal injury from arterial clamps. *Am J Surg* 1976;132:183–188.
23. Archie JP. Early postoperative femoral-distal bypass graft failure due to vascular clamp injury induced common femoral artery thrombosis. *American Surgeon* 1988;54:167–168.
24. Misare BD, Pomposelli FB, Gibbons GW, et al. Infrapopliteal bypasses to severely calcified, unclampable outflow arteries: two year results. *J Vasc Surg* 1996;24: 6–16.
25. Papanicolaou G, Zierler ER., Beach KW, et al. Hemodynamic parameters of failing infrainguinal bypass grafts. *Am J Surg* 1995;169:238–244.
26. Bandyk DF, Cato RF, Towne TB. A low flow velocity predicts failure of femorotibial bypass grafts. *Surgery* 1985;98:799–809.
27. Belkin M. The hemodynamics of vein graft stenosis. *Semin Vasc Surg* 1993;6:111–117.
28. Bandyk DF, Jorgensen RA, Towne JB. Intraoperative assessment of in-situ saphenous vein arterial grafts using pulsed Doppler spectral analysis. *Arch Surg* 1986;121: 292–299.
29. Bandyk DF, Johnson BL, Gupta AK, et al. Nature and management of duplex abnormalities encountered during infrainguinal vein bypass grafting. *J Vasc Surg* 1996;24:430–438.
30. Yu A, Gregory, D, Morrison L, et al. The role of intra-

operative duplex imaging in arterial reconstructions. *Am J Surg* 1996;171:500–501.

31. Harward TS, et al. Impact of angioscopy on infrainguinal graft patency. *Am J Surg* 1994;168:107–110.

32. Miller A, Campbell DR, Gibbons GW, et al. Routine intraoperative angioscopy in lower extremity revascularization. *Arch Surg* 1984;124:604–608.

33. Grundfest WS, Litvack F, Glick D, et al. Intraoperative Decision based on angioscopy in peripheral vascular surgery. *Circulation* 1988;78(suppl 1):113–117.

34. White GH, White RA, Kopchok GE, et al. Intraoperative video angioscopy compared with arteriography during peripheral vascular operations. *J Vasc Surg* 1987; 6:488–495.

35. Gilbertson JJ, Walsh DB, Zwolak RM, et al. A blinded comparison of angiography, angioscopy and duplex scanning in the intraoperative evaluation of in-situ saphenous vein bypass grafts. *J Vasc Surg* 1992;15: 121–129.

36. Miller A, Marcaccio EJ, Tannenbaum GA, et al. Comparison of angioscopy and arteriography for monitoring infrainguinal bypass vein grafts: results of a prospective randomized trial. *J Vasc Surg* 1993;17:382–398.

37. Marcaccio, EJ, Miller A, Tannenbaum GA, et al. Angioscopically directed interventions improve arm vein bypass grafts. *J Vasc Surg* 1993;17:994–1004.

38. Mehigian JT, Olcott C. Video angioscopy as an alternative to intraoperative arteriography. *Am J Surg* 1986; 152:134–145.

39. Fleisher HL, Thompson BW, McCowan TC, et al. Angioscopically monitored saphenous vein valvulotomy. *J Vasc Surg* 1986;4:360–364.

40. Sales CM, Marin ML, Veith FJ, et al. Saphenous vein angioscopy; a valuable method to detect unsuspected venous disease. *J Vasc Surg* 1993;19:992–1000.

41. Baxter BT, Rizzo RJ, Flinn WR, et al. A Comparative study of intraoperative angioscopy and completion arteriography following femorodistal bypass. *Arch Surg* 1990;125:997–1002.

42. Liebeman PR, Menzoian JO, Mannick JA, et al. Intraoperative arteriography in femoropopliteal and femorotibial bypass grafts. *Arch Surg* 1981;116: 1019–1021.

43. Bernhard VM. Patch versus no patch for closure of carotid endarterectomy. *Semin Vasc Surg* 1989;2:35–42.

44. Archie JP. Prevention of early stenosis and thromboses after carotid endarterectomy by saphenous vein patch angioplasty. *Stroke* 1986;17:901–905.

45. Deriu GP, Ballotta E, Bonavina L, et al. The rationale for patch angioplasty after carotid endarterectomy: early and long term follow-up. *Stroke* 1984;15: 972–979.

46. Katz MM, Jones GT, Degenhardt J, et al. The use of patch angioplasty to alter the incidence of carotid restenosis following thromboendarterectomy. *J Cardiovasc Surg* 1987;28:2–8.

47. Little JR, Bryerton BS, Furlan AF. Saphenous vein patch graft in carotid endarterectomy. *J Neurosurg* 1984;61:743–747.

48. Clagett GP, Patterson CB, Fisher DF, et al. Vein patch versus primary closures for carotid endarterectomy. *J Vasc Surg* 1989;9: 213–223.

49. Lord RSA, Raj TB, Stary DL, et al. Comparison of saphenous vein patch, polytetrafluoroethylene patch, and direct arteriotomy closure after carotid endarterectomy. *J Vasc Surg* 1989;9:521–529.

50. Eikelboom BC, Ackerstaff RG, Hoeneveld H, et al. Benefits of carotid patching: a randomized study. *J Vasc Surg* 1988;7:240–247.

51. Comerota AJ, Aldridge SA, Cohen G, et al. A strategy of aggressive regional therapy for acute iliofemoral venous thrombosis with contemporary venous thrombectomy or catheter directed thrombolysis. *J Vasc Surg* 1994;20:244–254.

52. Plate G, Einarsson E, Ohlin P, et al. Thrombectomy with temporary arteriovenous fistula: the treatment of choice in acute iliofemoral venous thrombosis. *J Vasc Surg* 1984;1:867–876.

PART III

Prevention and Treatment of Thromboembolic Disorders

Cardiovascular Thrombosis: Thrombocardiology and Thromboneurology, Second Edition,
edited by M. Verstraete, V. Fuster, and E. J. Topol,
Lippincott–Raven Publishers, Philadelphia © 1998.

21

Valvular Heart Disease and Prosthetic Heart Valves

James H. Chesebro and Valentin Fuster

Cardiovascular Institute, Mount Sinai School of Medicine,
New York, New York 10029

PATHOGENESIS AND RISK

As in other cardiovascular problems, antithrombotic therapy in patients with valvular heart disease and prosthetic heart valves is based on pathogenesis and risk (see Chapter 23) (1). Higher risk problems may require different therapy. The pathogenesis involves intracavitary mural thrombi in cardiac chambers, changes in rheology of blood flow with stasis activating the coagulation system or turbulent flow activating platelets, and differing substrates for thrombosis. The latter includes calcified or deendothelialized valve leaflets (which may expose subendothelial collagen), heterotopic or xenotopic valvular tissue, or prosthetic materials such as the sewing- associated vascular disease (2,3), Dacron rings common to all prosthetic valves (attracts acute platelet deposition immediately after valve replacement (4), or prosthetic structures of the valve that may vary in thrombogenicity. Prolene suture material appears to be the least thrombogenic of five different materials (5). The most highly thrombogenic substrate is thrombus itself, especially if acute embolism has exposed a fresh surface of the inner thrombus that contains thrombin adsorbed to fibrin (6,7). Thus, a recent thromboembolism always signifies a high risk of recurrent thromboembolism.

DEFINITION OF THROMBOEMBOLISM

Guidelines for reporting morbidity and mortality after cardiac valvular operations have been updated and clarified (8). Thromboembolism is a clinical diagnosis that occurs in the absence of infection; it is clinically manifest less frequently than the pathologic incidence (in part due to size of emboli and the organ involved), and 80 to 90% of the time is manifested in the brain or eye (7,9). The definition of thromboembolism to the brain or eye is a temporary or permanent neurologic deficit of sudden onset with focal motor weakness or visual deficit. Emboli may also involve the limbs, heart, kidneys, splanchnic bed, or spleen. Diagnosis should be by operation, autopsy, or clinical (8). Thromboemboli to the limbs are diagnosed by the presence of ischemic pain, paresthesias, pallor, and pulselessness. The presumed diagnosis of coronary emboli may be made on the basis of a myocardial infarction occurring in a patient under the age of 40, or in the presence of previously documented normal coronary arteries by angiography. The effects of thromboemboli may be categorized as: (a) minor or transient, (b) major with permanent residue, or (c) fatal. Unfortunately, these data have not often been recorded in published studies, but improvement has been occurring in quality peer reviewed journals. Because a stroke or permanent (or >3 weeks) neurologic deficit occurs in approximately half of thromboemboli to

the brain, and because some studies only record a permanent deficit as an embolic event (and disregard reversible ischemic neurologic deficit [RIND, lasts >24 hours <3 weeks] or transient ischemic attack [TIA, fully reversible within 24 hours]), the incidence of thromboemboli may be as much as 50% underestimated. Frequency and regularity of follow-up may also influence the identification of thromboembolic events. Patient questionnaires will also underestimate events compared with questionnaires plus interviews of the patient. Thus the incidence of thromboembolism may be difficult to measure and compare from study to study because of different or uncertain definitions of events, different methods of follow-up, and variable reporting of linearized or actuarial rates.

PRINCIPLES FOR ANTITHROMBOTIC THERAPY

Table 21-1 outlines clinical indications for anticoagulation in patients with valvular heart disease. In addition, the international normalized ratio (INR) for the standardization of prothrombin times is of great importance for achieving appropriate level of the anticoagulation (see Chapter 9) (49). The nomogram designed by Poller (49) is extremely useful in converting the observed prothrombin time ratio for different thromboplastins (which have different sensitivity) to the INR.

The therapeutic range for oral anticoagulation differs depending upon the thromboembolic risk and pathogenesis (based mainly on thrombogenicity of the substrate) (1) and especially the presence of associated vascular disease often found in patients over age 60 (2,3). Thus patients at high risk with valvular heart disease (those with previous thromboembolism) should have an INR of 2.5 to 3.5. For all other patients with valvular heart disease who are at medium risk, an INR of 2.0 to 3.0 is optimal (1,61). Patients with recurrent systemic thromboembolism in spite of adequate warfarin therapy may also receive aspirin 80-100 mg/day (50). Patients unable to take aspirin may increase warfarin dose to an

INR of 2.5-3.5, add dipyridamole 400 mg/day or ticlopidine 250 mg twice daily (62).

Clinical recommendations for the use of antithrombotic therapy can be classified into five levels as previously described (51).

Level I studies are randomized trials with a low false-positive or alpha error in which a convincing and statistically significant benefit for treatment is found with a 95% confidence interval for the difference well away from zero (such as a previous prospective randomized trial in aortocoronary bypass graft operation where the difference between treatment and placebo was highly significant, $p = 10^{-6}$ or 95% confidence interval 16% to 35%, which is well away from zero) (52). In addition, level I trials should have a low false-negative or β error with a high power or 95% confidence interval, which excludes any practical possibility of therapy being beneficial in a sufficiently large trial [such as the lack of benefit of sulfinpyrazone in patients with unstable angina in the trial by Cairns et al. (53), which excluded any practical possibility that sulfinpyrazone could halve the risk of myocardial infarction and cardiac death].

Level II studies are also randomized trials but have a high false-positive or α error, a high false-negative or β error (low power, such as five of the six trials with aspirin therapy after myocardial infarction that showed positive but statistically insignificant trends favoring aspirin), or both errors.

Level III studies are nonrandomized comparisons between patients (concurrent cohorts) who did and who did not receive antithrombotic therapy. Most of the studies in valvular heart disease and prosthetic heart valves are in this category.

Level IV studies are also nonrandomized comparisons between patients who did and who did not receive antithrombotic therapy. However, the groups are not concurrent in time but rather consist of a treatment group that is current and a control group that is historical or from a different time period. Most of the studies in patients with mitral valve disease are in this category.

Level V studies are case series without controls.

Grade A, B, or C recommendations are derived from level I to V studies. Grade A recommendations are supported by at least one and preferably more than one level I randomized trial. Grade B recommendations are supported by at least one level II randomized trial. Grade C recommendations are only supported by level III or IV studies, these are supported by an extremely high risk of thromboembolism in mitral stenosis being reduced to a very low risk of thromboembolism (<1% per year) in patients on adequate anticoagulation and by recent grade. A recommendations in nonvalvular atrial fibrillation are where there are five level I studies (44,54,55,56,57), one level II study (58), and a pooled analysis of the five trials (59) documenting the significant reduction in stroke by warfarin compared to placebo or control.

REPORTING OF THROMBOEMBOLISM

Reporting of thromboembolism has improved since criteria for high quality were outlined and discussed (8,103,104). A greater proportion of the ten criteria are addressed, but some of the last three or four criteria are less well adhered to. These factors facilitate a comparison of studies at different centers and include the following:

1. *Adequacy of follow-up.* This includes proportion of patients and duration of follow-up.
2. *Proportion of patients responding to specific questions.* This should also include frequency of follow-up, whether it was by questionnaire only or direct patient contact as well.
3. *Specific definition of thromboembolism.* Succinct definitions were given earlier and are discussed in more detail elsewhere (8,26,103).
4. *Categorization of thromboembolism:* (a) minor or transient, e.g., transient ischemic attack (TIA) or RIND; (b) major

or associated with a permanent neurologic deficit, myocardial infarction, or reoperation (or other significant therapeutic modality), or (c) lethal. Emboli to the retina or brain cause a residual deficit in about half the cases and are lethal in about 10% (9).

5. *Actuarial rate.* The incidence of thromboembolism or bleeding at a specific point in time should be provided in either tabular or graphic form or in the text. Data for at least 4 to 5 years of follow-up or beyond are preferable.

6. *Linearized rate.* This should be given or calculable as a percentage of events per year or events per 100 patient-years.

7. *Valve thrombosis.* This should be listed separately from thromboembolic events because it is often lethal and is also an indication of the durability of the valve.

8. *Duration of anticoagulation.* The proportion of patients who received anticoagulation for specified time intervals should be stated.

9. *Adequacy of control.* Prothrombin times need to be standardized to the INR in order to compare prothrombin times from different laboratories using thromboplastins of different sensitivities. The International Sensitivity Index of the thromboplastin should be stated, along with the INR of the targeted therapeutic range.

10. *Analysis of affect of anticoagulation.* Adequacy of anticoagulation should be compared with the incidence of thromboembolism. The proportion of prothrombin times within the defined therapeutic range, the proportion to low, and the proportion to high should be given for each group of patients. In addition, the prothrombin time at the time of thromboembolic or bleeding event should also be reported. The incidence of thromboembolism in patients who have a given proportion of prothrombin times in range is useful to report. The different intensities of anticoagulation and variability about the mean probably accounts for the great range in incidence of thromboembolism in reports of the same valve type. Recent data of more than 20,000 prothrombin times in more than 180 patients with a prosthetic valve for 5 to >20 years are showing that increased variability of prothrombin times adds to the risk of thromboembolism.

11. *Bleeding events.* Bleeding events should be defined and reported as in 5, 6, and 10, so as to give an appreciation for the incidence of bleeding and the relation to adequacy of anticoagulation. A major bleeding event is usually defined as an intracranial bleed or one that results in death or permanent injury (e.g., visual loss) or requires hospitalization or a blood transfusion.

VALVULAR HEART DISEASE

Incidence of Thromboembolism

In patients with valvular heart disease, the incidence of thromboembolism depends on the valve involved, the degree of left ventricular dysfunction, left atrial size, atrial fibrillation, and history of previous thromboembolism (11–18).

Mitral Stenosis

Mitral stenosis is the most common form of valvular disease causing thromboembolism. Associated mitral regurgitation may also be present. Thrombi are localized to either the left atrial appendage or the left atrial wall with about equal frequency. Thromboembolism is the presenting symptom in more than 10% of patients with mitral stenosis and may occur with all degrees of stenosis. A conservative incidence of thromboembolic events is >2% to 5% per year with up to 16% being fetal (11,12,17,19–24). Atrial fibrillation increases the risk of thromboembolism by 5- to 18-fold and thus to a severe level (11,12,14,18,25). As extrapolated from the Stroke Prevention in Atrial Fibrillation echocardiography substudy (SPAF-III), marked spontaneous echo contrast or smoke in the left atrium predicts high risk (12% per year) of thromboembolic events (65).

Mitral Regurgitation

The incidence of thromboembolism is 1% to 3% per year, which is less common than with mitral stenosis. But thromboembolism is higher in those with severe regurgitation or in those with associated mitral stenosis. It is especially associated with atrial fibrillation and reduced left ventricular function. With the latter three risks, the incidence is >4% of patients per year and involving at least 14% to 18% of patients (11,22,121). In 65 patients with severe mitral regurgitation followed for at least 10 years at the Mayo Clinic, thromboembolism occurred in 2.9% of patients per year (26). Thus patients with significant mitral regurgitation have at least a medium risk of thromboembolism and require anticoagulation for its prevention.

Mitral Valve Prolapse

Mitral valve prolapse is extremely common and occurs in 2% to 6% of the general population when diagnosed by auscultatory and echocardiographic criteria (27–29). Up to 17% of young women may have mitral valve prolapse (28). Although the relation between cerebral ischemia and mitral valve prolapse was proposed more than 20 years ago (30), it is difficult to establish a causal relation between valvular disease and cerebral ischemia in individual patients. More common causes of cerebral ischemia must be excluded before implicating mitral valve prolapse, especially in the elderly (31).

Patients with redundant mitral valve leaflets have the highest frequency of complications as shown in a long-term follow-up of 237 patients with mitral valve prolapse documented by echocardiography (29). Cerebral emboli occurred in 10 patients, of whom 2 had predisposing factors (infective endocarditis in one and left ventricular aneurysm with thrombus in another). In the remaining 8 pa-

tients, 6 had atrial fibrillation with left atrial enlargement; only 2 patients had no atrial fibrillation or other predisposing causes (1 with and 1 without redundant mitral valve leaflets).

Valvular thrombi are the most likely source of cerebral emboli in patients with mitral valve prolapse (27,30,32). Another source is left atrial thrombi or low left atrial appendage flow velocity in those with paroxysmal or chronic atrial fibrillation (65). Fortunately, massive cerebral infarction is uncommon in the absence of atrial fibrillation. Most cerebral emboli in patients with mitral valve prolapse are transient ischemic attacks or small strokes (33,34).

Aortic Valve Disease

Thromboembolism is much less common than in mitral valve disease and is most often associated with other risks such as coexistent mitral valve disease, atrial fibrillation, or endocarditis (35–37). The precise incidence is less certain. In 68 patients with significant aortic regurgitation followed at the Mayo Clinic, the incidence of thromboembolism was 0.8% per year and occurred in 4.4% of patients followed for at least 10 years (26).

In aortic stenosis, most emboli are calcareous, observed in the retinal arteries on funduscopic examinations, and may be clinically silent (38,39). The first indication of calcific aortic stenosis may uncommonly be an embolus. The risk of embolism is not increased with the severity of valvular stenosis. Emboli may be dislodged during cardiac catheterization or at surgery unless great care is taken. Platelet-fibrin thrombi may be seen on disrupted valvular endothelium in pathologic specimens (40). In aortic valve disease transient monocular blindness or retinal artery occlusion occurs more frequently than brain infarction. These clinical observations suggest that relatively small emboli are associated with calcific aortic stenosis (31). Echocardiography, especially transesophageal, may identify a shaggy appearance of calcification of the aortic valve leaflets.

RISK FACTORS FOR SYSTEMIC EMBOLISM

Atrial Fibrillation

Lone atrial fibrillation in the absence of cardiopulmonary disease or hypertension (even under treatment) in persons under age 60 accounts for only 2 to 3% of those with atrial fibrillation and does not significantly increase the risk of thromboembolism. Atrial fibrillation is the most important risk factor and marker for thromboembolism in chronic or paroxysmal atrial fibrillation (11–14,18,22,26,41,42). The frequency of atrial fibrillation greatly increases with age regardless of gender (43). Atrial fibrillation unrelated to valvular disease (nonvalvular atrial fibrillation) starts at a mean age of 64 years, affects 2% to 5% of the general population over 60, and is associated with a 5% to 7% yearly risk of thromboembolism (see Chapter 12) (18). In younger patients with valvular disease, atrial fibrillation is nearly always associated with mitral valve disease. Thromboembolism often occurs early after the onset of atrial fibrillation. In one study, 33% of thromboemboli occurred within the first month and 66% within 12 months of the onset of atrial fibrillation (11). Patients with paroxysmal atrial fibrillation are at equal risk of thromboembolism as those with chronic atrial fibrillation, even in patients without valvular disease (18,44). Atrial fibrillation greatly increases the risk of thromboembolism in patients with valvular disease. Thus it is critical to constantly look for atrial fibrillation by history or telephone monitoring and even anticipate it in those with a large left atrium.

Left Atrial Size

Patients with mitral valve disease have the most profound left atrial enlargement. However, after atrial fibrillation is established in mitral valve disease, the degree of enlargement as assessed by M-mode echocardiography is not an independent risk factor for thromboembolism (41). In nonvalvular atrial fibrillation, a retrospective study suggests that left atrial enlargement may increase the risk of stroke (15). A prospective study (Stroke Prevention in Atrial Fibrillation [SPAF] Study) found that both left atrial size (>2.4 cm/m^2) from M-mode echocardiograms and left ventricular dysfunction from 2-D echocardiograms (moderate to severe, global or regional, dysfunction) were significant predictors of thromboembolism in patients with nonvalvular atrial fibrillation (60). Thus left atrial enlargement in patients with sinus rhythm may indirectly lead to thromboembolism because of the predisposition to atrial fibrillation. This is why prophylactic anticoagulation may be started in patients with a very large left atrium.

Previous Embolism

Previous embolism, especially if recent, is a strong risk factor for subsequent thromboembolism, probably because residual thrombus is a highly thrombogenic substrate (6,7). The incidence of recurrent embolism in patients with valvular heart disease is approximately 10% per year, and overall, occurs in 30 to 75% of patients (11,13,23,45-47). Most recurrent thromboemboli occur within the first six months after the initial event (11,23). Mortality from recurrent emboli in patients with mitral stenosis may be as high as 42% (11,21). Thus, therapy in such patients should be designed as a high-risk category with a higher level of anticoagulation (INR 2.5-3.5) (1,61).

Other Factors

In nonvalvular atrial fibrillation hypertension (even under treatment), recent (within 3 months) heart failure and prior thromboembolism are clinical risk factors that define high risk (7% per year with one factor and 18% per year with two or more risk factors) and low risk of 2.5% per year (no risk factors, 1.4% per year if no diabetes) (64). Symptoms due to valvular disease or functional class do not predict the likelihood of thromboembolism (12,22). Nor does mitral valvotomy with relief of symptoms eliminate the risk of recurrent embolism (12,20). Low cardiac output is an important risk factor for thromboembolism and may in part be related to left ventricular dysfunction or a very large left atrium prone to atrial fibrillation and decreased flow velocities in the left atrial appendage (1,11,12,16,41,60,64). Although age appears to be an independent risk factor, this may be related to the higher incidence of atherosclerosis of the thoracic aorta and atrial fibrillation in the older age group (2,43,65). In mitral valve disease the initial thromboembolism is most common during the fourth decade of life, and at least 38% of patients will have had an embolism by the seventh decade (48) unless prophylactic therapy is started.

RECOMMENDATIONS FOR ANTITHROMBOTIC THERAPY

Mitral Valve Disease

Patients who are at risk for thromboembolism (Table 21-1) should be anticoagulated. Decisions for therapy are made somewhat easier by the recent trials in atrial fibrillation documenting the need for therapy in all patients with paroxysmal or chronic atrial fibrillation, even those without valvular heart disease (44,54,55,56,57,58,59,65). The older

patient with more marked disease is also at greater risk, partly because of the risk factors listed in Table 21-1, but also because of concomitant atherosclerotic vascular disease (2,18). Thus, a medium-risk patient with a thromboembolic event while on low-dose anticoagulation requires the level of anticoagulation recommended for high-risk patients.

Patients with valvular disease with no risk factors for thromboembolism have no greater risk for thromboembolism than from severe hemorrhage secondary to anticoagulant therapy (66). Thus, anticoagulant therapy is not appropriate in these low-risk patients. Although platelet inhibitor therapy with sulfinpyrazone has been reported to reduce systemic embolism (67), concomitant anticoagulant therapy was used in two thirds of the patients. Thus sulfinpyrazone was not adequately tested alone.

Mitral Valve Prolapse

The incidence of thromboembolism is extremely small, and therefore prophylactic therapy is not warranted unless risk factors are present (Table 21-1). After a mild or transient embolic event, initial treatment with oral anticoagulation is warranted for 3 to 6 months. If risks in Table 21-1 are not present, this may empirically be followed by a platelet inhibitor such as aspirin (80 to 325 mg per day). If present, anticoagulation is indicated. As previously mentioned, valvular thrombi

---

TABLE 21-1. *Valvular heart disease: indications for anticoagulation*

Medium Risk[a]
1A. Atrial fibrillation (chronic or paroxysmal) in mitral regurgitation or after anticoagulation for 1 year in mitral stenosis.
1B. Atrial fibrillation (chronic or paroxysmal) regardless of type or severity of valvular heart disease in patients over age 60 with one or more of following: (a) systolic blood pressure >160, (b) prior thromboembolism, (c) impaired left ventricular function (moderate/severe, global/regional), (d) women over age 75 years (60,63,64).
2. Sinus rhythm with a very large left atrium (>55 mm by M-mode echocardiography).
3. Presence of heart failure or severe left ventricular dysfunction.

High Risk[b]
4. Atrial fibrillation (chronic or paroxysmal) in mitral stenosis during the first year of anticoagulation.
5. History of previous systemic embolism.

From Chesebro et al., ref. 26, with permission.
[a]International normalized ratio = 2.0 to 3.0.
[b]International normalized ratio = 2.5 to 3.5.

are probably the most frequent cause of systemic embolism in these patients and such emboli are usually small. If the thromboembolism is large or recurs during antiplatelet therapy, the search for other causes and the use of long-term anticoagulant therapy is warranted.

Aortic Valve Disease

There are a few patients with aortic valve disease who have risk factors for thromboembolism (Table 21-1) and require oral anticoagulation. Most emboli in these patients are calcareous. Such emboli are not preventable, and if proven to originate from the aortic valve (which may be difficult) replacement may be justified for recurrent embolism. It is possible that turbulent flow may disrupt valvular endothelium even across a mildly abnormal aortic valve (or in a bicuspid valve) and stimulate platelet deposition (40). Thus some neurologic symptoms in patients with aortic stenosis may be from platelet emboli and warrant a trial of platelet inhibitor therapy. However, this hypothesis is untested. There are no data to support the routine use of platelet inhibitor therapy in these patients.

PROSTHETIC HEART VALVES

Incidence and Mechanisms

Patients with prosthetic heart valve replacement have a medium to high and long-term risk of thromboembolism (1,9,10). The proportion of patients free of thromboembolism decreases throughout the first and second decades after operation in spite of administration of oral anticoagulants. In the long-term follow-up of Starr-Edwards prosthetic valves, only 66% had no thromboembolism at 10 years and only 58% no thromboembolism at 15 years after operation (9). The lowest proportion of patients free of thromboembolism or thrombosis after mechanical valve replacement is 86% at 14 years (1.4% per year) after replacement with the St. Jude Medical prosthesis when intravenous heparin was started during the sixth postoperative hour and continued subcutaneously until oral anticoagulation was in the therapeutic INR range (68).

Pathogenesis Involves Platelets and Coagulation

Factors of perivalvular substrates (surgically exposed tissue and prosthetic material), blood flow rheology (stasis and turbulence), and blood coagulation (antithrombotic therapy, INR, and platelet inhibitor) contribute to valvular thrombus and thromboembolism (Table 21-2). Thrombosis begins during operation. The damaged perivalvular tissue and prosthetic materials lead to contact activation of the coagulation cascade with thrombin generation and platelet activation as soon as blood begins flowing across the valve (69–72). Thrombin may also be formed on

TABLE 21-2. *Prosthetic heart valves and systemic embolism pathophysiology and risk stratification*

	Thrombi			Emboli
Type	Substrate[a]	Flow[b]	Coagulation[c]	(Events per 100 patient-years[d]) No anticoagulation (anticoagulation)
Mitral mechanical	++	++	+	5 (2.5)
Aortic mechanical	++	+	+	4 (2)
Mitral bioprosthesis	+	+	0	2 (1)
Aortic bioprosthesis	+	0	0	1 (0.5)

[a]Perivalvular excision tissue, Dacron sewing ring, prosthesis, and suture (early).
[b]Atrial fibrillation (left atrium size), design of prosthesis (thrombosis-emboli).
[c]INR and platelet inhibitor drug and dose.
[d]Endpoint of thromboembolism.

platelet membranes (via the prothrombin activator complex, which accelerates thrombin generation 278,000-fold) after their adhesion and activation by a prosthetic surface. Thrombin is the most sensitive activator of platelets in the arterial circulation and also promotes fibrin-thrombus generation. It takes five times greater levels of thrombin inhibition to prevent platelet thrombi compared with fibrin thrombi (71). Thus, inhibition of both coagulation and platelets may be necessary to maximize antithrombotic effects with prosthetic heart valves. Since specific thrombin inhibition can totally prevent experimental arterial thrombus after deep injury and limit platelet deposition to a single layer, this type of therapy may be promising in the future (72).

In addition, both mechanical and bioprosthetic valves contain a Dacron sewing ring that may activate both the coagulation cascade and platelets. Indium-III-labeled platelets may be used experimentally with scintigraphy to image platelet deposition on this ring within the first 24 hours after operation when either a mechanical or a bioprosthetic valve is placed in the animal (4,69). Platelet-rich thrombi may be additionally stabilized by fibrin, which adsorbs thrombin and might further activate platelets. Stasis (spontaneous echo contrast) and decreased blood flow (in the left atrial appendage during atrial fibrillation or during low cardiac output states with left ventricular dysfunction) also promotes fibrin formation. Early thrombus formation causes increased thromboembolic risk early after prosthetic heart valve replacement (73–86).

A shortened platelet survival indicates an increased risk of thromboembolism and is frequently present in patients with prosthetic heart valve replacement (80–82). Decreased platelet survival directly relates to the surface area of the prosthetic valve. The aortic valve has a smaller surface area than the mitral. A shortened platelet survival correlates with increased risk of thromboembolism since this reflects ongoing platelet aggregation and deaggregation which may culminate in a clinical event (80,82). Platelet inhibitor therapy that corrects a shortened platelet survival appears to predict the effectiveness of this therapy in preventing thromboembolism and is the reason that dipyridamole at 400 mg per day was chosen as adjunctive therapy to anticoagulation (80–82).

Fibrinopeptide A is marker of in vivo thrombin activity as reflected by the conversion of fibrinogen to fibrin by thrombin. Elevated levels reflect ongoing conversion of fibrinogen to fibrin by thrombin an incomplete inhibition of coagulation. Because a five times greater level of thrombin inhibition is required to inhibit the formation of platelet thrombi compared to fibrin thrombi (71,72), inhibition of elevated levels of fibrinopeptide A does not necessarily reflect inhibition of platelet activity and the formation of platelet thrombi. The level of oral anticoagulation is inversely related to fibrinopeptide A levels in patients with mechanical and bioprosthetic heart valves. Fibrinopeptide A levels remain elevated above the normal for healthy subjects in patient with mechanical prosthetic heart valves receiving adequate oral anticoagulation (INR 3.0 to 4.5) (83). Patients with bioprosthetic heart valves in the mitral position treated with oral anticoagulation to the same INR have lower levels of fibrinopeptide A that do not significantly differ from normal. Lower levels of anticoagulation increase fibrinopeptide A (83). Studies of clinical outcome and risk of clinical outcome and risk of thromboembolism correlating with fibrinopeptide A levels have not been done. More thrombin inhibition is required to prevent platelet thrombi (71,72,83).

Risk Factors for Thromboembolism

There is a cumulative increase in risk of thromboembolism directly with time after operation. In addition, both patient factors and valve factors contribute to this risk (Table 21-3).

Valve Location

Patients with aortic valve replacement have the lowest risk of thromboembolism. Mitral valve replacement has a higher risk, and dou-

TABLE 21-3. *Risk factors for thromboembolism in patients with prosthetic heart valves*

Cumulative incidence increases directly with time
    after operation
Patient factors
  Valve location[a]
  Adequacy of anticoagulation (level and variability)
  Atrial fibrillation
  Sinus rhythm with large left atrium (>50 mm)
  Previous thromboembolism
  Left ventricular dysfunction
  Year of operation (nowadays operation is
    performed earlier in course of disease)
Valve factors
  Design: less turbulence and stasis
  Materials: less thrombogenic

From Chesebro et al., ref. 26, with permission.
[a]Aortic, mitral, or combined valve replacement.

ble valve replacement has a similar or higher risk. This increased risk may be in part related to the surface area of the prosthetic heart valve as well as to more advanced heart disease in those with double valve replacement. Thus there is a greater potential for left ven-tricular dysfunction and atrial fibrillation following double valve replacement.

Adequacy of Anticoagulation

Optimal anticoagulation is probably the most important factor in the prevention of thromboembolism (9,84–88,90). The optimal INR was defined by plotting the incidence of thromboembolic and bleeding events at the different INR intensities of anticoagulation (Fig. 21-1) (89). This also has a theoretical basis in the inverse relationship between fibrinopeptide A (reflecting thrombin activity) and the level of anticoagulation (83). Adequacy of anticoagulation is now defined by the prothrombin time INR (2.5 to 3.5 for mechanical valves and 2.0 to 3.0 for bioprosthetic valves) (62) and by the proportion of prothrombin times within these therapeutic ranges. In observing over 12,000 prothrombin times and the relationship to thromboembolism or bleeding (Table 21-4),

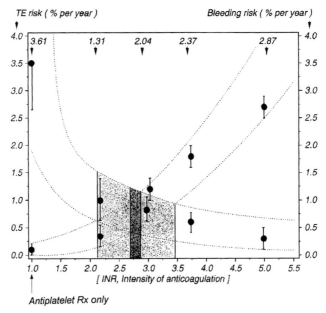

FIG. 21-1. Incidence of thromboembolic (TE) and bleeding events (*y* axis) with different intensities of oral anticoagulation (*x* axis). Patients with an INR of 1.0 were only taking a platelet inhibitor because of a contraindication to oral anticoagulation. The lowest incidence of both TE and bleeding complications occurred in the INR range of 2.2 to 3.5. The optimal range was calculated to be 2.7 to 2.9. (From Ionescu et al., ref. 75, with permission.)

TABLE 21-4. *Clinical events versus adequacy of prothrombin time*[a]

Event	Thromboembolism, percent patients with low prothrombin time (<1.5 times control)	Bleeding, percent patients with high prothrombin time (> 2.5 times control)
No	30	4
Yes (overall)	41	11
Yes (at time of event)	54	38

Adapted from Chesebro et al., ref. 10, with permission.
[a]Therapeutic prothrombin time (PT) is defined as 1.5 to 2.5 times control.

we observed that patients who had thromboembolism had a significantly greater proportion of low prothrombin times (41%) compared with those without thromboembolism (30%) and over half the time had a low prothrombin time at the time of the thromboembolic event. Likewise, patients who had a major bleeding episode had a significantly greater proportion of elevated prothrombin time (11%) compared with those who had no bleeding event (4% with elevated prothrombin times), and 38% of patients had an elevated prothrombin time at the time of the event (88).

In another study anticoagulation was defined as adequate if the prothrombin time were (on the average) above or equal to 1.5 times control value for the preceding year. Using these criteria, adequacy of anticoagulation reflected the incidence of thromboembolism in mitral valve replacement when adequate anticoagulation versus inadequate anticoagulation was considered. However, there is a trend but not a significant relationship between the adequacy of anticoagulation and the incidence of thromboembolism after aortic valve replacement (Table 21-5). The lack of difference for patients with aortic valve replacement may reflect the high flow across the aortic valve, which can predispose to thrombi consisting predominantly of platelets compared with fibrin thrombi that appears to be more prominent after mitral valve replacement. The extreme of inadequate anticoagulation is the use of no anticoagulation; combined aspirin alone in patients temporarily unable to take anticoagulants (Table 21-6). Observational studies after mechanical aortic valve replacement have shown an extremely high risk of thromboembolism in the absence of anticoagulation, documenting the need for oral anticoagulation after mechanical prosthetic valve replacements (Table 21-7). The lowest incidence of thromboembolism on platelet inhibitor therapy alone is in patients with the St. Jude Medical prosthesis (Fig. 21-1).

The variability in prothrombin times is probably as important as the intensity (88) because a high and equal number of emboli (4.0% and 3.0% per year in the moderate- and high-intensity groups, respectively) occurred whether the target prothrombin time

TABLE 21-5. *Starr-Edwards prosthesis: systemic embolism and adequacy of anticoagulation*[a]

Anticoagulation	% Events (patient-years)	
	MVR	AVR
Adequate τ	6.4	6.5
Inadequate	14.2	8.5
p Value	<0.01	NS

From Fuster et al., ref. 203, with permission from the American Heart Association, Inc.
[a]Rabbit brain thromboplastin ratio of 1.5 to 2.5 (international normalized ratio = 3.0 to 7.5): inadequate if less than the lower ratio.
AVR, aortic valve replacement; MVR, mitral valve replacement; NS, not significant.

TABLE 21-6. *Platelet inhibitors alone for mechanical prosthetic heart valves*

Study	Drug	Thromboembolism (%/year)
Salazar et al. (194)	Acetylsalicylic acid (1,000 mg/day)	29 pregnancy
Chaux et al. (117)	Acetylsalicylic acid (975 mg/day) Dipyridamole (275 mg/day)	7
Mok et al. (201)	Acetylsalicylic acid (1,000 mg/day); Dipyridamole (275 mg/day)	7

TABLE 21-7. *Thromboembolism in mechanical valve replacement*

		AVR/MVR			
		%/Year			
Study	Pt (no)	TE	Thromb	Bleed	Years of operation
Starr-Edwards valve					
Fessatidis, Hackett (104,105) (1987)	327/279	1.6[a]/1.2[a]	0/0	0.7/0.3	
AVR + MVR	46	5.6	0	0.4	1974–1983
Schoevaerdts (106)	–/549	–/3.1	–/0	–/1.1	1965–1985
Cobanoglu (107)	707/1	2.8/–	0/–	2.0/–	1965–1986
Bjork-Shiley valve					
Harjula (108)	–/176	–/2.5	–/0.4	–/0.5	1973–1982
Bloomfield (109)	100/122	1.4/5.0		1.5/1.5	1975–1979
Borkon (110)	266/–	1.4/–	0.2/–	6.2/–	1976–1981
Lindblom (111,112)	1573/	1.0[b]/2.2[b]	0.1/0.6	1.4/1.2	1969–1983
Thulin (113)	214/163	3.4/5.0	0/0		1982–1985
Milano (114)	147/	1.0/	0.1/	1.3/	1970–1985
Fessatidis (115)	–/331	–/0.4[a]	–/0	–/0.1	1973–1985
Vogt (137)	84	1.4	–	0.7	1981–1983
Bloomfield (116)	109/129	1.0/2.6	–	2.7/2.0	1975–1979
St. Jude valve					
Chaux (117)	73/90	1.3/2.3	0.3/0	–	1978–1982
AVR + MVR	25	3.7	–		
(antiplatelet Rx only)	12	6.5	–	–	
Kinsley (119)	335/330	2.5/2.7	0.1/0.8	–	1980–1984
AVR + MVR	126	1.7	0.4	–	Same
Nakano (120)	140/244	0.7/2.0	0.3/0.2	–	1978–1984
Montalescot (121) (1989)	49/–	0.93/-	–/0	3.3/–	1978–1981
Arom (122) (1989)	469/340	1.1/1.8	–/0.1	0.6	1977–1987
AVR + MVR	75	1.6	–		
Vogt (137) (1990)	94	2.0	–	1.7	1981–1983
Czer (123) (1990)	290/252	2.3/1.6	0.3/0.3	2.8/2.1	1978–1988
Kratz (124) (1993)	254/202	1.8/2.9	0.2/0.2	3.0	1982–1991
Fernandez (125) (1994)	611/490	2.2	0.2/0.2	3.0	1982–1991
Ibrahim (126) (1994)	578/440	2.4/4.4	0.1/0.1	1.7/2.8	1979–1992
Baudet (68)	773/207	0.84/1.8[c]	0.25/0.44	0.95/0.89	1978–1987
(if no ACRx) (118)	65/10	6.1/16.7	6.2/5.6	–	1978–1983
Omniscience valve (AV/MV)					
Callaghan (127)	76/102	3.1	0.6	2.6	1979–1985
Carrier (128)	33/72	3.0	0.8	3.4	1980–1984
Lillehei-Kastor valve					
Stewart (129)	273/–	1–5/–	0.2/–	2.0/–	1975–1984

[a]PT 2.5 to 4.0 times control ("standardized British corrected") in anticoagulation clinics.
[b]Excludes transient cerebral ischemic attacks.
[c]Thromboembolism undefined.
ACRx, oral anticoagulant therapy; AVR/MVR, aortic valve replacement/mitral valve replacement (the values in each column compare the number of cases in each group); bleed, bleeding episodes; Pt, patient; Rx, therapy; TE, thromboembolism; Thromb, thrombosis of valve.

ration was 1.5 ± 0.2 (INR 2.65) or 2.5 ± 0.2 (INR 9); 19 of the 33 emboli occurred when the prothrombin time ratio was <1.5 (approximately half in each group). Increased variability in prothrombin times over the long-term confirms an increased risk of thromboembolism in patients with prosthetic heart valves (91).

Only recently have a small number of studies begun to correlate the intensity of anticoagulation with the incidence of thromboemboli and bleeding after prosthetic heart valve replacement (Tables 21-4 and 21-8, Fig. 21-1). This helps to define the optimal INR range (Fig. 21-1). The intensity and variability of the prothrombin times are probably the major factors in the frequency of thromboembolism and will need to be recorded in future reports of prosthetic heart valves and the treatment of other thromboembolic problems. The intensity of prothrombin times with low variability may have accounted for the lower rates of thromboemboli in the studies by Fessatidis (Table 21-7) and Vallejo (Table 21-8).

Atrial Fibrillation

During valve replacement in the 1960s, this was not an independent risk factor for thromboembolism because nearly all patients with mitral valve replacement had atrial fibrillation owing to deferral of the operation until the later stages of the disease (9,84,86). Recent studies have shown the independent risk of thromboembolism by low flow in the left atrial appendage associated with atrial fibrillation (59,60,65). Thromboembolism from bioprosthetic valves may occur more often in patients with atrial fibrillation (78,93–97). Thus, because even paroxysmal atrial fibrillation increases the risk of stroke (44,54,55,59), it is important to observe for this during follow-up after valve replacement. Patients with atrial fibrillation for less than a year before operation are more likely to convert to sinus rhythm after operation, especially after hospital discharge. Up to one third of patients with atrial fibrillation before operation may convert to sinus rhythm after operation. Atrial fibrillation increases with age and thus should be closely looked for in patients over age 60, including those with aortic valve replacement (25). After aortic valve replacement, as many as 60% of patients over age 70 may have at least transient atrial fibrillation (98). In mitral disease, earlier operation may be justified to restore sinus rhythm and prevent or delay chronic atrial fibrillation, especially if valve reconstruction is undertaken (99–101). Patients with a large left atrium are at high risk

TABLE 21-8. *Thromboembolism in Medtronic Hall, St. Jude Medical, and Omnicarbon mechanical valve and targeted international normalized ratios*

		AVR/MVR					
					%/Year		
Study	Valve	Pt (no.)	Targeted INR	TE	Thromb	Bleed	Years of operation
Butchart (130) (1988)	MH	255/460	2.5–3.5	1.6/3.2	0/0	0.7	1979–1987
MVR + AVR		137	2.5–3.5	3.4	0	Same	
Antunes (131) (1988)	MH	257/386	Poor compliance (third world)	3.5/3.1	1.1/1.1	1.0/0.5	1980–1984
Vallejo (132) (1990)	MH	117/143	3.0–4.5	0.7/1.5	0.01	0.39	1981–1986
Acar (133) (1996)	SJ + O	179/9	2.0–3.0	3.1/–	1/188	11.2	1991–1994
	SJ + O	192/7	3.0–4.5	2.4/–	0/192	20.4	1991–1994

INR, international normalized ratio; AVR/MVR, aortic valve replacement/mitral valve replacement (the values in each column compare the number of cases in each group); Pt, patient; TE, thromboembolism; Thromb, thrombosis of valve; Bleed, bleeding episodes; MH, Medtronic Hall; SJ, St. Jude Medical; O, Omnicarbon.

of developing atrial fibrillation and thus should be anticoagulated.

Previous Thromboembolism

This indicates a high risk for subsequent thromboembolism, as previously noted. Thus all patients with this history should be anticoagulated after valve replacement regardless of type of valve or after mitral valve repair.

Left Ventricular Dysfunction

Patients with a dilated, poorly functioning left ventricle are at risk of thromboembolism even without valve replacement and thus require anticoagulation (16).

Year of Operation

An older year of operation (especially before 1980) usually places patients at a higher risk of thromboembolism because patients today undergo operation at an earlier stage of their disease (102,103), usually have better left ventricular function, a smaller left atrium, and a lower incidence of atrial fibrillation.

Valve Design and Materials

Older valves created greater turbulent flow and regions of enhanced platelet activation. Older valves also used more thrombogenic materials. Today valves are designed for less turbulent flow. Although materials are less thrombogenic, none of the mechanical valves can be used without anticoagulation. However, the St. Jude Medical prosthesis appears to have a lower risk of thromboembolism at the same level of anticoagulation (68,89).

MECHANICAL PROSTHETIC CARDIAC VALVES

Incidence of Thromboembolism

Reports of mechanical valve replacement are summarized in Table 21-7 for different valve types. The Starr-Edwards valve has the longest track record and very low rates of valve thrombosis. Even more recent models, when considered, have as low a rate of thromboembolism. The St. Jude valve appears to have the lowest rate of thromboembolism overall, but is not immune from valve thrombosis, especially when anticoagulants are not used. The Starr-Edwards, St. Jude, and Medtronic Hall valve (Table 21-7) appear to have the lowest rates of valve thrombosis. The Bjork-Shiley appears to have the highest risk of thrombosis.

The greatest difference in rates of thromboembolism appear to be related to the intensity and variability of anticoagulation, but this was seldom properly assessed. Only in recent studies has a targeted range for anticoagulation been stated (Table 21-8 and Fig. 21-1). For the St. Jude Medical prosthesis in the aortic, mitral, or both locations, the INR range of 2.2 to 3.5 resulted in the lowest rate of both thromboembolic and bleeding complications (Fig. 21-1) (89). The low-risk patient with a St. Jude or Omnicarbon mechanical prosthetic aortic valve replacement in normal sinus rhythm with a left atrial diameter <50 mm is the special case for lower dose oral anticoagulation to an INR of 2.0 to 3.0 (133,134). Reliable means for carrying out targeted goals for anticoagulation need to be implemented whether it be via anticoagulation clinics or a nurse or secretary specifically assigned to making sure that the patient has prothrombin times at least every 3 to 4 weeks (and contacts the physician with the results so that optimal control can be maintained). The importance of appropriately high levels of anticoagulation, close monitoring, and positive encouragement of reliable patients is suggested by the studies of Fessatidis and colleagues (104,105,115) (Table 21-7), and by the lower rate of thromboembolism for higher (and probably less variable) levels of anticoagulation achieved for the same valve type (Table 21-8 and Fig. 21-1). Randomized prospective trials comparing mechanical prosthetic heart valves (Table 21-9) may help define in vivo thrombogenicity of different valves. However, detailed information concerning the adequacy

TABLE 21-9. *Thromboembolism in trials of mechanical cardiac valves*

Study	Valve	Pt (no)	% Year TE		Thromb	Bleed	Years of operation
Randomized prospective studies							
Mikaeloff (135)	BS-MV	–/178	4.3		0.4	2.4	1979–1981
	SJM-MV	–/179	2.3		0.4	1.6	1979–1983
	SE-MV	65	5.3		0	1.6	1982–1983
	BS	160		1.3		–	1982–1987
Kuntze (136)	MHV	148		3.4		–	
	EDV	88		5.1		–	
Vogt (137)	BS	84	1.4		0	2.2	1981–1983
Nonrandomized, concomitant patients, same center							
Cortina (138)	BS	–/51	–/1.1		–/0	–/	1980–1983
	MHV	–/152	–/2/2		–/0.4	–/	
	OmS	–/65	–/4.5		–/3.1	–/	

BS, Bjork-Shiley; SJM, St. Jude Medical; SE, Starr-Edwards; MHV, Medtronic Hall Valve; EDV, Edwards Duromedics valve; OmS, Omniscience valve; Pt, Patient; TE, thromboembolism: Thromb, thrombosis of valve; Bleed, bleeding episodes: MV, mitral valve.

of anticoagulation within valve groups was not included in the reports cited in Table 21-9.

In our prospective study (10) of mechanical prosthetic valve replacement from 1979 to 1981 that involved mainly Starr-Edwards and Bjork-Shiley valves and a small number of St. Jude valves, the incidence of thromboembolism was low (1.2% to 1.8% per year) and did not differ among any of these valve types. The highest rates of thromboembolism occur during the first year after operation when there is probably more variability in anticoagulation, and fresh tissue injury at the valve excision site and prosthetic surfaces are exposed to flowing blood. Thus the greatest protection from thromboembolism is required during the first year. In addition, anticoagulation is essential for chronic prevention of thromboembolism and valve thrombosis. Platelet inhibitor therapy alone is not effective enough (117,118) and should only be used temporarily if anticoagulation needs to be interrupted.

Prospective Intervention Trials

Because oral anticoagulation cannot completely prevent thromboembolism in patients with mechanical heart valves (Tables 21-7 through 21-9), prospective randomized trials of oral anticoagulation with and without platelet inhibition have been conducted.

Dipyridamole has been approved by the U.S. Food and Drug Administration for the prevention of thromboembolism in conjunction with oral anticoagulation in patients with mechanical prosthetic heart valves. Dipyridamole has its best antiplatelet effect against prosthetic surfaces (139,140). Dipyridamole decreased the incidence of thromboembolism in mechanical prosthetic heart valves when added to oral anticoagulation compared to anticoagulation alone in five trials [one level I study (141) and four level II studies (10,142–144)] (Table 21-10). Although the level I study by Sullivan et al. has been criticized for not reporting levels of anticoagulation in both groups, more than 4,000 prothrombin times were subsequently collected for both groups and showed comparable levels of anticoagulation in each group (145). A dipyridamole dosage of 300 to 400 mg per day or 5 to 6 mg per day was chosen in these studies because this dosage maximally prolonged a shortened platelet survival in patients with prosthetic heart valve replacement (80,146). Aspirin was added to oral anticoagulation in four trials (10,50,147) and reduced thromboembolism. The only level I trial that used 100 mg aspirin per day added to warfarin showed a decisive reduction in major systemic embolism, nonfatal intracranial hemorrhage, or death from hemorrhage or vascular causes (50). The other trials were smaller,

TABLE 21-10. *Antithrombotic therapy in patients with mechanical prosthetic heart valves*

Study	Methods	Follow-up (yr)	Treatment group	Dose (mg/day)	Patient number	Thromboembolic events (%/yr)
Sullivan (141)	Prospective, randomized	1	A/C + placebo		84	14
			A/C + D	400	79	1
Kasahara (142)	Prospective, randomized	1–3 (mean 30 mo)	A/C		39	21
			A/C + D	400	40	5
Groupe PACTE (143)	Prospective, randomized	1	A/C		154	5
			A/C + D	300	78	4
Rajah (144)	Prospective, randomized	1 to 2	A/C		87	13
			A/C + D	300	78	4
Dale (92)	Prospective, randomized, blind	1	A/C + placebo		38	9
			A/C + ASA	1,000	39	2
Altman (147)	Prospective, randomized	2	A/C		65	20
			A/C + ASA	500	57	5

From Fuster and Chesebro, ref. 146, with permission from the Mayo Foundation.
A/C, anticoagulant; ASA, acetylsalicylic acid (aspirin); D, dipyridamole.

used a larger dose of aspirin which caused more bleeding, and had a smaller benefit. Thus in patients with mechanical heart valves and high-risk patients with prosthetic tissue valves, the addition of aspirin to warfarin therapy reduced mortality, particularly mortality from vascular causes, together with major systemic embolism (50).

BIOPROSTHETIC CARDIAC VALVES

Incidence of Thromboembolism

Thromboembolism after bioprosthetic valve replacement may be less common than after mechanical valve replacement in patients with similar degrees of anticoagulation (Tables 21-7 and 21-11). However, the incidence is extremely variable and may depend on the patient selection and severity of underlying disease (risk factors for thromboembolism) and the intensity and variability of anticoagulation used early after valve replacement when the risk of thromboembolism is extremely high. Previous (73–78) and more recent (79,157) studies have documented that the highest risk of thromboembolism is within the first 3 months after operation. In a randomized prospective trial of two different intensities of oral anticoagulation (INR 2.5 to

4.0 versus 2.0 to 2.25) for the first 3 months after operation, the incidence of thromboemboli was high and similar in both groups (12.1% per 3 months in the standard or higher intensity group and 12.8% per 3 months in the lower intensity group) (157). Oral anticoagulation was started when patients were able to take medications by mouth. Only low-dose subcutaneous heparin (5,000 U every 12 hours) was used early after operation for up to 7 days. No antiplatelet therapy was used.

By contrast, when subcutaneous heparin is started 6 hours after operation to prolong the activated partial thromboplastin time (APTT) to just beyond the upper limit of normal until the chest tubes are removed, and then the heparin is increased to prolong the activated partial thromboplastin time to 1.5 to 2 times control, and immediately followed by oral anticoagulation, the incidence of thromboembolism is extremely low after both aortic and mitral valve replacement in studies by Perier and colleagues (Table 21-11) and Baudet and colleagues (68,158). In a retrospective review we found a similar very high incidence of thromboembolism during the first 3 months (which was highest during the first 10 days) and a lower incidence during the next 4 to 12 years of 1.9% per year for aortic valve replacement (whether or not patients remained

TABLE 21-11. *Thromboembolism in bioprosthetic valve replacement*

Study	Pt (no)	Chronic ACRx (%)	TE	Thromb	Bleed	Year of operation
				%/Year		
			TE	Thromb	Bleed	
Porcine valve						
Burtolotti (148)	71	90	1.3	0	1.3	1970–1983
AVR + MVR						
Kimose (149)	–/188	100	0.5	0	1.2	1976–1986
Magilligan (150)	492/554	–	0.7	0	–	1971–1987
Second Generation						
Jamieson (151)	546/225	36[a]/52[a,b]	2.8/2.4	0.0	0.3/1.2	1981–1985
AVR + MVR	95	AF[c]	1.7	0	1.1	Same
Bovine pericardial valve						
Xiadong (152)	55/381	AF	0.41	0	–	1976–1985
Daeven (153)	220/121	171[b]/61[b]	0.6/2.2	0	–	1980–1985
AVR + MVR	63	49[b]	1.8	0	–	Same
Second Generation						
Revuelta (154)	89/27	36 (AF)[b]	1.2	0	–	1982–1986
Cosgrove (155)	310/	54[c]/–	1.6/–	0/–	1.0/–	1982–1985
Homograft Aortic Valve						
Matsuki (156)	555/–	–	0.34/0	–	–	1964–1986

[a]This percentage received anticoagulant or platelet inhibitor therapy.
[b]Short-term oral or antiplatelet Rx for 3 months.
[c]Short-term oral anticoagulant therapy in all for 2 to 6 months.

AF, chronic anticoagulant therapy if atrial fibrillation, large left atrium, intracardiac thrombus; AVR/MVR, atrial valve replacement/mitral valve replacement; Pt, patient; TE, thromboembolism; Thromb, thrombosis or valve; ACRx, oral anticoagulant activity.

on oral anticoagulation) and for mitral valve patients 1.2% per year if on oral anticoagulation and 4.3% per year if not anticoagulated (p < 0.05) (79). These studies suggest that more intense antithrombotic therapy is required very early (for 3 months) after operation and that chronic antithrombotic therapy should be continued thereafter.

No prospective randomized intervention trials for the prevention of thromboembolism have been done in patients with bioprosthetic heart valves except as part of a higher risk larger trial with mechanical valve patients (50). One level IV study involved young patients (mean age 44) who had mitral valve replacement with a porcine bioprosthesis and had atrial fibrillation; one group had valve replacement between 1975 and 1979, were treated with 1 g aspirin per day starting on the second postoperative day, and had an incidence of thromboemboli of 1.3% per year; the second group had valve replacement after 1979, were treated with 0.5 g aspirin every other day starting on the first postoperative day, and had an

incidence of thromboembolism of 0.3% per year. There was no control group. Thus aspirin alone may be effective, but requires further study. Aspirin alone was better than placebo in the SPAF study where enteric-coated aspirin at 325 mg per day significantly reduced stroke from 6.3% per year to 3.2% per year in patients with no significant valvular disease (44).

Thus it appears that valve location (aortic or mitral), adequacy of antithrombotic therapy, observation before or beyond the first 3 months after operation, and the presence of atrial fibrillation are all significant influences on the risk of thromboembolism after bioprosthetic valve replacement. These factors and the previous studies all provide knowledge of the pathogenesis and risk of thromboembolism and provide valuable information for the current recommendations that follow.

CURRENT RECOMENDATIONS

Recommendations for antithrombotic therapy for prosthetic valve replacement are out-

TABLE 21-12. *Antithrombotic therapy for prosthetic heart valves: current recommendations*

IN ALL PATIENTS, BEGIN HD WARFARIN STARTING 24 TO 48 HOURS AFTER OPERATION
(MAY START DOWN NASOGASTRIC TUBE). INR 2.5–3.5

Valve	Situations	Therapy
Mechanical	Routine	MD warfarin[a]
	High risk[b]	HD warfarin + ASA 80–100 mg/day or D 400 mg/day if intolerant of ASA
	Low risk (Bileaflet AV, NSR, LD, warfarin ACRx problems (bleeding or >75–80 years old)	If intolerant of D, HD warfarin[c] + Sulf 800 mg/day 1) LD warfarin[d] + ASA 80–100 mg/day or D 400 mg/day or if no warfarin 2) D 400 mg/day + ASA 80–100 mg/day or sulf 800 mg/day
	Recurrent embolism	Consider reoperation
Bioprosthetic	AVR routine-NSR	MD warfarin for 3 months, then ASA 80 mg/day
	MVR routine-NSR	MD warfarin[c] for 3 mo, then ASA 80 mg/day
	If AF or LS > 50 mm	LD warfarin ↓long-term
	If LA thrombus, previous TE, vascular disease	MD warfarin long-term + ASA 80–100 mg/day

[a]MD warfarin to prolong INR to 2.5 to 3.5.

[b]High risk includes patients with mechanical prosthetic valve implanted before 1980, previous thromboembolism, vascular disease, poor compliance, high variability in prothrombin times (INR <3.0 more than 40% of time), or patient population with an incidence of thromboembolism >2.0%/year on warfarin alone.

[c]High risk, thus higher dose (HD) warfarin to prolong INR to 3.0 to 4.0.

[d]Medium risk, thus lower dose (LD) warfarin to prolong INR to 2.0 to 3.0. ACRx, anticoagulant therapy; AF, atrial fibrillation; ASA, aspirin; AVR, aortic valve replacement; D, dipyridamole; LA, left atrium; MVR, mitral valve replacement; NSR, normal sinus rhythm; Sulf, sulfinpyrazine; TE, thromboembolism; INR, international normalized ratio.

lined in Table 21-12. Because platelet thrombus deposition (predominantly on the sewing ring) begins as soon as blood flows through the prosthetic valve and can be imaged within hours after operation by indium-III-platelet scintigraphy (4,69), antithrombotic therapy would ideally be started before operation and continued early after operation, but such studies have not yet been performed. Warfarin should be started within 24 to 48 hours after operation and administered at a dose sufficient to prolong the INR to 2.5 to 3.5. Warfarin should be continued indefinitely to prolong the INR to 2.5 to 3.5.

Therapy that needs testing in terms of benefit (antithrombotic) versus risk (hemorrhage) includes aspirin 160 mg down the nasogastric tube plus subcutaneous heparin 12,500 U starting 6 hours after operation in all patients for all types of prosthetic valves (it takes approximately 48 to 60 hours to reach therapeutic levels to maintain the activated partial thromboplastin time at 1.5 to 2.0, the upper limit of normal). Then subcutaneous heparin, 12,500 U every 12 hours, would be continued (adjusting to maintain the activated partial thromboplastin time at 1.5 to 2 times the upper limit of normal) until the time of hospital dismissal or until the prothrombin time has been in range with oral anticoagulation for approximately 3 to 5 days.

Patients with Mechanical Prosthetic Heart Valves

All patients should receive oral anticoagulants. Patients with a risk of thromboembolism (valve implanted before 1980, previous thromboembolism, vascular disease, anticoagulation decreased or stopped due to bleeding, poor patient compliance, high variability in prothrombin times, patient population with an incidence of thromboembolism >2.0% per year on warfarin alone) should have supplemental antithrombotic therapy with aspirin 80 to 100 mg per day or dipyridamole. There is a lower incidence of thromboembolism when dipyridamole is added to anticoagulation (see Table 21-1). The dipyridamole dosage 350 to 400 mg per day or 5 to

6 mg per kg per day (e.g., 75 mg three times a day with meals and 150 mg at bedtime) and should be added to warfarin therapy (grade A recommendation) in high-risk patients.

Approximately 5% to 10% of patients have intolerance to dipyridamole due to gastrointestinal upset or headache (10). The former may be diminished by administering therapy concomitantly with food or in a sustained release form (available in Europe and some other countries). The vasodilator effects (headaches) may also be diminished by slowing the absorption with food or slightly lowering the dose to see if symptoms are diminished. In an emergency, the vasodilator effects (such as angina from an overdose of dipyridamole) can be reversed immediately with intravenous aminophylline (50 to 100 mg infused over 1 to 2 minutes) (159).

In high-risk patients who remain intolerant of dipyridamole in spite of these measures, an alternative therapy is the addition of sulfinpyrazone (800 mg per day) to warfarin therapy. This is a grade C recommendation and is based on one level III study (69). Sulfinpyrazone has not been used in a randomized prospective trial. The study was uncontrolled and suggested that sulfinpyrazone was effective in certain patients, mainly those in whom it prolongs the shortened platelet survival. Sulfinpyrazone may prolong the prothrombin time in patients on warfarin (see Chapter 27). Thus, it should be checked more frequently after initiating this therapy. In patients with recurrent thromboemboli or who have significant vascular problems (biological tissue exposure to blood) which increase risk of thromboemboli, low-dose aspirin (80 mg per day) is beneficial (grade A recommendation) (50). For antipyrexia or analgesia, acetaminophen, sodium salicylate, or salsalate should be used rather than larger doses of aspirin.

In patients who have bleeding during anticoagulation when the prothrombin time is not beyond INR 4.5, we recommend evaluation for a secondary cause of bleeding (such as an underlying tumor or a low platelet count) and lower doses of warfarin, INR 2.0 to 3.0, in combination with dipyridamole or aspirin 80 to 100 mg per day. Bleeding is also more common after the initiation of anticoagulation since underlying lesions such as tumors may be revealed by the secondary bleed.

For patients unable to tolerate anticoagulation, we recommend a trial of dipyridamole (400 mg per day, as outlined) combined with aspirin 80 to 100 mg per day or sulfinpyrazone at 200 mg four times daily as empiric but temporary therapy. This therapy is not recommended indefinitely because antiplatelet therapy is not effective in the long term in patients with mechanical prosthetic cardiac valves (Tables 21-6 and 21-7). A patient who has recurrent thromboembolism while on adequate antithrombotic therapy with warfarin plus platelet inhibition should be seriously considered as a candidate for another valve replacement.

Bioprosthetic Cardiac Valve Replacement

Warfarin should be administered within 24 to 48 hours after operation at a dose to prolong the INR to 2.5 to 3.5 for 3 months. Patients at high risk (previous thromboembolism, vascular disease, or left atrial thrombus) should be continued on this dose of warfarin indefinitely and combined with aspirin 80 to 100 mg per day. Patients with paroxysmal or chronic atrial fibrillation, a large left atrium (>50 mm by M-mode echocardiography), or left ventricular dysfunction (ejection function <30% or fractional shortening <25% by echocardiography should be continued on warfarin to prolong the INR to 2.0 to 3.0. For patients with aortic or mitral valve replacement without the latter risk factors, aspirin (80 mg per day) may be continued indefinitely (grade C recommendation) as empiric therapy from one level IV study (160). Aspirin combined with warfarin may be needed for the first 10 to 90 days after operation and in patients who have associated aortocoronary bypass grafts, but additional studies are needed. Prospective randomized controlled trials are needed to determine the optimal antithrombotic therapy.

Prothrombin times should be monitored at least every 3 to 4 weeks in patients who are

TABLE 21-13. *Patient conditions can change warfarin dosage*

Decrease dose	Increase dose
↓Oral intake (postop)	↑Vitamin K intake
↓Vitamin K stores (recent A/C, NPO, antibiotics)	Leafy green vegetables (broccoli, lettuce, spinach)
Liver disease	
Hepatic congestion	
Renal disease (↓ or Δ albumin)	Green beans
Malignancy, sepsis	Cauliflower
Diarrhea, steatorrhea	Liver
Hypermetabolism (hyperthyroidism, fever)	Hypometabolism
Hereditary ↓ vitamin K clotting factors (hypothyroidism)	Hereditary resistance

A/C, anticoagulant therapy; NPO, nothing orally; postop, postoperatively; ↓, decrease; ↑, increase; Δ, changes.

stable and receiving therapy with warfarin. More frequent monitoring should be done whenever the prothrombin time is above or below the therapeutic range or whenever the patient's condition or therapy changes (Table 21-13) (see Chapter 27). Many drugs can alter the prothrombin time (see partial list in Chapter 27). Whenever any medication is added or deleted, always recheck the prothrombin time a week later. Close monitoring of therapy is important since increased variability appears related to increased risk of thromboembolism and probably bleeding. On the average, in a routine practice, 30% of prothrombin times may be too low, and 5% to 10% may be too high (10). Patients should avoid extremes in diet and try to keep green vegetable intake at a steady level because ingestion of vitamin K–containing food such as broccoli, lettuce, or other green vegetables can lower or normalize the prothrombin time (161).

Diagnosis and Treatment of Prosthetic Valve Thrombosis

Acute prosthetic valvular thrombosis is usually a medical emergency that carries a high risk of mortality unless diagnosed early and treated promptly. Thus, suspicion of the problem should be high, and urgent diagnosis is required. Mechanical prosthetic valvular thrombosis may occur at any time and is associated with inadequate anticoagulation in more than 50% to 70% of patients (162–174). Bioprosthetic valve thrombosis is uncommon, may occur especially during the early months

after operation, and appears preventable by therapy with warfarin (INR 2.5 to 3.5) for 3 months (98,158).

Symptoms vary from insidious and mild to abrupt circulatory failure. Any new or worsening symptoms require a thorough evaluation to exclude valve obstruction. Usual symptoms are new onset and progressive dyspnea, often for more than a week. New onset angina may occur in half of patients. Acute myocardial infarction is unusual (171). Many patients present in acute pulmonary edema or severe heart failure (162–168).

On physical examination most patients have pulmonary rales and may have signs of right heart failure such as edema, hepatomegaly, and elevated jugular venous pressure. A new murmur is present in 90% of these patients. Abnormal (absent or decreased) opening or closing clicks are present in 60%.

Rapid diagnosis is necessary and can be accomplished using Doppler echocardiography to measure transvalvular flow velocities for calculation of pressure gradients and measurements of pressure half-time to estimate valve area. These same techniques can substitute for cardiac catheterization and may also be used to monitor progress of thrombolysis if this therapy is chosen (166). Fluoroscopy, phonocardiography, and two-dimensional echocardiography are of limited value (164,168). However, some have found biplane cinefluoroscopy valuable for simple diagnosis of reduced disc/leaflet motion in patients with radiopaque disc valves (164,168).

Treatment is usually urgent valve replacement or debridement with a mortality risk of 8% to 50%. This risk is mainly related to preoperative functional class (18% for class IV and 5% for classes I to III) (163–165,167, 168a). Acute therapy has been reviewed (1686). In patients with tricuspid valve thrombosis or those at high surgical risk for left-sided valve replacement, thrombolysis of valvular thrombus may be considered (162,166).

For mitral or aortic valve thrombosis, duration of thrombolytic therapy has ranged from 5 to 95 hours, with success in 82% and emboli in 18% (162,170). Streptokinase and urokinase have been used most frequently. Streptokinase is often administered as a loading dose of 250,000 to 500,000 IU intravenously over 30 minutes followed by an infusion of 100,000 IU per hour for 9 to 96 hours or 150,000 IU per hour for 10 hours (162,166, 169,170,173). Urokinase may also be used in doses recommended for pulmonary embolism, 4,500 IU per kg per hour intravenous infusion over 12 to 24 hours without a loading dose (162). Tricuspid valve thrombosis has also been treated with a single intravenous dose of streptokinase (750,000 IU) over 20 minutes or recombinant tissue plasminogen activator (150 mg altephase intravenously over 8 hours ± an additional 50 mg intravenously over the next 8 hours, or 70 mg intravenously over 5 hours, or 10 mg bolus plus 40 mg intravenously over 2 hours along with simultaneous heparin (175–181). Because thrombolytic agents activate thrombin and platelets, simultaneous heparin infusion should be administered for 5 to 7 days, maintaining the activated partial thromboplastin time at 1.5 to 2 times control before switching to warfarin to maintain the INR at 3.0 to 4.5. Doppler echocardiography is an excellent method for monitoring progress and outcome of thrombolysis.

SPECIAL SITUATIONS

Patients with prosthetic cardiac valve replacement may develop four situations which could require alteration of their antithrombotic therapy.

Noncardiac Surgery

Discontinuation of anticoagulation for 5 to 10 days appears to carry a low risk for patients undergoing a noncardiac operation (181). In order to minimize risk, we recommend stopping warfarin 4 to 5 days before operation, continuing dipyridamole (400 mg per day, or starting it if it is not being administered), and starting a heparin infusion (to maintain the activated partial thromboplastin time at twice control) when the prothrombin time decreases to less than INR 2.0 to 2.5. The heparin infusion should be continued until 4 to 5 hours before operation. Subcutaneous heparin (15,000 U per day given in two or three divided doses) should be continued during and early after the operation, except in patients undergoing brain or intraocular operations. The heparin therapy should be increased as soon as possible to 12,500 U twice daily (and titrated to an activated partial thromboplastin time of twice control 6 to 12 hours after a dose), and warfarin therapy should be restarted as soon as possible after operation.

Prosthetic Valve Endocarditis

Patients with prosthetic valve endocarditis who are not receiving anticoagulant therapy have a 50% risk of thromboembolism to the brain (182–184). Anticoagulant therapy can probably decrease the incidence of thromboembolism by six- to ninefold, as suggested by three non-randomized clinical studies (182,183,185). Hemorrhage into the brain occurred in 14% of these patients, but the overall risk appears to be considerably lower with anticoagulation. Thus, we advise continuing therapeutic anticoagulation for the patient with prosthetic valve endocarditis as long as there is no clinical or laboratory evidence of intracranial hemorrhage or gastrointestinal bleeding. Patients should be switched to a heparin infusion therapy (APTT 1.5 to 2.0 × control) in the hospital for versatility in case emergency operation is required or significant bleeding occurs.

Anticoagulation After a Thromboembolic Event

The optimal time to start anticoagulation after a thromboembolic event to the brain has been controversial. A second embolism may occur early after the first event; thus immediate anticoagulation appears advisable. However, caution is advised because anecdotal reports and experimental studies suggest that immediate anticoagulation, especially in patients with a large embolic brain infarct, can result in secondary hemorrhages with increased morbidity. Data from 15 prospective and retrospective level V studies (31) suggest that approximately 12% of patients (range 0 to 22) with aseptic embolism to the brain from a cardiac source experience a second embolic event within 2 weeks. Early recurrence is evenly distributed over the initial 2 weeks at about 1% per day.

Recurrent thromboembolism appears to be decreased by immediate anticoagulation with heparin. In patients receiving anticoagulation, there was a reduction in early recurrent embolism within 14 days to about one third of that in patients who did not receive anticoagulants in six level III and level IV studies (31). A level II randomized trial (186) of 45 patients showed that patients who received anticoagulants had a lower recurrence rate of thromboembolism. However, another randomized study showed the opposite effect (187). There are large variations in the reported risk of cerebral hemorrhage after anticoagulating for embolic stroke. The risk of hemorrhages ranges from 0 to 24% (31). Details of intensity of anticoagulation are lacking for an analysis of risk.

A large brain infarct appears to place patients at a higher risk of hemorrhage when anticoagulated immediately after an embolic stroke. Spontaneous hemorrhagic transformation may be delayed for several days but occurs most frequently within 48 hours (31,188). A national conference on antithrombotic therapy has made recommendations concerning this delicate problem (31).

Immediate anticoagulation of small to moderate-sized embolic strokes appears advisable if computed tomographic (CT) scan of the head performed within 24 to 48 hours of the stroke does not indicate hemorrhage and if acute hypertension ($\geq 180/100$ mm Hg) is not present. The same principles apply for continuation of anticoagulation therapy in patients with a prosthetic heart valve who have an embolic stroke during long-term anticoagulant therapy. Patients with a large embolic infarct appear to be at special risk for delayed hemorrhagic transformation; thus anticoagulation is usually postponed for 5 to 7 days before restarting or initiating anticoagulation. This allows time to document that a repeat CT scan of the head does not show hemorrhagic transformation. An infusion of heparin is preferable to large boluses to avoid large swings in anticoagulation and APTT beyond 2.0 times the upper limit of normal. A therapeutic range of 1.5 to 2.0 times control is recommended for the APTT.

Antithrombotic Therapy During Pregnancy

Anticoagulant therapy in general during pregnancy is discussed in detail in Chapter 26. For women with a prosthetic cardiac valve and of childbearing age, education concerning pregnancy and anticoagulation is critical. Pregnancy should be well planned. Warfarin should be stopped as soon as possible after conception to avoid the teratogenic risk of warfarin that is especially prominent during the first trimester. Women who receive warfarin therapy at the time of conception and during the first trimester have a high fetal wastage. This wastage may be higher than 80% in women with multiple prosthetic heart valves (189). Exposure after the first trimester may also predispose to congenital anomalies. The major anomalies include nasal hypoplasia, stippling of bones (chondrodysplasia punctata or Conradi's syndrome), mental retardation, optic atrophy, microcephaly, and spasticity or hypotonia (189–193). Coumarin derivatives cross the placental barrier, anticoagulate the fetus, and can lead to hemorrhagic complications, especially at the time of delivery.

Anticoagulation should be switched from warfarin to subcutaneous heparin at the time of suspected conception, such as with flattening of the temperature curve at the time of anticipated ovulation, or at the time of a positive test for human chorionic gonadotropin, which can detect pregnancy 5 days before the missed menstrual period.

Administration of subcutaneous heparin should be continued throughout the first trimester. Some advocate continuation throughout the pregnancy to try to minimize any possible risk of congenital anomaly. Heparin therapy should be started at a minimum dose of 12,500 U every 12 hours following a bolus of 5,000 U intravenously to saturate intravascular binding sites and adjusted upward as necessary to maintain the APTT within 2.0 to 2.5 times control when drawn 6 to 12 hours after the previous dose. This appears to maintain good antithrombotic protection against thromboembolism (195). A target APTT of 1.5 to 2.5 times control appears too low (196); target should be 2.0 to 2.5 times control, which requires an average of 17,000 U every 12 hours. A tuberculin syringe with a 25-gauge needle and heparin in a concentration of 20,000 or 40,000 U per ml are convenient for repeated injection in the abdominal region with continued rotation of sites over the entire abdominal wall. A dose of 5,000 U of heparin every 12 hours is not sufficient for the prevention of thromboembolism in patients with prosthetic heart valves (193,197). Subcutaneous heparin should be continued through the first trimester, at which time oral anticoagulation can be restarted and continued through week 37 or until 1 to 2 weeks before anticipated delivery. At that time the patient should be switched to a heparin infusion, which is continued until the induction of labor. At labor the patient is switched to low-dose subcutaneous heparin, 5,000 U every 8 hours. Fortunately, heparin does not cross the placental barrier. Warfarin therapy should be restarted immediately after delivery. Nursing mothers can use warfarin because only an inactivate metabolite of warfarin is found in breast milk, and this does not change the pro-

thrombin time of the infant (198,199). To be certain that there is not an unusual situation, the infant should have a prothrombin time checked on one occasion after the nursing mother is on warfarin therapy and has been nursing the infant regularly.

A bioprosthetic heart valve is preferred for women of child-bearing age who wish to bear children because many do not require long-term anticoagulant therapy (i.e., assuming they have no other risk factors for thromboembolism). However, the risk of bioprosthetic calcification in women under age 35 and short durability of the bioprosthetic valve (10 to 15 years) have to be kept in mind. Platelet inhibitor drugs should be avoided as a routine during pregnancy because aspirin may cause premature closure of the ductus arteriosus. Dipyridamole and sulfinpyrazone have indeterminant effects on the fetus and are not approved for use during pregnancy. Maternal and fetal outcomes during pregnancy of women with prosthetic heart valves have been variable in reports (194,195,200). However, careful planning of conception and antithrombotic therapy appears extremely valuable for minimizing the risk to both mother and infant.

Because of more thromboembolic and bleeding complications associated with heparin targeted to an APTT of 1.5 to 2.5 times control (196) or during uncertain control (202), and because the incidence of warfarin embryopathy appears to be very low, recent reports are recommending continued warfarin therapy throughout pregnancy (196,202).

CONCLUSION

Patients at high risk for thromboembolism who require anticoagulation to an INR of 2.5 to 3.5 are those with mitral stenosis who are in the first year of anticoagulation for paroxysmal or chronic atrial fibrillation, mitral valve disease who are in the first year after a thromboembolic event, tilting disk or bileaflet mechanical prosthetic valve, or bioprosthetic heart valve during the first 3 months after operation. Patients with mechanical or bioprosthetic valve replacement who have coronary, peripheral, or cerebral vascular disease, prior thromboembolism, or left atrial thrombus should also receive aspirin 80 to 100 mg per day. Patients at medium risk who require anti-coagulation to an INR of 2.0 to 3.0 are those with (1) paroxysmal or chronic atrial fibrillation and (a) mitral regurgitation, (b) mitral stenosis after one year of anticoagulation, or (c) over age 60 with systolic blood pressure >160, prior thromboembolism, moderately or severely impaired left ventricular function, or women over age 75 years; (2) sinus rhythm with a very large left atrium (> 55 mm by M-mode echocardiography; (3) heart failure or severe left ventricular dysfunction; (4) bio-prosthetic heart valve replacement beyond 3 months after operation with atrial fibrillation or left atrial size >50 mm; or (5) bileaflet mechanical prosthetic aortic valve replacement in patient with sinus rhythm and left atrial size <50 mm.

Anticoagulation for patients with mechanical caged ball valve replacement is probably an INR of 3.0 to 4.0 (extrapolated from older studies using prothrombin ratios) along with aspirin 80 to 100 mg per day, but there are no randomized trials to support this. Optimal anti-coagulation for patients >75 years is probably at the lower end of the recommended range, and if this range is an INR of 2.0 to 3.0, a range of 1.7 to 2.0 may be protective and minimize the risk of bleeding. Patients with bioprosthetic valve replacement, no atrial fibrillation, prior thromboembolism, left ventricular dysfunction of enlarged left atrium, may be protected from thromboembolism by long-term aspirin alone, but a controlled trial is needed. The optimal supplemental antiplatelet therapy for patients with prior thromboembolism or associated vascular disease and whether all mechanical valve patients on antiplatelet therapy can have their INR lowered to 2.0 to 3.0 are uncertain and require further study.

REFERENCES

1. Stein B, Fuster V, Halperin JL, Chesebro JH. Antithrombotic therapy in cardiac disease. An emerging approach based on pathogenesis and risk. *Circulation* 1989;80:1501–1513.

2. Amarenco P, Duyckaerts C, Tzourio C, et al. The prevalence of ulcerated plaques in the aortic arch in patients with stroke. *N Engl J Med* 1992;326:221–225.
3. Toschi V, Gallo R, Lettino M, et al. Tissue factor modulates the thrombogenicity of human atherosclerotic plaques. *Circulation* 1997;95:594–599.
4. Dewanjee MK, Fuster V, Rao SA, Forshaw PL, Kaye MP. Noninvasive radioisotopic technique for detection of platelet deposition in mitral valve prostheses and quantitation of visceral microembolism in dogs. *Mayo Clin Proc* 1983;58:307–14.
5. Dahike H, Dociu N, Thurau K. Thrombogenicity of different suture materials as revealed by scanning electron microscopy. *J Biomed Mater Res* 1980;14:251–268.
6. Meyer BJ, Badimon JJ, Mailhac A, et al. Inhibition of growth of thrombus on fresh mural thrombus: targeting optimal therapy. *Circulation* 1994;90:2432–2438.
7. Liu CY, Nossel HL, Kaplan KL. The binding of thrombin to fibrin. *J Biol Chem* 1979;254:10421–10425.
8. Edmunds LH, Clark RE, Cohn LH, Grunkemeier GL, Miller DC, Weisel RD. Guidelines for reporting morbidity and mortality after cardiac valvular operations. *J Thorac Cardiovasc Surg* 1996;112:708–711.
9. Fuster V, Pumphrey CW, McGoon MD, Chesebro JH, Pluth JR, McGoon DC. Systemic thromboembolism in mitral and aortic Starr-Edwards prostheses: a 10-19 year follow-up. *Circulation* 1982;66(suppl I):I-157–161.
10. Chesebro JH, Fuster V, Elevback LR, et al. Trial of combined warfarin plus dipyridamole or aspirin therapy in prosthetic heart valve replacement: danger of aspirin compared with dipyridamole. *Am J Cardiol* 1983;51:1537–1541.
11. Szekely P. Systemic embolism and anticoagulant prophylaxis in rheumatic heart disease. *Br Med J* 1964;1:1209–1212.
12. Coulshed N, Epstein EJ, McKendrick CS, Galloway RW, Walker E. Systemic embolism in mitral valve disease. *Br Heart J* 1979;32:26–34.
13. Fleming HA, Bailey SM. Mitral valve disease, systemic embolism and anticoagulants. *Postgrad Med J* 1971;47:599–604.
14. Wolf PA, Dawber TR, Thomas HE Jr, et al. Epidemiologic assessment of chronic atrial fibrillation and risk of stroke: the Framingham Study. *Neurology* 1978;28:973–977.
15. Caplan LR, D'Crux I, Hier DB, Reddy H, Shah S. Atrial size, atrial fibrillation, and stroke. *Ann Neurol* 1986;19:158–161.
16. Fuster V, Gersh BJ, Giuliani ER, et al. The natural history of idiopathic dilated cardiomyopathy. *Am J Cardiol* 1981;47:525–531.
17. Pumphrey CW, Fuster V, Chesebro JH. Systemic thromboembolism in valvular heart disease and prosthetic heart valves. *Mod Concepts Cardiovasc Dis* 1982;51:131–136.
18. Chesebro JH, Fuster V, Halperin JL. Atrial fibrillation—risk marker for stroke. *N Engl J Med* 1990;323:1556–1558.
19. Askey JM, Berstein S. The management of rheumatic heart disease in relation to systemic arterial embolism. *Prog Cardiovasc Dis* 1960;3:220–232.
20. Deveral PB, Olley PM, Smith DR, Watson DA, Whitaker W. Incidence of systemic embolism before and after mitral valvotomy. *Thorax* 1968;23:530–536.

21. Abernathy WS, Willis PW. Thromboembolic complications of rheumatic heart disease. *Cardiovasc Clin* 1973;5:131–175.
22. Nielson GH, Galea EG, Hossack KF. Thromboembolic complications of mitral valve disease. *Aust NZ J Med* 1978;8:372–376.
23. Easton JD, Sherman DG. Management of cerebral embolism of cardiac origin. *Stroke* 1980;11:433–442.
24. Hart RG, Miller VT. Cerebral infarction in young adults: a practical approach. *Stroke* 1983;14:110–114.
25. Wolf PA, Abbott RD, Kannel WB. Atrial fibrillation: a major contributor to stroke in the elderly: the Framingham Study. *Arch Intern Med* 1987;147:1561–1564.
26. Chesebro JH, Adams PC, Fuster V. Antithrombotic therapy in patients with valvular heart disease and prosthetic heart valves. *J Am Coll Cardiol* 1986;8:41B–56B.
27. Barnett JH, Boughner DR, Taylor DW, et al. Further evidence relating mitral-valve prolapse to cerebral ischemic events. *N Engl J Med* 1980;302:139–144.
28. Savage DD, Garrison RJ, Devereaux RB, et al. Mitral valve prolapse in the general population. I. Epidemiologic features: the Framingham Study. *Am Heart J* 1983;106:571–576.
29. Nishimura RA, McGoon MD, Shub C, Miller FA, Ilstrup DM. Tajik Al. Echocardiographically documented mitral valve prolapse: long-term follow-up of 237 patients. *N Engl J Med* 1985;313:1305–1309.
30. Barnett HJM, Jones MW, Boughner DR, Kostuk WJ. Cerebral ischemic events associated with prelapsing mitral valve. *Arch Neurol* 1976;33:777–782.
31. Sherman DG, Dyken ML, Fisher M, Harrison MJG, Hart RG. Antithrombotic therapy for cerebrovascular disorders. *Chest* 1989;95(suppl):140S–155S.
32. Barnett HJ. Heart in ischemic stroke-a changing emphasis. *Neurol Clin* 1983;1:291–315.
33. Schnee MA, Bucal AA. Fatal embolism in mitral valve prolapse. *Chest* 1983;83:285–287.
34. Jackson AC, Boughner DR, Barnett HJ. Mitral valve prolapse and cerebral ischemic events in young patients. *Neurology* 1984;24:384–387.
35. Dry BTJ, Willius FA. Calcareous disease of the aortic valve: a study of 228 cases. *Am Heart J* 1939;17:138–157.
36. Kumpe CW, Bean WB. Aortic stenosis: a study of the clinical and pathologic aspects of 107 proved cases. *Medicine* 1948;27:139–185.
37. Rotman M, Morris JJ Jr, Behar VS, et al. Aortic valvular disease. Comparison of types and their medical and surgical management. *Am J Med* 1971;51:241–257.
38. Holley KE, Bahn RC, McGoon DC, Mankin HT. Spontaneous calcific embolization associated with calcific aortic stenosis. *Circulation* 1963;27:197–202.
39. Brockmeier LB, Adolph RJ, Gustin BW, Holmes JC, Sacks JG. Calcium emboli to the retinal artery in calcific aortic stenosis. *Am Heart J* 1981;101:32–37.
40. Stein PD, Sabbah HN, Pitha JV. Continuing disease process of calcific aortic stenosis. Role of microthrombi and turbulent flow. *Am J Cardiol* 1977;39:159–163.
41. Sherrid MV, Clark RD, Cohn K. Echocardiographic analysis of left atrial size before and after operation in mitral valve disease. *Am J Cardiol* 1979;43:171–178.
42. Rogers PH, Sherry S. Current status of antithrombotic therapy in cardiovascular disease. *Prog Cardiovasc Dis* 1976;19:235–253.
43. Kannel WB, Abbott RD, Savage DD, et al. Epidemiologic features of chronic atrial fibrillation. *N Engl J Med* 1982;306:1018–1022.
44. Stroke Prevention in Atrial Fibrillation Study Group Investigators. Preliminary report of the SPAF Study. *N Engl J Med* 1990;322:863–868.
45. Daley R, Mattingly TW, Holt CL, et al. Systemic arterial embolism in rheumatic heart disease. *Am Heart J* 1951;42:566–81.
46. Carter AB. Prognosis of cerebral embolism. *Lancet* 1965;2:514–519.
47. Darling RC, Austen WG, Linton RR. Atrial embolism. *Surg Gynecol Obstet* 1967;124:106–114.
48. Casella L, Abelmann WH, Ellis LB. Patients with mitral stenosis and systemic emboli. *Arch Intern Med* 1964;114:773–781.
49. Poller L. Simple nanogram for the derivation of international normalized ratios for the standardization of prothrombin time. *Thromb Haemost* 1988:60:18–20.
50. Turpie AGG, Gent M, Laupacis A, et al. A comparison of aspirin with placebo in patients treated with warfarin after heart valve replacement. *N Engl J Med* 1993;329:524–529.
51. Cook OJ, Guyatt GH, Laupacis A, Sackett DL, Goldberg RJ. Clinical recommendations using levels of evidence for antithrombotic agents. *Chest* 1995(suppl):227S–230S.
52. Chesebro IH, Fuster V, Eiveback LR, et al. Effect of dipyridamole and aspirin on late vein-graft patency after coronary bypass operations. *N Engl J Med* 1984;310:209–214.
53. Cairns JA, Gent M, Singer J, et al. Aspirin, sulfinpyrazone or both in unstable angina: results of a Canadian multicenter trial. *N Engl J Med* 1985;313:1369–1375.
54. Petersen P, Boysen G, Godtfredsen J, Andersen ED, Andersen B. Placebo controlled randomized trial of warfarin and aspirin for prevention of thromboembolic complications in chronic atrial fibrillation: the Copenhagen AFASAK Study. *Lancet* 1989;1:175–179.
55. Boston Area Anticoagulation Trial for Atrial Fibrillation Investigators. The effect of low-dose warfarin on the risk of stroke in patients with nonrheumatic atrial fibrillation. *N Engl J Med* 1990;323:1505–1511.
56. Ezekowitz MD, Bridgers SL, James KE, et al. Warfarin in the prevention of stroke associated with nonrheumatic atrial fibrillation. *N Engl J Med* 1992;327:1406–1412.
57. Stroke Prevention in Atrial Fibrillation Investigators. Warfarin vs aspirin for prevention of thromboembolism in atrial fibrillation: Stroke Prevention in Atrial Fibrillation II Study. *Lancet* 1994;343:687–691.
58. Connolly SJ, Laupacis A, Gent M, et al. Canadian Atrial Fibrillation Anticoagulation (CAFA) Study. *J Am Coll Cardiol* 1991;18:349–355.
59. Atrial Fibrillation Investigators. Risk factors for stroke and efficacy of antithrombotic therapy in atrial fibrillation: analysis of pooled data from five randomized control trials. *Arch Intern Med* 1994;154:1449–1457.
60. The Stroke Prevention in Atrial Fibrillation Investigators. Predictors of thromboembolism in atrial fibrillation: II. Echocardiographic features of patients at risk. *Ann Intern Med* 1992;116:6–12.
61. Dalen JE, Hirsh J. Fourth ACCP conference on antithrombotic therapy. *Chest* 1995;108(suppl):225S–522S.
62. Levine HJ, Pauker SG, Eckman MH. Antithrombotic

therapy in valvular heart disease. *Chest* 1995;108 (suppl):360S–370S.

63. Stroke Prevention in Atrial Fibrillation Investigators. Risk factors for thromboembolism during aspirin therapy in patients with atrial fibrillation: the stroke prevention in atrial fibrillation study. *J Stroke Cerebrovasc Dis* 1995;5:147–157.

64. The Stroke Prevention in Atrial Fibrillation Investigators. Predictors of thromboembolism in atrial fibrillation: I. Clinical features of patients at risk. *Ann Intern Med* 1992;116:1–5.

65. The Stroke Prevention in Atrial Fibrillation Investigators Committee on Echocardiography. Transesophageal echocardiographic correlates of thromboembolism in high-risk patients with nonvalvular atrial fibrillation. *Ann Intern Med.* In press.

66. Levine MN, Raskob G, Hirsh J. Hemorrhagic complications of long-term anticoagulant therapy. *Chest* 1989;95(suppl):26S–36S.

67. Steele P, Rainwater J. Favorable effect of sulfinpyrazone on thromboembolism in patients with rheumatic heart disease. *Circulation* 1980;62:462–465.

68. Baudet EM, Puel V, McBride JT, et al. Long-term results of valve replacement with the St. Jude Medical prosthesis. *J Thorac Cardiovasc Surg* 1995;109: 858–870.

69. Dewanjee MK, Trastek VF, Tago M, Kaye MP. Radioisotopic techniques for noninvasive detection of platelet deposition in bovine tissue mitral-valve prostheses and in vitro quantification of visceral microembolism in dogs. *Invest Radiol* 1984;6:535–542.

70. Forbes CD, Prentice CRM. Thrombus formation and artificial surfaces. *Br Med Bull* 1978;34:201–207.

71. Markwardt F, Kaiser B, Nowak G. Studies on antithrombotic effects of recombinant hirudin. *Thromb Res* 1989;54:377–388.

72. Heras M, Chesebro JH, Webster MWI, et al. Hirudin, heparin, and placebo during deep arterial injury in the pig: the in vivo role of thrombin in platelet-mediated thrombosis. *Circulation* 1990;82:1476–1484.

73. Pipkin RD, Buch WS, Fogarty TS. Evaluation of aortic valve replacement with a porcine xenograft without long-term anticoagulants. *J Thorac Cardiovasc Surg* 1976;71:179–186.

74. Stinson EB, Griepp RB, Oyer PE, Shumway NE. Long-term experience with porcine aortic valve xenografts. *J Thorac Cardiovasc Surg* 1977;73:54–63.

75. Ionescu MI, Pakrashi BC, Mary DAS, Bartek IT, Woolner GH, McGoon DC. Long-term evaluation of tissue valves. *J Thorac Cardiovasc Surg* 1974;68: 361–379.

76. Cevese PG. Long-term results of 212 xenograft valve replacement. *J Cardiovasc Surg* 1975;16:639–642.

77. Davila JC, Magilligan DJ, Lewis JW. Is the Hancock porcine valve the best cardiac valve substitute today? *Ann Thorac Surg* 1978;26:303–316.

78. Edmiston WA, Harrison EC, Duwick GF, Parnassus W, Lau FYK. Thromboembolism in mitral porcine valve recipients. *Am J Cardiol* 1978;41:508–511.

79. Heras M, Chesebro JH, Fuster V, et al. High risk of thromboemboli early after bioprosthetic cardiac valve replacement. *J Am Coll Cardiol* 1995;25:1111–1119.

80. Harker LA, Slichter SJ. Studies of platelet and fibrinogen kinetics in patients with prosthetic heart valves. *N Engl J Med* 1970;283:1302–1305.

81. Weily HS, Genton E. Altered platelet function in patients with prosthetic mitral valves: effects of sulfinpyrazone therapy. *Circulation* 1970;42:967–972.

82. Steele P, Rainwater J, Vogel R. Platelet suppressant therapy in patients with prosthetic cardiac valves: relationship of clinical effectiveness to alteration of platelet survival time. *Circulation* 1979;60:910–913.

83. Pengo V, Peruzzi P, Baca M, et al. The optimal therapeutic range for oral anticoagulant treatment as suggested by fibrinopeptide A (FPA) levels in patients with heart valve prosthesis. *Eur J Clin Invest* 1989;19: 181–184.

84. Friedli B, Aerichide N, Grondin P, Campeau L. Thromboembolic complications of heart valve replacement. *Am Heart J* 1971;81:702–708.

85. Gadboys HL, Litwak RS, Niemetz J, Wisch N. Role of anticoagulants in preventing embolization from prosthetic heart valves. *JAMA* 1967;202:134–138.

86. Cleland J, Molloy PJ. Thromboembolic complications of cloth-covered Starr-Edwards prostheses no. 2300 aortic and no. 6300 mitral. *Thorax* 1973;28:41–47.

87. Barnhorst DA, Oxman HA, Connolly DC, et al. Long-term follow up of isolated replacement of the aortic or mitral valve with the Starr-Edwards prosthesis. *Am J Cardiol* 1975;35:228–233.

88. Saour JN, Sieck JO, Mamo LAR, Gallus AS. Trial of different intensities of anticoagulation in patients with prosthetic heart valves. *N Engl J Med* 1990;322: 428–432.

89. Horstkotte D, Schulte HD, Bircks W, Strauer BE. Lower intensity anticoagulation therapy results in lower complication rates with the St. Jude Medical prosthesis. *J Thorac Cardiovasc Surg* 1994;107: 1136–1145.

90. Bjork VO, Henze A. Ten years experience with the Bjork-Shiley tilting disk valve. *J Thorac Cardiovasc Surg* 1979;78:331–342.

91. Huber KC, Gersh BJ, Bailey KR, Hodge DO, Chesebro JH. Variability in anticoagulation control predicts thromboembolism: a 23 year population based study [Abstract]. *Circulation* 1991;84(suppl II):I-356.

92. Dale J, Myhre E. Can acetylsalicylic acid alone prevent arterial thromboembolism? A pilot study in patients with aortic ball valve prosthesis. *Acta Med Scand* 1981;645(suppl):73–78.

93. Cohn LH, Koster JK, Meed RBB, Collins JJ. Long-term follow up of the Hancock bioprosthetic heart valve [Abstract]. *Circulation* 1979;60(suppl I):I-87.

94. Hetzer R, Hill JD, Kerth WJ, et al. Thromboembolic complications after mitral valve replacement with Hancock xenograft. *J Thorac Cardiovasc Surg* 1978; 75:651–688.

95. Oyer PE, Stinson ER, Griepp RB, Shumway NE. Valve replacement with the Starr-Edwards and Hancock prostheses. *Ann Surg* 1977;186:301–309.

96. Lakier JB, Khaja R, Magiligan DJ Jr, Goldstein S. Porcine xenograft valves: long-term (60-90 month) follow up. *Circulation* 1980;62:313–318.

97. Anderson ET, Hancock EWL. Long-term follow up of aortic valve replacement with the mesh aortic homograft. *J Thorac Cardiovasc Surg* 1976;72:150–156.

98. Douglas P, Hirshfeld JW, Edmunds LH. Clinical correlates of post-operative atrial fibrillation [Abstract]. *Circulation* 1984;70(suppl II):II-165.

99. Cohn LH, Alfred EN, Cohn LA, DiSesa VJ, Shemin

RJ, Collins JJ Jr. Long-term results of open mitral valve reconstruction for mitral stenosis. *Am J Cardiol* 1985;55:731–734.

100. Carpentier A, Chauvaud S, Fabiana JN, et al. Reconstructive surgery of mitral valve incompetence. *J Thorac Cardiovasc Surg* 1980;79:338–348.

101. Spencer FC, Colvin SB, Culliford AT, Isom OW. Experiences with the Carpentier techniques of mitral valve reconstruction in 103 patients (1980–1985). *J Thorac Cardiovasc Surg* 1985;90:341–350.

102. Macmanus Q, Grunkemeier GL, Lambert LE, Teply JF, Harlan BJ, Starr A. Year of operation as a risk factor in the late results of valve replacement. *J Thorac Cardiovasc Surg* 1980;80:834–841.

103. McGood DC. The risk of thromboembolism following valvular operations: how does one know? *J Thorac Cardiovasc Surg* 1984;88:782–786.

104. Hackett D, Fessatidis I, Saphsford R, Oakley C. Ten year clinical evaluation of Starr-Edwards 2400 and 1260 aortic valve prostheses. *Br Heart J* 1987;57:356–363.

105. Fessatidis I, Hackett D, Oakley CM, Sapsford RN, Bentall HH. Ten year clinical evaluation of isolated mitral valve and double-valve replacement with the Starr-Edwards prosthesis. *Ann Thorac Surg* 1987;43:368–372.

106. Schoevaerdts JC, el Gariani A, Lichtsteiner M, Jaumin P, Ponlot R, Chalant CH-H. Twenty years experience with the Model 6120 Starr-Edwards valve in the mitral position. *J Thorac Cardiovasc Surg* 1987;94:375–382.

107. Cobanoglu A, Fessler CL, Guvendik L, Grunkemeier G, Starr A. Aortic valve replacement with the Starr-Edwards prosthesis: a comparison of the first and second decades of follow-up. *Ann Thorac Surg* 1988;45:248–252.

108. Harjula A, Mattila S, Maamies T, et al. Long-term follow-up of Bjork-Shiley mitral valve replacement. 10 years experience. *Scand J Thorac Cardiovasc Surg* 1986;20:79–84.

109. Bloomfield P, Kitchin AH, Wheatley DJ, Walbaum PR, Lutz W, Miller HC. A prospective valuation of the Bjork-Shiley Hancock, and Carpentier-Edwards heart valve prostheses. *Circulation* 1986;73:1213–1222.

110. Borkon AM, Soule LM, Baughman KL, et al. Comparative analysis of mechanical and bioprosthetic valves after aortic valve replacement. *J Thorac Cardiovasc Surg* 1987;94:20–33.

111. Lindblom D. Long-term clinical results after aortic valve replacement with the Bjork-Shiley prosthesis. *J Thorac Cardiovasc Surg* 1988;95:658–667.

112. Lindblom D. Long-term clinical results after mitral valve replacement with the Bjork-Shiley prosthesis. *J Thorac Cardiovasc Surg* 1988;95:321–333.

113. Thulin LI, Bain WH, Huysmans HH, et al. Heart valve replacement with the Bjork-Shiley monostrut valve: early results of a multicenter clinical investigation. *Ann Thorac Surg* 1988;45:164–170.

114. Milano AD, Bortollotti U, Mazzucco A, Guerra F, Magni A, Gallucci V. Aortic valve replacement with the Hancock standard, Bjork-Shiley, and Lillehi-Kaster prostheses. A comparison based on follow-up from 1 to 15 years. *J Thorac Cardiovasc Surg* 1989;98:37–47.

115. Fessatidis JT, Vassiliadis KE, Monro JL, Ross JK, Shore DF, Drury PJ. Thirteen years evaluation of the Bjork-Shiley isolated mitral valve prosthesis. The Wessex experience. *J Cardiovasc Surg* 1989;30:957–965.

116. Bloomfield P, Wheatley DJ, Prescott RJ, Miller HC. Twelve-year comparison of a Bjork-Shiley mechanical heart valve with porcine bioprostheses. *N Engl J Med* 1991;324:573–579.

117. Chaux A, Czer LSC, Matloff JM, et al. The St. Jude Medical bileaflet valve prosthesis: a 5 year experience. *J Thorac Cardiovasc Surg* 1984;88:706–717.

118. Baudet EM, Oca CC, Roques XF, et al. A 5 1/2 year experience with the St. Jude Medical cardiac valve prosthesis: early and late results of 737 valve replacements in 671 patients. *J Thorac Cardiovasc Surg* 1985;90:137–144.

119. Kinsley RH, Antunes MJ, Colsen PR. St. Jude Medical valve replacement. *J Thorac Cardiovasc Surg* 1986;92:349–360.

120. Nakano K, Imamura E, Hashimoto A, et al. Six-year experience with the St. Jude Medical prosthesis: early and late results of 540 valves in 462 patients. *Jpn Circ J* 1987;51:275–283.

121. Montalescot G, Thomas D, Drobinski G, et al. Clinical and ultrasound results after aortic valve replacement: intermediate-term follow-up with the St. Jude Medical prosthesis. *Am Heart J* 1989;118:104–113.

122. Arom KV, Nicoloff DM, Kersten TE, Northrup WF III, Lindsay WG, Emery RW. Ten years experience with the St. Jude Medical valve prosthesis. *Ann Thorac Surg* 1989;27:831–837.

123. Czer LS, Chaux A, Matloff JM, et al. Ten-year experience with the St. Jude Medical valve for primary valve replacement. *J Thorac Cardiovasc Surg* 1990;100:44–55.

124. Kratz JM, Carwford FA, Sade RM, Crumbley AJ, Stroud MR. St. Jude prosthesis for aortic and mitral valve replacement: a ten-year experience. *Ann Thorac Surg* 1993;56:462–468.

125. Fernandez J, Laub GW, Adkins MS, et al. Early and late-phase events after valve replacement with the St. Jude Medical prosthesis in 1,200 patients. *J Thorac Cardiovasc Surg* 1994;107:394–406.

126. Ibrahim M, O Kane H, Cleland J, Gladstone D, Sarsam M, Patterson C. The St. Jude Medical prosthesis: a thirteen-year experience. *J Thorac Cardiovasc Surg* 1994;108:221–230.

127. Callaghan JC, Coles J, Damle A. Six year clinical study of use of the omniscience valve prosthesis in 219 patients. *J Am Coll Cardiol* 1987;9:240–246.

128. Carrier M, Martineau J-P, Bonan R, Pelletier LC. Clinical and hemodynamic assessment of the Omniscience prosthetic heart valve. *J Thorac Cardiovasc Surg* 1987;93:300–307.

129. Stewart S, Cianciotta D, Hicks GL, DeWeese JA. The Lillehei-Kaster aortic valve prosthesis. Long-term results in 273 patients with 1253 patient-years of follow-up. *J Thorac Cardiovasc Surg* 1988;95:1023–1030.

130. Butchart EG, Lewis PA, Grunkemeier GL, Kulatilake N, Breckenridge IM. Low risk of thrombosis and serious embolic events despite low-intensity anticoagulation. Experience with 1,004 Medtronic Hall valves. *Circulation* 1988;78(suppl I):I-66–77.

131. Antunes MJ, Wessels A, Sadowski RG, et al. Medtronic Hall valve replacement in a third-world population group. A review of the performance of

1000 prostheses. *J Thorac Cardiovasc Surg* 1988;95: 980–993.

132. Vallejo JL, Gonzales-Santos JM, Albertos J, et al. Eight years experience with the Medtronic Hall valve prosthesis. *Ann Thorac Surg* 1990;50:429–436.

133. Acar J, Boissel JP, Iung B, et al. AREVA: multicenter randomized comparison of low-dose versus standard-dose anticoagulation in patients with mechanical prosthetic heart valves. *Circulation* 1996;94:2107–2112.

134. Chesebro JH, Fuster V. Optimal antithrombotic therapy for mechanical prosthetic heart valves. *Circulation* 1996;94:2055–2056.

135. Mikaeloff PH, Jegaden O, Ferrini M, Coll-Mazzei J, Bonnefoy JY, Rumolo A. Prospective randomized study of St. Jude Medical versus Bjork-Shiley or Starr-Edwards 6120 valve prostheses in the mitral position. Three hundred and fifty-seven patients operated on from 1979 to December 1983. *J Cardiovasc Surg* 1989;30:966–975.

136. Kuntze CEE, Ebels T, Eijgelaar A, van der Heide JNH. Rates of thromboembolism with three different mechanical heart valve prostheses: randomised study. *Lancet* 1989;1:514–517.

137. Vogt S, Hoffmann A, Roth J, et al. Heart valve replacement with the Bjork-Shiley and St. Jude Medical prostheses: a randomized comparison in 178 patients. *Eur Heart J* 1990;11:583–591.

138. Cortina JM, Martinell J, Artiz V, Fraile J, Rabago G. Comparative clinical results with Omnisciene (STMI), Medtronic-Hall, and Bjork-Shiley convexo-concave (70 degrees) prostheses in mitral valve replacement. *J Thorac Cardiovasc Surg* 1986;91:174–183.

139. Nuutinen LS, Pihlajaniemi R, Saarela E, Karkola P, Hollmen A. The effect of dipyridamole on the thrombocyte count and bleeding tendency in open-heart surgery. *J Thorac Cardiovasc Surg* 1977;74:295–298.

140. Pumphrey CW, Fuster V, Dewanjee MK, Chesebro JH, Vlietstra RE, Kaye MP. Comparison of antithrombotic action of calcium antagonist drugs with dipyridamole in dogs. *Am J Cardiol* 1983;51:591–595.

141. Sullivan JM, Harken DE, Gorlin R. Pharmacologic control of thromboembolic complications of cardiac-valve replacement. *N Engl J Med* 1971;284:1391–1394.

142. Kasahara T. Clinical effect of dipyridamole ingestion after prosthetic heart valve replacement—especially on the blood coagulation system. *J Jpn Assoc Thorac Surg* 1977;25:1007–1021.

143. Groupe de Recherche PACTE. Prevention des accidents thromboemboliques systemiques chez les porteurs de prothesis valvulaires artificielles: essai cooperatif controle du dipyridamole. *Coeur* 1978;9:915–969.

144. Rajah SM, Sreeharan N, Joseph A, et al. A prospective trial of dipyridamole and warfarin in heart valve patients [Abstract]. *Acta Therapeutica* 1980;6(suppl 93):54.

145. Ranhosky A. Dipyridamole. *N Engl J Med* 1987;317:1734.

146. Fuster V, Chesebro JH. Antithrombotic therapy: current concepts of thrombogenesis: role of platelets. *Mayo Clin Proc* 1981;56:102–112.

147. Altman R, Boullon F, Rouvier J, et al. Aspirin and prophylaxis of thromboembolic complications in patients with substitute heart valves. *J Thorac Cardiovasc Surg* 1976;72:127–129.

148. Bortolotti U, Milano A, Thiene G, et al. Long-term dura-

bility of the Hancock porcine bioprosthesis following combined mitral and aortic valve replacement: an 11-year experience. *Ann Thorac Surg* 1987;44:139–144.

149. Kimose HH, Lund O, Ljungstrom B. Isolated mitral valve replacement with Carpentier-Edwards bioprosthesis: independent risk factors for long-term survival and prosthesis failure. *Thorac Cardiovasc Surg* 1989;37:135–142.

150. Magilligan DJ, Lewis JW, Stein P, Alam M. The porcine bioprosthetic heart valve: experience at 15 years. *Ann Thorac Surg* 1989;48:324–330.

151. Jamieson WRE, Munro AI, Miyagishima RT, et al. The Carpentier-Edwards supraannular porcine bioprosthesis. *J Thorac Cardiovasc Surg* 1988;96:652–666.

152. Xiaodong Z, Jiaqiang G, Yingchun C, Chengjun T. Ganxin2 X. Ten-year experience with pericardial xenograft valves. *J Thorac Cardiovasc Surg* 1988;95:572–576.

153. Daenen W, Noyez L, Lesaffre E, Goffin Y, Stalpaeri G. The Ionescu-Shiley pericardial valve results in 473 patients. *Ann Thorac Surg* 1988;46:536–541.

154. Revuelta JM, Bernal JM, Gutierrez JA, Gaite L, Alonso C, Duran CMG. Mitroflow heart valve: 5.5 years clinical experience. *Thorac Cardiovasc Surg* 1988:36:262–265.

155. Cosgrove DM, Lytle BW, Taylor PC, et al. Surgery for acquired heart disease: the Carpentier-Edwards pericardial aortic valve—ten year results. *J Thorac Cardiovasc Surg* 1995;110:651–662.

156. Matsuki 0, Robles A, Gibbs S, Bodnar E, Ross DN. Longterm performance of 555 aortic homografts in the aortic position. *Ann Thorac Surg* 1988;46:187–191.

157. Turpie AGG, Gunstensen J, Hirsh J, Nelson H, Gent M. Randomized comparison of two intensities of oral anticoagulant therapy after tissue heart valve replacement. *Lancet* 1988;1:1242–1245.

158. Perier P, Deloche A, Chauvaud S, et al. A 10-year comparison of mitral valve replacement with Carpentier-Edwards and Hancock porcine bioprostheses. *Ann Thorac Surg* 1989;48:54–69.

159. Gould KL. Noninvasive assessment of coronary stenose, by myocardial perfusion imaging during pharmacologic coronary vasodilation. 1. Physiologic basis and experimental validation. *Am J Cardiol* 1978;41:267–278.

160. Nunez L, Aguado G, Larrea JL, Celemin D, Oliver J. Prevention of thromboembolism using aspirin after mitral valve replacement with porcine bioprosthesis. *Ann Thorac Surg* 1984;37:84–7.

161. Kempin SJ. Warfarin resistance caused by broccoli. *N Engl J Med* 1983;308:1229–1230.

162. Lorient Roudaut MF, Ledain L, Roudaut R, Besse P, Boisscau MR. Thrombolytic treatment of acute thrombotic obstruction with disk valve prostheses: experience with 26 cases. *Semin Thromb Hemost* 1987;13:201–205.

163. Deviri E, Sareli P, Wisenbaugh T, Cronje SL. Obstruction of mechanical heart valve prostheses: clinical aspects and surgical management. *J Am Coll Cardiol* 1991;17:646–650.

164. Kontos GJ Jr, Schaff HV, Orszulak TA, Puga FJ, Pluth JR, Danielson GK. Thrombotic obstruction of disc valves: clinical recognition and surgical management. *Ann Thorac Surg* 1989;48:60–65.

165. Massad M, Fahl M, Slim M, et al. Thrombosed Bjork-

Shiley standard disc mitral valve prosthesis. *J Cardiovasc Surg* 1989;30:976–980.

166. Zoghbi WA, Desir RM, Rosen L, Lawrie GM, Pratt CM, Quinones MA. Doppler echocardiograph: application to the assessment of successful thrombolysis of prosthetic valve thrombosis. *J Am Soc Echocardiogr* 1989;2:98–101.

167. Montero CG, Mula N, Brugos R, Pradas R, Figuera D. Thrombectomy of the Bjork-Shiley prosthetic valves revisited: long-term results. *Ann Thorac Surg* 1989;48:824–828.

168a. Balram A, Kaul U, Rao R, et al. Thrombotic obstruction of Bjork-Shiley valves-diagnostic and surgical considerations. *Int J Cardiol* 1984;6:61–69.

168b. Lengyel M, Fuster V, Keltai M, et al. Guidelines for the management of left-sided prosthetic valve thrombosis. A role for thrombolytic therapy. *JACC* 1997;30(in press).

169. Tyagi S, Gambhir DS, Khalilullah M. Thrombolytic therapy for a thrombosed Bjork-Shiley mitral valve prosthesis. *Indian Heart J* 1988;40:507–508.

170. Graver LM, Gelber PM, Tyras DH. The risks and benefits of thrombolytic therapy in acute aortic and mitral prosthetic valve dysfunction: report of a case and review of the literature. *Ann Thorac Surg* 1988;46:85–88.

171. Quintanilia MA, Haque AK. Thrombotic obstruction of prosthetic aortic valve presenting as acute myocardial infarction. *Am Heart J* 1989;117:1378–1379.

172. Tapanainen J, Ikiiheimo M, Jouppila P, Kortelainen M-L, Salmela P. Thrombosis in a mechanical aortic valve prosthesis during subcutaneous heparin therapy in pregnancy: a case report. *Eur J Obstet Gynecol Reprod Biol* 1990;36:175–177.

173. Witchitz S, Veyrat C, Moisson P, Scheinman N, Rozenstajn L. Fibrinolytic treatment of thrombus on prosthetic heart valves. *Br Heart J* 1980;44:545–554.

174. Minami K, Horstkotte D, Schulte HD, Bircks W. Thrombosis of two St. Jude Medical prostheses in one patient after triple valve replacement. *Eur J Cardiothorac Surg* 1988;2:48–52.

175. Mosseri M, Galoon E, Gotsman MS, Rosenheck S, Milgarter E. Successful treatment of an immobile and thrombosed prosthetic tricuspid valve by fibrinolysis with a single dose of streptokinase. *Isr J Med Sci* 1988;24:114–116.

176. Cambier P, Mombaerts P, De Geest H, Cohen D, Van de Werf F. Treatment of prosthetic tricuspid valve thrombosis with recombinant tissue-type plasminogen activator. *Eur Heart J* 1987;8:906–909.

177. Prieto Palomino MA, Ruiz de Elvira MJ, Sanchez Llorente F, et al. Successful thrombolysis on a mechanical tricuspid prosthesis. *Eur Heart J* 1989;10:1115–1117.

178. Tischler MD, Lee RT, Kirshenbaum JM. Successful treatment of prosthetic tricuspid valve thrombosis with shortcourse recombinant tissue-type plasminogen activator. *Am Heart J* 1990;120:975–977.

179. Matsuda M, Matsuda Y, Okuda F, et al. Thrombolysis of tricuspid Bjork-Shiley prosthesis with tissue-type plasminogen activator. *Jpn Circ J* 1988;52:583–587.

180. Cohen ML, Barzilai B, Gutierrez F, Jaffe AS, Eisenberg P. Treatment of prosthetic tricuspid valve thrombosis with low-dose tissue plasminogen activator. *Am Heart J* 1990;120:978–980.

181. Tinker JH, Tarhan S. Discontinuing anticoagulant ther-
apy in surgical patients with cardiac valve prostheses: observations in 180 operations. *JAMA* 1978;239:738–739.

182. Garvey GJ, Neu HC. Infective endocarditis-an evolving disease. A review of endocarditis at the Columbia-Presbyterian Medical Center 1968-1973. *Medicine* 1978;57:105–127.

183. Wilson WR, Geraci JE, Danielson GK, et al. Anticoagulant therapy and central nervous system complications in patients with prosthetic valve endocarditis. *Circulation* 1978;57:1004–1007.

184. Block PC, DeSanctis RW, Weinberg AN, Austen WG. Prosthetic valve endocarditis. *J Thorac Cardiovasc Surg* 1970;60:540–548.

185. Karchmer AW, Dismukes WE, Buckley MJ, Austen WG. Late prosthetic valve endocarditis: clinical features influencing therapy. *Am J Med* 1978;64:199–200.

186. Cerebral Embolism Study Group. Immediate anticoagulation of embotic stroke: a randomized trial. *Stroke* 1983;14:668–676.

187. Lodder J, van der Lust PJ. Evaluation of the risk of immediate anticoagulant treatment in patients with embolic stroke of cardiac origin. *Stroke* 1983;14:42–46.

188. Cerebral Embolism Study Group. Immediate anticoagulation of embolic stroke: brain hemorrhage and management options. *Stroke* 1983;14:42–46.

189. Lutz DJ, Noller KL, Spitter JA, Danielson GK, Fish CR. Pregnancy and its complications following cardiac valve prostheses. *Am J Obstet Gynecol* 1978;131:460–468.

190. Bloomfield DK. Fetal deaths and malformations associated with the use of coumarin derivatives in pregnancy: a critical review. *Am J Obstet Gynecol* 1970;107:883–888.

191. Becker MH, Genieser NB, Finegold M, Miranda D, Spackman T. Chondrodysplasia punctata. Is maternal warfarin therapy a factor? *Am J Dis Child* 1975;129:356–359.

192. Shaul WL, Hall JG. Multiple congenital anomalies associated with oral anticoagulants. *Am J Obstet Gynecol* 1978;127:191–198.

193. Iturbe-Alessio I, Fonseca MDC, Mutchinik O, Santos MA, Zajaraias A, Salazar E. Risks of anticoagulant therapy in pregnant women with artificial heart valves. *N Engl J Med* 1986;315:1390–1393.

194. Salazar E, Zajaria A, Gutierrez N, Iturbe I. The problem of cardiac valve prostheses, anticoagulants, and pregnancy. *Circulation* 1984;70(suppl I):1-169–177.

195. Sareli P, England MJ, Berk MR, et al. Maternal and fetal sequelae of anticoagulation during pregnancy in patients with mechanical heart valve prostheses. *Am J Cardiol* 1989;63:1462–1465.

196. Salazar E, Izaguirre R, Verdejo J, Mutchinick O. Failure of adjusted doses of subcutaneous heparin to prevent thromboembolic phenomena in pregnant patients with mechanical cardiac valve prostheses. *J Am Coll Cardiol* 1996;27:1698–1703.

197. Wang RYC, Lee PK, Chow JSF, Chen WWC. Efficacy of low-dose, subcutaneously administered heparin in treatment of pregnant women with artificial heart valves. *Med J Aust* 1983;2:126–128.

198. Baty JD, Breckenridge A, Lewis PJ, et al. May mothers taking warfarin breast feed their infants? *Br J Clin Pharmacol* 1976;3:969.

199. O'Reilly RA, Aggeler PM. Determinants of the response to oral anticoagulant drugs in man. *Pharmacol Rev* 1970;22:35–96.

200. Vitali E, Donatelli F, Quaini E, Groppeli G, Pellegrini A. Pregnancy in patients with mechanical prosthetic heart valves: our experience regarding 98 pregnancies in 57 patients. *J Cardiovasc Surg* 1986;27:221–227.

201. Mok CK, Boey J, Wang R, et al. Warfarin vs dipyridamole-aspirin and pentoxifylline-aspirin for the prevention of prosthetic heart valve thromboembolism: a prospective randomized clinical trial. *Circulation* 1985;72:1059–1083.

202. Sbarouni E, Oakley CM. Outcome of pregnancy in women with valve prostheses. *Br Heart J* 1994;71:196–201.

Cardiovascular Thrombosis: Thrombocardiology and Thromboneurology, Second Edition,
edited by M. Verstraete, V. Fuster, and E. J. Topol,
Lippincott–Raven Publishers, Philadelphia © 1998.

22

Prosthetic Heart Valves

Eric G. Butchart

*Department of Cardiothoracic Surgery, University Hospital of Wales,
Cardiff CF4 4XW, United Kingdom*

Prosthetic heart valves have been used with increasing success to replace abnormal native valves for almost 40 years. From the earliest experiences with these devices it was soon apparent that prevention of thrombosis accumulation on what was in effect a large foreign body in the bloodstream would prove one of the greatest challenges for both design engineers and clinicians managing patients postoperatively. Many early designs failed catastrophically because of their extreme susceptibility to obstructive thrombosis despite anticoagulation (1). Gradually, with greater understanding of the different hemocompatibility of various materials and an appreciation of the importance of the washing effect of high-velocity blood flow for all parts of the prosthesis, more successful mechanical valve designs were introduced whose susceptibility to thrombus deposition was greatly reduced. Concurrently bioprosthetic valves made from animal tissue were also developed in the hope that they would be immune from the problem of thrombosis. Sadly, this proved not to be the case. Porcine valves in particular showed valve thrombosis rates without anticoagulation similar to the least thrombogenic mechanical valves with anticoagulation (2).

It must be acknowledged that all currently available replacement devices, whether mechanical or bioprosthetic remain imperfect in terms of thromboresistance. In the case of mechanical valves, the prosthetic surfaces are covered with a thin and constantly changing layer of plasma proteins to which variable numbers of platelets and leukocytes become transiently adherent (3). In the case of bioprostheses, the original endothelial (or mesothelial, in the case of pericardial valves) layer is lost during preparation and preservation, exposing basement membrane and collagen. Some degree of fibrous "sheathing" takes place and reendothelialization with host endothelium occurs after some years, but the latter is never complete and its anticoagulant function is uncertain (2).

Despite the imperfections of both mechanical and bioprosthetic valves, the majority of patients experience no thrombotic or embolic events during the lifespan of their prosthesis. Embolism after valve replacement is traditionally attributed to the prosthesis for reporting purposes (4) but this simplistic inculpation does nothing to advance our understanding of the mechanisms involved in a particular patient at a particular time. Unless the mechanisms are fully understood, it is impossible to devise appropriate prophylaxis and treatment. If stroke and valve thrombosis particularly are to be prevented it is insufficient to simply place the patient on anticoagulant therapy after valve replacement and "hope for the best."

THE SIGNIFICANCE OF EMBOLISM

In patients with prosthetic valves both mechanical and biological, embolic rates vary between zero and 4% per year following aortic valve replacement (AVR) and between 0.5% and 7.5% following mitral valve replacement (MVR) (5). Embolic incidence within groups of patients is often used as a means of attempting to distinguish between the effectiveness of different forms of treatment, particularly between different types of prosthesis (6,7) and between different regimens of antithrombotic management (7–10). However, follow-up methods and definitions have a huge effect on the recording of embolic events. Furthermore, in most series of prosthetic valves, the majority of events reported as embolism are cerebrovascular (6,11) and the authors conveniently assume not only that all events are embolic in etiology but that all the "emboli" originated from the prosthesis, despite the fact that many pathophysiologic mechanisms other than cardioembolism lead to cerebral infarction: in situ arterial thrombosis, artery-to-artery embolism, intrinsic small vessel vasculopathies, various types of arteritis, and global hypoperfusion (12). The proportion of cerebrovascular events due to embolism in patients with prosthetic valves is likely to be higher than in the general population (15%) (13) but logically cannot be 100%. Even when a cerebrovascular event is truly cardioembolic, it is usually uncertain as to whether the embolus originated from the prosthesis or from another site.

There is a "background incidence" of stroke and transient ischemic accident (TIA) in the general population, which gradually rises with age, reaching about 2% per year by the age of 80 in Western populations (14). This incidence may be reduced in some subgroups by anticoagulation (notably in patients with atrial fibrillation) but is never abolished (15–18). The presence of coronary disease increases the risk of stroke two-to threefold depending on age (19), whereas carotid disease and aortic atheroma increase the risk still further (20). In addition, hypertension, diabetes, increased left ventricular mass, and cigarette smoking each act as major independent stroke risk factors (21–25). Unless the prevalence of these risk factors is known in a series of prosthetic valve patients, it is impossible to interpret data on "embolism."

It is particularly meaningless to describe prosthetic valves or, indeed, therapeutic regimens as having "embolic rates." Only groups of patients have embolic rates or, more properly, cerebrovascular event rates, and these are determined not only by their type of prosthesis and their antithrombotic management but by their age, their stroke and cardiac risk factors, and by trigger factors for thrombosis. It is hence not surprising that there is as much variation in embolic rates between reported series of the same prosthesis as there is between different prostheses (5). Furthermore, meta-analysis of reported series (7) merely derives meaningless averages that do nothing to advance understanding of the underlying mechanisms that account for the differences.

Following AVR in a middle-aged and elderly population, the incidence of cerebrovascular events has been shown to be predominantly associated with established stroke risk factors, particularly hypertension and continued cigarette smoking (26), and to be relatively little influenced by differences in anticoagulation intensity (27). In a series based on the Medtronic Hall tilting disc valve, patients who were normotensive, in sinus rhythm, nondiabetic, and nonsmokers with no evidence of arterial disease suffered no cerebrovascular events during a 13-year follow-up period (26). Although it may not be possible to extrapolate these data to other types of prosthesis, this series serves to underline the importance of taking stroke risk factors into account when analyzing prosthetic valve data. The mechanism of cerebrovascular events in this series of patients after AVR remains speculative. The incidence among the patients with one or more stroke risk factors (2.1% per year) is in keeping with epidemiologic data on stroke in a similar group of subjects in the general population without prosthetic valves, although the possibility of some interaction between the prosthesis and stroke risk factors remains.

In patients with prosthetic heart valves, abnormal flow conditions imposed by the prosthesis coexist with disturbed flow conditions due to abnormal cardiac function and/or with irregular roughened arterial surfaces due to atheromatous plaques. The latter and the prothrombotic endothelial dysfunction that accompanies them (28,29) are in turn associated with well-established risk factors for arterial disease: hypertension, cigarette smoking, diabetes, and hyperlipidemia (30).

The abnormal flow conditions caused by prosthetic valves are of two types: relative stagnation and high-velocity disturbed flow causing high shear stress (31). Relative stagnation exists in areas of very low flow or even reversed flow adjacent to certain parts of the

prosthesis according to its particular design (e.g., the hinge pockets of a bileaflet valve and the concave outflow surfaces of a bioprosthesis) (32). High-shear stress occurs during forward flow and in mechanical valves during regurgitant flow when high-velocity jets of blood are forced through narrow gaps in the mechanism with the prosthesis in a closed position. The degree of shear stress also varies according to valve design (31). Relative stagnation in any part of the circulation increases the risk of thrombosis (33) but is particularly dangerous in proximity to an artificial surface (3). High-shear stress is also deleterious in that it induces platelet activation (34–36). Activated platelets may subsequently adhere to a prosthetic surface (37) or to an abnormal surface downstream from the prosthesis, e.g., an aortic atheromatous plaque, with subsequent microembolism (38) (Fig. 22-1).

Prostheses in different positions within the heart impose and are associated with different flow conditions that have implications for the mechanisms of thrombosis and embolism and for antithrombotic therapy. Aortic prostheses are associated with relatively little stagnation unless of inferior design or incorrectly implanted; the dominant feature rather is high-shear stress (31). In addition, many aortic

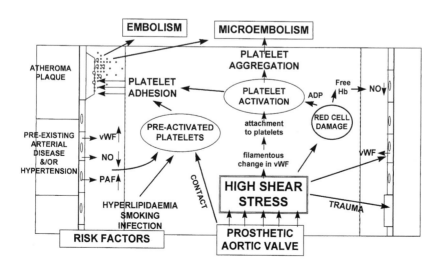

FIG. 22-1. Effect of high-shear stress in aortic valve replacement.

valves are implanted within aortas scarred by atherosclerosis. Mitral prostheses in contrast are associated with much more stagnation (32), not only because the velocity of forward flow is much lower, especially in atrial fibrillation, but because they are situated facing into the left atrium, which is itself an area of relative stagnation, in many cases of mitral valve disease, due to chamber enlargement and atrial fibrillation (33). Mitral valve disease is also usually associated with less arterial disease than aortic valve disease (26,39) (Fig. 22-2).

These fundamental differences result in a higher incidence of both valve thrombosis and embolism after mitral valve replacement MVR than after AVR (5). Because these complications are related to blood stagnation both in the left atrium and adjacent to the prosthesis, and because anticoagulation is particularly useful for reducing thrombosis under these conditions, a dose–response effect can be demonstrated with increasing intensity of anticoagulation (27). In contrast, embolism after AVR appears to be little influenced by the intensity of anticoagulation (27), suggesting a dominant effect of platelet activation and arterial disease (26). Several randomized trials have failed to detect any significant difference in embolic incidence with different intensities of anticoagulation in populations in which AVR and sinus rhythm predominated (8–10,40).

It can be concluded that in patients with prosthetic valves anticoagulation is of most value in preventing thrombosis on the prosthesis itself and within the left atrium and the embolism that arises from these sites, but it is of much less value in preventing "embolism" arising as the result of high-shear stresses or arterial disease or an interaction between the two (Fig. 22-3).

PROSTHETIC VALVE THROMBOSIS

Valve thrombosis is a potentially dangerous complication with a high mortality in most series. Among anticoagulated patients the incidence varies from zero to 0.5% per year in the aortic position and from zero to 3% per year in the mitral position (5). The risk of thrombosis is determined primarily by the inherent thrombogenicity of the individual type of prosthesis, which depends on construction materials, stagnation characteristics, and propensity for activating platelets, through the shear stresses it imposes on flowing blood (vide supra) (2). Other factors that increase thrombogenicity are poor hemodynamic performance with high transprosthetic gradient, especially in the mitral position (41), and susceptibility to tissue ingrowth, leading to progressive stenosis and interference with occluder movement (42–44).

The risk of valve thrombosis is secondarily determined by patient-related factors and anti-

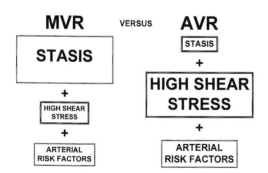

FIG. 22-2. Comparison of the dominant factors involved in determining thrombotic risk in mitral and aortic valve replacement.

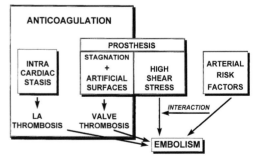

FIG. 22-3. The causes of embolism after valve replacement showing the limitations of anticoagulation.

coagulation management. Applying the principles of Virchow's triad (45), the patient-related factors comprise intracardiac flow conditions and the coagulability of the blood. Design-related stasis is present to a varied degree in different prostheses, including bioprostheses (32), and is enhanced by low intracardiac flow conditions, imposed either by low cardiac output (46,47) or by left atrial stasis (44). Advanced New York Heart Association (NYHA) class is a predisposing factor (48), and atrial fibrillation and left atrial enlargement are reported to increase the risk of mitral valve thrombosis with some prostheses (44).

Hypercoagulability almost certainly contributes to valve thrombosis, as both a risk factor and a trigger factor, but its importance as a significant contributor has probably been obscured in many series of prosthetic valve thrombosis by the dominant etiologic roles of prosthesis thrombogenicity and anticoagulation interruption and by the lack of thorough investigation for possible trigger factors. In prostheses of low thrombogenicity, valve thrombosis is a rare event (49) and consequently the search for contributing factors is likely to be more rewarding. A recent detailed analysis of cases of thrombosis of the Medtronic Hall valve suggests that prior pulmonary infection may be a trigger factor in some cases, especially when combined with interruption of anticoagulation (3). The prosthesis exists in a fragile equilibrium with the blood, always covered with a thin and constantly changing film of proteins (50). Raised plasma fibrinogen levels, consequent upon infection (51), are likely to lead to a greater proportion of fibrinogen in this surface film (3), especially in areas exposed to very low flow (50). The combination of the prothrombotic effects of leukocyte activation (52–54) with an alteration in the balance of the protein composition in the surface film may be sufficient to upset the equilibrium in favor of thrombus deposition. Hyperfibrinogenemia also enhances platelet aggregability (55) and increases plasma viscosity (56), especially in areas of relatively stagnant flow (57). Prothrombotic changes occurring in association

with pulmonary infection are particularly dangerous because of their close proximity upstream to the prosthesis.

The hypothesis of infection-triggered valve thrombosis is in accordance with infection as a trigger factor for cerebral infarction (58,59), with chronic inflammation as a risk factor for stroke and myocardial infarction (60), and with the winter preponderance of stroke and myocardial infarction in the general population (61–63) and of cerebrovascular events after MVR (39). The hyperfibrinogenemia associated with chronic infection and parasite infestation in sub-Saharan Africa (64) could be part of the explanation for the higher incidence of valve thrombosis in this region (65).

Anticoagulation interruption and complete absence of anticoagulation are clearly major contributors to many cases of valve thrombosis (47,66–70), but certainly not to all, reflecting the importance of other predisposing factors. Caution should be exercised in evaluating reports in which valve thrombosis is attributed to "inadequate" or "poorly controlled" anticoagulation, as these are meaningless terms unless accompanied by numerical definitions. Nevertheless, it is possible that a higher than expected incidence of valve thrombosis in a particular series results from choosing a target anticoagulation intensity that is too low for the prosthesis involved (vide infra).

ANTITHROMBOTIC MANAGEMENT

From the foregoing it is clear that effective antithrombotic management needs to involve much more than simply treating the patient with anticoagulants (71). Risk factors for thrombosis and underlying causes of hypercoagulability should be corrected if possible. Atrial fibrillation is associated with a fivefold increase in the risk of stroke (19) and it is important to try to restore sinus rhythm. Hypertension, obesity, and hyperlipidemia should be treated, cigarette smoking stopped, and advice given about diet, exercise, and the avoidance of potentially thrombogenic drugs (71). Hyperfibrinogenemia and other evidence of chronic inflammation should be sought and thoroughly investigated. If possible, the source of the inflammation should be treated or eliminated. If this is not possible, consideration should be given to fibrinogen-lowering drugs (72). All acute infections, but particularly respiratory infections, should be treated promptly.

Correcting these factors will substantially reduce the risk of thrombosis but will not eliminate the need for anticoagulation in the presence of a mechanical valve or remaining intracardiac conditions that favor thrombus deposition, i.e., atrial fibrillation, left atrial enlargement, or impaired left ventricular function. Indirect evidence of intracardiac stasis and a potentially thrombotic milieu obtained from the detection of spontaneous echo contrast and raised levels of coagulation activation peptides also indicates the need for anticoagulation (71).

Homografts and most bioprostheses in the aortic position do not require long-term anticoagulation, providing that the patient is in sinus rhythm and intracardiac conditions are relatively normal. However, there is evidence that anticoagulation for the first 3 months, until the sewing ring is endothelialized, reduces the higher incidence of embolism at this time (73). Most patients with mitral bioprostheses will require long-term anticoagulation at some stage because of the high prevalence of atrial fibrillation (74). For this reason, bioprostheses and homografts in the mitral position are of questionable value.

Choosing the Intensity of Anticoagulation

The role of the various components of the hemostatic system in thrombosis varies according to flow conditions (57), with the coagulation system playing a major role under stagnant "venous" conditions but a relatively minor role under conditions of high-shear stress where the actions of platelets, von Willebrand factor, and other adhesive proteins predominate, to enable the thrombus to resist the high-shear stresses (34,75). As a result, moderate- or low- intensity anticoagulation is effective under venous conditions but even high-intensity oral anticoagulation cannot totally abolish thrombosis, in the presence of powerful platelet activators such as collagen, under arterial conditions (76).

The flow conditions associated with mechanical valves (and, to a lesser extent, with bioprostheses) are a mixture of "arterial" and "venous" conditions (vide supra). As the dominant effect of anticoagulation is to inhibit thrombus deposition under "venous" conditions and on artificial surfaces, the prevention of valve thrombosis becomes the principal aim of anticoagulation, whereas minimization of embolism and bleeding are secondary objectives because neither can be completely prevented during anticoagulation.

Fibrin deposition under "stagnant" conditions is readily controlled by anticoagulation (76,77) and from basic principles one would anticipate that the less stagnant the flow conditions, the lower would be the intensity of anticoagulation required to control it. At the other extreme, a prosthesis with high stagnation characteristics or poor washing of some of its surfaces would probably need much higher intensity of anticoagulation. Examples of these two extremes can be found among different designs of tilting disc valves, with some designs clearly requiring a higher intensity of anticoagulation to prevent valve thrombosis than others (2,78). Similarly, in bileaflet valves, the design of the hinge pocket is critical in determining susceptibility to thrombosis because this area is particularly vulnerable to thrombus deposition (37) due to complex geometry and low-velocity forward flow (31). The blood path through the hinge needs both optimum washing and "wiping," i.e., full contact between the opposed moving surfaces throughout their excursion, to minimize the risk of thrombus deposition (79). Designs with more vulnerable hinge pockets may need higher intensities of anticoagulation.

It is thus important to distinguish between mechanical valves when making recommendations of anticoagulation intensity (78). Unfortunately, the widespread practice of categorizing mechanical heart valves according to their age (first generation, second generation, etc.) and/or their basic design (caged ball, tilting disc, bileaflet) for the purpose of making anticoagulation recommendations is too simplistic and likely to lead to inaccurate and dangerous generalizations (80,81). It cannot be assumed that all valves in a particular design category are of equal thrombogenicity or that a newly introduced design is necessarily less thrombogenic than an older design, as illustrated by the recent example of a new bileaflet valve that had to be withdrawn before early clinical trials were complete due to a high incidence of valve thrombosis (82). Hence data mainly based on one individual type of prosthesis cannot be extrapolated to other prostheses within the same broad design category, as in many recommendations (80,81).

Ideally, antithrombotic management in general and anticoagulation in particular should be both prosthesis-specific and patient-specific. Unfortunately, despite almost 40 years of experience with heart valve replacement, hard scientific data on which to base recommendations are remarkably few. Although much basic research has been performed on the factors that govern thrombus deposition on artificial surfaces in the bloodstream (Chapter 50), laboratory research directed to identifying the optimum anticoagulation intensity to prevent thrombus deposition on different materials under various flow conditions has never been performed. However, this type of experimental work has been performed on exposed subendothelium under simulated "venous" and "arterial" flow conditions at different anticoagulation intensities, showing that low-intensity anticoagulation is of value in reducing thrombus formation under conditions of low flow whereas even high-intensity anticoagulation cannot abolish the much smaller predominantly platelet thrombus formation that occurs at high flow rates (76). Although probably quantitatively different, it is likely that similar principles would apply to artificial surfaces. If so, the predominant effect of anticoagulation on prosthetic valves is likely to be in preventing thrombus formation in areas exposed to low flow, whereas the washing effect of high flow maintains the remainder of the prosthetic surface thrombus-free. Because the proportion of the prosthetic surface exposed to low flow varies from one design to another and because particular design characteristics (e.g., tortuous blood path, disturbed or reversed flow, or lack of wiping effect) may favor thrombus deposition, there is reason to be precise in specifying the optimum International Normalized Ratio (INR), if not for each prosthesis individually (the ideal), at least for groups of prostheses categorized by their thrombogenicity rather than by their year of introduction or superficial similarities (i.e., bileaflet, tilting disc, etc.) (71). Precision is important in recommending an optimum INR for each prosthesis under given clinical circumstances, not only to prevent thrombosis but also to avoid an unnecessarily high level of anticoagulation with its associated increased risk of bleeding (Chapter 51).

Several randomized trials of different levels of anticoagulation were performed in the late 1980s and early 1990s (Fig. 22-4) (8–10,40). Unfortunately, all of these trials either were methodologically flawed in one or more respects or addressed only a small subset of patients with prosthetic valves. All contained relatively small numbers of patients with short follow-up. One trial involved patients with bioprostheses who were anticoagulated for 3 months only (8). All other trials in patients with mechanical valves recruited patients with more than one type of prosthesis with insufficient numbers of each to enable subset analysis comparing one prosthesis with another (9,10,40). Other factors making interpretation of these trials difficult and diminishing their relevance in terms of answering basic questions were the use of antiplatelet agents in all patients in one trial (10), the use of unrealistically high-intensity anticoagulation for one group in another trial (9), and the exclusion of high-risk patients in the third trial (40). In patients who were predominantly in sinus rhythm (and, in one trial from Saudi Arabia, predominantly under the age of 30) (9), all that can be concluded from these trials

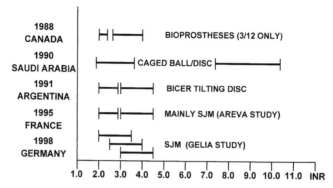

FIG. 22-4. Summary of randomized trials of different intensities of anticoagulation after heart valve replacement. Results from the GELIA study are expected in 1998. (Data from refs. 8, 9, 10, and 40.)

is that higher intensity anticoagulation caused more bleeding but did not significantly reduce the incidence of embolism in the categories of patients selected for the trials. This is scarcely surprising given the diverse etiology of ischemic cerebrovascular events (vide supra). In general, these trials do not help the clinician faced with the selection of the most appropriate anticoagulation intensity for each type of prosthesis under different clinical circumstances. The AREVA trial, for example, suggests that in patients in sinus rhythm with no risk factors for embolism, the St. Jude valve in the aortic position can be safely managed with an INR in the range 2.0 to 3.0 (40), but gives no guidance for the patient in atrial fibrillation and congestive cardiac failure with a St. Jude valve in the mitral position.

In the absence of clinically relevant guidance from randomized trials, it is necessary to work toward practical recommendations from basic principles. The principal aims of anticoagulation are to prevent thrombus formation on the prosthetic surface and in the left atrium and the embolism which can result from these sites (Fig. 22-3). Embolism arising as the result of high-shear stress and arterial disease, either separately or in combination, will not be significantly affected by anticoagulation. The sum total of embolism will thus only be minimized and not abolished by anticoagulation, and nothing is to be gained by raising the INR above that necessary to prevent left atrial thrombosis and prosthesis thrombosis.

If left atrial conditions are normal, with sinus rhythm, no significant left atrial enlargement, no mitral valve gradient, normal left ventricular function, and absence of spontaneous echo contrast (SEC), as a marker of relative stagnation, as in most AVR patients, the prosthesis becomes the determining factor in deciding the INR (Table 22-1) because anticoagulation is not required for abnormal left atrial conditions (71).

In the presence of abnormal left atrial conditions leading to relative stasis, such as atrial fibrillation, moderate to severe dilatation, significant mitral valve gradient (native or prosthetic), or impaired left ventricular function, especially when these lead to SEC, a minimum level of INR is required to combat the risk of left atrial thrombosis before considering the level for the prosthesis (72). A safe minimum level has never been determined in these circumstances, but it has been shown in previously unanticoagulated patients with rheumatic mitral valve disease that a mean INR of 3.0 is capable of halting the progression of established left atrial thrombosis and allowing its complete resolution by natural thrombolysis with the return of fibrinopeptide A levels to normal (83). This rather extreme test of the efficacy of anticoagulation almost certainly indicates that this intensity of anticoagulation is adequate for most adverse left atrial conditions, and indeed an INR around 3.0 is generally recommended for patients with mitral valve dis-

TABLE 22-1. *INR recommendations according to prosthesis thrombogenicity and intracardiac conditions*

	SR LA0 MVgr0 LVF+ SEC0	AF LA0 AVR LVF+ SEC0	AF LA + MVgr+ or MVR LVF↓ SEC+	AF LA++ CHF/CO↓ LVF↓↓ SEC++
Low-thrombogenicity prosthesis	2.5	2.5	3.0	3.5–4.0
High-thrombogenicity prosthesis	4.0	4.0	4.0	4.0–4.5

SR, sinus rhythm; AF, atrial fibrillation; LA0, normal-sized left atrium; LA+ and LA++, enlarged and grossly enlarged left atrium; MVgr0, no significant mitral valve gradient; AVR, aortic valve replacement; MVR, mitral valve replacement; MVgr+, significant mitral valve gradient; CHF, congestive heart failure; CO↓, low cardiac output; LVF+, normal left ventricular function; LVF↓ and LVF↓↓, impaired and severely impaired left ventricular function; SEC0, SEC+, and SEC++, spontaneous echo contrast in left atrium absent, present, and gross, respectively.

ease without a prosthesis (84). If atrial fibrillation is the only adverse factor, the left atrial size is normal, and there is no mitral valve disease, low-intensity anticoagulation (mean INR around 2.0) is sufficient to lower prothrombin fragment F_{1+2} levels to below normal and provide effective embolic prophylaxis (85,86). If lone atrial fibrillation coexists with AVR, the prosthesis should be the determining factor in deciding the INR. At the other end of the spectrum, the dangerous combination of atrial fibrillation, severe left atrial enlargement, and severely impaired left ventricular function is additive or multiplicative in determining embolic risk (87). On basic principles it may be prudent to aim for a higher INR under these circumstances (3.5 to 4.0), although there are no data to confirm this recommendation (88,89).

The correct INR is the lowest value that confers adequate risk protection. If a combination of left atrial factors is abnormal, an INR of 3.0 should be the minimum intensity. The thrombogenicity of the prosthesis only becomes the determining factor when left atrial conditions are normal or when it exceeds the thrombogenic potential of adverse left atrial conditions.

Prosthetic valves vary in their susceptibility to thrombosis when exposed to hypercoagulable conditions or reduced anticoagulation. This thrombogenicity is difficult to define precisely in numerical terms but can be expressed in approximate terms graphically by relating throm-

bosis rate per 100 patient years to anticoagulation intensity (Fig. 22-5) (78). Valve A in the figure represents a low-thrombogenicity prosthesis requiring only low-intensity anticoagulation to remain free of thrombosis under most conditions, whereas valve C represents a high-thrombogenicity prosthesis in which the risk of valve thrombosis cannot be totally eliminated even with high-intensity anticoagulation. Examples from the literature can be found that correspond approximately to points on these curves, although for most prostheses insufficient published data on INR levels exist to allow construction of a curve (2,78).

For low-thrombogenicity prostheses an INR of 2.5 is sufficiently high to prevent valve thrombosis in the absence of abnormal intracardiac conditions (49). For prostheses of high thrombogenicity, aiming for an INR of 4.0 gives a greater margin of protection, allowing for the fact that variability in INR level is the rule rather than the exception in most patients (78). Two examples at either end of the scale of thrombogenicity illustrate the danger of attempting to categorize prostheses by superficial design similarities. The Medtronic Hall valve is a tilting disc prosthesis with a very low susceptibility to thrombosis (49), even under the very testing conditions found in developing countries (90) where anticoagulation is at best highly erratic or intermittent and at worst absent altogether (65). The thrombosis resistance of this prosthesis approximates to the curve for valve A in Fig. 22-5. It can thus be categorized in Table 22-1 as a low-thrombogenicity prosthesis. At the other end of the scale, another tilting disc valve, the Omniscience valve, has a high susceptibility to valve thrombosis when exposed to low-intensity anticoagulation (2). It can be characterized by the curve for valve C in Fig. 22-5 and should therefore be considered a high-thrombogenicity prosthesis in Table 22-1.

Bileaflet valves also vary in their susceptibility to thrombosis. The Medtronic Parallel valve (now withdrawn from the market) (82) would probably correspond to valve C in Fig. 22-5, whereas other bileaflet valves probably occupy intermediate positions between valves A and C. Among the available bileaflet valves, the St. Jude Medical valve is probably the least susceptible to valve thrombosis (91,92) and should be categorized as a low-thrombogenicity prosthesis in Table 22-1. All bioprostheses can also be included in the low-thrombogenicity prostheses category in Table 22-1 (78).

Because data on many types of prosthetic valve are sparse or even absent, cardiac surgeons and physicians supervising anticoagulation control will need to exercise judgment based on unpublished information in deciding the appropriate category for these prostheses

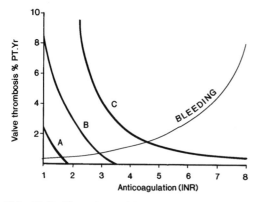

FIG. 22-5. Thrombogenicity curves of three hypothetical valves, relating valve thrombosis rate to anticoagulation intensity. See text for explanation. (From Butchart, ref. 78, with permission.)

in Table 22-1. Newly introduced prostheses present a particular problem. In this situation it is probably safer to err on the side of higher rather than lower anticoagulation until data become available to make a judgment on thrombogenicity. The advent of more sophisticated anticoagulation control (Chapter 51) and the introduction of patient-controlled home prothrombin monitoring to provide more stable INR levels may eventually allow some revision of INR recommendations to be made in the direction of lower intensity.

Anticoagulation and Antiplatelet Therapy

Antiplatelet therapy alone has been shown to give inadequate protection against left atrial thrombosis, mechanical valve thrombosis, and cardiogenic embolism in all age groups, including children (66,85,93–96), especially in the presence of atrial fibrillation (85,97). Aspirin alone has been recommended as long-term prophylaxis for patients with bioprostheses to minimize platelet adhesion (98), but in vitro studies have shown no significant decrease in platelet adherence to bioprosthetic cusps in media containing therapeutic levels of aspirin (99), and it is likely that any therapeutic benefit of aspirin in patients with bioprostheses is mediated through its effect on associated nonprosthetic risk factors (vide infra).

The combination of anticoagulation and an antiplatelet agent is widely prescribed for patients with prosthetic valves but uncertainty exists about the indications, the most useful antiplatelet agent, and the dosage. Aspirin is the most commonly prescribed antiplatelet agent but its mechanism of action is insufficiently focused to enable a strong therapeutic benefit to be envisaged in relation to mechanical valves. ADP-dependent shear-induced platelet aggregation is not significantly inhibited by aspirin (100) and experimental work on animals shows that aspirin does not prevent platelet adhesion to prosthetic surfaces (101). The most important disadvantage of aspirin is the increased risk of bleeding in comparison to anticoagulation alone. The risk needs to be evaluated in the context of a "background incidence" of major bleeding in the general population aged 60+ of 0.7 to 1.6% per year (17,102,103) and bleeding rates reported in the literature for mechanical valves predominantly in the range 1% to 3% per year with a mean of about 2% per year (5). The risk of major bleeding with aspirin rises with increasing dose of aspirin and with increasing intensity of anticoagulation (Fig. 22-6) (104–111), reaching 14% per year with high-dose aspirin and high-dose anticoagulation (104,111). The combination of low-dose aspirin (75 mg per day) with an INR of 1.5 is reported to carry a low risk of bleeding (112), but higher doses of aspirin (325 mg per day), when combined with an INR even as low as 1.2 to 1.3, cause major bleeding at a rate of 2.4% per year (110).

In evaluating clinical trials of aspirin in patients with prosthetic valves, it is important to

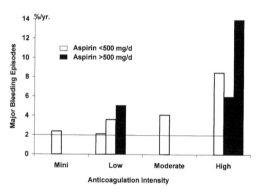

FIG. 22-6. Rate of major bleeding in combined anticoagulation and aspirin therapy according to aspirin dose and anticoagulation intensity. Data from refs. 104–111. Bleeding rates from refs. 104 and 106 have been arbitrarily included in the high- intensity group; in ref. 106, although the mean INR was stated to be around 3.0, the bleeding rate of 6.6% per year in the control group is typical of high-intensity anticoagulation; in ref. 104 the anticoagulation intensity was not stated in INR terms but an assessment of anti-coagulation practice in Nordic countries based on above-average bleeding rates concluded that intensity was too high (ref. 111). The line drawn through 2% per year represents the average bleeding rate with anticoagulation alone in reported mechanical valve series.

appreciate that an apparent benefit may be due to an action on concomitant arterial risk factors rather than an action on factors associated with the prosthesis itself. In the mid-1970s, two randomized studies comparing anticoagulation alone with anticoagulation plus aspirin both showed significantly fewer embolic events among patients treated with aspirin (104,113). These two studies were limited mainly to aortic valve replacement with Starr Edwards valves. No information was given in either study about concomitant arterial disease in the two groups of patients. This omission may be relevant because "arterial" risk factors have been shown to be major determinants of embolic risk following aortic valve replacement particularly (26), and aspirin is known to be effective in reducing the incidence of stroke and TIA in the general population, in the presence of arterial risk factors (114,115). The incidence of gastrointestinal bleeding was 4 to 5.5 times higher in the aspirin groups (104,113) and in one study the overall incidence of major bleeding was 14% per year (104). In another study in which almost half of patients had mitral prostheses, no benefit in thromboprophylaxis was demonstrated from the combination of aspirin and warfarin (105), but the incidence of serious bleeding with this combination was four times higher than warfarin alone or warfarin plus dipyridamole (105).

A randomized, double-blind, placebo-controlled trial to assess the efficacy of aspirin plus warfarin after valve replacement appeared to show a benefit from the addition of aspirin, but only when the non-hemorrhagic adverse outcomes were combined as "vascular" events and/or deaths (106). In this trial, 35% of the patients had ischemic heart disease and almost half the "vascular" deaths were due to myocardial infarction or "acute heart failure." Most of these deaths were in the placebo group. Aspirin is of proven benefit in ischemic heart disease and in stroke prevention in the presence of arterial risk factors (115). It seems likely, therefore, that the greatest impact of aspirin in this particular trial was on the patients who would have suffered a vascular event or death whether they had a prosthetic valve or not. Major bleeding in the aspirin-treated group occurred at the rate of 8.5% per year, about four times higher than that reported in most series of prosthetic valves treated with anticoagulation alone (5). It is of great concern that this trial is now widely quoted as evidence in support of the routine addition of aspirin to anticoagulation for isolated valve replacement not only in middle-aged and elderly patients (80) but in young women during pregnancy also (116).

The only other antiplatelet agent that has been evaluated in clinical trials in combination with anticoagulation is dipyridamole. It inhibits ADP-induced aggregation in vivo (although not in vitro), possibly by augmenting the effect of nitric oxide (117) and inhibits platelet adhesion to artificial surfaces in animal experiments (101), both potentially useful mechanisms for patients with prosthetic valves. Several studies have demonstrated a therapeutic benefit with this drug in patients with prosthetic valves (118). No information was provided about concomitant arterial risk factors, but because dipyridamole is thought to be ineffective in the prevention of stroke and myocardial infarction in the general population (119) and because reduction in platelet adherence to artificial surfaces has been demonstrated in animals (101), it is probable that the therapeutic benefit was real. However, all of these studies were performed many years ago predominantly on patients with caged ball valves. The caged ball valve is unique in that it combines high shear stresses (and associated ADP release) with a zone of stagnation at the apex of the cage (31), favoring the adhesion of activated platelets. From its mode of action, a theoretical benefit could be anticipated from dipyridamole with this particular prosthesis. There are no studies that have examined the effect of dipyridamole in patients with modern tilting disc and bileaflet valves.

Further clinical trials of antiplatelet drugs are required with specific types of prosthetic valve, but ideally should be limited to patients without concomitant arterial disease. Alterna-

tively, arterial disease and other risk factors should be allowed for in the analysis. Agents particularly worthy of further trials because of their modes of action are dipyridamole, molsidomine, ticlopidine (and the related compound clopidogrel), and the newer glycoprotein IIb/IIIa inhibitors (71,120) (see also Chapter 8).

Until appropriate clinical trials have been performed, the exact role of antiplatelet therapy remains unclear. In balancing the increased risk of intracerebral hemorrhage (ICH) associated with the combination of aspirin and anticoagulation (121) against a possible decreased risk of ischemic stroke, it is important to appreciate that ICH produces much greater disability than ischemic stroke and carries a much poorer prognosis, with a 1-year survival of only 23% in the 65 to 74 year age group in comparison to 81% for ischemic stroke (122). In patients with low thrombogenicity prostheses with no arterial disease, antiplatelet therapy probably has no advantage. In patients with arterial disease, diabetes, or inability to stop cigarette smoking, aspirin may reduce the risk of nonprosthetic arterial thrombosis and embolism (71). However, ideally it should only be used in low dose and in combination with low-intensity anticoagulation in order to reduce the risk of bleeding. In practical terms this may limit its use to patients with low thrombogenicity prostheses (Table 22-1).

Caged ball valves require special consideration because of their unique "self-cleaning" mechanism with a tendency to shed thrombus on the struts of the cage by repetitive ball contact. Obstructive valve thrombosis is consequently uncommon and not clearly related to anticoagulation intensity (5). Based on its mode of action and the evidence of efficacy referred to above, dipyridamole can probably be recommended for patients with caged ball valves in conjunction with moderate intensity anticoagulation (INR 3.0 to 4.0).

Antiplatelet agents are often prescribed for prosthetic valve patients after they have suffered one or more cerebrovascular events, but there is no evidence that antiplatelet agents are effective in secondary prevention and no effort should be spared in investigating the underlying cause of the events (71).

Anticoagulation During Noncardiac Surgery

There is a widespread view among noncardiac surgeons that it is necessary to discontinue oral anticoagulation prior to any surgical procedure. This attitude is particularly prevalent in the United States, where high-intensity anticoagulation has been used for many years, and is based on reports of excessive intraoperative bleeding and wound hematomas in some patients in whom high-intensity oral anticoagulation was continued (123).

Anticoagulation interruption in a patient with a prosthetic heart valve is potentially hazardous. The hazard of prosthetic valve thrombosis is of much greater concern than that of embolism, on which estimates of the risk of anticoagulation interruption are often based (124). Prosthetic valve thrombosis is associated with a very high mortality, partly because its development is often insidious, with eventual presentation in extremis some weeks after a period of anticoagulation interruption. Most reported series of prosthetic valve thrombosis show that in the absence of tissue ingrowth as a predisposing factor, anticoagulation interruption (usually for another surgical procedure) is a major trigger factor for valve thrombosis (47,67–70). The risk is higher for patients with mitral prostheses (123), for patients with congestive heart failure (125), and for patients with more thrombogenic prostheses (Fig. 22-5).

Anticoagulation interruption results in a period of rebound hypercoagulability during the first 4 days after withdrawal, with levels of factor VII and factor IX rising more rapidly than those of protein C and protein S, creating an imbalance between coagulation factors and natural anticoagulants, maximal at 1 week (126). Superimposing the prothrombotic response to any major surgical operation upon this rebound hypercoagulability further increases the risk of thrombosis.

Because of the high mortality of prosthetic valve thrombosis most cardiac surgeons have a different perspective to general surgeons and hematologists on the debate about anticoagulation interruption, preferring to have anticoagulation continued wherever possible (127). It is preferable to discuss any proposed surgical procedure with the patient's cardiac surgeon before proceeding. For many minor operations, including dental surgery (128) and ophthalmic surgery (129), and for some abdominal operations (130), low-intensity anticoagulation (INR 2.0) may be continued with no significant increased risk of bleeding. However, if the patient is also taking aspirin, this should be stopped 1 week before surgery to allow normally functioning platelets to be produced. In abdominal operations intravenous warfarin can be given until normal gastrointestinal absorption returns. Most cardiac surgeons are accustomed to performing major operations on patients with an INR in the region of 2.0 and in the majority of patients find that there is no important effect on intraoperative bleeding. Surgical procedures associated with large raw surfaces or large skin flaps may bleed more with continued anticoagulation and require more critical risk assessment. If it is necessary to reduce the INR intraoperatively or postoperatively, fresh frozen plasma should be used in preference to vitamin K, as the latter will make re-anticoagulation difficult for some days.

Anticoagulation During Pregnancy

Anticoagulation management during pregnancy is discussed in detail in Chapter 44, but as in the preceding section of this chapter, a cardiac surgeon's perspective may differ from that of a hematologist. Because valve thrombosis is such a catastrophic complication with a high mortality, its prevention must be accorded the highest priority. It is widely believed that all prosthetic valves are at increased risk of thrombotic obstruction during pregnancy (131), but a survey of anticoagulant practice during pregnancy among several European centers has shown that the problem of valve thrombosis is largely confined to patients who have been switched from oral anticoagulants to heparin (132). Other authors have reported similar findings (133,134). Heparin is known to be relatively less effective during pregnancy (135–137), so that in order to achieve the same degree of anticoagulation, the heparin dosage must be gradually increased as pregnancy advances, and very carefully monitored for its efficacy, particularly in the last trimester (135). Failure to prescribe adequate doses of heparin probably accounts for most cases of valve thromboses that occur on heparin therapy.

There are other disadvantages to heparin. Long-term heparin anticoagulation is inconvenient and is associated with a 10% to 12% risk of maternal hemorrhage (132), a 2% risk of osteoporotic vertebral fractures (139), and a 27% to 33% risk of an abnormal outcome of pregnancy (stillbirth or prematurity) (132, 138). The alternative of maintaining oral anticoagulation throughout pregnancy is not without risk to the pregnancy and the fetus but the data in the literature need to be interpreted according to the intensity of oral anticoagulation and dosage of warfarin employed. As with hemorrhagic events elsewhere in the body, the risk of maternal hemorrhage is closely related to the intensity of anticoagulation. With low-intensity oral anticoagulation (INR 2.0 to 2.5), the risk of antepartum hemorrhage is 0 to 2% (140,141). Similarly, in patients who have continued on oral anticoagulants until the time of delivery, the risk of peripartum hemorrhage appears to be low. In one series with a target INR of 2.0 to 2.5 there were no cases of excessive bleeding with vaginal delivery (141).

Similarly, taking into account the series that have reported warfarin embryopathy according to anticoagulation intensity (133, 140,141), there is a strong suggestion that embryopathy is dose-related with a very low risk using low-intensity anticoagulation and low-dose warfarin (140). The availability of modern low-thrombogenicity prostheses that can be safely maintained on low-intensity oral anticoagulation (INR 2.5) throughout pregnancy should preclude the need for heparin therapy at any stage of pregnancy. The advice to switch to heparin in the first trimester is often impractical as many women in developing countries, where the problem is commonest, do not seek medical advice until after the first trimester.

It has recently been proposed that aspirin should be added to the anticoagulant regime during pregnancy (116), but this suggestion is not supported by any data showing that this combination is either safe or effective during pregnancy. Given the known increased risk of bleeding when aspirin is combined with anticoagulation and given the lack of data to show that aspirin helps to prevent valve thrombosis, it seems particularly dangerous to advise its routine use during pregnancy.

MANAGEMENT OF OBSTRUCTIVE VALVE THROMBOSIS

The symptoms of obstructive valve thrombosis are often insidious, developing over weeks or even months as thrombus slowly accumulates (2). Progression of symptoms tends to be more rapid with bileaflet valves than with tilting disc valves as even small quantities of thrombus at the hinge points of a bileaflet valve can immobilize both leaflets. With prostheses of this type symptoms tend to develop over days rather than weeks, even when cases of obstruction of one leaflet only are included in the comparison (2). When considering the diagnosis of valve thrombosis, it is important to remember that even bioprosthetic valves are not immune to obstructive thrombosis. Confirmation of the diagnosis of valve thrombosis is usually readily accomplished with transesophageal echocardiography (TEE). In tilting disc and bileaflet valves with radiopaque occluders, impaired occluder movement is also detectable by fluoroscopy (142).

The choice of treatment between surgery and thrombolytic therapy depends on the underlying cause and the age and extent of the thrombus. If obstruction is due to a combination of tissue ingrowth and thrombosis, thrombolysis will not be successful. Similarly, long-standing thrombosis with successive layers of thrombus deposition with a firm, rubbery consistency is resistant to thrombolysis. If valve thrombosis appears primarily related to the high thrombogenicity of the particular type of prosthesis and occurs despite well-controlled anticoagulation, it is better to take the opportunity to replace the prosthesis with another of lower thrombogenicity in order to prevent recurrence of the problem. It is logical therefore to consider thrombolytic therapy only in patients with recent thrombosis related to nonexistent or inadequate anticoagulation or to temporary factors that have increased coagulability. Factors favoring a successful outcome include preservation of some degree of occluder mobility (143), aortic position (144), hemodynamic stability (142), and bileaflet valve thrombosis because the volume of thrombus causing reduced occluder movement is often quite small (70). However, even under these relatively favorable circumstances, thrombolysis gives imperfect results with incomplete restoration of leaflet motion in some patients and a risk of rethrombosis (70). One series has reported delayed full opening of bileaflet valve leaflets days to months after initial partial success in some patients (144). Overall, series of unselected patients have reported high rates of recurrent or residual thrombosis (38%), an incidence of embolism of about 18%, and 30% mortality following surgery for failed thrombolytic therapy (145). There are no randomized studies and individual series are difficult to compare because of differences in selection criteria, thrombolytic therapy, type of prosthesis, size and maturity of thrombus, and NYHA class at the time of treatment.

The reason for the recent resurgence of interest in thrombolytic therapy has been lower cost, particularly in developing countries (144), and lower mortality rates in comparison to those quoted for reoperation in some older series (70,142). However, the mortality of reoperation is closely related to the NYHA class at the time of surgery (146), and with the ever increasing availability of TEE to facili-

tate early diagnosis, patients with valve thrombosis should not be allowed to deteriorate to the extent that they are in extremis prior to surgery. "Elective" reoperation on valve thrombosis in its early stages should be a low-risk procedure. The slower progression of symptoms of valve thrombosis in tilting disc and caged ball valves in comparison to bileaflet valves may give an additional margin of safety in this respect (2).

If reoperation is performed a choice must be made between thrombectomy and replacement. If valve thrombosis is due to non-existent anticoagulation or to other factors that have increased coagulability on a transient basis, thrombectomy may be sufficient, providing that access to both surfaces of the prosthesis is good enough to permit complete removal of all thrombus. Thrombectomy is easiest to perform on tilting disc valves in the aortic position, especially if they can be rotated within the housing to allow thorough inspection of the subvalvular area. Results with aortic prosthesis thrombectomy are correspondingly better (142). Mitral prostheses are more difficult to visualize adequately as large quantities of thrombus may remain hidden on the ventricular surface of the prosthesis. If visualization cannot be improved by a supplementary transaortic approach and the prosthesis cannot be rotated to facilitate inspection, it is safer to replace it.

If anticoagulation has been well controlled in a range appropriate to the thrombogenicity of the prosthesis and there is no evidence that transient or correctable hypercoagulability or tissue ingrowth has contributed to valve thrombosis, it must be assumed that the thrombogenicity of the prosthesis is the primary cause and it should be replaced with a less thrombogenic valve.

CONCLUSION

Prosthetic heart valves vary in their susceptibility to valve thrombosis according to subtle differences in design and, in terms of thrombogenicity, cannot be classified by their braod design categories (e.g., tilting disc, bileaflet, etc.). Other factors contributing to the risk of valve thrombosis include intracardiac flow conditions, tissue ingrowth, coagulability of the blood, and anticoagulation management. Most events classified as embolism are cerebrovascular events of diverse etiology and many are closely related to known stroke risk factors and arterial disease. Anticoagulation reduces the risk of valve thrombosis and intracardiac thrombosis under conditions of relative stagnation and the embolism which arises from these sources. In contrast, it has little effect on embolism and cerebrovascular events related to shear stress–induced platelet activation and arterial disease. Stroke risk factor management is therefore of equal importance to anticoagulation management. As far as possible, anticoagulation intensity (measured in terms of INR) should be adjusted to intracardiac conditions and prosthesis thrombogenicity and should therefore be both patient-specific and prosthesis-specific.

Uncertainties still exist about the optimum INR range for many types of prosthesis and about the role of antiplatelet therapy. Further research is required in these areas, in parallel with efforts to unravel underlying mechanisms responsible for triggering thrombosis and embolism at a particular moment in time. In particular, infection as a trigger factor for thrombosis requires further investigation.

REFERENCES

1. Lefrak EA, Starr A. Historic aspects of cardiac valve replacement. In: *Cardiac Valve Prostheses.* New York: Appleton-Century-Crofts, 1979;3–37.
2. Butchart EG. Thrombogenicity, thrombosis and embolism. In: Butchart EG, Bodnar E (eds). *Current Issues in Heart Valve Disease: Thrombosis, Embolism and Bleeding.* London: ICR, 1992;172–205.
3. Butchart EG. Fibrinogen and leukocyte activation— the keys to understanding prosthetic valve thrombosis? *J Heart Valve Dis* 1997;6:9–16.
4. Edmunds LH Jr, Clark RE, Cohn LH, Grunkemeier GL, Miller DC, Weisel RD. Guildines for reporting morbidity and mortality after cardiac valvular operations. *J Thorac Cardiovasc Surg* 1996;112:708–711.
5. Grunkemeier GL, Starr A, Rahimtoola SH. Prosthetic heart valve performance: long-term follow-up. *Curr Prob Cardiol* 1992;17:331–406.
6. Edmunds LH Jr. Thrombotic and bleeding complications of prosthetic heart valves. *Ann Thorac Surg* 1987;44:430–445.
7. Cannegieter SC, Rosendall FR, Briët E. Thromboembolic and bleeding complications in patients with mechanical heart valve prostheses. *Circulation* 1994;89: 635–641.
8. Turpie AGG, Gunstensen J, Hirsh J, Nelson H, Gent M. Randomised comparison of two intensities of oral anticoagulation therapy after tissue heart valve replacement. *Lancet* 1988;1:1242–1245.
9. Saour JN, Sieck JO, Mamo LAR, Gallus AS. Trial of different intensities of anticoagulation in patients with prosthetic heart valves. *N Engl J Med* 1990;322: 428–432.
10. Altman R, Rouvier J, Gurfinkel E, et al. Comparison of two levels of anticoagulation therapy in patients with substitute heart valves. *J Thorac Cardiovasc Surg* 1991;101:427–431.
11. Cerebral Embolism Task Force. Cardiogenic brain embolism. The second report of the Cerebral Embolism Task Force. *Arch Neurol* 1989;46:727–743.
12. Bamford J, Sandercock P, Dennis M, Burn J, Warlow C. Classification and natural history of clinically identifiable subtypes of cerebral infarction. *Lancet* 1991; 337:1521–1526.
13. Hart RG. Prevention and treatment of cardioembolic stroke. In: Furlan AJ (ed). *The Heart and Stroke.* London: Springer, 1987;117–138.
14. Bamford J, Warlow CP. Stroke and TIA in the general population. In: Butchart EG, Bodnar E (eds). *Current Issues in Heart Valve Disease: Thrombosis, Embolism and Bleeding.* London: ICR, 1992; 3–15.
15. Lundstrom T, Ryden L. Haemorrhagic and thromboembolic complications in patients with atrial fibrillation on anticoagulant prophylaxis. *J Intern Med* 1989;225:137–142.
16. Petersen P, Boysen G, Godtfredsen J, Andersen ED, Andersen B. Placebo-controlled, randomised trial of warfarin and aspirin for prevention of thromboembolic complications in chronic atrial fibrillation. The Copenhagen AFASAK study. *Lancet* 1989;1:175–179.
17. Stroke Prevention in Atrial Fibrillation Study Group Investigators. Preliminary report of the Stroke Prevention in Atrial Fibrillation Study. *N Engl J Med* 1990; 322:863–868.
18. Connolly SJ, Laupacis A, Gent M, Roberts RS, Cairns JA, Joyner C. Canadian Atrial Fibrillation Anticoagulation (CAFA) Study. *J Am Coll Cardiol* 1991;18: 349–355.
19. Wolf PA, Abbott RD, Kannel WB. Atrial fibrillation as an independent risk factor for stroke: the Framingham Study. *Stroke* 1991;22:983–988.
20. Jones EF, Kalman JM, Calafiore P, Tonkin AM, Donnan GA. Proximal aortic atheroma—an independent risk factor for cerebral ischaemia. *Stroke* 1995;26: 218–224.
21. Wolf PA, Kannel WB, Cupples LA, DíAgostino RB. Risk factor interaction in cardiovascular and cerebrovascular disease. In: Furlan AJ (ed). *The Heart and Stroke.* London: Springer, 1987;331–355.
22. MacMahon S, Peto R, Cutler J, et al. Blood pressure, stroke and coronary heart disease;part 1, prolonged differences in blood pressure: prospective observational studies corrected for the regression dilution bias. *Lancet* 1990;335:765–774.
23. Bowler JV, Hachinski V. Epidemiology of cerebral infarction. In: Gorelick PB (ed). *Atlas of Cerebrovascu-*

lar Disease. Philadelphia: Current Medicine, 1996;
1.2–1.22.

24. Manolio TA, Kronmal RA, Burke GL, O'Leary DH, Price TR. Short-term predictors of incident stroke in older adults. *Stroke* 1996;27:1479–1486.

25. Shinton R, Beevers G. Meta-analysis of relation between cigarette smoking and stroke. *Br Med J* 1989;298:789–794.

26. Butchart EG, Moreno de la Santa P, Rooney SJ, Lewis PA. Arterial risk factors and ischaemic cerebrovascular events after aortic valve replacement. *J Heart Valve Dis* 1995;4:1–8.

27. Butchart EG, Lewis PA, Bethel JA, Breckenridge IM. Adjusting anticoagulation to prosthesis thrombogenicity and patient risk factors: recommendations for the Medtronic Hall valve. *Circulation* 1991;84(suppl 3):III-61–III-69.

28. Harrison DG, Minor RL, Guerra R, Wuillen JE, Sellke FW. Endothelial dysfunction in atherosclerosis. In: Rubanyi GM (ed). *Cardiovascular Significance of Endothelium-Derived Vasoactive Factors.* Mount Kisco, NY: Futura, 1991;263–280.

29. Burrig KF. The endothelium of advanced arteriosclerotic plaques in humans. *Arterioscler Thromb* 1991;11:1678–1689.

30. Packham MA, Kinlough-Rathbone RL. Mechanisms of atherogenesis and thrombosis. In: Bloom AL, Forbes CD, Thomas DP, Tuddenham EGD (eds). *Haemostasis and Thrombosis* (3rd ed). Edinburgh: Churchill Livingstone, 1994;1107–1138.

31. Yoganathan AP, Wick TM, Reul H. The influence of flow characteristics of prosthetic valves on thrombus formation. In: Butchart EG, Bodnar E (eds). *Current Issues in Heart Valve Disease: Thrombosis, Embolism and Bleeding.* London: ICR, 1992;123–148.

32. Jones M, Eidbo EE. Doppler color flow evaluation of prosthetic mitral valves: experimental epicardial studies. *J Am Coll Cardiol* 1989;13:234–240.

33. Yasaka M, Beppu S. Hypercoagulability in the left atrium, Part II: Coagulation factors. *J Heart Valve Dis* 1993;2:25–34.

34. Ruggeri ZM. Mechanisms of shear-induced platelet adhesion and aggregation. *Thromb Haemost* 1993;70:119–123.

35. Alkhamis TM, Beissinger RL, Chediak J. Artificial surface effect on red blood cells and platelets in laminar shear flow. *Blood* 1990;75:1568–1575.

36. Kroll MH, Hellums JD, McIntyre LV, Schaefer Al, Moake JL. Platelets and shear stress. *Blood* 1996;88:1525–1541.

37. Okazaki Y, Wika KE, Matsuyoshi T, et al. Platelets deposited early postoperatively on the leaflet of a mechanical valve in sheep without postoperative anticoagulants or antiplatelet agents. *ASAIO J* 1996;42:M750–M754.

38. Janicek MJ, van den Abbeele AD, DeSisto WC, et al. Embolization of platelets after endothelial injury to the aorta in rabbits. Assessment with 111Indium-labelled platelets and angiography. *Invest Radiol* 1991;26:655–659.

39. Butchart EG, Moreno de la Santa P, Rooney SJ, Lewis PA. The role of risk factors and trigger factors in cerebrovascular events after mitral valve replacement: implications for antithrombotic management. *J Cardiovasc Surg* 1994;9(suppl):228–236.

40. Acar J, Iung B, Biossell JP, et al. AREVA: multicenter randomized comparison of low-dose versus standard-dose anticoagulation in patients with mechanical prosthetic heart valves. *Circulation* 1996;94:2107–2112.

41. Roberts WC, Morrow AG. Mechanisms of left atrial thrombosis after mitral valve replacement: pathologic findings indicating obstruction to left atrial emptying. *Am J Cardiol* 1966;18:497–503.

42. Yoganathan AP, Corcoran WH, Harrison EC, Carl JR. The Bjork-Shiley aortic prosthesis: flow characteristics, thrombus formation and tissue overgrowth. *Circulation* 1978;58:70–76.

43. Deviri E, Sareli P, Wisenbaugh T, Cronje SL. Obstruction of mechanical heart valve prostheses: clinical aspects and surgical management. *J Am Coll Cardiol* 1991;17:646–650.

44. Renzulli A, De Luca L, Caruso A, Verde R, Galzerano D, Cotrufo M. Acute thrombosis of prosthetic valves: a multivariate analysis of the risk factors for a life threatening event. *Eur J Cardiothorac Surg* 1992;6:412–421.

45. Virchow R. Gesammelte abhandlungen zur Wissenschaftlichen medizin. IV Thrombose und embolie. *Gefassentzundung und Septische Infektion.* Frankfurt: Meidinger, 1856.

46. Hetzer R, Hill DJ, Kerth WJ, Wilson AJ, Adappa MG, Gerbode F. Thrombosis and degeneration of Hancock valves: clinical and pathological findings. *Ann Thorac Surg* 1978;26:317–322.

47. Cohn LH, Allred EN, DiSesa VJ, Sawtelle K, Shemin RJ, Collins JJ Jr. Early and late risk of aortic valve replacement: a 12 years concomitant comparison of the porcine bioprosthetic and tilting disc prosthetic aortic valves. *J Thorac Cardiovasc Surg* 1984;88:695–705.

48. Ryder SJ, Bradley H, Brannan JJ, Turner MA, Bain WH. Thrombotic obstruction of the Bjork-Shiley valve: the Glasgow experience. *Thorax* 1984;39:487–492.

49. Butchart EG, Lewis PA, Grunkemeier GL, Kulatilake N, Breckenridge IM. Low risk of thrombosis and serious embolic events despite low-intensity anticoagulation: experience with 1,004 Medtronic Hall valves. *Circulation* 1988;78(suppl I):I-66–I-77.

50. Vroman L. Protein/surface interaction. In: Szycher M (ed). *Biocompatible Polymers, Metals and Composites.* Lancaster, PA: Technomic, 1983;81–88.

51. Lowe GDO. Rheology of disease. In: Lowe GDO (ed). *Clinical Blood Rheology* (vol 2). Boca Raton: CRC Press, 1988;89–111.

52. Edwards RL, Rickles FR. The role of leukocytes in the activation of blood coagulation. *Semin Hematol* 1992;29:202–212.

53. Bazzoni G, Dejana E, Maschio AD. Platelet-neutrophil interactions. Possible relevance in the pathogenesis of thrombosis and inflammation. *Haematologica* 1991;76:491–499.

54. Cerletti C, Evangelista V, De Gaetano G. Polymorphonuclear leucocyte-dependent modulation of platelet function: relevance to the pathogenesis of thrombosis. *Pharmacol Res* 1992;26:261–268.

55. Landolfi R, De Cristofaro R, DeCandida E, Rocca B, Bizzi B. Effect of fibrinogen concentration on the velocity of platelet aggregation. *Blood* 1991;78:377–381.

56. Lowe GDO, Barbenel JC. Plasma and blood viscosity.

In: Lowe GDO (ed). *Clinical Blood Rheology* (vol 1). Boca Raton: CRC Press, 1988; 11–44.

57. Slack SM, Cui Y, Turitto VT. The effects of flow on blood coagulation and thrombosis. *Thromb Haemost* 1993;70:129–134.

58. Syrjanen J, Valtonen VV, Iivanainen M, Kaste M, Huttunen JK. Preceding infection as an important risk factor for ischaemic brain infarction in young and middle aged patients. *Br Med J* 1988;296:1156–1160.

59. Grau AJ, Buggle F, Heindl S, et al. Recent infection as a risk factor for cerebrovascular ischaemia. *Stroke* 1995;26:373–379.

60. Ridker PM, Cushman M, Stampfer MJ, Tracy RP, Hennekens CH. Inflammation, aspirin, and the risk of cardiovascular disease in apparently healthy men. *N Engl J Med* 1997;336:973–979.

61. Bull GM, Morton J. Environment, temperature and death rates. *Age Ageing* 1978;7:210–224.

62. Ricci S, Celani MG, Vitali R, La Rosa F, Righetti E, Duca E. Diurnal and seasonal variations in the occurrence of stroke: a community based study. *Neuroepidemiology* 1992;11:59–64.

63. Woodhouse PR, Khaw KT, Plummer M, Foley A, Meade TW. Seasonal variations of plasma fibrinogen and factor VII activity in the elderly: winter infections and death from cardiovascular disease. *Lancet* 1994; 343:435–439.

64. Meade TW, Stirling Y, Thompson SG, et al. An international and interregional comparison of haemostatic variables in the study of ischaemic heart disease. *Int J Epidemiol* 1986;15:331–336.

65. Williams MA. Anticoagulation in developing countries. In: Butchart EG, Bodnar E (eds). *Current Issues in Heart Valve Disease: Thrombosis, Embolism and Bleeding.* London: ICR, 1992;362–368.

66. Ribeiro PA, Al Zaibag M, Idris M, et al. Antiplatelet drugs and the incidence of thromboembolic complications of the St Jude Medical aortic prosthesis in patients with rheumatic heart disease. *J Thorac Cardiovasc Surg* 1986;91:92–98.

67. Lindblom D. Long-term clinical results after aortic valve replacement with the Bjork-Shiley prosthesis. *J Thorac Cardiovasc Surg* 1988;95:658–667.

68. Kontos GJ, Schaff HV, Orszulak TA, Puga FJ, Pluth JR, Danielson GK. Thrombotic obstruction of disc valves: clinical recognition and surgical management. *Ann Thorac Surg* 1989;48:60–65.

69. Massad M, Fahl M, Slim M, et al. Thrombosed Bjork-Shiley standard disc mitral valve prosthesis. *J Cardiovasc Surg* 1989;30:976–980.

70. Silber H, Khan SS, Matloff JM, Chaux A, De Robertis M, Gray R. The St. Jude valve: thrombolysis as the first line of therapy for cardiac valve thrombosis. *Circulation* 1993;87:30–37.

71. Butchart EG. Thrombogenesis and its management. In Acar J, Bodnar E (eds). *Textbook of Acquired Heart Valve Disease.* London, ICR, 1995;1048–1120.

72. Ernst E, Resch KL. Therapeutic interventions to lower plasma fibrinogen concentration. *Eur Heart J* 1995; 16(suppl A):47–53.

73. Heras M, Chesebro JH, Fuster V, et al. High risk of thromboemboli early after bioprosthetic cardiac valve replacement. *J Am Coll Cardiol* 1995;25:1111–1119.

74. Myken PSU, Caidahl K, Larsson S, Berggren HE. Ten-year experience with the Biocor porcine bioprosthesis in the mitral position. *J Heart Valve Dis* 1995;4:63–69.

75. Bloom AL. Physiology of blood coagulation. *Haemostasis* 1990;20(suppl 1):14–29.

76. Inauen W, Bombeli T, Baumgartner HR, Haeberli A, Straub PW. Effects of the oral anticoagulant phenprocoumon on blood coagulation and thrombogenesis induced by rabbit aorta subendothelium exposed to flowing human blood: role of dose and shear rate. *J Lab Clin Med* 1991;118:280–288.

77. Hirsh J. Effectiveness of anticoagulants. *Semin Thromb Hemost* 1986;12:21–37.

78. Butchart EG. Prosthesis-specific and patient-specific anticoagulation. In: Butchart EG, Bodnar E (eds). *Current Issues in Heart Valve Disease: Thrombosis, Embolism and Bleeding.* London: ICR, 1992;293–317.

79. Gross JM, Shu MCS, Dai FF, Ellis J, Yoganathan AP. A microstructural flow analysis within a bileaflet mechanical heart valve hinge. *J Heart Valve Dis* 1996;5: 581–590.

80. Stein PD, Alpert JS, Copeland J, Dalen JE, Goldman S, Turpie AGG. Antithrombotic therapy in patients with mechanical and biological prosthetic heart valves. *Chest* 1995;108(suppl):s371–s379.

81. Cannegieter SC, Rosendaal FR, Wintzen AR, van der Meer FJM, Vandenbrouke JP, Briët E. Optimal oral anticoagulant therapy in patients with mechanical heart valves. *N Engl J Med* 1995;333:11–17.

82. Bodnar E. The Medtronic parallel valve and the lessons learned. *J Heart Valve Dis* 1996;5:572–573.

83. Yasaka M, Yamaguchi T, Miyashita T, Tsuchiya T. Regression of intracardiac thrombus after cardioembolic stroke. *Stroke* 1990;21:1540–1544.

84. Gohlke-Barwolf C, Acar J, Burckhardt D, et al. Guidelines for prevention of thromboembolic events in valvular heart disease. *J Heart Valve Dis* 1993;2: 398–410.

85. Kistler JP, Singer DE, Millenson MM, et al. Effects of low intensity anticoagulation on level of activity of the hemostatic system in patients with atrial fibrillation. *Stroke* 1993;24:1360–1365.

86. Boston Area Anticoagulation Trial for Atrial Fibrillation Investigators: The effect of low-dose warfarin on the risk of stroke in patients with non-rheumatic atrial fibrillation. *N Engl J Med* 1990;323:1505–1511.

87. Stroke Prevention in Atrial Fibrillation Investigators: Predictors of thromboembolism in atrial fibrillation: II. Echocardiographic features of patients at risk. *Ann Intern Med* 1992;116:6–12.

88. Lip GYA. Intracardiac thrombus formation in cardiac impairment: the role of anticoagulant therapy. *Postgrad Med J* 1996;72:731–738.

89. Cleland JGF, Cowbrun PJ, Falk RH. Should all patients with atrial fibrillation receive warfarin? Evidence from randomized clinical trials. *Eur Heart J* 1996;17: 674–681.

90. Antunes MJ, Wessels A, Sadowski RG, et al. Medtronic Hall valve replacement in a third world population group. *J Thorac Cardiovasc Surg* 1988;95: 980–993.

91. Bodnar E. Mechanical valves. In: Acar J, Bodnar E (eds). *Textbook of Acquired Heart Valve Disease.* London: ICR, 1995;965–1001.

92. Akins CW. Results with mechanical cardiac valvular prostheses. *Ann Thorac Surg* 1995;60:1836–1844.

93. Myers ML, Lawrie GM, Crawford ES, et al. The St.

Jude valve prosthesis: analysis of the clinical results in 815 implants and the need for systemic anticoagulation. *J Am Coll Cardiol* 1989;13:57–62.

94. Moggio RA, Hammond GL, Stansel HC Jr, Glen WWL. Incidence of emboli with cloth covered Starr-Edwards valve without anticoagulation and with varying forms of anticoagulation. *J Thorac Cardiovasc Surg* 1978;75:296–299.

95. Mok DK, Boey J, Wang R, et al. Warfarin versus dipyridamole-aspirin and pentoxifyllin-aspirin for the prevention of prosthetic heart valve thromboembolism: a prospective randomized clinical trail. *Circulation* 1985;82:1059–1063.

96. Elliott MJ, Young C. Anticoagulation in children. In: Butchart EG, Bodnar E (eds). *Current Issues in Heart Valve Disease:* Thrombosis, Embolism and Bleeding. London: ICR, 1992;346–355.

97. Dale J, Myhre E. Can acetylsalicylic acid alone prevent arterial thromboembolism? A pilot study in patients with aortic ball valve prostheses. *Acta Med Scand* (suppl):1981;645:73–78.

98. Nunez L, Aguado GM, Larrea JL, Celemin D, Oliver J. Prevention of thromboembolism using aspirin after mitral valve replacement with porcine bioprostheses. *Ann Thorac Surg* 1984;37:84–87.

99. Magilligan DJ, Oyama C, Klein S, Riddle JM, Smith D. Platelet adherence to bioprosthetic cardiac valves. *Am J Cardiol* 1984;53:945–949.

100. Moake JL, Turner NA, Stathopoulos NA, Nolasco L, Hellums JD. Shear-induced platelet aggregation can be mediated by vWF released from platelets, as well as by exogenous large or unusually large vWF multimers, requires adenosine diphosphate, and is resistant to aspirin. *Blood* 1988;71:1366–1374.

101. Harker LA, Hanson SR, Kirkman TR. Experimental arterial thromboembolism in baboons: mechanisms, quantitation and pharmacologic prevention. *J Clin Invest* 1979;64:559–569.

102. Sixty Plus Reinfarction Study Research Group. Risk of long-term oral anticoagulant therapy in elderly patients after myocardial infarction. *Lancet* 1982;1:64–68.

103. European Atrial Fibrillation Trial Study Group. Secondary prevention in non-rheumatic atrial fibrillation after transient ischaemic attack or minor stroke. *Lancet* 1993;342:1255–1262.

104. Dale J, Myhre E, Storstein O, Stormorken H, Efskind L. Prevention of arterial thromboembolism with acetylsalicyclic acid: a controlled clinical study in patients with aortic ball valves. *Am Heart J* 1977;94:101–111.

105. Chesebro JH, Fuster V, Elveback LR, et al. Trial of combined warfarin plus dipyridamole or aspirin therapy in prosthetic heart valve replacement: danger of aspirin compared with dipyridamole. *Am J Cardiol* 1983;51:1537–1541.

106. Turpie AGG, Gent M, Laupacis A, et al. A comparison of aspirin with placebo in patients treated with warfarin after heart valve replacement. *N Engl J Med* 1993;329:524–529.

107. Albertal J, Sutton M, Pereyra D, et al. Experience with moderate intensity anticoagulation and aspirin after mechanical valve replacement. A retrospective, non-randomized study. *J Heart Valve Dis* 1993;2:302–327.

108. Hurlen M, Erikssen J, Smith P, Arnesen H, Rollag A.

Comparison of bleeding complications of warfarin and warfarin plus acetylsalycic acid: a study in 3166 outpatients. *J Intern Med* 1994;236:299–304.

109. Altman R, Rouvier J, Gurfinkel E, Scazziota A, Turpie AGG. Comparison of high-dose with low-dose aspirin in patients with mechanical heart valve replacement treated with oral anticoagulant. *Circulation* 1996;94:2113–2116.

110. Stroke Prevention in Atrial Fibrillation Investigators. Adjusted-dose warfarin versus low-intensity, fixed-dose warfarin plus aspirin for high risk patients with atrial fibrillation: Stroke Prevention in Atrial Fibrillation III randomised clinical trial. *Lancet* 1996;348:633–638.

111. Jorgensen T, Danneskiold-Samsoe B, Godtfredsen J, Jespersen J. *Anticoagulation Therapy in the Nordic Countries.* Copenhagen: Danish Hospital Institute, 1995.

112. Meade TW, Roderick PJ, Brennan PJ, Wilkes HC, Kelleher CC. Extracranial bleeding and other symptoms due to low dose aspirin and low intensity oral anticoagulation. *Thromb Haemost* 1992;68:1–6.

113. Altman R, Boullon F, Rouvier J, Raca R, de la Fuente L, Favaloro R. Aspirin and prophylaxis of thromboembolic complications in patients with substitute heart valves. *J Thorac Cardiovasc Surg* 1976;72:127–129.

114. Miller VT, Rothrock JF, Pearce LA, Feinberg WM, Hart RG, Anderson DC. Ischaemic stroke in patients with atrial fibrillation: effect of aspirin according to stroke mechanism. *Neurology* 1993;43:32–36.

115. Antiplatelet Trialists' Collaboration. Collaborative overview of randomised trials of antiplatelet therapy—I: prevention of death, myocardial infarction, and stroke by prolonged antiplatelet therapy in various categories of patients. *Br Med J* 1994;308:81–106.

116. Ginsberg JS, Hirsh J. Use of antithrombotic agents during pregnancy. *Chest* 1995;198(suppl):s305–s311.

117. Bult H, Fret HRL, Jordaens FH, Herman AG. Dipyridamole potentiates platelet inhibition by nitric oxide. *Thromb Haemost* 1991;66:343–349.

118. Fuster V, Israel DH. Platelet inhibitor drugs after prosthetic heart valve replacement. In: Butchart EG, Bodnar E (eds). *Current Issues in Heart Valve Disease: Thrombosis, Embolism and Bleeding.* London: ICR, 1992;247–262.

119. Fitzgerald GA. Dipyridamole. *N Engl J Med* 1987;316:1247–1257.

120. Schafer AI. Antiplatelet therapy. *Am J Med* 1966;101:199–209.

121. Thrift AG, Donnan GA, McNeil JJ. Epidemiology of intracerebral haemorrhage. *Epidemiol Rev* 1995;17:361–381.

122. Taylor TN, Davis PH, Torner JC, Holmes J, Meyer JW, Jacobson MF. Lifetime cost of stroke in the United States. *Stroke* 1996;27:1459–1466.

123. Katholi RE, Nolan SP, McGuire LB. Living with prosthetic heart valves: subsequent noncardiac operations and the risk of thromboembolism or haemorrhage. *Am Heart J* 1976;92:162–167.

124. Kearon C, Hirsh J. Management of anticoagulation before and after elective surgery. *N Engl J Med* 1997;336:1506–1511.

125. Carter SA, McDevitt E, Gatje BW, Wright IS. Analysis of factors affecting the recurrence of thromboembolism off and on anticoagulation therapy. *Am J Med* 1958;25:43–51.

126. Grip L, Blomback M, Chulman S. Hypercoagulable state and thromboembolism following warfarin withdrawal in post-myocardial infarction patients. *Eur Heart J* 1991;12:1225–1233.

127. Bryan AJ, Butchart EG. Prosthetic heart valves and anticoagulant management during non-cardiac surgery. *Br J Surg* 1995;82:577–578.

128. McIntyre H. Management, during dental surgery, of patients on anticoagulants. *Lancet* 1966;2:99–100.

129. Robinson GA, Nylander A. Warfarin and cataract extraction. *Br J Ophthalmol* 1989;73:702–703.

130. Rustad H, Myrhe E. Surgery during anticoagulant treatment: the risk of increased bleeding on oral anticoagulant treatment. *Acta Med Scand* 1963;173:115–119.

131. Oakley CM. Anticoagulation during pregnancy. In: Butchart EG, Bodnar E (eds). *Current Issues in Heart Valve Disease: Thrombosis, Embolism and Bleeding.* London: ICR, 1992;339–345.

132. Sbarouni E, Oakley CM. Outcome of pregnancy in women with valve prostheses. *Br Heart J* 1994;71: 196–201.

133. Iturbe-Alessio I, Fonseca MC, Mutchinik O, Santos MA, Zajarias A, Salazar E. Risks of anticoagulant therapy in pregnant women with artificial heart valves. *N Engl J Med* 1986;315:1390–1393.

134. Wang RYC, Lee PK, Chow JSF, Chen WWC. Efficacy of low dose, subcutaneously administered heparin in treatment of pregnant women with artificial heart valves. *Med J Aust* 1983;2:126–128.

135. Bonnar J. Long-term self-administered heparin therapy for prevention and treatment of thromboembolic complications of pregnancy. In: Kakkar VV, Thomas DP (eds). *Heparin: Chemistry and Clinical Usage.* London: Academic, 1976;247–260.

136. Whitfield LR, Lele AS, Levy G. Effect of pregnancy on the relationship between concentration and anticoagulant action of heparin. *Clin Pharmacol Ther* 1983; 34:23–28.

137. Kaplan KL, Owen J. Plasma levels of platelet secretory proteins. *Crit Rev Oncol Hematol* 1986;5:235–255.

138. Hall JG, Pauli RM, Wilson KM. Maternal and fetal sequelae of anticoagulation during pregnancy. *Am J Med* 1980;68:122–140.

139. Dahlman TC. Osteoporotic fractures and the recurrence of thromboembolism during pregnancy and the puerperium in 184 women undergoing thromboprophylaxis with heparin. *Am J Obstet Gynecol* 1993;168: 1265–1270.

140. Cotrufo M, de Luca TSL, Calabro R, Mastrogiovanni G, Lama D. Coumarin anticoagulation during pregnancy in patients with mechanical valve prostheses. *Eur J Cardiothorac Surg* 1991;5:300–305.

141. Sareli P, England MJ, Berk MR, et al. Maternal and fetal sequelae of anticoagulation during pregnancy in patients with mechanical heart valve prostheses. *Am J Cardiol* 1989;63:1462–1465.

142. Hausmann D, Mugge A, Daniel WG. Valve thrombosis: diagnosis and management. In: Butchart EG, Bodnar E (eds). *Current Issues in Heart Valve Replacement: Thrombosis, Embolism and Bleeding.* London: ICR, 1992;387–401.

143. Vitale N, Renzulli A, Cerasuolo F, et al. Prosthetic valve obstruction: thrombolysis versus operation. *Ann Thorac Surg* 1994;57:365–370.

144. Reddy NK, Padmanabhan TNC, Singh S, et al. Thrombolysis in left-sided prosthetic valve occlusion: immediate and follow-up results. *Ann Thorac Surg* 1994;58: 462–471.

145. Graver LM, Gelber PM, Tyras DH. The risks and benefits of thrombolytic therapy in acute aortic and mitral prosthetic valve dysfunction: report of a case and review of the literature. *Ann Thorac Surg* 1988;46: 85–88.

146. Butchart EG, Breckenridge IM. The timing of prosthetic valve reoperations based on an analysis of risk factors. *Z Kardiol* 1986;75 (suppl 2):155–159.

Cardiovascular Thrombosis: Thrombocardiology and Thromboneurology, Second Edition,
edited by M. Verstraete, V. Fuster, and E. J. Topol,
Lippincott–Raven Publishers, Philadelphia © 1998.

23

Thrombosis in the Cardiac Chambers: Ventricular Dysfunction and Atrial Fibrillation

Jonathan L. Halperin and *Palle Petersen

*Cardiovascular Institute, Mount Sinai Medical Center, New York, New York, 10029; and
Department of Neurology, Hvidovre Hospital, DK-2650 Hvidovre, Denmark

CARDIOGENIC THROMBOEMBOLISM

Epidemiology

Cardioembolic Stroke

Cardiogenic cerebral embolism is the mechanism responsible for approximately 20% of ischemic strokes—nearly 100,000 strokes each year among North Americans, and more than a million worldwide. These ischemic episodes derive from a diversity of cardiac disorders (Fig. 23-1). There is a history of nonvalvular atrial fibrillation in about half of cases, valvular heart disease in a quarter, and left ventricular mural thrombus in almost a third (1). In the absence of antithrombotic therapy, the risk of stroke associated with atrial fibrillation is 5 to 6 events per 100 patient-years, at least five times the rate among comparably aged patients without this cardiac rhythm disturbance, accumulating to a 35% lifetime risk of stroke. The risk is directly related to age,

such that over half of strokes occur in patients >75 years old (2–4). As for emboli of left ventricular origin, 60% are associated with acute myocardial infarction (5). Intracavitary thrombus occurs in about one third of patients in the first 2 weeks following anterior myocardial infarction and in an even greater proportion of those with large infarcts involving the left ventricular apex (1–4). Clinically evident cerebral infarction occurs in approximately 10% of patients with left ventricular thrombus following myocardial infarction in the absence of anticoagulant therapy (6). Trials of thrombolytic therapy suggest a lower incidence of left ventricular thrombus formation (7–9), but this is controversial (10). The remainder of ventricular thrombi occur in patients with chronic ventricular dysfunction resulting from coronary disease, hypertension, or other forms of dilated cardiomyopathy who face a persistent risk of stroke and systemic embolism.

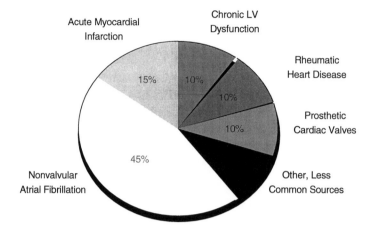

Acute Myocardial Infarction

Chronic LV Dysfunction

Rheumatic Heart Disease

Prosthetic Cardiac Valves

Other, Less Common Sources

Nonvalvular Atrial Fibrillation

15%

10%

10%

10%

45%

FIG. 23-1. Cardiac conditions associated with cerebral embolism. (From Cerebral Embolism Task Force, ref.1, with permission.)

Asymptomatic Cerebral Ischemia

Although clinical stroke in patients with cardiogenic embolism is typically associated with substantial acute neurologic deficit and often with lasting functional disability, the incidence of subclinical "silent" strokes is not precisely known. Such events are usually identified as small subcortical hypodense zones on computed cerebral tomography, though silent cortical infarction or large deep areas of infarction have been reported in up to 10% of patients with atrial fibrillation (11). Histopathologic confirmation that these infarcts are ischemic is lacking, and although this seems a likely etiology there is no proof that cardiogenic thromboembolism is responsible. One series of studies found minor silent cerebral infarcts in 48% of 29 patients with chronic atrial fibrillation present for at least 1 year (12), but a lower rate among patients with paroxysmal atrial fibrillation (13). Another study found the incidence of silent infarction to be 58% in patients with chronic and 38% in those with paroxysmal atrial fibrillation (14). Interpretation of these data is hampered by uncertainty about the prevalence of asymptomatic cerebral infarction in older persons without atrial fibrillation, though the prevalence of prior silent stroke in acute stroke patients is reportedly about 10% (15,16). Embolism arising from the cardiac chambers may contribute to the problem of multi-infarct dementia among the elderly, taking an uncounted toll on cognitive function (3–5).

Extracranial Systemic Embolism

More than 90% of clinically recognized cardioembolic events involve the brain, reflecting both the high relative sensitivity of cerebral tissue to ischemia and the biophysics of the arterial circulation. Other regions of the systemic circulation are not spared, particularly the abdominal viscera and the extremities. Acute arterial occlusive events may involve virtually any arterial bed, and limb ischemia, renal, splenic, mesenteric, and coronary embolism have been frequently described. Among patients with arterial embolism complicating myocardial infarction, multiple sites are involved in approximately 20% of cases, and a similar proportion is likely in patients with other conditions predisposing to thromboembolism derived from the cardiac chambers.

Pathogenesis of Thrombus in the Cardiac Chambers

The pathogenesis of intracavitary mural thrombosis follows the triad of precipitating factors established over a century ago by Virchow: endothelial injury, a zone of circulatory stasis, and a hypercoagulable state (17). Shortly after the onset of acute myocardial infarction, leukocyte infiltration separates endothelial cells from their basal lamina (18), exposing subendothelial tissue to intracavitary blood and creating a nidus for thrombus development. Endocardial abnormalities have been identified histologically in specimens from patients with left ventricular aneurysm (19) and in patients with idiopathic dilated cardiomyopathy (20). Experimental and clinical studies have emphasized the importance of wall motion abnormalities in the development of left ventricular mural thrombus, and stasis of blood in regions of akinesia or dyskinesia seems the essential factor (21–23). Stasis is similarly important in the development of atrial thrombus when effective mechanical atrial activity is impaired, as occurs in atrial fibrillation, atrial enlargement, mitral stenosis, and cardiac failure (24). Stasis brings about conditions of low shear rate, and deposition of fibrin plays the predominant pathogenetic role in the development of intracavitary thrombus. In patients with acute myocardial infarction, the incidence of thromboembolism is related to plasma fibrinogen level, suggesting a hypercoagulable tendency in this condition. The surface of fresh thrombus is highly thrombogenic, and a local hypercoagulable state may be heightened in the milieu of endocardial injury (25).

Both thrombin formation and platelet activation have been implicated in the process of mural thrombus formation. Like collagen, thrombin is a powerful activator of platelet aggregation. Since platelets and the coagulation system are closely interrelated in the genesis of left ventricular mural thrombosis, both platelet inhibitor and anticoagulant medication have potential roles for the prevention of thrombus and associated embolic phenomena. Abnormal endocardial tissue surfaces, including myxomatous or fibrotic mitral valve leaflets, mitral annular dilatation or calcification, damaged chordae tendinea, and other lesions, may stimulate platelet aggregation and the coagulation system. Alterations in hemostatic function have been identified in patients with nonvalvular atrial fibrillation (whether or not they have sustained prior ischemic stroke), including higher plasma concentrations of von Willebrand factor, factor VIIIc, fibrinogen, the fibrinolytic product D-dimer, and proteins related to activated platelets (β-thromboglobulin, and platelet factor 4) have been found compared with age- and gender-matched patients with prior stroke and sinus rhythm as well as with healthy control subjects (26). These biochemical changes may be either a cause or an effect of ongoing thrombosis in patients with atrial fibrillation, but correlations with morphologic evidence of thrombus formation or with clinical thromboembolic risk have not yet been established.

Mechanisms of Stroke

Embolism originating from the cardiac chambers involves both the regional stasis, and procoagulant factors that favor thrombus formation, and the dynamic forces of the circulation responsible for the migration of thrombotic material into the systemic circulation. In patients with atrial fibrillation, thrombus is most frequently detected in the left atrial appendage; in cases of left ventricular aneurysm, stasis favors thrombus formation within a circulatory cul-de-sac near the cardiac apex. Isolation of thrombus in these regions from dynamic circulatory forces protects against embolic migration (27). However, in the early phase after acute myocardial infarction, or in patients with thrombus in the body of the left atrium rather than in the appendage, exposure of thrombus to intracardiac blood flow raises the risk of embolism. In short, factors leading to thrombus formation are not the same as those which produce systemic embolism, a paradox that must not be neglected in the selection of therapeutic options (28).

The etiologies of ischemic stroke in patients with atrial fibrillation or left ventricular dysfunction are diverse, ranging from embolism of distant stasis-related thrombus in the left atrium or left ventricle, to thrombotic complications of associated cerebrovascular disease (1). Beyond primary thrombotic mechanisms, coexisting atherosclerotic lesions in the aorta, extracranial or intracranial arteries may reduce cerebral perfusion by direct obstruction or as a result of thrombus formation provoked by exposure of lipid material and subintimal vascular collagen (29). In stenotic lesions of the carotid arteries, exposure of extracellular matrix leads to thrombus formation, as contrasted with lipid-rich plaques in the thoracic aorta that are similar to coronary artery lesions with a propensity to ulceration. The prevalence of atherosclerotic carotid artery disease is twice as high in patients with atrial fibrillation as in age-matched controls (30), but only one in four patients with atrial fibrillation and stroke has significant carotid disease apparent on ultrasound examination (31). Arguably, these contrasting figures point to a cardioembolic mechanism of stroke in patients with atrial fibrillation, despite coexisting vascular disease. Furthermore, patients with chronic left ventricular dysfunction often have a history of atherosclerosis, hypertension, or other disorders independently associated with disease of the extracranial or intracranial cerebral vasculature.

Clinical estimates of the incidence of symptomatic cardiogenic embolism as the etiology of stroke in patients with atrial fibrillation vary widely and are difficult to verify, but are generally in excess of 50% (4,32,33). Ischemic cerebrovascular disease and intracranial hemorrhage account for an uncertain proportion of strokes in patients with potential sources of cardiogenic thromboembolism. In clinical practice, determination of the etiology of any given stroke is often difficult, although angiographic, CT, and magnetic resonance imaging (MRI) features may be characteristic. Diagnosis is often based in large measure on the perceived embolic risk attributed to the nature of coexisting heart disease as well as on the identification of carotid or vertebrobasilar artery lesions, which may also respond favorably to antithrombotic medication.

Stroke Related to Other Abnormalities of the Atria

Acute ischemic stroke of cryptogenic origin often results in a search for sources of cardiogenic embolism. Previously unrecognized atrial fibrillation is disclosed during cardiac rhythm monitoring in some 20% to 25% of such cases. Transesophageal echocardiography and autopsy studies have identified patent foramen ovale, the most common postnatal residuum of the fetal circulation, occurring in up to 27% of otherwise normal hearts in one series (34). However, the prevalence of this anatomic finding is significantly greater in individuals younger than 55 years with stroke than in those without cerebral infarction (40% as compared with 10%) and the difference is even greater among those without other identified stroke etiology (35). The mechanism of stroke in these cases is thought to involve paradoxical embolism of thrombus formed in the peripheral venous system rather than in the cardiac chambers. Aneurysmal deformity of the interatrial septum has been recognized with increased frequency as the advent of transesophageal echocardiography and may be associated with an increased risk of ischemic stroke, but the mechanism of this association is not clear and may involve coexisting conditions such as patent foramen ovale or atrial fibrillation rather than thrombus formation on the surface of the aneurysm itself (36).

ATRIAL FIBRILLATION

Stratification of Thromboembolic Risk

Patients at High Risk: Valvular Heart Disease

Patients with atrial fibrillation associated with rheumatic valvular heart disease or prosthetic heart valves face a particular danger of stroke and systemic embolism: thromboembolic event rates of at least 8-10%/year, 17 times that of patients in normal sinus rhythm in the Framingham Heart Study (37) and high enough to justify in the minds of most clinicians the hemorrhagic risks associated with maintenance oral anticoagulant therapy with coumarin drugs, even in the absence of randomized trials (38).

Among patients with nonvalvular atrial fibrillation, the risk is greatest when stroke or systemic embolism has occurred within the previous 2 years; in such cases the risk of recurrent stroke exceeds 10% per year (39). The mechanism of this incremental risk is not clear, but it may relate either to the potential for the surface of more recently formed thrombus to stimulate additional coagulation, or to the contribution of other clinical factors such as hypertensive or atherosclerotic vascular disease to ischemic events.

Several reports suggest that patients with atrial fibrillation in the setting of thyrotoxicosis, often associated with decompensated congestive heart failure, are also at high risk (averaging 14% over varying periods of observation) (40–42), though the mechanism underlying this enhanced embolic potential is not clear (40,43,44). The notion of increased thromboembolic risk in thyrotoxic atrial fibrillation has been challenged on the basis of comparison between these patients and those with thyrotoxicosis in sinus rhythm. A logistic regression analysis found only age to be an independent predictor of cerebral ischemic events (42); although 13% of patients with atrial fibrillation had ischemic cerebrovascular events (6.4% per year), compared with 3% of those in normal sinus rhythm (1.7% per year) (38–41), there was no adjustment for duration of observation or time to event. Discounting transient ischemic attacks, the increased risk of stroke in patients with atrial fibrillation reached statistical significance (p = 0.03) (42). Although it remains controversial as to whether patients with atrial fibrillation associated with thyrotoxicosis are at increased risk of thromboembolic cerebrovascular events (45), consensus has emerged favoring treatment with anticoagulant medication in the absence of a specific contraindication, at least until a euthyroid state has been restored and congestive heart failure has been corrected.

Patients at Low Risk: Lone Atrial Fibrillation

On the other end of the thromboembolic risk spectrum are patients younger than 60 years with "lone" atrial fibrillation with no history, symptoms, signs, or echocardiographic evidence of associated cardiopulmonary disease (between 2.7% and 11.4% of cases of atrial fibrillation in the Framingham Heart Study) (46). Kopecki described a cohort of 99 such patients extending over nearly 15 years, in which the incidence of stroke was 0.4% year and mortality 0.1% per year, not significantly greater than rates in patients with normal sinus rhythm (47). Because lone atrial fibrillation defined in this way is associated with a very low risk of stroke, factors other than the rhythm disturbance itself must contribute to thromboembolic events. Atrial fibrillation then represents a marker of associated cardiovascular pathology that combines with advanced age, hypertension, and congestive heart failure to substantially increase the risk of cerebral ischemia (48).

Risk Stratification of Nonvalvular Cardiac Disease

A large number of patients with nonvalvular atrial fibrillation are at intermediate risk of thromboembolism, averaging about 5% per year. The range of risk is relatively wide (from <3 to well over 10% per year), reflecting the diversity of this population and accounting for controversy about chronic antithrombotic therapy. Within this broad spectrum, subgroups of atrial fibrillation patients at relatively greater or lesser risk have been defined on the basis of clinical and echocardiographic features. Subpopulations with relatively high or low absolute rates of stroke have been defined, determining which atrial fibrillation patients gain the greatest benefit from chronic anticoagulation with coumarin drugs, offsetting their risk, expense, and inconvenience. Because etiologic classification of ischemic strokes based on clinical features is imperfect and not adequately validated, risk stratification is presently based on combined analysis of all ischemic strokes rather than those specifically of cardioembolic origin (49).

Schemes for stratification of risk in patients with atrial fibrillation have been pursued extensively using clinical and echocardiographic parameters (50–58). A collaborative analysis of the control groups of five prospective studies provides the most reliable basis for risk stratification available, and the results are outlined in Fig. 23-2 (48,49). Both continuous and paroxysmal patterns of atrial fibrillation carry approximately equal thromboembolic risk (48, 49,51). Other studies support the notion that stroke in patients with atrial fibrillation is directly related to coexistent heart disease, hypertension, age, and perhaps female gender (52,53). Patients <65 years of age with atrial fibrillation who have no other risk factors for thromboembolism have an annual stroke rate of about 1% per year; the rate rises to >8% per year in those over 75 years of age with even a single risk factor (47). Patients under age 75 years without a history of thromboembolism, hypertension, or congestive heart failure had a stroke rate <1% per year, even in the absence of antithrombotic therapy (48). The clinical variables are independently predictive of thromboembolic risk and clinically useful to characterize atrial fibrillation patients with high and low risks for stroke.

Risk factors *(control groups)*	*Relative risk*
• Previous stroke or TIA	2.5
• History of hypertension	1.6
• Advanced age (continuous)	1.4 / 10y
• Diabetes mellitus	1.7
• Congestive heart failure	1.4

FIG. 23-2. Risk factors for thromboembolism in patients with nonvalvular atrial fibrillation. Collaborative analysis of five primary prevention trials of antithrombotic therapy. (From Kopecky et al., ref. 47, with permission.)

Role of Echocardiography

Precordial Echocardiography

Aside from the identification of mitral stenosis, the main echocardiographic correlate of thromboembolic risk in patients with atrial fibrillation is impairment of left ventricular systolic function (50,59), which may promote stasis of blood within the left atrium in the presence of atrial fibrillation. Enlargement of the left atrium, seemingly a correlate of stasis within the atrial appendage, has some predictive value as a marker of stroke risk (60–62), but left ventricular dysfunction is a more powerful predictor of stroke risk in patients not given antithrombotic medication (63). Most studies have focused on the diameter of the left atrium in the anteroposterior dimension, as measured by M-mode echocardiography, and this enlarges progressively with the duration of atrial fibrillation (64–67). One report identified mitral annular calcification as an additional echocardiographic risk factor, but this has not been confirmed in other studies (68). Precordial echocardiographic findings can be combined with clinical risk stratifiers to identify atrial fibrillation patients without risk factors, who are at very low inherent risk of thromboembolism (50).

Transesophageal Echocardiography

Transesophageal echocardiography (TEE) more frequently identifies potential sources of cerebral embolism in patients with acute brain infarction than transthoracic echocardiography (69), particularly thrombus in the left atrial appendage. When standards for acquisition and interpretation are carefully applied, this technique provides a unique diagnostic window for evaluating the left atrium, left atrial appendage, and thoracic aorta, and also appears more sensitive for detection of spontaneous echo contrast, which is associated with circulatory stasis and thrombus formation (70). In a study of patients with atrial fibrillation at high risk of stroke based on age, gender, prior thromboembolism, and/or left ventricular dysfunction, TEE features associated with subsequent ischemic events were abnormalities of the left atrial appendage (reduced emptying velocity, dense spontaneous echo contrast, or manifest thrombus) or complex atherosclerotic lesions of the proximal aorta (71). TEE findings support the view that multiple mechanisms are responsible for thromboembolism in patients with nonvalvular atrial fibrillation, involving thrombus formation in the cardiac chambers, as well as extracardiac vascular disease.

Antithrombotic Therapy

To the extent that stasis-related thrombi are responsible for ischemic stroke in patients with atrial fibrillation, administration of anticoagulant medication such as warfarin or other coumarin derivatives represents a logical preventive approach. The presence of endothelial lesions in the heart or blood vessels that might be a nidus for thrombus formation raises the likelihood of a response to platelet inhibitors such as aspirin (30). The differential responses to warfarin and aspirin in recent clinical trials of antithrombotic therapy in patients with cardiac sources of embolism may reflect, in part, the relative predominance of these etiologic properties.

Before data from randomized trials became available, only patients with mitral stenosis, prosthetic heart valves, or a history of systemic embolism in the previous 2 years were regularly treated with antithrombotic agents for prevention of subsequent stroke (72–74). Numerous nonrandomized and uncontrolled trials suggested that anticoagulation reduced the rates of embolism and death in patients with rheumatic valvular disease by about 25% (38), and based on known embolic risk and on results of clinical trials, chronic anticoagulation to prolong the prothrombin time International Normalized Ratio (INR) to 2.0–3.0 is highly effective for primary prevention of stroke in these patients (41). The natural history of lone atrial fibrillation suggests that for patients under the age of 60 years without organic heart disease the hazards of chronic anticoagulation outweigh its potential benefits

(45). Until recently, however, there were no data available from randomized trials to balance the benefits of antithrombotic therapy against attendant hemorrhagic risks.

Clinical Trials of Antithrombotic Medication

Five randomized clinical trials using prothrombin time INR ranges between approximately 1.8 and 4.2 showed a mean reduction in initial ischemic stroke of nearly 70% in patients assigned anticoagulation; on-therapy analysis indicated an even greater benefit (65,75–77). The incremental risk of severe bleeding was <1% per year among anticoagulated patients, a selected group followed carefully according to clinical trial protocols. Whether such low bleeding risks can be achieved in general clinical practice is an important and unresolved issue. Low-intensity anticoagulation (INR 2 to 3) clearly confers benefit (2,48), and warfarin is highly effective in subgroups of atrial fibrillation patients who carry a high inherent risk of thromboembolism (Fig. 23-2) (2,48).

The safety and tolerability of chronic anticoagulation to conventional levels has not been well defined among patients over 75 years old, who account for nearly half of atrial fibrillation–associated strokes. All but one of the anticoagulation trials enrolled atrial fibrillation patients about a decade younger (4). The single placebo-controlled trial involving atrial fibrillation patients with a mean age of 75 years reported an overall withdrawal rate from anticoagulation of 38% after a year, and the attrition rate among the oldest patients may have been even higher (78). The risk of major hemorrhage during anticoagulation (INR range 2.0 to 4.5, mean 2.7) in another trial was substantially greater among atrial fibrillation patients older than 75 years than among younger patients anticoagulated to similar intensities (79). While the elderly have a greater risk of atrial fibrillation–associated stroke, the benefit of anticoagulation is offset somewhat by this greater toxicity, and the inability of the very elderly to sustain chronic anticoagulation is a noteworthy finding of several trials (73,74).

The efficacy of aspirin for stroke prevention in atrial fibrillation patients is more controversial (4). The effect of aspirin in doses between 75 and 325 mg per day has been assessed in three placebo-controlled trials with a statistically significant pooled risk reduction of about 25% (range 14% to 44%) in aspirin-treated patients (4,73) (80). Aspirin was less effective than warfarin in two of these trials analyzed along intention-to-treat paradigms and according to on-treatment (efficacy) analysis of the third (66,73,74). A trial of antithrombotic therapy for secondary prevention of recurrent stroke in patients with atrial fibrillation and recent nondisabling ischemic stroke or transient ischemic attack found warfarin substantially more effective than placebo (event rates 4% per year and 12% per year, respectively; hazard ratio 0.34; 95% CI 0.20 to 0.57), whereas aspirin appeared relatively ineffective (81). In terms of absolute event rates, nine vascular events (mainly strokes) are prevented for every 100 patients treated with anticoagulation for a year. Aspirin was a safer, though less effective, alternative when anticoagulation was contraindicated, preventing four vascular events each year for every 100 treated patients, compared with placebo. There is no compelling evidence that the specific dose of aspirin between 75 and 325 mg per day confers more or less benefit, though the individual

trial results suggest greater efficacy at the higher dosage. Aspirin efficacy was inexplicably linked to patient age, exerting substantial prophylactic effect against thromboembolism only among patients younger than 75 years old in the SPAF-I study (Fig. 23-3). Aspirin thus appears active, especially for primary prevention of stroke in atrial fibrillation patients, but less uniformly effective than warfarin. Aspirin is inexpensive, easily administered, and produces less bleeding toxicity than anticoagulation in elderly patients (Fig. 23-4) (74).

A randomized trial (SPAF-III) comparing adjusted-dose warfarin (target INR 2 to 3) to low-intensity warfarin (INR 1.2 to 1.5) plus aspirin (325 mg daily) in patients at high intrinsic risk of thromboembolism was stopped at an interim analysis due to the lack of efficacy of combination therapy. Anticoagulation intensity in the combination therapy arm yielded high stroke rates similar to those expected during treatment with aspirin alone (Fig. 23-5). Another study comparing combinations of aspirin and warfarin with either agent alone (AFASAK-2) was stopped when these results became available because of concern about the ethics of treatment other than warfarin in high-risk patients (82).

A Dutch primary prevention trial involving use of aspirin and anticoagulant medication for nonvalvular atrial fibrillation in general

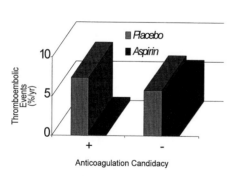

FIG. 23-3. Differential effect of aspirin in relation to patient age in the Stroke Prevention in Atrial Fibrillation (SPAF-I) study.

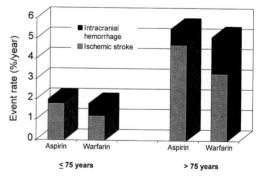

FIG. 23-4. Comparison of total stroke event rates during treatment with aspirin or warfarin in the Stroke Prevention in Atrial Fibrillation (SPAF-II) study.

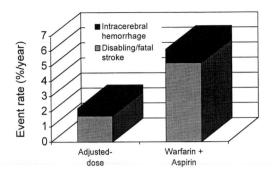

FIG. 23-5. CNS event rates during treatment of high-risk atrial fibrillation patients with warfarin (INR 2 to 3) compared with a fixed low-dose combination of warfarin plus aspirin in the Stroke Prevention in Atrial Fibrillation (SPAF-III) study.

practice (PATAF) has ended. A preliminary report of results in 729 patients (55% females) followed a mean of 2.7 years indicated that there were no significant differences in event rates between 141 patients assigned to aspirin, 122 patients assigned to warfarin at target INR 1.1 to 1.6, and 131 patients given warfarin at target INR 2.5 to 3.5 (83a). The overall event rates were low, perhaps due to recruitment in a population served by general practitioners; this combined with the number of treatment arms seems to have yielded limited statistical power for comparison of the therapeutic strategies.

In Italy, the SIFA study compared the platelet inhibitor indobufen (100 to 200 mg bid) with warfarin (INR 2.0 to 3.5) in patients with atrial fibrillation and recent cerebral ischemic events. After 12 months the rate of the primary event constellation (nonfatal stroke including intracerebral hemorrhage, pulmonary or systemic embolism, myocardial infarction, and vascular death) was 10.6% in those assigned to indobufen (95% CI 7.7 to 13.5) and 9.0% in the warfarin group (95% CI 6.3 to 11.8), a statistically insignificant difference between treatments. Extracerebral bleeding was uncommon and limited to the warfarin group (83b). The results of another multicenter Italian trial (MIWAF) comparing conven-

tional warfarin therapy (INR 2.0 to 3.0) with a fixed low dose of warfarin (1.25 mg daily) are expected late in 1997 (84).

Anticoagulation for Cardioversion to Sinus Rhythm

Although spontaneous termination of episodes of atrial fibrillation among patients in whom fibrillation is paroxysmal is not associated with increased risk of thromboembolism (85), the incidence of stroke within the first several days following successful electrical reversion to sinus rhythm by direct-current countershock is between 5% and 7%, and this risk may be lowered by anticoagulant therapy (86–88). In the largest series, involving 437 patients with a variety of atrial arrhythmias, 58% of whom had underlying rheumatic heart disease, anticoagulant therapy was not randomized. Those receiving anticoagulants prior to electrical cardioversion had ischemic events at a rate of 0.8 incident per 100 successful conversions, compared with 5.3% in those not anticoagulated (p = 0.016), despite the greater prevalence of rheumatic heart disease, congestive heart failure, prior embolism, and cardiac enlargement among those receiving anticoagulants (86,87). Half of the thromboembolic events occurred in patients with nonrheumatic cardiac disorders. The substantial reduction in the incidence of presumed embolic events has led to the recommendation that warfarin (INR 2.0 to 3.0) be prescribed for 3 to 4 weeks prior to cardioversion (89,90). Awareness of the risk of thromboembolism may contribute to event detection under these circumstances, or patients at greater intrinsic risk of thromboembolism (such as those with left ventricular dysfunction) may more frequently be candidates for cardioversion. Although atrial stunning at the moment of termination of atrial fibrillation may be associated with a transiently increased risk of thrombus formation, there is no intuitive reason to believe that rates of thromboembolism differ between spontaneous, chemical, or electrical means of cardioversion. It is also likely that the risk of stroke at the time of cardioversion is still linked to the intrinsic cardiovascular factors which contribute to risk on a chronic basis.

Serial transesophageal echocardiography of patients with nonvalvular atrial fibrillation after initial identification of atrial thrombus has documented resolution of thrombus over 4 weeks of anticoagulation with warfarin (91). These observations support the use of anticoagulant medication for a period of 3 to 4 weeks prior to cardioversion. And both because restoration of atrial mechanical function may be delayed after sinus rhythm appears on the surface electrocardiogram and because of the possibility that atrial fibrillation may recur, anticoagulation is generally continued for a similar period (3 to 4 weeks) after successful direct-current cardioversion. But the risk of thrombus formation may be greatest in the moments after the countershock is delivered, when transesophageal echocardiography has demonstrated that a period of atrial quiescence occurs associated with stasis manifested by the appearance of spontaneous echo contrast in the left atrium and appendage (92). The implication is that antithrombotic therapy should be most intensive during rather than only before and after cardioversion, and heparin might be administered intravenously at that time in a dose sufficient to prolong the activate partial thromboplastin time (APTT) to 1.5 to 2.0 times the control value.

LEFT VENTRICULAR DYSFUNCTION

Stratification of Thromboembolic Risk

Acute Myocardial Infarction

Without antithrombotic therapy or thrombolytic reperfusion, left ventricular mural thrombus develops in 20% of cases of acute myocardial infarction, 40% of anterior infarcts, and 60% of those large anterior infarcts that involve the ventricular apex and produce peak serum creatine kinase concentrations >2,000 U/L. Autopsy studies after fatal myocardial infarction, representing the largest infarcts, have found the incidence of mural thrombus in the range of 40% to 70% when anticoagulant therapy was not given (93–96), but this incidence is substantially reduced (to 22% to 24%) by anticoagulant treatment (97,98).

Over 90% of ventricular thrombus associated with acute myocardial infarction occurs when apical akinesis or hypokinesis enlarges the zone of intraventricular stasis. A propensity to thrombus formation probably begins at the onset of myocardial necrosis, when endocardial inflammation creates a thrombogenic surface (99). Although thrombus most often develops within the first 10 days (100), the tendency to coagulation along the endocardial surface persists over a period of 1 to 3 months, during which the risk of thrombosis remains related to the amount of myocardium damaged (87).

Stroke or systemic embolism occurs in up to 12% of all patients with acute myocardial infarction. The rate is higher in those with anterior than inferior infarcts and may reach 20% of those with the large anteroapical infarcts cited above (101). Cerebral embolism occurs clinically in about 10% of patients with echocardiographically evident mural thrombus associated with acute myocardial infarction. The incidence of embolism is highest during the period of active thrombus formation in the first 1 to 3 months, yet the embolic risk remains substantial even beyond the acute phase in patients with persistent myocardial dysfunction, congestive heart failure, or atrial fibrillation.

Most studies suggest that prognosis for survival of patients developing left ventricular mural thrombus in the course of acute myocardial infarction is less favorable than for those who do not have this echocardiographic finding (88) (102). This has been attributed to larger infarct size in patients with thrombus development and the association with anterior rather than inferior infarction site, and it is not clear as to whether mural thrombus formation constitutes an independent risk factor for mortality (103). In some studies, however, the prognosis for survival has actually been better in patients with evidence of thrombus formation and the risk of stroke was no greater than in those without thrombus, leading to the conclusion that thrombus may offer a protective effect and that antithrombotic medication may not be needed (104). Early in-hospital mortality may be greater in patients without thrombus than in those in whom thrombus occurs because nearly detectable thrombotic masses do not always develop before the sixth day, so that patients at highest risk may not survive long enough for ventricular thrombus to form. Although thrombus remains echocardiographically apparent for a year after myocardial infarction in over one third of patients in whom the diagnosis is initially made, and evidence of thrombus persists for 2 years in about one fourth of cases, relatively few of these persistent thrombi are associated with late embolic events. The implied benignity of the echocardiographic finding of left ventricular thrombus formation after myocardial infarction in some series may reflect the limited number of cases of large anterior infarction (89).

Chronic Ventricular Dysfunction

In patients with very localized forms of chronic left ventricular dysfunction following ventricular aneurysm formation beyond 3 months of myocardial infarction, thrombus can be identified in almost half the cases by echocardiography or other imaging techniques, but the incidence of systemic embolism is relatively low—no more than 1 event per 100 patient-years (105). On the other hand, when left ventricular systolic function is more diffusely reduced as occurs in dilated cardiomyopathy, the risk of cerebral embolism is greater, in the range of 3% to 4% per year (106). This points again to the balance between the effect of regional circulatory stasis, which favors thrombus formation within the aneurysmal cavity, and the isolation from the dynamic forces of the circulation, which protects against embolic migration. In contrast, protrusion and mobility of the thrombotic mass in the ventricular chamber are associated with much greater embolic potential (107).

Identification of Left Ventricular Thrombus

Transthoracic Echocardiography

Despite the availability of alternative methods for detection of left ventricular thrombi, echocardiography performed serially at selected intervals in the postinfarction period has been established as the best available means of cardiac imaging to define the natural history of left ventricular thrombi and the response to therapy. Echocardiography also helps characterize thrombus size, shape, mobility, site of attachment, and adjacent regional left ventricular wall thickness and function (93,100,108,109) features related to the risk of thromboembolic events including ischemic stroke. Spatial Doppler flow patterns of intracavitary blood, which are associated with left ventricular thrombus formation following infarction, may elucidate mechanisms of thrombus formation and the potential for embolism (110). Serial echocardiographic studies of patients with acute myocardial infarction have been consistent with respect to the incidence of ventricular thrombi. The sensitivity and specificity of echocardiography for the detection of left ventricular thrombi range from 77% to 95% and 86% to 94%, respectively (111–115). The coefficient of correlation with autopsy series has been reported in the range of 0.85, but these analyses tend to overrepresent larger infarcts and may not apply to thrombus that develops clinically in less catastrophic cases (87).

There is no consensus regarding echocardiographic criteria by which left ventricular mural thrombus may be defined, but those proposed by Asinger are most widely cited (116). These include detection of an echodense mass in the left ventricular cavity on at least two views distinguished from adjacent endocardium in a region of asynergy. The resolution of two-dimensional transthoracic echocardiography identifies thrombus larger than that sufficient to inflict extensive embolic—usually cerebral—tissue damage.

While more than one third of patients with acute anterior myocardial infarction develop left ventricular thrombus, this complication occurs in <5% of those with inferior infarction (Table 23-1). In those with large infarcts, up to two thirds of thrombi are visible echocardiographically within 48 hours of hospital presentation (96,106,117), and the vast majority form within the first 2 weeks (97,118). About one fourth of cases of ventricular mural thrombus are identified in the first 24 hours after acute myocardial infarction, 50% are detected within the first 2 to 3 days, 75% within the first 6 days, and the remainder by the end of 2 weeks (88,102, 119,120). Spontaneous resolution of thrombus occurs at a rate of 20% to 30% per year, and this process can be accelerated with anticoagulant therapy (88,96,98,121–123).

Early echocardiographic appearance of ventricular intracavitary thrombus is associated with a greater risk of systemic embolism and generally worse prognosis than those that develop later in the course, perhaps due to the greater extent of myocardial damage in the early cases (119), and this risk persists well beyond the acute phase following infarction (88,119,124). Echocardiographic features that increase the probability of embolism include protrusion and mobility of intracavitary thrombus as determined in multiple views.

Spontaneous echo contrast, seen most often in dilated cardiac chambers with reduced blood flow, appears to reflect platelet aggregation within areas of blood stasis in the ventricular cavity adjacent to a thrombogenic mural surface and may represent a thrombogenic state (125,126). Left ventricular spatial flow patterns identified by Doppler echocardiography exhibit some predictive capacity for thrombus formation (103,104) but remain abnormal even beyond 3 months of acute myocardial infarction.

Other Imaging Techniques

Although transesophageal echocardiography is superior to transthoracic imaging for the detection of left atrial thrombus, this technique has not been validated for the diagnosis of left ventricular thrombus. Contrast ventriculography appears to have a lower sensitivity and specificity than echocardiography for the detection of left ventricular mural thrombus and carries the risk of inducing embolism by mechanical dislodgement of thrombotic material. [111]Indium-labeled platelet scintigraphy requires a latency period of 48 to 72 hours for detection of intracardiac thrombus (127) to allow sufficient platelet accumulation on the surface of a ventricular thrombus to permit imaging, but false-positive results appear less frequently than with echocardiographic imaging and it has been hypothesized that the method may identify thrombotically active masses prone to embolism (128). The diagnostic accuracy and clinical usefulness of "ultrafast" gated cardiac CT and MRI for detection of ventricular thrombus in patients with myocardial infarction is emerging but there has as yet been no satisfactory demonstration of the superiority of these methods

TABLE 23-1. *Incidence of left ventricular thrombus following myocardial infarction*

		Anterior infarction			Inferior infarction		
Author	Total cases	Cases	Thrombi	%	Cases	Thrombi	%
Asinger (116)	70	35	12	34	35	0	0
Friedman (152)	52	21	8	38	13	2	15
Weinreich (87)	261	130	44	34	131	2	2
Visser (153)	96	65	21	32	31	1	3
Johannessen (154)	90	53	15	28	28	0	0
Gueret (155)	90	46	21	46	44	0	0
Nihoyannopoulos (104)	87	53	21	40	34	0	0
Keren (156)	198	124	38	31	74	0	0
Total	944	527	180	34	390	5	1

for selection of patients requiring more intensive forms of antithrombotic therapy (129).

Antithrombotic Therapy

Acute Myocardial Infarction

Because stasis predominantly activates the coagulation system leading more to fibrin formation than platelet aggregation in the pathogenesis of ventricular thrombus, anticoagulant drugs have long been the principal therapeutic agents. Over the past 20 years three large trials involving patients with acute inferior and anterior myocardial infarctions concluded that initial treatment with heparin followed by administration of oral coumarin drugs reduced the occurrence of cerebral embolism from 3% to 1% when compared with no anticoagulation (Table 23-2). Differences were statistically significant in two of the studies, with a concordant trend in the third (130–132). Four randomized studies involving patients with acute myocardial infarction have addressed the relationship of echocardiographically detected left ventricular

thrombus and cerebral embolism (133–136). In aggregate, thrombus formation was reduced by more than 50% with anticoagulation; individually, however, each trial had insufficient sample size to detect significant differences in embolism.

The anticoagulant heparin is commonly given parenterally from the time of diagnosis of anterior infarction until the presence or absence of thrombus is investigated by two-dimensional echocardiography, and an oral antithrombotic medication regimen is then substituted (for about 3 months) based on the results of the ultrasound examination and other clinical circumstances. Two randomized trials (137,138) have documented that therapeutic anticoagulation reduces the incidence of left ventricular thrombi complicating anterior myocardial infarction in the initial hospital period (1 to 2 weeks postinfarction) by about 50%, and several studies suggest acceleration of thrombus resolution with anticoagulation (118,122–124). Furthermore, anticoagulant therapy reduces the incidence of systemic (97,124,131) and cerebral (139) embolism in patients with left ventricular

TABLE 23-2. *Myocardial infarction, ventricular thrombus, and embolism*

Author	Anticoagulation	Thrombus detected	Follow-up	LVT	Embolism	%
Tramarin (122)		4 weeks	11 months			
	–			17	0	0
	+			17	0	0
Keating (124)		2 weeks	11 months			
	–			5	3	60
	+			9	0	0
Weinreich (87)		1–3 weeks	15 months			
	–			14	3	22
	+			25	0	0
Asinger (116)		7 days	9 months			
	–			2	0	0
	+			7	0	0
Turpie (137)		10 days	6 months			
	–			8	0	0
	+			30	0	0
Visser (101)		2–3 days	12 months			
	–			10	1	10
	+			11	1	9
Domenicucci (118)		12 days	14 months			
	–			59	5	8
Nihoyannopoulos (104)		6 days	39 months			
	–			21	0	0
Keren (128)		10 months	29 months			
	–			26	6	23

thrombi in the early phase after myocardial infarction.

The therapeutic effects of aspirin administration to reduce the rates of reinfarction, stroke, and mortality in survivors of acute myocardial infarction have been documented in a number of trials, but the use of platelet inhibitors to reduce the incidence of left ventricular thrombi has not been studied extensively. Clinical investigation using [111]indium platelet imaging to assess the effect of aspirin on the hematologic activity of left ventricular thrombi has yielded conflicting results (77,114). One trial involving a small number of patients found aspirin superior to no treatment in effecting regression of left ventricular thrombi (95), and a single nonrandomized study found aspirin effective for reducing thromboembolic events in patients with dilated cardiomyopathy (140). However, several other studies found there to be no influence of aspirin on the incidence of left ventricular thrombus (95,141,142). A study comparing aspirin, anticoagulants, and placebo in patients with echocardiographically documented left ventricular thrombus found anticoagulants and aspirin to be associated with equal rates of thrombus resolution (123).

Published guidelines endorsed by a consensus of the American Heart Association and American College of Cardiology recommend pre-discharge echocardiography for patients with acute anterior myocardial infarction at risk for developing left ventricular thrombus (143). Based on available clinical trial results, class I recommendations have been promulgated for oral anticoagulant treatment of patients with echocardiographically detected left ventricular thrombi after anterior myocardial infarction. There is no consensus, however, regarding the duration of anticoagulant treatment (143). The persistence of stroke risk for several months after infarction in these patients can be surmised from aggregate results of a number of studies, but alternative antithrombotic regimens have not been systematically evaluated. The risk of thromboembolism seems to decrease beyond the first 3 months, and in patients with chronic ventric-

ular aneurysm the risk of embolism is comparatively low, even though intracavitary thrombi occur frequently in this condition.

In patients without echocardiographically evident thrombus at the time of hospital discharge, the most pressing clinical question is whether anticoagulation, administration of a platelet inhibitor, or some combination of both approaches is most effective for preventing the development of thrombosis and embolism. Two studies from which data have been reported on the occurrence of thrombus following hospital discharge seem concordant in finding left ventricular thrombus in approximately 10% of patients with anterior Q-wave infarcts not given anticoagulants following discharge. Although the number of patients anticoagulated was too small to permit firm conclusions, no patient developed thrombus.

Regarding the intensity of anticoagulation for prevention of left ventricular mural thrombus formation in patients with acute myocardial infarction, Turpie et al. (137) described a randomized prospective trial involving 221 patients with acute anterior myocardial infarction who did not receive thrombolytic agents in the acute phase, where subcutaneous administration of calcium heparin in a dose of 12,500 U every 12 hours offered greater benefit for prevention of left ventricular mural thrombus during the first 10 days than the lower dosage of 5,000 U every 12 hours conventionally given for prevention of venous thrombosis. Thrombus was detected echocardiographically in 11% of the group given the higher heparin dose, compared with 32% of those receiving the lower dose (p = 0.0004). This beneficial effect correlated strongly with plasma heparin activity. The overall incidence of nonhemorrhagic stroke in the early period following infarction was just under 1% in those initially treated with high-dose heparin and close to 4% in the low-dose group (p = 0.17), but insufficient event rates may have been why there was no significant difference in embolic complications. Hemorrhagic complications were equally common in both treatment groups in this study.

In the SCATI (Studio sulla Calciparina nell'Angina e nella Trombosi Ventricolare nell'Infarto) randomized trial of 771 patients with acute myocardial infarction, 433 were given the thrombolytic agent streptokinase (1.5 million U over 1 hour) (138). Half received heparin (12,500 U every 12 hours) and the others no heparin. Of the 235 cases of initial anterior infarction, satisfactory two-dimensional echocardiographic examinations were obtained both early after admission and near the time of discharge in 200. The predischarge echocardiograms showed a significantly lower incidence of left ventricular thrombus in those receiving heparin (18%) than in the control group (37%; p < 0.01). The earlier echocardiogram was obtained within 24 hours of admission in 86% of patients, at which time 20 (18%) of those assigned to receive heparin and 13 (14%) of those in the control group showed evidence of thrombus—not a significant difference. Among those free of early echocardiographically manifest thrombus, 6% of those treated with heparin developed thrombus by the time of the predischarge examination, compared with 26% of the controls (relative risk 0.17, 95% confidence interval 0.06 to 0.47; p < 0.0002). However, it is not clear as to what proportion of these patients were given thrombolytic therapy and whether this intervention affected the rate of development of ventricular thrombus. Stroke occurred in two patients in the control group, and both had echocardiographic evidence of mural thrombus; no strokes were detected in the treated patients. One fatal cerebral hemorrhage occurred in a patient in the heparin group.

It is clear from these studies that early administration of intravenous or high-dose subcutaneous heparin is effective in reducing the incidence of left ventricular thrombus formation, detected echocardiographically, in patients with acute anterior myocardial infarction. It is less clear as to whether this form of therapy will reduce the occurrence of systemic arterial embolism because the rate of such events has been too small in these studies to detect any effect of anticoagulant treatment. Administration of heparin is generally begun immediately after the onset of infarction and continue for a period of about 10 days. It is not appropriate to await the results of echocardiographic examination before instituting antithrombotic therapy because treatment is most effective when given as early as possible in the course of acute infarction and delay might result in reduced efficacy. Furthermore, echocardiography within the first 24 hours after the onset of infarction may fail to detect early thrombus formation and later studies may detect thrombus too late to avoid embolic complications.

In some patients—those, for example, with ventricular mural thrombus identified by echocardiography or large akinetic regions—heparin therapy may be followed by warfarin. Therapy with warfarin is associated with resolution of echocardiographic features of left ventricular thrombus following myocardial infarction in the majority of cases, and the oral anticoagulant is usually stopped after 1 to 3 months unless the risk of thromboembolism remains elevated as a result of heart failure, impaired left ventricular function, or persistent echocardiographic evidence of mural thrombus.

Whether thrombolytic therapy reduces the likelihood of developing ventricular thrombus is still uncertain. Anticoagulation designed to prevent acute coronary reocclusion following thrombolytic therapy may prevent intracavitary thrombus, and reduction in infarct size makes mural thrombus formation less likely. Natarajan et al. (7) described 45 patients with acute myocardial infarction evolving mean serum creatine kinase concentrations of about 1,000 U, half of whom were given streptokinase and half no antithrombotic therapy. Echocardiography between the seventh and tenth days found apical wall motion abnormalities in all cases. Thrombus formed in 44% of the control group (a surprisingly high prevalence given the modest enzyme levels) but in none of those given the thrombolytic agent. In the considerably larger Thrombolysis in Myocardial Infarction (TIMI) study, echocardiograms were obtained 48 to 72 hours after hospitalization in 96 patients with acute myocardial infarction, 43 of whom had received tissue plasminogen activator, 22 streptokinase, and 31 no thrombolytic agents; all were treated with subcutaneous heparin (5,000 U every 12 hours) (144). Infarcts were anterior in about 45% of the cases, and peak serum creatine kinase activity averaged 2,683 U in those given no thrombolytic agents. Left ventricular thrombus was identified in 33% of anterior infarcts, compared with only 4% of inferior infarcts, and rates of thrombus formation were approximately 30% lower in patients who were given lytic therapy than in those who were not. Thrombus was present in 19% of those given tissue plasminogen activator, 5% of patients receiving streptokinase and 23% of those given neither; these did not represent statistically significant differences. No emboli were detected in the entire series. In yet another series (145), left ventricular thrombus was less prevalent after streptokinase treatment of the acute infarction, but left ventricular thrombus was detected in 70% of the control group and ejection fractions were lower. It may turn out, therefore, that left ventricular thrombus relates more to residual systolic myocardial function than to whether or not thrombolytic treatment is employed.

No trial of sufficient size has yet established the role of thrombolytic or platelet inhibitor therapy for prevention of left ventricular thrombus formation following acute myocardial infarction. Kouvaris et al. (123) randomly assigned 60 patients to an oral anticoagulant regimen (prothrombin time ratio 1.6 to 2.0), aspirin (650 mg daily), or no antithrombotic medication. After 16 months of observation, reduction in size or resolution of echocardiographically manifest thrombus occurred in 15% of patients given the anticoagulant, 13% of those given aspirin, and only 4% of those in the control group (p < 0.04). Once again, the size of the population studied was inadequate to produce firm conclusions, but the results support the use of some form of antithrombotic therapy over none at all. In the Second International Study of Infarct Survival (ISIS-2) (112) of 17,187 patients, use of

aspirin, 160 mg daily reduced the frequency of clinical stroke by >40% during the initial hospital period, although this includes both hemorrhagic and ischemic brain events. A meta-analysis of individual small studies supports mainly the effectiveness of anticoagulant medication (odds ratios: 0.32 with anticoagulant therapy, 0.65 with thrombolytic therapy, and 1.43 with platelet inhibitor therapy compared with respective control groups) (10).

Quantifying the persistent risk of thromboembolic events in those who survive myocardial infarction with chronic left ventricular dysfunction is one of the most vexing problems facing physicians caring for these patients. For the majority of patients with long-standing ventricular dysfunction related to either dilated cardiomyopathy or coronary disease, there is the need to determine the optimum type and dosage of antithrombotic medication. The roles of echocardiography and other imaging technology for selecting patients at high risk of embolic complications for prophylactic treatment are only beginning to unfold. Beyond the problem of left ventricular thromboembolism, patients with myocardial infarction present a complex situation in which antithrombotic therapy may have implications for prevention of future coronary events. The question of the best approach to prevention of both left ventricular thrombus and complications of underlying coronary atherosclerotic disease is still unsettled. As the use of aspirin in patients with acute and chronic forms of ischemic heart disease may increase the risk of bleeding in patients given anticoagulants in conventional doses, physicians face a dilemma: Aspirin may be recommended for prevention of coronary complications, but this may not avoid cardiogenic embolism.

Chronic Left Ventricular Aneurysm

In the chronic phase after myocardial infarction, left ventricular mural thrombus may persist or form anew within the cavity of a dyskinetic ventricular aneurysm. In contrast to acute myocardial infarction, the incidence of embolism in patients with chronic left ventricular aneurysm is significantly lower (0.35% per year) (106). The reasons for this difference are probably twofold. First, thrombus formed early after acute infarction is usually mobile and friable, and protrudes into the ventricular cavity, whereas thrombus in chronic aneurysms is laminated and more adherent to the endocardium. Second, thrombus sequestered within an aneurysmal sac devoid of contractile fibers is less prone to propulsion into the ventricular outflow tract. Although some investigators (97) have found a persistent risk of embolism in postinfarction patients, it was not the presence of an aneurysm but rather the mobility and protrusion of thrombus that predicted embolic events. Patients with remote infarction and chronic left ventricular aneurysm are therefore at lower risk of embolism than patients in whom thrombus develops in the setting of acute infarction. Even within this subset, however, the question of whether anticoagulants should be given to patients with echocardiographic evidence of mobile or protruding thrombus remains unanswered.

Chronic Ischemic Heart Disease Following Myocardial Infarction

The Warfarin Reinfarction Study (WARIS) (146) examined the response to warfarin in comparison with placebo among 1,214 survivors of initial myocardial infarction age 75 years or younger followed for a mean of 37 months. Mortality was reduced by 24% (p = 0.26) with sustained anticoagulation in the range of 2.8 to 4.8 INR, and the incidence of recurrent infarction was reduced by 43% (p = 0.0001). The rate of stroke was also significantly reduced by 61%, from 41 events among patients assigned to placebo to 16 in those assigned to warfarin (p = 0.0001). Studies were not performed to detect left ventricular mural thrombus; there was no attempt to determine stroke mechanism, and many of these events may have been related to hemorrhage or atherothrombotic phenomena rather

than to cardiogenic embolism. Similar results were reported in the ASPECT study (147).

The safety and efficacy of platelet inhibitor therapy has not been directly compared with adjusted-dose warfarin following acute myocardial infarction in a trial of sufficient scope. The value of anticoagulant therapy for prevention of recurrent coronary events, coupled with its effectiveness for prevention of mural thrombosis and probable efficacy for prevention of systemic embolism, would make this an appealing option for survivors of acute myocardial infarction were it not for the hemorrhagic risks associated with long-term treatment and the inconvenience of prothrombin time monitoring. Accordingly, there has arisen great interest in the potential use of lower intensity anticoagulant therapy and combinations of an anticoagulant with platelet inhibitory agents such as aspirin. The Coumadin-Aspirin Reinfarction Study (CARS) compared combinations of low fixed doses of aspirin plus warfarin against aspirin alone in nearly 9,000 patients with acute myocardial infarction and found no difference in the rate of recurrent myocardial infarction while the rate of ischemic stroke was slightly lower in those taking aspirin monotherapy. Adjusted-dose warfarin was not included and neither the incidence of ventricular thrombus nor the etiology of stroke was determined (148).

Dilated Cardiomyopathy

Postmortem (116) and echocardiographic (117) studies have found a high prevalence of right and left ventricular mural thrombus in patients with idiopathic dilated cardiomyopathy (over 50% and 36%, respectively). Blood stasis and low shear rate present in a dilated, hypocontractile ventricle lead to activation of coagulation processes. Since the mural thrombus is not mechanically isolated as occurs in a ventricular aneurysm, embolism of thrombotic material may occur. In one retrospective study, patients treated with anticoagulants had no evidence of systemic embolism, whereas those not anticoagulated had an embolic rate of 3.5% per year (106). In the absence of a prospective trial of antithrombotic therapy in patients with idiopathic dilated cardiomyopathy, this evidence supports chronic warfarin administration, particularly in those with overt heart failure or atrial fibrillation. For cases of chronic dilated cardiomyopathy associated with advanced coronary atherosclerotic heart disease remote from acute myocardial infarction, there are no studies on which to base a decision regarding the use of anticoagulant medication over or a platelet inhibitor such as aspirin either for the purpose of preventing systemic embolism or mortality related to a recurrent ischemic event.

CONCLUSION

Within the cardiac chambers, stasis of blood flow causes coagulation to predominate over platelet activation as the principal mechanism of thrombus formation, and anticoagulant therapy alone seems most appropriate in management of these patients. At highest risk are patients with atrial fibrillation and prior embolism; at somewhat lower but yet substantial risk are those with mitral stenosis or prosthetic heart valves. Patients at medium risk are those immediately following large anterior myocardial infarction and uncompensated dilated cardiomyopathy. For these groups, there is sufficient evidence to indicate chronic anticoagulation. Some patients with nonvalvulopathic atrial fibrillation also benefit from warfarin therapy, but subgroups within this population have not yet been sufficiently defined. At lowest risk are patients with lone atrial fibrillation without overt heart disease and those with chronic left ventricular aneurysm who do not require anticoagulants.

Atrial fibrillation is now recognized as a major risk factor for the development of ischemic stroke, particularly among elderly patients. But the rhythm disturbance represents a marker of associated cardiovascular pathology that may be more directly at the root of many cases of stroke than cardioembolic mechanisms alone. The effectiveness and relative safety of chronic anticoagulant therapy with

warfarin has now been validated in six separate clinical trials, supporting a thrombotic mechanism for most of the strokes that occur in patients with atrial fibrillation, and the success of therapy with aspirin in some patients suggests that administration of this platelet inhibitor might be sufficient for selected individuals with nonvalvular atrial fibrillation. Goals for the future include continued collaborative analysis by investigators involved with ongoing and completed trials to further stratify patients in terms of the relative risk of stroke based on the etiology of the dysrhythmia and associated clinical conditions. Such efforts have already enlarged the available data pool, allowing inferences about the optimal type and intensity of antithrombotic therapy (Fig. 23-6). A longer range view includes the development and testing of even more effective strategies of antithrombotic therapy, comparison of strategies of rate control versus rhythm control (cardioversion and antiarrhythmic therapy) in terms of resultant thromboembolism, and evaluation of other therapeutic modalities directed at control of hypertension and hyperlipidemia in terms of their impact on rates of ischemic stroke (14). For the moment, however, physicians are faced with the challenge of identifying patients with atrial fibrillation who benefit from anticoagulant or aspirin therapy, and to supervise treatment closely to avoid both the scourges of hemorrhage and stroke (Fig. 23-7).

The best approach to prevention of embolism in patients with acute myocardial infarction cannot yet be defined on the basis of sound data, but it seems reasonable to administer heparin to those with large anterior infarcts during the early phase (15). Among the many questions left unanswered is whether to regularly perform investigations like echocardiography to detect left ventricular thrombus. Another is how long to continue prophylactic anticoagulant medication in patients without thrombus formation and when to withdraw anticoagulant medication when thrombus is identified, i.e., at the time of the patient's discharge from hospital or after 3 months. A third issue is whether thrombolytic therapy

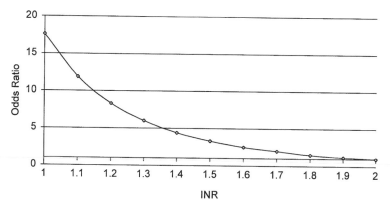

FIG. 23-6. Odds of developing ischemic stroke in relation to intensity of anticoagulation.

will reduce the likelihood of developing ventricular thrombus in the first place. Then there is the problem of quantifying the persistent risk of thromboembolic events in those who survive myocardial infarction with chronic left ventricular dysfunction (6).

In addition to addressing the problem of left ventricular thromboembolism, antithrombotic therapy may have implications for prevention of future coronary events in patients with myocardial infarction. The best approach to prevention of both left ventricular thrombus and complications of underlying coronary atherosclerotic disease remains to be defined on the basis of a prospective clinical trial, which might not only compare the safety and efficacy of aspirin and warfarin but consider as well the potential advantages of a combi-nation of low doses of both forms of antithrombotic medication.

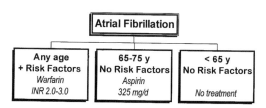

FIG. 23-7. Current guidelines for antithrombotic therapy in patients with atrial fibrillation. Risk factors include: mitral stenosis, prosthetic heart valve, congestive heart failure, previous stroke or transient cerebral ischemic attack, hypertension, coronary artery disease, diabetes, thyrotoxicosis.

REFERENCES

1. Cerebral Embolism Task Force. Cardiogenic brain embolism: the second report of the Cerebral Embolism Task Force. *Arch Neurol* 1989;46:727–743.
2. Kannel WB, Abbott RD, Savage DD, McNamara PM. Epidemiologic features of chronic atrial fibrillation: the Framingham Study. *N Engl J Med* 1982;306:1018–1022.
3. Wolf PA, Abbott RD, Kannel WB. Atrial fibrillation: a major contributor to stroke in the elderly: the Framingham Study. *Arch Intern Med* 1987;147:1561.
4. Halperin JL, Hart RG. Atrial fibrillation and stroke: new ideas, persisting dilemmas [Editorial]. *Stroke* 1988;19:937–941.
5. Sherman DG, Dyken ML, Fisher M, Harrison MJG, Hart RG. Cerebral embolism. *Chest* 1986;89(suppl):82S–98S.
6. Fuster V, Halperin JL. Left ventricular thrombi and cerebral embolism. *N Engl J Med* 1989;320:392–394.
7. Natarajan D, Hotchandani RK, Nigam PD. Reduced incidence of left ventricular thrombi with intravenous streptokinase in acute anterior myocardial infarction: prospective evaluation by cross-sectional echocardiography. *Int J Cardiol* 1988;20:201–207.
8. Held AC, Gore JM, Paraskos J, et al. Impact of thrombolytic therapy on left ventricular mural thrombi in acute myocardial infarction. *Am J Cardiol* 1988;62:310–311.
9. Eigler N, Maurer G, Shah PK. Effect of early systemic thrombolytic therapy on left ventricular mural thrombus formation in acute anterior myocardial infarction. *Am J Cardiol* 1984;54:261–263.
10. Vaitkus PT, Barnathan ES. Do anticoagulants, thrombolytics or antiplatelet agents reduce the incidence of left ventricular thrombus after anterior myocardial infarction? *J Am Coll Cardiol* 1991;17(suppl 2):146A.
11. Feinberg WM, Seeger JF, Carmody RF, Anderson DC, Hart RG, Pearce LA. Epidemiologic features of asymptomatic cerebral infarction in patients with non-

valvular atrial fibrillation. *Arch Intern Med* 1990;150: 2340–2344.

12. Petersen P, Madsen EB, Brun B, Pedersen F, Glydensted C, Boysen G. Silent cerebral infarction in chronic atrial fibrillation. *Stroke* 1989;18:1098–1100.

13. Petersen P, Pedersen F, Johnsen A, et al. Cerebral computed tomography in paroxysmal atrial fibrillation. *Acta Neurol Scand* 1989;79:482–486.

14. Sasaki W, Yanagisawa S, Maki K, Onodera A, Awagi T, Kanazawa T. High incidence of silent small cerebral infarction in patients with atrial fibrillation. *Circulation* 1987;76:104.

15. Chodosh EH, Foulkes MA, Kase CS, et al. Silent stroke in the NINCDS Stroke Data Bank. *Neurology* 1988;38:1674–1679.

16. Kase CS, Wolf PA, Chodosh EH, et al. Prevalence of silent stroke in patients presenting with initial stroke: the Framingham Study. *Stroke* 1989;20:850–852.

17. Virchow R. *Gesammelte Abhandlungen zur Wissenschaftlichen Medicine.* Frankfurt: Meidinger, 1856;219–732.

18. Johnson RC, Crissman RS, Didio LJA. Endocardial alterations in myocardial infarction. *Lab Invest* 1979;40: 183–193.

19. Hochman JS, Platia EB, Bulkley BH. Endocardial abnormalities in left ventricular aneurysms: a clinicopathologic study. *Ann Intern Med* 1984;100:29–35.

20. Roberts WC, Siegel RJ, McManus BM. Idiopathic dilated cardiomyopathy: analysis of 152 necropsy patients. *Am J Cardiol* 1987;60:1340–1355.

21. Mikell FL, Asinger RW, Elsperger KJ, Anderson WR, Hodges M. Regional stasis of blood in the dysfunctional left ventricle: echocardiographic detection and differentiation from early thrombosis. *Circulation* 1982;66:755–763.

22. Asinger RW, Mikell FL, Elsperger J, Hodges M. Incidence of left ventricular thrombosis after acute transmural myocardial infarction: serial evaluation by two-dimensional echocardiography. *N Engl J Med* 1981; 305:297–302.

23. Weinrich DJ, Burke JF, Pauletto FJ. Left ventricular mural thrombi complicating acute myocardial infarction: long term follow-up with serial echocardiography. *Ann Intern Med* 1984;100:789–794.

24. Shresta NK, Moreno FL, Narciso FV, Torres L, Calleja HB. Two-dimensional echocardiographic diagnosis of left atrial thrombus in rheumatic heart disease: a clinicopathologic study. *Circulation* 1983;67:341–347.

25. Fulton RM, Duckett K. Plasma-fibrinogen and thromboemboli after myocardial infarction. *Lancet* 1976;2: 1161–1164.

26. Gustafsson C, Blomback M, Britton M, Hamsten A, Svensson J. Coagulation factors and the increased risk of stroke in nonvalvular atrial fibrillation. *Stroke* 1990; 21:47–51.

27. Cabin HS, Roberts WC. Left ventricular aneurysm, intra-aneurysmal thrombus and systemic embolus in coronary heart disease. *Chest* 1980;77:586–590.

28. Fuster V, Halperin JL. Left ventricular thrombi and cerebral embolism: an emerging approach [Editorial]. *N Engl J Med* 1989;320:392–394.

29. Stein B, Fuster V, Halperin JL, Chesebro JH. Antithrombotic therapy in cardiac disease: an emerging approach based on pathogenesis and risk. *Circulation* 1989;80:1501–1513.

30. Tegeler CH. Stroke Prevention in Atrial Fibrillation Study Carotid Stenosis Study Group: carotid stenosis in atrial fibrillation. *Neurology* 1989;39(suppl):159.

31. Weinberger J, Rothlauf EB, Materese E, Halperin JL. Noninvasive evaluation of the extracranial carotid arteries in patients with cerebrovascular events and atrial fibrillation. *Arch Intern Med* 1988;148:1785–1788.

32. D'Olhaberriague L, Hernandez-Vidal A, Molina L, et al. A prospective study of atrial fibrillation and stroke. *Stroke* 1989;20:1648–1652.

33. Bogousslavsky J, vanMelle G, Regli F, Kappenberger L. Pathogenesis of anterior circulation stroke in patients with nonvalvular atrial fibrillation: the Lausanne Stroke Registry. *Neurology* 1990;40:1046–1050.

34. Hagen PT, Scholz DG, Edwards WD. Incidence and size of patent foramen ovale during the first 10 decades of life: an autopsy study of 965 normal hearts. *Mayo Clin Proc* 1984;59:17–20.

35. Lechat P, Mas JL, Lascault G, et al. Prevalence of patent foramen ovale as a risk factor for stroke. *N Engl J Med* 1988;318:1148–1152.

36. Cabanes L, Mas JL, Cohen A, et al. Atrial septal aneurysm and patent foramen ovale as risk factors for cryptogenic stroke in patients less than 55 years of age: a study using transesophageal echocardiography. *Stroke* 1993;24:1865–1873.

37. Wolf PA, Dawber TR, Thomas HE, Kannel WB. Epidemiologic assessment of chronic atrial fibrillation and risk of stroke: the Framingham Study. *Neurology* 1978;28:973–977.

38. Levine HJ, Pauker SG, Eckman MH. Antithrombotic therapy in valvular heart disease. *Chest* 1995;108 (suppl):360S–370S.

39. Sherman DG, Dyken ML, Gent, M, Harrison MJG, Hart RG, Mohr JP. Antithrombotic therapy for cerebrovascular disorders: an update. *Chest* 1995;108 (suppl):444S–456S.

40. Hurley DM, Hunter AN, Hewett MJ, et al. Atrial fibrillation and arterial embolism in hyperthyroidism. *Aust NZ J Med* 1981;11:391.

41. Yuen RWM, Gutteridge DH, Thompson PL, et al. Embolism in thyrotoxic atrial fibrillation. *Med J Aust* 1979;1:630.

42. Staffurth JS, Gibberd MC, Tang Fui SN. Arterial embolism in thyrotoxicosis with atrial fibrillation. *Br Med J* 1977;2:688.

43. Bar-Sela S, Ehrenfeld M, Eliakim M. Arterial embolism in thyrotoxicosis with atrial fibrillation. *Arch Intern Med* 1981;141:1191.

44. Petersen P, Hansen JM. Stroke in thyrotoxicosis with atrial fibrillation. *Stroke* 1988;19:15.

45. Petersen P. Thromboembolic complications in atrial fibrillation. *Stroke* 1990;21:4–13.

46. Brand FN, Abbott RD, Kannel WB, et al. Characteristics and prognosis of lone atrial fibrillation: 30-year follow-up in the Framingham Study. *JAMA* 1985;254: 3449.

47. Kopecky SL, Gersh BJ, McGoon MD, et al. The natural history of lone atrial fibrillation: a population-based study over three decades. *N Engl J Med* 1987;317:669.

48. Chesebro JH, Fuster V, Halperin JL. Atrial fibrillation—Risk marker for stroke. *N Engl J Med* 1990;323: 1556–1558.

49. Hart RG, Halperin JL. Atrial fibrillation and stroke: revisiting the dilemmas. *Stroke* 1994;25:1337–1344.

50. Atrial Fibrillation Investigators. Risk factors for stroke and efficacy of antithrombotic therapy in atrial fibrillation: analysis of pooled data from five randomized controlled trials. *Arch Intern Med* 1994;154: 1449–1457.

51. Stroke Prevention in Atrial Fibrillation Investigators: predictors of thromboembolism in atrial fibrillation: I. Clinical features of patients at risk. *Ann Intern Med* 1992;116:1–5.

52. Stroke Prevention in Atrial Fibrillation Investigators: predictors of thromboembolism in atrial fibrillation: II. Echocardiographic features of patients at risk. *Ann Intern Med* 1992;116:6–12.

53. Moulton AW, Singer DE, Haas JS. Risk factors for stroke in patients with nonrheumatic atrial fibrillation: a case-control study. *Am J Med* 1991;91:156–161.

54. Cabin HS, Clubb KS, Hall C, Perlmutter RA, Feinstein AR. Risk for systemic embolization of atrial fibrillation without mitral stenosis. *Am J Cardiol* 1990;65: 1112–1116.

55. Flegel KM, Hanley J. Risk factors for stroke and other embolic events in patients with nonrheumatic atrial fibrillation. *Stroke* 1989;20:1000–1004.

56. Wiener I. Clinical and echocardiographic correlates of systemic embolization in nonrheumatic atrial fibrillation. *Am J Cardiol* 1987;59:177.

57. Aronow WS, Gutstein H, Hsieh FY. Risk factors for thromboembolic stroke in elderly patients with chronic atrial fibrillation. *Am J Cardiol* 1989;63:366–367.

58. Petersen P, Kastrup J, Helweg-Larsen S, Boysen G, Godtfredsen J. Risk factors for thromboembolic complications in chronic atrial fibrillation. *Arch Intern Med* 1990;150:819–821.

59. Blackshear JL, Pearce LA, Asinger RW, et al. Mitral regurgitation protects against thromboembolic events in patients with atrial fibrillation. *Am J Cardiol* 1993;72:840–843.

60. Wiener I, Hafner R, Nicolai M, et al. Clinical and echocardiographic correlates of systemic embolism in nonrheumatic atrial fibrillation. *Am J Cardiol* 1987; 59:177.

61. Caplan LR, D'Cruz I, Hier DB, et al. Atrial size, atrial fibrillation and stroke. *Ann Neurol* 1986;19:158.

62. Tegeler CH, Hart RG. Atrial size, atrial fibrillation, and stroke. *Ann Neurol* 1987;21:315–316.

63. Rosenthal MS, Halperin JL. Thromboembolism in nonvalvular atrial fibrillation: the answer may be in the ventricle. *Int J Cardiol* 1992;37:277–282.

64. Presti CF, Asinger RW, Goldman ME. Comparative measurements of the left atrium in patients with constant vs. intermittent nonvalvulopathic atrial fibrillation. *Circulation* 1988;78:600.

65. Ruocco NA, Most AS. Clinical and echocardiographic risk factors for systemic embolization in patients with atrial fibrillation in the absence of mitral stenosis. *J Am Coll Cardiol* 1986;7:165A.

66. Benjamin EJ, Levy D, Plehn JF, Belanger AJ, D'Agostino RB, Wolf PA. Left atrial size: an independent risk factor for stroke. The Framingham Study. *Circulation* 1989;80:615.

67. Petersen P, Kasrtrup J, Brinch K, Boysen G, Godtfredsen J. Relation between left atrial dimension and duration of atrial fibrillation. *Am J Cardiol* 1987;60: 382–384.

68. The Boston Area Anticoagulation Trial for Atrial Fib-

rillation Investigators: the effect of low-dose warfarin on the risk of stroke in patients with nonrheumatic atrial fibrillation. *N Engl J Med* 1990;323:1505–1511.

69. Daniel WG, Angermann C, Engberding, et al. Transesophageal echocardiography in patients with cerebral ischemic events and arterial embolism: the European multicenter study. *Circulation* 1989;80(suppl 4):II-473.

70. Stroke Prevention in Atrial Fibrillation Investigators Committee on Echocardiography: transesophageal echocardiography in atrial fibrillation: standards for acquisition and interpretation and assessment of interobserver variability. *J Am Soc Echocardiogr* 1996;9: 556–566.

71. Stroke Prevention in Atrial Fibrillation Investigators Committee on Echocardiography. Transesophageal echocardiographic correlates of thromboembolism in high-risk patients with atrial fibrillation. In press.

72. Coulshed N, Epstein EJ, McKenrick CS, Galloway RW, Walker E. Systemic embolism in mitral valve disease. *Br Heart J* 1970;32:26.

73. Sage JI, Van Uitert RL. Risk of recurrent stroke in patients with atrial fibrillation and nonvalvular heart disease. *Stroke* 1983;14:537.

74. Hart RG, Coull BM, Hart PD. Early recurrent embolism associated with nonvalvular atrial fibrillation. *Stroke* 1983;14:688–693.

75. Stroke Prevention in Atrial Fibrillation Study Investigators. Stroke Prevention in Atrial Fibrillation Study: final results. *Circulation* 1991;84:527–539.

76. Connolly SJ, Laupacis A, Gent M, Roberts RS, Cairns JA, Joyner C. Canadian atrial fibrillation anticoagulation (CAFA) study. *J Am Coll Cardiol* 1991; 18:349–355.

77. Ezekowitz MD, Bridgers SL, James KE, et al. Warfarin in the prevention of stroke associated with atrial fibrillation. *N Engl J Med* 1992;327:1406–1412.

78. Petersen P, Boysen G, Godtfredsen J, Anderson ED, Andersen B. Placebo-controlled, randomized trial of warfarin and aspirin prevention of thromboembolic complications in chronic atrial fibrillation. *Lancet* 1989;1:175–179.

79. Stroke Prevention in Atrial Fibrillation Investigators. A comparison of warfarin with aspirin for prevention of arterial thromboembolism in atrial fibrillation: results of the stroke prevention in atrial fibrillation II study. *Lancet* 1994;343:687–691.

80. Petersen P, Boysen G. Prevention of stroke in atrial fibrillation. *N Engl J Med* 1990;323:482.

81. EAFT Study Group. European atrial fibrillation trial: secondary prevention of vascular events in patients with nonrheumatic atrial fibrillation and a recent transient ischemic attack or minor ischemic stroke. *Lancet* 1993;324:1255–1261.

82. Koefoed BG, Gullov AL, Petersen P. The Copenhagen Atrial Fibrillation, Aspirin and Anticoagulant Therapy study (AFASAK 2): methods and design. *J Thrombos Thrombolys* 1995;2:125–130.

83a. Primary preventive effects of anticoagulants and acetylsalicylic acid on arterial thromboembolism in patients with non-valvular atrial fibrillation in general practice (PATAF). *Stroke* 1993;10:1619.

83b. Morocutti C, Amabile G, Fattaposta F, et al. Indobufen versus warfarin in the secondary prevention of major vascular events in nonrheumatic atrial fibrillation. *Stroke* 1997;28:1015–1021.

84. Pengo V, Barbero F, Zasso A, Biasiolo A, Nante G, Dalla Volta S. A trial of fixed minidose warfarin in non-rheumatic atrial fibrillation: MIWAF. In: *Proceedings of the IVth International Symposium on Heart–Brain Interactions*. Bologna, Italy 1996:116.

85. Petersen P, Godtfredsen J. Embolic complications in paroxysmal atrial fibrillation. *Stroke* 1986;17:622.

86. Stein B, Halperin JL, Fuster V. Should patients with atrial fibrillation be anticoagulated prior to and chronically following cardioversion? In: Cheitlin MD (ed). *Dilemmas in clinical cardiology*. Philadelphia: FA Davis, 1990;231–247.

87. Bjerkelund CJ, Orning OM. An evaluation of DC shock treatment of atrial arrhythmias: immediate results and complications in 437 patients, with long term results in the first 290 of these. *Acta Med Scand* 1968; 184:481.

88. Bjerkelund CJ, Orning OM. The efficacy of anticoagulant therapy in preventing embolism related to DC electrical conversion of atrial fibrillation. *Am J Cardiol* 1969;23:208.

89. Weinberg DM, Mancini GBJ. Anticoagulation for cardioversion of atrial fibrillation. *Am J Cardiol* 1989; 63:745–746.

90. Arnold AZ, Mick MJ, Mazurek RP, Loop FD, Trohman RG. Rose of prophylactic anticoagulation for direct current cardioversion in patients with atrial fibrillation or atrial flutter. *J Am Coll Cardiol* 1992;19:851–855.

91. Collins LJ, Silverman DI, Douglas PS, Manning WJ. Cardioversion of nonrheumatic atrial fibrillation: reduced thromboembolic complications with 4 weeks of precardioversion anticoagulation are related to atrial thrombus resolution. *Circulation* 1995;92:156–159.

92. Fatkin D, Kuchar DL, Thorburn CW, Fenely MP. Transesophageal echocardiography before and during direct current cardioversion of atrial fibrillation: evidence for "atrial stunning" as a mechanism of thromboembolic complications. *J Am Coll Cardiol* 1994; 23:307–316.

93. Asinger RW, Mikell FL, Elsperger J, Hodges M. Incidence of left ventricular thrombosis after acute transmural myocardial infarction: serial evaluation by two-dimensional echocardiography. *N Engl J Med* 1981; 305:297–302.

94. Weinrich DJ, Burke JF, Pauletto FJ. Left ventricular mural thrombi complicating acute myocardial infarction: long term follow-up with serial echocardiography. *Ann Intern Med* 1984;100:789–794.

95. Funke Kupper AJ, Verheugt FWA, Peels CH. Left ventricular thrombus incidence and behavior studied by serial two-dimensional echocardiography in acute anterior myocardial infarction: left ventricular wall motion, systemic embolism and oral anticoagulation. *J Am Coll Cardiol* 1989;13:1514–1520.

96. Halperin JL, Fuster V. Left ventricular thrombus and stroke after myocardial infarction toward prevention on perplexity? *J Am Coll Cardiol* 1989;14:912–914.

97. Veterans Administration Cooperative Study Investigators: anticoagulants in acute myocardial infarction: results of a cooperative clinical trial. *JAMA* 1973;225: 724–729.

98. Hilden T, Iversen K, Raaschou F, et al. Anticoagulants in acute myocardial infarction. *Lancet* 1961;2: 327–331.

99. Johnson RC, Crissman RS, Didio LJA. Endocardial alterations in myocardial infarction. *Lab Invest* 1979;40: 183–193.

100. Jugdutt BI, Sivaram CA, Wortman C, Trudell C, Penner P. Prospective two-dimensional echocardiographic evaluation of left ventricular thrombus and embolism after acute myocardial infarction. *J Am Coll Cardiol* 1989;13:554–64.

101. Visser CA, Kan G, Meltzer RS, Lie KI, Durer D. Long-term follow-up of left ventricular thrombus after acute myocardial infarction: a two-dimensional echocardiographic study in 96 patients. *Chest* 1984;86: 532–536.

102. Spirito P, Bellotti P, Chiarella F, Domenicucci S, Sementa A, Vecchio C. Prognostic significance and natural history of left ventricular thrombi in patients with acute anterior myocardial infarction: a two-dimensional echocardiographic study. *Circulation* 1985;72: 774–780.

103. Haugland JM, Asinger RW, Mikell FL, Elsperger J, Hodges M. Embolic potential of left ventricular thrombus detected by two-dimensional echocardiography. *Circulation* 1984;70:588–598.

104. Nihoyannopoulos P, Smith GC, Maseri A, Foale RA. The natural history of left ventricular thrombus in myocardial infarction: a rationale in support of masterly inactivity. *J Am Coll Cardiol* 1989;14:903–911.

105. Lapeyre AC, Steele PP, Kazmier FJ, Chesebro JH, Vliestra RE, Fuster V. Systemic embolism in chronic left ventricular aneurysm: incidence and the role of chronic anticoagulation. *J Am Coll Cardiol* 1985;6: 534–538.

106. Fuster V, Gersh BJ, Giuliani ER, Tajik AJ, Brandenburg RO, Frye RL. The natural history of idiopathic dilated cardiomyopathy. *Am J Cardiol* 1981;47:525–531.

107. Visser CA, Kan G, Meltzer RS, et al. Embolic potential of left ventricular thrombus after myocardial infarction: a two-dimensional echocardiographic study of 119 patients. *J Am Coll Cardiol* 1985;5:1276–1280.

108. Meltzer RS, Visser CA, Fuster V. Intracardiac thrombi and systemic embolization. *Ann Intern Med* 1986;104:689–98.

109. Johannessen KA, Nordrehaug JE, von der Lippe G, Vollset SE. Risk factors for embolisation in patients with left ventricular thrombi and acute myocardial infarction. *Br Heart J* 1988;60:104–10.

110. Maze SS, Kotler MN. Parry WR. Flow characteristics in the dilated left ventricle with thrombus: qualitative and quantitative Doppler analysis. *J Am Coll Cardiol* 1989;13:873–881.

111. Delemarre BJ, Visser CA, Bot H, Dunning AJ. Prediction of apical thrombus formation in acute myocardial infarction based on left ventricular spatial flow pattern. *J Am Coll Cardiol* 1990;15:355–360.

112. DeMaria AN, Bommer W, Neumann A, et al. Left ventricular thrombi identified by cross-sectional echocardiography. *Ann Intern Med* 1979;90:14.

113. Visser CA, Kan G, David GK, Lie KI, Kurrer D. Two-dimensional echocardiography in the diagnosis of left ventricular thrombus: a prospective study of 67 patients with anatomic validation. *Chest* 1983;83: 228–232.

114. Stratton JR, Lighty GW, Pearlman AS, Ritchie JL. Detection of left ventricular thrombus by two-dimensional echocardiography: sensitivity, specificity, and causes of uncertainty. *Circulation* 1982;66:156–166.

115. Visser C, Roelandt J. Left ventricular thrombus. *Echocardiography* 1985;2:245–255.
116. Asinger RW, Mikell FL, Sharma B, Hodges M. Observations on detecting left ventricular thrombus with two-dimensional echocardiography: emphasis on avoidance of false positives. *Am J Cardiol* 1981;47:145–156.
117. Vecchio C, Chiarella F, Lupi G, Bellotti P, Domenicucci S. Left ventricular thrombus in acute myocardial infarction after thrombolysis: a GISSI-2 connected study. *Circulation* 1991;84:512–19.
118. Domenicucci S, Bellotti P, Chiarella F, Lupi G, Vecchio C. Spontaneous morphologic changes in left ventricular thrombi: a prospective two-dimensional echocardiographic study. *Circulation* 1987;75:737–743.
119. Fuster V, Halperin JL. Left ventricular thrombi and cerebral embolism. *N Engl J Med* 1989;320:392–394.
120. Stratton JR, Resnick AD. Increased embolic risk in patients with left ventricular thrombi. *Circulation* 1987;75:1004–1011.
121. Stratton JR, Nemanich JW, Johannessen KA, Resnick AD. Fate of left ventricular thrombi in patients with remote myocardial infarction or idiopathic cardiomyopathy. *Circulation* 1988;78:1388–1393.
122. Tramarin R, Pozzoli M, Febo O, et al. Two-dimensional echocardiographic assessment of anticoagulant therapy in left ventricular thrombosis early after acute myocardial infarction. *Eur Heart J* 1986;7:482–492.
123. Kouvaris G, Chronopoulos G, Soufras G, et al. The effects of long-term antithrombotic treatment on left ventricular thrombi in patients after acute myocardial infarction. *Am Heart J* 1990;119:73–78.
124. Keating EC, Gross SA, Schlamowitz RA, et al. Mural thrombi in myocardial infarction: prospective evaluation by two-dimensional echocardiography. *Am J Med* 1983;74:989–995.
125. Mahoney C, Evans JM, Spain C. Spontaneous contrast and circulating platelet aggregates. *Circulation* 1989;80:1.
126. deBelder MA, Tourikis L, Leech G, Camm AJ. Spontaneous contrast echos are markers of thromboembolic risk in patients with atrial fibrillation. *Circulation* 1989;80:1.
127. Ezekowitz MD, Wilson DA, Smith EO, et al. Comparison of indium-111 platelet scintigraphy and two-dimensional echocardiography in the diagnosis of left ventricular thrombi. *N Engl J Med* 1982;306:1509–1513.
128. Penny WJ, Chesebro JH, Heras M, Fuster V. Antithrombotic therapy for patients with cardiac disease. *Curr Probl Cardiol* 1988;13:464–469.
129. Sechtem U, Theissen P, Heindel W, et al. Diagnosis of left ventricular thrombi by magnetic resonance imaging and comparison with angiocardiography, computerized tomography and echocardiography. *Am J Cardiol* 1989;64:1195–1199.
130. Veterans Administration Cooperative Study Investigators: anticoagulants in acute myocardial infarction: results of a cooperative clinical trial. *JAMA* 1973;225:724–729.
131. Working Party on Anticoagulant Therapy in Coronary Thrombosis: assessment of short term anticoagulant administration after cardiac infarction: report of the Working Party on Anticoagulant Therapy in Coronary Thrombosis to the Medical Research Council. *Br Med J* 1969;1:335–342.
132. Drapkin A, Merskey C. Anticoagulant therapy after acute myocardial infarction: relation of therapeutic benefit to patient's age, sex and severity of infarction. *JAMA* 1972;222:541.
133. Nordrehaug JE, Johennessen K-A, von der Lippe G. Usefulness of high-dose anticoagulants in preventing left ventricular thrombus in acute myocardial infarction. *Am J Cardiol* 1985;55:1491–1493.
134. Davis MJE, Ireland MA. Effect of early anticoagulation on the frequency of left ventricular thrombi after anterior wall acute myocardial infarction. *Am J Cardiol* 1986;57:1244–1247.
135. Gueret P, Dubourg O, Ferrier E, Farcot JC, Rigaud M, Bourdarias JP. Effects of full-dose heparin anticoagulation on the development of left ventricular thrombosis in acute transmural myocardial infarction. *J Am Coll Cardiol* 1986;8:419–426.
136. Arvan S, Boscha K. Prophylactic anticoagulation for left ventricular thrombi after acute myocardial infarction: a prospective randomized trial. *Am Heart J* 1987;113:688–693.
137. Turpie AGG, Robinson JG, Doyle DJ, et al. Comparison of high-dose with low-dose subcutaneous heparin to prevent left ventricular mural thrombosis in patients with acute transmural anterior myocardial infarction. *N Engl J Med* 1989;320:352–57.
138. The SCATI (Studio sulla Calciparin nell'Angina e nella Thrombosi Ventriculare nell'Infarto) group. Randomised controlled trial of subcutaneous calcium-heparin in acute myocardial infarction. *Lancet* 1989;2:182–86.
139. Cairns JA, Lewis HD, Meade TM, Sutton GC, Theroux P. Antithrombotic agents in coronary artery disease. *Chest* 1995;108 (suppl):380S–400S.
140. Dunkman WB, Johnson GR, Carson PE, Bhat G, Farrell L, Cohn J. Incidence of thromboembolic events in congestive heart failure. *Circulation* 1993;87(suppl VI):94–101.
141. Johanessen KA, Stratton JR, Taulow E, Osterud B, von der Lippe G. Usefulness of aspirin plus dipyridamole in reducing left ventricular thrombus formation in anterior wall acute myocardial infarction. *Am J Cardiol* 1989;63:101–102.
142. Funke Kupper AJ, Verheugt FWA, Peels CH, Gelma TW, den Hollander W, Roos JP. Effect of low dose acetylsalicylic acid on the frequency and hematologic activity of left ventricular thrombus in anterior wall acute myocardial infarction. *Am J Cardiol* 1989;63:917–20.
143. American College of Cardiology/American Heart Association guidelines for the early management of patients with acute myocardial infarction. *Circulation* 1990;82:664–707.
144. Held AC, Gore JM, Paraskos J, et al. Impact of thrombolytic therapy on left ventricular mural thrombi in acute myocardial infarction. *Am J Cardiol* 1988;62:310–311.
145. Eigler N, Maurer G, Shah PK. Effect of early systemic thrombolytic therapy on left ventricular mural thrombus formation in acute anterior myocardial infarction. *Am J Cardiol* 1984;54:261–263.
146. Smith P, Arnesen H, Holme I. The effect of warfarin on mortality and reinfarction after myocardial infarction. *N Engl J Med* 1990;323:147–152.
147. ASPECT Research Group. Effect of long-term oral an-

ticoagulant treatment on mortality and cardiovascular morbidity after myocardial infarction. *Lancet* 1994; 343:499–503.

148. The CARS Investigators. Randomized double-blind study of fixed low-dose warfarin plus aspirin in post-myocardial infarction patients: the Coumadin Aspirin Reinfarction Study (CARS). *Lancet* 1997;350: 389–396.

149. Stroke Prevention in Atrial Fibrillation Investigators: a differential effect of aspirin in the Stroke Prevention in Atrial Fibrillation Study. *J Stroke Cerebrovasc Dis* 1993;3:181–188.

150. Hylek EM, Singer DE. An analysis of the lowest effective intensity of prophylactic anticoagulation for patients with nonrheumatic atrial fibrillation. *N Engl J Med* 1996;335:540–546.

151. Laupacis A, Albers G, Dalen J, Dunn M, Feinberg W, Jacobson A. Antithrombotic therapy in atrial fibrillation. *Chest* 1995;108:352S–359S.

152. Friedman MJ, Carlson K, Marcus FI, Woolfenden JM. Clinical correlations in patients with acute myocardial infarction and left ventricular thrombus detected by two-dimensional echocardiography. *Am J Med* 1982; 72:894–898.

153. Visser CA, Kan G, Meltzer RS, Lie KI, Durrer D. Long-term follow-up of left ventricular thrombus after acute myocardial infarction: a two-dimensional echocardiographic study in 96 patients. *Chest* 1984; 86:532–536.

154. Johannessen KA, Nordehaug JE, von der Lippe G. Left ventricular thrombosis and cerebrovascular accident in acute myocardial infarction. *Br Heart J* 1984; 51:553–556.

155. Gueret P, Dubourg O, Ferrier A, Farcot JC, Rigaud M, Bourdarias JP. Effects of full-dose heparin anticoagulation on the development of left ventricular thrombosis in acute transmural myocardial infarction. *J Am Coll Cardiol* 1986;8:419–426.

156. Keren A, Goldberg S, Gottlieg S, et al. Natural history of left ventricular thrombi: their appearance and resolution in the posthospitalization period of acute myocardial infarction. *J Am Coll Cardiol* 1990;15:790–800.

Cardiovascular Thrombosis: Thrombocardiology and Thromboneurology, Second Edition,
edited by M. Verstraete, V. Fuster, and E. J. Topol,
Lippincott–Raven Publishers, Philadelphia © 1998.

24

Unstable Angina

David J. Moliterno and *Marc Cohen

*Department of Cardiology, The Cleveland Clinic Foundation, Cleveland, Ohio 44195; and
*Department of Medicine (Cardiology), Allegheny University of the Health Sciences,
Philadelphia, Pennsylvania 19102*

Unstable angina is part of the acute coronary syndromes and is adjacent to non-Q-wave myocardial infarction and slightly more distantly related to Q-wave myocardial infarction. At the interface between unstable angina and myocardial infarction, these two entities become nearly indistinct as most features related to diagnosis, pathophysiology, and treatment are shared. Indeed, the phrase "unstable angina," first used decades ago (1,2), describes a symptom complex intermediate between stable angina and myocardial infarction. Other terms used to describe unstable angina also exemplify its unpredictability and its close apposition to myocardial infarction: intermediate coronary syndrome and preinfarction angina (2–5). The importance of recognizing unstable angina as an acute coronary syndrome is important because it can have a relatively high morbidity and mortality, similar to that of acute myocardial infarction. This chapter will review unstable angina, its variable presentation and outcome, and contemporary strategies for prevention and treatment of this often atherothrombotic disorder.

Clinically, the acute coronary syndromes are the leading causes of hospitalizations for adults in the United States. The incidence of unstable angina is increasing, and reportedly nearly a million hospitalizations each year in the United States are with a primary diagnosis of unstable angina. A similar number of unstable angina episodes likely occur outside the hospital setting and are unrecognized or managed in the outpatient setting. With heightened public awareness, improved survival following myocardial infarction, and an increasing proportion of the population being of advanced age, this number should continue to rise despite primary and secondary prevention measures. Several studies have suggested that the incidence of unstable angina has steadily increased to exceed that of acute myocardial infarction (Fig. 24-1) (6).

The diversity of conditions leading to unstable angina as well as the varying symptoms upon presentation have made the definition and classification of unstable angina difficult (7). Braunwald (8) suggested a classification scheme based on angina severity, clinical eti-

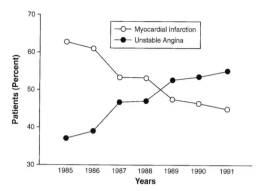

FIG. 24-1. The relative proportion of patients (%) admitted to the coronary care unit of the Montreal Heart Institute from 1985 through 1991 with a diagnosis of unstable angina and myocardial infarction. As can be seen, the proportion of patients with unstable angina steadily increased over this interval to slightly exceed that of myocardial infarction. In the United States currently, the incidence of myocardial infarction and unstable angina is believed similar, though patients with infarction are more frequently hospitalized. (From Théroux and Liddon, ref. 6, with permission.)

ology, intensity of antianginal therapy, and presence of electrocardiographic changes (Table 24-1). Patients in class I have new or accelerated exertional angina, whereas those in class II have subacute (> 48 hours since last pain) or class III acute ≤ 48 hours since last pain) rest angina. Among 3,000 consecutive 1996 hospital admissions for unstable angina in the United States, the Global Unstable Angina Registry and Treatment Evaluation (GUARANTEE) study reported that one third of patients had new or accelerated symptoms associated with exertion, whereas two thirds had rest angina (9). This distinction is impor-

tant because patients with exertional angina may have a gradual worsening of an underlying atherosclerotic coronary arterial narrowing as opposed to those with rest angina who have an abrupt reduction in myocardial perfusion due to a ruptured plaque. The precipitant or clinical circumstances associated with unstable angina are also used to classify patients and are categorized as type A, secondary (e.g., anemia, fever, hypoxia); B, primary; or C, postinfarction (<2 weeks after infarction). Intensity of antianginal therapy is subclassified as 1, no treatment; 2, usual oral therapy; and 3, intense therapy, such as intravenous nitroglycerin. A patient with atherosclerotic heart disease and acute chest pain during minimal activity or at rest while taking usual medical therapy would be categorized as class $IIIB_2$. This is by far the most common presentation, representing roughly half of all unstable angina hospitalizations (9).

PATHOPHYSIOLOGY

Supply Demand Mismatch

To better understand the prevention and treatment of unstable angina, the underlying pathophysiology must first be considered. The myocardial ischemia of unstable angina, like all causes of tissue ischemia, results from excessive demand or inadequate supply of nutrients, primarily oxygen. Excess demand from increased myocardial workload (heart rate × systolic pressure product) or wall stress is responsible for nearly all cases of stable angina and perhaps one third of unstable angina episodes. For example, in Braunwald

TABLE 24-1. *Braunwald classification of unstable angina*

Severity	①	I	Symptoms with exertion
		II	Symptoms at rest: subacute (between 2 and 30 days prior)
		III	Symptoms at rest: acute (within prior 48 hours)
Precipitant	②	A	Secondary
		B	Primary
		C	Postinfarction
Therapy present during symptoms	③	1	No treatment
		2	Usual angina therapy
		3	Maximal therapy

class I unstable angina, stable symptoms accelerate and become more intense, frequent, or easily provoked, and this is from heightened demands outstripping myocardial blood supply. Conversely, inadequate supply alone is responsible for few cases of stable angina and roughly two thirds of unstable angina episodes. The etiology of the supply–demand mismatch can be classified as primary or secondary. Primary causes of ischemia are from obstructive coronary lesions. Secondary causes are varied, extrinsic to the coronary arterial bed, and are responsible for <10% of unstable angina episodes. These precipitants of myocardial ischemia usually increase myocardial demands in the presence of otherwise noncritical coronary artery stenoses. Listed in Table 24-2 are examples of secondary disorders that increase myocardial oxygen demand (e.g., fever, thyrotoxicosis, cocaine) or decrease oxygen supply (e.g., hypoxemia, anemia) and potentially cause unstable angina.

Plaque Disruption

Braunwald class II and III unstable angina are usually the result of reduction in coronary arterial perfusion associated with atherosclerotic plaque disruption and thrombosis. The fatty streak is the earliest lesion of athero-

TABLE 24-2. *Secondary causes of myocardial ischemia*

Increased myocardial oxygen demand
  Fever
  Tachyarrhythmias
  Malignant hypertension
  Thyrotoxicosis
  Pheochromocytoma
  Cocaine
  Amphetamines
  Aortic stenosis
  Supravalvular aortic stenosis
  Obstructive cardiomyopathy
  Aortovenous shunts
  High-output states
  Congestive failure
Decreased oxygen supply
  Anemia
  Hypoxemia
  Polycythemia

Adapted from Théroux and Liddon, ref. 6.

sclerosis and is the result of intimal accumulation of foam cells, which are lipid-laden macrophages, and smooth muscle cells. The oxidized low-density lipoprotein cholesterol (LDL-C) within foam cells is cytotoxic, procoagulant, and chemotactic. Through platelet adhesion and monocyte and smooth muscle cell recruitment, growth factors are secreted and collagen, elastin, and glycoproteins are produced. These structural proteins surround the accumulating and decaying foam cells and form the fibromuscular cap covering the plaque's lipid core. As the atherosclerotic plaque grows, production of macrophage proteases (10) and neutrophil elastases (11) within the plaque can cause thinning of the fibromuscular cap. This, in combination with heightened circumferential wall stress and blood flow shear stress, can lead to plaque fissuring or rupture, especially at the junction of the cap and the vessel wall (Fig. 24-2).

The degree or extent of plaque disruption occurs over a spectrum, with the most minor fissuring being occult and moderate to large disruptions leading to severe unstable angina or acute infarction. In minor fissures, the area of damage is limited, coronary flow remains brisk, accumulation of thrombus does not occur, and the lesion heals uneventfully. Falk and others (12,13) have histologically and angiographically demonstrated that coronary stenoses of unstable angina are the result of repeated episodes of plaque ulceration and healing with a resultant gradual increase in plaque volume. During vessel wall repair, the lesion may increase its fibrous content (organization of thrombus) thereby limiting future disruptions. Whether or not vessel occlusion occurs depends on many factors, including the extent of vessel disruption, rheology of blood, platelet aggregability, and the balance of endogenous hemostatic and thrombolytic factors.

Thrombosis

The thrombotic process following plaque rupture (detailed in Chapter 2) is multistaged and begins with the exposure of subendothelial constituents. These components (e.g., col-

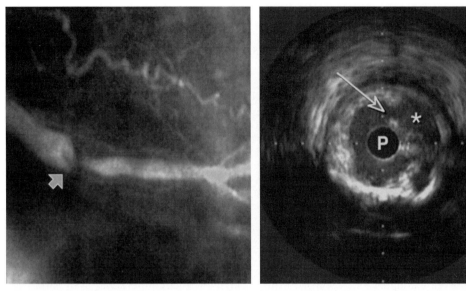

A   B

FIG. 24-2. A: Angiography of the right coronary artery in a patient with unstable angina reveals a focal stenosis with an adjacent area of haziness *(wide arrow).* **B:** By intravascular ultrasound a ruptured atherosclerotic plaque can be seen. The ultrasound probe (P) is against the fibromuscular cap which was overlying the atherosclerotic plaque (*). The site of rupture *(thin arrow)* can be identified at the shoulder of the cap as it joins the vessel wall.

lagen, von Willebrand factor, and fibronectin) are recognized by platelet surface receptors (primarily glycoprotein Ib) and platelet adhesion and activation occurs. As platelets adhere to the vessel wall, they become activated. During activation platelets secrete a host of substances from their α granules that lead to vasoconstriction, chemotaxis, mitogenesis, and activation of neighboring platelets (14) (Fig. 24- 3). These are the processes that must be addressed in the treatment of unstable angina. The released platelet substances include thromboxane A_2, serotonin, fibrinogen, plasminogen activator inhibitor–1 (PAI-1), and growth factors. Platelet activation leads to the recruitment and "functionalization" of glycoprotein IIb/IIIa integrins or specialized surface receptors that mediate aggregation (platelet–platelet binding). Aggregated platelets accelerate the production of thrombin by providing the surface for the binding of cofactors required for the conversion of prothrombin to thrombin. In a reciprocating fashion, thrombin is a potent agonist for further platelet activation, and it stabilizes the throm-

bus by converting fibrinogen to fibrin. Sherman et al. (15) performed angioscopy in 10 patients with unstable angina. Distinctive intimal abnormalities were observed in all patients, 4 of whom had complex plaque morphology and 7 (70%) had identifiable thrombus. Patients with accelerating symptoms had complex plaque morphology, whereas those with rest angina consistently had intracoronary thrombus. The nonocclusive thrombus of unstable angina can become transiently or persistently occlusive. Depending on the duration of occlusion, the presence of collateral vessels, and the area of myocardium perfused, recurrent unstable angina, non-Q-wave or Q-wave infarction can result.

Several investigations have been performed to assess serologic factors associated with hemostasis and endogenous thrombolysis. Wilensky and colleagues (16) measured fibrinopeptide A (the polypeptide fragment cleaved from fibrinogen when thrombin converts it to fibrin) among 70 patients with stable angina, unstable angina, or noncardiac chest pain. Compared to patients with stable

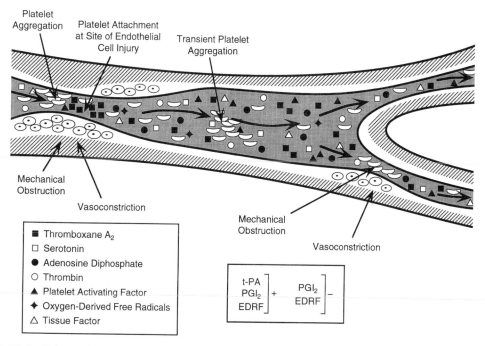

FIG. 24-3. Schematic diagram of mechanism underlying primary acute coronary syndromes. At the site of atherosclerotic plaque (anatomic obstruction) endothelial injury is present. This in combination with the release of vasoactive and platelet activating substances such as thromboxane A2, serotonin, thrombin, and adenosine diphosphate (ADP) causes a physiologic obstruction superimposed on the anatomic obstruction. Platelet activation and aggregation can occur as a result of these substances or in response to exposure of the subendothelial matrix following plaque fissuring or rupture. Platelets release additional vasoactive factors and fibrinogen which, in turn, leads to further vasoconstriction, platelet activation, thrombin formation, and potentially vessel obstruction. (Adapted from Willerson et al., ref. 26, with permission.)

angina or non- cardiac chest pain, those with unstable angina on average had substantially higher levels ($p < 0.002$). Merlini et al. (17) showed elevations in prothrombin fragment 1+2 and fibrinopepetide A among patients with unstable angina and myocardial infarction compared to a healthy control group. Interestingly, when studied months following the acute coronary syndrome persistent elevations in F 1+2 were still present while the fibrinopeptide A levels normalized. Théroux et al. (18) also reported acutely elevated fibrinopeptide A in unstable angina; Kruskal et al. (19) found increased levels of D dimer; and Zalewski et al. (20) reported increased levels of PAI-1 activity. These observations support the concept that thrombin activity is heightened in many patients with unstable

angina. On the other hand, other investigations have not found heightened levels or activities of hemostatic factors in patients with unstable angina. Explanations for these seemingly inconsistent findings include the heterogeneous population of patients with unstable angina, the relatively small thrombus burden present in some lesions, and the transient nature to these hemostatic factors. For example, Alexopoulos et al. (21) reported no difference in D-dimer or PAI-1 levels among patients with unstable angina compared to control when measure within 24 hours of the last episode of pain. In contrast, the positive findings for D dimer reported by Kruskal (19) were from samples collected within minutes of symptoms. Finally, in many patients heightened platelet activity may be more etio-logically important than fibrin formation.

As mentioned, in acute coronary syndromes platelets aggregate in response to exposed vessel wall collagen or local aggregants (thromboxane, adenosine diphosphate) and when activated release vasoactive substances that promote vasoconstriction (thromboxane, platelet factor 4) and thrombosis (PAI-1) (20). Fitzgerald et al. (22), measuring levels of thromboxane metabolites among subjects with coronary artery disease, found the highest levels in those with unstable angina. Eighty-four percent of episodes of chest pain were associated with phasic increases in excretion of thromboxane, suggesting a close temporal relation between platelet activation and clinical events. Heightened platelet activation occurs to some extent in all patients with thrombus-related unstable angina or acute infarction.

Vasoconstriction and Cyclic Flow Variation

Continuous monitoring in patients with unstable angina at rest has revealed that many first display a decrease in coronary sinus blood flow, followed by typical electrocardiographic changes of ischemia and then chest discomfort. Therefore, in response to chest pain, heart rate and systolic arterial pressure may rise (23,24). These episodes of ischemia, as well as those documented by Holter monitoring (25), resolve minutes later and may recur cyclically during disease instability. Episodic platelet aggregation at the site of coronary stenoses has been shown responsible for the cyclic flow reduction and transient myocardial ischemia in animal models (Fig. 24- 3) (26). In short, most subjects with rest angina have recurrent, transient reduction in coronary blood supply secondary to vasoconstriction and thrombus formation at the site of atherosclerotic plaque rupture. These events occur as a complex interaction among the vascular wall, leukocytes, platelets, and atherogenic lipoproteins.

Coronary Anatomy

Angiographic studies in patients with unstable angina have differed greatly regarding the observed presence and severity of coronary atherosclerosis, thrombosis, and irregular lesion morphology. The seeming inconsistency of these reports, which has fueled disagreement among investigators, is also understandable when considering the diversity of patients falling under the definition of unstable angina as well as the timing and limitations of arteriography. The reported presence of thrombus at coronary angiography in patients with unstable angina has ranged widely from <10% (27) among those with chest pain within the previous month to >50% (28–30) among those with rest angina within the preceding 24 hours. Twenty-nine percent of unstable angina subjects in the TIMI IIIA angiographic trial were found to have apparent thrombus, whereas an additional group of patients were categorized as having possible thrombus. In the setting of myocardial infarction the incidence of angiographically demonstrable thrombus steadily decreases in the hours to days following the acute event, remaining evident in 40% to 50% of subjects at 2 weeks. It is not surprising, therefore, that thrombus is present in many patients with Braunwald class C unstable angina (i.e., that occurring within 2 weeks of infarction) and in others spontaneous thrombolysis may occur. In most subjects with acute coronary syndromes, the inciting pathophysiologic event is an occlusive coronary arterial thrombus, but in some of these individuals endogenous thrombolysis occurs within minutes, thereby avoiding myocardial cell necrosis. In addition to rapid endogenous lysis of the thrombus, additional reasons that a number of unstable angina subjects do not have angiographic evidence of thrombus are likely the limitations of angiography and the multifaceted etiology of this syndrome.

TREATMENT AND OUTCOME

Medical Therapy

Since there is significant overlap in the pathophysiology of unstable angina and acute myocardial infarction, there are many similarities in treatment strategies. Because the pathophysiologic cornerstone of acute coronary syndromes is the formation of thrombus, treatment can be directed at platelets, thrombin, fibrin, and other coagulation factors. The respective categories of therapy are (a) antiplatelet agents (Chapter 8), such as aspirin, ticlopidine, and potent platelet glycoprotein IIb/IIIa inhibitors, (b) antithrombins (Chapters 9 to 12), such as heparin, factor Xa inhibitors, and hirudin, (c) fibrinolytic agents or plasminogen activators (Chapter 17), and (d) inhibitors of vitamin K–dependent coagulation proteins (Chapter 16), such as warfarin. Since inhibitors of the vitamin K–dependent factors usually takes days to become effective, they are less clinically important in the unstable phase of acute coronary syndromes. Rather, most patients presenting with unstable angina or infarction will receive a combination of rapid-acting anticoagulant therapies, such as intravenous heparin and oral aspirin.

Antiplatelets

The benefit of aspirin therapy alone or in combination with heparin in the treatment of unstable angina has been proven in several randomized trials. Aspirin, a cyclooxygenase and hydroperoxidase inhibitor, blocks synthesis of thromboxane A_2 and hinders platelet aggregation from some but not all stimuli. In the landmark study by Théroux and colleagues (31) entitled "Aspirin, Heparin, or Both to Treat Acute Unstable Angina," there was a significant reduction in cardiac death or myocardial infarction from 11.9% in the placebo group, to 3.3% with aspirin alone, and 1.6% with the combination of aspirin and heparin (p = 0.0042). The Research Group on Instability in Coronary Artery Disease in Southeast Sweden (RISC) (32) demonstrated a 57% (p = 0.033) reduction in myocardial infarction and death with aspirin therapy compared with placebo, whereas intermittent intravenous heparin showed no significant influence on these endpoints. One-year follow-up of these patients continued to show nearly a 50% reduction (p < 0.0001) in death and MI in aspirin-treated patients compared with placebo (33). While the dose of aspirin and the duration of follow-up varied in each of these studies, a substantial reduction in relative risk of adverse cardiac events was consistently seen. Based on pooled data from >2,000 patients (31,33–35) (Table 24-3), the occurrence of infarction or death was reduced from 11.8% (control) to 6.0% (aspirin).

Ticlopidine, a recently popularized antiplatelet agent due to its use following intracoronary stent implantation, inhibits ADP-mediated platelet aggregation (36) and antagonizes the interaction of fibrinogen with the platelet's IIb/IIIa receptor (37). While these mechanisms are distinctly different from the actions of aspirin and require 48–72 hours to become clinically manifest (38), available data suggest ticlopidine to be similarly effective to aspirin in reducing adverse cardiac events in unstable angina. Balsano et al. (39) reported the use of ticlopidine in a randomized study of 652 patients with unstable angina. Nonfatal infarction and vascular death were reported in 13.6% of control sub-

TABLE 24-3. *Randomized trials of aspirin for patients with acute coronary syndromes*

| Study/author | Patients | Aspirin | | MI or death | | | |
		Duration (mo)	Daily dose (mg)	Control (%)	Aspirin (%)	Relative risk (%)	p
Unstable angina trials							
Lewis (35)	1266	3	324	10.1	5.0	–51	<0.001
Cairns (34)	278	24	1300	14.1	11.5	–20	0.008
Théroux (31)	239	<1	650	11.9	3.3	–72	0.012
Wallentin (33)	288	3	75	17.6	7.4	–58	0.004
Pooled	2071			11.8	6.0	–49	<0.001

jects and 7.3% of patients receiving ticlopidine, or a 46% risk reduction (p = 0.009). Considering available trial data with aspirin or ticlopidine compared with placebo, the Antiplatelet Trialists' Collaboration reported on seven trials including 4,018 patients. The occurrence of adverse vascular events (myocardial infarction, stroke, or vascular death) was reduced by 35% by antiplatelet therapy (14.1% versus 9.1%, p < 0.001) (40).

The newest and most promising family of antiplatelet agents is the glycoprotein IIb/IIIa receptor inhibitors. As noted, platelet aggregation can be initiated by a number of pathways. However, the final common pathway of aggregation—irrespective of how it is initiated—involves the binding of the IIb/IIIa receptors of adjacent platelets by an interposing fibrinogen molecule. By blocking IIb/IIIa receptors, platelet aggregation can be effectively prevented. Many antagonists to the glycoprotein IIb/IIIa receptor were recently developed and are being used for acute coronary syndromes during percutaneous coronary revascularization. Several clinical studies have been completed for the use of intravenous IIb/IIIa inhibitors for in-hospital management of unstable angina and acute myocardial infarction.

Platelet IIb/IIIa inhibitors have been most widely studied in the setting of percutaneous coronary revascularization, where activated platelets are known to cause abrupt vessel closure. Several studies, including the Evaluation of c7E3 for the Prevention of Ischemic Events (EPIC) (41) and Evaluation of PTCA to Improve Long-Term Outcomes by c7E3 Glycoprotein Receptor Blockade (EPILOG) (42) trials, have included a large number of patients with unstable angina (43). Although the overall cohort receiving c7E3 (abciximab) in these trials had a dramatic reduction in the occurrence of death or myocardial infarction following angioplasty or atherectomy, an even greater benefit was extended to those with a recent acute coronary syndrome. Compared to placebo, those with unstable angina who received abciximab as bolus plus infusion had a 70% reduction in death, myocardial infarc-

tion, or urgent revascularization in the first 30 days of follow-up (Fig. 24-4) (43).

The Canadian Lamifiban study was a phase II, dose-exploring study of 365 patients with unstable angina who were randomized in a double-blind fashion to IIb/IIIa therapy or placebo (44). Aspirin was given to all patients, and heparin was given to a minority of patients (at the discretion of the primary physician). Lamifiban, a small molecule, nonpeptide, highly specific inhibitor for the IIb/IIIa receptor, was used as bolus plus infusion, with the infusion doses ranging from 1 μg per minute to 5 μg per minute for 72 hours. At 30-day follow-up those assigned to high-dose lamifiban (4 μg or 5 μg per minute) had a 70% reduction in the composite of death and myocardial infarction compared with placebo (8.1% versus 2.5%) (Fig. 24-5). A phase IIIa study of lamifiban in unstable angina, Platelet IIb/IIIa Antagonism for the Reduction of Acute Coronary Syndrome Events in a Global Organization Network (PARAGON), with 2,282 patients was recently completed. Patients were randomized to low-dose or high-dose lamifiban versus placebo and subrandomized to heparin or heparin-placebo. At 30-day follow-up, the occurrence of death and myocardial infarction was modestly lowered (12%) only among the low-dose (1 μg per minute) lamifiban group compared with placebo (11.7% versus 10.3%). By 6 months, however, both doses of lamifiban had lower rates of death or myocardial infarction. This reduction remained greatest (29% lower) for low-dose therapy compared with placebo (Fig. 24-6). Subsequently, similar results were reported with another short-acting, nonpeptide, IIb/IIIa inhibitor, tirofiban. Patients in the Platelet Receptor Inhibition for Ischemic Syndrome Management (PRISM) study (n = 3,231) were randomized to tirofiban (0.15 μg per kg per minute) or heparin for 48 hours. A similar study, involving patients with more severe unstable angina (recurrent episodes of ischemia or enzymatic evidence of infarction), the Platelet Receptor Inhibition for Ischemic Syndrome Management in Patients Limited by Unstable Signs and

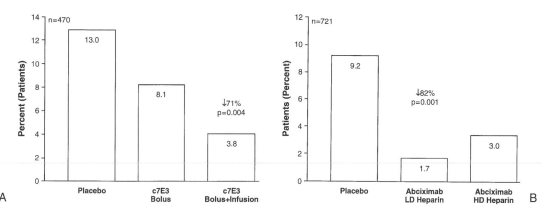

FIG. 24-4. Percentage of unstable angina patients with death, myocardial infarction or need for urgent angioplasty or bypass surgery in the first 30 days of the Evaluation of c7E3 for the Prevention of Ischemic Events (EPIC) trial **(A)** and the percent of patients with death or myocardial infarction in the first 30 days of the Evaluation of PTCA to Improve Long-Term Outcomes by c7E3 Glycoprotein Receptor Blockade (EPILOG) **(B)** trials. In both studies, potent platelet inhibition with abciximab produced a striking reduction in ischemic events among patients with unstable angina. (Data from EPIC and EPILOG Investigators, refs. 41 and 42; and Lincoff et al., ref. 43.)

Symptoms (PRISM PLUS), randomized 1,915 patients to tirofiban (0.15 μg per kg per minute), heparin (APTT twice control), or heparin plus tirofiban (0.10 μg per kg per minute). Both PRISM and PRISM PLUS showed a significant reduction in the composite of death or myocardial infarction early (2 and 7 days, respectively) with a smaller but persistent reduction in the composite at 30 days (19% and 29%, respectively) (Fig. 24-6). Finally, the PURSUIT trial has completed enrollment with 10,948 patients randomized to Integrilin versus placebo, with all patients receiving aspirin and heparin. A 10% reduction (15.7% vs. 14.2%) in death or MI was observed for treated patients at 30 days.

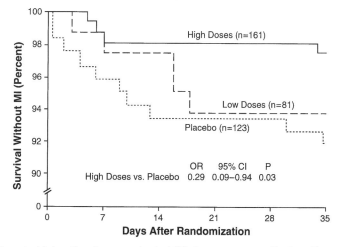

FIG. 24-5. Likelihood of infarction-free survival at 30 days among patients with unstable angina receiving placebo, or lamifiban infusion at low-dose (1 or 2 μg per minute) or high-dose (4 or 5 μg per minute). Those assigned to a high dose of lamifiban had the best outcome. (From Théroux et al., ref. 44, with permission.)

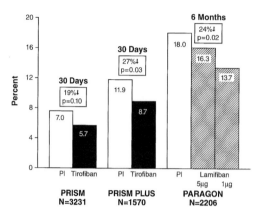

FIG. 24-6. Death or myocardial infarction. With the use of potent platelet IIb/IIIa antagonist, several recent unstable angina trials have demonstrated a significant reduction in the composite of death and myocardial infarction at 30 days and 6 months. In the Platelet Receptor Inhibition for Ischemic Syndrome Management (PRISM) and the Platelet Receptor Inhibition for Ischemic Syndrome Management in Patients Limited by Unstable Signs and Symptoms (PRISM PLUS) studies, patients received tirofiban alone for 48 hours (PRISM) or in combination with heparin for 72 hours (PRISM PLUS) and demonstrated significant in-hospital benefit and at late follow-up. In the Platelet IIb/IIIa Antagonism for the Reduction of Acute Coronary Syndrome Events in A Global Organization Network (PARAGON) study a significant reduction in events was present for patients receiving low-dose lamifiban at 6 months.

Antithrombins

Thrombin, an end-product of the coagulation mechanism, initiates transformation of fibrinogen to a fibrin clot and activates platelets. Its antagonist, antithrombin III, is the major endogenous inhibitor of the coagulation cascade and is the essential cofactor for heparin. Heparin is a mucopolysaccharide which forms a heparin-antithrombin III complex increasing antithrombin activity over a thousand fold. Clinically, many trials have been performed using heparin in unstable angina. The first unstable angina study, comparing heparin, atenolol, or both against placebo, demonstrated a risk reduction of in-hospital myocardial infarctions by nearly 80%. Similar results were observed in the study by Théroux et al. study-

ing aspirin and heparin therapies in unstable angina (31). In addition to an 85% relative risk reduction in myocardial infarction among those treated with heparin, the incidence of refractory angina decreased from 22.9% to 8.5%. Despite these studies, others have been unable to clearly demonstrate a benefit of heparin in the setting of concomitant aspirin therapy (32,45,46). Oler and colleagues performed a meta-analysis of 6 trials with over 1300 patients who were treated with heparin (APTT 1.5-2x control) in addition to 75 to 650 mg aspirin per day. With the addition of heparin there was a trend (p=0.06) for a lower rate of the composite of death or myocardial infarction during inpatient therapy (relative risk=0.67, Fig. 24-7) though this was lost at follow-up weeks to months later (relative risk=0.82) (47). When more potent antiplatelet therapy is utilized, such as the IIb/IIIa inhibitors studied in PARAGON and PRISM, the modest benefit of heparin therapy is even further attenuated.

Direct thrombin inhibitors (e.g., hirudin, efegatran, argatroban) and low molecular weight heparin (e.g., enoxaparin, dalteparin)

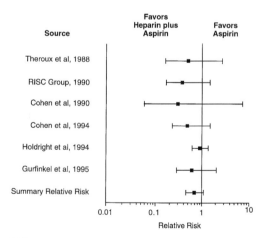

FIG. 24-7. Relative risk and 95% confidence intervals for the addition of heparin to aspirin therapy in randomized trials of unstable angina. In the meta-analysis of 6 trials, there was a trend (p = 0.06) showing benefit with regimen of heparin plus aspirin compared to aspirin therapy alone. (From Oler A, et al., ref. 47, with permission.)

have been more recently studied in acute coronary syndromes. These agents may help avoid important limitations of heparin therapy— bleeding, monitoring extent of anticoagulation, and lack of efficacy against clot-bound. The limitations of heparin are a result of the relatively narrow therapeutic window to balance its bleeding risk with its efficacy as an antithrombin. For example, in the GUSTO I and II trials there were consistent relationships between bleeding, subsequent ischemic events, and prolongation of APTT. Granger et al. (48) showed that an APTT of 50 to 75 seconds (which is best attained with weight-adjusted heparin dosing) was associated with the lowest adverse event rates (Fig. 24-8). In contrast, using modestly higher antithrombin doses, such as in GUSTO-IIa (49), a higher targeted prolongation of APTT (60-85 seconds) was associated with an increased rate of transfusions, serious bleeding events, and hemorrhagic stroke. The reasons for the disassociation between safety and efficacy of higher doses of heparin in acute coronary syndromes may be secondary to heparin's actions as an indirect thrombin inhibitor, and this is evidenced by findings of persistent thrombin generation and activity during heparin therapy (50,51).

The anti-thrombin effect of heparin is lost when thrombin is bound to fibrin or the endothelium, and heparin can be inactivated by platelet factor 4 and heparinases. Low molecular weight or fractionated heparins have more inhibitory activity against factor Xa and are less inactivated by platelet factor 4. Direct anti-thrombins are effective against free as well as bound thrombin, and they do not require antithrombin III as a cofactor. Hirudin, a direct thrombin antagonist derived from the leech *Hirudo medicinalis*, is the most potent naturally-occurring anticoagulant. Hirudin was compared to heparin for all acute coronary syndromes in the GUSTO-IIb study among 12,142 patients, and the rate of death or (re)infarction was slightly reduced (9.8% to 8.9%, OR=0.89, p=0.058).

Low molecular weight heparins have been studied in unstable angina in Efficacy and Safety of Subcutaneous Enoxaparin in Non-Q wave Coronary Events (ESSENCE) study (52) and the FRISC study. In ESSENCE, 3171 patients with unstable angina or non-Q-wave myocardial infarction were randomized to LMWH (enoxaparin) or unfractionated heparin for 2 to 8 days. At 30-day follow-up the rate of death, (re)infarction, and recurrent ischemia was reduced 15% (23.3% to 19.8%, p=0.017)(Fig. 24-9) by enoxaparin. The rate of death or (re)infarction was reduced 20% (p=0.081). In the Fragmin during Instability

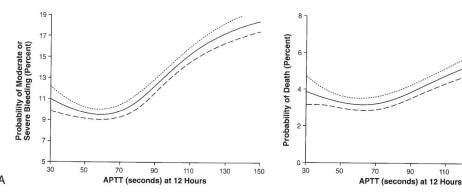

FIG. 24-8. A: Association between moderate and severe bleeding and the activated partial thromboplastin time (APTT) measured 12 hours after enrollment into the Global Utilization of Streptokinase and t-PA for Occluded Coronary Arteries (GUSTO-I) trial. The lowest bleeding rate was observed for APTT's from 50 to 70 seconds. This same range was associated with the lowest probability of death **(B)** at 30-day follow-up. (From Granger et al., ref. 48, with permission.)

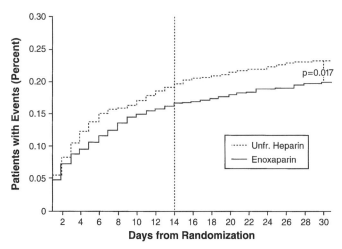

FIG. 24-9. Cumulative event curves for unfractionated heparin and low molecular weight heparin (enoxaparin) in the ESSENCE trial. At 30-day follow-up there were significantly fewer episodes of the ischemic composite including death, myocardial infarction, or recurrent angina. (From Cohen et al., ref. 52.)

in Coronary Artery Disease (FRISC) study, 1506 patients with non-ST segment elevation acute coronary syndromes were randomized to placebo or dalteparin at high dose for 6 days and then moderate dose for 5-6 weeks (53). A substantial reduction in death or myocardial infarction was observed at 6 days, though this was attenuated at 40 days. At 150-day follow-up, no difference in these end-points was observed between treatment groups (Fig. 24-10). In summary, in unstable angina the substantial early benefit from aspirin (35-50% reduction in death or infarction) can be slightly improved with unfractionated heparin and moderately improved with more potent antithrombins (fractionated heparin or direct thrombin inhibitors) or more potent antiplatelets (GP IIb/IIIa inhibitors).

Thrombolytic Therapy

Since coronary thrombus formation is known to be pathophysiologically responsible for many cases of unstable angina, and thrombolytic therapy is of clear benefit in the setting of myocardial infarction, thrombolysis for unstable angina seems intuitive. The earliest trials of thrombolytic agents in unstable angina were without control populations and demonstrated little benefit. These were followed by angiographic trials of intracoronary thrombolysis in acute coronary syndromes and revealed angiographic improvement, however, without substantial clinical benefit. A number of placebo-controlled trials have been performed with intravenous thrombolytic agents used in conjunction with aspirin and heparin (54-67). The results from these trials, assessing the inci-

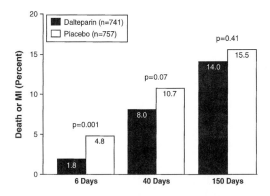

FIG. 24-10. Reduction in the occurrence of death or myocardial infarction over time in the Fragmin during Instability in Coronary Artery Disease (FRISC) study. A marked reduction in adverse events was observed early, though this was attenuated at late follow-up. (Data from FRISC Group, ref. 53, with permission.)

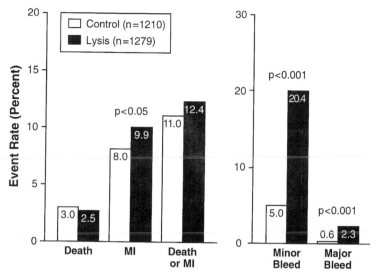

FIG. 24-11. Combining data from 14 randomized placebo-controlled trials of thrombolytic therapy in unstable angina, there was a paradoxically higher rate of myocardial infarction among those assigned to thrombolysis. There was also a marked increase in the occurrence of major bleeding and blood transfusions in the thrombolytic group. (Data from Moliterno et al., ref. 68, with permission.)

dence of non-fatal infarctions and death, vary substantially. Three of the four largest trials did observe a tendency for more non-fatal infarctions among subjects receiving thrombolytic therapy. While none of these differences was strongly powered, a formal meta-analysis (68) of nearly 2500 patients demonstrated a paradoxically higher ($p<0.05$) rate of non-fatal infarction or the combination of death and infarction (12.4% vs 11.0%) among subjects receiving thrombolysis. The risk of major bleeding events was also higher among patients receiving thrombolytic therapy (Fig. 24-11). The reasons for this may include the paradoxically heightened thrombosis-potential associated with thrombolytic therapy due to exposure of clot-bound thrombin and activation of platelets (Fig. 24-12).

Antianginals

The obvious goal of therapy is to reverse the oxygen supply-demand mismatch by minimizing requirements and maximizing delivery of tissue nutrients. Secondary precipitants, such as anemia, hypoxemia, and thyroid

dysfunction are clinically important in a small number of unstable angina patients (5-10%) and should be sought after and corrected. Specific therapy for primary causes of ischemia should be directed at each pathophysiologic origin. Nitrates, the oldest category of antianginals, remain the therapeutic mainstay for patients with acute coronary syndromes. Regardless of administration route —topically, sublingually, orally or intravenously— they ameliorate several pathways of angina and reduce the incidence of symptomatic ischemia (69). Through endothelium-independent smooth muscle relaxation in the vasculature, nitrates lower systemic arterial pressure and decrease venous return to the heart, both of which reduce myocardial wall stress. Similarly, nitrates are excellent coronary vasodilators and dilate "fixed" stenoses as well as abate "reactive" stenoses, e.g. vasoconstriction and vasospasm. Recent study of platelet function in whole blood found intravenous nitroglycerin to inhibit aggregation, an effect that was substantial and rapidly reversible (70). Other possible beneficial effects or nitroglycerin include an increase in coronary

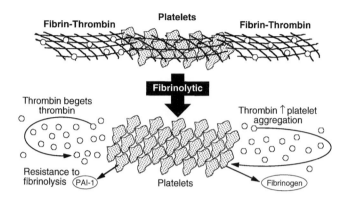

FIG. 24-12. Schematic of thrombus associated with acute myocardial infarction. In addition to fibrin strands, the thrombus is composed of many components, including thrombin and activated platelets. Clot-bound thrombin is not inactivated by heparin–antithrombin III complexes and can lead to further production of thrombin and activate platelets. Activated platelets can also accelerate the production of thrombin and release factors associated with thrombosis and rethrombosis (plasminogen-activated inhibitor–1, thromboxane, and fibrinogen).

collateral blood flow (71) and a favorable redistribution of regional flow (72). Important caveats to nitrate therapy include rapid (< 24 hour) development of drug tolerance with continuous therapy (i.e., without a nitrate-free interval) and reported induction of heparin resistance (73,74). Long-acting forms of oral nitrates have become popular recently, but should be reserved for patients with stable symptoms. Data demonstrating a reduction in cardiac events with nitrate therapy are lacking. So, too, are data for the timing, route, and duration of therapy for nitrates in acute coronary syndromes. Despite this, clinical experience and targeting known pathophysiologic mechanisms have kept nitrates at the forefront of unstable angina therapy.

Beta-adrenergic blocking agents, like nitrates, serve a number of important roles in the treatment of myocardial ischemia. There main function, blocking adrenergic receptors, serves to blunt heart rate increases which occur in response to physical exertion, chest pain, or as a reflex to vasodilators. In addition, beta blockers decrease blood pressure and myocardial contractility, each thereby lowering myocardial oxygen demands. Clinical trials of beta-adrenoreceptor blockers in the setting of stable and unstable angina have shown decrease in both ischemic symptoms

and occurrence of myocardial infarctions (75). Another potential benefit of beta-adrenergic blocking agents is inhibition of platelet aggregation which has been observed in several in vitro studies (76,77). Infrequent situations of angina where beta blocker therapy should be avoided include non-ischemic exacerbation of heart failure, cocaine-induced coronary vasoconstriction (78), and vasospastic angina (79). Beta-blockers should be used cautiously or avoided in those susceptible to reactive (bronchospastic) airway disease. Cardioselective beta-blockers, such as metoprolol and atenolol, are preferred to the nonselective beta-blockers since they produce fewer unwanted (non-cardiac) effects.

Calcium channel antagonists are effective in lowering blood pressure and decreasing chest pain frequency in patients with stable angina. They are generally considered safe as long as the patient does not have important systolic ventricular dysfunction. The use of short-acting calcium channel antagonists in the treatment of unstable angina has produced mixed results, which is not surprising considering similarly diverse results found in the treatment of post-infarction subjects. By partially blocking the flux of calcium ions into muscle cells, calcium channel blockers cause relaxation of vascular smooth muscle and the myocardium.

Like other vasodilators, these effects intuitively decrease myocardial oxygen consumption. Some calcium channel blockers, such as verapamil and diltiazem cause reduction in heart rate, whereas, nifedipine may actually lead to a reflex increase in heart rate. The Holland Interuniversity Nifedipine/metoprolol Trial (HINT) (75) was a double-blind, placebo-controlled, randomized study of medical therapies in 515 subjects with unstable angina. Among subjects receiving nifedipine without pretreatment or concomitant beta blocker therapy, the event ratio of recurrent ischemia or infarction was 1.15 relative to placebo. When nifedipine was used in combination with metoprolol or initiated in patients already receiving beta-blockade, respective cardiac event ratios were 0.80 and 0.68 compared to placebo. Diltiazem, on the other hand, was shown to be equally effective to propranolol in reducing episodes of symptomatic ischemia and produced a similar long-term outcome regarding cardiovascular events (80). The newest calcium channel antagonists, nicardipine and amlodipine, reportedly have minimal to no cardiodepressant or chronotropic effects, so that they can more

safely be used in combination with beta-blockers or used in patients with known chronic heart failure (81).

Combinations of these several classes of antianginals are reportedly similar or superior to monotherapy (75,82) and likely for patients with an acute coronary syndrome, a combination of all three agents is optimal. In summary, the medical therapies of unstable angina need to be directed at each of the known underlying precipitants of ischemia: thrombus (antiplatelet and antithrombins); vasoconstriction (nitrates and calcium channel inhibitors); and increased rate-pressure product and myocardial workload (nitrates, calcium channel blockers, and beta-adrenergic blockers); while thrombolytic therapy should be avoided. The relative benefit of these therapies has been projected from a number of pooled studies (83) as seen in Fig. 24-13.

Hypolipidemic Agents

In addition to lowering plasma lipoprotein levels, hypolipidemic and antioxidant thera-

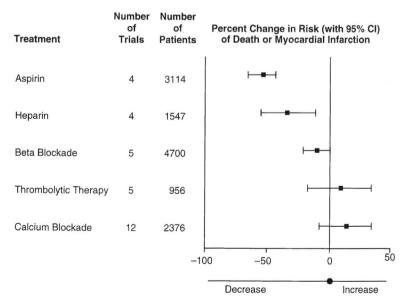

FIG. 24-13. Percent change in the risk of death or myocardial infarction from pooled data involving major therapies for unstable angina. (Adapted from Granger and Califf, ref. 83., with permission.)

pies have other reported benefits to vascular biology. HMG Co-A Reductase inhibitors have a direct antiproliferative effect on endothelial and smooth muscle cells (84), and antioxidants remove free radicals, reduce platelet aggregation, and modulate prostaglandin and leukotriene synthesis (85). While no hypolipidemic agent has been tested in large-scale clinical trial specifically for the treatment of unstable angina, many trials have been completed among patients with known ischemic heart disease. In these trials, hypolipidemic agents employed over a several year period resulted in a 30% reduction in the occurrence of ischemic cardiovascular events (86-88). For example, the Scandinavian Simvastatin Survival Study (4S) (89) randomized 4,444 patients with angina or history of myocardial infarction to simvastatin or placebo. At an average follow-up of over 5 years, in addition to a reduction in the need for myocardial revascularization among those receiving simvastatin, there was a 41% reduction in cardiac mortality and a 38% reduction in definite myocardial infarction (Fig. 24-14). These therapies should likely be used for the long-term management of most patients with pri-

mary unstable angina. For the acute treatment of fixed underlying atherosclerotic coronary arterial stenosis, invasive cardiac procedures may be needed.

Invasive Procedures

The percent of patients with unstable angina or myocardial infarction who undergo cardiac catheterization is similar. Also consistent among the acute coronary syndromes is that approximately 40% of patients undergo coronary revascularization in the days to weeks following presentation. Uniquely different between these coronary syndromes is that patients with acute myocardial infarction are more likely to undergo percutaneous angioplasty, whereas those with unstable angina undergo percutaneous and surgical revascularization with a similar frequency. This is likely due to the ability of angioplasty to restore coronary perfusion promptly and with relative safety compared to emergent bypass surgery in the setting of infarction. The more challenging question in unstable angina is whether an aggressive strategy of early catheterization and revascularization in all pa-

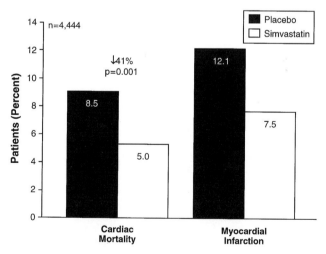

FIG. 24-14. A marked reduction in cardiac mortality and the occurrence of definite myocardial infarction was noted in the Scandinavian Simvastatin Survival Study (4S) at 5-year follow-up for those assigned to lipid-lowering therapy. (Data from Scandinavian Simvastatin Survival Study Group, ref. 89.)

tients is beneficial overall. Some have proposed such a strategy, whereas others have only referred those patients with recurrent ischemic symptoms or a significantly positive stress test to angiography and revascularization. There are data to suggest that angioplasty performed in the acute setting of myocardial ischemia results in a heightened rate of abrupt vessel closure, stent thrombosis, myocardial infarction, and overall ischemic events (90,91); however, the introduction of platelet IIb/IIIa inhibitors may have ameliorated this.

The TIMI-IIIB study directly assessed the use of an early aggressive angiography-revascularization strategy versus a conservative strategy for unstable angina. This study included 1,473 patients, half of whom had angiography and revascularization performed within 48 hours of admission unless contraindicated. The remaining patients were managed conservatively, and underwent angiography and revascularization only for definitive indications: recurrent ischemia or ventricular arrhythmias, depressed left ventricular function, or a functional study indicating high risk for an ischemic event. At 42-day follow-up, 15.5% of the aggressive strategy group had died, a non-fatal myocardial infarction, or a positive stress test compared with 17.7% of those assigned to the conservative treatment group (p=0.26). Interestingly, despite being assigned to a conservative approach, 64% of this group underwent angiography and 49% underwent myocardial revascularization during the first 6 weeks. Those assigned to the conservative treatment strategy were also more likely to be rehospitalized and took more antianginals compared with the aggressive treatment strategy group. Compared to the overall study group, a post-hoc analysis revealed patients above the age of 65 years to benefit from an aggressive treatment approach. More recently, preliminary reports (1997 American College of Cardiology Scientific Session) from the Veterans Affairs Non-Q-Wave Infarction Strategies In-Hospital (VANQWISH) study and the Organization of the Assessment of Strategies for Ischemic Syndromes (OASIS) registries support the conservative strategy approach. At 1-year follow-up of 920 patients randomized between treatment strategies, the occurrence of all-cause mortality was 30% greater among those assigned to the aggressive treatment group in VANQWISH. Likewise in OASIS registry, patients with a non-ST elevation acute ischemic syndrome who were treated by an aggressive revascularization approach had a lower rate of recurrent angina at 6 months, but had a higher rate of cardiovascular death or infarction.

OUTCOME

Bleeding Events

Considering outcome, the safety of therapies employed can be judged by the incidence of complications, such as bleeding and stroke since much of the pharmacologic thrust targets platelets and the coagulation cascade. Transfusions are given to 5% to 10% of hospitalized patients with acute coronary syndromes. Among patients with electrocardiographic evidence of ischemia at rest, either Braunwald class II-III unstable angina or acute myocardial infarction, transfusions are consistently seen used in 10% of patients (92). Severe bleeding, usually defined as >5 g of hemoglobin loss or bleeding that results in hemodynamic compromise, occurs at a lower frequency (1% to 1.5%). Among patients with coronary artery disease, patients with unstable angina are more likely to be elderly and have slightly higher systolic blood pressure; these are also known risk factors for intracranial hemorrhage. The rate of all strokes (hemorrhagic and nonhemorrhagic) is ≤1% in most unstable angina studies. Aspirin does not significantly increase the risk of serious bleeding or stroke, whereas increased dose of heparin is associated with increased bleeding as previously mentioned. The platelet glycoprotein IIb/IIIa inhibitors are associated with increased bleeding at vascular access sites and the gastrointestinal tract, but are not independently associated with an increased risk of stroke.

Death and (Re)infarction

Because the course of unstable angina can be unpredictable and potentially life threatening, the level of care or aggressiveness of approach needs to be carefully established. In previous studies the incidence of myocardial infarction in the early weeks following hospitalization was approximately 10% and the incidence of death 4%. Even using more contemporary strategies, the TIMI IIIB (66) data reveal a 6-week rate of non-fatal myocardial infarction of 5.4% and death of 2.4%. Similarly, the overall rate of death or myocardial infarction at 30 days in GUSTO-IIb was 9.4% and the rate of stroke was 1%. With these important adverse cardiac events in mind, an assertive approach should be initially taken in all patients to ameliorate ongoing or recurrent myocardial ischemia. The outcome for patients with the most abnormal presenting electrocardiograph (ST-segment depression with T-wave inversion) have an outcome similar to patients with acute infarction. Other predictors for long-term outcome for those with unstable angina include age, underlying left ventricular systolic function, and extent of coronary artery disease.

CONCLUSION

Unstable angina belongs to the continuum of the acute coronary syndromes because of shared pathophysiology, evaluation, and treatments with it and non-Q-wave and Q-wave myocardial infarction. While the etiology and definition of unstable angina can be broad, an atherothrombotic coronary arterial plaque is present in many cases of unstable angina. Especially among patients with recurrent ischemia or frank electrocardiographic evidence of ischemia (ST-depression in combination with T-wave inversion) morbidity and mortality are heightened. Patients with unstable angina have inconsistent results with thrombolytic therapy, but the majority of these patients have a worsened outcome than those not receiving thrombolysis. In contrast, a substantial reduction in death, myocardial infarction, and overall vascular mortality is provided to unstable angina patients when given antiplatelet therapy. Beyond the 35-50% reduction in death and myocardial infarction with aspirin or ticlopidine, the new potent antiplatelet IIb/IIIa inhibitors extend this benefit moderately further. New direct antithrombins and low molecular weight heparins also extend the anticoagulant benefit to this group of patients by providing an early reduction in the adverse event rate.

While patients with unstable angina are in general older, more likely to have comorbidities, multivessel coronary artery disease, and previous myocardial revascularization compared with other cardiac patients, medical and revascularization therapies continue to become more aggressive since outcome still needs substantial improvement. There is little doubt that with further tailoring and refinement of diagnostic tests as well as antiplatelet, antithrombin, and antianginal therapies, treatment benefits can be improved. For the future, in addition to the long-term benefit provided by hypolipidemic agents, intermediate and long-term administration of antithrombin and more potent anti-platelet therapies are being tested.

REFERENCES

1. Conti CR, Greene B, Pitt B, et al. Coronary surgery in unstable angina pectoris. *Circulation* 1971;44:II-154.
2. Fowler NO. Preinfarction angina: a need for an objective definition and for a controlled clinical trial of its management. *Circulation* 1971;44:755–758.
3. Wood P. Acute and subacute coronary insufficiency. *Br Med J* 1961;I:1779–1782.
4. Vakil RJ. Preinfarction syndrome: management and follow-up. *Am J Cardiol* 1964;14:55–63.
5. Scanlon PJ, Nemickas R, Moran JF, et al. Accelerated angina pectoris: clinical hemodynamic, arteriographic, and therapeutic experience in 85 patients. *Circulation* 1973;47:19–26.
6. Théroux P, Liddon RM. Unstable angina: pathogenesis, diagnosis and treatment. *Curr Probl Cardiol* 1993;18: 157–231.
7. Fuster V, Chesebro JH. Mechanisms of unstable angina. *N Engl J Med* 1986;315:1023–1024.
8. Braunwald E. Unstable angina. A classification. *Circulation* 1989;80:410–414.
9. Moliterno DJ, Aguirre FV, Cannon CP, et al., for the GUARANTEE Investigators. The Global unstable angina registry and treatment evaluation. *Circulation* 1996;94:I-195.

10. Aceti A, Taliani G, de Bac C, Sebastiani A. Monocyte activation and increased procoagulant activity in unstable angina. *Lancet* 1990;336:1444–1446.

11. Dinerman JL, Mehta JL, Saldeen TGP, et al. Increased neutrophil elastase release in unstable angina pectoris and acute myocardial infarction. *J Am Coll Cardiol* 1990;15:1559–1563.

12. Falk E. Unstable angina with fatal outcome: dynamic coronary thrombosis leading to infarction and/or sudden death. *Circulation* 1985;71:699–708.

13. Moise A, Théroux P, Taeymans Y, et al. Unstable angina and progression of coronary atherosclerosis. *N Engl J Med* 1983;309:685–689.

14. Coller B. The role of platelets in arterial thrombosis and the rationale for blockade of platelet GP IIb/IIIa receptors as antithrombotic therapy. *Eur Heart J* 1995;16 (suppl L):11–15.

15. Sherman CT, Litvack F, Grundfest W, et al. Coronary angioscopy in patients with unstable angina pectoris. *N Engl J Med* 1986;315:913–919.

16. Wilensky R, Bourdillon P, Vix V, Zeller J. Intracoronary artery thrombus formation in unstable angina: a clinical, biochemical and angiographic correlation. *J Am Coll Cardiol* 1993;21:692–699.

17. Merlini P, Bauer K, Oltrona L, et al. Persistent activation of coagulation mechanism in unstable angina and myocardial infarction. *Circulation* 1994;90:61–68.

18. Théroux P, Latour J, Leger-Gauthier C, DeLara J. Fibrinopeptide A and platelet factor levels in unstable angina pectoris. *Circulation* 1987;75:156–162.

19. Kruskal JB, Commerford PJ, Franks JJ, Kirsch RE. Fibrin and fibrinogen-related antigens in patients with stable and unstable coronary artery disease. *N Engl J Med* 1987;309:1361–1365.

20. Zalewski A, Shi Y, Nardone D, et al. Evidence for reduced fibrinolytic activity in unstable angina at rest. *Circulation* 1991;83:1685–1691.

21. Alexopoulos D, Ambrose JA, Stump D, et al. Thrombosis-related markers in unstable angina pectoris. *J Am Coll Cardiol* 1991;17:866–871.

22. Fitzgerald DJ, Roy L, Catella F, Fitzgerald GA. Platelet activation in unstable coronary disease. *N Engl J Med* 1986;315:983–989.

23. Chierchia S, Brunelli C, Simonetti I, Lazzari M, Maseri A. Sequence of events in angina at rest: primary reduction in coronary flow. *Circulation* 1980;61:759–768.

24. Davies GJ, Bencivelli W, Fragasso G, et al. Sequence and magnitude of ventricular volume changes in painful and painless myocardial ischemia. *Circulation* 1988;78:310–319.

25. Gottlieb SO, Weisfeldt ML, Ouyang P, Mellits ED, Gerstenblith G. Silent ischemia as a marker for early unfavorable outcomes in patients with unstable angina. *N Engl J Med* 1986;314:1214–1219.

26. Willerson JT, Golino P, Eidt J, Campbell WB, Buja LM. Specific platelet mediators and unstable coronary artery lesions experimental evidence and potential clinical implications. *Circulation* 1989;80:198–205.

27. Vetrovec GW, Cowley MJ, Overton H, Richardson DW. Intracoronary thrombus in syndromes of unstable myocardial ischemia. *Am Heart J* 1981;102:1202–1208.

28. Freeman MR, Williams AE, Chisholm RJ, Armstrong PW. Intracoronary thrombus and complex morphology in unstable angina. *Circulation* 1989;80:17–23.

29. Capone G, Wolf NM, Meyer B, Meister SG. Frequency of intracoronary filling defects by angiography in angina pectoris at rest. *Am J Cardiol* 1985;56:403–406.

30. Gotoh K, Minamino T, Katoh O, et al. The role of intracoronary thrombus in unstable angina: angiographic assessment and thrombolytic therapy during ongoing anginal attacks. *Circulation* 1988;77:526–534.

31. Théroux P, Ouimet H, McCans J, et al. Aspirin, heparin, or both to treat acute unstable angina. *N Engl J Med* 1988;319:1105–1111.

32. The RISC Group. Risk of myocardial infarction and death during treatment with low dose aspirin and intravenous heparin in men with unstable coronary artery disease. *Lancet* 1990;336:827–830.

33. Wallentin LC, and the Research Group on Instability in Coronary Artery Disease in Southeast Sweden. Aspirin (75 mg/day) after an episode of unstable coronary artery disease: long-term effects on the risk for myocardial infarction, occurrence of severe angina and the need for revascularization. *J Am Coll Cardiol* 1991;18:1587–1593.

34. Cairns JA, Gent M, Singer J, et al. Aspirin, sulfinpyrazone, or both in unstable angina. *N Engl J Med* 1985;313:1369–1375.

35. Lewis HDJ, Davis JW, Archibald DG, et al. Protective effects of aspirin against acute myocardial infarction and death in men with unstable angina. *N Engl J Med* 1983;309:396–403.

36. Maffrand J, Bernat A, Delebasse D, Defreyen G, Cazenave J, Gordon J. ADP plays a key role in thrombogenesis in rats. *Thromb Haemost* 1988;59:225–230.

37. De Minno G, Cerbone A, Mattioli P, Turco S, Iovine C, Mancini M. Functionally thrombosthenic state in normal platelets following the administration of ticlopidine. *J Clin Invest* 1985;75:328–338.

38. Panak E, Maffrand J, Picard-Fraire C, Vallee E, Blanchard J, Roncucci R. Ticlopidine: a promise for the prevention and treatment of thrombosis and its complications. *Haemostasis* 1983;13(suppl 1):1–54.

39. Balsano F, Rizzon P, Violi F, et al., and the Studio della Ticlopidina nell'Angina Instabile Group. Antiplatelet treatment with ticlopidine in unstable angina. A controlled multicenter clinical trial. *Circulation* 1990;82:17–26.

40. Antiplatelet Trialists' Collaboration. Collaborative overview of randomised trials of antiplatelet therapy - I. Prevention of death, myocardial infarction, and stroke by prolonged antiplatelet therapy in various categories of patients. *Br Med J* 1994;308:81–106.

41. The EPIC Investigators. Use of a monoclonal antibody directed against the glycoprotein IIb/IIIa receptor in high-risk coronary angioplasty. *N Engl J Med* 1994;330:956–961.

42. The EPILOG Investigators. Platelet glycoprotein IIb/IIIa receptor blockade and low-dose heparin during percutaneous coronary revascularization. *N Engl J Med* 1997;336:1689–1696.

43. Lincoff AM, Califf RM, Anderson K, et al. Evidence for prevention of death and myocardial infarction with platelet membrane glycoprotein IIb/IIIa receptor blockade by abciximab (c7E3Fab) among patients with unstable angina undergoing percutaneous coronary revascularization. *J Am Coll Cardiol* 1997;30:149–156.

44. Théroux P, Kouz S, Roy L, et al., on behalf of the Investigators. Platelet membrane receptor glycoprotein

IIb/IIIa antagonism in unstable angina. The Canadian Lamifiban Study. *Circulation* 1996;94:899–905.

45. Holdright D, Patel D, Cunningham D, et al. Comparison of the effect of heparin and aspirin versus aspirin alone on transient myocardial ischemia and in-hospital prognosis in patients with unstable angina. *J Am Coll Cardiol* 1994;24:39–45.

46. Wallis DE, Boden WE, Califf R, et al. Failure of adjuvant heparin to reduce myocardial ischemia in the early treatment of patients with unstable angina. *Am Heart J* 1991;122:949–954.

47. Oler A, Whooley MA, Oler J, Grady D. Adding heparin to aspirin reduces the incidence of myocardial infarction and death in patients with unstable angina: a meta-analysis. *JAMA* 1996;276:811–815.

48. Granger CB, Hirsh J, Califf RM, et al., for the GUSTO Trial Investigators. Activated partial thromboplastin time and outcome after thrombolytic therapy for acute myocardial infarction: results from the GUSTO trial. *Circulation* 1996;93:870–878.

49. The Global Use of Strategies to Open Occluded Coronary Arteries (GUSTO) IIa Investigators. Randomized trial of intravenous heparin versus recombinant hirudin for acute coronary syndromes. *Circulation* 1994;90: 1631–1637.

50. Merlini P, Bauer K, Oltrona L, et al. Thrombin generation and activity during thrombolysis and concomitant heparin therapy in patients with acute myocardial infarction. *J Am Coll Cardiol* 1995;25:203–209.

51. Granger CB, Becker R, Tracy RP, et al., for the GUSTO hemostasis substudy group. Thrombin generation, inhibition and clinical outcomes in patients with acute myocardial infarction treated with thrombolytic therapy and heparin: results from the GUSTO trial. *J Am Coll Cardiol.* In press.

52. Cohen M, Demers C, Gurfinkel E, et al. A comparison of low-molecular-weight heparin with unfractionated heparin for unstable coronary artery disease. *N Engl J Med* 1997;337:447–452.

53. Fragmin during Instability in Coronary Artery Disease (FRISC) Group. Low-molecular-weight heparin during instability in coronary disease. *Lancet* 1996;347: 561–568.

54. Ardissino D, Barberis P, De Servi S, et al. Recombinant tissue-type plasminogen activator followed by heparin compared with heparin alone for refractory unstable angina pectoris. *Am J Cardiol* 1990;66:910–914.

55. Bär F, Verheugt F, Materne P, et al. Thrombolysis in patients with unstable angina improves the angiographic but not the clinical outcome: results of UNASEM, a multicenter, randomized, placebo-controlled, clinical trial with anistreplase. *Circulation* 1992;86:131–137.

56. Charbonnier B, Bernadet P, Schiele F, Thery C, Bauters C. Intravenous thrombolysis by recombinant plasminogen activator (rt-PA) in unstable angina. A multicenter study versus placebo. *Arch Maladies du Coeur des Vaisseaux* 1992;85:1471–1477.

57. Freeman MR, Langer A, Wilson RF, Morgan CD, Armstrong PW. Thrombolysis in unstable angina. Randomized double-blind trial of t-PA and placebo. *Circulation* 1992;85:150–157.

58. Gold HK, Coller BS, Yasuda T, et al. Rapid and sustained coronary artery recanalization with combined bolus injection of recombinant tissue-type plasminogen activator and monoclonal antiplatelet GP IIb/IIIa antibody in a canine preparation. *Circulation* 1988;77:670–677.

59. Karlsson J, Berglund U, Bjorkholm A, Ohlsson J, Swahn E, Wallentin L, for the TRIC Study Group. Thrombolysis with recombinant human tissue-type plasminogen activator during instability in coronary artery disease: effect on myocardial ischemia and need for coronary revascularization. *Am Heart J* 1992;124:1419–1426.

60. Neri Serneri G, Gensini GF, Poggesi L, et al. Effect of heparin, aspirin, or alteplase in reduction of myocardial ischaemia in refractory unstable angina. *Lancet* 1990; 335:615–618.

61. Nicklas JM, Topol EJ, Kander N, et al. Randomized, double-blind, placebo-controlled trial of tissue plasminogen activator in unstable angina. *J Am Coll Cardiol* 1989;13:434–441.

62. Roberts MJD, McNeil AJ, Wilson DCM, et al. Double-blind randomized trial of alterplase versus placebo in patients with chest pain at rest. *Eur Heart J* 1993;14: 1536–1542.

63. Saran RK, Bhandari K, Narain VS, et al. Intravenous streptokinase in the management of a subset of patients with unstable angina: a randomized controlled trial. *Int J Cardiol* 1990;28:209–213.

64. Schreiber TL, Macina G, McNulty A, et al. Urokinase plus heparin versus aspirin in unstable angina and non-Q-wave myocardial infarction. *Am J Cardiol* 1989;64: 840–844.

65. Scrutinio D, Biasco MG, Rizzon P. Thrombolysis in unstable angina: results of clinical studies. *Am J Cardiol* 1991;68:99B–104B.

66. The TIMI IIIB Investigators. Effects of tissue-type plasminogen activator and a comparison of early invasive and conservative strategies in unstable angina and non-Q-wave myocardial infarction: results of the TIMI IIIB trial. *Circulation* 1994;89:1545–1556.

67. Williams DO, Topol EJ, Califf RM, et al. Intravenous recombinant tissue-type plasminogen activator in patients with unstable angina pectoris. *Circulation* 1990;82: 376–383.

68. Moliterno DJ, Sapp SK, Topol EJ. The paradoxical effect of thrombolytic therapy for unstable angina: meta-analysis. *J Am Coll Cardiol* 1994;23:288A.

69. Curfman GD, Heinsimer JA, Lozner EC, Fung H-L. Intravenous nitroglycerin in the treatment of spontaneous angina pectoris: a prospective, randomized trial. *Circulation* 1983;67:276–282.

70. Diodati J, Theroux P, Latour JG, Lacoste L, Lam JYT, Waters D. Effects of nitroglycerin at therapeutic doses on platelet aggregation in unstable angina pectoris and acute myocardial infarction. *Am J Cardiol* 1990;66: 683–688.

71. Cohen MV, Downey JM, Sonnenblick EH, Kirk ES. The effects of nitroglycerin on coronary collaterals and myocardial contractility. *J Clin Invest* 1973;52:2836–2847.

72. Bache RJ, Ball RM, Cobb FR, Rembert JC, Greenfield JC. Effects of nitroglycerin on transmural myocardial blood flow in the unanesthetized dog. *J Clin Invest* 1975;55:1219–1228.

73. Becker RC, Corrao JM, Bovill EG, et al. Intravenous nitroglycerin-induced heparin resistance: a qualitative antithrombin III abnormality. *Am Heart J* 1990;119: 1254–1261.

74. Habbab MA, Haft JI. Heparin resistance induced by intravenous nitroglycerin. *Arch Intern Med* 1987;147:857–860.

75. Lubsen J, Tijssen JGP, for the HINT Research Group. Efficacy of Nifedipine and Metoprolol in the treatment of unstable angina in the coronary care unit: findings from the Holland Interuniversity Nifedipine/Metoprolol Trial (HINT). *Am J Cardiol* 1987;60:18A–25A.

76. Gasser JA, Betterridge DJ. Comparison of the effects of carvedilol, propranolol, and verapamil on in vitro platelet function in healthy volunteers. *J Cardiovasc Pharmacol* 1991;18 (suppl 4):S29–34.

77. Ondriasova E, Ondrias K, Stasko A, Nosal R, Csollei J. Comparison of the potency of five potential beta-adrenergic blocking drugs and eight calcium channel blockers to inhibit platelet aggregation and to perturb liposomal membranes prepared from platelet lipids. *Physiol Res* 1992;41:267–272.

78. Lange RA, Cigarroa RG, Flores ED, Hillis LD. Potentiation of cocaine-induced coronary vasoconstriction by beta-adrenergic blockade. *Ann Intern Med* 1990;112:897–903.

79. Robertson RM, Wood AJJ, Vaughn WK, et al. Exacerbation of vasotonic angina pectoris by propranolol. *Circulation* 1982;65:281–285.

80. Théroux P, Taeymans Y, Morissette D, Bosch X, Pelletier GB, Waters DD. A randomized study comparing propranolol and diltiazem in the treatment of unstable angina. *J Am Coll Cardiol* 1985;5:717–722.

81. Packer M, O'Connor C, Ghali J, et al. Effect of amlodipine on morbidity and mortality in severe chronic heart failure. *N Engl J Med* 1996;335:1107–1114.

82. Lubsen J. Medical management of unstable angina. What have we learned from the randomized trials. *Circulation* 1990;82:82–87.

83. Granger CB, Califf RM. Stabilizing the unstable artery. In: Califf R, Mark D, Wagner G (eds). *Acute Coronary Care* (2nd ed). St. Louis: Mosby-Year Book, 1995;525–541.

84. Constantinescu DE, Banka VS, Tulenko TN. Lovastatin inhibits proliferation of arterial smooth muscle and endothelial cells. Indication in atherosclerosis and prevention of restenosis. *Eur Heart J* 1992;13:82.

85. Godfried S, Deckelbaum L. Natural antioxidants and restenosis after percutaneous transluminal coronary angioplasty. *Am Heart J* 1995;129:203–210.

86. Brown G, Albers JJ, Fisher LD, et al. Regression of coronary artery disease as a result of intensive lipid-lowering therapy in men with high levels of apolipoprotein B. *N Engl J Med* 1990;323:1289–1298.

87. Blankenhorn DH, Azen SP, Kramsch DM, et al. Coronary angiographic changes with lovastatin therapy: the Monitored Atherosclerosis Regression Study (MARS). *Ann Intern Med* 1993;119:969–976.

88. Watts GF, Lewis B, Brunt JNH, et al. Effects on coronary artery disease of lipid-lowering diet, or diet plus cholestyramine, in the St. Thomas' Atherosclerosis Regression Study (STARS). *Lancet* 1992;339:563–569.

89. Scandinavian Simvastatin Survival Study Group. Randomised trial of cholesterol lowering in 4444 patients with coronary heart disease: the Scandinavian Simvastatin Survival Study (4S). *Lancet* 1994;344:1383–1389.

90. Ellis S, Roubin G, King SB III, et al. Angiographic and clinical predictors of acute closure after native vessel angioplasty. *Circulation* 1988;77:372–379.

91. Mak KH, Belli G, Ellis SG, Moliterno DJ. Subacute stent thrombosis: current issues and future directions. *J Am Coll Cardiol* 1996;27:494–503.

92. The Global Use of Strategies to Open Occluded Coronary Arteries (GUSTO) IIb Investigators. A comparison of recombinant hirudin with heparin for the treatment of acute coronary syndromes. *N Engl J Med* 1996;335:775–782.

Cardiovascular Thrombosis: Thrombocardiology and Thromboneurology, Second Edition, edited by M. Verstraete, V. Fuster, and E. J. Topol, Lippincott–Raven Publishers, Philadelphia © 1998.

25

Antithrombotic Agents in the Secondary and Primary Prevention of Cardiovascular Diseases in High and Usual Risk Individuals

Patricia R. Hebert, *Paul M. Ridker, †Valentin Fuster, and ‡Charles H. Hennekens

*Departments of Preventive Medicine and Medicine, Vanderbilt University School of Medicine, Nashville, Tennessee 37232; *Department of Medicine, Brigham and Women's Hospital, Boston, Massachusetts 02167; †Cardiovascular Institute, Mount Sinai Medical Center, New York, New York 10029; and ‡Harvard Medical School, Boston, Massachusetts 02115*

Antithrombotic therapies, both antiplatelet and anticoagulant, have been used to treat a wide range of occlusive vascular diseases. In this chapter, we review the evidence on the effects of antiplatelet and anticoagulant therapies on subsequent cardiovascular disease events in patients with a history of prior occlusive cardiovascular diseases (secondary prevention) and of aspirin in apparently healthy individuals (primary prevention). The evidence of efficacy of antithrombotic agents in patients with unstable angina or those with evolving acute myocardial infarction (MI) are covered in other chapters.

ANTIPLATELET AND ANTICOAGULANT THERAPY IN SECONDARY PREVENTION

Antiplatelet Therapy

Evidence for the efficacy of antiplatelet drugs in secondary prevention comes primar-ily from an overview of the randomized trials conducted by the worldwide Antiplatelet Trialists' (APT) Collaboration (1,2). The overview was first published in 1988 (1) and updated in 1994 (2). By the late 1980s, 25 trials of antiplatelet therapy in the secondary prevention of cardiovascular disease had been conducted (3–33), which included approximately 29,000 patients. Ten trials included about 18,000 patients with a history of MI (3–15); 13 had been conducted among about 9,000 patients with a history of stroke or transient ischemic attack (TIA) (16–31); and two included about 2,000 patients with unstable angina (32,33). The trials tested aspirin, dipyridamole (Persantine), sulfinpyrazone (Anturane), or suloctidil, either alone or in combination. The overview, or meta-analysis, of all trials of secondary prevention provides more statistically stable estimates (i.e., less variability due to chance fluctuations in the data) than the individual trials of antiplatelet therapy (Table 25-1) (1).

TABLE 25-1. *Effects of antiplatelet therapy versus control in all high-risk patients[a]: updated Antiplatelet Trialists' Overview*

Endpoint	% Odds reduction ± SD
Any important vascular event (MI, stroke, or vascular death)	27 ± 2
Nonfatal MI	35 ± 4
Nonfatal stroke	31 ± 5
Vascular death	18 ± 3

[a]All high-risk patients include those with: (1) an acute MI, (2) a past history of MI, (3) a past history of stroke or transient ischemic attack, or (4) some other relevant medical history (unstable angina, stable angina, vascular surgery, angioplasty, atrial fibrillation, valvular disease, peripheral vascular disease, etc.).

In the initial overview, the three main endpoints examined were nonfatal MI, nonfatal stroke, and total cardiovascular death. For each of these endpoints, highly significant reductions were observed (p < 0.0001) in those allocated to antiplatelet treatment as compared to controls. As expected in these high-risk populations, the proportion of deaths attributed to noncardiovascular diseases was small and was not significantly affected by antiplatelet therapy. Therefore, a favorable effect on total mortality (p < 0.0001) was also observed. Specifically, when all available trials were considered, for subsequent nonfatal MI, there was a highly significant 32 ± 5% reduction in risk (p < 0.00001); furthermore, the reductions were similar in magnitude and significance in the trials of patients with coronary (31% reduction) and cerebrovascular (35% reduction) disease. For total cardiovascular mortality, there was a statistically significant (p < 0.003) 15% reduction, which was the same for the coronary and cerebrovascular trials. Finally, there was also a significant (p < 0.0001) 25% reduction in risk of developing any important vascular event (a combined endpoint that included nonfatal MI, nonfatal stroke, or vascular death).

With respect to the different antiplatelet drugs tested, there was no clear evidence that aspirin plus dipyridamole was any more effective than aspirin alone. The indirect comparison between the two risk reductions was not significant and the combined results of the direct comparisons indicated no differ-

ence. There was also no evidence that aspirin in daily doses of 900 to 1500 mg was any more effective in reducing vascular events than 300 mg, the lowest dose tested.

Although the initial APT overview provided reliable evidence of the benefits of antiplatelet therapy in individuals with a prior MI, unstable angina, stroke, and TIAs, it did not assess whether such treatment would benefit other patient populations at high risk for occlusive vascular disease, including those with chronic stable angina, peripheral vascular disease, or undergoing revascularization procedures. The initial overview also did not address the question of the benefits of antiplatelet therapy in subgroups of high-risk patients, such as women or the elderly, or in those with hypertension or diabetes.

To address these questions, in 1994 the updated APT overview included data from a much broader range of high-risk patients (2). This overview utilized data from 174 trials of prolonged antiplatelet therapy (for 1 month or longer) and involved over 70,000 patients with prior cardiovascular disease, more than twice the number included in the original overview. When all high-risk patients were considered together, there were statistically significant reductions of 27% for all important vascular events (MI, stroke, or vascular death), 35% for nonfatal MI, 31% for nonfatal stroke, and 18% for vascular death. For patients with a prior history of cardiovascular disease, antiplatelets were estimated to prevent from 35 to 40 events per 1,000 patients treated.

With respect to the new patient populations, there were approximately 22,000 patients included in the updated overview at high risk for occlusive vascular events due to atrial fibrillation, valve surgery, peripheral vascular disease, unstable or chronic stable angina, and coronary revascularization (either coronary artery bypass graft or percutaneous transluminal coronary angioplasty). In these high-risk patients, antiplatelet therapy was associated with statistically significant decreases of 32% in both recurrent MI and subsequent vascular events.

The updated overview also provides reliable evidence that antiplatelet therapy of high-risk patients produces reductions in vascular events of similar sizes in middle-aged (<65 years of age) and elderly patients (≥65 years), in men and women, in hypertensive and non-hypertensive patients, and in patients with and without diabetes.

Aspirin was examined in the updated overview in doses ranging from 75 to 1500 mg per day. As was the case in the initial overview, there was no evidence that higher doses were any more effective than lower doses in reducing the risk of occlusive vascular disorders. Whereas 300 mg was the lowest dose of aspirin tested in the initial overview, the updated analyses included randomized trials involving approximately 5,000 patients that tested a daily dose of 75 mg. When analyzed separately, patients assigned to this far lower dose experienced a statistically significant 29% reduction in subsequent vascular events (p < 0.0001). Furthermore, the hypothesized mechanism for aspirin's benefit on the risks of occlusive vascular events is based on its ability to inhibit platelet aggregation (Fig. 25-1). Basic research findings demonstrate that in platelets, small amounts of aspirin irreversibly acetylate the active site of cyclooxygenase, which is required for the production of thromboxane A_2, a powerful promoter of aggregation (34). This effect is so pronounced that higher doses of aspirin appear to provide no additional benefit. It has been hypothesized that far higher doses may even reverse this tendency as a result of the activation of reversible vessel wall enzymes. Based on these basic research findings, as

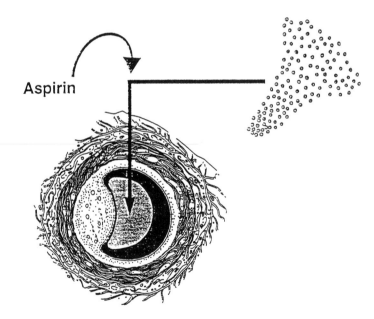

FIG. 25-1. Platelet adhesion is the first step in the initiation of thrombus formation. This is followed by platelet activation and the release of a number of mediators, including arachidonic acid, the next step in the initiation of thrombus formation. Arachidonic acid released from platelets is converted to thromboxane A2 by the enzyme cyclooxygenase. Thromboxane A2 is an extremely potent inducer of platelet aggregation, which is the third and final step in the initiation of thrombus formation. Thromboxane A2 is also a vasoconstrictor. A single dose of aspirin irreversibly acetylates cyclooxygenase and thereby inhibits platelet production of thromboxane A2. Although aspirin may also inactivate cyclooxygenase in other cells, they recover rapidly and synthesize new cyclooxygenase. Platelets, which lack nuclei, cannot synthesize new cyclooxygenase and remain inactive for the rest of their life span. Even a low dose of aspirin can thereby inhibit the initiation of intravascular thrombus formation, the crucial event in unstable angina and myocardial infarction.

well as the fact that side effects of aspirin are dose-related, daily doses of 50 to 80 mg of aspirin have been recommended for long-term secondary prevention of cardiovascular disease (35).

In addition to the antiplatelet drugs tested in the original overview, the updated analysis also included three trials that tested ticlopidine versus aspirin. Ticlopidine is a thienopyridine derivative that inhibits ADP-induced platelet aggregation (36), whose primary indication is the prevention of stroke. In the updated analysis, as was the case in the initial overview, no significant differences were demonstrated in the effectiveness of the various antiplatelet agents. However, because differences in the effectiveness of antiplatelet regimens are smaller and more difficult to detect than differences between antiplatelet versus no-antiplatelet treatment, the possibility of a small advantage of one type of agent versus another cannot be excluded. With respect to adverse effects, the most serious side effect of ticlopidine is neutropenia, which occurs in about 2.4% of treated patients and warrants careful monitoring (37). Diarrhea and skin rashes are other common side effects of ticlopidine, whereas gastrointestinal distress and bleeding occur more frequently with aspirin.

Since the publication of the updated overview, a randomized trial of clopidogrel versus aspirin in patients at high risk of ischemic events (CAPRIE) has also been reported (38). Clopidogrel is a new thienopyridine derivative chemically related to ticlopidine but with reportedly fewer side effects. In this study, 19,185 patients with atherosclerotic vascular disease (e.g., ischemic stroke, recent MI, or peripheral vascular disease) were randomly assigned to either clopidogrel (75 mg daily) or aspirin (325 mg daily). The mean follow-up was 1.9 years and the major outcome assessed a combined endpoint of ischemic stroke, MI, or vascular death. The annual rate of these events was 5.32% in the clopidogrel-treated patients and 5.83% in the aspirin-treated patients, representing an 8.7% (95% CI 0.3–16.5%) reduction in risk in favor of clopi-

dogrel. As regards side effects, participants on clopidogrel had a higher frequency of severe rash (0.26% versus 0.10%, p = 0.02) and severe diarrhea (0.23% versus 0.11%, p = 0.08). Patients assigned to aspirin had more severe upper gastrointestinal discomfort (1.23% versus 0.97%, p = 0.096) and gastrointestinal bleeds (2.66% versus 1.99%, p = 0.05). There was also a possible small but nonsignificant increase in the frequency of intracranial hemorrhages in the aspirin-treated group (0.49% versus 0.35%, p = 0.23). There was no evidence of excess neutropenia in the clopidogrel as compared to the aspirin-treated patients.

Glycoprotein IIb/IIIa integrin antagonists are also a new class of antiplatelet drug that appear promising (39). However, at this time, initial short-term testing has been limited to intravenous administration in patients undergoing high-risk coronary interventions, as well as patients with unstable angina and acute MI (39–41). No prevention trials with oral agents of this class have been reported.

Anticoagulant Therapy

The efficacy of anticoagulant therapy in the secondary prevention of MI has also been documented. The risk reductions in recurrent MI achieved with anticoagulants as compared to placebo are similar in size (about 30% to 35%) to those achieved with antiplatelet drugs. Trials comparing anticoagulants to antiplatelet therapy have not found significant differences in reinfarction or death. However, the risk of serious bleeds is higher with anticoagulants than with aspirin.

In the Dutch Sixty Plus Study (42), patients over age 60 who were already receiving warfarin following myocardial infarction were randomized to continued warfarin therapy or to placebo. After an average follow-up period of 2 years, there was a 43% reduction in mortality associated with warfarin (p = 0.02) and a 51% reduction in nonfatal reinfarction (p < 0.01). Rates of intracranial hemorrhage were increased in the warfarin group (1.6% versus 0.2%), although total stroke rates were similar between therapies.

The Warfarin and Reinfarction Study (WARIS) was a randomized double-blind placebo-controlled trial of warfarin (target International Normalized Ratio [INR] of 2.8 to 4.8) in 1,214 patients 75 years of age or younger enrolled at a mean of 27 days post MI (43). Patients were instructed to avoid aspirin during the trial. At a mean of 37 months of treatment and follow-up, there was a 34% reduction (95% CI: 19–54%) in risk of recurrent MI in the warfarin-treated as compared to the placebo group. The risks of death and of stroke were also significantly decreased by 24% and 55%, respectively, in the warfarin-treated group. With respect to side effects, serious bleeds including five hemorrhagic strokes occurred in 13 of the warfarin-treated patients (0.6% per year) as compared to none in the placebo group.

Two randomized trials have compared anticoagulant to antiplatelet therapy in secondary prevention of MI. The German-Austrian Myocardial Infarction Study (GAMIS) randomized 946 men and women, 45 to 75 years of age, between 38 and 42 days post MI to open label phenprocoumon (target INR of 2.5 to 5.0), aspirin (1.5 g per day), or aspirin placebo (45). At 2 years follow-up, there were no significant differences between the phenprocoumon and aspirin groups in the incidence of fatal plus nonfatal coronary events (32 in the phenprocoumon versus 24 in the aspirin group, $p = 0.28$) or total deaths (39 versus 27, $p = 0.13$). With respect to side effects, there were no significant differences in the frequency of hemorrhages. Twelve patients in the phenprocoumon and nine in the aspirin group had bleeds ($p = 0.52$), none of which were fatal. The Enquete de Prevention Secondaire de l'Infarctus du Myocarde (EPSIM) trial randomized 4,303 men and women at an average of 11.4 days post MI to oral anticoagulants (adjusted for a prothrombin time between 25% and 35% of normal) or aspirin (0.5 g three times a day) (45). At 2 years follow-up, there were no significant differences in coronary events (20 in the oral anticoagulant versus 32 in the aspirin group, $p = 0.076$) or in total deaths (8.4% in both treatment groups). With respect to side effects, there were more bleeds in the anticoagulant group and more gastric disorders in the aspirin group. One hundred and four patients (16%) in the anticoagulant group and 35 in the aspirin group (5%) experienced bleeds ($p < 0.001$). Twenty-one of these in the anticoagulant group and five in the aspirin group were severe bleeds ($p < 0.001$). Gastritis and peptic ulcer were more common in those in the aspirin group (4 versus 18, $p < 0.001$).

Randomized trials currently underway will also examine the efficacy of warfarin plus aspirin as compared to aspirin alone in the secondary prevention of MI. The major difficulty with such combined regimens is an increased frequency of bleeding that may be minimized by using low-dose aspirin with less intense warfarin therapy. The Coronary Artery Reinfarction Study (CARS) randomized 9,000 patients to one of three treatment regimens: aspirin 160 mg per day, aspirin 80 mg per day plus warfarin 3 mg per day, or aspirin 80 mg per day plus warfarin 1 mg per day (46). In preliminary analyses of this trial, aspirin plus warfarin has not proven to be a superior treatment to aspirin alone. Another ongoing Veterans Administration trial (CHAMPS) is randomizing 4,000 patients to receive either aspirin 160 mg per day or aspirin 80 mg per day plus warfarin to achieve a target INR of 1.5 to 2.5. Final reports from these two trials should provide information about both the efficacy and safety of combined aspirin plus warfarin regimens in the secondary prevention of MI.

ASPIRIN THERAPY IN PRIMARY PREVENTION

Whereas aspirin therapy is clearly indicated for all patients suffering acute MI as well as all who have had a prior MI or other manifestations of atherosclerotic disease (secondary prevention), the balance of benefits and risks in apparently healthy individuals (primary prevention) is less clear. This is due to the availability of data from only two randomized trials as well as the far lower risk of cardiovascular disease in apparently healthy individuals. Because side effects of aspirin are dose-related and similar in high- and low-risk patients, direct evidence concerning benefits and risks in primary prevention are even more crucial (47).

The U.S. Physicians' Health Study (48) used a 2×2 factorial design to test simultaneously the effects of aspirin in reducing cardiovascular disease and that of β-carotene in the prevention of cancer. A total of 22,071 male physicians, aged 40 to 84 years, were randomized to receive either aspirin 325 mg on alternate days, β-carotene 50 mg on alternate days, both active treatments, or both placebos. The aspirin component of the trial was terminated early after an average follow-up of 60.2 months due to the emergence of a statistically extreme benefit on risk of MI. Treatment with aspirin resulted in a 44% reduction in the risk of a first MI (p < 0.00001), with significant benefits on both fatal and nonfatal events. As regards stroke, although there were insufficient numbers of events on which to base firm conclusions, there was no evidence of a benefit. There was, in fact, a possible but nonsignificant 19% increase (110 in the aspirin versus 92 in the placebo group) in risk of nonfatal confirmed stroke. This was attributable primarily to a slight increase in hemorrhagic stroke, which was based on small numbers and did not achieve statistical significance. For cardiovascular mortality, the numbers of events were too small to draw firm conclusions, but there was also no significant difference (81 aspirin versus 83 placebo confirmed cardiovascular deaths).

The other primary prevention trial was conducted among 5,139 British male physicians aged 50 to 78 years (49). The British Doctors' Trial tested a daily dose of 500 mg of aspirin and the control group was simply instructed to avoid aspirin and aspirin-containing compounds. After 6 years of treatment and follow-up, there were no significant differences between the treatment groups in nonfatal myocardial infarction, nonfatal stroke, vascular death, or a combined endpoint of all important vascular events.

An overview of the U.S. and British trials was performed to consider the primary prevention trial data in aggregate (50) (Table 25-2). Because the U.S. trial was so much larger, the overview demonstrated a highly significant 32% reduction in risk of first nonfatal MI (p < 0.00002). In terms of absolute risk reductions, it was estimated in the updated APT overview that approximately four events are prevented for each 1,000 apparently healthy individuals treated (2). With respect to the effects of aspirin on stroke and vascular deaths, there were too few endpoints on which to draw firm conclusions regarding the effects of aspirin in primary prevention.

To date, the two randomized trials of aspirin in primary prevention have been in men. The available data on aspirin use in apparently healthy women comes from observational studies. The findings of these studies are inconsistent, with two studies suggesting benefit (51,52) and two reporting no apparent effect (53,54). A currently ongoing large-scale trial begun in 1992, the Women's Health Study (55), will assess the benefits and risks

TABLE 25-2. *Aspirin in primary prevention: U.S. Physicians' Health Study and British Doctors' Trial*

Endpoint	Percent reduction ± SD among those assigned aspirin		
	U.S. Physicians' Health Study	British Doctors' Trial	Overview
Nonfatal MI	39 ± 9	3 ± 19	32 ± 8
Nonfatal stroke	↑19 ± 15	↑13 ± 24	↑18 ± 13
Total vascular mortality	2 ± 15	7 ± 14	5 ± 10
Important vascular events	18 ± 7	4 ± 12	13 ± 6

↑, Nonsignificant increased risk among aspirin-allocated subjects.

of low- dose aspirin in apparently healthy women. Approximately 40,000 women, aged 45 years and older, have been randomized to either aspirin 100 mg on alternate days or placebo. The trial is also testing vitamin E (600 IU on alternate days) in the primary prevention of cancer and cardiovascular disease. Aspirin and warfarin are being evaluated in primary prevention in the Thrombosis Prevention Trial, a randomized trial of low-dose aspirin (75 mg daily) and low-intensity oral anticoagulation with warfarin (INR 1.5) in men aged 45 to 69 in the United Kingdom who are at high risk of ischemic heart disease (56).

CONCLUSION

Antiplatelet therapy, chiefly with aspirin, has clear benefits in secondary prevention for patients who have suffered a prior cardiovascular event. A recent updated overview of antiplatelet trials in secondary prevention showed that when all high-risk patients were considered, there were statistically significant reductions of 27% for all important vascular events (MI, stroke, or vascular death), 35% for nonfatal MI, 31% for nonfatal stroke, and 18% for vascular death. The updated overview also indicated that the benefits in secondary prevention extend to a far broader range of patients than was previously demonstrated. Significant benefits not only accrue to survivors of an MI, stroke, or TIA, but also to patients with peripheral vascular disease, atrial fibrillation, chronic stable angina, or valvular disease, as well as those undergoing revascularization procedures. Moreover, these benefits were observed in high-risk patients regardless of their age or gender or the presence of hypertension or diabetes. At present, daily doses of 50 to 80 mg of aspirin may be appropriate for long-term secondary prevention in all patients with prior episodes of occlusive vascular disease in the heart and peripheral arteries. For stroke, the fact that benefits on subsequent stroke are similar for coronary heart disease patients given low doses and stroke and TIA patients given high doses suggests that lower doses may suffice.

On the other hand, the pathophysiology of stroke may differ in patients with prior coronary versus cerebrovascular disease. If so, then higher doses, which cause more side effects, may nonetheless be warranted in cerebrovascular disease patients.

The more widespread use of aspirin in secondary prevention would avoid perhaps 10,000 premature deaths each year in the United States. As regards the approved professional labeling indications for aspirin, in the 1980s the U.S. Food and Drug Administration approved labeling of aspirin for patients with prior myocardial infarction and unstable angina, as well as for men with prior transient ischemic attacks. In January 1997, at a joint meeting of the FDA's Nonprescription Drugs and Cardiovascular and Renal Drugs Advisory Committees, the members voted to recommend that the FDA expand the professional labeling indication for aspirin to include women as well as men with prior transient ischemic attacks, patients with prior occlusive stroke or chronic stable angina, and those who have undergone arterial revascularization procedures (either bypass surgery or percutaneous transluminal angioplasty).

With respect to comparisons of the effects of different antiplatelet therapies in the secondary prevention of cardiovascular disease, no clear differences were demonstrated in either the original or updated overview between aspirin and other antiplatelets (including sulfinpyrazone, combined aspirin and dipyridamole, or ticlopidine). However, very recently, and notwithstanding the fact that more testing is needed, a randomized trial of clopidogrel versus aspirin in secondary prevention indicated a small but significant advantage of clopidogrel over aspirin in reducing risk of a combined endpoint of ischemic stroke, MI, or vascular death. In addition, a new class of antiplatelet drug, GP IIb/IIIa integrin antagonists, appears promising, although testing at this time has been limited to intravenous administration in patients undergoing high-risk coronary interventions or those with unstable angina or acute MI.

While anticoagulants have also been shown to be of net benefit in the secondary prevention of cardiovascular disease, they are associated with more bleeding than is aspirin. Further, trials comparing anticoagulants (warfarin) with aspirin have not found significant differences in risks of reinfarction or death. There are, however, currently ongoing trials assessing the efficacy of low-dose aspirin plus low-intensity warfarin as compared to aspirin alone in prevention of recurrent MI in individuals who have survived an initial MI.

For primary prevention, the risk of a first MI in men is reduced conclusively by about a third by the use of low-dose aspirin. As expected, the absolute risk reduction, about four events per 1,000 patients treated, is much smaller than that achieved with treatment in secondary prevention Further, the evidence for stroke and vascular mortality remains inconclusive due to inadequate numbers of endpoints in both the primary prevention trials and their overviews. In addition, there are no data of randomized trials conducted in women. Thus, policy recommendations must await the accrual of a sufficient totality of evidence from the Women's Health Study and the Thrombosis Prevention Trial. In the meanwhile, primary aspirin prophylaxis may be considered as an individual clinical judgment by the health care provider for patients whose risk of first MI is sufficiently high to justify possible side effects of long-term aspirin use. For primary prevention, a daily dose of 50 to 80 mg seems sufficient to achieve the benefit and minimize side effects. Aspirin should always be considered an adjunct rather than an alternative to treating or eliminating other risk factors for cardiovascular disease, including cigarette smoking, elevated cholesterol levels, and hypertension.

Summary of Key Concepts

Certainties

Antiplatelets (namely aspirin) have clear benefits for secondary prevention of MI in patients who have suffered a prior cardiovascular event. Considering all high-risk patients together, treatment yields reductions of about one third in nonfatal stroke, one third in nonfatal MI, and one sixth in vascular death.

Anticoagulants have also been demonstrated to have clear benefits for secondary prevention of MI. However, the net benefit is less clear than with antiplatelets, due at least in part to the higher risk of bleeding.

For primary prevention, risk of a first MI is reduced conclusively by about a third by the use of low-dose aspirin.

Uncertainties

A recent randomized trial of clopidogrel versus aspirin in secondary prevention indicated that clopidogrel was marginally more effective than aspirin in reducing a combined endpoint of ischemic stroke, MI, or vascular death. Specifically, with randomization of nearly 20,000 patients, there was a small reduction in the annual rate of this combined endpoint among those receiving clopidogrel compared with aspirin (5.32% versus 5.83%), with a modest p value of 0.043. As no serious complications were reported, this medication can be considered an equivalent alternative to aspirin. Ongoing and planned trials will provide additional comparisons of the benefit-to-risk ratios of various antiplatelet regimens in secondary prevention.

Future Topics

For primary prevention of cardiovascular disease, whether there are beneficial effects of low-dose aspirin on stroke and vascular mortality remains inconclusive due to inadequate numbers of these events in the randomized trials that have been conducted to date or their overviews.

For primary prevention of cardiovascular disease, whether the beneficial results obtained in clinical trials of men are generalizable to women is also uncertain.

REFERENCES

1. Antiplatelet Trialists' Collaboration. Secondary prevention of vascular events by prolonged antiplatelet therapy. *Br Med J* 1988;296:320–331.

2. Antiplatelet Trialists' Collaboration. Collaborative overview of randomized trials of antiplatelet therapy—I. Prevention of death, myocardial infarction, and stroke by prolonged antiplatelet therapy in various categories of patients. *Br Med J* 1994;308:81–106.

3. Schoenberger J and the Aspirin Myocardial Infarction Study Research Group. A randomized, controlled trial of aspirin in persons recovered from myocardial infarction. *JAMA* 1980;243:661–669.

4. Klimt CR, Knatterud GL, Stamler J, Meier P. Persantine-aspirin reinfarction study, part II: secondary prevention with persantine and aspirin. *J Am Coll Cardiol* 1986;7:251–269

5. Krol WF and the Persantine-Aspirin Reinfarction Study Research Group. Persantine and aspirin in coronary heart disease. *Circulation* 1980;62:449–461.

6. Krol WF, Klint CR, Morledge J, Haberman S, Stamler J, for the Persantine-Aspirin Reinfarction Study Research Group. Persantine-aspirin reinfarction study: design, methods and baseline results. *Circulation* 1980;62(suppl II):II-1–II-22.

7. Elwood PC, Sweetnam PM. Aspirin and secondary mortality after myocardial infarction. *Lancet* 1979;2:1313–1315.

8. Sherry S, Gent M, Lilienfeld A, McGregor M, Mustard F, Yu P, and the Anturane Reinfarction Trial Research Group. Sulfinpyrazone in the prevention of sudden death after myocardial infarction. *N Engl J Med* 1980;302:250–256.

9. Stamler J, Berge KG, Berkson DM, and the Coronary Drug Project Research Group. Aspirin in coronary heart disease. *J Chron Dis* 1976;29:625–642.

10. Vogel G, Fischer C, Huyke R. Prevention of reinfarction with acetylsalicylic acid. In: Breddin K, Loew D, Ueberla K, Dorndorf W, Marx R (eds). *Prophylaxis of venous, peripheral, cardiac and cerebral vascular diseases with acetylsalicylic acid.* Stuttgart: Schattauer, 1981;123–128.

11. Elwood PC, Cochrane AL, Burr ML, et al. A randomized controlled trial of acetylsalicylic acid in the secondary prevention of mortality from myocardial infarction. *Br Med J* 1974;1:436–440.

12. Elwood PC. Trial of acetylsalicylic acid in the secondary prevention of mortality from myocardial infarction. *Br Med J* 1981;282:481.

13. Polli EE, Cortellaro M. The Anturan reinfarction study. In: Polli EE, Cortellaro M (eds). *Secondary prevention of ischaemic cardiac events: present status and new perspectives.* Berne: Hans Huber, 1983;51–60.

14. Polli E, Cortellano M, Baroni L, et al. Anturan Reinfarction Italian Study: Sulphinpyrazone in post-myocardial infarction. *Lancet* 1982;1:237–242.

15. Breddin K, Loew D, Lechner K, Ueberla K, Walter E. Secondary prevention of myocardial infarction: a comparison of acetylsalicylic acid, placebo and phenprocoumon. *Haemostasis* 1980;9:325–344.

16. Lowenthal A, Dom L, Moens E, and the European Stroke Prevention Study Group. European stroke prevention study: principal end points. *Lancet* 1987;2:1351–1354.

17. Peto R, Warlow C, and the UK-TIA Study Group. United Kingdom transient ischaemic attack (UK-TIA) aspirin trial: interim results. *Br Med J* 1988;296:316–320.

18. Bousser MG, Eschwege E, Haguenau M, Lefauconnier JM, Touboul D, Touboul PJ. Essai cooperatif controle "AICLA": Prevention secondaire des accidents ischemiques cerebraux lies a l'atherosclerose par l'aspirine et le dipyridamole. *Rev Neurol (Paris)* 1981;5:333–341.

19. Bousser MG, Eschwege E, Haguenau M. AICLA controlled trial of aspirin and dypridamole in the secondary prevention of atherothrombotic cerebral ischemia. *Stroke* 1983;14:5–14.

20. Barnett HJM, Gent M, Sackett DL, and the Canadian Cooperative Study Group. A randomized trial of aspirin and sulfinpyrazone in threatened stroke. *N Engl J Med* 1978;299:53–59.

21. Britton M, Helmers C, Samuelsson K. High dose salicylic acid after cerebral infarction [Abstract]. *Stroke* 1986;17:132.

22. Britton M, Helmers C, Samuelsson K. High dose salicylic acid after cerebral infarction. A Swedish co-operative study. *Stroke* 1987;18:325–334.

23. Gent M, Blakely JA, Hachinski V, et al. A secondary prevention, randomized trial of suloctidil in patients with a recent history of thromboembolic stroke. *Stroke* 1985;16:416–423.

24. Guiraud-Chaumeil B, Rascol A, David J, Boneu B, Clanet M, Bierme R. Prevention des recidives des accidents vasculaires cerebraux ischemiques per les anti-aggregants plaquettaires. *Rev Neurol (Paris)* 1982;138:367–385.

25. Fields WS, Lemak NA, Frankowski RF, Hardy RJ. Controlled trial of aspirin in cerebral ischemia. *Stroke* 1977;8:301–316.

26. Fields WS, Lemak NA, Frankowski RF, Hardy RJ. Controlled trial of aspirin in cerebral ischemia. *Stroke* 1978;9:309–318.

27. Blakely JA. A prospective trial of sulphinpyrazone and survival after thrombotic stroke [Abstract]. *Thromb Diathesis Haemorrhagica* 1979;42:161.

28. Sorensen PS, Pedersen H, Marquardsen J, et al. Acetylsalicylic acid in the prevention of stroke in patients with reversible cerebral ischaemic attacks: a Danish cooperative study. *Stroke* 1983;14:15–22.

29. Acheson J, Danta G, Hutchison EC. Controlled trial of dipyridamole in cerebral vascular disease [Abstract]. *Br Med J* 1969;1:614–615.

30. Robertson JT, Dugdale M, Salky N, Robinson H. The effect of a platelet inhibiting drug in the therapy of patients with transient ischaemic attacks and strokes. *Thromb Diatheses Haemorrhagica* 1975;34:598.

31. Reuther R, Dorndorf W. Aspirin in patients with cerebral ischaemia and normal angiograms: the results of a double blind trial. In: Breddin K, Dorndorf W, Loew D, Marx R (eds). *Acetylsalicylic acid in cerebral ischaemia and coronary heat disease.* Stuttgart: Schattauer Verlag, 1978;97–106.

32. Lewis HD Jr, David JW, Archibald DG, et al. Protective effects of aspirin against myocardial infarction and death in men with unstable angina: results of a Veterans Administration cooperative study. *N Engl J Med* 1983;309:396–405.

33. Cairns JA, Gent M, Singer J, et al. Aspirin, sulfinpyrazone or both in unstable angina. *N Engl J Med* 1985;313:1369–1375.

34. Moncada S, Vane JR. Archidonic acid metabolites and the interactions between platelets and blood-vessel walls. *N Engl J Med* 1979;300:1142–1147.

35. Hennekens CH. Update on aspirin in the primary and secondary prevention of CV disease. *Hospital Med* 1997;January:15–21.

36. Hass WK, Easton JD (eds). *Ticlopidine, platelets and vascular disease.* New York: Springer-Verlag, 1993.

37. Moloney BA. An analysis of the side-effects of ticlopidine. In: Hass WK, Easton JD (eds). *Ticlopidine, platelets and vascular disease.* New York: Springer-Verlag, 1993;117–139.

38. CAPRIE Steering Committe. A randomized, blinded, trial of clopidogrel versus aspirin in patients at risk of ischaemic events (CAPRIE). *Lancet* 1996;348:1329–1338.

39. Topol EJ. Novel antithrombotic approaches to coronary artery disease. *Am J Cardiol* 1995;75:27B–33B.

40. Topol EJ, Califf RM, Weisman HF, et al., on behalf of the EPIC investigators. Randomized trial of coronary intervention with antibody against platelet IIb/IIIa integrio for reduction of clinical restenosis: results at six monts. *Lancet* 1994;343:881–886.

41. Verheugt FWA. In search of a superaspirin for the heart. *Lancet* 1997;349:1409–1410.

42. Sixty Plus Reinfarction Study Research Group. A double-blind trial to assess long-term anticoagulant therapy in elderly patients after myocardial infarction. *Lancet* 1980;2:989–993.

43. Smith P, Arnesen H, Holme I. The effect of warfarin on mortality and reinfarction. *N Engl J Med* 1990;323: 147–152.

44. Breddin D, Loew D, Lechner K, et al. The German-Austrian Aspirin Trial. A comparison of aspirin, placebo and phenprocoumon in secondary prevention of myocardial infarction. *Circulation*(suppl V) 1980;62:V63–V72.

45. The EPSIM Research Group. A controlled comparison of aspirin and oral anticoagulants in prevention of death after myocardial infarction. *N Engl J Med* 1982;307: 701–708.

46. Goodman SG, Langer A, Durica SS, et al. Safety and anticoagulation effect of a low-dose combination of warfarin and aspririn in clinically stable coronary artery disease. *Am J Cardiol* 1994;74:657–661.

47. Hennekens CH, Buring JE, Sandercock P, Collins R, Peto R. Aspirin and other antiplatelet agents in the secondary and primary prevention of cardiovascular disease. *Circulation* 1989;80:749–756.

48. The Steering Committee of the Physicians Health Study Research Group. Final report on the aspirin component of the Physicians' Health Study. *N Engl J Med* 1989; 321:129–135.

49. Peto R, Gray R, Collins R, et al. A randomized trial of the effects of proplylactic daily aspirin in British male doctors. *Br Med J* 1988;296:313–316.

50. Hennekens CH, Peto R, Hutchison GB, Doll R. An overview of the British and American aspirin studies. *N Engl J Med* 1988;318:923–924.

51. Boston Collaborative Drug Surveillance Group. Regular aspirin intake and acute myocardial infarction. *Br Med J* 1974;1:440–443.

52. Manson JE, Stampfer MJ, Colditz GA, et al. A Prospective study of aspirin use and primary prevention of cardiovascular disease in women. *JAMA* 1991;266:521–527.

53. Hammond EC, Garfinkel L. Aspirin and cornary heart disease: findings of a prospective study. *Br Med J* 1975;2:269–271.

54. Paganini-Hill A, Chao A, Ross RK, Henderson BE. Aspirin use and chronic diseases: a cohort study of the elderly. *Br Med J* 1989;299:1247–1250.

55. Buring JE, Hennekens CH, for the Women's Health Study Research Group. Women's Health Study: rational and background. *J Myocard Ischemia* 1992;4:30–40.

56. Meade TW, Wilkes HC, Stirling Y, Brennan PJ, Kelleher C, Browne W. Randomized controlled trial of low dose warfarin in the primary prevention of ischaemic heart disease in men at high risk: design and pilot study. *Eur Heart J* 1988;9:836–843.

*Cardiovascular Thrombosis: Thrombocardiology
and Thromboneurology, Second Edition,*
edited by M. Verstraete, V. Fuster, and E. J. Topol,
Lippincott–Raven Publishers, Philadelphia © 1998.

26

Acute Phase Treatment of Myocardial Infarction: Selecting Patients for Thrombolysis

Frans J. Van de Werf and *Eric J. Topol

*Department of Cardiology, University Hospital Gasthuisberg, B-3000 Leuven, Belgium; and
Department of Cardiology, The Cleveland Clinic Foundation, Cleveland, Ohio 44195

Thrombolytic therapy has become standard treatment in the majority of patients with a suspected acute myocardial infarction. Tens of thousands of patients have been studied in megatrials that have unequivocally identified coronary artery reperfusion in general and thrombolysis more particularly as the mainstay of acute treatment of patients with this disease.

As with most diseases, development of an effective treatment for acute myocardial infarction was contingent on understanding its pathophysiology. The key concepts of thrombotic occlusion as the direct cause of an acute myocardial infarction and the possibility of myocardial salvage by restoration of coronary flow fostered a decade of clinical research in thrombolytic therapy (1). Although thrombolysis is one of the best studied therapeutic strategies of modern medicine, many uncertainties still remain with regard to the selection of patients for this type of treatment. In this chapter, we present guidelines for selecting patients with an acute myocardial infarction for thrombolysis and for selecting the most appropriate thrombolytic agent and absolute and relative contraindications for this type of therapy.

SELECTING PATIENTS FOR THROMBOLYSIS

The Time Window for Treatment

An overview of nearly all placebo-controlled trials of intravenous thrombolytic therapy by the Fibrinolytic Therapy Trialists (FTT) Collaborative Group, encompassing almost 60,000 patients, has clearly shown that thrombolytic therapy is beneficial in patients with suspected acute myocardial infarction admitted to the hospital within 12 hours after the onset of symptoms (2). Among the 45,000 patients presenting with ST-segment elevations or bundle-branch block, highly significant absolute mortality reductions of 30 per 1,000 for patients presenting within 6 hours and of about 20 per 1,000 for those presenting between 6 and 12 hours after the onset of symptoms have been clearly demonstrated. In patients presenting 13 to 18 hours after the onset of infarction, a statistically uncertain benefit of about 10 lives saved per 1,000 was found. The results of this overview indicate an almost straight-line relationship between absolute mortality reduction and delay from onset of infarction up to 21 hours after onset with every additional hour of delay associated with a reduction in the benefit of about 1.6 (standard deviation 0.6) lives per 1,000 patients (Fig. 26-1).

This FTT analysis probably underestimates the benefit of early thrombolysis because, as pointed out by Rawles, this analysis is heavily weighted by patients treated too late for myocardial salvage to have been the mechanism of benefit (3). For patients treated within the time window of 0 to 2.5 hours, Rawles calculated a possible maximum benefit of about 34 lives per 1,000 patients per hour of earlier treatment (3). In an analysis performed by Boersma et al. (4), the benefit of thrombolytic

therapy was significantly higher in patients presenting within 2 hours after the onset of symptoms as compared with those presenting later: 44% versus 20% (p = 0.001) (Fig. 26-2). Boersma et al. concluded that the relationship between treatment delay and absolute reduction in early mortality is better described by a nonlinear than a linear regression equation (Fig. 26-3), further supporting the concept of a first golden hour.

Many investigators have studied prehospital administration of thrombolytic agents. The feasibility, safety, and time-saving value (about 2 hours with domiciliary and 1 hour with mobile care thrombolysis) have been demonstrated in well-designed trials (the European Myocardial Infarction Project [EMIP] [5]; the Myocardial Infarction Triage and Intervention Project [MITI] [6]; and the Grampian Region Early Anistreplase Trial [GREAT] [7]). Although in all these trials the mortality rates were lower with prehospital administration, in none of the trials did the difference reach statistical significance. Nevertheless, a meta-analysis (8) of the three trials mentioned above and of five other smaller trials clearly showed the cumulative salutary impact of prehospital thrombolysis with a significant reduction in early mortality

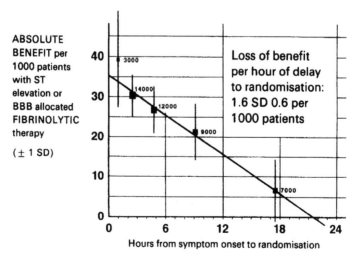

FIG. 26-1. Absolute reduction in 35-day mortality versus delay from symptom onset to randomization (thrombolysis versus placebo) among 45,000 patients with ST-segment elevation or bundle-branch block. (Data from the FTT analysis, ref. 2, with permission.)

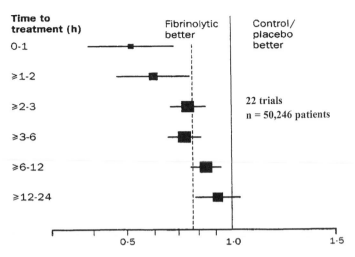

FIG. 26-2. Proportional effect of thrombolytic therapy versus placebo on 35-day mortality according to treatment delay. (From Boersma et al., ref. 4, with permission.)

of 16.7% and 18 lives saved per 1,000 patients treated as compared with hospital thrombolysis. The relationship between duration of symptoms and clinical outcome described above is supported by data from studies that examined the relationship between treatment delay and reduction in infarct size. For example, in a study of 432 patients presenting within 6 hours of the onset of symptoms of first acute myocardial infarction, the myocardial area at risk before thrombolysis has been estimated from the number and height of the ST-segment elevations on the admission electrocardiogram and compared with the final infarct size after treatment measured with thallium 201 scintigraphy (9). In this study, each 30-minute treat-

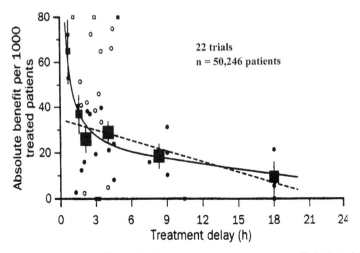

FIG. 26-3. Absolute 35-day mortality reduction versus treatment delay. Full dots, information from trials included in the FTT analysis (2); open dots, information from additional trials; black squares, average effects in six time-to-treatment groups (areas of squares inversely proportional to variance of absolute benefit described). (From Boersma et al., ref. 4, with permission.)

ment delay was associated with an increase in infarct size of 1%. After 4 hours there was no difference in final infarct size between treated patients and patients who did not receive thrombolysis (Fig. 26-4). Similarly, in the MITI trial (6), very early treatment (within less than 70 minutes of symptom onset) was associated with a marked attenuation of infarct size.

In conclusion, all patients with an acute myocardial infarction presenting to the hospital within 12 hours of symptom onset (and with ST-segment elevation or bundle-branch block, see next section) have a significantly reduced mortality when given thrombolytic therapy. The sooner thrombolysis is started the greater the benefit. In very early treated patients, an infarction can be aborted with successful thrombolysis. There are no (statistically) convincing data supporting the use of thrombolytic therapy in patients after 12 hours, although a mortality reduction of 10 per 1,000 patients in those presenting between 12 and 18 hours is possible. It is likely that during the first 2 to 3 hours successful thrombolysis saves about 30 lives per 1,000 patients treated. Therefore, in rural regions where important transport delays exist, prehospital thrombolysis is probably beneficial provided that experienced personnel is available on the

ambulance and that an electrocardiogram can be taken and analyzed.

The Presenting Electrocardiogram

As shown by the FTT analysis (2), the benefit of thrombolysis is larger in patients with ST-segment elevations or bundle-branch block on admission (Fig. 26-5). A greater absolute mortality reduction was observed in patients with ST-segment elevations in the anterior leads than in those with inferior ST-segment elevations (3.7% versus 0.9% at 35 days). In this analysis no significant mortality reduction has been observed among patients with ST-segment depression. On the contrary, among the patients with ST-segment depression on admission mortality at 35 days was nonsignificantly higher after thrombolysis (15.2%) than in similar control patients (13.8%), representing a 13% proportional increase with 99% confidence intervals ranging from a 12% reduction to an increase of 44%. As a consequence of this and other trial results (Thrombolysis in Myocardial Infarction [TIMI IIIB] [10]), patients without ST-segment elevations on admission are currently not being given thrombolytic therapy. A possible explanation for the ineffectiveness of thrombolysis or even for a worse outcome in this category of

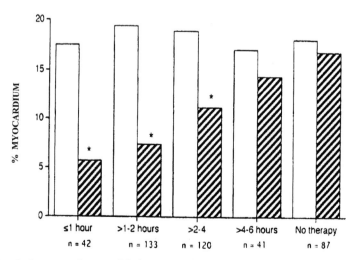

FIG. 26-4. Estimated myocardium at risk (*open bars*) calculated from the number and height of the ST-segment elevations on admission (Aldrich score) and final infarct size (*hatched bars*) after thrombolysis measured with thallium 201 scintigraphy. (Data from Raitt et al., ref. 9.)

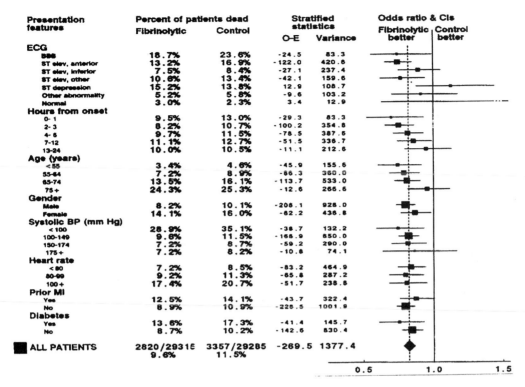

FIG. 26-5. Proportional effects of thrombolytic therapy on 35-day mortality subdivided by presentation features. (From the FTT Collaborative Group, ref. 2, with permission.)

patients is the plasmin-mediated procoagulant effects of fibrinolytic therapy. After lysis of the fibrin network by plasmin there is exposure of thrombin and enhanced thrombin activity (11,12). Exposed thrombin is one of the most potent activators of platelets and, autocatalytically, stimulates further thrombin formation. Thus, it is possible that in some patients the nonobstructive mural thrombus on the ruptured plaque could progress to occlusion during thrombolysis. The policy of withholding thrombolysis from patients without ST-segment elevations can be criticized. Patients with unstable coronary syndromes and ST-segment depression on admission are a very heterogeneous group. Some of these patients with ST-segment depression in the anterior leads may actually be developing a true transmural posterior infarction. The presence of ST-segment elevations in the posteriorly recorded leads V7–V8 and of prominent R waves in leads V1–V2 can be

helpful in making the diagnosis of a true posterior infarction. Other patients may develop a non–Q-wave infarction or may have unstable angina without myocardial cell necrosis. In general, the deeper the ST-segment depression and the greater the number of leads with ST-segment depression, the greater the likelihood of developing myocardial necrosis (13). In view of these considerations, it is not so surprising that among the 528 patients with confirmed non–Q-wave infarction and with ST-segment depression of ≥2 mm on admission who participated in the Late Assessment of Thrombolytic Efficacy (LATE) study, mortality rates were significantly lower in those who received thrombolysis: 8.6% versus 16.6% at 35 days (p < 0.006) and 20.1% versus 31.9% at 1 year (p < 0.006) (14) (Fig. 26-6). Thus, the overall outcomes observed after thrombolysis in the FTT analysis may well represent the net result of a benefit in patients with a non–Q-wave (or a

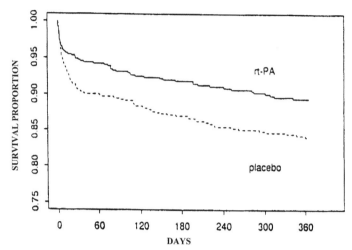

FIG. 26-6. Cumulative 1-year survival rates in patients with non–Q-wave myocardial infarction treated with rt-PA (*solid lines*) or placebo (*dashed lines*) in the LATE study. (From Langer et al., ref. 14, with permission.)

transmural posterior) myocardial infarction and a harm in patients with unstable angina. New prospective trials are required to evaluate the possible benefit of thrombolysis in patients with ST-segment depression and confirmed acute myocardial infarction. In the absence of these results, the administration of thrombolytic therapy in selected patients with important ST-segment depression (≥ 2 mm) may be justified, especially in those thought to have an evolving posterior wall infarction and in whom no invasive procedures can be performed.

In the FTT overview, about 2,000 patients with bundle-branch block were randomized and mortality rates among these patients were high (2), supporting the knowledge that (new) bundle-branch block is usually associated with extensive myocardial necrosis and/or a previous myocardial infarction. Although left bundle-branch block but not right bundle-branch block may obscure the diagnosis of acute myocardial infarction, no distinction was made in the FTT analysis between both conduction abnormalities. Hence, the differential effect of thrombolysis on both conduction disturbances, complicating an acute myocardial infarction, is unknown. The GUSTO-I investigators have identified electrocardiographic criteria on admission that significantly increase the likeli-

hood of acute myocardial infarction in patients with left bundle-branch block (15). These electrocardiographic criteria are elevation of the ST segment of 1 mm or more that are in the same direction of the QRS complex; ST-segment depression of 1 mm or more in leads V1, V2, or V3; and ST-segment elevations of 5 mm or more that are in the opposite direction from the QRS complex.

In conclusion, patients with ischemic chest pain presenting with ST-segment elevations or bundle-branch block accompanied by ST-segment changes are the ideal candidates for thrombolysis in the absence of contraindications. Although the benefit of thrombolytic therapy is greater in patients with anterior infarction, in patients with inferior infarction the benefit from this therapy outweighs the risks. In selected patients presenting with typical symptoms and with ST-segment depression of ≥ 2 mm thrombolytic therapy may be beneficial as well, especially if true posterior wall infarction is likely. More studies in patients with ST-segment depressions are needed.

Age

As shown in GUSTO-I, older patients have a higher-risk profile with regard to baseline clin-

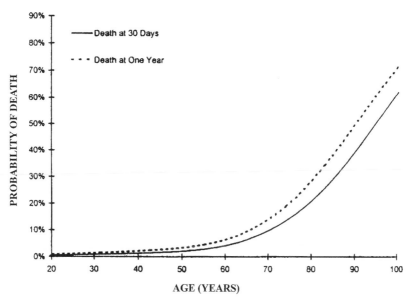

FIG. 26-7. Probability of death at 30 days and 1 year as a function of age in GUSTO-I. (From White et al., ref. 17, with permission.)

ical and angiographic characteristics (16,17). Even in the era of reperfusion therapy, advanced age remains the single most important independent risk factor predicting early and late mortality (18). In GUSTO-I, in which all patients received thrombolytic therapy, mortality rates at 30 days ranged from 1.1% in patients more than 45 years of age to more than 20% in those over 75 years of age (16–18). The probability of 30-day and 1-year mortality as a function of age in this trial is shown in Fig. 26-7. A striking increase in the risk for early and late death is observed in the elderly.

In earlier, placebo-controlled trials of thrombolytic therapy, advanced age was often an exclusion criterion because of concerns about the risk of intracranial hemorrhage. Nevertheless, data from five placebo-controlled trials indicate a greater absolute reduction in mortality with thrombolysis in elderly patients as compared with younger patients: 2.1 lives saved per 100 patients under the age of 65 years versus 4.2 lives saved per 100 patients over the age of 65 years (19).

In the GUSTO-I trial, not only mortality but also the incidence of major complications such as stroke (both hemorrhagic and non-

hemorrhagic), shock, bleeding, and reinfarction increased dramatically with age as shown in Table 26-1 (17). Despite these high event rates, recent analyses from GUSTO-I and other trials indicate that thrombolytic therapy is nevertheless very cost effective in the elderly (20,21).

In conclusion, advanced age should not be considered a contraindication for thrombolysis. Severe hypertension and other comorbidity associated with an increased risk of (intracranial) bleeding must be taken into account when deciding whether to give thrombolysis to elderly patients with a suspected acute myocardial infarction.

Gender

Women experience myocardial infarction an average of 10 years later than men, but after menopause the rates become increasingly similar, and by 70 to 75 years of age the rates are almost the same. The higher prevalence of female gender in elderly patients with acute myocardial infarction is illustrated in the data from the GUSTO-I trial. The proportions of female patients in the different age categories

TABLE 26-1. *Major clinical events after thrombolysis in different age categories in the GUSTO-I trial*

	Age (years)			
	<65 (n = 24,708)	65–74 (n = 11,201)	75–85 (n = 4,625)	>85 (n = 412)
In-hospital mortality, n (%)	2.8	9.1	19.1	27.9
30-day mortality, n (%)	3.0	9.5	19.6	30.3
Stroke, n (%)	0.8	2.1	3.4	2.9
Hemorrhagic	0.3	1.0	1.6	1.7
Nonhemorrhagic	0.4	0.9	1.3	0.5
Hemorrhagic conversion	0.1	0.1	0.2	0.1
Unknown	0.04	0.1	0.4	0.5
Nonfatal, disabling	0.3	0.7	0.9	0.7
Death or stroke, n (%)	3.6	10.7	21.0	31.6
Death or hemorrhagic stroke, n (%)	3.2	9.9	20.0	30.8
Death or nonfatal disabling stroke, n (%)	3.3	10.2	20.5	31.1
Bleeding, n (%)	9.5	15.8	20.5	23.1
Severe	0.8	1.6	2.5	1.7
Moderate	8.7	14.2	18.0	21.4

Data from White et al., ref. 17, with permission.

in GUSTO-I were less than 65 years, 27%; 65 to 74 years, 33%; 75 to 85 years, 44%; and more than 85 years, 56% (17). Thrombolytic therapy reduces mortality in both women and men. In the FTT analysis the proportional reduction in mortality among women was slightly smaller (12% versus 19% in men), but the absolute reduction was almost identical for both sexes (around 2%) (2).

In the GUSTO-I study, in which all patients were given thrombolytic therapy, female sex had only a borderline significant relation (p = 0.043) with 30-day mortality (18), and beyond 30 days no gender-specific differences in outcome could be demonstrated after adjustments for baseline risk factors (Fig. 26-8) (22). Similarly, in the GISSI-2/International Study Group trial, after adjusting for worse baseline characteristics, women had the same mortality rate as men (23–25). In this trial, thrombolytic therapy in women was associated with a significantly higher incidence of hemorrhagic stroke (adjusted odds ratio of 1.72 with 95% confidence interval [CI] of 1.04 to 2.85) (25). In the larger GUSTO-I trial, however, female sex was not retained as an independent risk factor for hemorrhagic stroke, although women in this trial also were much more likely to experience intracranial hemorrhage than men (26).

The prognostic information already contained in the combination of age, weight and blood pressure (three significant, independent predictors of intracranial hemorrhage in GUSTO-I) can explain the lack of a consistent, independent association between female gender and hemorrhagic stroke despite a striking univariable relationship (26).

In conclusion, the early and long-term benefits of thrombolytic therapy are equal in both sexes. Due to a lower weight and, often, an advanced age, in association with a higher blood pressure, female patients with an acute myocardial infarction have a higher risk for intracranial hemorrhage as compared with men, although the absolute increase is small. This should not be a reason for withholding thrombolytic therapy from women with an acute myocardial infarction.

Diabetes

Diabetic patients with acute myocardial infarction have a worse prognosis (27). They are less likely to be treated with thrombolytic agents because of concerns about the increased risk of retinal and other bleeding complications.

In the FTT overview, the excess of stroke and major bleeds associated with fibrinolytic therapy was only slightly higher in diabetic

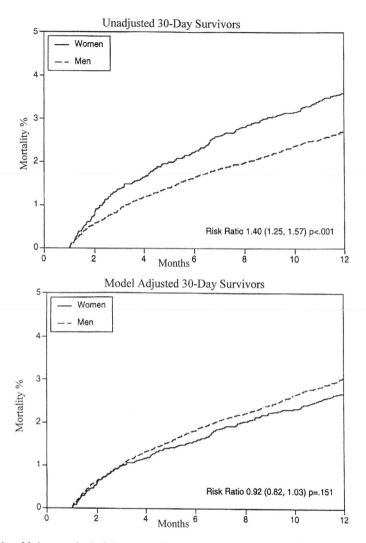

FIG. 26-8. Kaplan-Meier survival plots comparing women versus men who had survived the first 30 days. **Upper panel:** unadjusted. **Lower panel:** adjusted for baseline characteristics and 30-day mortality according to the model of Lee et al. (From Moen et al., ref. 22, with permission.)

patients (2). Also in the GISSI-2/International Study Group trial the incidence of these complications was similar among diabetic and nondiabetic patients (28).

With regard to efficacy, the proportional and absolute reductions in mortality with thrombolysis were slightly and nonsignificantly greater among diabetic patients in the FTT analysis: 21.4% and 3.7% versus 14.7% and 1.3%, respectively (2). In addition, it has been shown in the GUSTO-I angiographic substudy that thrombolytic therapy is equally efficacious in restoring early coronary artery patency in patients with and without diabetes (29). Nevertheless, despite thrombolytic therapy, mortality rates among diabetic patients remain high, and even after adjusting for both clinical and angiographic variables, diabetes remains an independent determinant of early mortality (29). A higher reocclusion rate and a reduced hyperkinesis in the noninfarcted zone after acute coronary occlusion may contribute to the increased prevalence of heart failure and mortality observed in diabetics (29).

In conclusion, diabetic patients with an acute myocardial infarction are at least equally good candidates for thrombolytic therapy as are nondiabetics. There is no convincing evidence that the risk of bleeding is higher in diabetic patients as compared with similar nondiabetic patients. Despite effective treatment with fibrinolytic agents, diabetics have a worse clinical outcome.

Shock

Cardiogenic shock is considered to be an indication for primary angioplasty due to concerns that thrombolytic therapy might be ineffective (30,31). In the GISSI-I study (32), hospital mortality rates in patients in Killip class IV were high (70.0%), with no difference between control patients and patients treated with streptokinase (69.9% versus 70.1%, respectively).

Also in the FTT overview (2), although the numbers are small, patients with both systolic blood pressure of less than 100 mmHg and heart rate over 100 beats/min were at high risk, with a lower 35-day mortality rate in those given thrombolytic therapy than in control patients: 53.8% (71 of 132) versus 61.1% (88 of 144). This difference was not statistically significant.

In conclusion, patients in cardiogenic shock should undergo primary angioplasty if this procedure can be performed by an experienced team without delay. If immediate primary angiography is not possible, thrombolytic therapy (preferably a nonfibrin-specific agent such as streptokinase) should be given to patients in cardiogenic shock.

Hypertension

A history of hypertension and high systolic or diastolic blood pressure on admission are associated with an increased risk of bleeding complications, especially intracranial hemorrhage. In the GUSTO-I trial, hypertension (in the past or at the time of enrollment) was not an exclusion criterion. A systolic blood pres-

sure of ≥180 mmHg, unresponsive to therapy, at entry was considered to be a relative contraindication to enrollment, but the final decision whether or not to enroll was left to the investigator. Data from this trial indicate that in patients with an acute myocardial infarction and a high systolic blood pressure at entry, the risk for death was similar to that in normotensive patients (excluding patients with systolic blood pressure of less than 120 mmHg, in whom the risk for death was higher) (33).

The risk for intracranial hemorrhage, however, increased with systolic blood pressure. There was no threshold for this effect, but at systolic blood pressures of ≥170 mmHg, the probability curve became steeper (Fig. 26-9). For example, the incidence of intracranial hemorrhage in patients with a systolic blood pressure on entry of ≥175 mmHg was 1.71%, which is more than twice the rate observed in patients with a normal systolic blood pressure on admission.

The effect of elevated diastolic blood pressures at entry on clinical outcomes in GUSTO-I was less striking. There was a slight increase in the rates of intracranial hemorrhage with increasing diastolic blood pressure, whereas no significant changes in mortality were observed with diastolic blood pressures ≥100 mmHg (33).

In contrast to patients with a high systolic blood pressure at entry, patients with a previ-

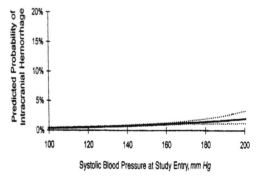

FIG. 26-9. Predicted probabilities (*solid line*) with 95% CIs (*dashed lines*) for intracranial hemorrhage within 30 days as a function of systolic blood pressure at entry. (From Aylward et al., ref. 33, with permission.)

ous history of hypertension represent a higher risk group (higher age, more females, higher incidence of diabetes, and Killip class greater than I) and therefore have a worse clinical outcome after thrombolysis. This worse clinical outcome includes both a higher cardiac death rate and higher total and hemorrhagic stroke rates (33).

In conclusion, patients with an acute myocardial infarction and a markedly elevated systolic blood pressure on admission have an increased risk for hemorrhagic stroke. The reduction in cardiac mortality after thrombolysis is the same as in normotensive patients. In patients at low risk of dying from cardiac causes but with very elevated systolic blood pressures, the risk for stroke after thrombolysis may outweigh the reduction in cardiac mortality and morbidity. Whether acute treatment of high blood pressure on admission reduces the risk for stroke after thrombolysis is unknown and needs further study.

Prior Coronary Bypass Surgery

Few data exist on the effect of intravenous thrombolysis in patients with acute myocardial infarction and previous coronary bypass surgery. In the GUSTO-I trial, prior coronary bypass surgery was an independent clinical predictor of 30-day mortality, reflecting the increased presence of multivessel disease and impaired left ventricular function in this subpopulation of patients with an acute myocardial infarction (18). Furthermore, a lower 90-minute coronary artery patency rate after thrombolysis and higher rates of reocclusion may contribute to the increased mortality rates observed in these patients as reviewed by Zahger et al. (34). The less favorable response to intravenous thrombolysis in patients with prior coronary bypass surgery may be due to larger thrombi in those cases in which a vein graft is the culprit vessel. This also may explain the greater benefit observed with a more potent thrombolytic agent (alteplase) in these patients in GUSTO-I (35).

In conclusion, patients with prior coronary bypass surgery and an acute myocardial infarc-tion may benefit from thrombolysis, although the results are inferior to those in patients without such a history. Comparative trials with other (mechanical) reperfusion strategies are lacking.

CONTRAINDICATIONS FOR THROMBOLYTIC THERAPY

With increasing knowledge of the benefits and risks of thrombolysis, the indications for this therapy have broadened over the years. Many more patients are now given thrombolytic therapy than 10 years ago. Nevertheless, there are still a number of absolute and relative contraindications for this type of reperfusion therapy. They are listed in Table 26-2. It is very unlikely that any of these contraindications will disappear from the list in the future because of the inherent risk of bleeding complications associated with fibrinolytic therapy. Because of this risk, alternative reperfusion strategies, without fibrinolytic agents, are likely to be used more frequently in the near future in patients at high risk for bleeding complications. An increasing number of hospitals in the Western world have the capacity of performing primary angioplasty, which has recently been shown to provide a modest clinical advantage over current thrombolytic therapy (36,37). Furthermore, it has been shown in a number of pilot studies that high bolus doses of heparin and of the glycoprotein IIb/IIIa recep-

TABLE 26-2. *Contraindications for thrombolytic therapy*

Absolute
Active internal bleeding
Aortic dissection
History of hemorrhagic stroke
History of intracranial or spinal disease (e.g., neoplasm, aneurysm, AV fistula)
Recent head trauma
Recent major surgery
Relative
Severe uncontrolled hypertension
Active peptic ulcer
Pericarditis
Bleeding diathesis
Use of oral anticoagulants
Pregnancy
Recent puncture of a noncompressible vessel
Prolonged resuscitation with chest trauma
Recent retinal laser treatment

tor antagonist abciximab alone are able to restore coronary blood flow in patients with an acute myocardial infarction, most likely by facilitating endogenous fibrinolysis (38,39). In patients with an increased risk of bleeding complications in whom primary angioplasty cannot be performed for logistic reasons, antithrombotic therapy alone or in association with a markedly reduced dose of a thrombolytic agent may represent an effective and safe reperfusion strategy. Large studies with this new pharmacologic reperfusion strategy are needed before its potential value can be fully evaluated.

SELECTING THE MOST APPROPRIATE THROMBOLYTIC AGENT

Many new thrombolytic agents will reach the market in the coming years, such as mutants of alteplase (reteplase, lanetoplase, TNK-tPA), recombinant pro-urokinase (saruplase), recombinant staphylokinase, and vampire bat plasminogen activator. At present the two most frequently used agents are streptokinase and alteplase. Streptokinase is a bacterial protein produced by streptococci. It is the first thrombolytic agent that has been given intravenously to large numbers of patients with acute myocardial infarction and the prototype of the so-called non–fibrin-specific agents. Alteplase and recombinant tissue plasminogen activator, a human protein produced by recombinant DNA technology, is much more expensive. It is the natural plasminogen activator of the human body and markedly more fibrin specific than streptokinase. It induces more early coronary artery recanalization (40), but its use is also associated with a greater incidence of intracranial hemorrhage (16,23,24). Although the selection of a particular thrombolytic agent is of marginal importance compared with the need to start reperfusion therapy as quickly and widely as possible, some general principles can be given.

Patients previously treated with immunogenic agents such as streptokinase, acylated plasminogen–streptokinase complex (AP-SAC), or staphylokinase should not be treated twice with the same agent because of the presence of neutralizing antibodies and, therefore, the risk for allergic reactions and reduced efficacy.

Patients with large amounts of ischemically jeopardized myocardium will derive the most benefit from agents with enhanced clot dissolution capacity such as alteplase. This is especially true when treatment can be given within the first hours after the onset of symptoms and when an increased risk for intracranial hemorrhage is absent.

Although data are limited, there is some evidence for preferring a non–fibrin-specific agent like streptokinase in patients in Killip class IV. Both the GISSI-2/International Study Group trial (23) and the GUSTO-I trial (16) have shown significantly lower mortality rates with streptokinase as compared with the fibrin-specific agent alteplase. The reasons for these observations are unclear. One possible explanation, supported by experimental data, is that a sufficient high coronary perfusion pressure is needed for local fibrin-specific dissolution of coronary artery clots, whereas the induction of a general plasma lytic state with subsequent local clot lysis can occur at low arterial blood pressures. The lowered blood viscosity with streptokinase due to massive fibrinogen consumption may be another explanation. As mentioned above, primary angioplasty is the reperfusion strategy of choice in patients with cardiogenic shock.

Although few data are available, patients with prior coronary bypass surgery and an acute myocardial infarction appear to derive a greater benefit from thrombolysis if a more potent, fibrin-specific agent like alteplase is given (35). The large thrombus volume in occluded vein grafts is the most likely explanation for this observation.

CONCLUSION

Despite the dramatic reductions in mortality demonstrated in large trials, thrombolytic therapy is still underused in patients with acute myocardial infarction as shown by numerous national surveys throughout the world. Concerns about bleeding complications, especially hemorrhagic stroke, are the main reason for withholding thrombolytic therapy. These and other hazards are small compared with the life-saving potential of thrombolysis. A proper selection of patients is of great importance for optimizing the cost-benefit ratio of this therapy.

REFERENCES

1. Van de Werf F, Califf RM, Armstrong PW, et al. on behalf of the GUSTO-I Steering Committee. Progress culminating from ten years of clinical trials on thrombolysis for acute myocardial infarction. *Eur Heart J* 1995; 16:1024–1026.
2. Fibrinolytic Therapy Trialists (FTT) Collaborative Group. Indications for fibrinolytic therapy in suspected acute myocardial infarction: collaborative overview of early mortality and major morbidity results from all randomized trials of more than 1,000 patients. *Lancet* 1994;343:311–322.
3. Rawles J. What is the likely benefit of earlier thrombolysis. *Eur Heart J* 1996;17:991–995.
4. Boersma E, Maas ACP, Deckers JW, Simoons ML. Early thrombolytic treatment in acute myocardial infarction: reappraisal of the golden hour. *Lancet* 1996; 348:771–775.
5. The European Myocardial Infarction Project Group. Prehospital thrombolytic therapy in patients with suspected acute myocardial infarction. *N Engl J Med* 1993;329:383–389.
6. Weaver WD, Cerqueria M, Hallstrom AP, et al. for the Myocardial Infarction Triage and Intervention Project Group. Prehospital-initiated vs hospital-initiated thrombolytic therapy. *JAMA* 1993;270:1211–1216.
7. GREAT Group. Feasibility, safety, and efficacy of domiciliary thrombolysis by general practitioners. *Br Med J* 1992;305:548–553.
8. Fath-Ordoubadi F, Al-Mohammad A, Heuns TY, Beatt KJ. Pre-hospital thrombolysis: does it save extra lives compared to hospital thrombolysis? An overview of randomized trials [Abstract]. *Eur Heart J* 1995;16 (suppl):123.
9. Raitt MH, Maynard C, Wagner GS, Cerqueria MD, Selvester RH, Weaver WD. Relation between symptom duration before thrombolytic therapy and final myocardial infarct size. *Circulation* 1996;93:45–53.
10. The TIMI IIIB Investigators. Effects of tissue plasminogen activator and a comparison of early invasive and conservative strategies in unstable angina and non-Q wave myocardial infarction. Results of the TIMI IIIB trial. *Circulation* 1994;89:1545–1556.
11. Rapold HJ, Brimaudo V, Declerck PJ, Kruithof KO, Bachmann F. Plasma levels of plasminogen activator inhibitor type 1, B-thromboglobulin and fibrinopeptide A before, during and after treatment of acute myocardial infarction with alteplase. *Blood* 1991;78:1490–1495.
12. Rapold HJ, de Bono DP, Arnold AER, et al. Plasma fibrinopeptide A levels in patients with acute myocardial infarction treated with alteplase. Correlation with concomitant heparin, coronary artery patency and recurrent ischemia. *Circulation* 1992;85:928–934.
13. Lee HS, Cross SJ, Rawles JM, Jennings KP. Patients with suspected myocardial infarction who present with ST depression. *Lancet* 1993;342:1204–1207.
14. Langer A, Goodman SG, Topol EJ, et al. Late assessment of thrombolytic efficacy (LATE) study: prognosis in patients with non-Q wave myocardial infarction. *J Am Coll Cardiol* 1996;27:1327–1332.
15. Sgarbossa EB, Ponski SL, Barbapelata, et al. for the GUSTO-I Investigators. Electrocardiographic diagnosis of evolving acute myocardial infarction in the presence of left bundle-branch block. *N Engl J Med* 1996;344: 481–487
16. GUSTO Investigators. An international randomized trial comparing four thrombolytic strategies for acute myocardial infarction. *N Engl J Med* 1993;329: 673–682
17. White HD, Barbash GI, Califf RM, et al. for the GUSTO-I Investigators. Age and outcome with contemporary thrombolytic therapy:results from the GUSTO-I trial. *Circulation* 1996;94:1826–1833.
18. Lee KL, Woodlief LH, Topol EJ, et al. Predictors of 30-day mortality in the era of reperfusion for acute myocardial infarction. Results from an international trial of 41,021 patients. *Circulation* 1995;91:1659–1668
19. Gurwitz JH, Goldberg RJ, Gore JM. Coronary thrombolysis for the elderly. *JAMA* 1991;265:1720–1723.
20. Krumhorz HM, Pastermak RC, Weinstein MC, et al. Cost-effectiveness of thrombolytic therapy with streptokinase in elderly patients with suspected acute myocardial infarction. *N Engl J Med* 1992;327:7–13.
21. Mark DB, Hlatky MA, Califf RM, et al. Cost-effectiveness of thrombolytic therapy with tissue plasminogen activator versus streptokinase for acute myocardial infarction: results from the GUSTO randomized trial. *N Engl J Med* 1995;322:1418–1424.
22. Moen EK, Asher CR, Miller DP, et al. Long-term follow-up of gender-specific outcomes after thrombolytic therapy for acute myocardial infarction from the GUSTO-I trial. *J Women's Health* 1997;6:285–293.
23. International Study Group. In-hospital mortality and clinical course of 20,981 patients with suspected acute myocardial infarction randomized between alteplase and streptokinase with or without heparin. *Lancet* 1990; 336:71–75.
24. Gruppo Italiano per lo Studio della Sopravvivenza nell Infarto Miocardico. GISSI-2: a factorial randomized trial of alteplase versus streptokinase and heparin versus no heparin among 12,490 patients with acute myocardial infarction. *Lancet* 1990;336:65–71.
25. White HD, Barbash GI, Modan M, et al. for the Investigators of the International Tissue Plasminogen Activator/Streptokinase Mortality Study. After correcting for worse baseline characteristics, women treated with thrombolytic therapy for acute myocardial infarction have the same mortality and morbidity as men except for a higher incidence of hemorrhagic stroke. *Circulation* 1993;88:2097–2103.
26. Gore JM, Granger CB, Simoons ML, et al. Stroke after thrombolysis: mortality and functional outcomes in the GUSTO-I trial. *Circulation* 1995;92:2811–2818.
27. Garcia MJ, McNamara PM, Gordon T, Kannel WB. Morbidity and mortality in diabetics in the Framingham

population: sixteen year follow-up study. *Diabetes* 1974;23:105–111.

28. Barbash GI, White HD, Modan M, Van de Werf F, for the Investigators of the International Tissue Plasminogen Activator/Streptokinase Mortality Trial. Significance of diabetes mellitus in patients with acute myocardial infarction receiving thrombolytic therapy. *J Am Coll Cardiol* 1993;22:707–713.

29. Woodfield SL, Lundergan CF, Reimer JS, et al. Angiographic findings and outcome in diabetic patients treated with thrombolytic therapy for acute myocardial infarction: the GUSTO-I experience. *J Am Coll Cardiol* 1996;28:1661–1669.

30. Lange RA, Hillis LD. Immediate angioplasty for acute myocardial infarction. *N Engl J Med* 1993;328:726–728.

31. Holmes DR, Bates ER, Kleiman NS, et al. Contemporary reperfusion therapy for cardiogenic shock: the GUSTO-1 trial experience. *J Am Coll Cardiol* 1995;26:668–674.

32. GISSI (Gruppo Italiano per lo Studio della Streptochinasi nell Infarto miocardico). Effectiveness of intravenous thrombolytic treatment in acute myocardial infarction. *Lancet* 1986;1:397–401.

33. Aylward PE, Wilcox RG, Horgan JH, et al. Relation of increased arterial blood pressure to mortality and stroke in the context of contemporary thrombolytic therapy for acute myocardial infarction. *Ann Intern Med* 1996;125:891–900.

34. Zahger D, Cercek B, Cannon CP, Jordan M, Shah PK, for the TIMI-4 Investigators. Thrombolytic therapy for acute myocardial infarction in patients with prior coronary bypass surgery: results from the thrombolysis in myocardial infarction (TIMI) 4 trial. *Thromb Thrombolysis* 1995;2:45–50.

35. DeFranco AC, Abramouritz B, Kirchbaum D, Topol EJ. Substantial (threefold) benefit of accelerated t-PA over standard thrombolytic therapy in patients with prior bypass surgery and acute MI:results of GUSTO trial [Abstract]. *J Am Coll Cardiol* 1994;23:345.

36. The GUSTO-IIb Angioplasty Substudy Investigators. An international randomized trial of 1138 patients comparing primary coronary angioplasty versus tissue plasminogen activator for acute myocardial infarction. *N Engl J Med* 1997;336:1621–1628.

37. Weaver WD, Simes RJ, Betriu A, et al. Primary coronary angioplasty vs intravenous thrombolysis for treatment of acute myocardial infarction: a quantitative overview of their comparative effectiveness. *JAMA* 1997 (in press).

38. Cigarroa JE, Ferrell MA, Collen D, Leinbach RC. Enhanced endogenous coronary thrombolysis during acute myocardial infarction following selective platelet reception blockade with ReoPro [Abstract]. *Circulation* 1996;94(suppl I):1–563.

39. Verheugt FWA, Marsh RC, Veen G, Bronzwaer JGF, Zijlstra FJ. Megadose bolus heparin as first treatment for acute myocardial infarction: results of the HEAP pilot study [Abstract]. *Eur Heart J* 1996;17(suppl):122.

40. GUSTO Angiographic Investigators. The effects of tissue plasminogen activator, streptokinase, or both on coronary-artery patency, ventricular function, and survival after acute myocardial infarction. *N Engl J Med* 1993;329:1615–1622.

*Cardiovascular Thrombosis: Thrombocardiology
and Thromboneurology, Second Edition,*
edited by M. Verstraete, V. Fuster, and E. J. Topol,
Lippincott–Raven Publishers, Philadelphia © 1998.

27

Prehospital Management of Acute Myocardial Infarction

Christopher P. Cannon

*Cardiovascular Division, Brigham and Women's Hospital,
Boston, Massachusetts 02115*

Aggressive management of acute myocardial infarction leads to improved outcome. This involves both the administration of reperfusion therapy to patients with ST-segment elevation myocardial infarction (STEMI), as well as the treatment with early defibrillation of sudden cardiac death, which account for more than half of the deaths from acute myocardial infarction. In addition, other medical therapies (e.g., aspirin, β-blockers) are beneficial. Many of these therapies are highly time dependent: most sudden deaths occur within 1 hour of onset of symptoms; treatment with reperfusion therapy is beneficial within 12 hours but is more beneficial the earlier it is administered.

Thus, the focus of prehospital management is on rapid identification and treatment of patients with acute myocardial infarction. However, there are many components to time delays between the onset of symptoms of acute myocardial infarction and the start of cardiac monitoring (and defibrillation if needed) or the achievement of reperfusion of the oc-

cluded infarct-related artery (1). Time delays exist with both patient and the medical system aspects of the prehospital time delays, with patient delays being the most important. This chapter will focus on the prehospital aspects of management of acute myocardial infarction, including (a) the rationale for early defibrillation and rapid reperfusion in acute myocardial infarction, (b) the factors related to time delays in patient presentation to the hospital, (c) strategies for reducing time delays (both patient and medical system delays; e.g., patient education, early defibrillation for cardiac arrest, prehospital electrocardiograms [ECGs], and treatment with thrombolysis).

Overall, the goals of prehospital management of acute myocardial infarction are as follows:

1. Patient notifies the medical system soon after the onset of symptoms.
2. Rapid transport and early cardiac monitoring and defibrillation should be avail-

able, usually via emergency medical services (EMS).

3. Patients with acute myocardial infarction are identified as STEMI versus non-STEMI.

4. Reperfusion therapy be initiated as soon as possible (either prehospital or in-hospital) for STEMI.

REPERFUSION THERAPY: THE EARLY OPEN ARTERY THEORY

The early open artery theory is the paradigm by which thrombolytic therapy is understood to be beneficial in acute myocardial infarction: early achievement of an open infarct-related artery is associated with improved outcome (2). Beginning with animal studies (3), the initial angiographic studies in patients using intracoronary streptokinase (4,5), and numerous other angiographic studies over the subsequent 15 years (6–16) have all lent strong support to this theory. In an overview of all the angiographic studies that used the TIMI flow grading system (17) comprising over 4,200 patients, patients with a patent infarct-related artery 90 minutes after treatment with thrombolysis had a 50% lower mortality compared with patients with a persistently occluded artery (p < 0.00001) (18). Furthermore, patients who achieved TIMI grade 3 flow (an open artery with normal perfusion) at 90 minutes had a 66% lower mortality (3.6%) compared with patients with TIMI grade 0 or 1 flow (an occluded artery, p < 0.00001) (18). Thus, the focus of acute myocardial infarction management has turned to rapid achievement of reperfusion of the infarct-related artery.

IMPORTANCE OF TIME TO TREATMENT

Because achievement of early infarct-related artery patency has been shown to be perhaps the most important goal in acute myocardial infarction management, one method of achieving an early open artery is to begin thrombolytic therapy earlier. As such, time

can be considered an adjunctive agent in a thrombolytic or reperfusion regimen (1). The importance of rapid time to treatment was highlighted by the first mega-trial, GISSI-1, which found that streptokinase led to a 19% reduction in mortality compared with placebo (19). However, patients who were treated within 1 hour from the onset of chest pain had a 50% reduction in mortality (19). The TIMI 2 trial extended these observations and found that for each hour earlier that a patient was treated, there was a decrease in the absolute mortality rate by 1% (20), which translates

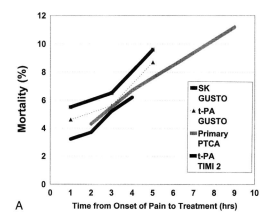

A

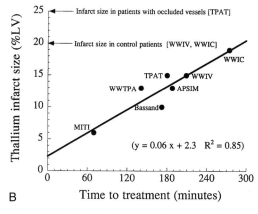

B

FIG. 27-1. A: Relationship between time to treatment and mortality for thrombolytic therapy and primary angioplasty. (From Cannon and Braunwald, ref. 41, with permission.) **B:** Relationship between time to treatment and infarct size. (From Martin and Kennedy, ref. 79, with permission.)

into an additional 10 lives saved per 1,000 patients treated (Fig. 27-1) (18). This has recently been observed in the GUSTO-I trial (21,22) and in an initial series of patients treated with primary percutaneous transluminal coronary angioplasty (PTCA) (23).

The mechanism of benefit of rapid time to treatment fits the paradigm of the open artery theory. Rapid time to treatment has been shown to be associated with reduced infarct size (Fig. 27-1) and improved left ventricular function (24,25). Thus, earlier treatment with either thrombolysis or primary angioplasty is associated with improved survival, emphasizing the need to speed treatment (26). With this goal in mind, rapid identification and transportation of the myocardial infarction patient to the hospital have been the focus of prehospital management.

CARDIAC ARREST/ SUDDEN CARDIAC DEATH

It is important to remember, however, that for the approximately 1.25 million people who experience an acute myocardial infarction each year, nearly 500,000 die, and half of these deaths occur before the patient arrives at the hospital (27,28). These sudden cardiac deaths usually occur within 1 hour of the onset of symptoms of acute myocardial infarction and are frequently due to malignant ventricular arrhythmias (28). Therefore, before one would be able to receive reperfusion therapy, one must survive the prehospital phase. Thus, the second major focus of prehospital management is to provide early monitoring, defibrillation, and advanced cardiac life support if needed.

Witnessed cardiac arrest victims have a significantly better survival rate than those who suffer unwitnessed cardiac arrest (29–31). It has been observed that most survivors of cardiac arrest are patients whose collapse is witnessed by a bystander, who receive cardiopulmonary resuscitation (CPR) within 4 to 5 minutes, and who receive advanced cardiac life support (ACLS) care (e.g., defibrillation, intubation, drug therapy)

within the first 10 minutes (29–31). Time, measured in minutes, becomes a critical determinant in the outcome of cardiac arrest victims (Fig. 27-2).

The American Heart Association has proposed the concept of a "chain of survival" for victims of cardiac arrest (32). The chain of survival has four components:

1. Early access to the EMS system.
2. Early CPR either by bystanders or first-responder rescuers.
3. Early defibrillation by first responders, emergency medical technicians (EMTs), paramedics, or nurses and physicians if they are on the scene.
4. Early ACLS.

Each link in the chain must be strong to ensure maximal survival rates for those who experience out-of-hospital cardiac arrest. The chain of survival also can be applied to individuals with symptoms and signs of an acute myocardial infarction or other acute coronary syndromes. Systems designed to reduce the time to defibrillation, CPR, and the arrival of ACLS-certified paramedics have been shown to be beneficial (Fig. 27-2) (30,31). Expanding this paradigm may be possible using automated external defibrillators (AEDs) or the full range of emergency vehicles (33). AEDs now permit basic-level EMTs, fire rescue personnel, and first responders as well as the traditional ACLS (paramedic) providers to defibrillate the patient (33). Thus, by expanding the availability of early defibrillation, it may be possible to resuscitate more myocardial infarction patients, who would then become potential candidates for reperfusion therapy.

National Heart Attack Alert Program

In recognition of these needs to expand the use of known therapies for acute myocardial infarction, such as thrombolysis and early defibrillation, the National Heart, Lung, and Blood Institute launched the National Heart Attack Alert Program (NHAAP) in June of 1991. The NHAAP is a national

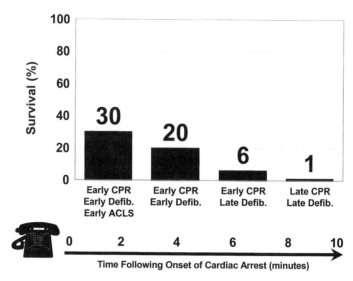

FIG. 27-2. Relationship of time to treatment and mortality for defibrillation and early cardiopul-monary resuscitation in cardiac arrest. (Data from Eisenberg et al., refs. 30 and 31.)

education effort to promote the rapid identi-fication and treatment of acute myocardial infarction, with the overriding goal of reduc-ing mortality and morbidity from acute my-ocardial infarction, including sudden death. The NHAAP has divided the aspects of acute myocardial infarction management into three phases, which provide a basis for improving care in the prehospital and hospital phase of management (Fig. 27-3).

Phase I: Patient/bystander recognition and ac-tion. The patient must recognize the symp-toms and signs of a possible heart attack and seek help immediately (34,35).

Phase II: Prehospital action. The EMS staff should be dispatched appropriately and re-spond in the shortest time possible, trans-porting the patient and providing life-sus-taining measures if needed (36–38).

Phase III: Hospital action. The emergency de-partment staff of the hospital receiving the patient must be prepared to rapidly diag-nose acute myocardial infarction (39) and initial reperfusion (and other) therapy as appropriate (40).

In addition, the fourth phase in actually achieving an open infarct-related artery, the

ultimate goal of reperfusion therapy, is the time from initiating therapy to achieving reperfusion (1,40,41).

PATIENT DELAYS

Studies of treatment delay document that the most common reason for delay is the pa-tient not seeking care promptly (42). The me-dian time delay in seeking care after the onset of symptoms of acute myocardial infarction ranges from 2 to 6.4 hours (43). In the prethrombolytic era, an overview of 16 stud-ies noted that the median time delay was ap-proximately 3 hours (44). The median time delay to treatment with thrombolysis in the National Registry of Myocardial Infarction was 2.2 hours, although presentation after 6 hours was the most common reason for not treating with thrombolytic therapy (42). In the TIMI 9 Registry of patients with ST-segment elevation myocardial infarction, 12% of pa-tients could not be treated with thrombolysis because of presentation more than 12 hours after the onset of symptoms (45). Conversely, few patients are treated within the first hour from onset of symptoms: only 3% of patients

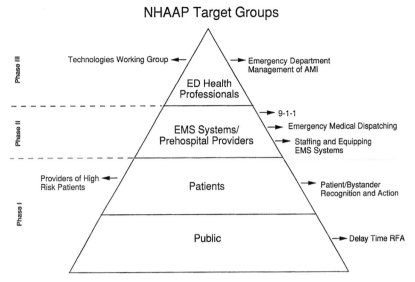

FIG. 27-3. The National Heart Attack Alert Program. Three phases of acute myocardial infarction management and target groups for educational messages on the importance of rapid treatment of acute myocardial infarction.

in the Global Utilization of Streptokinase and Tissue Plasminogen Activator for Occluded Coronary Arteries (GUSTO) trial (46), 3% in the TIMI II trial (47), and 11% in the Gruppo Italiano per lo Studio della Streptochinasi nell' Infarto Miocardico (GISSI) I trial (19) were treated within the first hour of symptom onset.

TABLE 27-1. *Factors affecting prehospital delay in patients with symptoms and signs of acute myocardial infarction*

Factors contributing to increased delay
Older age
Female gender
African-American race
Low socioeconomic status
Low emotional or somatic awareness
History of angina, diabetes, or both
Consulting a spouse or other relative
Consulting a physician
Self-treatment
Factors contributing to decreased delay
Hemodynamic instability
Large infarct size
Sudden onset of severe chest pain
Recognition by patient that symptoms are heart related
Consulting a friend, coworker, or stranger

From Dracup et al., ref. 35, with permission.

Factors Related to Patient Delays

What factors are responsible for patient delays? Table 27-1 shows the various demographic and clinical factors related to increased time to presentation (35). Older age (48–51) and female gender (50,52–54) are associated with increased delay in presenting to the hospital with acute myocardial infarction. Only preliminary information is available at present, but delays appear to be considerably greater in blacks (54–56) and were up to 11.9 hours in one study in the inner city (55). Low socioeconomic status appears to increase delays (57), although not in all studies (58).

Several clinical characteristics also affect delay time. Severe chest pain is associated with reduced delay times, but only if it is sudden in onset (54) or accompanied by hemodynamic instability (49,50). Unfortunately, patients with a history of angina or diabetes are more likely to delay than patients without these conditions (50,52). Amazingly, patients already diagnosed with coronary artery disease, heart failure, or prior myocardial infarction have the same or greater delay times as those without prior coronary artery disease (43,48).

Other health-care system factors play a role. If patients call a physician, delay times are significantly increased (54,59). Such delays are feared to increase as health management organizations increasingly insist that patients contact their primary care physician before presenting to the emergency department. On the other hand, if patients consult a friend, coworker, or stranger, they present to the emergency department more quickly than if they consult a family member/significant other (35,54), potentially because family members/significant others are more easily dissuaded by the patient from calling 9-1-1 than are nonrelatives (54). Many aspects of these delays can potentially be modified, which will hopefully translate into improved outcome.

Transport/EMS Delays

Prehospital delay times—those associated with the transport of the patient by ambulance or private vehicle—add only an average of 7 to 22 minutes to the delay time. In rural areas, much longer delays are common (60,61). However, use of 9-1-1 to access EMS has been shown to decrease time to reperfusion with thrombolytic therapy by as much as 60 minutes for individuals with symptoms and signs of an acute myocardial infarction, compared with patients who transport themselves (24). Unfortunately, only half of the patients with symptoms of a heart attack use the EMS system (62). In addition, EMS is currently only available in 83% of the United States (36). In addition, poor coordination between EMS and other first response groups, such as fire rescue squads, may lead to inadvertent delays, which emphasizes the need for good community planning in the prehospital EMS to eliminate such delays.

IMPROVING TIME TO TREATMENT AND SURVIVAL

Reducing Patient Delays

The first component of reducing time delays is improving patient awareness of acute myocardial infarction symptoms. Two approaches can be taken. One is to educate the general public (people at risk for, but without, prior coronary artery disease). The other is to educate patients with stable coronary artery disease, i.e., those at highest risk for a subsequent myocardial infarction, a much smaller group of patients.

Public awareness campaigns aimed at encouraging patients who are experiencing chest pain or cardiac symptoms to rapidly seek medical advice appear to improve the time between onset of symptoms and presentation to the medical facility (63,64). Gaspoz and colleagues conducted a public campaign in the Geneva area and found a significant reduction in the median time of onset of pain to hospital arrival although this reduction was only 25 minutes (p < 0.001) (63). The mean time was reduced by approximately 3 hours (p < 0.001) (63). However, there was an early, transient increase in the number of patients presenting to the hospital with noncardiac chest pain. Blohm et al. also found that the median time delay was reduced by approximately 40 minutes, from 3 hours to 2 hours and 20 minutes during the public media campaign (p < 0.001) (64). Importantly, they documented a reduction in infarct size as measured by maximum creative phosphokinase (CPK) (64). Thus, public campaigns appear to be beneficial based on these initial studies.

However, because only limited information is available about the type of messages to be used and the overall effectiveness of such public campaigns, the NHAAP is currently sponsoring a randomized trial called REACT (Rapid Early Access to Coronary Treatment), which studies ways to best accomplish broadbased public awareness campaigns. However, many different strategies may work in different communities. For example, an effective public campaign in New York City might be very different from that in a rural area. Given the intuitive benefits of public awareness, many hospitals are currently "reaching out" with public service messages for heart attack awareness.

Patient's Name: _____

Physicians now have treatments that can stop heart attacks and lessen damage to the heart. To make sure you can benefit from these treatments, you need to act promptly if you begin to experience symptoms that might signal a heart attack.

What To Do If You Think You Are Having a Heart Attack

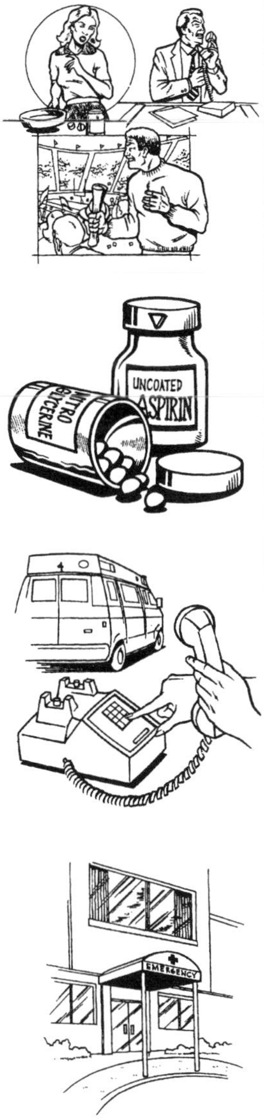

1. **This is what you may feel:**
   - ❏ Chest pain or discomfort
   - ❏ Left arm pain
   - ❏ Pain radiating to your neck or jaw
   - ❏ Shortness of breath
   - ❏ Sweating
   - ❏ Upset stomach
   - ❏ Discomfort in the area between your breastbone and navel
   - ❏ A sense of dread
   - ❏ Other: _____
     _____

2. **Medication instructions:**
   - ❏ Chew one 325 mg. tablet of uncoated (nonenteric) aspirin
   - ❏ Place one tablet of nitroglycerin under your tongue as soon as you feel discomfort. Take a second tablet if the discomfort does not go away in 5 minutes. Take a third tablet after 5 more minutes if the discomfort does not go away.
   - ❏ Other: _____
     _____

3. **If the symptoms stop, call your physician at:** _____

4. **If symptoms continue for more than 15 minutes, call the emergency medical services phone number below. (Often this is 9-1-1, but you should check to make sure.)**

   At home, the emergency phone number is: _____

   At work, the emergency phone number is: _____

   At _____ , the emergency phone number is:
   _____

5. **Know the location of the nearest 24-hour emergency department.**

   At home, the closest emergency department is: _____

   At work, the closest emergency department is: _____

   At _____ , the closest emergency department is:
   _____

Signed: _____ M.D./ R.N.

Place this form next to the phone, near your other emergency numbers!

FIG. 27-4. Patient advisory form. Instructions for patients on what to do in case of acute myocardial infarction symptoms. (From Dracup et al., ref. 80, with permission.)

Patient Education

The other approach to reducing patient delays during the acute myocardial infarction phase is to focus the resources of educational materials on patients with coronary artery disease, a much smaller number compared with the general public. By educating patients with stable coronary artery disease, or other significant risk factors for acute myocardial infarction (e.g., peripheral vascular disease, diabetes, etc.) they may present earlier to the hospital and have improved outcomes. The NHAAP recommends that in both inpatient and outpatient settings, primary care physicians (and specialists) provide patients and their family members with advice about what actions to take in response to symptoms of an acute myocardial infarction (or unstable angina) (35). The discussion should include mention of the emotional aspects (e.g., fear and denial) that patients and those around them may experience in the acute myocardial infarction setting, as well as barriers that may be associated with the health-care delivery system (e.g., distance to the hospital or cost issues) (35). Assistance from other health-care providers (e.g., nurses) should be solicited to initiate, reinforce, and supplement the counseling. A patient advisory form is shown in Fig. 27-4 as an aid to providers in counseling their high-risk patients about these issues (35).

Physicians' offices and clinics should devise a system to triage patients rapidly when they call or walk in seeking advice for possible acute myocardial infarction symptoms (35). Further research is needed to learn more about effective counseling strategies, symptom manifestation in high-risk groups including women and minorities, and health-care delivery systems that enhance access to timely care for acute myocardial infarction patients (34).

Another practical issue is education of spouses. Because family members can frequently be dissuaded by the patient from calling 9-1-1 (54), it is important to educate spouses and other family members of the signs and symptoms of acute myocardial infarction and to emphasize that they perform the action plan in Fig. 27-4. This can be done in a physician's office during regular follow-up visits for patients with stable coronary artery disease.

Reducing Transport and EMS Delays

The next component of reducing time delays is focused on reducing transportation times. Amazingly, only 50% of patients present to the emergency department by ambulance (62). Because patients not transported by EMS do not have the benefit of cardiac monitoring and defibrillation in case of lethal arrhythmia, such patients do not receive optimal care. In addition, because use of the 9-1-1 EMS system has been shown to reduce time to treatment with thrombolysis (65), an ongoing goal is to make it available throughout the United States (36). Furthermore, it is being proposed that the number of defibrillators, including automatic external defibrillators, should be expanded greatly to allow public access to early defibrillation (33).

The next component of reducing time delays is focused on speeding response times for EMTs, which has been a continuing priority in the United States and elsewhere. Reducing response times is critical to improving outcomes for patients in cardiac arrest (30,31). In addition, improved dialogue and communication between emergency medical technicians and hospital emergency departments has speeded the time to evaluation and treatment in many hospitals (65). The NHAAP has made recommendations for improving prehospital systems and preparation of EMS personnel (36–38).

Community Planning

Taking a broader view than just EMS, one must recall that there are numerous providers of prehospital care and new concerns regarding where patients should be sent. Fire rescue vehicles provide a large proportion of prehospital care throughout the country, even in cities such as Boston where there are full EMS systems. Thus, in 1980 the American Heart Association proposed that the entire community be considered a "coronary care unit" (66). The rationale for this is that because heart attacks occur at home, at work, and in the community, and people die without potentially life-saving care, identification and treatment of acute myocardial infarction (and sudden death in particular) as well as acute coronary syndromes in general, should be community concerns. Therefore, it is critical that communities develop an action plan to ensure a consistent, appropriate, and coordinated response to the needs of patients who will be accessing their community's coronary care system and to educate patients and the public of the need for early and appropriate treatment. In addition, with the changes in health-care insurance and preferred providers, some groups are proposing modifications in the long-standing policy that acute myocardial infarction patients are transported to the nearest hospital. On the other hand, transport of very high risk acute myocardial infarction patients (e.g., those with cardiogenic shock or contraindications to thrombolysis) to a tertiary care facility with angioplasty facilities does appear to be medically sound. However, the criteria and action plan for such a policy need to be developed. The NHAAP has made recommendations on the essential components of a community plan to ensure that a seamless response to the acute cardiac patient is as efficient as the response on the emergency department/hospital level (67).

Prehospital ECGs

Prehospital ECGs are another component of prehospital care that have been shown to decrease time to treatment (65,68–71) and be associated with a lower mortality rate in one study (72). Prehospital ECGs involve both the performance of the ECG in the field, but also with transmission via fax to a physician for interpretation (65,68). By this means, rapid identification of patients with acute ST elevation myocardial infarction is possible, and early evidence indicates that this speeds treatment and may improve outcome of patients with acute myocardial infarction (24,65,68). Interestingly, the time component that is reduced is the in-hospital time to treatment (i.e., the "door-to-needle" time). Because the ECG is already obtained, and the patient is identified as an ST elevation myocardial infarction patient, there are no time delays in obtaining a history (or in performing an ECG), and in some cases, thrombolytic therapy could be readied at the bedside before the patient actually arrived in the emergency department. Kereiakes and colleagues carried out a randomized trial and observed that patients who had a prehospital ECG obtained and transmitted to the emergency department had a significantly reduced door-to-needle time (30 versus 50 minutes, p = 0.004) (70).

A recent study of 66,995 patients in the multicenter National Registry of Myocardial Infarction 2 Trial found that prehospital ECGs were associated with a 10-minute decrease in door-to-needle time with thrombolysis (p < 0.001) and a 23-minute decrease in door-to-balloon time (p < 0.001) (72). In addition, patients who had a prehospital ECG performed were significantly more likely to receive reperfusion therapy, and more importantly, they had reduced mortality. In patients with a prehospital ECG, mortality was 8% compared with 12% for those without a prehospital ECG. Even after correcting for differences in baseline characteristics in a multivariate model, the performance of a prehospital ECG was associated with improved survival (odds ratio 0.83, 95% confidence interval 0.71 to 0.96, p = 0.01) (72). This study provides evidence that first, the prehospital ECG is an excellent rapid marker of acute myocardial infarction that helps alert the health professionals to treatment options (e.g., thrombolysis). This also suggests that other tests, such as a rapid bedside troponin T measurement (73,74) or other technologies (39), might also assist in early management of patients with acute myocardial infarction. Second, by performing the ECG early in the course of the evaluation of the patient, the presence of ST segment elevation can help physicians focus on acute myocardial infarction rather than other diagnoses. Thus, healthcare systems need to consider equipping and training the EMS personnel to perform prehospital ECGs.

Prehospital Thrombolysis

Although performance of a prehospital ECG is helpful, actual treatment with thrombolytic therapy in the prehospital setting offers the potential of very rapid treatment. Because the EMTs in an ambulance only have to drive to the patient's home or location (and not also back to the hospital), it eliminates nearly half of the transportation time. The diagnostic tests must still be performed, but with training, these can be accomplished rapidly. Several trials of prehospital treatment with thrombolytic therapy has shown reductions in both time to treatment and mortality, especially in rural areas (75,76).

The Myocardial Infarction and Triage Intervention (MITI) trial compared prehospital versus hospital administration of thrombolytic therapy in the Seattle area (24). Patients who were treated in the prehospital phase had a significant reduction in the time to treatment with thrombolytic therapy by 33 minutes (p < 0.001) (24). Although mortality

was 31% lower, it was not a significant difference in this small trial (24). The GREAT trial, conducted in a rural area in England, compared prehospital or "home" thrombolysis to hospital-initiated thrombolytic therapy and documented a greater than 2 hour time savings by treatment with thrombolysis at home (75). Importantly, this 2-hour savings in time to treatment was associated with a 50% reduction in mortality. At 1 year, mortality was 21.6% for patients treated in hospital compared with 10.4% for patients at home (p = 0.007) (75).

The European Myocardial Infarction Project was a large randomized trial of prehospital versus hospital-based thrombolytic therapy (76). A total of 5,469 patients were randomized during prehospital administration of anistreplase or administration of thrombolytic therapy at the hospital. They achieved a 55-minute reduction in time to treatment with prehospital thrombolysis that was associated with a strong trend toward reduction in the overall 30-day mortality rate from 11.1% to 9.7% (p = 0.08) (76). Importantly, cardiovascular mortality was reduced from 9.8% to 8.3% (p = 0.05) (76). An overview of all the major prehospital thrombolysis trials is shown in Fig. 27-5. When looking at the total experience, prehospital treatment was associated with a 17% reduction in mortality (p = 0.03)

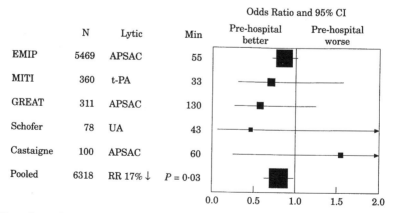

FIG. 27-5. Mortality reduction with prehospital thrombolysis. (Reproduced from Topol, ref. 81, with permission.)

(76). One rule of thumb sometimes used is that if prehospital thrombolysis can reduce time to treatment by at least 50 to 60 minutes, it is probably beneficial. However, if only 10 to 20 minutes can be saved, hospital-based thrombolysis is probably just as effective.

Prehospital Aspirin

Given the benefits of aspirin in acute myocardial infarction, and those of rapid time to treatment with thrombolysis, it has been thought that prehospital aspirin might improve outcome. However, one study found no benefit of prehospital aspirin versus administration of aspirin in the hospital (77). On the other hand, overall use of aspirin is lower than what is optimal, ranging from as low as 63% in one study (42) to only 87% in others (45,78). Thus, standardized protocols or "checklists" that include aspirin in the prehospital phase will ensure that aspirin is not overlooked.

CONCLUSION

The field of prehospital management of acute myocardial infarction has expanded rapidly in the past several years. It includes involving the patients in their management by trying to educate them about the importance of rapid presentation to the emergency department for evaluation in case of acute myocardial infarction. It also involves improving the EMS response times, which are critical in providing early defibrillation to patients with acute myocardial infarction complicated by ventricular fibrillation. In addition, emerging evidence supports the prehospital performance of ECGs to rapidly identify patients who will benefit from reperfusion therapy. Prehospital thrombolysis also appears to be beneficial, especially in areas where transport delays are long.

What is less clear is exactly how to convey the message to patients and the general public about the importance of getting to the hospital quickly. The National Institutes of Health–sponsored REACT trial should soon provide some answers. With all the changes in the health-care system, community planning seems to be needed to coordinate EMS and other prehospital systems, but exactly how this will take place is not yet clear. In the area of early defibrillation, there is growing interest in the expanded use of automatic external defibrillators, which do not require EMS personnel, in order to provide true public access to early defibrillation. It remains to be seen whether this expanded availability of defibrillation via AEDs will lead to improved survival. Hopefully, this will be assessed either in a trial or in monitoring in a clinical effectiveness assessment of death rates pre- and post-their availability. Given the apparent benefit of prehospital ECGs, an area for future research is to investigate whether other markers of acute myocardial infarction, such as a bedside assay for troponin T or I, could be used to rapidly identify and prompt early treatment of acute myocardial infarction patients. For prehospital thrombolysis, it is not clear how much of a time savings is needed in order for it to translate into clinical benefit. The field has evolved rapidly, but many interesting questions remain regarding how to implement prehospital thrombolysis and the magnitude of benefit of these promising new ways of improving the outcome of patients with acute myocardial infarction.

REFERENCES

1. Cannon CP, Antman EM, Walls R, Braunwald E. Time as an adjunctive agent to thrombolytic therapy. *J Thromb Thrombolysis* 1994;1:27–34.
2. Braunwald E. The open-artery theory is alive and well—again. *N Engl J Med* 1993;329:1650–1652.
3. Reimer KA, Lowe JE, Rasmussen NM, Jennings RB. The wavefront phenomenon of ischemic cell death. 1. Myocardial infarct size vs. duration of coronary occlusion in dogs. *Circulation* 1977;56:786–794.
4. Rentrop KP, Blanke H, Karsch KR, Kreuzer H. Initial experience with transluminal recanalization of the recently occluded infarct-related coronary artery in acute myocardial infarction. Comparison with conventionally treated patients. *Clin Cardiol* 1979;2:92–105.
5. Ganz W, Buchbinder N, Marcus H, et al. Intracoronary thrombolysis in evolving myocardial infarction. *Am Heart J* 1981;101:4–13.
6. Stadius ML, Davis K, Maynard C, Ritchie JL, Kennedy JW. Risk stratification for 1 year survival based on characteristics identified in the early hours of acute myocardial infarction. *Circulation* 1986;74:701–711.

7. Dalen JE, Gore JM, Braunwald E, et al. Six- and twelve-month follow-up of the Phase I Thrombolysis in Myocardial Infarction (TIMI) Trial. *Am J Cardiol* 1988;62:179–185.

8. Belenkie I, Thompson CR, Manyari DE, et al. Importance of effective, early and sustained reperfusion during acute myocardial infarction. Am J Cardiol 1989;63:912–916.

9. Flygenring BP, Sheehan FH, Kennedy JW, Dodge HT, Braunwald E, for the TIMI Investigators. Does arterial patency 90 minutes following thrombolytic therapy predict 42 day survival? [Abstract]. *J Am Coll Cardiol* 1991;17(suppl A):275.

10. Karagounis L, Sorensen SG, Menlove RL, Moreno F, Anderson JL, for the TEAM-2 Investigators. Does thrombolysis in myocardial infarction (TIMI) perfusion grade 2 represent a mostly patent artery or a mostly occluded artery? Enzymatic and electrocardiographic evidence from the TEAM-2 study. *J Am Coll Cardiol* 1992;19:1–10.

11. Anderson JL, Karagounis LA, Becker LC, Sorensen SG, Menlove RL, for the TEAM-3 Investigators. TIMI perfusion grade 3 but not grade 2 results in improved outcome after thrombolysis for myocardial infarction: ventriculographic, enzymatic and electrocardiographic evidence from the TEAM-3 study. *Circulation* 1993; 87:1829–1839.

12. Cannon CP, McCabe CH, Diver DJ, et al. Comparison of front-loaded recombinant tissue-type plasminogen activator, anistreplase and combination thrombolytic therapy for acute myocardial infarction: results of the Thrombolysis in Myocardial Infarction (TIMI) 4 trial. *J Am Coll Cardiol* 1994;24:1602–1610.

13. Cannon CP, McCabe CH, Henry TD, et al. A pilot trial of recombinant desulfatohirudin compared with heparin in conjunction with tissue-type plasminogen activator and aspirin for acute myocardial infarction: results of the Thrombolysis in Myocardial Infarction (TIMI) 5 Trial. *J Am Coll Cardiol* 1994;23:993–1003.

14. Lincoff AM, Topol EJ, Califf RM, et al. Significance of a coronary artery with thrombolysis in myocardial infarction grade 2 flow "patency" (outcome in the Thrombolysis and Angioplasty in Myocardial Infarction (TAMI) trials). *Am J Cardiol* 1995;75:871–876.

15. The GUSTO Angiographic Investigators. The comparative effects of tissue plasminogen activator, streptokinase, or both on coronary artery patency, ventricular function and survival after acute myocardial infarction. *N Engl J Med* 1993;329:1615–1622.

16. Simes RJ, Topol EJ, Holmes DR, et al. Link between the angiographic substudy and mortality outcomes in a large randomized trial of myocardial reperfusion. Importance of early and complete infarct artery reperfusion. *Circulation* 1995;91:1923–1928.

17. TIMI Study Group. The Thrombolysis in Myocardial Infarction (TIMI) trial; phase I findings. *N Engl J Med* 1985;312:932–936.

18. Cannon CP, Braunwald E. GUSTO, TIMI and the case for rapid reperfusion. *Acta Cardiol* 1994;49:1–8.

19. Gruppo Italiano per lo Studio della Streptochinasi nell'Infarto Miocardico (GISSI). Effectiveness of intravenous thrombolytic treatment in acute myocardial infarction. *Lancet* 1986;1:397–401.

20. Timm TC, Ross R, McKendall GR, Braunwald E, Williams DO, and the TIMI Investigators. Left ventricular function and early cardiac events as a function of time to treatment with t-PA: a report from TIMI II [Abstract]. *Circulation* 1991;84:II-230.

21. Topol EJ, Califf RM, Lee KL, on behalf of the GUSTO Investigators. More on the GUSTO trial [Letter]. *N Engl J Med* 1994;331:277–278 (errata *N Engl J Med* 1994; 331:687 and 1994;331:1323).

22. Newby LK, Rutsch WR, Califf RM, et al. Time from symptom onset to treatment and outcomes after thrombolytic therapy. *J Am Coll Cardiol* 1996;27:1646–1655.

23. O'Keefe JH, Rutherford BD, McConahay DR, et al. Early and late results of coronary angioplasty without antecedent thrombolytic therapy for acute myocardial infarction. *Am J Cardiol* 1989;64:1221–1230.

24. Weaver WD, Cerqueira M, Hallstrom AP, et al. Prehospital-initiated vs hospital-initiated thrombolytic therapy. Myocardial Infarction Triage and Intervention Trial. *JAMA* 1993;270:1211–1216.

25. Weaver WD. Time to thrombolytic treatment: factors affecting delay and influence on outcome. *J Am Coll Cardiol* 1995;25(suppl):3–9.

26. Cannon CP. Time to treatment: a crucial factor in thrombolysis and primary angioplasty. *J Thromb Thrombolysis* 1996;3:249–256.

27. American Heart Association. *1997 Heart and Stroke Statistical Update.* American Heart Association, Dallas 1997.

28. National Heart Lung and Blood Institute. *Morbidity and Mortality: Chartbook on Cardiovascular, Lung and Blood Diseases.* Bethesda, MD: US Department of Health and Human Services, Public Health Service, National Institute of Health, 1992.

29. Weaver WD, Cobb LA, Hallstrom AP, Fahrenbruch C, Copass MK, Ray R. Factors influencing survival after out-of-hospital cardiac arrest. *J Am Coll Cardiol* 1986; 7:752–757.

30. Eisenberg MS, Horwood BT, Cummins RO, Reynolds-Haertle R, Hearne TR. Cardiac arrest and resuscitation: a tale of 29 cities. *Ann Emerg Med* 1990;19:179–186.

31. Eisenberg MS, Cummins RO, Damon S, Larsen MP, Hearne TR. Survival rates from out-of-hospital cardiac arrest: recommendations for uniform definitions and data to report. *Ann Emerg Med* 1990;19:1249–1259.

32. Cummins RO, Ornato JP, Thies WH, Pepe PE. Improving survival from sudden cardiac death: the chain of survival concept. *Circulation* 1991;83:1832–1847.

33. Weisfelt ML, Kerber RE, McGoldrick RP, et al. American Heart Association report on the Public Access Defibrillation Conference, December 8–10, 1994. *Circulation* 1995;92:2740–2747.

34. National Heart Attack Alert Program Coordinating Committee Access to Care Subcommittee. *Patient/Bystander Recognition and Action: Rapid Identification and Treatment of Acute Myocardial Infarction.* NIH Publication No. 93-3303. Bethesda: U.S. Department of Health and Human Services, Public Health Service, National Institutes of Health, National Heart, Lung, and Blood Institute, 1995;2.

35. Dracup K, Alonzo AA, Atkins JM, et al. The physician's role in minimizing prehospital delay in patients at high risk for acute myocardial: recommendations from the National Heart Attack Alert Program. *Ann Intern Med* 1997;126:645–651.

36. National Heart Attack Alert Program Coordinating Committee Access to Care Subcommittee. 9-1-1: rapid

identification and treatment of acute myocardial infarction. *Am J Emerg Med* 1995;13:188–195.

37. National Heart Attack Alert Program Coordinating Committee Access to Care Subcommittee. Staffing and equipping emergency medical services systems: rapid identification and treatment of acute myocardial infarction. *Am J Emerg Med* 1995;13:58–65.

38. National Heart Attack Alert Program Coordinating Committee Access to Care Subcommittee. Emergency medical dispatching: rapid identification and treatment of acute myocardial infarction. *Am J Emerg Med* 1995;13:67–73.

39. Selker HP, Zalenski RJ, Antman EM, et al. An evaluation of technologies for identifying acute cardiac ischemia in the emergency department: a report from a National Heart Attack Alert Working Group. *Ann Emerg Med* 1997;29:13–87.

40. National Heart Attack Alert Program Coordinating Committee—60 Minutes to Treatment Working Group. Emergency department: rapid identification and treatment of patients with acute myocardial infarction. *Ann Emerg Med* 1994;23:311–329.

41. Cannon CP, Braunwald E. Time to reperfusion: the critical modulator in thrombolysis and primary angioplasty. *J Thromb Thrombolysis* 1996;3:109–117.

42. Rogers WJ, Bowlby LJ, Chandra NC, et al. Treatment of myocardial infarction in the United States (1990 to 1993). Observations from the National Registry of Myocardial Infarction. *Circulation* 1994;90:2103–2114.

43. Dracup K, Moser DK. Treatment-seeking behavior among those with signs and symptoms of acute myocardial infarction. *Heart Lung* 1991;20:570–575.

44. Ridker PM, Manson JE, Goldhaber SZ, Hennekens CH, Buring JE. Comparison of delay times to hospital presentation for physicians and nonphysicians with acute myocardial infarction. *Am J Cardiol* 1992;70:10–3.

45. Cannon CP, Henry TD, Schweiger MJ, et al. Current management of ST elevation myocardial infarction and outcome of thrombolytic ineligible patients: results of the multicenter TIMI 9 Registry [Abstract]. *J Am Coll Cardiol* 1995;(special issue):231–232.

46. The GUSTO Investigators. An international randomized trial comparing four thrombolytic strategies for acute myocardial infarction. *N Engl J Med* 1993;329:673–682.

47. TIMI Study Group. Comparison of invasive and conservative strategies after treatment with intravenous tissue plasminogen activator in acute myocardial infarction. Results of the Thrombolysis in Myocardial Infarction (TIMI) Phase II trial. *N Engl J Med* 1989;320:618–627.

48. Yarzebski J, Goldberg RJ, Gore JM, Alpert JS. Temporal trends and factors associated with extent of delay to hospital arrival in patients with acute myocardial infarction: the Worcester Heart Attack study. *Am Heart J* 1994;128:255–263.

49. Maynard C, Althouse R, Olsufka M, Ritchie JL, Davis KB, Kennedy JW. Early versus late hospital arrival for acute myocardial infarction in the Western Washington thrombolytic therapy trials. *Am J Cardiol* 1989;63:1296–1300.

50. Turi AG, Stone PH, Muller JE, et al. Implications for acute intervention related to time of hospital arrival in acute myocardial infarction. *Am J Cardiol* 1986;58:203–209.

51. Weaver WD, Litwin PE, Martin JS, et al. Effect of age on use of thrombolytic therapy and mortality in acute myocardial infarction. *J Am Coll Cardiol* 1991;18:657–662.

52. Meischke H, Eisenberg MS, Larsen MP. Prehospital delay interval for patients who use emergency medical services: the effect of heart-related medical conditions and demographic variables. *Ann Emerg Med* 1993;22:1597–1601.

53. Cunningham MA, Lee TH, Cooke EF, et al. The effect of gender on the probability of myocardial infarction among emergency department patients with acute chest pain: a report from the Multicenter Chest Pain Study Group. *J Gen Intern Med* 1989;4:392–398.

54. Alonzo AA. The impact of the family and lay others on care-seeking during life-threatening episodes of suspected coronary artery disease. *Soc Sci Med* 1986;22:1297–1311.

55. Clark LT, Bellan SV, Shah AH, Feldman JG. Analysis of prehospital delay among inner-city patients with myocardial infarction: implications for therapeutic intervention. *J Natl Med Assoc* 1992;84:931–937.

56. Cooper RS, Simmons B, Castaner A, Prasad R, Franklin C, Ferlinz J. Survival rates and prehospital delay during myocardial infarction among black persons. *Am J Cardiol* 1986;65:1411–1415.

57. Ghali JK, Cooper RS, Kowatly I, Liao Y. Delay between onset of chest pain and arrival to the coronary care unit among minority and disadvantaged patients. *J Natl Med Assoc* 1993;85:180–184.

58. Crawford SL, McGraw SA, Smith KW, McKinlay JB, Pierson JE. Do blacks and whites differ in their use of health care for symptoms of coronary heart disease? *Am J Public Health* 1994;84:957–964.

59. Gray D, Keating NA, Murdock J, Skene AM, Hampton JR. Impact of hospital thrombolysis policy on out-of-hospital response to suspected myocardial infarction. *Lancet* 1993;341:654–657.

60. Gillum RF, Feinleib M, Margolis JR, Fabsitz RR, Brasch RC. Delay in the prehospital phase of acute myocardial infarction: lack of influence on incidence of sudden death. *Arch Intern Med* 1976;136:649–654.

61. Weilgosz AT, Nolan RP, Earp JA, Biro E, Wielgosz MB. Reasons for patients' delay in response to symptoms of acute myocardial infarction. *Can Med Assoc* 1988;139:853–857.

62. Ho MT, Eisenberg MS, Litwin PE, Schaeffer SM, Damon SK. Delay between onset of chest pain and seeking medical care: the effect of public education. *Ann Emerg Med* 1989;18:727–731.

63. Gaspoz JM, Unger PF, Urban P, et al. Impact of a public campaign on pre-hospital delay in patients reporting chest pain. *Heart* 1996;76:150–155.

64. Blohm M, Herlitz J, Hartford M, et al. Consequences of a media campaign focusing on delay in acute myocardial infarction. *Am J Cardiol* 1992;69:411–413.

65. Weaver WD, Eisenberg MC, Martin JS, et al. Myocardial Infarction Triage and Intervention Project—phase I: patient characteristics and feasibility of prehospital initiation of thrombolytic therapy. *J Am Coll Cardiol* 1990;15:925–931.

66. McIntyre KM. Cardiopulmonary resuscitation and the ultimate coronary care unit. *JAMA* 1980;244:510–511.

67. National Heart Attack Alert Program Coordinating Committee Access to Care Subcommittee. Community planning considerations for ensuring access to timely and appropriate care of patients with acute coronary syndromes. *J Thromb Thrombolysis* (in press).

68. Karagounis L, Ipsen SK, Jessop MR, et al. Impact of field-transmitted electrocardiography on time to in-hospital thrombolytic therapy in acute myocardial infarction. *Am J Cardiol* 1990;66:786–791.

69. Aufderheide TP, Hedley GE, Thakur RK, et al. The diagnostic impact of prehospital 12-lead electrocardiography. *Ann Emerg Med* 1990;19:1280–1287.

70. Kereiakes DJ, Gibler WB, Martin LH, Pieper KS, Anderson LC, and the Cincinnati Heart Project Study Group. Relative importance of emergency medical system transport and the prehospital electrocardiogram on reducing hospital time delay to therapy for acute myocardial infarction: a preliminary report from the Cincinnati Heart Project. *Am Heart J* 1992;123:835–840.

71. Lambrew CT, Weaver WD, French WJ, Bowlby L, Rubison M, for the National Registry of Myocardial Infarction (NRMI). Impact of hospital protocols on time to treatment with thrombolytic therapy (door to drug time) [Abstract]. *J Am Coll Cardiol* 1994;(special issue):14.

72. Canto JG, Rogers WJ, Bowlby LJ, et al. The prehospital electrocardiogram in acute myocardial infarction: is the full potential being realized? *J Am Coll Cardiol* 1997;29:498–505.

73. Antman EM, Grudzien C, Sacks DB. Evaluation of a rapid bedside assay for detection of serum cardiac troponin T. *JAMA* 1995;273:1279–1282.

74. Antman EM, Sacks D, Rifai N, et al. Time to positivity of a rapid bedside assay for troponin T predicts prognosis in unstable angina: findings in TIMI 11A [Abstract]. *Circulation* 1996;94(suppl I):322–323.

75. Rawles J, on behalf of the GREAT Group. Halving of mortality at 1 year by domiciliary thrombolysis in the Grampian Region Early Anistreplase Trial (GREAT). *J Am Coll Cardiol* 1994;23:1–5.

76. The European Myocardial Infarction Project Group. Prehospital thrombolytic therapy in patients with suspected acute myocardial infarction. *N Engl J Med* 1993;329:383–389.

77. Greenbaum R, Flaherty M, Chan KL, Shanit D. Failure to improve outcome in suspected acute myocardial infarction by pre-hospital administration of aspirin [Abstract]. *J Am Coll Cardiol* 1996;27(suppl A):11.

78. Ellerbeck EF, Jencks SF, Radford MJ, et al. Quality of care for medicare patients with acute myocardial infarction. A four-state pilot study from the Cooperative Cardiovascular Project. *JAMA* 1995;273:1509–1514.

79. Martin GV, Kennedy JW. Choice of thrombolytic agent. In: Julian DG, Braunwald E (ed). *Management of Acute Myocardial Infarction.* London: Saunders, 1994;71–105.

80. Dracup K, Alonzo AA, Atkins JM, et al. For the Working Group on Educational Strategies to Prevent Prehospital Delay in Patients at High Risk for Acute Myocardial Infarction: educational strategies to prevent prehospital delay in patients at high risk for acute myocardia. *J Thromb Thrombolysis* (in press).

81. Topol EJ. Early myocardial reperfusion: an assessment of current strategies in acute myocardial infarction. *Eur Heart J* 1996;17(suppl E):42–48.

*Cardiovascular Thrombosis: Thrombocardiology
and Thromboneurology, Second Edition,*
edited by M. Verstraete, V. Fuster, and E. J. Topol,
Lippincott–Raven Publishers, Philadelphia © 1998.

28

CCU Treatment of Acute Myocardial Infarction

Karl-Ludwig Neuhaus, Uwe Zeymer, and *Harvey D. White

*Medizinische Klinik II, Städtische Kliniken Kassel, D-34125 Kassel, Germany; and
Department of Cardiology, Green Lane Hospital, Auckland 1003, New Zealand

Acute myocardial infarction remains one of the most common causes of death in the Western world. Its prevalence is increasing in the developing world as the incidence of smoking increases, fat consumption increases, and the amount of exercise decreases (1). Most infarctions are due to rupture or fissuring of atherosclerotic plaques with exposure or release of thrombogenic factors, including tissue factor, as well as resultant platelet adhesion, aggregation, and thrombus formation (2). Rupture often occurs in lipid-rich, nonhemodynamically significant plaques. The superimposed thrombus may be occlusive, usually resulting in Q-wave infarction, or nonocclusive, usually resulting in a non–Q-wave infarction.

Mortality remains high despite major advances in medical therapy, including the administration of aspirin and thrombolytic therapy. Most deaths occur in the community, a third within the first hour, and the 28-day mortality rate remains about 50% (3). Among patients

eligible for thrombolytic therapy in the trial situation, the 1-month mortality rate may be as low as 6.3% (4). However, only about 50% of patients with acute infarction are eligible for thrombolytic therapy (5), and in routine clinical practice the rate of ineligibility may be higher than in a trial situation. Also, treatments that have been shown to be effective such as aspirin and thrombolytic therapy are still underutilized (6).

This chapter will concentrate on treatments that have been proven effective, with emphasis on evidence from clinical trials. We will also express our opinions on the numerous situations for which there are few randomized trial data available. The role of thrombolytic and antithrombotic therapy will not be discussed.

GENERAL MANAGEMENT

Relief of pain and anxiety should be the first priority. Triage should be rapid. An electrocardiogram should be performed within 10 minutes of the patient first being seen, aspirin should be given immediately, and, if the patient is thrombolytic eligible, administration of thrombolytic therapy should be begun within 15 to 30 minutes. Routine oxygen therapy has not been shown to be beneficial unless hypoxemia is present, but most coronary care units routinely administer oxygen in the first few hours.

Antiplatelet Agents

The Second International Study of Infarct Survival (ISIS-2) showed that patients randomized to receive 160 mg of aspirin had a 20% reduction in mortality at 35 days (7). Although the relative benefit was not related to the delay from the onset of chest pain, the absolute benefit may be larger in patients treated earlier, and it is recommended that patients be given aspirin as soon as possible.

In an overview of all the available trials, the Antiplatelet Trialists showed that long-term aspirin therapy resulted in a 10% to 15% reduction in mortality and a 20% to 30% reduction in reinfarction after 2 years (8). It is recommended that chronic low-dose aspirin therapy be continued indefinitely in all patients without contraindications.

β-Blockers

A number of trials have shown that intravenous administration of β-blockers reduces mortality by approximately 13% (9) and reduces the incidence of ventricular fibrillation and reinfarction (10). The major mechanism of benefit in these studies was reduction of cardiac rupture (11). However, these trials were conducted before the widespread use of aspirin and thrombolytic therapy, and a similar mortality benefit has not been shown in patients receiving thrombolytic therapy. Drugs that reduced the heart rate by more than 10 beats/min resulted in a greater mortality reduction than drugs with intrinsic sympathomimetic effects (Fig. 28-1).

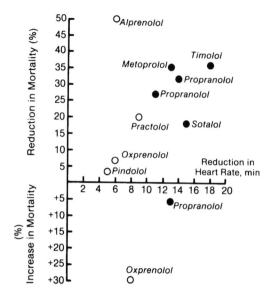

FIG. 28-1. Mortality reduction with β-blocker therapy. The effects seem to be less with oxprenolol and pindalol, both of which have sympathomimetic effects.

In the Thrombolysis in Myocardial Infarction (TIMI-IIB) study (12), 1,430 patients were randomized to receive either immediate intravenous metoprolol or oral metoprolol delayed by 6 days. Recurrent ischemia and infarction were reduced at 6 days and at 6 weeks by immediate metoprolol, but there was no effect on mortality or on the incidence of cardiac rupture. At 1 year there was no effect on reinfarction. It could be argued that the early effect on recurrent ischemia and infarction also might have been achieved by administration of metoprolol on day 1 or 2, and that the lack of effect on overall mortality could be due to a type 2 error.

It seems reasonable to recommend intravenous β-blockers for patients ineligible to receive thrombolytic therapy, but because of possible hypotensive effects, this should be delayed until after the administration of angiotensin-converting enzyme (ACE) inhibitors in patients with previous infarction, anterior infarction, or heart failure. The data are not sufficiently compelling to make a firm recommendation for treatment of thrombolytic-eligible patients.

The role of oral β-blocker therapy in prolonging life after recovery from acute myocardial infarction has been evaluated in trials involving more than 18,000 patients. A meta-analysis showed a reduction in mortality of 23% (10) and a reduction in nonfatal recurrent infarction of 26%. In the Metoprolol in Acute Myocardial Infarction (MIAMI) trial, mortality increased in patients in whom metoprolol was stopped after 7 years (13). It is therefore recommended that oral β-blocker therapy be continued indefinitely in all patients without contraindications.

Angiotensin-Converting Enzyme Inhibitors

ACE inhibitors block the renin-angiotensin system, which is activated early after infarction, particularly in patients with large infarcts. These agents reduce infarct scar expansion, left ventricular remodeling, shape changes, and left ventricular dilatation, which is the most important long-term adverse prognostic factor after acute myocardial infarction (14). ACE inhibitors also have been shown to produce coronary dilatation and to have local tissue effects.

In approximately 95,000 randomized patients, early administration of ACE inhibitors in the first few hours after the onset of myocardial infarction has been shown to save five lives at 1 month for every 1,000 patients treated (15–18). This benefit also was shown in patients treated with aspirin, β-blockers, or thrombolytic therapy.

In the Fourth International Study of Infarct Survival (ISIS-4), 28% of the mortality reduction was achieved on days 0 to 1, and in the Gruppo Italiano per lo Studio della Sopravvivenza nell'Infarto Miocardico (GISSI-3) study, 44% of the mortality reduction occurred on days 0 to 1. The effect is larger (more than 10 lives saved per 1,000 patients treated) in patients with anterior infarction, heart failure, or a history of previous infarction. There is a cost of about a 3% incidence of hypotension requiring cessation of therapy if the lower limit of systolic blood pressure for

administration is 90 to 100 mmHg, as in the ISIS-4 trial (15). The Survival of Myocardial Infarction Long-Term Evaluation (SMILE) study (19) randomized patients within 24 hours of the onset of symptoms of anterior infarction who did not receive thrombolytic therapy to receive zofenopril or control treatment. At 6 weeks there was a 25% reduction in mortality from 6.5% to 4.9%.

A number of trials have evaluated treatment after 48 hours. The Trandolapril Cardiac Evaluation Study (TRACE) (20) selected patients for randomization on the basis of echocardiographic evidence of impaired left ventricular function 3 to 7 days after infarction. Over 4 years, mortality was reduced by 22%. The Acute Infarction Ramipril Efficacy (AIRE) study (21) randomized patients with clinical evidence of heart failure to receive ramipril or placebo 3 to 10 days after infarction. There was a 27% reduction in mortality at 15 months. The Survival and Ventricular Enlargement (SAVE) trial (22) randomized patients with ejection fractions of less than 40% 3 to 16 days after infarction to receive captopril or placebo. At 42 months there was a 19% reduction in mortality. The survival curves did not diverge until about 12 months. Interestingly, there was also no effect on fatal and nonfatal reinfarction, suggesting that ACE inhibitors might reduce the incidence of plaque rupture or slow the atherosclerotic process.

Therapy could be begun selectively (for patients with anterior infarction, previous infarction, or heart failure) or nonselectively, i.e., in all patients 1 to 2 hours after administration of thrombolytic therapy or intravenous β-blockers if the systolic blood pressure was ≥105 mmHg. Our approach is to use selective therapy. Assessment of left ventricular function (invasively or noninvasively) should be done before hospital discharge, and ACE inhibitors should be commenced in patients with ejection fractions of less than 50%.

Nitrates

Sublingual nitroglycerin should be administered for the relief of ischemia. Intravenous nitroglycerin is also useful in patients with recurrent ischemia but is limited by the rapid development of tolerance within 24 hours (23). In addition to dilating the epicardial coronary arteries, increasing collateral blood flow, dilating the pulmonary veins, and decreasing ventricular preload, nitrates also have antiplatelet effects. They have been shown to reduce infarct size, left ventricular remodeling, dilatation, and heart failure and to increase collateral blood flow (24,25). Several recent large trials have assessed the effects on mortality and have shown no beneficial effects. The ISIS-4 trial randomized 58,000 patients to receive either oral controlled-release mononitrate or placebo for 4 weeks beginning soon after the onset of infarction. About 54% of patients received nontrial intravenous nitrates. Perhaps not surprisingly, there was no reduction in mortality (7.2% with placebo versus 7.0% with nitrates) (15). The GISSI-3 trial randomized 20,000 patients to receive either control therapy or intravenous nitrates followed by 10 mg of transdermal nitroglycerin daily for 6 weeks. There was also a high rate of crossover (43%) to active intravenous nitrate therapy. The mortality rate was 6.9% in the control patients and 6.5% in those who received nitrates (16). Nitrates were generally well tolerated in these trials. Nitrates are recommended for patients with continuing ischemia or heart failure.

Calcium-Channel Blockers

Use of calcium-channel blockers in the acute phase of infarction is not recommended and may in fact be harmful (26). Overviews show a trend toward increased mortality without any reduction in reinfarction. Diltiazem has been shown to reduce reinfarction in patients with non–Q-wave infarction, normal left ventricular function, and no heart failure (26). However, this was a retrospective subgroup analysis, and long-term follow-up showed no beneficial effect (27). In the Danish Verapamil Infarction (DAVIT-II) trial (28), verapamil therapy begun 1 to 3 weeks

after infarction reduced mortality by 9% (p = NS).

Antiarrhythmic Agents

The incidence of ventricular fibrillation after arrival in hospital has been reported to be between 2% and 7% (29,30), and more than 80% of episodes occur during the first 4 hours. Meta-analysis of randomized trials of various antiarrhythmic agents suggest that class I agents are of no benefit and may in fact be harmful, whereas class II and III agents may be beneficial (31). This has led to recommendations that class I agents, particularly lignocaine, should not be used prophylactically (32), and controversy continues in the absence of compelling evidence from large clinical trials regarding the role of class II agents such as sotalol and class III agents such as amiodarone.

The trials with lignocaine were conducted before the widespread use of aspirin and thrombolytic therapy and were generally of inadequate sample size. The incidence of ventricular fibrillation may be higher when thrombolytic therapy is given very early (33). It is of considerable interest that in GUSTO-I and GUSTO-IIb combined, patients receiving prophylactic lignocaine had a lower risk of death at 24 hours (odds ratio 0.81, 95% confidence interval 0.67 to 0.97) and a trend toward a lower death rate at 30 days (odds ratio 0.92, 95% confidence interval 0.82 to 1.02).

Cardiogenic Shock

Cardiogenic shock is responsible for most deaths during acute myocardial infarction. In the GUSTO-I study it was responsible for 58% of the 30-day mortality (34). The historic mortality rate for cardiogenic shock is between 80% and 90%. In the Fibrinolytic Therapy Trialists' overview, administration of thrombolytic therapy to patients with a systolic blood pressure of less than 100 mmHg and a heart rate of more than 100 beats/min resulted in 70 lives saved per 1,000 patients treated (35). Patients randomized to receive streptokinase rather than tissue-type plasminogen activator (t-PA) have had a lower mortality in two trials (4,36,37). Recent thrombolytic trials such as GUSTO (34) have reported lower mortality rates than the historic controls (58% at 30 days), but these results may reflect patient selection.

Seventeen studies have reported the results of angioplasty in a total of 453 patients with cardiogenic shock. Angioplasty resulted in a mortality rate of 46% (38–40). There have been 19 reports involving a total of 323 patients who have undergone bypass surgery for cardiogenic shock, with a pooled mortality rate of 32% (41). All of these studies were confounded by a selection bias. The Should We Emergently Revascularize Occluded Coronaries for Cardiogenic Shock (SHOCK) trial registry, completed in 1992 and 1993 (42) reported a mortality rate in unselected patients of 66%.

It appears from all of these studies that achievement of infarct artery patency is important in improving survival. Inotropic drugs such as dopamine and adrenaline are important in management but are unlikely to have a major impact on survival. Intra-aortic balloon pumping (IABP) is highly effective in stabilizing patients (43) but has not been shown to prolong life. A randomized trial evaluating IABP after thrombolytic therapy is ongoing. The results of the SHOCK trial, comparing revascularization (angioplasty or surgery) with intensive medical therapy (including thrombolysis and IABP), are awaited.

Mechanical Complications

Myocardial rupture from acute myocardial necrosis may affect the left ventricular free wall, leading to cardiac tamponade, the intraventricular septum causing a septal defect, or a papillary muscle causing acute mitral insufficiency. Echocardiography has become the primary diagnostic tool for all types of rupture.

Free wall rupture is almost invariably a fatal event, occurring predominantly in first myocardial infarctions in the elderly without preceding angina (44). The typical clinical presentation is recurrence of pain and ST-segment changes followed by circulatory collapse and electromechanical dissociation (45). The only therapeutic option is immediate surgical repair, which is rarely feasible. Only anecdotal survival has been reported, mostly in patients with subacute rupture (46).

Ventricular and papillary rupture result in acute volume overload of the infarcted left ventricle, usually followed by overt pulmonary congestion or edema. The therapy of choice is to reduce left ventricular afterload to the minimal tolerated level in order to decrease shunt and regurgitant volume. The vasodilator of choice is sodium nitroprusside. Intra-aortic balloon pumping is especially useful as a bridge to definitive treatment by surgical repair. The timing of surgery has been a matter of debate (47). In the experience of the authors, however, early operation is mandatory in all patients in whom pulmonary congestion does not respond readily to pharmacotherapy.

The timing of myocardial rupture has been greatly modified by thrombolytic therapy. In the prefibrinolytic era, rupture typically occurred between days 2 and 7 after acute infarction, whereas after thrombolysis the vast majority of ruptures occur within 24 hours after treatment (48).

Assessment of Reperfusion

The standard for the assessment of reperfusion is direct angiographic visualization of the infarct-related coronary artery. The TIMI flow grade (49) has been the generally accepted measure for describing the quality of antegrade flow beyond the infarct-related lesion and has been shown to closely correlate with survival in several thousand patients (50,51). A major drawback of angiography is the invasive nature of the investigation, which precludes its routine use because it is unavailable to most patients and carries an increased risk of bleeding, especially during thrombolytic treatment. Other indices of reperfusion, such as the rate of enzyme increase and resolution of ST elevation, have therefore been extensively investigated (52).

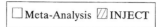

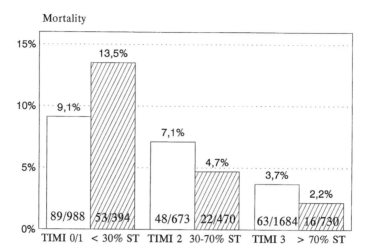

FIG. 28-2. Influence of TIMI flow grade after 90 minutes and ST-segment resolution after 180 minutes on in-hospital (30-day) mortality. Angiographic data were derived from a meta-analysis of angiographic trials and ST-resolution data from the electrocardiographic substudy of the INJECT trials. (Data from Schröder et al., ref. 53.)

The sensitivity and specificity of enzyme kinetics for the prediction of early and complete reperfusion in the individual patient are limited, and their predictive value can be improved only to a limited extent by inclusion of symptom relief (52). Furthermore, apart from myoglobin, the release of most enzymes is too slow to help in decision making with regard to reperfusion strategies. The most widely used, CKMB, takes up to 14 hours to reach its peak serum level in the case of early reperfusion, and even longer when the infarct artery remains occluded. Similar rates of increase are observed for troponins, which make these enzymes unsuitable for assessment of early reperfusion.

ST-segment resolution, which can be readily obtained in all patients presenting with ST elevation, has been shown to correlate at least as well to in-hospital mortality as does the TIMI flow grade (Fig. 28-2). Large, randomized trials have reported an extremely low mortality rate in patients with complete ST resolution, but those without ST resolution 3 hours after treatment onset have an eightfold death rate

(53,54). However, there is a significant proportion of patients with an intermediate extent of ST resolution, in whom the predictive value of this index is rather weak and insufficient when making decisions for the individual patient. Furthermore, at least one third of all patients with acute myocardial infarction do not present with ST elevation, which is a clear disadvantage when compared with enzyme analyses.

In summary, both enzyme and ST analysis are strong indicators of reperfusion and clinical outcome when patient groups are under consideration, e.g., in trials comparing different medical strategies. In the individual patient, decisions regarding therapeutic options, e.g., rescue angioplasty for presumably failed thrombolysis, remain a matter of clinical judgment rather than being guided by reperfusion indices.

REVASCULARIZATION AFTER LYSIS

Angioplasty after Successful Thrombolysis

After successful thrombolysis, a significant residual stenosis is found in the infarct-related

TABLE 28-1. *Meta-analysis of randomized trials comparing routine angioplasty (PTCA) after thrombolysis with a conservative strategy*

	Patients (n)		Death		Death or reinfarction	
PTCA regimen	PTCA	Conservative	PTCA	Conservative	PTCA	Conservative
Immediate PTCA	783	785	7.2%	6.5%	11.9%	13.1%
Early PTCA	2,506	2,504	5.2%	4.8%	12.1%	11.5%
Elective PTCA	252	254	3.6%	2.8%	12.7%	7.9%

coronary artery in more than 90% of patients. In order to prevent reocclusion and reinfarction, routine angioplasty has been attempted in a series of randomized trials. The timing of the intervention varied from immediate to early (1 to 2 days) or delayed (1 to 2 weeks) after thrombolysis. However, in none of these trials was routine angioplasty beneficial with regard to mortality or reinfarction (55). Instead, a nonsignificant trend toward a worse outcome in the aggressively treated groups has been observed (Table 28-1). Routine angioplasty after successful thrombolysis has therefore been abandoned. Angioplasty is now restricted to patients in whom it is clinically indicated, especially in those with recurrent angina, reinfarction, or hemodynamic instability.

Angioplasty after Failed Thrombolysis (Rescue Angioplasty)

Infarct artery patency is a powerful predictor of outcome in patients with acute myocardial infarction (51). For persistent occlusion of the infarct-related artery despite thrombolytic therapy, rescue angioplasty has been proposed to achieve coronary artery patency. Although successful angioplasty after failed thrombolysis seems to be beneficial and may improve clinical outcome, an unsuccessful attempt is associated with an exceedingly high mortality rate of up to 40% (56,57). The potential harm from unsuccessful procedures might therefore outweigh the benefit from successful ones. Furthermore, only 80% to 90% of patients with failed thrombolysis are suitable for rescue angioplasty. The average success rate is in the 80% range, and reocclusion occurs in about 20% of these patients.

The only randomized study of meaningful size to evaluate rescue angioplasty was conducted in 151 patients who presented within 8 hours of the onset of symptoms of their first anterior myocardial infarction and whose left anterior descending coronary artery was still occluded more than 90 minutes after the initiation of thrombolysis. The intervention was successful in 92% of the patients allocated to angioplasty. The combined endpoint of death or severe heart failure within 30 days occurred in 6% and 17% (p = 0.05) after angioplasty and conservative treatment, respectively. Although there was no difference in the resting left ventricular ejection fraction, the left ventricular ejection fraction during exercise was significantly better in the intervention group (58).

The decision for rescue angioplasty should be based on an individual assessment of symptoms, signs of ischemia on the electrocardiogram, and presence of hemodynamic instability. The benefit of successful rescue angioplasty must be weighed against the potential harm from an unsuccessful attempt, especially in hemodynamically stable patients with smaller infarcts or those with complete relief of symptoms after thrombolysis.

Coronary Artery Bypass Grafting after Thrombolysis

About 10% to 20% of patients with acute myocardial infarction are currently referred for coronary artery bypass grafting (4) for one of the following reasons: persistent or recurrent chest pain despite thrombolysis or angioplasty; coronary artery anatomy unsuitable for angioplasty (e.g., left main stenosis or diffuse triple-vessel disease); or a complication of acute myocardial infarction such as ventricular septal rupture or severe mitral regurgitation due to papillary muscle dysfunction. Patients with significant residual stenoses and recurrent angina after successful thrombolysis, who for anatomic reasons are more suitable for surgical revascularization than for angioplasty, have undergone coronary artery surgery with quite a low mortality rate. When surgery is performed urgently for active and ongoing ischemia or cardiogenic shock, operative mortality increases substantially (59). Nevertheless, surgical revascularization may improve the prognosis of patients with cardiogenic shock due to acute myocardial infarction, but the favorable results reported from shock registries may be confounded by a significant selection bias (42).

Patients who are referred urgently for bypass surgery within 6 to 12 hours after thrombolysis should receive aprotinin and fresh frozen plasma to correct their coagulation system deficit and minimize the requirements for blood transfusion.

PRIMARY ANGIOPLASTY

The first large series of patients treated with primary angioplasty for acute myocardial infarction were published in the early 1980s (60). The rationale of primary angioplasty was to increase the patency rate of the infarcted vessel, reduce the incidence of reocclusion, and avoid the risk of severe bleeding complications associated with thrombolysis.

With primary angioplasty, the initial success rate, in terms of early infarct vessel patency, is about 90%, with reocclusion rates comparable with those observed after thrombolysis. It was introduced as routine clinical practice in many interventional departments worldwide after three papers on direct angioplasty appeared in a 1993 issue of the *New England Journal of Medicine* (61–63). However, there is still controversy as to whether primary angioplasty, as a general treatment strategy, is superior to thrombolysis (Fig. 28-3). The first randomized trials comparing thrombolysis with primary angioplasty

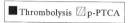

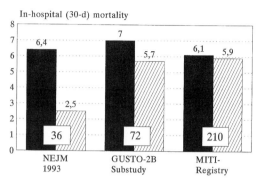

FIG. 28-3. Comparison of in-hospital (30-day) mortality after thrombolysis and primary angioplasty for acute myocardial infarction. The numbers in the bars represent the total number of deaths observed in the studies. (Data from Gibbons et al., ref. 61; Grines et al., ref. 62; Zijlstra et al., ref. 63; GUSTO IIb, ref. 64; and Every et al., ref. 65.)

showed a better outcome after angioplasty with regard to mortality, intracerebral bleeding, and reinfarction. In contrast, the larger GUSTO-IIb angioplasty substudy, comparing primary angioplasty and thrombolysis with front-loaded t-PA in over 1,000 patients, showed no significant difference in 30-day mortality (5.7% with angioplasty versus 7.0% with t-PA), but there was a marginally significant difference in the combined endpoint of death, nonfatal reinfarction, and nonfatal disabling stroke (9.6% with angioplasty versus 13.7% with t-PA) (64). At 6-month follow-up, the differences in favor of angioplasty were almost halved and were no longer significant (10.6% with angioplasty versus 8.2% with t-PA). The MITI registry (65), which may reflect everyday clinical practice more closely than a randomized trial, showed no benefit of direct angioplasty over thrombolysis in more than 3,000 patients.

Therefore, the evidence presented as yet does not justify a general recommendation to treat every patient with acute myocardial infarction by angioplasty rather than thrombolysis. Primary angioplasty should certainly be used in patients with contraindications against thrombolytic therapy or a high risk of intracerebral bleeding. In cardiogenic shock, successful angioplasty seems to improve the outcome (42). However, the true impact of immediate angioplasty in cardiogenic shock can only be estimated from randomized studies that are currently underway.

FAILED REPERFUSION AND RECURRENT ISCHEMIA

After 15 years of intensive investigation aimed at improving the efficacy of intravenous thrombolysis in acute myocardial infarction, there is still a significant failure rate in terms of early, complete, and sustained reperfusion. Depending on the thrombolytic agent, the dose, the dosing regimen, and the timing of patency assessment, the proportion of unsuccessful treatments ranges from about 65% for streptokinase to about 40% for reteplase (41). These percentages refer to the incidence of TIMI-3 flow measured angiographically 90 minutes after the onset of treatment, and they clearly indicate the unsatisfactory efficacy of contemporary fibrinolytic therapy and the need for improvement. This has become more evident with the advent of primary angioplasty as an alternative reperfusion strategy, although the 95% success rates reported in early, relatively small randomized trials have not been fully confirmed in the larger, more recent trials such as GUSTO-IIb, where the TIMI-3 rates after angioplasty were only about 75% (64).

Several mechanisms contribute to an eventual failure of thrombolysis to reopen an infarct-related acute coronary occlusion:

- In up to 10% of all cases the occlusion may not be thrombotic at all, but rather caused by a spontaneous coronary dissection and/or intramural hemorrhage, or prolonged coronary artery spasm.
- In cardiogenic shock or severe hemodynamic compromise, perfusion pressures may not be adequate to achieve sufficient local concentrations of the thrombolytic agent, especially when the site of the occlusion is at the blind end of an unbranched segment of the artery.
- The composition of the clot may be unsuitable for fibrinolysis; for example, platelet-rich clots are known to be resistant to plasmin.
- Even in the case of successful clot lysis, adequate reperfusion may not occur due to the "no reflow" phenomenon, which has been attributed to myocardial edema or microvascular damage after prolonged periods of ischemia.

The rate of TIMI-3 flow is lower after streptokinase or urokinase than with t-PA or its analogues when treatment is begun more than 3 hours after treatment onset, reflecting the decreasing efficacy of these compounds in older clots and more cross-linked fibrin. Fixed doses have almost exclusively been used, although a significant decrease in early patency and TIMI-3 flow rates with most thrombolytics has been reported with increasing patient weight.

Attempts to increase the efficacy of thrombolysis by improvements in concomitant treatment, without increasing the risk of bleeding, have yielded mixed results. Hirudin, as a more specific thrombin inhibitor than heparin, has not fulfilled its promise in major clinical trials, at least as an adjunct to t-PA (66,67). The value of more potent platelet inhibition by selective glycoprotein IIb/IIIa receptor blockade remains to be determined in the setting of acute myocardial infarction and thrombolysis.

Recurrent ischemia after successful thrombolysis occurs in 5% to 10% of patients during the hospital stay (4). A lower incidence has been reported after direct angioplasty, which may indicate the need for reassessment of its value in the prevention of these adverse events, although former trials consistently showed no clinical benefit from routine use of angioplasty after thrombolysis.

RECOMMENDATIONS

The patient should immediately be given 150 to 300 mg of aspirin to chew (if it is enteric-coated) or to swallow, and aspirin ther-apy should be continued indefinitely. Routine prophylactic lignocaine is not recommended in patients who are ineligible for thromboly-sis. Thrombolytic-ineligible patients and those in cardiogenic shock should be consid-ered for primary angioplasty and, in centers experienced in primary angioplasty, this is an alternative approach for thrombolytic-eligible patients provided they can be treated within 60 minutes of arrival. Intravenous heparin is recommended for thrombolytic-treated pa-tients and for thrombolytic-ineligible patients with anterior infarction. Intravenous β-block-ers should be given to thrombolytic-ineligible patients and considered for thrombolytic-eli-gible patients. Oral β-blockers should be ad-ministered long-term in all patients without contraindications.

ACE inhibitors should be begun within 1 to 2 hours of admission in patients with left ven-tricular failure, anterior infarction, or a history of previous infarction if the systolic blood pressure is ≥105 mmHg. ACE inhibitors also should be begun as soon as possible in patients with ejection fractions of less than 50%. Ni-trates are not recommended for routine use ex-cept for relief of ischemia. Calcium-channel blockers are not recommended for routine use in patients with Q-wave or non–Q-wave infarc-tion and should be considered third-line ther-apy after β-blockers and nitrates for treatment of angina. Oral anticoagulants are recom-mended for patients with echocardiographic evidence of left ventricular thrombus. All pa-tients should have assessment of primary risk factors and treatment as appropriate, as well as cardiac rehabilitation if it is available.

CONCLUSION

The management of acute myocardial in-farction has changed dramatically over the past decade. The goal of therapy is to achieve rapid, complete, and sustained reperfusion of the infarct-related artery as soon as possible. Intravenous thrombolytic therapy currently achieves this in just over half the patients who receive it. Angioplasty could potentially achieve this more efficiently, but it is limited by availability, and the achievement of epicar-dial blood flow may not necessarily translate into myocyte nutritional blood flow due to the no reflow phenomenon. Antithrombotic ther-apy to reduce reocclusion, ACE inhibitors to reduce remodeling and left ventricular dilata-tion, β-blockers to reduce myocardial de-mands, cardiac rupture and arrhythmias, and nitrates to reduce ischemia all play major roles in the modern, comprehensive strategy for the management of patients with acute myocardial infarction. Primary prevention through modifi-cation of risk factors continues to be the most important strategy to affect the overall commu-nity impact of myocardial infarction. New ther-apies are urgently needed to reduce still further the rates of mortality and morbidity.

REFERENCES

1. Pearson TA. Global perspectives on cardiovascular dis-ease. *Evidence-Based Cardiovasc Med* 1997;April:4–6.
2. Davies MJ, Woolf N, Robertson WB. Pathology of acute myocardial infarction with particular reference to oc-clusive coronary thrombi. *Br Heart J* 1976;38:659–664.
3. WHO MONICA project. Myocardial infarction and coronary deaths in the World Health Organization MONICA project: registration procedures, event rates, and case-fatality rates in 38 populations from 21 coun-tries in four continents. *Circulation* 1994;90:583–612.
4. The GUSTO Investigators. An international randomized trial comparing four thrombolytic strategies for acute myocardial infarction. *N Engl J Med* 1993;329:673–682.
5. French JK, Williams BF, Hart HH, et al. Prospective evaluation of eligibility for thrombolytic therapy in acute myocardial infarction. *Br Med J* 1996;312:1637–1641.
6. Ketley D, Woods KL. Impact of clinical trials on clini-cal practice:example of thrombolysis for acute myocar-dial infarction. *Lancet* 1993;342:891–894.
7. ISIS-2 (Second International Study of Infarct Survival) Collaborative Group. Randomised trial of intravenous streptokinase, oral aspirin, both, or neither among 17,187 cases of suspected acute myocardial infarction: ISIS-2. *Lancet* 1988;2:349–360.
8. Secondary prevention of vascular disease by prolonged antiplatelet treatment. Antiplatelet Trialists' Collabora-tion. *Br Med J Clin Res Ed* 1988;296:320–331.
9. Held PH, Yusuf S. Effects of beta-blockers and calcium channel blockers in acute myocardial infarction. *Eur Heart J* 1993;14(suppl F):18–25.
10. Yusuf S, Peto R, Lewis J, Collins R, Sleight P. Beta blockade during and after myocardial infarction: an overview of the randomized trials. *Prog Cardiovasc Dis* 1985;27:335–371.
11. ISIS-1 (First International Study of Infarct Survival) Collaborative Group. Mechanisms for the early mortal-ity reduction produced by beta-blockade started early in

acute myocardial infarction:ISIS-1 [erratum *Lancet* 1988;2:292]. *Lancet* 1988;1:921–923.

12. Roberts R, Rogers WJ, Mueller HS, et al. Immediate versus deferred β-blockade following thrombolytic therapy in patients with acute myocardial infarction: results of the thrombolysis in myocardial infarction (TIMI) II-B study. *Circulation* 1991;83:422–437.

13 Olsson G, Oden A, Johansson L, Sjogren A, Rehnqvist N. Prognosis after withdrawal of chronic postinfarction metoprolol treatment: a 2–7 year follow-up. *Eur Heart J* 1988;9:365–372.

14. White HD, Norris RM, Brown MA, Brandt PWT, Whitlock RML, Wild CJ. Left ventricular end-systolic volume as the major determinant of survival after recovery from myocardial infarction. *Circulation* 1987;76:44–51.

15. ISIS-4 (Fourth International Study of Infarct Survival) Collaborative Group. ISIS-4: a randomised factorial trial assessing early oral captopril, oral mononitrate, and intravenous magnesium sulphate in 58,050 patients with suspected acute myocardial infarction. *Lancet* 1995;345:669–685.

16. Gruppo Italiano per lo Studio della Sopravvivenza nell'Infarto Miocardico. GISSI-3: effects of lisinopril and transdermal glyceryl trinitrate singly and together on 6-week mortality and ventricular function after acute myocardial infarction. *Lancet* 1994;343:1115–1122.

17. Swedberg K, Held P, Kjekshus J, et al. Effects of the early administration of enalapril on mortality in patients with acute myocardial infarction: results of the Cooperative New Scandinavian Enalapril Survival Study II (CONSENSUS II). *N Engl J Med* 1992;327:678–684.

18. Chinese Cardiac Study Collaborative Group. Oral captopril versus placebo among 13,634 patients with suspected acute myocardial infarction: interim report from the Chinese Cardiac Study (CCS-1). *Lancet* 1995;345:686–687.

19. Ambrosioni E, Borghi C, Magnani B. The effect of the angiotensin-converting-enzyme inhibitor zofenopril on mortality and morbidity after anterior myocardial infarction. The Survival of Myocardial Infarction Long-Term Evaluation (SMILE) Study Investigators. *N Engl J Med* 1995;332:80–85.

20. Kober L, Torp Pedersen C, Carlsen JE, et al. A clinical trial of the angiotensin-converting-enzyme inhibitor trandolapril in patients with left ventricular dysfunction after myocardial infarction. Trandolapril Cardiac Evaluation (TRACE) Study Group. *N Engl J Med* 1995;333:1670–1676.

21. The Acute Infarction Ramipril Efficacy (AIRE) Study Investigators. Effect of ramipril on mortality and morbidity of survivors of acute myocardial infarction with clinical evidence of heart failure. *Lancet* 1993;342:821–828.

22. Pfeffer MA, Braunwald E, Moyé LA, et al. Effect of captopril on mortality and morbidity in patients with left ventricular dysfunction after myocardial infarction: results of the survival and ventricular enlargement trial. *N Engl J Med* 1992;327:669–677.

23. Meredith IT, Alison JF, Zhang FM, Horowitz JD, Harper RW. Captopril potentiates the effects of nitroglycerin in the coronary vascular bed. *J Am Coll Cardiol* 1993;22:581–587.

24. Jugdutt BI, Warnica JW. Intravenous nitroglycerin therapy to limit myocardial infarct size, expansion, and complications: effect of timing, dosage, and infarct lo-

cation [erratum *Circulation* 1989;79:1151]. *Circulation* 1988;78:906–919.

25. Bussmann WD, Passek D, Seidel W, Kaltenbach M. Reduction of CK and CK-MB indexes of infarct size by intravenous nitroglycerin. *Circulation* 1981;63:615–622.

26. Gibson RS, Boden WE, Theroux P, et al. Diltiazem and reinfarction in patients with non–Q-wave myocardial infarction. Results of a double-blind, randomized, multicenter trial. *N Engl J Med* 1986;315:423–429.

27. Wong SC, Greenberg H, Hager WD, Dwyer EM. Effects of diltiazem on recurrent myocardial infarction in patients with non–Q wave myocardial infarction. *J Am Coll Cardiol* 1992;19:1421–1425.

28. Danish Study Group on Verapamil in Myocardial Infarction. Effect of verapamil on mortality and major events after acute myocardial infarction (the Danish Verapamil Infarction Trial II–DAVIT II). *Am J Cardiol* 1990;66:779–785.

29. Lawrie DM, Higgins MR, Godman MJ, Oliver MF, Julian DG, Donald KW. Ventricular fibrillation complicating acute myocardial infarction. *Lancet* 1968;2:523–528.

30. Volpi A, Maggioni A, Franzosi MG, Pampallona S, Mauri F, Tognoni G. In-hospital prognosis of patients with acute myocardial infarction complicated by primary ventricular fibrillation. *N Engl J Med* 1987;317:257–261.

31. Teo KK, Yusuf S, Furberg CD. Effects of prophylactic antiarrhythmic drug therapy in acute myocardial infarction. An overview of results from randomized controlled trials. *JAMA* 1993;270:1589–1595.

32. Ryan TJ, Anderson JL, Antman EM, et al. ACC/AHA Guidelines for the management of patients with acute myocardial infarction: a report of the American College of Cardiology/American Heart Association Task Force on Practice Guidelines (Committee on Management of Acute Myocardial Infarction). *J Am Coll Cardiol* 1996;28:1328–1428.

33. Boissel JP, Castaigne A, Mercier C, Lion L, Leizorovicz A. Ventricular fibrillation following administration of thrombolytic treatment. The EMIP experience. European Myocardial Infarction Project. *Eur Heart J* 1996;17:213–221.

34. Holmes DR, Califf RM, Van de Werf F, et al. Difference in countries' use of resources and clinical outcome for patients with cardiogenic shock after myocardial infarction: results from the GUSTO Trial. *Lancet* 1997;349:75–78.

35. Fibrinolytic Therapy Trialists' (FTT) Collaborative Group. Indications for fibrinolytic therapy in suspected acute myocardial infarction: collaborative overview of early mortality and major morbidity results from all randomised trials of more than 1000 patients. *Lancet* 1994;343:311–322.

36. Gruppo Italiano per lo Studio della Sopravvivenza nell'Infarto Miocardico. GISSI-2: a factorial randomised trial of alteplase versus streptokinase and heparin versus no heparin among 12,490 patients with acute myocardial infarction. *Lancet* 1990;336:65–71.

37. The International Study Group. In-hospital mortality and clinical course of 20,891 patients with suspected acute myocardial infarction randomised between alteplase and streptokinase with or without heparin. *Lancet* 1990;336:71–75.

38. O'Neill WW. Angioplasty therapy of cardiogenic

shock: are randomized trials necessary? *J Am Coll Cardiol* 1992;19:915–917.

39. Bates ER, Topol EJ. Limitations of thrombolytic therapy for acute myocardial infarction complicated by congestive heart failure and cardiogenic shock. *J Am Coll Cardiol* 1991;18:1077–1084.
40. Himbert D, Juliard JM, Steg PG, Karrillon GJ, Aumont MC, Gourgon R. Limits of reperfusion therapy for immediate cardiogenic shock complicating acute myocardial infarction. *Am J Cardiol* 1994;74:492–494.
41. Hochman JS. Cardiogenic shock:can we save the patient? *ACC Educational Highlights* 1996;12:1–5.
42. Hochman JS, Boland J, Sleeper LA, et al. Current spectrum of cardiogenic shock and effect of early revascularization on mortality. Results of an International Registry. SHOCK Registry Investigators. *Circulation* 1995; 91:873–881.
43. Scheldt S, Wilner G, Mueller H, et al. Intra-aortic balloon counterpulsation in cardiogenic shock. *N Engl J Med* 1973;288:979–984.
44. Lukac P, Kofler K, Waldhor T, Steinbach K. Epidemiology of heart wall rupture during acute infarction. *Z Kardiol* 1996;85:776–781.
45. Figueras J, Curos A, Cortadellas J, Soler-Soler J. Reliability of electromechanical dissociation in the diagnosis of left ventricular free wall rupture in acute myocardial infarction. *Am Heart J* 1996;131:861–864.
46. Aliabadi D, Roldan CA, Pett S, Follis F, Holland M. Percutaneous cardiopulmonary support for the management of catastrophic mechanical complications of acute myocardial infarction. *Cathet Cardiovasc Diagn* 1996; 37:223–226.
47. Lemery R, Smith HC, Giuliani ER, Gersh BJ. Prognosis in rupture of the ventricular septum after acute myocardial infarction and role of early surgical intervention. *Am J Cardiol* 1992;70:147–151.
48. Becker RC, Gore JM, Lambrew C, et al. A composite view of cardiac rupture in the United States National Registry of Myocardial Infarction. *J Am Coll Cardiol* 1996;27:1321–1326.
49. The TIMI Study Group. The Thrombolysis in Myocardial Infarction (TIMI) Trial: phase I findings. *N Engl J Med* 1985;312:932–936.
50. Simes RJ, Topol EJ, Holmes DR, et al. Link between the angiographic substudy and mortality outcomes in a large randomized trial of myocardial reperfusion: importance of early and complete infarct artery reperfusion. *Circulation* 1995;91:1923–1928.
51. Granger CB, White HD, Bates ER, Ohman EM, Califf RM. A pooled analysis of coronary arterial patency and left ventricular function after intravenous thrombolysis for acute myocardial infarction. *Am J Cardiol* 1994;74: 1220–1228.
52. Califf RM, O'Neil W, Stack RS, et al. Failure of simple clinical measurements to predict perfusion status after intravenous thrombolysis. *Ann Intern Med* 1988;108: 658–662.
53. Schröder R, Wegscheider K, Schröder K, Dissmann R, Meyer-Sabellek W. Extent of early ST segment elevation resolution: a strong predictor of outcome in patients with acute myocardial infarction and a sensitive measure to compare thrombolytic regimens: a substudy of the International Joint Efficacy Comparison of Thrombolytics (INJECT) Trial. *J Am Coll Cardiol* 1995;26: 1657–1664.

54. Neuhaus KL, Molhoek P, Tebbe U, Jessel A, Zeymer U, Schröder R. Early resolution of ST segment elevation is a strong predictor of cardiac 30-day mortality from AMI. Results of the HIT-4 ECG substudy. *Eur Heart J* (in press).
55. Michels KB, Yusuf S. Does PTCA in acute myocardial infarction affect mortality and reinfarction rates? A quantitative overview (meta-analysis) of the randomized clinical trials. *Circulation* 1995;91:476–485.
56. Ellis SG, Van de Werf F, Ribeiro-daSilva E, Topol EJ. Present status of rescue coronary angioplasty:current polarization of opinion and randomized trials. *J Am Coll Cardiol* 1992;19:681–686.
57. McKendall GR, Forman S, Sopko G, Braunwald E, Williams DO. Value of rescue percutaneous transluminal coronary angioplasty following unsuccessful thrombolytic therapy in patients with acute myocardial infarction. Thrombolysis in Myocardial Infarction Investigators. *Am J Cardiol* 1995;76:1108–1111.
58. Ellis SG, da Silva ER, Heyndrickx G, et al. Randomized comparison of rescue angioplasty with conservative management of patients with early failure of thrombolysis for acute anterior myocardial infarction. *Circulation* 1994;90:2280–2284.
59. Gersh BJ, Chesebro JH, Braunwald E, et al. Coronary artery bypass graft surgery after thrombolytic therapy in the Thrombolysis in Myocardial Infarction Trial, Phase II (TIMI II). *J Am Coll Cardiol* 1995;25:395–402.
60. Hartzler GO, Rutherford BD, McConahay DR, et al. Percutaneous transluminal coronary angioplasty with and without thrombolytic therapy for treatment of acute myocardial infarction. *Am Heart J* 1983;106:965–973.
61. Gibbons RJ, Holmes DR, Reeder GS, et al. Immediate angioplasty compared with the administration of a thrombolytic agent followed by conservative treatment for myocardial infarction. *N Engl J Med* 1993;328: 685–691.
62. Grines CL, Browne KF, Marco J, et al. A comparison of immediate angioplasty with thrombolytic therapy for acute myocardial infarction. *N Engl J Med* 1993;328: 673–679.
63. Zijlstra F, de Boer MJ, Hoorntje JC, Reiffers S, Reiber JHC, Suryapranata H. A comparison of immediate coronary angioplasty with intravenous streptokinase in acute myocardial infarction. *N Engl J Med* 1993;328:680–684.
64. The Global Use of Strategies to Open Occluded Coronary Arteries in Acute Coronary Syndromes (GUSTO IIb) Angioplasty Substudy Investigators. A clinical trial comparing primary coronary angioplasty with tissue plasminogen activator for acute myocardial infarction. *N Engl J Med* 1997;336:1621–1628.
65. Every NR, Parsons LS, Hlatky M, Martin JS, Weaver WD, for the myocardial infarction triage and intervention investigators. A comparison of thrombolytic therapy with primary coronary angioplasty for acute myocardial infarction. *N Engl J Med* 1996;335:1253–1260.
66. The Global Use of Strategies to Open Occluded Coronary Arteries (GUSTO) IIb Investigators. A comparison of recombinant hirudin with heparin for the treatment of acute coronary syndromes. *N Engl J Med* 1996;335: 775–782.
67. Antman EM, for the TIMI 9B Investigators. Hirudin in acute myocardial infarction: Thrombolysis and Thrombin Inhibition in Myocardial Infarction (TIMI) 9B Trial. *Circulation* 1996;94:911–921.

Cardiovascular Thrombosis: Thrombocardiology
and Thromboneurology, Second Edition,
edited by M. Verstraete, V. Fuster, and E. J. Topol,
Lippincott–Raven Publishers, Philadelphia © 1998.

29

Adjunctive Antithrombotic Treatment to Thrombolysis in Acute Myocardial Infarction

David A. Vorchheimer and *David W. M. Muller

*Cardiovascular Institute, Mount Sinai Medical Center, New York, New York 10029; and
Department of Cardiology, St. Vincent's Hospital, Darlinghurst NWS 2010, Australia

Pathologic and angiographic observations derived from clinical trials of acute myocardial infarction have firmly established the crucial role of thrombosis in the pathogenesis of acute myocardial infarction. Reperfusion therapy is designed to dissolve or remove thrombotic material at the site of atherosclerotic plaque rupture, as well as to restore blood flow. In the Global Use of Strategies to open Occluded Coronary Arteries-I (GUSTO-I) study, mortality at 24 hours (1) and 30 days (2) was related to the adequacy of angiographic patency at 90 minutes; this benefit was sustained at 1 year (3).

Recombinant tissue plasminogen activator (t-PA) restores complete patency in just over one half of patients, whereas streptokinase achieves this goal in less than one third (4). Partial reperfusion (i.e., Thrombolysis in

Myocardial Infarction-2 [TIMI-2] flow) confers a worse prognosis than no reperfusion in the early setting, suggesting that partial reperfusion results in additional damage to the left ventricle (1). Furthermore, not all arteries opened after thrombolytic therapy remain open: reocclusion after thrombolytic therapy occurs in approximately 5% to 10% of cases during the hospital stay and in up to 30% within the first year (5). Reocclusion of an artery initially reperfused is associated with a substantial increase in early mortality (6). Approximately 50% of reocclusions are clinically silent (6). Even aggressive approaches to prevent reocclusion, such as a strategy of routine early angiography and angioplasty after thrombolysis, do not prevent recurrent ischemia, reinfarction, or death (7).

After successful thrombolysis, a residual thrombus may remain. This thrombus constitutes a powerful stimulus to rethrombosis (8). Active thrombin and factor X, liberated from within the thrombus during thrombolysis, are partly rebound to the fibrin remnants. Platelets are activated and accumulate. Platelets adhering to the reforming thrombus release vasoconstrictors, which causes arterial spasm, increased shear forces, endothelial dysfunction, and further platelet deposition. Although all thrombolytic agents can activate platelets indirectly by generating plasmin (9), streptokinase may even activate platelets directly, possibly by the binding of streptokinase-specific antibody complexes to platelets (10). At clinically used doses needed to achieve coronary reperfusion, streptokinase is associated with much higher systemic plasmin activity than the more fibrin-specific thrombolytic t-PA. Moreover, streptokinase induces a more prolonged systemic plasmin activity than does t-PA because of the longer half-life of the streptokinase–plasminogen complex. Plasmin, released from the lysing clot, activates blood coagulation, leads to thrombin generation, and aggregates platelets (11). The administration of thrombolytic therapy to patients results in increases in thrombin generation (12) (as measured by elaboration of prothrombin fragment 1.2) and thrombin activity (13) (as measured by plasma levels of fibrinopeptide A, which is released from fibrin by the action of thrombin). Activation of procoagulant markers during thrombolytic therapy in a clinical trial was associated with failed reperfusion and increased mortality (14). Treatment with heparin prevented thrombin activation, but not thrombin generation (15). Numerous studies have examined the effects of adjunctive antithrombin therapy for patients with acute myocardial infarction.

ADJUNCTIVE ANTITHROMBIN THERAPY IN ACUTE MYOCARDIAL INFARCTION TREATED WITHOUT THROMBOLYSIS

A large number of trials of heparin followed by oral anticoagulant therapy were conducted before the thrombolytic era. Many of these were not randomized, properly controlled, or sufficiently large to detect a significant treatment effect. Three trials were of sufficient size to evaluate treatment effect. Anticoagulation was initiated relatively late (72 hours), and the quality and measurement of anticoagulant effect was uncertain. In the Medical Research Trial, short-term anticoagulation reduced mortality from 18.2% to 16.2%, and reinfarction from 13.0% to 9.7% (p = NS) (16). In the Bronx Municipal Hospital study, treatment with heparin followed by phenindione reduced the case mortality from 21.2% to 14.9% (p < 0.05) (17). In the Veterans Administration Cooperative Study, in-hospital all-cause mortality was reduced from 11.2% to 9.6% (p = NS) in the anticoagulation group (18). In a meta-analysis of all six randomized trials of anticoagulants in acute myocardial infarction conducted before 1977, the pooled analysis showed a 21% reduction in mortality, from 19.6% to 15.4% (p < 0.05) (19).

ADJUNCTIVE ANTITHROMBIN THERAPY IN ACUTE MYOCARDIAL INFARCTION TREATED WITH THROMBOLYSIS

Patency Studies

In the Thrombolysis and Angioplasty in Myocardial Infarction 3 (TAMI-3) trial, administration of a 10,000-U heparin bolus, initiated 20 minutes after lysis and not followed by a continuous infusion, did not improve 90-minute patency when compared with t-PA alone (20). In a study by Bleich and colleagues, 83 patients receiving t-PA were randomized to heparin (5,000 U intravenous bolus followed by 1,000 U/hr infusion) or to placebo. Angiographic patency at a mean of 57 hours was 71% in the heparin-treated group, but only 44% in the no heparin group (21). In the Heparin-Aspirin Reperfusion Trial (HART), patency was 82% for patients receiving t-PA with bolus and intravenous heparin, compared with 51% in patients treated with t-PA and 80 mg aspirin (22). In the

HART study, coronary patency was related to adequacy of anticoagulation as determined by prolongation of the activated partial thrombo-plastin time (APTT) value: patients with an APTT value less than 45 seconds had a pa-tency rate of 45% (TIMI 2 or 3), whereas pa-tients with APTT values greater than 60 sec-onds had a 95% TIMI 2 or 3 patency rate. In the European Cooperative Study Group Study, of 652 patients who all received t-PA and aspirin, angiography at 81 hours showed slightly, but significantly, improved patency with heparin compared with placebo (83% versus 75%, p = 0.01) (23).

To synthesize the results of these trials, it appears that the greatest benefit for heparin is seen in the absence of aspirin therapy, such as was seen in the Bleich trial; when an adequate dose of aspirin is administered in conjunction with the thrombolytic agent, the heparin ben-efit is small (ECSG-6 trial), and when a low and potentially suboptimal aspirin dose is given, the heparin benefit is intermediate (HART). Patency trials examining intra-venous heparin in addition to aspirin and streptokinase, or anistreplase (24) (DUCCS-1), showed no benefit with heparin. In the lat-ter trial, withholding intravenous heparin was associated with a 46% reduction in bleeding complications.

The value of oral anticoagulation started 48 hours after successful thrombolysis was examined in the APRICOT trial (25). In 300 patients with patent infarct-related arteries 48 hours after thrombolysis, no difference in re-occlusion at 3 months was apparent between patients treated with aspirin, warfarin, or nei-ther (25% versus 30% versus 32%). An event-free clinical course was observed in 93% of patients treated with aspirin, 82% of those treated with warfarin, and 76% of those given placebo (p < 0.001 for aspirin versus placebo, p < 0.05 for aspirin versus warfarin). These data suggest that long-term oral anticoagu-lation with warfarin has little to offer over oral aspirin. Its use postinfarction should therefore be confined to patients at risk for peripheral thromboembolism from ventricular mural thrombi.

Mortality Trials

In the ISIS-2 pilot study (26), intravenous heparin was associated with a nonsignificant decrease in reinfarction, but no decrease in mortality. The subsequent ISIS-2 trial was an open-label, randomized trial using a 2 × 2 fac-torial design of four treatment groups: (a) 1.5 million units (MU) intravenous streptokinase over 60 minutes, (b) 162.5 mg oral aspirin/day for 30 days, (c) both treatments, (d) neither treatment. Although the trial did not include protocol-mandated heparin, nearly two thirds of patients enrolled in this study received some form of heparin in a nonrandomized manner: 5-week mortality was highest in pa-tients who received no heparin (9.8%), inter-mediate in those treated with subcutaneous heparin (7.6%), and lowest in those who re-ceived intravenous heparin in addition to streptokinase and aspirin (6.4%) (27). Two large trials were designed to specifically ad-dress the value of adjunctive heparin with thrombolytic therapy. The GISSI-2 trial (28) used a 2 × 2 factorial design to randomize pa-tients to intravenous t-PA or streptokinase, as well as to 12,500 U heparin subcutaneously or no heparin beginning 12 hours after random-ization. Among the entire 20,891 patients en-rolled in GISSI-2 and the International t-PA/SK Mortality Trial (29), there was no difference in mortality between heparin and no heparin groups. In ISIS-3, patients were also randomized to 12,500 U of subcutaneous unfractionated heparin every 12 hours. Thirty-five day mortality was comparable in both groups (30). However, 17% of patients enrolled in the placebo group crossed over at the discretion of the treating physician and re-ceived heparin. A pooled analysis combining the results of these two trials showed a 35-day mortality rate of 10.2% in the placebo group compared with 10.0% in the heparin group (p = NS) (30).

The failure of these large trials to demon-strate a significant benefit from heparin led to examination of design features of the trial to account for the trial results. Heparin therapy was initiated relatively late in both trials (first dose administered at 4 hours in ISIS-3, and at 12 hours in the International t-PA/SK Mortality Trial). The dose administered was relatively conservative, and the subcutaneous route of administration would have produced only minimal anticoagulation, with delayed onset of therapeutic effect. Studies of the time course of APTT prolongation have shown that the peak level of anticoagulation achieved by a dose of subcutaneous heparin occurs 4 hours after injection and that maximal APTT prolongation only occurs after repetitive doses of heparin (31). The GUSTO-I trial was partially designed to address questions regarding the role of subcutaneous versus intravenous heparin. Among 20,251 patients treated with streptokinase plus aspirin, half were randomized to subcutaneous heparin (12,500 U twice daily beginning 4 hours after the start of the thrombolytic infusion), and half to intravenous heparin (5,000-U bolus begun immediately, followed by a continuous infusion of 1,000 U/hr adjusted to maintain a target APTT of 60 to 85 seconds). All 10,396 patients receiving t-PA also received intravenous heparin; t-PA plus subcutaneous heparin was not investigated. In the streptokinase arms, the 30-day mortality rates were 7.2% with subcutaneous heparin and 7.4% with intravenous heparin (p = NS); in the t-PA plus intravenous heparin group, the mortality rate was 6.3% (32).

Two recent overviews have examined the role of heparin in acute myocardial infarction. An analysis of the six randomized trials comparing intravenous heparin to no heparin after thrombolysis concluded that available data were insufficient to support or refute the use of routine intravenous heparin (33). Among the 1,735 patients pooled together, in-hospital mortality was 5.1% for patients allocated to intravenous heparin versus 5.6% for controls, corresponding to absolute difference of five deaths per 1,000 patients treated. No evidence for reduction in reinfarction and recurrent ischemia was seen, although a nonsignificant trend toward increased risk of intracranial bleeding and stroke, as well as a clear increase in any bleeding, was noted for patients allo-

cated to heparin. No significant difference was observed in the effect of heparin between patients receiving streptokinase or t-PA, or between those who did and did not receive aspirin. The investigators noted that to have adequate statistical power to detect a 10% relative risk reduction in mortality would require the randomization of 40,000 to 50,000 patients in a two-arm trial of heparin versus no heparin. In a systematic overview of 26 studies of anticoagulant versus placebo, the investigators concluded that the available clinical evidence from randomized trials does not justify the routine addition of either intravenous or subcutaneous heparin to aspirin, regardless of which fibrinolytic therapy is used (34). In the absence of aspirin, anticoagulant therapy reduced mortality by 25% (from 14.9% to 11.4%, 2p = 0.002). However, in the presence of aspirin, heparin reduced mortality by only 6% (from 9.1% to 8.6%, 2p = 0.03); this finding was only just conventionally significant. Effects of similar size were seen with the different anticoagulant regimens studied (i.e., intravenous versus subcutaneous, high dose versus low dose). A small nonsignificant excess of stroke and a definite excess of major bleeding was seen with heparin (1.0% versus 0.7%, 2p < 0.0001). Most of the evidence pooled in this analysis comes from the aforementioned GISSI-2 and ISIS-3 studies, in which heparin began relatively late. The GUSTO-I study (which did not directly compare heparin with control) was not included in this analysis.

ADJUNCTIVE NOVEL THROMBIN INHIBITORS

Numerous novel thrombin inhibitors are under investigation (see Chapter 6). Only those agents evaluated in human trials will be summarized here. Direct thrombin inhibitors have been extensively studied in recently completed clinical trials. Pilot data obtained from dose-ranging studies such as TIMI-5 (35) (hirudin with t-PA) and TIMI-6 (36) (hirudin with streptokinase) were encouraging. Two trials were launched to compare heparin to hirudin as adjunctive treatments to thrombolysis. Both studies used a single high dose of hirudin (the highest dose used in TIMI-5) as well as aggressive weight-adjusted heparin dosing. Both TIMI 9A (37) and GUSTO IIa (38) were terminated prematurely by their data and safety monitoring committees because of an excess of intracerebral hemorrhage in both the heparin and hirudin arms. Both studies subsequently resumed with lower doses of anticoagulation. In GUSTO IIb, among the 4,131 patients with ST-segment elevation (74% of whom received thrombolysis, consisting of t-PA in 70% of patients and streptokinase in 30%), 30-day death and myocardial infarction occurred in 11.3% of the heparin group and 9.9% of the hirudin group (p = NS) (39). In TIMI 9B, the composite primary endpoint occurred in 11.9% of the heparin-treated patients and 12.9% of the hirudin-treated patients (p = NS) (40). Mechanistic differences between heparin and hirudin have been invoked to explain the failure of hirudin to demonstrate superiority in clinical trials, despite its superior thrombin inhibition. A current view is that although hirudin is more potent than heparin as a thrombin inhibitor, heparin is the more effective inhibitor of procoagulant (prothrombin) activation and thrombin generation (41). As discussed above, during thrombolysis, thrombin is elaborated. This thrombin is inhibited by hirudin; however, small amounts of fibrin-bound thrombin may be transiently protected from the action of hirudin and could lead to further fibrin production, platelet activation, and thrombus formation. Studies of hemostatic markers of thrombin generation (fibrinopeptide A) and thrombin activation (prothrombin fragment 1.2) support the view that heparin is more effective at inhibiting thrombin generation than hirudin and does so at equivalent levels of thrombin activity (42). The direct thrombin inhibitor hirulog was evaluated in the recently completed HERO Trial (43). Four hundred twelve patients admitted within 12 hours of onset of acute myocardial infarction received aspirin and streptokinase and were randomized to intravenous heparin, or to one of two doses of hirulog.

TIMI-3 flow at 90 minutes was highest in the high-dose hirulog group (48%), slightly lower in the low-dose hirulog group (46%), and lowest in the heparin arm (35%), (heparin versus hirulog, p = 0.024). The study was not powered to examine clinical endpoints.

At present, the combination of direct thrombin inhibitors with streptokinase appears most promising. In the aforementioned GUSTO IIb trial, compared with patients treated with streptokinase plus heparin, patients treated with streptokinase plus hirudin had a substantial reduction in the composite endpoint of mortality and nonfatal reinfarction at 24 hours (5.1% versus 2.0%, p = 0.009) and 30 days (14.4% versus 8.6%, p = 0.004). No differences were seen between the heparin- and hirudin-treated patients in the t-PA group (44). The ongoing HERO-2 trial will enroll 17,000 patients to further explore this question.

Several other specific thrombin inhibitors are the subject of ongoing clinical trials. Argatroban, a nonpeptide arginine derivative, has been evaluated in two multicenter, randomized, controlled trials as adjunctive therapy to thrombolysis for acute myocardial infarction. In the Argatroban in Myocardial Infarction (AMI) Study, 910 patients received low-dose argatroban (1.0 mg/kg/min), high-dose argatroban (3.0 mg/kg/min), or placebo for 48 to 72 hours (45). All patients received aspirin and streptokinase (1.5 MU over 45 to 60 minutes). Angiography, performed in a subgroup of 180 patients, showed no difference in the incidence of TIMI grade 3 flow rate at 90 minutes for the overall population, but significantly better complete patency (as measured by frame counting) in patients presenting within 3 hours of symptom onset who were treated with high-dose argatroban. At 30 days, there was no difference in clinical event rate for the overall population, but a trend toward a better outcome in patients treated within 3 hours with high-dose argatroban. Other ongoing argatroban studies include the 1,200 patient ARGAMI trial and the MINT trial, which was terminated after recruitment of 120 patients.

The combination of efegatran (given intravenously for 72 to 96 hours) and streptokinase was evaluated in 247 patients in a randomized, open-label, dose-ranging study (46). Clinical and angiographic outcomes of patients receiving the combination were compared with those of patients receiving t-PA and intravenous heparin. In a second dose-ranging study, heparin or escalating doses of efegatran (0.3 to 1.2 mg/kg/hr) were compared in 330 patients with acute myocardial infarction (47). Clinical results of these two trials should soon be available. Two additional thrombin receptor antagonists, napsagatran and inogatran, have been characterized but not yet tested clinically as adjunctive treatments to thrombolysis for acute myocardial infarction.

<u>CLASS I</u> (Evidence and /or general agreement that treatment is beneficial, useful, and effective)
1. Patients undergoing percutaneous and/or surgical revascularization

<u>CLASS II</u> (Conflicting evidence and/or divergence of opinion about the usefulness/efficacy of a treatment)

<u>CLASS IIa</u> (Weight of evidence/opinion is in favour of usefulness/efficacy)

1. Intravenously in patients undergoing reperfusion therapy with alteplase (tPA). *Comment: The recommended regimen is 70 U/kg as a bolus at initiation of alteplase infusion, then an initial maintenance dose of approximately 15 U/kg/hr, adjusted to maintain aPTT at 1.5 to 2.0 times control (50-75 seconds) for 48 hours. Continuation of heparin beyond 48 hours should be restricted to patients at high risk for systemic or venous thromboembolism.*

2. Subcutaneously (7500U twice daily) (intravenous heparin is an acceptable alternative) in all patients not treated with thrombolytic therapy who do not have a contraindication to heparin. In patients who are at high risk for systemic emboli (large or anterior MI, atrial fibrillation, previous thrombus or known left ventricular thrombus), intravenous heparin is preferred.

3. Intravenously in patients treated with nonselective thrombolytic agents (streptokinase, anistreplase, urokinase) who are at high risk for systemic emboli (large or anterior MI, atrial fibrillation, previous thrombus or known left ventricular thrombus). *Comment: It is recommended that heparin be withheld for 4 hours and that aPTT testing begin at that time. Heparin should be started when the aPTT returns to less than 2 times control (about 70 seconds), then infused to keep the aPTT 1.5-2.0 times control (initial infusion rate about 1000 U/hr). After 48 hours, a change to subcutaneous heparin, warfarin, or aspirin alone should be considered.*

<u>CLASS IIb</u> (Usefulness/efficacy is less well established by evidence/options)

1. Patients treated with nonselective thrombolytic agents (streptokinase, anistreplase, urokinase), not at high risk, subcutaneous heparin 7500 U to 12500 U twice a day until completely ambulatory.

<u>CLASS III</u> (Conditions for which there is evidence and/or general agreement that treatment is not useful/effective and in some cases may be harmful)l.

1. Routine intravenous heparin with 6 hours to patients receiving a nonselective fibrinolytic agent (streptokinase, anistreplase, urokinase) who are not at high risk for systemic embolism.

FIG. 29-1. ACC/AHA recommendations for heparin use in acute myocardial infarction. (Modified from Ryan et al., ref. 51.)

Finally, low molecular weight heparins have several potential advantages over unfractionated heparin, including a more predictable anticoagulant effect, resistance to inhibition by activated platelets, and reduced need for monitoring. Among patients with a recently diagnosed acute myocardial infarction treated with streptokinase, extending the anticoagulant effect of heparin by continuous treatment with low molecular weight heparin for an additional 25 days prevented recurrent ischemic events in the month after initiating therapy, and this effect was sustained over 6 months (48). Low molecular weight heparins have not been used together with thrombolytic therapy in large trials. In one small study, systemic factor Xa and thrombin activity after thrombolytic therapy for acute myocardial infarction was uninfluenced by prethrombolytic administration of either dalteparin or unfractionated heparin (49).

RECOMMENDATIONS FOR ANTITHROMBOTIC THERAPY

Although considerable controversy exists regarding some aspects of adjunctive antithrombotic therapy with thrombolysis, recent practice guidelines published by the American College of Chest Physicians (50) and the American College of Cardiology/ American Heart Association (51) offer physicians a current consensus view and a practical approach (Fig. 29-1). In patients who receive thrombolysis, recommendations for adjunctive heparin differ depending on the thrombolytic agent. In patients given t-PA, high-dose intravenous heparin (70 to 75 U/kg bolus started immediately, followed by continuous infusion at 15 U/kg/hr, approximately 1,000 to 1,200 U/hr) should be maintained to a target APTT of 1.5 to 2.0 times control for 48 hours. Given the absence of randomized data showing evidence for benefit of any adjunctive heparin regimen administered with streptokinase (and the other nonselective agents, anistreplase and urokinase), neither intravenous nor subcutaneous heparin is routinely recommended. Intravenous heparin (begun 4 hours after lytic therapy and started when the APTT is less than twice control) is indicated for patients at high risk for embolism, such as those with large or anterior myocardial infarction, atrial fibrillation, previous embolus, or documented left ventricular thrombus. For such high-risk patients who received t-PA, the intravenous heparin infusion may be continued beyond 48 hours for those at high risk for coronary artery reocclusion or converted to a subcutaneous regimen for those at persistent risk of systemic embolization. The target APTT level in patients treated with thrombolytic therapy remains somewhat controversial. Prior attempts to achieve enhanced lysis with aggressive anticoagulation (target APTT 60 to 90 seconds), such as were used in the weight-adjusted nomograms in the aforementioned GUSTO IIa and TIMI 9A trials, resulted in the premature termination of these studies due to an excessive rate of intracerebral hemorrhage in the heparin-treated groups. More recent information identified a somewhat lower APTT (target 50 to 75 seconds) as the optimal range (52). For patients who do not receive thrombolysis who do not have a contraindication to heparin, intravenous or subcutaneous heparin is recommended; the intravenous route is preferred for high-risk patients (as defined above).

ADJUNCTIVE ANTIPLATELET THERAPY

As noted above, platelet activation plays a critical role not only in the initial formation of intracoronary thrombus after plaque rupture, but also in reocclusion after successful spontaneous or pharmacologically mediated thrombolysis. Activated platelets provide several cofactors necessary for maximal expression of prothrombinase activity (53), optimize the activity of coagulation cascade enzymes on their surface membrane (54), and protect these enzymes from circulating inhibitors (54). Several factors released from activated platelets, including platelet factor 4 and heparitinase, also degrade heparin and limit its effectiveness in preventing thrombus propagation and reoc-

clusion (55). The administration of thrombolytic therapy for acute myocardial infarction
increases the extent of platelet activation by
releasing thrombin from dissolving clot
(12,56), and by inducing the release of
platelet-activating factor (57). This is true for
both fibrin-specific (13,58) and nonspecific
(9,10) lytic agents. Thus, measures to inhibit
platelet activation should clearly be an integral
part of every reperfusion strategy.

CLINICAL TRIALS OF ADJUNCTIVE ANTIPLATELET THERAPY

Aspirin and Other Inhibitors of Platelet Activation

The importance of aspirin, and antiplatelet
therapy in general, in the management of
acute myocardial infarction was highlighted
in the Second International Study of Infarct
Survival Collaborative Group (ISIS-2) trial
(27). In this randomized, placebo-controlled
trial, the 5-week mortality rate was reduced
by 21% in patients treated with aspirin alone
(160 mg/day), by 26% in those treated with
streptokinase alone, and by 42% in those
treated with both streptokinase and aspirin.
On the basis of these results, and the fact that
aspirin is inexpensive and well tolerated, it is
strongly recommended that all patients presenting with definite or suspected acute myocardial infarction should receive soluble aspirin (at least 160 mg) as soon as possible.
Nevertheless, aspirin usage remains relatively
low in some patient groups, particularly the
elderly (59).

Aspirin exerts its antiplatelet effect by irreversibly acetylating the enzyme cyclooxygenase, thereby inhibiting the production of
thromboxane A_2 (and prostacyclin) for the life
of the platelet. Thromboxane A_2, which is synthesized in response to a number of stimuli,
promotes platelet aggregation. Because
thromboxane A_2 is only one of a very large
number of platelet agonists, the ability of aspirin to prevent platelet activation, adhesion,
and aggregation is limited. The combination
of aspirin with ticlopidine or clopidogrel, a

ticlopidine analogue, offers the potential for
broader spectrum platelet inhibition than can
be achieved with aspirin alone (60). Ticlopidine and clopidogrel block adenosine diphosphate–mediated platelet activation by selectively and irreversibly binding to its platelet
receptor. Data from clinical trials suggest that
these agents may play a useful role in preventing thrombotic complications after percutaneous coronary interventions (61,62), and perhaps in acute myocardial infarction. A third
group of antiplatelet agents includes ridogrel,
a specific inhibitor of thromboxane A_2 synthase and, to a lesser extent, of the thromboxane A_2 receptor. This has the theoretical advantage over aspirin of avoiding the
potentially detrimental effects of inhibition of
prostacyclin synthesis. To date, however, clinical experience with this drug, particularly in
the setting of acute myocardial infarction, is
limited (63,64). In an experimental study (65),
the combination of t-PA with hirulog and ridogrel appeared to enhance thrombolytic efficacy and prevent reocclusion in a canine
model of acute myocardial infarction. In one
clinical study, however, ridogrel did not improve 90-minute patency when compared with
aspirin (63). Finally, prostacyclin analogues
have been used as adjunctive antiplatelet
agents with thrombolytic therapy for acute
myocardial infarction (66–68). Intracoronary
prostaglandin E_1 increased the rate of reperfusion and reduced the incidence of reocclusion
in patients treated with intracoronary streptokinase (68). Similarly, beraprost, a stable analogue of prostacyclin, reduced the incidence of
reocclusion after successful t-PA–mediated
reperfusion in a canine model of acute myocardial infarction (67). However, intravenous
prostacyclin did not increase the efficacy of
alteplase in the TAMI-4 study (66).

Inhibition of Platelet Adhesion

Once activated, initial binding of platelets
to injured endothelium involves the interaction between a multivalent molecule (von
Willebrand factor) and both subendothelial
components of the vessel wall and specific

platelet receptors, particularly under conditions of high shear stress. The platelet receptors include glycoprotein (GP)Ib and GPIIb/IIIa. Blockade of the von Willebrand-GPIb binding domain with a recombinant peptide fragment (VCL) has been shown to abolish platelet-mediated cyclic flow variations in the injured coronary arteries of nonhuman primates (69) and to enhance the thrombolytic efficacy of t-PA in dogs with acute myocardial infarction induced by coronary electrical injury (70). To date, however, inhibitors of the GPIb receptor have not been tested as adjuncts to thrombolysis in clinical trials.

Monoclonal Antibody to GPIIb/IIIa Receptor

The final common pathway for platelet aggregation is activation of the GPIIb/IIIa receptor. Platelet activation results in activation and externalization of the membrane receptor, which allows platelet aggregation to occur by cross-linking of adjacent receptors with fibrinogen. Since 1983, a number of inhibitors of the GPIIb/IIIa receptor have been developed and used in clinical trials (71). The first of these, 7E3, was developed as a murine monoclonal antibody (72). To reduce the potential for immunologic reactions to the drug, the murine Fc fragment was removed and was replaced by the human constant immunoglobulin G Fab region to form a chimera known as c7E3 Fab or abciximab (71).

Abciximab has now undergone extensive clinical testing. In a series of landmark studies, abciximab therapy given as a bolus of 0.25 mg/kg with a subsequent 12-hour infusion (10 mg/min) was shown to markedly reduce ischemic complications after percutaneous coronary interventions (73,74) both during the initial hospital stay and during a 6-month follow-up. Flow cytometry studies have suggested that one potential explanation for this prolonged benefit of abciximab is that the drug remains membrane bound for several weeks. One possible explanation is that the drug may be displaced from the membrane of one platelet to that of a younger platelet, thereby perpetuating the antiplatelet effect longer than expected from the known survival of the original platelet population.

The potential for synergism between GPIIb/IIIa inhibition and thrombolytic therapy was initially evaluated in the TAMI-8 pilot study (75). In this open-labeled trial, 60 patients were randomly assigned to receive the murine monoclonal antibody m7E3 Fab in increasing doses 3, 6, or 15 hours after the administration of t-PA (100 mg over 3 hours) for acute myocardial infarction. Abciximab was given as a bolus only in doses ranging from 0.1 to 0.25 mg/kg. Ten patients who received t-PA alone were included as control patients. Platelet aggregation was almost completely inhibited with the highest doses of abciximab. In 43 patients who underwent coronary angiography, the infarct-related artery was patent (TIMI 3 flow) in 56% of control patients compared with 92% of patients treated with m7E3Fab at a mean of 121 hours. In addition to this greater infarct vessel patency, there was a trend toward less frequent recurrent ischemia in patients who received abciximab.

Major bleeding was frequent in both groups in the TAMI-8 study. The potential for life-threatening bleeding is clearly a major concern with this combination of powerful antithrombotic compounds. It should be noted that in the TAMI-8 study (75), heparin was given at conventional doses when the m7E3 was started late (15 hours) after the t-PA, and was reduced to a 2,500 unit bolus and infusion of 800 U/hr when the study drug was initiated 3 or 6 hours after t-PA. In the PROLOG and EPILOG trials (76,77), it was demonstrated that the incidence of major bleeding could be substantially reduced by lowering the dose of heparin from 100 U/kg to 70 U/kg without reducing the short-term therapeutic efficacy of the abciximab. Thus, it may be possible to substantially reduce the dose of heparin given to patients receiving combined abciximab and thrombolytic therapy as a means of reducing the potential for hemorrhagic side effects.

Experimental studies suggest that it also may be possible to reduce the dose of thrombolytic therapy without reducing thrombolytic efficacy. Although abciximab has no direct intrinsic thrombolytic activity, it does appear to have some disaggregatory activity and can lead to dissolution of platelet-rich thrombi when given without thrombolytic therapy, perhaps by displacing fibrinogen from the platelet membrane. Furthermore, abciximab also binds to and inactivates vitronectin. Because vitronectin is required for binding of plasminogen activator 1 (PAI-1) to the endothelium, abciximab may indirectly augment plasminogen activator activity by inhibiting PAI-1 activation.

Consistent with these observations are those of Gold and colleagues, who examined the ability of abciximab to achieve reperfusion in the absence of concomitant thrombolytic therapy in an open-chested canine model of acute myocardial infarction and in patients undergoing primary angioplasty for acute myocardial infarction (78). In the 13 patients studied (78), bolus abciximab alone achieved TIMI grade 2 or 3 flow in seven patients (54%) within 10 minutes of administration, and an increase in TIMI flow by at least one grade in 11 patients (85%). Similarly, a very high early patency rate has been observed in the first 100 patients enrolled in the TIMI 14 trial of low-dose fibrinolytic therapy and full-dose abciximab. Thus, this may be an effective means of achieving lysis of platelet-rich thrombi in acute myocardial infarction with a considerably lower risk of bleeding. On the basis of these observations, larger randomized clinical trials of low-dose fibrinolytic therapy with full-dose abciximab are planned. Further data on the role of abciximab in the setting of acute myocardial infarction will also soon be available from the RAPPORT trial, a 500-patient randomized controlled trial of primary angioplasty with or without adjunctive abciximab.

Peptide Inhibitors of GPIIb/IIIa Receptor

A second class of IIb/IIIa receptor antagonists was developed after the screening of a number of naturally occurring GPIIb/IIIa an-

tagonists (such as the pit viper venoms) demonstrated homology for a three-amino acid domain that was responsible for their antiplatelet activity (79). These compounds had in common an arginine-glycine-aspartate (RGD) sequence typically occurring in linear arrays up to 100 amino acids in length. Integrelin is a synthetic, cyclic heptapeptide with a KGD (lysine-arginine-aspartate) sequence that has greater specificity for the fibrinogen binding region of the GPIIb/IIIa receptor than the RGD peptides. It has a rapid onset of action and a half-life of 1.5 to 2 hours. Thus, in contrast to abciximab, integrelin is a competitive inhibitor with very high specificity for the GPIIb/IIIa receptor and a rapid onset and short duration of activity.

Clinical trials of integrelin have evaluated its efficacy in unstable angina (80), elective percutaneous coronary interventions (81), and acute myocardial infarction (82). In the latter trial (82), 180 patients were assigned to one of six doses of integrelin or placebo, with a bolus dose ranging from 36 to 180 mg/kg and an infusion rate ranging from 0.2 to 0.75 mg/kg/min. Heparin was given to all patients as a bolus dose of 40 U/kg and an infusion of 15 U/kg/hr adjusted to maintain the APTT at two to 2.5 times the baseline level. The study was conducted in two phases, the first 132 patients as an open-label dose ranging study, and the next 48 patients as a double-blind, randomized study using the highest integrelin dose. t-PA was given to all patients according to the accelerated regimen (32). Thus, in contrast to the TAMI-8 study (75), in the integrelin trial, the heparin dose was lower and was weight adjusted, accelerated t-PA was given, the integrelin was given as a bolus and a 24-hour infusion, and it was given within 30 minutes of the initiation of the thrombolytic infusion.

When compared with patients treated with no integrelin, those receiving the highest dose of integrelin had a higher 90 minute patency (TIMI-3 flow: 66% versus 39%, $p = 0.006$) and a shorter median time to ST-segment recovery (65 versus 116 minutes, $p = 0.05$), with no increase in the frequency of bleeding. Platelet function studies showed that the highest dose of integrelin achieved maximal platelet inhibition 2 to 6 hours after the integrelin bolus, and platelet aggregation was inhibited by more than 70% at 24 hours. Four hours after cessation of the infusion, platelet activity had returned to normal in all patient groups.

Concern has been raised about the adequacy of the dosing regimen in this and other clinical trials of integrelin (83). Currently, in contrast to the in vitro assays available for abciximab therapy, there is no method available for directly determining receptor occupancy of the competitive GPIIb/IIIa inhibitors. Normally, RGD binding sites bind calcium, which must be displaced by the adhesive proteins or receptor antagonist. In the presence of a calcium chelating agent (e.g., citrated blood), in vitro tests of drug efficacy may overestimate the therapeutic efficacy of a given drug dose. Thus, although in vitro assays suggested a desired biologic effect of integrelin, this may have been a misrepresentation of the true degree of platelet inhibition.

Nonpeptide GPIIb/IIIa Antagonists

The third group of compounds that inhibit the platelet GPIIb/IIIa receptor are small, nonpeptide molecules that bind to the RGD recognition site of the GPIIb/IIIa receptor. Clinical testing of several of these compounds has now been completed. Tirofiban, a tyrosine derivative, was shown in one study to be highly effective during the periprocedural period in the setting of high-risk percutaneous coronary intervention for unstable angina or acute myocardial infarction (84). In two additional studies, prolonged infusion of tirofiban reduced ischemic complications and death in patients admitted with unstable angina or non–Q-wave myocardial infarction (45,85). To date, tirofiban has not been evaluated in a clinical study as an adjunct to thrombolytic therapy for the management of acute myocardial infarction.

A second nonpeptide inhibitor of the GPIIb/IIIa receptor is lamifiban. In a double-blind, dose-ranging clinical trial, lamifiban reduced ischemic events in patients with unstable angina both during the infusion and at 1 month with only a small increase in the incidence of bleeding (86). A larger, 9,000 patient study of lamifiban for unstable angina (PARAGON) is currently underway (87). The combination of lamifiban with thrombolytic therapy for acute myocardial infarction was tested in the recently completed PARADIGM trial (88). Patients who presented within 12 hours of the onset of chest pain were randomly assigned to receive lamifiban (400-mg bolus followed by 1.5 mg/min infusion for 24 hours) in combination with either streptokinase or t-PA. Angiography was not performed routinely, but continuous 12-lead electrocardiographic monitoring was used as a surrogate for patency at 90 minutes (89). In a preliminary report from the first 150 patients, ST segments returned toward baseline (less than 200 mV) more frequently in the lamifiban group than in the control group (77% versus 56%, p = 0.019), with no difference in the frequency of major bleeding (2% versus 4%, p = NS) or need for blood transfusion (12% versus 10%, p = NS).

The third nonpeptide GPIIb/IIIa agent currently undergoing evaluation in early clinical trials is xemilofiban, an orally active agent. Xemilofiban offers the potential for prolonged, potent antiplatelet therapy, not only during the acute phase of thrombolysis, but also during the convalescent phase during which the risk of reocclusion remains high. Important interactions between intravenously administered antagonists such as abciximab and xemilofiban have been noted (90), suggesting that careful pharmacodynamic studies will be necessary before trials of xemilofiban and thrombolytic therapy can be performed. Nonetheless, larger scale clinical trials of xemilofiban are currently planned.

CONCLUSION

Successful reperfusion therapy requires both successful thrombolysis and long-term maintenance of patency by prevention of reocclusion. The combination of a fibrinolytic agent with a potent inhibitor of platelet aggregation is likely to achieve optimal rates of reperfusion without reocclusion. Whether the newer antithrombin therapies will prove to be superior to heparin, and whether better inhibitors of thrombin generation and activity will be synergistic with the antiplatelet agents remains to be seen. However, it is highly likely that the combination of one or more of these agents, in appropriate doses, will achieve far greater patency rates than have been achieved to date, with a reduced incidence of serious hemorrhagic side effects.

REFERENCES

1. Kleiman NL, White HD, Ohman EM, et al. Mortality within 23 hours of thrombolysis for acute myocardial infarction. *Circulation* 1994;90:2658–2665.
2. Simes RJ, Topol EJ, Holmes DR, et al. The link between the angiographic substudy and mortality outcomes in a large randomized trial of myocardial reperfusion: the importance of early and complete infarct artery reperfusion. *Circulation* 1995;91:1923–1928.
3. Califf RM, White HD, Van der Werf F, et al. One year results from the Global Utilization of Streptokinase and t-PA for Occluded Coronary Arteries (GUSTO-I) trial. *Circulation* 1996;94:1233–1238.
4. GUSTO-I Angiographic Investigators. The effect of tissue plasminogen activator, streptokinase, or both on coronary artery patency, ventricular function, and survival after acute myocardial infarction. *N Engl J Med* 1993;329:1615–1622.
5. Verheugt FWA, Meijer A, Lagrand WK, van Eenige MJ. Reocclusion: the flip side of coronary thrombolysis. *J Am Coll Cardiol* 1996;27:766–773.
6. Ohman EM, Califf RM, Topol EJ, et al. Consequences of reocclusion after successful reperfusion therapy in acute myocardial infarction. *Circulation* 1990;82: 781–791.
7. The TIMI Study Group. Comparison of invasive and conservative strategies after treatment with intravenous tissue plasminogen activator in acute myocardial infarction. *N Engl J Med* 1989;320:618–627.
8. Topol EJ. Reperfusion for acute myocardial infarction: 1997 and beyond. *Cleveland Clin J Med* 1997;64:9–12.
9. Fitzgerald DJ, Catella F, Roy L, FitzGerald GA. Marked platelet activation in vivo after intravenous streptokinase in patients with acute myocardial infarction. *Circulation* 1988;77:142–150.
10. Vaughn DE, Van Houtte E, Declerck PJ, Collen D. Streptokinase-induced platelet aggregation: prevalence and mechanism. *Circulation* 1991;84:84–91.
11. Niewiarowski S, Senyi AF, Gillies P. Plasmin-induced platelet aggregation and platelet release reaction: effects on hemostasis. *J Clin Invest* 1973;52:1647–1659.
12. Eisenberg PR, Sobel BE, Jaffe AS. Activation of prothrombin accompanying thrombolysis with recombinant tissue-type plasminogen activator. *J Am Coll Cardiol* 1992;19:1065–1069.
13. Owen J, Friedman KD, Grossman BA, Wilkins C, Berke AD, Powers ER. Thrombolytic therapy with tissue plasminogen activator or streptokinase induces transient thrombin activity. *Blood* 1988;72:616–620.
14. Scharfstein JS, Abedschein DR, Eisenberg PR. Usefulness of fibrinogenolytic and procoagulant markers during thrombolytic therapy in predicting clinical outcomes in acute myocardial infarction. *Am J Cardiol* 1996;78:503–510.
15. Merlini PA, Bauer KA, Oltrona L, et al. Thrombin generation and activity during thrombolysis and concomitant heparin therapy in patients with acute myocardial infarction. *J Am Coll Cardiol* 1995;25:203–209.
16. BMJ Working Party. Assessment of short-term anticoagulant administration after cardiac infarction: report of the Working Party on Anticoagulant Therapy in Coronary Thrombosis to the Medical Research Council. *Br Med J* 1969;1:335–342.
17. Drapkin A, Merskey C. Anticoagulant therapy after acute myocardial infarction: relation of therapeutic benefit to patient's age, sex, and severity of infarction. *JAMA* 1972;222:541–548.
18. Veterans Administration Cooperative Study. Anticoagulants in acute myocardial infarction: results of a cooperative clinical trial. *JAMA* 1973;225:724–729.
19. Chalmers TC, Matta RJ, Smith JJ, Kunzler AM. Evidence favoring the use of anticoagulants in the hospital phase of acute myocardial infarction. *N Engl J Med* 1977;297:1091–1096.
20. Topol EJ, George BS, Kereiakes DJ, et al. A randomized controlled trial of intravenous tissue plasminogen activator and early intravenous heparin in acute myocardial infarction. *Circulation* 1989;79:281–286.
21. Bleich SD, Nichols TC, Schumacher RR, Cooke DH, Tate DA, Teichman SL. Effect of heparin on coronary arterial patency after thrombolysis with tissue plasminogen activator in acute myocardial infarction. *Am J Cardiol* 1990;66:1412–1417.
22. Hsia J, Hamilton WP, Kleiman N, Roberts R, Chaitman BR, Ross AM. A comparison between heparin and low-dose aspirin as adjunctive therapy with tissue plasminogen activator for acute myocardial infarction. Heparin-Aspirin Reperfusion Trial (HART) Investigators. *N Engl J Med* 1990;323:1433–1437.
23. de Bono DP, Simoons ML, Tijssen J, et al. Effect of early intravenous heparin on coronary patency, infarct size, and bleeding complications after alteplase thrombolysis: results of a randomized double blind European Cooperative Study Group trial. *Br Heart J* 1992;67:122–128.
24. O'Connor CM, Meese R, Carney R, et al. A randomized trial of intravenous heparin in conjunction with anistreplase (anisoylated plasminogen streptokinase activator complex) in acute myocardial infarction: the Duke University Clinical Cardiology Study (DUCCS) 1. *J Am Coll Cardiol* 1994;23:11–18.
25. Meijer A, Verheugt FWA, Werter CJPJ, Lie KI, van der Pol JMJ, van Eenige MJ. Aspirin versus coumadin in the prevention of reocclusion and recurrent ischemia after successful thrombolysis: a prospective placebo-controlled angiographic study. Results of the APRICOT Study. *Circulation* 1993;87:1524–1530.
26. The ISIS Pilot Study Investigators. Randomized factorial trial of high dose intravenous streptokinase, or oral aspirin and of intravenous heparin in acute myocardial infarction. *Eur Heart J* 1987;8:634–642.

27. ISIS-2 Collaborative Group. Randomised trial of intravenous streptokinase, oral aspirin, both or neither among 17,187 cases of suspected acute myocardial infarction: ISIS-2. *Lancet* 1988;2:349–360.

28. Gruppo Italiano per lo Studio della Sopravvivenza nell'Infarto miocardico. GISSI-2: a factorial randomised trial of alteplase versus streptokinase and heparin versus no heparin among 12,490 patients with acute myocardial infarction. *Lancet* 1990;336:65–71.

29. The International Study Group. In-hospital mortality and clinical course of 20,891 patients with suspected acute myocardial infarction randomised between alteplase and streptokinase with or without heparin. *Lancet* 1990;336:71–75.

30. ISIS-3 (Third International Study of Infarct Survival) Collaborative Group. ISIS-3: a randomised comparison of streptokinase vs tissue plasminogen activator vs anistreplase and of aspirin plus heparin vs aspirin alone among 41,299 cases of suspected acute myocardial infarction. *Lancet* 1992;339:753–770.

31. Prins MH, Hirsh J. Heparin as an adjunctive treatment after thrombolytic therapy for acute myocardial infarction [Abstract]. *Am J Cardiol* 1991;67:3–11.

32. The GUSTO Investigators. An international randomized trial comparing four thrombolytic strategies for acute myocardial infarction. *N Engl J Med* 1993;329:673–682.

33. Mahaffey KW, Granger CB, Collins R, et al. Overview of randomized trials of intravenous heparin in patients with acute myocardial infarction treated with thrombolytic therapy. *Am J Cardiol* 1996;77:551–556.

34. Collins R, MacMahon S, Flather M, et al. Clinical effects of anticoagulant therapy in suspected acute myocardial infarction: systematic overview of randomized trials. *Br Med J* 1996;313:652–659.

35. Cannon CP, McCabe CH, Henry TD, et al. A pilot trial of recombinant desulfatohirudin compared with heparin in conjunction with tissue-type plasminogen activator and aspirin for acute myyocardial infarction: results of the Thrombolysis in Myocardial Infarction (TIMI) 5 trial. *J Am Coll Cardiol* 1994;23:993–1003.

36. Lee LV. Initial experience with hirudin and streptokinase in acute myocardial infarction: results of the Thrombolysis in Myocardial Infarction (TIMI 6) Trial. *Am J Cardiol* 1995;75:7–13.

37. Antman EM, for the TIMI 9A Investigators. Hirudin in acute myocardial infarction: safety report from the Thrombolysis and Thrombin Inhibition in Myocardial Infarction (TIMI) 9A Trial. *Circulation* 1994;90:1624–1630.

38. Global Use of Strategies to open Occluded Coronary Arteries (GUSTO IIa) Investigators. Randomized trial of intravenous heparin versus recombinant hirudin for acute coronary syndromes. *Circulation* 1994;90:1631–1637.

39. The GUSTO IIb Investigators. A comparison of recombinant hirudin with heparin for the treatment of acute coronary syndromes. *N Engl J Med* 1996;335:775–782.

40. Antman EM, for the TIMI 9B Investigators. Hirudin in acute myocardial infarction: Thrombolysis and Thrombin Inhibition in Myocardial Infarction (TIMI 9B) Trial. *Circulation* 1996;94:911–921.

41. Loscalzo J. Thrombin inhibitors in fibrinolysis: a Hobson's choice of alternatives [Editorial]. *Circulation* 1996;94:863–865.

42. Zoldhelyi P, Janssens S, Lefevre G, Collen D, van der

Werf F, for the GUSTO IIa Investigators. Effect of heparin and hirudin (CGP 39393) on thrombin generation during thrombolysis for acute myocardial infarction [Abstract]. *Circulation* 1995;92(suppl I):470.

43. White HD, for the Hirulog Early Reperfusion/Occlusion (HERO) Trial Investigators. A randomised, double blind comparison of hirulog versus heparin in patients receiving streptokinase and aspirin for acute myocardial infarction. Presented at the 45th Annual Scientific Session of the American College of Cardiology, Orlando, Florida, March 1996.

44. Metz BK, Granger CB, White HW, Simes J, Topol EJ. Streptokinase and hirudin reduces death and reinfarction in acute myocardial infarction: results from GUSTO-IIb [Abstract]. *Circulation* 1996;94:430.

45. Theroux P. Platelet receptor inhibition for ischemic syndrome management (PRISM-PLUS) trial. Presented at the 46th American College of Cardiology Meeting, Anaheim, CA, March 1997.

46. Weaver WD, Fung A, Lorch G, et al. Efegatran and streptokinase vs. t-PA and heparin for treatment of acute MI [Abstract]. *Circulation* 1996;94(suppl 1):430.

47. Ohman EM, Slovak JP, Anderson RL, et al. Potent inhibition of thrombin with efegatran in combination with t-PA in acute myocardial infarction: results of a multicenter randomized dose ranging trial [Abstract]. *Circulation* 1996;94(suppl 1):430.

48. Glick A, Kornowski R, Michowich Y, et al. Reduction of reinfarction and angina with use of low molecular weight heparin administered prior to streptokinase in patients with acute myocardial infarction. *Am J Cardiol* 1996;77:1145–1148.

49. Nilsen DWT, Goransson L, Larsen AI, Hetland O, Kierulf P. Systemic thrombin generation and activity resistant to low molecular weight heparin administered prior to streptokinase in patients with acute myocardial infarction. *Thromb Haemost* 1997;77:57–61.

50. Cairns JA, Lewis HDJ, Meade TW, Sutton GC, Theroux P. Antithrombotic agents in coronary artery disease. Fourth ACCP Consensus Conference on Antithrombotic Therapy. *Chest* 1995;108(suppl):380–400.

51. Ryan TJ, Anderson JL, Antman EM, et al. ACC/AHA guidelines for the management of patients with acute myocardial infarction: a report of the American College of Cardiology/American Heart Association Task Force on Practice Guidelines (Committee on Management of Acute Myocardial Infarction). *J Am Coll Cardiol* 1996;28:1328–1428.

52. Granger CB, Hirsh J, Califf RM, et al. Activated partial thromboplastin time and outcome after thrombolytic therapy for acute myocardial infarction. Results from the GUSTO-I trial. *Circulation* 1996;93:870–878.

53. Rosing J, van Rijn JLML, Bevers EM, van Dieijon G, Cofurius P, Zwaal RFA. The role of activated platelets in prothrombin and factor X activation. *Blood* 1985;65:319–332.

54. Teitch JM, Rosenberg RM. Protection of factor Xa from neutralization by heparin-antithrombin complex. *J Clin Invest* 1983;71:1383–1387.

55. Eitzman DT, Chi L, Saggin L, Schwartz RS, Lucchesi BR, Fay WP. Heparin neutralization by platelet-rich thrombi: role of platelet factor 4. *Circulation* 1994;89:1523–1529.

56. Hung DT, Vu T-KH, Wheaton VI, et al. "Mirror image" antagonists of thrombin-induced platelet activation

based on thrombin receptor structure. *J Clin Invest* 1992;89:444–450.

57. Montrucchio G, Bergerone BF, Alloatti G, et al. Streptokinase induces intravascular release of platelet-activating factor in patients with acute myocardial infarction and stimulates its synthesis by cultured human endothelial cells. *Circulation* 1993;88:1476–1483.

58. Kerins DM, Roy L, FitzGerald GA, Fitzgerald DJ. Platelet and vascular function during coronary thrombolysis with tissue-type plasminogen activator. *Circulation* 1989;80:1718–1725.

59. Krumholz HM, Radford MJ, Ellerbeck EF, et al. Aspirin in the treatment of acute myocardial infarction in elderly Medicare beneficiaries: patterns of use and outcomes. *Circulation* 1995;92:2841–2847.

60. Herbert JM, Bernat A, Sainte-Marie M, Dol F, Rinaldi M. Potentiating effect of clopidogrel and SR 46349, a novel 5-HT2 antagonist, on streptokinase-induced thrombolysis in the rabbit. *Thromb Haemost* 1993;69:268–271.

61. Hall P, Nakamura S, Maiello L, et al. A randomized comparison of combined ticlopidine and aspirin therapy versus aspirin therapy alone after successful intravascular ultrasound-guided stent implantation. *Circulation* 1996;93:215–222.

62. Schomig A, Neumann FJ, Kastrati A, et al. A randomized comparison of antiplatelet and anticoagulant therapy after the placement of coronary artery stents. *N Engl J Med* 1996;334:1084–1089.

63. Tranchesi B, Pileggi F, Vercammen E, van der Werf F, Verstraete M. Ridogrel does not increase the speed and rate of coronary recanalization in patients with myocardial infarction treated with alteplase and heparin. *Eur Heart J* 1994;15:660–664.

64. van der Wieken LR, Simoons ML, Laarman GJ, et al. Ridogrel as an adjunct to thrombolysis in acute myocardial infarction. *Int J Cardiol* 1995;52:125–34.

65. Yao S-K, Ober JC, Ferguson JJ, et al. Combination of inhibition of thrombin and blockade of thromboxane A2 synthetase and receptors enhances thrombolysis and delays reocclusion in canine coronary arteries. *Circulation* 1992;86:1993–1999.

66. Topol EJ, Ellis SG, Califf RM, et al. Combined tissue-type plasminogen activator and prostacyclin therapy for acute myocardial infarction. *J Am Coll Cardiol* 1989;14:877–884.

67. Saito T, Saitoh S, Asakura T, Kanke M, Owada K, Marutama Y. Prostacyclin analogue, beraprost, sustains recanalization duration after thrombolytic therapy in acute myocardial infarction. *Int J Cardiol* 1993;38:225–233.

68. Sharma B, Wyeth RP, Gimenez HJ, Franciosa JA. Intracoronary prostaglandin E1 plus streptokinase in acute myocardial infarction. *Am J Cardiol* 1986;58:1161–1166.

69. McGhie AI, McNatt J, Ezov N, et al. Abolition of cyclic flow variations in stenosed, endothelium-injured coronary arteries in nonhuman primates with a peptide fragment derived from human plasma von Willebrand factor-glycoprotein Ib binding domain. *Circulation* 1994;90:2976–2981.

70. Yao S-K, Ober JC, Garfinkel LI, et al. Blockade of platelet membrane glycoprotein Ib receptors delays intracoronary thrombogenesis, enhances thrombolysis, and delays coronary artery reocclusion in dogs. *Circulation* 1994;89:2822–2828.

71. Lefkovits J, Plow EF, Topol EJ. Platelet glycoprotein IIb/IIIa receptors in cardiovascular medicine. *N Engl J Med* 1995;332:1553–1559.

72. Coller BS, Scudder LE, Beer J, et al. A murine monoclonal antibody that completely blocks the binding of fibrinogen to platelets produces a thrombasthenic-like state in normal platelets and binds to glycoproteins IIb and/or IIIa. *J Clin Invest* 1983;72:325–338.

73. Topol E, Califf R, Weisman H, et al. Randomized trial of coronary intervention with antibody against platelet IIb/IIIa integrin for reduction of clinical restenosis: results at six months. *Lancet* 1994;343:881–886.

74. The EPIC Investigators. Use of a monoclonal antibody directed against the platelet glycoprotein IIb/IIIa receptor in high risk coronary angioplasty. *N Engl J Med* 1994;330:956–61.

75. Kleiman NS, Ohman EM, Califf RM, et al. Profound inhibition of platelet aggregation with monoclonal antibody 7E3 Fab after thrombolytic therapy: results of the Thrombolysis in Myocardial Infarction (TAMI) 8 pilot study. *J Am Coll Cardiol* 1993;22:381–389.

76. Lincoff AM, Tcheng JE, Califf RM, et al. Standard versus low-dose weight-adjusted heparin in patients treated with the platelet glycoprotein IIb/IIIa receptor antibody fragment abciximab (c7E3Fab) during percutaneous coronary revascularization. *Am J Cardiol* 1997;79:286–291.

77. The EPILOG Investigators. Platelet glycoprotein IIb/IIIa receptor blockade and low-dose heparin during percutaneous coronary revascularization. *NEJM* 1997;336:1689–1696.

78. Gold HK, Garabedian HD, Dinsmore RE, et al. Restoration of coronary flow in myocardial infarction by intravenous chimeric 7E3 antibody without exogenous plasminogen activators: observations in animals and humans. *Circulation* 1997;95:1755–1759.

79. Dennis MS, Henzel WJ, Pitti RM, et al. Platelet glycoprotein IIb-IIIa protein antagonists from snake venoms: evidence for a family of platelet-aggregation inhibitors. (ArgGlyAsp/ fibrinogen receptor/ tigramin/echistatin/ kistrin). *Proc Natl Acad Sci U S A* 1989;87:2471–2475.

80. Schulman SP, Goldschmidt-Clermont PJ, Topol EJ, et al. Effects of Integrelin, a platelet glycoprotein IIb/IIIa receptor antagonist, in unstable angina: a randomized multicenter trial. *Circulation* 1996;94:2083–2089.

81. Tcheng JE, Harrington RA, Kottke-Marchant K, et al. Multicenter, randomized, double-blind, placebo-controlled trial of the platelet integrin glycoprotein IIb/IIIa blocker integrelin in elective coronary intervention. *Circulation* 1995;91:2151–2157.

82. Ohman EM, Kleiman NS, Gacioch G, et al. Combined accelerated tissue-plasminogen activator and platelet glycoprotein IIb/IIIa integrin receptor blockade with integrelin in acute myocardial infarction: results of a randomized, placebo-controlled, dose ranging trial. *Circulation* 1997;95:846–854.

83. Tcheng JE. Glycoprotein IIb/IIIa receptor inhibitors: putting the EPIC, IMPACT II, RESTORE, and EPILOG trials in perspective. *Am J Cardiol* 1996;78(suppl 3A):35–40.

84. The RESTORE Investigators. Effects of platelet glycoprotein IIb/IIIa blockade with Tirofiban on adverse cardiac events in patients with unstable angina or acute myocardial infarction undergoing coronary angioplasty. *Circulation* 1997;96:1445–1453.

85. White HD, for the PRISM trialists. Randomised trial of tirofiban and heparin versus heparin alone in patients with unstable angina and non-Q wave infarction. Presented at the 46th American College of Cardiology Meeting, Anaheim, CA, March 1997.

86. Theroux P, Kouz S, Roy L, et al. Platelet membrane receptor glycoprotein IIb/IIIa antagonism in unstable angina: the Canadian Lamifiban Study. *Circulation* 1996;94:899–905.

87. PARAGON Investigators. A randomized trial of potent platelet IIb/IIIa antagonism, heparin, or both in patients with unstable angina: the PARAGON Study [Abstract]. *Circulation* 1996;94:553.

88. Moliterno DJ, Harrington RA, Krucoff MW, et al. More complete and stable reperfusion with platelet IIb/IIIa antagonism plus thrombolysis for AMI: the PARADIGM Trial [Abstract]. *Circulation* 1996;94:553.

89. Krucoff MW, Croll MA, Pope JE, et al. Continuous 12-lead ST-segment recovery analysis in the TAMI-7 study: performance of a noninvasive method for real-time detection of failed myocardial reperfusion. *Circulation* 1993;88:437–446.

90. Kereiakes DJ, Runyon JP, Kleiman NS, et al. Differential dose-response to oral xemilofiban after antecedent intravenous abciximab: administration for complex coronary intervention. *Circulation* 1996;94:906–910.

Cardiovascular Thrombosis: Thrombocardiology and Thromboneurology, Second Edition, edited by M. Verstraete, V. Fuster, and E. J. Topol, Lippincott–Raven Publishers, Philadelphia © 1998.

30

Complications of Lytic and Antithrombotic Therapy in Acute Myocardial Infarction

Christopher B. Granger and *Maarten L. Simoons

*Department of Medicine, Duke University Medical Center, Durham, North Carolina 27705; and
Department of Cardiology, Erasmus University Rotterdam, 30159 GD Rotterdam, The Netherlands

Thrombolytic therapy combined with aspirin reduces short- and long-term mortality for patients with acute myocardial infarction (1–3). It does so, however, with a small but significant risk of hemorrhage, particularly intracranial hemorrhage. This risk of intracranial hemorrhage may influence the decision about whether thrombolytic therapy should be used and which agent should be selected. The likelihood of both intracranial hemorrhage (4,5) and overall mortality (6) can now be estimated for individual patients to help make clinical decisions (7). In several instances, testing of more potent thrombolytic or antithrombotic regimens has resulted in an unacceptably increased risk of intracranial hemorrhage (8–10). With even more potent antithrombotic therapies likely in the future, risk–benefit assessment may become increasingly important.

HEMORRHAGE

Not surprisingly, the major complication of thrombolytic and antithrombotic therapies is hemorrhage. The current treatment of many patients with acute myocardial infarction—thrombolytic therapy, aspirin, heparin, and early cardiac catheterization with the use of abciximab and ticlopidine when stents are used—produces a substantial risk of hemorrhage. Thrombolytic therapy causes bleeding primarily by dissolving fibrin in hemostatic clots, although there is also degradation of factors V and VIII and circulating fibrinogen, especially with streptokinase, to cause a systemic hypocoagulable state (11). Moreover, fibrin degradation products interfere with fibrin polymerization and can interfere with platelet function.

It was hoped that fibrin-specific thrombolytic agents such as alteplase, which have greater activity in converting plasminogen to plasmin at the fibrin clot surface and which cause only a modest decrease in circulating fibrinogen, would reduce the risk of bleeding. This has not been the case. The fact that alteplase confers only a slightly lower rate of noncerebral hemorrhage and a higher rate of intracranial hemorrhage than does streptokinase suggests that the main mechanism for hemorrhage, especially intracranial hemorrhage, is local lysis of fibrin in the hemostatic plug rather than effects of a systemic hypocoagulable state.

Intracranial Hemorrhage

Intracranial hemorrhage is the most feared complication of thrombolytic therapy, occurring in 0.3–1.0% of patients (1,5,12–15). Although the type of stroke was not carefully documented in most of the early thrombolytic trials, probable cerebral hemorrhage occurred in 0.4% of patients treated with thrombolytic therapy compared with 0.01% of placebo-treated patients in the Fibrinolytic Therapy Trialists Collaboration overview (1). The intracranial hemorrhage rates from each of the major placebo-controlled thrombolytic trials (Table 30-1) vary widely (16–22), which may be due in part to underreporting. Only in the more recent trials has computed tomography or magnetic resonance imaging been systematically obtained and reviewed for most suspected strokes, showing intracranial hemorrhage rates in the 0.4% to 0.9% range (Table 30-2) (5,14,23–25). The incidence may be even higher in unselected populations not enrolled in trials, as suggested by the 1.0% rate in a registry conducted in the Netherlands in 1988–1989 (15). It should be appreciated that the total number of strokes is only slightly increased with fibrinolytic therapy (3.9 per 1,000 patients treated) (1). In fact, the number of embolic strokes is reduced, almost balancing the excess hemorrhagic strokes.

The pathophysiology of intracranial hemorrhage after thrombolysis remains poorly understood. The finding that more potent, fibrin-specific agents are more likely to cause intracranial hemorrhage suggests that the main mechanism is dissolving hemostatic plugs in the cerebral vasculature. It appears that a variety of underlying vascular lesions in the brain, as well as more intense anticoagulant regimens, place patients at higher risk for cerebral hemorrhage, including amyloid angiopathy (26), identified as a factor associated with intracranial hemorrhage both with (27,28) and without thrombolysis (29,30). Brain lesions distinct from the hemorrhage, such as old lacunar infarcts, are common findings among patients with intracranial hemorrhage (31). Even minor head trauma, with relatively little disruption of cerebral vessels, appears to increase the risk of hemorrhage (32).

TABLE 30-1. *Intracranial hemorrhage in randomized, controlled thrombolytic trials of over 1,000 patients*

Trial	Agent	Intracranial hemorrhage rate, % (n/n)	
		Thrombolytic	Control
GISSI-1 (16)	Streptokinase	0.14% (8/5,860)	0% (0/5,852)
ISIS-2 (17)	Streptokinase	0.08% (7/8,592)	0% (0/8,595)
ISAM (18)	Streptokinase	0.47% (4/859)	0% (0/882)
EMERAS*a* (19)	Streptokinase	0.81% (18/2,234)	0.18% (4/2,259)
ASSET (20)	Alteplase	0.28% (7/2,512)	0.08% (2/2,493)
LATE (21)	Alteplase	0.85% (24/2,836)	0.21% (6/2,875)
AIMS (22)	Anistreplase	0.32% (2/624)	0.12% (1/634)
Pooled		0.30% (70/23,517)	0.06% (13/23,590)
95% CI		0.23–0.37%	0.03–0.09%

*a*Probable intracranial hemorrhage.

TABLE 30-2. *Intracranial hemorrhage rates in comparative thrombolytic trials*

Trial (reference)	n	Rate (n)	n	Rate (n)	Difference
		Streptokinase		Alteplase[a]	Alteplase versus streptokinase
GISSI-2/ International Study (14)	10,396	0.29% (30)	10,372	0.42% (44)	+0.23%
ISIS-3 (23)	12,848	0.30% (39)	12,841	0.72% (92)	+0.42%
GUSTO-I (5)	20,213	0.51% (104)	10,376	0.70% (73)	+0.19%
		Streptokinase		Reteplase	Reteplase versus streptokinase
INJECT (24)	3,006	0.37% (11)	3,004	0.77% (23)	+0.40%
		Alteplase		Reteplase	Reteplase versus alteplase
GUSTO-III (25)	4,921	0.87%	10,138	0.91%	+0.04%

[a]Alteplase 100 mg over 3 hours in GISSI-2, duteplase 0.6 MU/kg over 4 hours in ISIS-3, alteplase 100 mg over 90 minutes in GUSTO-I.

The median time of onset of intracranial hemorrhage is 10 to 15 hours after thrombolysis, and about 75% occur within 24 hours (5,12). Decreased consciousness is the most common initial symptom (26). The most common sites of hemorrhage are the major cerebral lobes, occurring in 70% to 80% of patients (26,31), with the second most common location being cerebellar. The average volume of hemorrhage is about 60 ml, or about the size of an egg (31), and about 15% to 20% of patients with intracranial hemorrhage have subdural blood (alone or in addition to the intracerebral blood). Nearly half have intraventricular blood. A substantial percentage (30%) have more than one location of blood collection, suggesting a diffuse underlying process predisposing to hemorrhage.

Reported rates of 30-day mortality after intracranial hemorrhage have averaged in the 50% to 70% range (5,14,15,33). Of the survivors, 63% have moderate or severe disability, and 33% have either mild or no disability (5). Therefore, only 13% of all patients with intracranial hemorrhage survive without significant disability. These patients with only mild or no disability had similar quality-of-life measures as did patients who did not have strokes, based on structured interviews (5).

Hemorrhage Other than Intracranial

Reported overall hemorrhage rates in thrombolytic trials are difficult to interpret because of varying definitions, intensities of data collection, thresholds for transfusion, and use of invasive procedures, including coronary artery bypass surgery. In randomized controlled trials of thrombolytic therapy, there was a two- to threefold higher incidence of major hemorrhage with thrombolysis, from 0.4% to 1.1%. Major hemorrhage is generally defined as bleeding that is considered life threatening or that requires transfusion (1). Most of the placebo-controlled trials used neither routine aspirin nor heparin. At the other end of the spectrum, patients in the early TIMI (34) and TAMI (35) trials, which included full-dose intravenous heparin and early angiography, were transfused 20% to 30% of the time. Most bleeding in these trials was associated with invasive procedures or bypass surgery, and bleeding was related to lower fibrinogen (35) and higher fibrin-degradation product levels (34). In the TIMI-II trial, in which patients were randomized to catheterization the first day versus a conservative approach, major bleeding (defined as a decrease in hemoglobin of 5 g/dl) was more common with the invasive approach (18.5% versus 12.8%, p < 0.001) (36). Bleeding was related to extent of fibrinogen breakdown, peak alteplase level, and prolonged activated partial thromboplastin time (APTT). The most common non–surgery-related hemorrhage site was a hemoglobin decrease without identified source (1.5%), followed by catheterization site (1.2%), gastrointestinal

(0.7%), other puncture site (0.5%), and genitourinary (0.2%).

In the GUSTO-I trial, 1.1% of patients had severe bleeding (resulting in hemodynamic compromise requiring intervention), and an additional 11.4% had moderate bleeding (requiring transfusion) (37). Events were most often related to bypass surgery (3.6%) or groin procedure (2.0%), or were gastrointestinal in nature (1.0%).

Bleeding Rates According to Thrombolytic Agent

Intracranial Hemorrhage

Although alteplase was first thought to be safer with regard to hemorrhage because of its fibrin specificity, it has been associated with a consistently greater (0.2% to 0.4% higher) risk of intracranial hemorrhage, perhaps related to greater thrombolytic potency (Table 30-2) (38). Anistreplase appears to confer a risk of intracranial hemorrhage more similar to that with alteplase than with streptokinase (23). Reteplase carries a higher rate of intracranial hemorrhage than does streptokinase (24) and a rate similar to that with alteplase in the doses used (Table 30-2).

Both the dose and speed of thrombolytic administration are related to intracranial hemorrhage risk. In the TIMI-II trial, a dose of 150 mg of alteplase was prematurely discontinued because of an unacceptably high rate of intracranial hemorrhage (8,39). Combining all 908 patients from the pilot and main TIMI-II trials treated with 150 mg alteplase over 6 hours, 14 intracranial hemorrhages occurred (1.5%). The intracranial hemorrhage rate decreased to 0.4% when the dose was reduced to 100 mg, although this may have been partly due to the adoption of more restrictive entry criteria (12). Of the 729 patients randomized to a lower dose of alteplase (0.8 mg/kg, maximum dose 80 mg), 0.55% had intracranial hemorrhage (40), somewhat lower than the average rate across trials with the 100-mg dose. The highest dose (50 mg) of a tissue plasminogen activator mutant (TNK-t-PA) was stopped early, when three of 78 patients experienced intracranial hemorrhage (41). In the COBALT study, two 50-mg boluses of alteplase conferred a nonsignificantly higher risk of intracranial hemorrhage than did accelerated alteplase (42).

Hemorrhage Other than Intracranial

In contrast to the increased risk of intracranial hemorrhage with alteplase, non-intracranial bleeding is consistently reduced with alteplase and other fibrin-specific agents (such as reteplase) compared with streptokinase (Table 30-3) (23–25,37,43). Both alteplase and reteplase confer a 15% to

TABLE 30-3. *Hemorrhage rates (other than intracranial) in comparative thrombolytic trials*

Trial	n	Major hemorrhage[a] (n)	n	Major hemorrhage[a] (n)	Difference
		Streptokinase		Alteplase[b]	Alteplase versus streptokinase
GISSI-2 (43)	10,386	0.9% (96)	10,372	0.6% (64)	−0.3%
ISIS-3 (23)	13,607	0.9% (118)	13,569	0.8% (109)	−0.1%
GUSTO-I (37)	20,196	12.9% (2,611)	10,366	11.1% (1,155)	−1.8%
		Streptokinase		Reteplase	Reteplase versus streptokinase
INJECT (24)	3,006	1.0%	3,004	0.7%	−0.3%
		Alteplase		Reteplase	Reteplase versus alteplase
GUSTO-III (25)	4,921	6.8%	10,138	6.9%	+0.2%

[a]Major hemorrhage is defined as receiving or requiring transfusion.
[b]Alteplase 100 mg over 3 hours in GISSI-2, duteplase 0.6 MU/kg over 4 hours in ISIS-3, alteplase 100 mg over 90 minutes in GUSTO-I.

20% relative reduction in major hemorrhage compared with streptokinase.

Bleeding Rates According to Type and Intensity of Anticoagulation and Antiplatelet Therapy

Intracranial Hemorrhage

Without thrombolytic therapy, patients with acute coronary syndromes treated with aspirin, heparin, or both do have a detectable, albeit small, risk of intracranial hemorrhage. In the FTT overview, there were only 16 probable or definite intracranial hemorrhages in more than 29,000 control patients for a rate of 0.05%, with a 95% confidence interval (CI) of 0.03% to 0.08% (1). With full-dose aspirin and intravenous heparin (without thrombolytic therapy), none of 4,343 patients with unstable angina or non–Q-wave myocardial infarction enrolled in the GUSTO-IIb trial had intracranial hemorrhage (95% CI <0.07%) (44). Also in the ESSENCE trial of 3,171 patients with unstable angina or non–Q-wave myocardial infarction, no patient randomized to the low molecular weight heparin enoxaparin experienced intracranial hemorrhage (45). A reasonable estimate of the risk of intracranial hemorrhage with aspirin and full-dose intravenous heparin, then, is one in 2,000 patients.

With the more potent antithrombin agent hirudin, even without thrombolytic therapy there was a 0.1% incidence of intracranial hemorrhage, with a 95% CI of 0.01% to 0.2% (44).

The addition of heparin or other antithrombin agents to thrombolytic therapy increases the risk of intracranial hemorrhage (46). In ISIS-3, there was a 0.15% absolute increase in definite intracranial hemorrhage with subcutaneous heparin 12,500 U twice a day (p < 0.05) (23). In GUSTO-I, full-dose intravenous heparin compared with subcutaneous heparin conferred a 0.11% higher rate of intracranial hemorrhage, which was not statistically significant (5). The addition of conventional-dose aspirin to thrombolytic therapy does not substantially increase the risk of intracranial hemorrhage (17).

Both the dose of heparin and its effect as measured by APTT are related to the risk of intracranial hemorrhage after thrombolysis (Fig. 30-1) (47). Two later trials used modestly higher doses of heparin after thrombolytic therapy. Patients who weighed ≥80 kg received 1,300 U (compared with 1,000 U in GUSTO-I) of heparin each hour, and the target APTT range was increased to 60 to 90 seconds. This resulted in a 10-second increase in the median APTT in the early hours and a doubling in the rate of intracranial hemorrhage, to 1.5% (Table 30-4). In GUSTO-IIb and TIMI-9B, which reduced the initial heparin infusion dose to that used in GUSTO-I (1,000 U/hr for all patients), the median APTT decreased by 15 to 20 seconds, and the intracranial hemorrhage rate decreased to 0.7%.

Several trials have reported a substantially higher risk of intracranial hemorrhage with hirudin and other direct thrombin inhibitors when given with thrombolysis (9,10,48,49). When the dose of hirudin was reduced by 50%, reinfarction was significantly reduced with hirudin compared with heparin (50), with no increased risk of intracranial hemorrhage (Table 30-4). The APTT with hirudin correlated with the risk of intracranial hemorrhage, similar to heparin.

Hemorrhage Other than Intracranial

The addition of heparin to thrombolytic therapy increases the risk of overall bleeding. The addition of 12,500 U twice daily of subcutaneous heparin in ISIS-3 (23) and GISSI-2 (43) increased the major bleeding incidence from 0.7% to 1.0% (p < 0.001). In one overview, intravenous heparin increased the overall bleeding rate from 16% to 23% (odds ratio 1.55; 95% CI, 1.2 to 2.0) (46). Another overview found an excess of three to 13 major hemorrhages per 1,000 patients treated (51). Not only does heparin increase the risk of bleeding, but higher dose intravenous heparin also increases risk over lower–dose, subcuta-

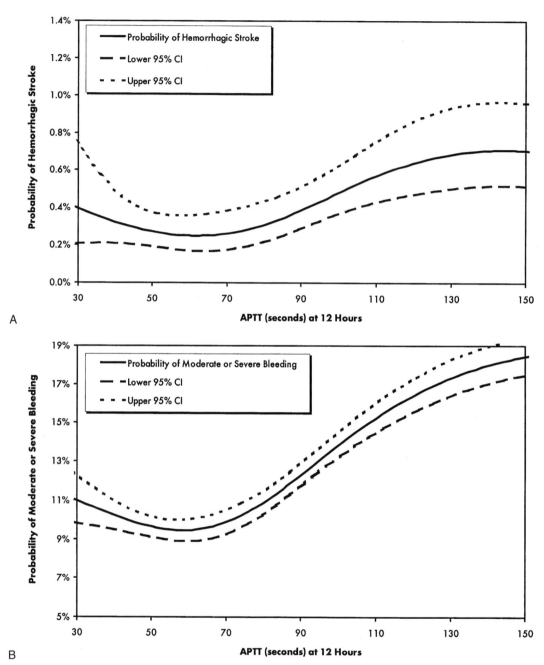

FIG. 30-1. Predicted probability and 95% CIs of intracranial hemorrhage **(A)** and of moderate and severe bleeding **(B)** according to activated partial thromboplastin time (APTT) at 12 hours among patients treated with thrombolytic therapy and intravenous heparin in the GUSTO-I trial. (From Granger et al., ref. 47, with permission.)

TABLE 30-4. *Rates of intracranial hemorrhage (ICH) and corresponding activated partial thromboplastin times (APTT) among patients treated with thrombolytic therapy, comparison of TIMI-9, GUSTO-II, and GUSTO-I*

Trial	Hirudin dose	12-hour APTT[a]	ICH rate, % (n/n)	Heparin dose	12-hour APTT[a]	ICH rate, % (n/n)
GUSTO-IIa (9)	0.6 mg/kg bolus	95 s	1.9% (13/677)	5,000 U bolus	85 s	1.2% (8/660)
TIMI-9A (10)	0.2 mg/kg/hr infusion	90 s	1.7% (6/345)	1,000–1,300 U/hr infusion	90 s	1.9% (7/368)
Combined			1.9% (19/1,022) 95% CI: 1.0–2.7%			1.5% (15/1,028) 95% CI: 0.7–2.2%
GUSTO-IIb (50)	0.2 mg/kg bolus	77 s	0.6% (11/1,731)	5,000 U bolus	65 s	0.6% (10/1,727)
TIMI-9B (50)	0.1 mg/kg/hr infusion	75 s	0.4% (6/1,474)	1,000 U/hr infusion	70 s	0.9% (13/1,456)
Combined			0.5% (17/3,205) 95% CI: 0.3–0.8%			0.7% (23/3,183) 95% CI: 0.4–1.0%
GUSTO-I (5) (223/31,115)				5,000 U bolus	78 s	0.7%
				1,000 U/hr infusion[a]		95% CI: 0.6–0.8%

[a]Median APTT, either actual or estimated from ranges.

neous heparin, from 11.8% to 14.0% (p = 0.0001) (37). Moreover, among patients treated with intravenous heparin, a higher degree of heparin effect as measured by APTT is associated with a higher risk of bleeding. Above an APTT of about 75 seconds, there is a 1% increased risk of moderate or severe bleeding for every 7-second increase in APTT (Fig. 30-1) (47).

As with unfractionated heparin, the risk of hemorrhage with low molecular weight heparin is related to dose. In the TIMI-11a trial (52), an open-label, dose-ranging study of enoxaparin for patients with unstable angina or non–Q-wave myocardial infarction, the major hemorrhage rate was 6.5% for patients receiving 1.2 mg/kg twice daily compared with 1.9% for 1.0 mg/kg twice daily. The anti-Xa levels of patients who bled were higher than those of patients without bleeding. The 1-mg/kg, twice-daily dose was compared with conventional unfractionated heparin in the randomized, placebo-controlled ESSENCE trial. Major bleeding was similar at that dose of enoxaparin, at 6.5% compared with 7.0% with unfractionated heparin, p = 0.57 (45).

Similar to heparin, the risk of hemorrhage with hirudin appears to be related to dose and anticoagulant effect. High-dose hirudin was associated with twice the rate of major spontaneous, nonintracranial hemorrhage (7.0% versus 3.0% with heparin, p = 0.02) (10). Reduced doses of hirudin were associated with similar rates of serious hemorrhage (1.2% versus 1.1%) and a modest increase in moderate hemorrhage (8.8% versus 7.7%, p = 0.03) compared with heparin (Table 30-4) (44,53).

Hemorrhage with Glycoprotein IIb/IIIa Inhibitors

The initial experience with glycoprotein (GP)IIb/IIIa antagonists was associated with a significant excess of major and minor bleeding in patients undergoing angioplasty (54). This excess was reduced and even disappeared in later studies through reduction of the heparin dose and meticulous care of the arterial puncture sites (55–57). In patients undergoing angioplasty, treatment with different GPIIb/IIIa blockers in association and aspirin and heparin was associated with a 0.2% risk of intracranial hemorrhage. This risk is slightly but not significantly higher than that of patients treated with aspirin and heparin only (58). In patients with unstable angina, with or without heparin, the risk of intracranial hemorrhage did not appear to be increased with tirofiban (59). Combination therapy with GPIIb/IIIa receptor blockers and thrombolytic therapy might be associated with a marked increase in bleeding risk, unless the dosage of either is reduced, but little information is available for such combination therapy (60).

Prediction of Hemorrhage

Intracranial Hemorrhage

Two predictive models of intracranial hemorrhage after thrombolytic therapy have been developed from large databases (4,5). Factors found to be independently associated with risk are shown in Fig. 30-2.

Older age is the most important predictor of intracranial hemorrhage (4,5,61,62), with a rapid increase in risk over the age of 65 years, increasing to about 2% at age 80 years (Fig. 30-3) (5). However, even though the risk of intracranial hemorrhage increases substantially with age, the absolute reduction in mortality also increases with age (1,6). Thus, the overall impact of thrombolysis compared with control (1) and of more aggressive thrombolytic therapy versus less aggressive (63) is generally favorable in the elderly.

Lower body weight is the second most important predictor of intracranial hemorrhage (4,15), even with alteplase given in a weight-adjusted manner (Fig. 30-3) (5). The higher risk of intracranial hemorrhage with lower body weights and at higher doses of thrombolytics and anticoagulants reinforces the rationale for weight-adjusted dosing of potent antithrombotic agents.

High blood pressure at presentation is a consistent, important predictor of intracranial hemorrhage (61,62,64). Different cut-off values have been applied, such as systolic blood pressure 170 mmHg or a diastolic 95 mmHg (4), but the relationship between blood pressure and risk is continuous, without a clear inflexion point at which risk abruptly increases (64). A small study suggested that "excess pulse pressure" may play an important role in determining risk (65), but later experience (5) has shown that it is the absolute value of both the diastolic and systolic pressures, not the difference between the two, that is critical. Whether lowering blood pressure in hypertensive patients before treatment reduces risk is not known, but doing so would be prudent.

The patient presenting with infarction and marked hypertension has a relatively low risk of death and thus may derive a limited benefit from thrombolysis. If the risk of intracranial hemorrhage outweighs the survival benefit, then direct angioplasty or even conservative medical management could be in the patient's best interest (64), but few such patients have been enrolled. The use of more aggressive, more potent thrombolytic regimens—alteplase versus streptokinase, or combined alteplase streptokinase versus either alone—is, not surprisingly, associated with a higher risk of intracranial hemorrhage. These four factors (age, weight, hypertension at presentation, and type of thrombolytic agent) can be used in a simple way to estimate the risk of intracranial hemorrhage for individual patients in the clinical setting (4).

History of cerebrovascular disease, either stroke or transient ischemic attack, has been associated with intracranial hemorrhage in two trials (5,12). Guidelines suggest that recent stroke should be an exclusion criterion for thrombolysis because such patients have been excluded from many clinical trials (2). Yet, there are no direct data to determine the degree of increased risk with recent stroke, and it is not known whether a remote stroke confers less risk than a recent stroke.

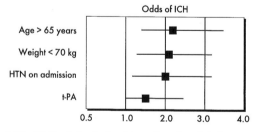

FIG. 30-2. Adjusted odds ratios for risk factors predictive of intracranial hemorrhage (ICH). HTN, hypertension; t-PA, alteplase. (Adapted from Simoons et al., ref. 4, with permission.)

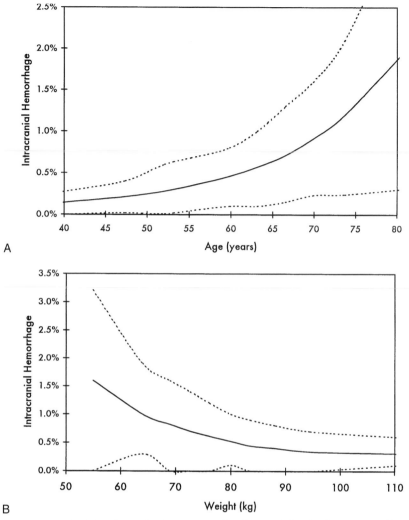

FIG. 30-3. Predicted probability (*solid line*) and 95% CIs (*dashed lines*) of intracranial hemorrhage according to patient age **(A)** and weight **(B)** in the GUSTO-I trial. (From Gore et al., ref. 5, with permission.)

Female sex, found to be an independent predictor in the GISSI 2/International Study (66), was also a significant univariable predictor in other studies, but not after adjustment for age, weight, and blood pressure (4,5). Use of warfarin upon presentation, found to be an important independent predictor in the Netherlands registry report (15), was not an independent predictor in a larger, pooled analysis (4). The use of calcium blockers was associated with increased risk in the TIMI-II trial (12), and the use of beta-blockers was associated with decreased risk (12), although neither of these observations was later confirmed (5).

Additional independent risk factors for intracranial hemorrhage include recent minor head or facial trauma and dementia (32). A history of facial or head trauma within the previous 2 weeks carried a 7.6-fold increased risk of intracranial hemorrhage (95% CI: 2.9 to 20), and dementia carried a 3.4-fold increased risk (95% CI: 1.2 to 10).

Hemorrhage Other than Intracranial

Three predictive models of noncerebral hemorrhage based on thrombolytic trial databases have been published (Table 30-5) (35–37). Because the GUSTO-I model contains nearly 50 times as many patients with bleeding as the other two models combined, this model is likely to be the most reliable for predicting the risk of bleeding. The most important predictors are the performance of invasive procedures (including bypass surgery), advanced age, lower body weight, and female sex.

In GUSTO-I, patients experiencing moderate or severe hemorrhage were an average 5 years older than those without bleeding, and age was the most important predictor after taking into account whether procedures were performed (Fig. 30-4) (37). Among patients not undergoing procedures in the GUSTO trial, the risk of bleeding increased by 40% for every 10 additional years of age (37).

Similarly, with every 10-kg decrease in weight there is a 30% increase in risk of hemorrhage (Fig. 30-4) (37). Women have nearly twice the risk of men, even after adjustment for other variables (36,37).

History of hypertension has been identified in most (15,35,37) but not all (67) studies as a risk factor for bleeding, albeit relatively less important (37).

Patients of African ancestry had a 30% higher risk of hemorrhage than did other

TABLE 30-5. *Baseline patient predictors of bleeding complications from multivariable logistic regression models*

	TAMI (35)	TIMI (36)	GUSTO-I (37)
Patients in the model	386	1,424	40,903
Patients (n) with hemorrhage[a]	14% (55)	7% (58)	12.6% (5,154)
Angiography	100% (acute)	50% within 42 days	55% in-hospital
Predictors of bleeding			
Bypass surgery	Bleeding (no. 1 predictor)	Not reported	Bleeding (no. 1 predictor); $\chi^2 = 775^b$; OR = 3.8–7.2
Angiography or angioplasty	All patients underwent angiography	Bleeding (angiography) (p < 0.001)	Bleeding $\chi^2 = 48$; OR = 1.2–1.6
Advanced age	Blood loss (p = 0.095)	Bleeding (invasive strategy arm)[c] (p < 0.001)	Bleeding (no. 1 nonprocedure predictor); $\chi^2 = 267$; OR = 1.4/10 yr
Lower body weight	Bleeding (p = 0.02)	Combined major and minor bleeding (p < 0.001)	Bleeding (no. 2 nonprocedure predictor); $\chi^2 = 218$; OR = 1.3/10 kg
Female sex	Increased blood loss (p = 0.01)	Combined major and minor bleeding (p < 0.001)	Bleeding (no. 3 nonprocedure predictor); $\chi^2 = 136$; OR = 1.7
African ancestry	Not evaluated	Not evaluated	Bleeding; $\chi^2 = 42$; OR =1.9
History of hypertension	Blood loss (p = 0.091)	Bleeding (p < 0.001), OR =3.2	Bleeding; $\chi^2 = 11$; OR =1.1
Cardiac decompensation	Not evaluated	Bleeding (p < 0.04), OR = 2.0	Bleeding, patients without invasive procedures; $\chi^2 = 30$
Low fibrinogen	Increased blood loss (p = 0.005)	Combined major and minor bleeding (p = 0.001)	Not evaluated
Platelet count ≤100,000/ml	Not evaluated	Bleeding (p < 0.001), OR = 7.5	Not evaluated
Alteplase level ≥1,500 ng/ml	Not evaluated	Bleeding (p < 0.001), OR =3.3	Not evaluated

[a]Major bleeding in TIMI and TAMI; moderate or severe bleeding in GUSTO-I.
[b]χ^2 >6 corresponds to p < 0.05; the greater the χ^2, the more statistically significant the predictive power.
[c]Conservative strategy patients received 100 mg alteplase.

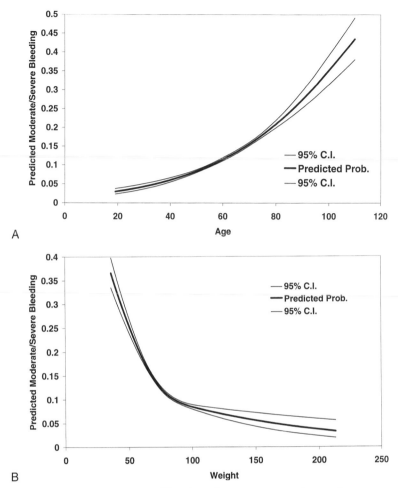

FIG. 30-4. Predicted probability and 95% CIs of moderate or severe hemorrhage according to patient age in years **(A)** and weight in kg **(B)** in the GUSTO-I trial. (From Berkowitz et al., ref. 37, with permission.)

races in GUSTO-I (37), largely confined to alteplase-treated patients. This may relate to an increased sensitivity to alteplase with greater fibrinogen breakdown and higher fibrin degradation product levels and transfusion rates (68). Fibrinogen depletion has been shown to be related to bleeding risk (35,36). Other factors related to an increased risk of hemorrhage include thrombocytopenia (36,69) and higher blood alteplase levels (36).

The GUSTO-I model has been translated into a simple "probability chart" tool for clinicians to predict the risk of moderate or severe

hemorrhage for patients undergoing thrombolytic therapy (Fig. 30-5) (37).

Special Patient Situations

There has been concern over the use of thrombolytic therapy for certain subsets of patients with acute infarction because of a possible increased risk of hemorrhage. For example, despite concern that thrombolysis after cardiopulmonary resuscitation could result in severe bleeding from chest trauma or severe cerebral ischemia and intracranial hemorrhage, among the total of 135 patients an-

1. Find Points for Each Risk Marker									
Age		Weight		Diastolic BP		Pulse		Miscellaneous Factors	
Years	Points	kg	Points	mm Hg	Points	Beats	Points	Factor	Points
30	18	140	35	140	13	40	4	Female sex	12
40	27	120	43	120	17	80	8	African ancestry	10
50	36	100	52	100	21	120	12	Current smoking	8
60	45	80	61	80	25	160	16	Hypertension	7
70	54	60	74	60	30	200	19	Prior angina	3
80	63	40	87					Prior MI	2
90	72								

Killip Class	Alteplase	Streptokinase + SQ heparin	Streptokinase + IV heparin	
I	32	38	43	
II	39	46	50	
III	48	53	57	
IV	55	60	65	

2. Sum Points For All Risk Factors

_____ + _____ + _____ + _____ + _____ + _____ = _____

Age   Weight   Diastolic BP   Pulse   Misc Factors   Killip class/Lytic   Point Total

3. Look Up Risk Corresponding to Point Total					
Points	Probability	Points	Probability	Points	Probability
182	10%	228	30%	257	50%
210	20%	243	40%		

FIG. 30-5. Algorithm to assess the risk of moderate or severe bleeding after thrombolytic therapy. BP, blood pressure; MI, myocardial infarction; SQ, subcutaneous; IV, intravenous. (Adapted from Berkowitz et al., ref. 37, with permission.)

alyzed, none experienced moderate or severe bleeding attributable to the resuscitation (70–72). Two of these reports included patients who had received prolonged resuscitation. Thus, the risk of serious bleeding from cardiopulmonary resuscitation seems low and generally should not deter thrombolysis.

Menstruating women compose another patient population in which the perceived risk of serious bleeding has deterred treatment. In a series of 12 women who were menstruating at the time of their infarctions, three required transfusion (73). There was no serious or life-threatening bleeding. Accordingly, menstruation should not be a contraindication to thrombolysis for women with a substantial anticipated benefit from reperfusion therapy.

Ocular bleeding resulting in serious disability or loss of visual acuity is extremely rare, occurring in none of the 6,000+ patients with diabetes in GUSTO-I, of which an estimated 300 had proliferative retinopathy (74). Therefore, diabetic retinopathy generally should not preclude patients from receiving thrombolysis.

Management of Hemorrhage

Optimal management of bleeding after thrombolysis is based on early identification and local control of bleeding, prompt resuscitation when needed, and reversing the underlying causes (Fig. 30-6) (11). Generally, the heparin effect should be immediately reversed with protamine, particularly in patients with a severe, abrupt-onset neurologic deficit within the first 24 hours after thrombolysis, while obtaining computed tomographic imaging of the head.

For suspected serious bleeding, two large-bore, intravenous lines should be placed, and fluid and packed red-cell transfusions should be started for hemodynamic instability. Local measures, such as manual pressure, should be used to control the bleeding. Anticoagulants and antiplatelet drugs should be discontinued, and protamine should be considered to reverse the heparin effect. A milligram of protamine sulfate neutralizes about 90 U of heparin, so that a typical patient on intravenous heparin might require an initial protamine

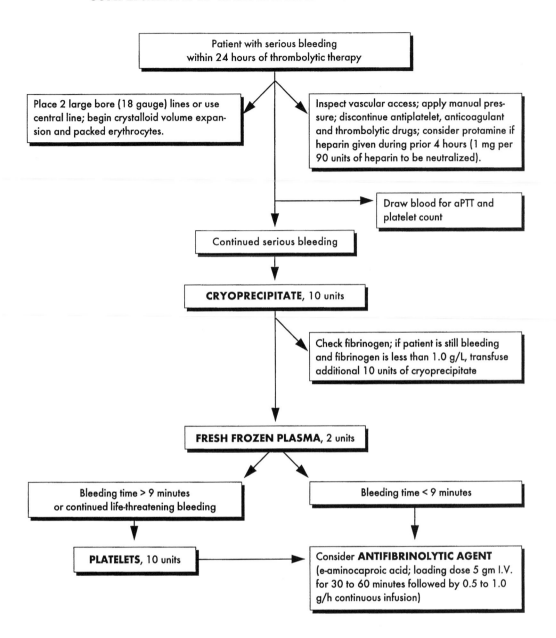

Steps are sequential. Each step is made with the presumption that the patient is still bleeding.

FIG. 30-6. Algorithm for bleeding management in patients with serious bleeding after thrombolytic therapy. (Adapted from Sane et al., ref. 11, with permission.)

dose of about 20 to 30 mg. An APTT should be drawn, which will reflect both the heparin effect and the systemic fibrinolytic state.

If bleeding continues early after thrombolysis, 10 U of cryoprecipitate could be given to replace fibrinogen and factor VIII, both of which are degraded by activated plasmin. Transfusion to a fibrinogen level of at least 1.0 g/L and factor VIII activity of at least 30% should be sufficient for hemostasis. Once fibrinogen levels are replete, fresh frozen plasma can be used as a source of factors V and VIII.

Platelet dysfunction is common among patients who have been given thrombolytic therapy, because of the inhibitory effect of fibrin degradation products and concomitant aspirin use (11). For patients with life-threatening bleeding, even for those with normal platelet counts, platelet transfusions should be considered.

Use of the antifibrinolytic lysine-analogue agents, such as ε-aminocaproic acid, is generally reserved for severe bleeding early after thrombolysis that is not controlled otherwise. These agents, which inhibit lysine-binding sites (where plasmin binds to fibrin), carry a risk of severe and refractory thrombosis, especially in patients with disseminated intravascular coagulation (75), diabetes, or previous protamine exposure.

An important clinical issue confronting the physician caring for a patient who has experienced intracranial hemorrhage after thrombolytic therapy is whether the chance of meaningful survival is high enough to warrant continued aggressive care. Four independent predictors of mortality may help to predict outcomes: lower Glasgow Coma Scale score, shorter time to stroke symptom onset, larger volume of hemorrhage on brain imaging, and advanced age (76). The role of neurosurgical evacuation of intracranial hemorrhage after thrombolysis is controversial. In one observational study, neurosurgical evacuation was associated with better survival, especially for cerebellar hemorrhages (77), even after adjustment for other prognostic variables.

IMMUNOLOGIC COMPLICATIONS

Both streptokinase and anistreplase, which are derived from group C streptococci, have the potential to cause immunologic reactions. Alteplase and reteplase, being derived from the human plasminogen activator protein, are not antigenic. Because of the ubiquitous nature of *Streptococcus,* nearly everyone has some circulating level of *Streptococcus* antibody (78,79).

Accurate determination of the true incidence of allergy to streptokinase is difficult, because symptoms of allergy and anaphylaxis are often indistinguishable from the fever, hypotension, wheezing, and shortness of breath that can occur from the infarction itself. In another trial, mild allergic reactions were reported in about 4% of patients treated with streptokinase (17,80). True anaphylactic shock is rare, ranging from 0.1% to 0.7% (16,80).

The likelihood of developing allergic reactions does not appear to be closely related to the baseline immunoglobulin G antistreptokinase antibodies (79), and there was no relationship in GUSTO-I between allergic reactions and reduced efficacy of streptokinase (81). Other immunologic reactions, such as serum sickness (82), renal injury (83), and lung injury (84), have been reported but are uncommon. Because about 50% of patients treated with streptokinase will have significant levels of neutralizing antibodies for at least 4 years (85), alteplase or reteplase has been recommended for such patients if they suffer a new infarction during this time.

Hypotension may occur in about 6% of patients who receive streptokinase (86), likely the result of kallikrein activation and release of bradykinin.

EARLY HAZARD AND MYOCARDIAL RUPTURE

Thrombolytic therapy reduces overall mortality, and more potent thrombolytics reduce mortality further than less potent therapy (87), including on the first day. However, there is evidence of increased mortality and myocardial rupture on the first day after thrombolysis.

The Fibrinolytic Therapy Trialists collaborative overview (1) reported five additional deaths per 1,000 patients among thrombolytic-treated versus control patients during the first day after thrombolytic therapy, primarily in patients presenting late after symptom onset. Although cause of death was not systematically documented, evidence suggests that these excess deaths were related to either proven or suspected myocardial rupture (88,89). Whether the early hazard of thrombolysis reflects a true, increased risk, the first day or a shift to earlier occurrence (of an overall lower incidence) of death in the thrombolytic arm is not known.

MAKING CLINICAL DECISIONS BY BALANCING RISK AND BENEFIT

In clinical practice, the benefits of thrombolysis outweigh the risk in almost all patients. However, it is prudent to consider direct angioplasty when available in patients at increased risk for major bleeding, particularly intracranial bleeding. Using data from different trials, a set of tables has been developed for easy and rapid assessment of the expected benefit of thrombolysis in a given patient, as well as the expected risk for intracranial hemorrhage. The benefit is expressed as the expected gain in life expectancy after reperfusion therapy. These tables may be used to assess the expected net clinical benefit (increased survival minus intracranial hemorrhage risk) and to select the optimal (most cost-efficient) mode of reperfusion therapy in a patient with specific features (7,90).

CONCLUSION

The overall benefits of thrombolytic and antithrombotic therapy for acute myocardial infarction have been well established, but they come at a price of serious bleeding, especially intracranial hemorrhage, in a subset of patients. Accurate assessment of risk with baseline prognostic variables can help the physician decide which patients are at high enough risk to warrant alternative, lower risk treatments. Ongoing research will help develop strategies associated with a lower risk of serious hemorrhage as well as better, clinically relevant tools to enable physicians to balance risk and benefit for individual patients.

REFERENCES

1. Fibrinolytic Therapy Trialists' (FTT) Collaborative Group. Indications for fibrinolytic therapy in suspected acute myocardial infarction: collaborative overview of early mortality and major morbidity results from all randomised trials of more than 1000 patients. *Lancet* 1994; 343:311–322.
2. Ryan TJ, Anderson JL, Antman EM, et al. ACC/AHA Guidelines for the management of patients with acute myocardial infarction: executive summary. A report of the American College of Cardiology/American Heart Association Task Force on practice guidelines (Committee on Management of Acute Myocardial Infarction). *Circulation* 1996;94:2341–2350.
3. Task Force on the Management of Acute Myocardial Infarction of the European Society of Cardiology. Acute myocardial infarction: pre-hospital and in-hospital management. *Eur Heart J* 1996;17:43–63.
4. Simoons ML, Maggioni AP, Knatterud G, et al. Individual risk assessment for intracranial haemorrhage during thrombolytic therapy. *Lancet* 1993;342:1523–1528.
5. Gore JM, Granger CB, Sloan MA, et al. Stroke after thrombolysis: mortality and functional outcomes in the GUSTO-I trial. *Circulation* 1995;92:2811–2818.
6. Lee KL, Woodlief LH, Topol EJ, et al. Predictors of 30-day mortality in the era of reperfusion for acute myocardial infarction: results from an international trial of 41,021 patients. *Circulation* 1995;91:1659–1668.
7. Boersma H, van der Vlugt JJ, Arnold AER, Deckers JW, Simoons ML. Estimated gain in life expectancy: a simple tool to select optimal reperfusion treatment in individual patients with evolving myocardial infarction. *Eur Heart J* 1996;17:64–75.
8. Braunwald E, Knatterud GL, Passamani E, Robertson TL, Solomon R. Update from the thrombolysis in myocardial infarction trial [Abstract]. *J Am Coll Cardiol* 1987;10:970.
9. The Global Use of Strategies to Open Occluded Coronary Arteries (GUSTO) IIa Investigators. Randomized trial of intravenous heparin versus recombinant hirudin for acute coronary syndromes. *Circulation* 1994;90: 1631–1637.
10. Antman EM, for the TIMI 9A Investigators. Hirudin in acute myocardial infarction: safety report from the Thrombolysis and Thrombin Inhibition In Myocardial Infarction (TIMI) 9A trial. *Circulation* 1994;90: 1624–1630.
11. Sane DC, Califf RM, Topol EJ, Stump DC, Mark DB, Greenberg CS. Bleeding during thrombolytic therapy for acute myocardial infarction: mechanisms and management. *Ann Intern Med* 1989;111:1010–1022.
12. Gore JM, Sloan M, Price TR, et al. Intracerebral hemorrhage, cerebral infarction, and subdural hematoma after acute myocardial infarction and thrombolytic therapy in the Thrombolysis In Myocardial Infarction study: Thrombolysis In Myocardial Infarction, Phase II, pilot and clinical trial. *Circulation* 1991;83:448–459.
13. Maggioni AP, Franzosi MG, Farina ML, et al. Cerebrovascular events after myocardial infarction: analysis of the GISSI trial. *Br Med J* 1991;302:1428–1431.
14. Maggioni AP, Franzosi MG, Santoro E, et al. The risk of stroke in patients with acute myocardial infarction after thrombolytic and antithrombotic treatment. *N Engl J Med* 1992;327:1–6.
15. de Jaegere PP, Arnold AA, Balk AH, Simoons ML. Intracranial hemorrhage in association with thrombolytic therapy: incidence and clinical predictive factors. *J Am Coll Cardiol* 1992;19:289–294.

16. Gruppo Italiano per lo Studio della Streptochinasi nell'Infarto Miocardico (GISSI). Effectiveness of intravenous thrombolytic treatment in acute myocardial infarction. *Lancet* 1986;1:397–402.

17. ISIS-2 (Second International Study of Infarct Survival) Collaborative Group. Randomised trial of intravenous streptokinase, oral aspirin, both, or neither among 17,187 cases of suspected acute myocardial infarction: ISIS-2. *Lancet* 1988;2:349–360.

18. The ISAM Study Group. A prospective trial of intravenous streptokinase in acute myocardial infarction (ISAM). Mortality, morbidity, and infarct size at 21 days. *N Engl J Med* 1986;314:1465–1471.

19. EMERAS (Estudio Multicentrico Estreptoquinasa Republicas de America del Sur) Collaborative Group. Randomised trial of late thrombolysis in patients with suspected acute myocardial infarction. *Lancet* 1993;342: 767–772.

20. Wilcox RG, von der Lippe G, Olsson CG, Jensen G, Skene AM, Hampton JR. Trial of tissue plasminogen activator for mortality reduction in acute myocardial infarction. Anglo-Scandinavian Study of Early Thrombolysis (ASSET). *Lancet* 1988;2:525–530.

21. LATE Study Group. Late assessment of thrombolytic efficacy (LATE) study with alteplase 6–24 hours after onset of acute myocardial infarction. *Lancet* 1993;342: 759–766.

22. AIMS Trial Study Group. Effect of intravenous APSAC on mortality after acute myocardial infarction: preliminary report of a placebo-controlled clinical trial. *Lancet* 1988;1:545–549.

23. ISIS-3 (Third International Study of Infarct Survival Collaborative Group). ISIS-3: a randomised comparison of streptokinase vs. tissue plasminogen activator vs. anistreplase and of aspirin plus heparin vs. aspirin alone among 41,299 cases of suspected acute myocardial infarction. *Lancet* 1992;339:753–770.

24. International Joint Efficacy Comparison of Thrombolytics. Randomised, double-blind comparison of reteplase double-bolus administration with streptokinase in acute myocardial infarction (INJECT): trial to investigate equivalence. *Lancet* 1995;346:329–336.

25. The Global Use of Strategies to Open Occluded Infarct Arteries (GUSTO-III) Investigators. An international, multicenter, randomized comparison of reteplase and tissue plasminogen activator for acute myocardial infarction. *N Engl J Med* 1997;337:1118–1123.

26. Sloan MA, Price TR, Petito CK, et al. Clinical features and pathogenesis of intracerebral hemorrhage after rt-pa and heparin therapy for acute myocardial infarction: the thrombolysis in myocardial infarction (TIMI) II pilot and randomized clinical trial combined experience. *Neurology* 1995;45:649–658.

27. Ramsey DA, Penswick JL, Robertson DM. Fatal streptokinase-induced intracerebral hemorrhage in amyloid angiopathy. *Can J Neurol Sci* 1990;17:336–341.

28. LeBlanc R, Haddad G, Robitaille Y. Cerebral hemorrhage from amyloid angiopathy and coronary thrombolysis. *Neurosurgery* 1992;31:586–590.

29. Itoh Y, Yamada M, Hayakawa M, Otomo E, Miyatake T. Cerebral amyloid angiopathy: a significant cause of cerebellar as well as lobar cerebral hemorrhage in the elderly. *J Neurol Sci* 1993;116:135–141.

30. Kalyan-Raman UP, Kalyan-Raman K. Cerebral amyloid angiopathy causing intracranial hemorrhage. *Ann Neurol* 1984;16:321–329.

31. Gebel JM, Sila CA, Sloan MA, Granger CB, Mahaffey KW, Weisenberger J. Hemorrhagic stroke complicating coronary arterial thrombolysis in the GUSTO-I trial. Presented at the 21st International Joint Conference on Stroke and Cerebral Circulation, San Antonio, Texas, January 1996.

32. Granger C, White H, Simoons M, et al. Risk factors for stroke following thrombolytic therapy: case-control study from the GUSTO trial [Abstract]. *J Am Coll Cardiol* 1995;25:232A.

33. Kase CS, Pessin MS, Zivin JA, et al. Intracranial hemorrhage after coronary thrombolysis with tissue plasminogen activator. *Am J Med* 1992;92:384–390.

34. Rao AK, Pratt C, Berke A, et al. Thrombolysis in Myocardial Infarction (TIMI) trial—Phase 1; hemorrhagic manifestations and changes in plasma fibrinogen and the fibrinolytic system in patients treated with recombinant tissue plasminogen activator and streptokinase. *J Am Coll Cardiol* 1988;11:1–11.

35. Califf RM, Topol EJ, George BS, et al. Hemorrhagic complications associated with the use of intravenous tissue plasminogen activator in treatment of acute myocardial infarction. *Am J Med* 1988;85:353–359.

36. Bovill EG, Terrin ML, Stump DC, et al. Hemorrhagic events during therapy with recombinant tissue-type plasminogen activator, heparin, and aspirin for acute myocardial infarction. *Ann Intern Med* 1991;115: 256–265.

37. Berkowitz SD, Granger CB, Pieper KS, et al. Incidence and predictors of bleeding after contemporary thrombolytic therapy for myocardial infarction. *Circulation* 1997;95:2508–2516.

38. Granger CB, Becker R, Tracy RP, et al. Thrombin generation, inhibition and clinical outcomes in patients with acute myocardial infarction treated with thrombolytic therapy and heparin: results from the GUSTO trial. *J Am Coll Cardiol* 1997 (in press).

39. TIMI Study Group. Comparison of invasive and conservative strategies after treatment with intravenous tissue plasminogen activator in acute myocardial infarction. Results of the Thrombolysis in Myocardial Infarction (TIMI) phase II trial. *N Engl J Med* 1989;320:618–627.

40. The TIMI IIIB Investigators. Effects of tissue plasminogen activator and a comparison of early invasive and conservative strategies in unstable angina and non–Q-wave myocardial infarction: results of the TIMI IIIB trial. *Circulation* 1994;89:1545–1556.

41. Braunwald E. TIMI-10B preliminary results. TIMI 10-B Investigators Meeting, Boston, Massachusetts, June 1997.

42. The COBALT Investigators. A comparison of continuous infusion of alteplase with double–bolus administration for acute myocardial infarction. *N Engl J Med* 1997;337:1124–1130.

43. Gruppo Italiano per lo Studio della Sopravvivenza nell'Infarto Miocardico. GISSI-2: a factorial randomised trial of alteplase versus streptokinase and heparin versus no heparin among 12,490 patients with acute myocardial infarction. *Lancet* 1990;336:65–71.

44. The Global Use of Strategies to Open Occluded Coronary Arteries (GUSTO) IIb Investigators. A comparison of recombinant hirudin with heparin for the treatment of acute coronary syndromes. *N Engl J Med* 1996;335: 775–782.

45. Cohen M, Demers C, Gurfinkel EP, et al. A comparison of low-molecular-weight heparin with unfractionated

heparin for unstable angina coronary artery disease. Efficacy and Safety of Subcutaneous Enoxaparin in Non–Q Wave Coronary Events Study Group (ESSENCE). *N Engl J Med* 1997;337:447–452.

46. Mahaffey KW, Granger CB, Collins R, et al. Overview of randomized trials of intravenous heparin in patients with acute myocardial infarction treated with thrombolytic therapy. *Am J Cardiol* 1996;77:551–556.

47. Granger CB, Hirsh J, Califf RM, et al. Activated partial thromboplastin time and outcome after thrombolytic therapy for acute myocardial infarction: results from the GUSTO-I trial. *Circulation* 1996;93:870–878.

48. Neuhaus KL, von Essen R, Tebbe U, et al. Safety observations from the pilot phase of the randomized r-Hirudin for Improvement of Thrombolysis (HIT-III) study: a study of the Arbeitsgemeinschaft Leitender Kardiologischer Krankenhausarzte (ALKK). *Circulation* 1994;90:1638–1642.

49. Ohman EM. PRIME preliminary results. Presented at the 69th Scientific Sessions of the American Heart Association, New Orleans, Louisiana, November 10–13, 1996.

50. Simes RJ, Granger CB, Antman EM, Califf RM, Braunwald E, Topol EJ. Impact of hirudin versus heparin on mortality and (re)infarction in patients with acute coronary syndromes: a prospective meta-analysis of the GUSTO-IIb and TIMI 9b trials [Abstract]. *Circulation* 1996;94:I-430.

51. Collins R, MacMahon S, Flather M, et al. Clinical effects of anticoagulant therapy in suspected acute myocardial infarction: systematic overview of randomised trials. *Br Med J* 1996;313:652–659.

52. Antman EM, McCabe CH, Marble SJ, et al. Dose ranging trial of enoxaparin for unstable angina: results of TIMI 11A [Abstract]. *Circulation* 1996;94:I-554.

53. Antman EM. Hirudin in acute myocardial infarction—thrombolysis and thrombin in myocardial infarction (TIMI) 9B trial. *Circulation* 1996;94:911–921.

54. EPIC Investigators. Use of a monoclonal antibody directed against the platelet glycoprotein IIb/IIIa receptor in high-risk coronary angioplasty. *N Engl J Med* 1996;330:956–961.

55. The CAPTURE Investigators. Randomised placebo-controlled trial of abciximab before and during coronary intervention in refractory unstable angina: the CAPTURE study. *Lancet* 1997;349:1429–1435.

56. Tcheng JE. Glycoprotein IIb/IIIa receptor inhibitors: putting the EPIC, IMPACT II, RESTORE, and EPILOG trials into perspective. *Am J Cardiol* 1996;78:35–40.

57. The EPILOG Investigators. Randomised placebo-controlled trial of effect of eptifibatide on complications of percutaneous coronary intervention—IMPACT-II. *Lancet* 1997;349:1422–1428.

58. Deckers J, Califf RM, Topol EJ, Tcheng JE, Simoons ML. Use of abciximab [ReoPro(R)] is not associated with an increase in the risk of stroke: overview of three randomized trials [Abstract]. *J Am Coll Cardiol* 1997;29:241.

59. Alexander K, Barsness GW, Miller JM, Tung CY. Session highlights from the American College of Cardiology meeting. March 16–19, 1997. *Am Heart J* 1997;134:138–154.

60. Ohman EM, Kleiman NS, Gacioch G, et al. Combined accelerated tissue-plasminogen activator and platelet glycoprotein IIb/IIIa integrin receptor blockade with integrelin in acute myocardial infarction: Results of a randomized, placebo-controlled, dose-ranging trial. *Circulation* 1997;95:846–854.

61. Anderson JL, Karagounis L, Allen A, Bradford MJ, Menlove RL, Pryor TA. Older age and elevated blood pressure are risk factors for intracerebral hemorrhage after thrombolysis. *Am J Cardiol* 1991;68:166–170.

62. O'Connor CM, Califf RM, Massey EW, et al. Stroke and acute myocardial infarction in the thrombolytic era: clinical correlates and long-term prognosis. *J Am Coll Cardiol* 1990;16:533–540.

63. White HD, Barbash GI, Califf RM, et al. Age and outcome with contemporary thrombolytic therapy: results from the GUSTO-I trial. *Circulation* 1996;94:1826–1833.

64. Aylward PE, Wilcox RG, Horgan JH, et al. Relation of increased arterial blood pressure to mortality and stroke in the context of contemporary thrombolytic therapy for acute myocardial infarction. *Ann Intern Med* 1996;125:891–900.

65. Selker HP, Beshansky JR, Schmid CH, et al. Presenting pulse pressure predicts thrombolytic therapy-related intracranial hemorrhage: thrombolytic predictive instrument (TPI) project results. *Circulation* 1994;90:1657–1661.

66. White HD, Barbash GI, Modan M, et al. After correcting for worse baseline characteristics, women treated with thrombolytic therapy for acute myocardial infarction have the same mortality and morbidity as men except for a higher incidence of hemorrhagic stroke. *Circulation* 1993;88:2097–2103.

67. Wall TC, Califf RM, Ellis SG, et al. Lack of impact of early catheterization and fibrin specificity on bleeding complications after thrombolytic therapy. The TAMI Study Group. *J Am Coll Cardiol* 1993;21:597–603.

68. Sane DC, Stump DC, Topol EJ, et al. Racial differences in responses to thrombolytic therapy with recombinant tissue-type plasminogen activator. Increased fibrin(ogen)olysis in blacks. The Thrombolysis and Angioplasty in Myocardial Infarction Study Group. *Circulation* 1991;83:170–175.

69. Harrington RA, Sane DC, Califf RM, et al. Clinical importance of thrombocytopenia occurring in the hospital phase after administration of thrombolytic therapy for acute myocardial infarction. *J Am Coll Cardiol* 1994;23:891–898.

70. Tenaglia AN, Califf RM, Candela RJ, et al. Thrombolytic therapy in patients requiring cardiopulmonary resuscitation. *Am J Cardiol* 1991;68:1015–1019.

71. Scholz KH, Tebbe U, Herrmann C, et al. Frequency of complications of cardiopulmonary resuscitation after thrombolysis during acute myocardial infarction. *Am J Cardiol* 1992;69:724–728.

72. van Campen LC, van Leeuwen GR, Verheugt FW. Safety and efficacy of thrombolysis for acute myocardial infarction in patients with prolonged out-of-hospital cardiopulmonary resuscitation. *Am J Cardiol* 1994;73:953–955.

73. Karnash SL, Granger CB, White HD, et al. Treating menstruating women with thrombolytic therapy: insights from the Global Utilization of Streptokinase and Tissue Plasminogen Activator for Occluded Coronary Arteries (GUSTO-I) trial. *J Am Coll Cardiol* 1995;26:1651–1656.

74. Mahaffey KW, Granger CB, Stebbins AL, Califf RM, GUSTO-I Investigators. Diabetic retinopathy should not be a contraindication to thrombolytic therapy: quantifi-

cation of risk of 6011 patients [Abstract]. *Circulation* 1995;92(suppl):I-417.

75. Naeye RL. Thrombotic state after a hemorrhagic diathesis, a possible complication of therapy with epsilon-amino caproic acid. *Blood* 1962;19:694–701.

76. Sloan MA, Sila CA, Mahaffey KW, et al. Prediction of 30-day mortality among patients with thrombolysis-related intracranial hemorrhage. *Circulation* 1997 (in press).

77. Mahaffey KW, White HD, Granger CB, et al. Neurosurgical evacuation for intracranial hemorrhage associated with improved outcome in GUSTO [Abstract]. *J Am Coll Cardiol* 1995;25:232–233.

78. Vaughan DE, Van Houtte E, Declerck PJ, Collen D. Streptokinase-induced platelet aggregation. *Circulation* 1991;84:84–91.

79. Lynch M, Pentecost BL, Littler WA, Stockley RA. Overt and subclinical reactions to streptokinase in acute myocardial infarction. *Am J Cardiol* 1994;74:849–852.

80. The GUSTO Investigators. An international randomized trial comparing four thrombolytic strategies for acute myocardial infarction. *N Engl J Med* 1993;329:673–682.

81. Tsang TSM, Califf RM, Stebbins AL, et al. Incidence and impact on outcome of streptokinase allergy in the GUSTO-I trial. *Am J Cardiol* 1997;79:1232–1235.

82. Toty WG, Romano T, Bemian GM, Gilula LA, Sherman LA. Serum sickness following streptokinase therapy. *Am J Radiol* 1982;138:143–144.

83. Murray N, Lyons J, Chappell M. Crescentic glomerulonephritis: a possible complication of streptokinase treatment for myocardial infarction. *Br Heart J* 1986;56:483–485.

84. Le SP, Chatterjee K, Wolfe CL. Adult respiratory distress syndrome following thrombolytic therapy with APSAC for acute myocardial infarction. *Am Heart J* 1992;123:1368–1369.

85. Elliott JM, Cross DB, Cederholm-Williams SA, et al. Neutralizing antibodies to streptokinase four years after intravenous thrombolytic therapy. *Am J Cardiol* 1993;71:640–645.

86. Lew AS, Laramee P, Cercek B, Shah PK, Ganz W. The hypotensive effect of intravenous streptokinase in patients with acute myocardial infarction. *Circulation* 1985;72:1321–1326.

87. Kleiman NS, White HD, Ohman EM, et al. Mortality within 24 hours of thrombolysis for myocardial infarction: the importance of early reperfusion. *Circulation* 1994;90:2658–2665.

88. Honan MB, Harrell FE Jr, Reimer KA, et al. Cardiac rupture, mortality and the timing of thrombolytic therapy: a meta-analysis. *J Am Coll Cardiol* 1990;16:359–367.

89. Becker RC, Gore JM, Lambrew C, et al. A composite view of cardiac rupture in the united states national registry of myocardial infarction. *J Am Coll Cardiol* 1996;27:1321–1326.

90. Simoons ML, Arnold AER. Tailored thrombolytic therapy. A perspective. *Circulation* 1993;88:2556–2564.

Cardiovascular Thrombosis: Thrombocardiology and Thromboneurology, Second Edition, edited by M. Verstraete, V. Fuster, and E. J. Topol, Lippincott–Raven Publishers, Philadelphia © 1998.

31

Antithrombotic Treatment in the Chronic Phase of Myocardial Infarction

Pål J. Smith

Department of Medicine, Baerum Hospital, N-13555 Baerum, Norway

Deterioration of stable ischemic heart disease may follow progression of atherosclerosis, formation of platelet aggregates, and coronary thrombosis. The association of thrombosis and atherosclerosis has long been recognized (1), and the presence of fibrin and other components of the clotting system in human atherosclerotic plaques has been documented (2), suggesting that development and progression of atherosclerotic lesions may be accelerated and amplified by activation of the clotting cascade (see Chapter 3).

Despite improved therapy during the acute and subacute phase of myocardial infarction the past decade, the risk of recurrent events remains high. The stabilized annual mortality rate 6 months after an acute event is about four to eight times that faced by a comparable noncoronary population (3). Although the short-term prognosis after myocardial infarction has improved considerably since 1960, positive changes in long-term prognosis in the regular clinical context still need verification (4). Antithrombotic therapy may be beneficial in preventing further cardiovascular attacks because thrombosis plays a major role in is-

chemic heart disease. This chapter deals with the rationale for antithrombotic therapy after myocardial infarction and the experiences from clinical trials. The large long-term trials are the primary focus of this review, although some studies with follow-up of less than 1 year have been briefly assessed to complete the picture.

GOALS OF ANTITHROMBOTIC THERAPY

The aims of antithrombotic therapy after myocardial infarction are to reduce or prevent (a) cardiac chamber thrombus formation and (b) recurrence of myocardial infarction and death. The notion that antithrombotic therapy retards progressive atherothrombosis is interesting, but has yet to be confirmed. For practical reasons, only oral antithrombotic drugs are feasible for long-term treatment. Up to now, only antiplatelet agents and anticoagulants (coumarins) have been orally active. This will change in the future as orally active specific thrombin inhibitors and inhibitors of factor Xa become available.

CLINICAL TRIAL EVALUATION

The validity of any trial is contingent upon adequate design, randomization, proper control, and a sufficient sample size. Whether all-cause mortality or cardiovascular mortality is the more appropriate endpoint may be debatable. On one hand, death is not necessarily a measure of thrombus formation. Sudden cardiac death is thought to be due principally to arrhythmias, even though some data suggest an association of sudden death with thrombosis (5). On the other hand, the results of a meta-analysis of six primary prevention trials suggested that coronary heart disease mortality tended to be lower in men on lipid-lowering agents, but that all-cause mortality did not decline because of an increase in deaths from external causes (6). Thus, to cover the possibility of a harmful effect of the drug, all-cause mortality should always be considered, particularly when long-term drug administration is involved. The assessment of a trial also should take beginning and duration of therapy into account. A short-term effect does not necessarily imply that it will be sustained. The effect of concomitant drugs is important; for instance, an unequivocal effect on mortality has been demonstrated by β-blockade after myocardial infarction (7). Studies have suggested, albeit weakly, an antiplatelet action of unselective β-receptor antagonists (8). Thus, chances are that weak platelet inhibitors might not add benefit to that brought about by a β-blocker. Finally, extrapolating from the study population may not be justified in trials where only fractions of the screened population have been entered into the study.

ANTITHROMBOTIC DRUGS

Platelet Inhibitors

Sulfinpyrazone

Two studies have evaluated the prophylactic effect of platelet inhibition by a daily dose of 800 mg sulfinpyrazone after myocardial infarction (9,10) (Table 31-1). The Anturane Reinfarction Trial (9) randomized 1,629 patients who had survived acute myocardial infarction by 25 to 35 days to sulfinpyrazone or matching placebo. The study was heavily criticized

TABLE 31-1. *Distribution of endpoints in the different antiplatelet trials according to treatment groups*

Study (year)	Reference	Treatment time (months)	Treatment type		Mortality (%)		Nonfatal MI (%)		Nonfatal CVA (%)		Averted events[a]
			C	T	C	T	C	T	C	T	
Sulfinpyrazone											
ART	9	16	783	775	6.3	4.1	3.5	1.3	—	—	4.3
ARIS	10	19	362	365	5.5	5.2	7.7	3.2	1.6	0.2	6.2
Ticlopidine/ Clopidogrel											
STAI	13	6	338	314	4.7	2.5	8.9	4.8	—	—	6.3
CAPRIE[b]	14	23	9,586	9,599	6.1	5.8	3.1	2.6	5.5	5.0	1.3
Aspirin/ Dipyridamole											
ELWOOD	15	12	624	615	9.7	7.6	—	—	—	—	2.1
CDPA	16	22	771	758	8.3	5.8	4.1	3.6	1.0	1.1	2.9
ELWOOD	17	12	850	832	14.8	12.3	7.4	3.7	—	—	6.2[c]
GAMIS	18	24	309	317	10.3	8.5	5.1	3.4	—	—	3.5[c]
AMIS	19	36	2,257	2,267	9.7	10.7	9.4	7.7	2.0	1.1	1.6
PARIS I	20	41	406	1,620[d]	12.8	10.6	9.9	7.4	2.0	1.1	5.6
PARIS II	21	23	1,565	1,563	7.2	7.1	4.5	2.1	2.1	1.3	3.3

MI, recurrent myocardial infarction; CVA, cerebrovascular attacks; C, control group; T, treatment group.
[a]Total death, nonfatal myocardial reinfarction, and nonfatal stroke averted per 100 patients treated for 0.5 to 3.5 years.
[b]Aspirin was control.
[c]On treatment analysis.
[d]Combined active treatment arms.

because of both design and analysis, and the U.S. Food and Drug Administration even published a formal critique of the study (11). Another trial was reported by the Anturan Reinfarction Italian Study Group (10). After an average 19 months of follow-up, mortality was similar in the two groups. However, the rate of combined fatal and nonfatal myocardial reinfarction was 3.2% in the actively treated group as compared with 7.7% in the control group. Due to the controversial findings, sulfinpyrazone has never come into common use.

Dipyridamole

Experience with this agent as monotherapy after myocardial infarction relates to one study only. No benefit was found of dipyridamole 400 mg daily compared with placebo, neither in terms of prevention of thromboembolic complications nor myocardial reinfarction or death (12). However, the study groups were small, and follow-up lasted only 1 month.

Ticlopidine and Clopidogrel

No large-scale trial on ticlopidine has been carried out in the postmyocardial infarction setting. One study including patients with unstable angina has been reported (13) (Table 31-1). Patients were observed for 6 months. Altogether, 652 patients (25% of those screened) were randomized either to conventional therapy (β-blocker, calcium-channel blocker, or nitrates or to conventional therapy plus ticlopidine 250 mg twice daily. The risk of vascular death and fatal myocardial infarction was reduced (16 events among the control group versus eight in the ticlopidine group), but the reduction was statistically not significant. However, total events (also including nonfatal reinfarction) was 13.6% in the conventionally treated group as compared with 7.3% in the ticlopidine group, which was statistically significant. Three nonfatal strokes occurred in the control group as compared with none in the ticlopidine group.

CAPRIE was a randomized, blinded trial designed to investigate the relative efficacy of clopidogrel (75 mg once daily) and aspirin (325 mg once daily) in reducing the risk of a composite cluster of ischemic events, including vascular death (14). The study population comprised subgroups of patients with recent iscemic stroke, recent myocardial infarction, and symptomatic peripheral arterial disease. A total of 19,185 patients were randomized, with more than 6,300 in each clinical subgroup. Follow-up lasted for 1 to 3 years. Intention-to-treat analysis in the overall population showed that the annual risk of an event in the clopidogrel group was 5.3% as compared with 5.8% in the aspirin group (Table 31-1). However, for patients with myocardial infarction, the average event rate per year was 5% in the clopidogrel group, as compared with 4.8% in the aspirin group. A test of heterogeneity suggested that true treatment effect might not be identical across the three subgroups (14).

Aspirin

Long-Term Clinical Trials on Aspirin

Seven randomized studies (15–21), involving 620 to 4,524 patients, have evaluated the prophylactic effect of aspirin in the long-term setting after myocardial infarction (Table 31-1). The time between the index infarction and onset of treatment varied considerably across these studies—from one study including most of the patients within 1 week, to that including the majority of the participants after more than 5 years. The earliest trial administered a daily dose of 300 mg aspirin, whereas larger doses (900 to 1,500 mg daily) were used in subsequent trials.

In 1974 Elwood randomized 1,239 men to receive either aspirin 300 mg daily or placebo an average of 10 weeks after acute myocardial infarction (15). Average length of follow-up was 12 months. Ten percent of those entered were withdrawn during the study. More deaths were observed in the placebo group than in the aspirin group. However, the difference did not attain statistical significance. No other endpoints were studied.

In the Coronary Drug Project Aspirin study of 1,529 men, mortality in the aspirin group was 5.8% as compared with 8.3% in the placebo group over 22 months (16). More than 5 years had elapsed since the index infarction in the majority of patients. The mortality rate in the control group was low. No important benefit was found pertaining to reinfarction or stroke. All patients in this trial had received either dextrothyroxine or varying doses of estrogen as part of another study, the Coronary Drug Project, for some time between the index infarction and recruitment. Although the hormone medication was discontinued 6 to 25 months before enrollment into the aspirin study, a general conclusion regarding the impact of this treatment cannot be made.

A follow-up study by Elwood and colleagues in 1979 was conducted in 1,682 patients (17). The majority of patients were included within 1 week after the qualifying infarction. A reduction in risk of death by aspirin by 17.3% was found, but again this reduction was not statistically significant. Data on reinfarctions were limited and uncertain according to the authors.

The German-Austrian trial (18) investigated three treatment arms: aspirin 1,500 mg daily or matching placebo, and an open group receiving oral anticoagulants (reviewed later in this chapter). Total mortality was 8.5% in the aspirin group and 10.3% in the placebo group, a reduction of 17% by aspirin. Neither this difference nor the difference in reinfarction or stroke was statistically conclusive.

The Aspirin Myocardial Infarction Study, sponsored by The National Heart, Lung and Blood Institute, involved 4,524 men and women recruited 8 weeks to 5 years after an acute myocardial infarction (19). The test medication consisted of 1,000 mg aspirin daily or matching placebo. Mortality from any cause after an average of 36 months was 10.7% in the aspirin group and 9.7% in the placebo group. The difference was not statistically significant. When fatal endpoints other than total mortality were analyzed, there again was no evidence of a benefit by aspirin. Both the incidence of recurrent nonfatal myocardial infarction and stroke was lower among

those taking aspirin (Table 31-1), but due to a large number of significance tests performed during and after follow-up, the authors correctly stated that "exact statements of statistical significance are impossible to make in this situation."

Dipyridamole was added to aspirin in two studies. The Persantine-Aspirin Reinfarction Study (20) had three arms consisting of one group receiving dipyridamole plus aspirin, one group receiving aspirin alone, and one placebo group (Table 31-1). The 1,759 men and 267 women were entered into the trial 2 months to 5 years after the qualifying infarction and were allocated to treatment with 972 mg aspirin daily (n = 810), 972 mg aspirin plus dipyridamole 225 mg daily (n = 810), or placebo matching the aspirin group (n = 406). Mean follow-up was 41 months. All-cause mortality in the placebo group was 12.8% compared with 10.5% in the group assigned to aspirin alone, and 10.7% in the group taking the combination of dipyridamole and aspirin. Regarding reinfarction and stroke rates, only small reductions by aspirin or the combined treatment were found (Table 31-1). A follow-up study with a two-group design was published in 1986 (21). In this study, 3,128 patients were entered within 4 weeks to 4 months after myocardial infarction. The test medication was aspirin 330 mg plus dipyridamole 75 mg three times daily or matching placebo medication. Mean observation time was 23 months. There was no difference in total mortality or stroke, whereas a significant reduction in nonfatal myocardial reinfarction was observed (4.5% in the control group vs. 2.1% in the actively treated group).

Short-Term Clinical Trials on Aspirin

ISIS-2 was a large trial of intravenous streptokinase or placebo and aspirin 162.5 mg/day or placebo in 17,187 patients with suspected myocardial infarction and symptoms of less than 24 hours duration (median 5 hours) (22). Aspirin or placebo was given for 5 weeks. Median follow-up was 15 months. Mortality was 9.4% with aspirin as compared with 11.8% with placebo, which was highly statistically significant. Aspirin also significantly reduced the risk of reinfarction (1% versus 2% in the placebo group) and nonfatal stroke (0.3% versus 0.6%).

A comparative study between aspirin 75 mg daily or matching placebo for up to 1 year and intermittent injections of intravenous heparin (7,500 U every 4 hours) or matching placebo for 5 days was reported by the Swedish RISC group in 1990 (23). Eligible for the study were patients with unstable angina and non–Q-wave myocardial infarction. The risk of death and recurrent myocardial infarction was reduced by aspirin; after 3 months the risk ratio was 0.36 (95% confidence interval [CI] 0.23 to 0.57). Reduction was seen in both unstable angina and myocardial infarction.

Side Effects by Platelet Inhibitors

Treatment with aspirin and the combination of aspirin with dipyridamole resulted in a raised frequency of side effects. Dipyridamole, either alone or combined with aspirin, was associated with increased incidences of headache. The rate of gastrointestinal symptoms was almost doubled in studies using a daily dose of 1,000 mg aspirin or more (17–19). Bleeding complications occurred chiefly in the gastrointestinal tract and pre-sented as hematemesis, bloody stool, and black tarry stool (Table 31-2).

Few and only minor adverse reactions were observed in the trial on ticlopidine and the RISC study (13,23). Those observed were mild gastrointestinal disorders and rash. No bleeding disorders were reported.

In the CAPRIE study (14) there were more patients with intracranial hemorrhage and gastrointestinal bleeding in the group who took aspirin than among those who were assigned to therapy with clopidogrel (Table 31-2).

A daily dose of 50 mg aspirin, or 400 mg dipyridamole or the two agents in a combined formulation, or placebo was used in a four-arm study in the secondary prevention of ischemic stroke (European Stroke Prevention Study) (24). Patients were observed for 2 years. All-site moderate and severe bleeding was significantly more common in patients who took aspirin in comparison with placebo or dipyridamole (3%, 1%, and 1%, respectively).

Meta-analysis of Platelet Inhibitors

In 1994 the Antiplatelet Trialists' Collaboration Group pooled the results of all platelet inhibitor trials on postmyocardial infarction treatment (25). The results favors aspirin over placebo with a reduction in cardiovascular mortality at 2 years (aspirin 13% and control

TABLE 31-2. *Distribution of fatal and serious nonfatal bleedings as reported in platelet inhibitor studies*

Study	Reference	ASA (mg/day)	DP and clopidogrel[a] (mg/day)	% Fatal		% Nonfatal		% Combined	
				C	T	C	T	C	T
ELWOOD I	15	300	—	—	—	—	—	—	—
CDPA	16	972	—	—	—	4.6	6.2	4.6	6.2
ELWOOD II	17	900	—	—	—	0.4	0.9	0.4	0.9
GAMIS	18	1,500	—	—	—	0.0	2.9	0.0	2.9
AMIS	19	1,000	—	—	—	4.9	8.2	4.9	8.2
PARIS I	20	972	225	—	—	1.7	3.4	1.7	3.4
PARIS II	21	972	225	—	—	0.9	1.5	0.9	1.5
CAPRIE[a]	14	325	75	—	—	1.6	1.4[b]		

DP, dipyridamole.
[a]Clopidogrel 75 mg versus aspirin 325 mg daily.
[b]Clopidogrel.

17%). Furthermore, a reduction in recurrent nonfatal reinfarction (34%) and reduction in nonfatal strokes (25%) by aspirin was observed. Moreover, pooling of data from 39 trials on ticlopidine versus control showed a significant reduction in vascular events by 33%. However, these trials were not performed in the postmyocardial infarction setting.

Conclusions Pertaining to Platelet Inhibitors

No aspirin trial alone has produced evidence in terms of a statistically significant reduction in total mortality in favor of aspirin over placebo. In contrast, reduction in the risk of recurrent myocardial infarction has been more promising. The pooling of all available data shows a reduction in cardiovascular mortality by platelet inhibitors by an order of magnitude of 13%. Furthermore, a reduction in nonfatal reinfarction by 34% and a reduction in the incidence of nonfatal stroke by 25% is demonstrable (25). Because small absolute reductions may suggest a great relative reduction if the incidence rate in the control group is low, avoided events per 100 patients treated may be a more informative way to assess the benefit of treatment. Table 31-1 suggests that long-term treatment with platelet inhibitors avoids two to six major events per 100 treated patients, when treatment is given for from 1 to 3.5 years. The associated risk for serious bleeding varies considerably across the studies, probably due to different criteria. Apparently gastrointestinal bleeding has not been separated from gastrointestinal symptoms in many studies, and only one study explicitly reports that no bleedings were fatal (18). Table 31-2 contains data on bleeding as provided in the different study reports. An attempt has been made to include in this summary only those bleeding episodes reported by the authors as being clinically important. It appears that aspirin doubles the risk of significant bleeding. All aspirin trials in patients after myocardial infarction used doses varying from 300 to 1,500 mg daily. Intermediate (160 mg) and low-dose aspirin as used in studies during and after the acute phase of unstable coronary disease causes less gastrointestinal upset and less occult blood loss (Table 31-2). At present the optimum dose of aspirin for secondary prevention after acute myocardial infarction is not firmly established.

ANTICOAGULANT DRUGS

Heparin

Clinical Trials on Heparin

The long-term effect of heparin after myocardial infarction has been investigated in one trial (26). A total of 3,859 patients were screened and 728 eventually entered into this study. The patients were recruited 6 to 18 months after myocardial infarction and randomly assigned to a daily subcutaneous injection of 12,500 IU unfractionated heparin daily for an average of 23 months, or no heparin. More than 30% of those assigned to heparin and more than 40% of those allocated to the control group took antiplatelet agents concurrently. Heparin treatment reduced the cumulative mortality rate by 34% on an intention-to-treat basis (not significant) and by 48% on an "on-treatment" basis (p < 0.05). The accumulated reinfarction rate was significantly lower in the heparin group (1.3%) as compared with the control group (3.5%). Only minor side effects were encountered.

In the Fragmin during Instability in Coronary Artery Disease (FRISC) study, patients with unstable angina or non–Q-wave myocardial infarction were randomly assigned to treatment with either low molecular weight heparin (dalteparin) or placebo injections (27). The study treatment was administered in addition to conventional treatment with aspirin and was commenced within 72 hours after admission to hospital. Follow-up lasted 150 days, whereas treatment was given for 35 to 45 days. At 6 days the rate of death and recurrent myocardial infarction was lower in the dalteparin group than in the placebo group (1.8% versus 4.8%; risk ratio 0.37; 95% CI 0.20 to 0.68). The difference persisted through day 40, whereas no significant difference was present after 4 to 5 months. There was no difference between the treatment groups with regard to major bleeding.

In the ESSENCE trial (28), the effect of low molecular weight heparin (enoxaparin) was compared with unfractionated intravenous heparin in patients with either unstable angina or non–Q-wave myocardial infarction. Preliminary data suggest a significant reduction at 2 to 8 days by enoxaparin. The TIMI IIB trial is testing a longer duration of treatment with enoxaparin versus standard intravenous heparin.

These studies provide evidence of a benefit of heparin after myocardial infarction. Despite the appeal of a fixed-dose regimen of subcutaneous heparin, with no need for laboratory control, the parenteral route is probably less feasible than orally administered drugs in a long-term setting.

Oral Anticoagulants

Clinical Trials

A vast number of trials have been performed in this field. However, of the 19 randomized clinical trials on long-term oral anticoagulants after myocardial infarction performed up to 1990, only three were of sufficient size and design to permit appropriate interpretation (Table 31-3). The British Med-

ical Research Council Trial (BMRC) (29), was a double-blinded comparison of a high-dose (anticoagulant group) with a very low dose of phenindione. The size of the background population is unknown. Patients were randomized within 4 to 6 weeks of infarction and observed for at least 2 years. Although both mortality (7.7% in the high-dose group versus 11.7% among the control group) and nonfatal reinfarction (13.3% in the high-dose group versus 36.7% in the control group) was reduced by anticoagulation, only the difference for myocardial reinfarction attained statistical significance. The incidence of thromboembolic morbidity, including pulmonary embolism and stroke, was low and did not permit separate assessment.

The Veterans Administration Trial entered 747 patients within 21 days of the acute event (30). Patients allocated to anticoagulation received bishydroxycoumarin. The anticoagulated group had fewer deaths and reinfarctions than did the placebo group during the 3 years of follow-up (p < 0.01), but the difference was less pronounced at 5 years. Patients in the anticoagulant group were less frequently hospitalized for recurrent myocardial infarction than were those taking placebo (66 versus 92 events). A reduction in other thromboembolic events also was seen (17 in the anticoagulant group and 39 among those assigned to placebo).

TABLE 31-3. *Distribution of endpoints in the different anticoagulant trials*

Study (year)	Reference	Treatment time (months)	Treatment type		Mortality (%)		Nonfatal MI (%)		Nonfatal CVA (%)		Averted events[a]
			C	T	C	T	C	T	C	T	
Heparin											
IHS	26	23	365	363	6.3	4.1	3.5	1.3[b]	—	—	4.3
Oral anticoagulants											
BMRC	29	>24	188	195	11.1	7.6	36.7	13.3	—	—	26.9
VAT	30	24–60	350	385	32.6	31.2	20.8	15.5	—	—	6.7
60+	31	24	439	439	15.7	11.6	8.4	4.1	3.4	1.3	10.5
WARIS	32	37	607	607	20.2	15.4	12.3	6.2	7.2	3.2	14.9
ASPECT	33	37	1,704	1,700	11.1	10.0	11.8	5.3	3.2	1.6	9.2

[a]Total deaths, nonfatal myocardial reinfarction, and nonfatal stroke averted per 100 patients treated for 6 months to 5 years.
[b]On treatment data.

The design of the Sixty Plus Trial was different from that of the others (31). This study entered patients over 60 years of age who had already been treated with oral anticoagulants (acenocoumarin or phenprocoumon) for at least 6 months, median 6 years. The patients received either continued anticoagulation or matching placebo. The difference in total mortality (51 deaths in the anticoagulant group versus 69 in the control group) attained borderline statistical significance. Those who continued anticoagulation fared considerably better with respect to total reinfarction (29 in the actively treated as compared with 64 in the placebo group), a difference yielding statistical significance. Notably, intracranial events due to any cause was impressively reduced by anticoagulation (12 in the anticoagulant group versus 20 in the control group).

The design of this trial did cause some concern, and critics argued that the study had just demonstrated the risk of stopping anticoagulant therapy in subjects who apparently had benefited from such therapy over the years.

Trials in the 1990s: WARIS and ASPECT

The WARIS trial was planned and designed as a response to the debate on long-term oral anticoagulation after the Sixty Plus study. It was a prospective, double-blind, placebo-controlled study, and evidence of success or failure was based primarily on the total death rate (32). Other endpoints were recurrent myocardial infarction and cerebrovascular accidents. Treatment allocation was stratified for chronic β-blockade.

Chronic atrial fibrillation, left ventricular mural thrombi, or a high risk for thromboembolic disease other than myocardial infarction were generally considered as indications for long-term anticoagulation.

A total of 1,918 eligible patients were identified, of whom 1,214 (63%) were entered into the study. Overall duration on test medication averaged 37 months. Endpoints were taken to be related to trial medication if occurring within 28 days after stopping test medication. For the intention-to-treat analy-

sis, all events after randomization were counted. The target range of anticoagulation was 2.8 to 4.8 INR (international normalized ratio), which is equivalent to a prolongation of 1.5 to two times control using a typical North American thromboplastin reagent.

Total mortality was reduced significantly by anticoagulation (from 20.2% in the control group to 15.4% in the warfarin group), and so also was the total reinfarction rate (20.4% versus 13.5%). Nonfatal reinfarction on treatment occurred in 12.3% of the patients in the placebo group compared with 6.2% of those in the warfarin group. An appreciable reduction in the number of stroke was noted in the warfarin group as compared with the placebo group (7.2 versus 3.2%). Four fatal intracerebral hemorrhages occurred in warfarin-treated patients, whereas no fatal thromboembolic strokes were observed. By contrast, no fatal hemorrhagic strokes and 10 fatal thromboembolic strokes were seen in patients taking placebo.

The Dutch ASPECT study was a randomized, placebo-controlled trial involving 3,404 hospital survivors of myocardial infarction (33). Its design was basically identical to that of the WARIS study. Patients were entered into the study within 6 weeks of discharge and randomly assigned to treatment with either vitamin K antagonists (nicoumalone or phenprocoumon) or placebo. The target range of prothrombin time was 2.8 to 4.8 INR, similar to that observed in the WARIS trial. Follow-up averaged 37 months. Anticoagulant therapy led to fewer deaths among patients randomized to placebo, even though the hazard ratio of 0.90 was statistically not significant. However, the effect on event rates of nonfatal recurrent myocardial infarction and stroke was more impressive (Table 31-3).

Quality of Anticoagulant Control

In a review of all prospective randomized trials to assess the effect of long-term anticoagulation in patients with coronary artery disease, Loeliger demonstrated a correlation between level and stability of anticoagulation

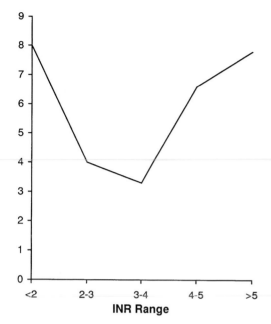

FIG. 31-1. INR specific event rates (events per 100 patient years) for bleeding and thromboembolic events combined at given levels of anticoagulation in the ASPECT study. (Data from Azar et al., ref. 35.)

on bleeding and thromboembolic complications, the optimal intensity of long-term anticoagulation in patients after myocardial infarction lies between 2.0 and 4.0 INR (Fig. 31-1). This is in keeping with previous proposed levels of intensity (36) and close to the quality of control achieved in the BMRC, Sixty Plus, WARIS, and ASPECT studies (29,31–33).

Meta-analysis of Oral Anticoagulants

In 1994 Yusuf et al. pooled the data from 16 randomized trials on oral anticoagulants published after 1960. The authors concluded that treatment with anticoagulants does reduce major vascular events (mortality, recurrent myocardial infarction, and stroke) to a substantial degree (37). Thus, mortality was significantly lowered (odds ratio 0.80; 95% CI 0.72, 0.89), as was relapsing myocardial infarction (odds ratio 0.55; 95% CI 0.49, 0.67).

Side Effects

This risk of bleeding in anticoagulation is related to the intensity of anticoagulation (38). Table 31-4 contains data on major bleeding complications in the anticoagulant trials. The low risk of bleeding in the WARIS Study, amounting to a combined incidence of serious bleeding of 0.6 per 100 years at risk, may be due to at least two important factors. First, the prothrombin time reagent used for all controls in the WARIS Study is extremely sensitive at the therapeutic level. By contrast, a number of North American thromboplastin

with degree of benefit. The more intensive regimens apparently achieved the better results (34). The ASPECT group attempted to define the optimal intensity of anticoagulation required to prevent both bleeding and thromboembolic events (35). They calculated incidence rates for either type of event associated with a specific normalized ratio. The numerator included events occurring at given INRs, and the denominator consisted of the total observation time. Giving equal weight

TABLE 31-4. *Frequency of fatal and serious nonfatal bleedings reported in studies on oral anticoagulants*

Study	Reference	% Fatal		% Nonfatal		% Combined	
		C	T	C	T	C	T
BMRC	29	0	0.5	0.0	8.2	0.0	8.7
VAT	30	0	1.0	2.8	15.0	2.8	16.0
60+	31	0	1.1	1.1	5.0	1.1	6.1
WARIS	32	0	0.4	0.0	1.3	0.0	1.7
ASPECT	33	0	0.6	1.1	3.8	1.1	4.4

C, control group; T, treatment group.

reagents have shown less sensitivity to the reduction of vitamin K–dependent clotting factors (39). Relatively insensitive reagents may lead to overdosing and may increase the risk of bleeding (39). Compared with the Sixty Plus and ASPECT studies, fewer patients in the WARIS study exhibited INR values exceeding the upper therapeutic limit during follow-up.

In their overview of oral anticoagulant trials Yusuf et al. also looked into bleeding complications (37). As expected, there were significantly more major bleeds among patients treated with anticoagulants than in those receiving placebo, but still there was a substantial benefit in terms of patients treated without complications.

Conclusions Pertaining to Oral Anticoagulants

Eight single studies, three of which involved heparin, and an overview (37) on 16 oral anticoagulant trials have been reviewed. For long-term purposes, the orally administered drugs are the most suitable. The three most recently published studies on oral anticoagulation—the Sixty Plus trial, the WARIS study, and the ASPECT trial—all meet the methodologic requirements for modern clinical trials: large sample size, double-blind placebo-controlled design, and analysis according to the intention-to-treat principle. As of yet, the WARIS study is the only study on any antithrombotic regimen proving efficacy by reduction of all-cause mortality (32). However, all studies showed a statistically significant reduction in relapsing myocardial infarction. The findings of the WARIS trial are supported not only by trends in other anticoagulant trials (29–31,33), but the findings are also remarkably similar to results of analyses of aggregated data (37). Moreover, the effect of anticoagulation was demonstrable even when a vast proportion of the patients received concurrent β-blockade, as seen in the Sixty Plus, WARIS, and ASPECT studies. Thrombolysis came into common use after the WARIS study but was used in 25% of the

patients in the ASPECT study. As seen in Table 31-3, anticoagulant therapy averts four to 26 events per 100 patients treated for 2 to 3 years. Given the results from the trials applying the most adequate control (29,31,33), avoidance of 10 to 14 events seems to be a realistic benefit. With reasonable management of the anticoagulant therapy, especially with the use of suitable control methods, the incidence of bleeding may be kept at a low level.

Aspirin Versus Anticoagulants

Two studies have compared aspirin and oral anticoagulants. Both were conducted in an unblinded fashion. In the GAMIS (German-Austrian Myocardial Infarction Study) 946 patients were randomized to treatment with phenprocoumon, aspirin, or placebo (18). This study was basically a study on aspirin with a matching placebo group, but an open anticoagulant group was also included. Patients were enrolled within 5 to 6 weeks after the index infarction and allocated to aspirin or matching placebo or anticoagulants aiming at a prolongation of the prothrombin time from 2.1 to 4.8 INR. No statistically significant difference was detectable between the groups, neither for the endpoint mortality, nor for reinfarction.

In the E.P.S.I.M study (40), 1,303 patients were entered an average of 11 days after myocardial infarction and allocated at random to anticoagulant therapy or aspirin in an unblinded fashion. Patients assigned to aspirin received 500 mg daily, whereas those in the anticoagulant group received a dosage of oral anticoagulants aiming for a prothrombin time range of 25% to 35% of normal. Mean follow-up was 29 months. More patients in the aspirin group than in the anticoagulant group were withdrawn during the study (139 versus 82). There were 67 deaths in the anticoagulant group and 72 in those taking aspirin. The rate of reinfarction was higher (n = 32) in the aspirin group than in the anticoagulant group (n = 20), but neither difference was statistically significant. The accomplished level of anticoagulation was clearly suboptimal by recommended standards (36).

For obvious reasons it is difficult to compare the pharmacotherapeutic potential and safety of drugs as observed in different trials. Even though populations at different risk have been studied, the present data suggest a superiority of anticoagulants compared with antiplatelet drugs, with more deaths and morbidity averted by anticoagulants (Tables 31-1 and 31-3). The presentations based on odds ratios provide no information on the amount of avoided events. Nevertheless, three out of four anticoagulant trials exhibit greater reductions in mortality and reinfarction than all antiplatelet studies. Notably, the 95% CI for the WARIS study is the only one not to include the possibility of an adverse effect regarding mortality. As for the endpoint myocardial reinfarction, the anticoagulant studies yield CIs that are narrower and indicate more of a benefit than do the antiplatelet studies. This superiority is plausibly explained by evidence indicating that thrombin is probably the most potent platelet-aggregating agent in vivo (41). Moreover, the type of thrombus differs between patients with unstable angina and those with acute myocardial infarction. The former patients mainly have thrombi consisting of platelets, whereas those with acute myocardial infarction mainly have thrombi consisting of fibrin (42). Thus, after myocardial infarction, antiplatelet agents would be less effective due to the lesser thrombogenic importance of platelets.

As outlined in Tables 31-2 and 31-4, the risk of hemorrhage resulting from anticoagulant therapy appears to be only slightly increased as compared with the risk of bleeding induced by aspirin.

The goal of the Coumadin Aspirin Reinfarction Study (CARS) was to compare low-dose coumadin plus aspirin (80 mg) with aspirin (160 mg) alone. The study was conducted in a large number of centers across the United States and Canada and closed in February 1996. The primary endpoint was the combined rate of nonfatal myocardial infarction, ischemic stroke, and cardiovascular death. The results are not yet formally published, but a preliminary report was presented at the hotline session at the annual American College of Cardiology meeting in 1996. There was no benefit of adding a fixed dose of warfarin (1 or 3 mg, respectively) to a low-dose of aspirin as compared with a traditional dose of aspirin in this study.

FUTURE DIRECTIONS/ FUTURE ANSWERS

Two questions need to be examined in greater detail:

1. What is the relative efficacy of aspirin, or other platelet inhibitors, compared with oral anticoagulants in a head-to-head comparison?
2. Does low-dose aspirin, combined with oral anticoagulants at a lower level of anticoagulation, offer any advantage over either therapy alone?

Two running trials may answer these questions. The Combination Hemotherapy and Mortality Prevention (CHAMP) trial is a study under the Veterans Affairs Cooperative Studies Program. Its primary endpoint is total mortality. Patients are randomized to either aspirin 162 mg daily or aspirin 81 mg daily plus warfarin with a target INR of 1.5 to 2.5. This study completed inclusion by fall 1996. The mean follow-up is planned to be 4 years.

The Norwegian Warfarin Aspirin Reinfarction Study (WARIS II) has a three-arm design and, similar to the CHAMP trial, addresses the period after acute myocardial infarction. Patients are assigned to either warfarin alone (target INR 2.8 to 4.2), aspirin alone (160 mg daily), or a combination of aspirin and warfarin (aspirin 75 mg daily, INR 2.0 to 2.5). The primary endpoint is the composite endpoint of death, nonfatal myocardial infarction, and nonfatal stroke. WARIS II is expected to complete enrollment of the planned 3,606 patients early in 1998. The last included patient will be observed for 2 years.

CONCLUSION

Each patient should have an individually tailored therapy after myocardial infarction.

TABLE 31-5. *Elements to be considered in evaluation of randomized clinical trials*

1. Are the results valid?
    Were patients randomized?
    Intention-to-treat analysis?
    Blinded endpoint evaluation?
2. Is the treatment effect clinically important?
    Were both statistical and clinical significance considered?
    Were all clinically relevant outcomes reported?
3. Are the results relevant to my patient?
    Were the study patients recognizably similar to my own?
    Is the therapeutic maneuver feasible in my practice?

Adapted from Cook et al., ref. 43.

Cook et al. have summed up important elements of a valid and useful clinical trial (43) (Table 31-5). Using these rules of single controlled studies and meta-analyses, the cornerstones of secondary prevention remain antithrombotic therapy, a β-blocker, and cholesterol-lowering therapy. As for antithrombotic therapy, aspirin and oral anticoagulants are the drugs of choice for the majority of cases. New agents will have to prove their efficacy and safety against these two in properly designed clinical trials. Some data suggest that oral anticoagulants may be considerably more effective than aspirin in the long-term setting. One explanation may be that the type of thrombus differs. Thrombi in patients with unstable angina mainly consist of platelets, whereas thrombi in patients with acute myocardial infarction mainly consist of fibrin. Hence, extrapolation of effects of antiplatelet therapy in patients with unstable angina, or a pathophysiologically similar condition, to patients with myocardial infarction may be basically wrong. The concept of a fixed low dose of an anticoagulant in combination with a low dose of aspirin as studied in the CARS study is unpromising. The ongoing CHAMP and WARIS II studies investigate the effect of aspirin versus the combined therapy of aspirin and warfarin (CHAMP) and aspirin, warfarin, and a combination arm (WARIS II). These data will provide urgently needed information about the relative efficacy of the different treatment modalities.

REFERENCES

1. Smith EB, Staples EM, Dietz HS. Role of endothelium in seqestration of lipoprotein and fibrinogen in aortic lesions, thrombi, and graft pseudo-intimas. *Lancet* 1979;2:812–816.
2. Smith EB, Staples EM. Haemostatic factors in human aortic intima. *Lancet* 1981;1:1171–1174.
3. Furberg CD. Secondary prevention trials after acute myocardial infarction [Abstract]. *Am J Cardiol* 1987;60:28–32.
4. De Vreede JJM, Gorgels APM, Verstraaten GMP, et al. Did prognosis after acute myocardial infarction change during the past 30 years? A meta-analysis. *J Am Coll Cardiol* 1991;18:698–706.
5. Davies MJ, Thomas A. Thrombosis and acute coronary artery lesions in sudden cardiac ischemic death. *N Engl J Med* 1984;310:1137–1140.
6. Muldoon MF, Manuck SB, Matthews KA. Lowering cholesterol concentration and mortality: a quantitative review of primary prevention trials. *Br Med J* 1990;301:309–314.
7. The Norwegian Multicenter Study Group. Timolol-induced reduction in mortality and reinfarction in patients surviving acute myocardial infarction. *N Engl J Med* 1981;304:801–807.
8. Weksler BB, Gillick M, Pink J. Effect of propranolol on platelet function. *Blood* 1977;49:185–196.
9. The Anturane Reinfarction Trial Research Group. Sulfinpyrazone in the prevention of sudden death after myocardial infarction. *N Engl J Med* 1980;302:250–256.
10. Anturan Reinfarction Italian Study. Sulphinpyrazone in post-myocardial infarction. *Lancet* 1982;1:237–242.
11. Temple R, Pledger GW. The FDA's critique of the Anturane Reinfarction Trial. *N Engl J Med* 1980;303:1488–1492.
12. Gent AE, Brook CGD, Foley TH, Miller TN. Dipyridamole: a controlled trial of its effect in acute myocardial infarction. *Br Med J* 1968;4:366–368.
13. Balsano F, Rizzon P, Violi F, et al. Antiplatelet treatment with ticlopidine in unstable angina. *Circulation* 1990;82:17–26.
14. CAPRIE Steering Committee. A randomized, blinded trial of clopidogrel versus aspirin in patients at risk of ischaemic events (CAPRIE). *Lancet* 1996;348:1329–1339.
15. Elwood PC, Cochrane AL, Burr ML, et al. A randomized controlled trial of acetyl salicylic acid in the secondary prevention of mortality from myocardial infarction. *Br Med J* 1974;1:436–440.
16. The Coronary Drug Project Research Group. Aspirin in coronary Heart disease. *J Chron Dis* 1976;29:625–642.
17. Elwood PC, Sweetnam PM. Aspirin and secondary mortality after myocardial infarction. *Lancet* 1979;2:1313–1315.
18. Breddin K, Loew D, Lechner K, Überla K, Walter E. Secondary prevention of myocardial reinfarction: a comparison of acetylsalicylic acid, placebo and phenprocoumon. *Haemostasis* 1980;9:325–344.

19. Aspirin Myocardial Infarction Study Research Group. A randomized, controlled trial of aspirin in persons recovered from myocardial infarction. *JAMA* 1980;243:661–669.

20. The Persantine-Aspirin Reinfarction Study Research Group. Persantine and aspirin in coronary heart disease. *Circulation* 1980;62:449–461.

21. Klimt CR, Knatterud GL, Stamler J, Meier P. Persantine-aspirin reinfarction study. Part II. Secondary prevention with Persantine and aspirin. *J Am Coll Cardiol* 1986;7:251–269.

22. ISIS-2 Collaborative Group. Randomised trial of intravenous streptokinase, oral aspirin, both or neither among 17,187 cases of suspected acute myocardial infarction. *Lancet* 1988;2:349–360.

23. The RISC group. Risk of myocardial infarction and death during treatment with low dose aspirin and intravenous heparin in men with unstable coronary artery disease. *Lancet* 1990;336:827–830.

24. Diener HC, Cunha L, Forbes C, Silvenius J, Smets P, Lowenthal A. European Stroke Study 2. Dipyridamole and acetylsalicylic acid in the secondary prevention of stroke. *J Neurol Sci* 1996;143:1–13.

25. Antiplatelet Trialists' Collaboration. Collaborative overview of randomised trials of antiplatelet therapy-I: prevention of death, myocardial infarction, and stroke by prolonged antiplatelet therapy in various categories of patients. *Br Med J* 1994;308:81–106.

26. Serneri GGN, Gensini GF, Carnovali M, Rovelli F, Pirelli S, Fortini A. Effectiveness of low-dose heparin in prevention of myocardial reinfarction. *Lancet* 1987;1:937–942.

27. FRISC Study Group. Low-molecular-weight heparin during instability in coronary artery disease. *Lancet* 1996;347:561–568.

28. Cohen M, Demers C, Gurfinkel E, Fromell G, Langer A, Turpie A, for the Essence Group. Primary end-point analysis from the ESSENCE trial. *Circulation* 1996;94(suppl I):554.

29. British Medical Research Council. An assessment of long-term anticoagulant administration after cardiac infarction. *Br Med J* 1964;2:837–843.

30. Ebert RV, Borden CW, Hipp HR, et al. Long-term anticoagulant therapy after myocardial infarction. *JAMA* 1969;207:2263–2267.

31. The Sixty Plus Reinfarction Study Research Group. A double-blind trial to assess long-term oral anticoagulant therapy in elderly patients after myocardial infarction. *Lancet* 1980;2:989–993.

32. Smith P, Arnesen H, Holme I. The effect of warfarin on mortality and reinfarction after myocardial infarction. *N Engl J Med* 1990;323:147–152.

33. ASPECT Research Group. Effect of long-term anticoagulant treatment on mortality and cardiovascular morbidity after myocardial infarction. *Lancet* 1994;343:499–503.

34. Loeliger EA. Oral anticoagulation in patients surviving myocardial infarction. A new approach to old data. *Eur J Clin Pharmacol* 1984;26:137–139.

35. Azar AJ, Cannegieter SC, Deckers JW, et al. Optimal intensity of oral anticoagulation after myocardial infarction. *J Am Coll Cardiol* 1996;27:1349–1355.

36. Loeliger EA. The optimal therapeutic range in oral anticoagulation. History and proposal. *Thromb Haemost* 1979;42:1141–1152.

37. Yusuf S, Michaelis W, Hua A, et al. Effects of oral anticoagulants on mortality, reinfarction and stroke after myocardial infarction. *Circulation* 1995;92(suppl I):343.

38. Landefeld CS, Goldman L. Major bleeding in outpatients treated with warfarin: incidence and prediction by factors known at the start of outpatient therapy. *Am J Med* 1989;87:144–152.

39. Hirsh J. Substandard monitoring of warfarin in North-America. *Arch Intern Med* 1992;152:257–258.

40. The E.P.S.I.M. Research Group. A controlled comparison of aspirin and oral anticoagulants in prevention of death after myocardial infarction. *N Engl J Med* 1982;307:701–708.

41. Mustard JF, Packham MA. Factors influencing platelet function: adhesion, release and aggregation. *Pharmacol Rev* 1970;22:97–187.

42. Kragel AH, Gertz SD, Roberts WC. Morphologic comparison of frequency and types of acute lesions in the major epicardial coronary arteries in unstable angina pectoris, sudden coronary death and myocardial infarction. *J Am Coll Cardiol* 1991;18:801–808.

43. Cook DJ, Gayatt GH, Laupacis A, Sackett DL. Rules of evidence and clinical recommendations on the use of antithrombotic agents. *Chest* 1992;102(suppl):305–311.

Cardiovascular Thrombosis: Thrombocardiology
and Thromboneurology, Second Edition,
edited by M. Verstraete, V. Fuster, and E. J. Topol,
Lippincott–Raven Publishers, Philadelphia © 1998.

32

Coronary Artery Bypass Surgery: Antithrombotic Therapy

James H. Chesebro and *Steven Goldman

*Cardiovascular Institute, Mount Sinai School of Medicine, New York, New York 10029; and
Department of Cardiology, Tucson Veterans Administration Medical Center, Tucson, Arizona 85723

PATHOGENESIS OF OCCLUSION

The pathogenesis of acute and chronic occlusion of aortocoronary vein grafts is depicted in Fig. 32-1A and B (1). Acute intraoperative angioscopy of vein grafts showed that only intraluminal examination may show technical faults in suturing at the distal anastomosis; this may occur in up to 20% of grafts and may cause low flow and increased risk for early occlusion (2). Disease of vein grafts is a form of accelerated atherosclerosis that begins with acute vascular injury, thrombin generation mural thrombosis, and smooth muscle cell proliferation (1). Injury to the vein graft, which begins with the endothelium, results from procurement of vein from the leg (Fig. 32-2A), surgical handling, delays before insertion in the aortocoronary position, the type and temperature of preservation solution, and the increased shear forces of the pulsatile arterial system (3,4). As soon as blood flows

through the vein graft, immediate platelet deposition occurs (Fig. 32-2D), with formation of mural thrombus that is evident histologically in three quarters of vein grafts in animals or patients who die within 24 hours of operation (3–6). The internal mammary artery is more protected (technically and genetically) from generalized injury and platelet deposition because of less extensive surgical handling, previous adaptation to arterial shear forces, and partially intact vasa vasorum.

With vascular injury there is thrombin generation, platelet deposition and secretion of growth and chemotactic factors for smooth muscle cells, monocytes, and leukocytes. Vascular injury also may induce expression of growth factors (such as platelet-derived growth factor [PDGF] and basic fibroblast growth factor [bFGF]) and tissue factor (which may initiate mural thrombosis) during the first 1 to 48 hours (7–10). Type II injury (endothelial denudation) occurs throughout

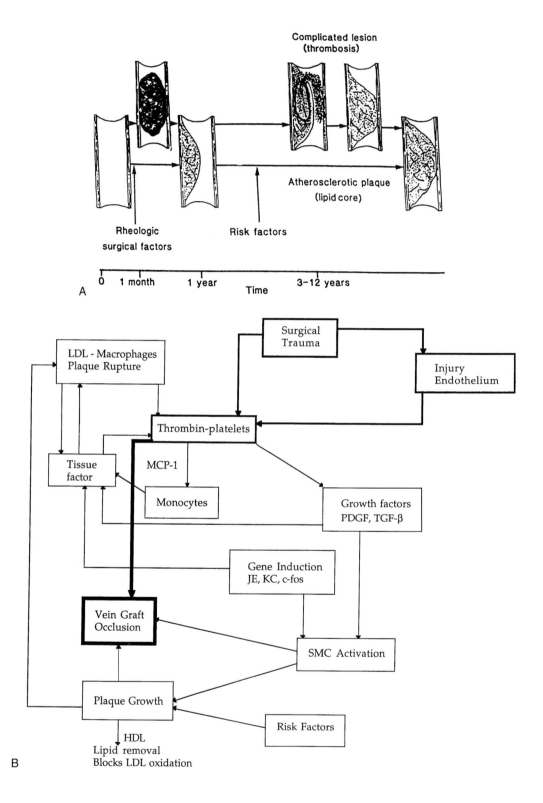

the vein graft (Fig. 32-2A), and type III, deep injury occurs at the anastomotic sites. Vein graft distension to high pressures is no longer performed because of the added injury from this stretch response and evidence that this stimulates marked medial smooth muscle cell proliferation within 48 hours (11,12). Immunohistologic staining of saphenous vein graft segments after removal from the leg shows positive staining for tissue factor and thrombin at the vascular wall–lumen interface (unpublished data, Fig. 32-2B and C).

Thrombosis

Platelet deposition within vein grafts begins during the operation as soon as blood flows throughout the graft (Fig. 32-2D). This information led to the approach that maximal antithrombotic protection should be started perioperatively to protect high-risk vein grafts in which blood flow is low (especially 40 ml/min) or the distal coronary artery is small (less than 1.5 mm) (3,5,13). Occlusion within the first month after operation is related to thrombosis, which is in part due to the grafted

artery, technical problems, injury, and associated atherosclerosis of the grafted artery (2,4,14). The extent of asymptomatic mural thrombus within the vein graft is underestimated at angiography unless it is quite extensive (4,34).

Smooth Muscle Cell Proliferation

Smooth muscle cell proliferation is evident histologically about a month after operation and is the main cause of occlusion 1 to 12 months after operation (1,14–16). Experimentally, smooth muscle cell proliferation can be divided into three phases. In phase I, there is medial smooth muscle cell hyperplasia that peaks at 48 hours, appears to be due to vascular stretching and injury, appears closely related to bFGF, is probably not related to platelets, but may be enhanced by thrombin (8,11,12,17–20). During phase II (4 to 14 days) or the intermediate phase, smooth muscles cells migrate from media to intima and proliferate within the intima (7,17). Smooth muscle cell migration and intimal proliferation are separable phenomena. Both may de-

---

FIG. 32-1. A: Stages of atherosclerotic vein graft disease are depicted. Stage I involves acute injury and thrombosis within the first month after operation and appears related to surgical and rheologic factors. Stage II occurs mainly between 1 and 12 months and involves accelerated smooth muscle cell proliferation and matrix synthesis. Stage III involves lipid incorporation into the vein graft wall and atherosclerotic plaque formation with rupture of the complicated lesion and subsequent thrombosis. (Modified from Fuster and Chesebro, ref. 76, with permission.) **B:** Pathogenesis of acute and late vein graft occlusion. The final pathway of both types of occlusion involves thrombin and platelets. The acute occlusion pathway within the first month is outlined in bold and involves surgical factors relating to endothelial injury of the vein graft and platelet deposition, which is more prominent in regions of deeper injury, especially at the distal anastomotic sites where sheer forces are higher as the vein joins a smaller coronary artery lumen. Over the first year in stage II with gene induction and growth factor release, including those from platelets and mural thrombus, there is smooth muscle cell activation and proliferation with formation of extracellular matrix, all of which contributes to vein graft occlusion. Few macroscopic changes occur between the first and third years. Lipid entry into the vein graft wall begins to be evident by year 3 and marks the beginning of stage III with formation of a complex lesion, which may disrupt and lead to spontaneous deep injury and acute thrombosis. Tissue factor is produced by macrophages and smooth muscle cells in the complex lesion and greatly contributes to thrombogenicity. LDL cholesterol may become oxidized and also activates macrophages. HDL cholesterol may remove lipid from the vein graft wall, blocks oxidation of LDL, and carries an important inhibitor of coagulation called tissue factor pathway inhibitor (TFPI) which inhibits the interaction between tissue factor and activated factor VII early in the coagulation cascade. Thus, particular attention is given to reducing all risk factors and especially lowering LDL cholesterol and increasing HDL cholesterol.

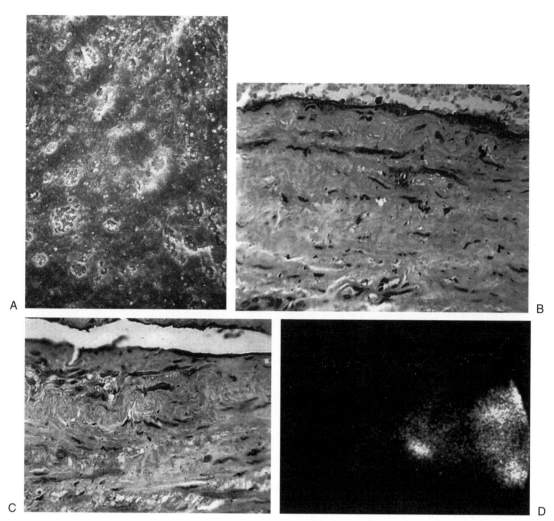

FIG. 32-2. A: Scanning electron microscopy of endothelial cell surface of human saphenous vein segment fixed immediately after dissected in situ and excised from vascular bed in leg. Note diffuse and extensive endothelial cell injury. **B** and **C:** Photomicrograph of human saphenous vein segment fixed immediately after dissection in situ and excision. Immunohistochemical staining with **(B)** tissue factor monoclonal antibody coupled to streptavidin and shows tissue factor presence on the venous wall–lumen interface. (Courtesy of John T. Fallon, MD, PhD.) α-thrombin monoclonal antibody coupled to streptavidin and shows α-thrombin presence on the venous wall–lumen interface **(C)**. (Courtesy of John T. Fallon, MD, PhD.) **D:** Indium 111 platelet scintigram of canine thorax showing the aortocoronary vein graft 24 hours after operation. This documents the significant platelet deposition early after operation. Indium 111 platelet deposition begins to increase as soon as blood starts to flow through the vein graft. (From Fuster et al., ref. 5, with permission.)

pend on platelets and PDGF; however, more growth factors (including bFGF, which is not platelet derived) also cause proliferation (7,19). In phase III (more than 14 days) or late smooth muscle cell proliferation, there is intimal hypertrophy and production of extracellu-lar matrix (17,21–24). Porcine studies in our laboratory suggest that deep arterial injury with mural thrombus leads to greater smooth muscle cell proliferation than does mild injury with a single layer of platelets (22). Likewise, therapy that reduces mural thrombus in vein grafts or coronary arteries reduces intimal thickening (4,15,23). Regrowth of endothelium may reduce but does not eliminate proliferation; endothelium regulates proliferation via synthesis of inhibitors or facilitators of growth (17). The process of accelerated atherosclerosis and smooth muscle cell proliferation was recently reviewed (1,24).

The stages of accelerated atherosclerosis in vein grafts are depicted in Fig. 32-1A. In stage I there is thrombosis, which usually occurs during the first few weeks. The stage of rapid proliferation begins within a month, is probably greater within the early months, but appears to mature over the first year. Few changes occur during the second and third year. Beyond the third year, lipid incorporation becomes evident with formation of complex atherosclerotic lesions which contain a lipid core. Mechanisms contributing to this are outlined in Fig. 32-1B and have been reviewed (1,24,25). Lipid entry into the vessel wall attracts monocytes with conversion to macrophages that engulf lipid and evolve into foam cells. Foam cells also may develop from lipid incorporation by smooth muscle cells. The lipid core attracts more monocytes, which also invade the fibrous cap covering the lipid pool. It appears that the fibrous cap becomes thinner with dissolution of the collagen matrix by macrophage metalloproteinases. This results in rupture of the fibrous cap and acute thrombus formation (1,24,25). The presence of coronary risk factors increases the likelihood of complex lesion formation, plaque rupture, and associated thrombosis. These risk factors include lipids [increased low-density lipoprotein (LDL) cholesterol, triglycerides, and lipoprotein(a), decreased high-density lipoprotein (HDL) cholesterol], cigarette smoking, diabetes, and hypertension (26–33). Continued smoking is particularly associated with thrombus in vein grafts (30,31). Thrombus in vein grafts is most frequently observed 5 to 10 years after operation (32). Thrombus is associated with a ruptured plaque or an aneurysmal dilatation. By 5 to 10 years after operation, clinical problems are related equally to atherosclerosis in vein grafts and progression of the underlying coronary artery disease (26,27).

Prevalence of Vein Graft Occlusion

In the first few weeks after operation, as many as 10% to 15% of patients may have one or more vein graft occlusions. This may be reduced by 50% to 70% with appropriately administered antithrombotic therapy (34–36). At one year, 10% to 25% of grafts may be occluded. This may be reduced by 30% to 56% with antithrombotic therapy. These occlusions may involve 40% to 50% of patients, and antithrombotic therapy may reduce this to 21% to 53% of patients with one or more occlusions (37–41). Variability in rates of occlusion with therapy may in part be related to operative techniques, underlying disease, arterial rheology (flow and lumen diameter), and arterial substrates exposed with the operation (28,29,34,35–38). Beyond 1 year, the occlusion rate is 2% to 4% per year over the first 5 years, when 35% of vein grafts may be occluded. By 10 years after operation, approximately 50% of vein grafts are occluded (42–45). The marked decrease in occlusion of the internal mammary artery graft probably relates in part to decreased injury at the time of operation with partial preservation of the vasa vasorum and the inherent decreased risk of arteriosclerotic involvement of this artery (29,44).

RATIONALE FOR OPTIMAL ANTITHROMBOTIC THERAPY

Because platelet deposition starts as soon as blood flows through the vein graft, perioperative antithrombotic therapy is critical for its reduction. This was shown experimentally (4,5) before designing large trials for the prevention of aortocoronary vein graft occlusion (34,35). Reduction of acute thrombus with perioperative antiplatelet therapy also significantly reduced subsequent intimal proliferation 2 to 3 months after operation or angioplasty (Fig. 32-3) (15,23). Thus antithrombotic therapy can intervene in stage I of vein graft dis-

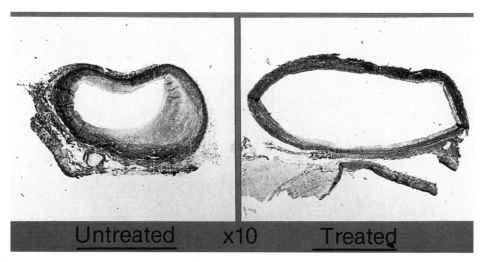

FIG. 32-3. Representative histologic cross-sections for distal vein grafts at 3 months after operation in a control group on the left (shows eccentric intimal proliferation) and from animal treated with anti-platelet therapy on the right (shows minimal eccentric proliferation).

ease (Fig. 32-1). This has been confirmed in several clinical trials (34–38,60,61). Success is not achieved when therapy is started too late, as shown by an earlier trial which started therapy 3 to 4 days after operation (46), compared to ≤2 days (34–37,47–52).

Dipyridamole by itself does not significantly reduce platelet deposition or mural thrombus formation on the deeply injured artery, but it does reduce platelet deposition on artificial surfaces (53). Thus, it is not surprising that three studies have not shown additional benefit of dipyridamole added to aspirin over aspirin alone (35,36,39,40,54).

The use of compounds during or soon after operation that block fibrinolysis or increase coagulation factors such as aprotinin or desmopressin (desamino-8-arginine vasopressin, DDAVP), may enhance mural thrombosis in vein grafts; although these compounds may not increase early overt occlusion, they may increase the risk of late vein graft disease. This danger is real: thrombosis enhances intimal proliferation (3,4,15, 22,23), and thrombosis and thrombolysis are simultaneous and dynamic processes that start as soon as the vein graft is placed. More preclinical animal studies are required with

aprotinin or infusion of factor VIII and von Willebrand factor (to mimic desmopressin, which does not have an effect in animals) to quantitatively determine if platelet deposition and mural thrombus are increased in vein grafts with this type of therapy.

Platelet Inhibitor Therapy

Dosages of platelet inhibitor therapy were originally chosen on the basis of prolongation of a shortened platelet survival in humans and their ability to significantly reduce quantitative indium 111–labeled platelet deposition in animals (4,5,55–58). This led to the dosages used in the two major platelet inhibitor trials in coronary bypass operations (34,35,37,38). The conduct of these trials also was based on the principles learned from animal studies and discussed above. In these trials, angiography was performed both early (1 week) and late (1 year) after operation.

In the Mayo Clinic Study, angiography was performed in 88% of patients early after operation (median 8 days), and the results are summarized in Fig. 32-4. The 70% reduction in vein graft occlusion was present in more than 50 subgroups, including patients at

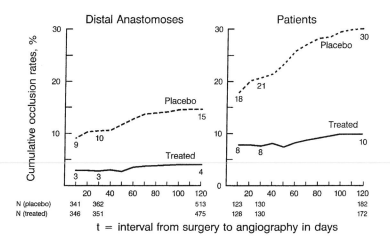

t = interval from surgery to angiography in days

FIG. 32-4. Occlusion rate of vein graft–coronary artery distal anastomoses totally occluded on angiography at t days after operation (for group difference, p value, and 95% CIs were as follows: at t = 10, p = 0.003, 5–22%; at t = 30, p = 0.0004, 7–23%; at t = 120, p < 10^{-6}, 14–30%) **(left)**. The range of t was 7 to 180 days. The occlusion rates did not change from 120 to 180 days after operation, when only six more patients underwent angiography. N = total number of distal anastomoses **(left)** or patients **(right)** in treated and placebo groups at 10, 30, and 120 days after operation. (From Chesebro et al., ref. 34, with permission.)

higher and lower risk for occlusion as determined by vein graft blood flow, coronary artery lumen diameter, or presence or absence of endarterectomy (34). In the Veterans Administration Cooperative Study, early catheterization was performed a mean of 9 days after operation and within 60 days in 72% of patients. These results are summarized in Fig. 32-5. There was no significant difference in early vein graft occlusion in any of the aspirin-containing drug regimens. Sulfinpyrazone was of borderline benefit and resulted in transient renal insufficiency in 5.3% of patients (35).

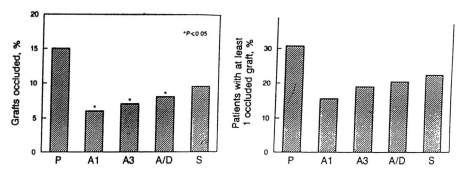

FIG. 32-5. Left: Percentage of occluded grafts in each treatment group from Veterans Administration Trial. P, placebo; A1, aspirin once daily; A3, aspirin three times daily; A/D, aspirin/dipyridamole; S, sulfinpyrazone. *p < 0.05 refers to comparison between each treatment group and placebo by cluster analysis. The 95% CIs of the differences are as follows: A1 versus P, 8.4% (1.7, 15.0 CIs); A3 versus P, 7.2% (0.5, 13.8 CIs); A/D versus P, 6.8% (0.1, 13.4 CIs); S versus P, 5.1% (-1.6, 11.8 CIs). **Right:** Percentage of patients with at least one occluded graft. The 95% CIs of the differences are as follows: A1 versus P, 13.4% (-0.2, 27.1 CIs); A3 versus P, 11.2% (-2.5, 24.9 CIs); A/D versus P, 9.2% (-4.5, 22.9 CI); S versus P, 8.1% (-5.5, 21.9 CI). (From Goldman et al., ref. 35, with permission.)

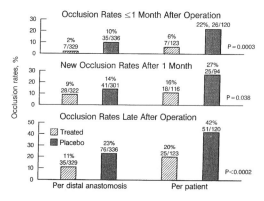

FIG. 32-6. Occlusion rates for all types of vein grafts. The rates are expressed per distal anastomosis and per patient (proportion with at least one occlusion). Occlusion is shown as events occurring within 1 month (95% CIs for the per patient difference, 8–24%), as new events occurring beyond 1 month (in distal anastomoses and patients without occlusion within 1 month of operation) from angiography performed 1 year later (per patient, p = 0.048; 95% CIs for the difference, 0–22%), and as events at a median of 1 year after operation (95% CIs for the per patient difference, 11–34%). These subsets include only patients who had angiography within 1 month of operation and again 1 year later. Below each percentage is shown the ratio of distal anastomoses or patients with occlusion to total distal anastomoses or patients. (From Chesebro et al., ref. 37, with permission.)

ministration Cooperative Study, new occlusions from 9 days after operation to 1 year later occurred in just under 10% of grafts; this was not significantly different in treated or control groups. This difference from the Mayo Clinic Study may relate to patient compliance or the extent to which risk factors were modified. The overall rates of occlusion of vein grafts at 1 year after operation in the Veterans Administration Cooperative Study are summarized in Fig. 32-7. The proportion of patients with one or more occlusions 1 year after operation was 44% in the placebo group compared with 35% in the treated group (p = 0.10). Angiography was performed late after operation in 65% of the patients (38). Thus, there do not appear to be significant differences between aspirin-containing regimens for treatment of patients with aortocoronary bypass graft operation. Other early studies confirmed the benefit of antiplatelet therapy (47–51). Aortocoronary artery vein graft occlusion rates are similar in the most recent large trials, and no therapy has proven superior to aspirin alone (39–41).

Perioperative Bleeding

In the Mayo Clinic Study, aspirin was started 7 hours after operation. There was no

In the Mayo Clinic Study, new occlusion of vein grafts beyond the first month after operation and up to 1 year after operation in patients with all types of grafts (proven to be patent by angiography at early study) is shown in the middle panel of Fig. 32-6 (occlusion of distal anastomoses on the left and by patients with one or more occlusions on the right). There was a significant reduction in new occlusions from 27% of patients in the placebo group to 16% in the treated group. Overall, 1 year after operation, 25% of grafts were occluded in the placebo group compared with 11% in the treated group; this involved 47% of patients with one or more occlusion in the placebo group compared with 22% in the treated group. Eighty-four percent of patients were studied late after operation (37). In the Veterans Ad-

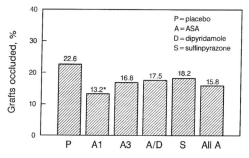

FIG. 32-7. Bar graph of percentage of occluded graphs in each treatment group and overall for aspirin from the Veterans Administration Cooperative Study one year after operation. A1 versus P, 9.4% difference (95% CIs: 0.0, 18.7); A3 versus P, 5.8% difference (95% CIs: -3.6, 15.2); A/D versus P, 5.1% difference (95% CIs: -4.2, 14.5); S versus P, 4.6% difference (95% CIs: -4.9, 13.8); all versus P, 6.8% difference (p = 0.029). (From Goldman et al., ref. 38, with permission.)

difference in chest-tube blood loss, transfusion requirements for red cells, platelets or fresh frozen plasma, or reoperation for bleeding (4% to 5% of patients in each group) (34). In the Veterans Administration Cooperative Study, preoperative aspirin was associated with a significant increase in chest-tube blood loss to slightly over 1,100 ml in the worst of three aspirin groups compared with slightly over 800 ml in the placebo group. In addition, 6.1% of patients underwent reoperation for bleeding in the preoperative aspirin group compared with 1.9% of patients in the placebo and sulfinpyrazone groups (35).

The Veterans Administration Cooperative Study Group has compared preoperative versus postoperative administration of aspirin (325 mg versus placebo the night before) (59). All patients received aspirin 325 mg 6 hours after operation and daily thereafter. Angiography was performed in 72% of patients an average of 8 days after operation. Vein graft occlusion was similar in both groups (7.4% with preoperative aspirin versus 7.8% without). In the group taking preoperative aspirin, none of 22 distal anastomoses in Y grafts were occluded compared with 7% of 43 distal anastomoses in the nonaspirin group. In addition, in the preoperative aspirin group, none of 131 internal mammary artery grafts were occluded compared with 2.4% in 125 internal mammary artery grafts in the nonaspirin group. These results in internal mammary artery grafts were of borderline significance and were retrospective observations that warrant a further prospective study. The median blood loss 35 hours after operation was 1,150 ml in the preoperative aspirin group compared with 1,045 ml in the nonaspirin group. Red cell transfusion was 900 ml versus 725 ml, and reoperation for bleeding was 6.3% versus 2.4% in the preoperative aspirin versus nonaspirin groups, respectively (59).

Aspirin 325 mg/day has been administered as early as 1 hour after operation down the nasogastric tube and compared with placebo (60). Vein graft angiography performed in 97% of patients a median of 7 days after operation showed occlusion in 1.6% of distal anastomoses in the aspirin group and 6.2% in the placebo group with no difference in chest-tube blood loss or blood transfusion requirements between groups. The reoperation rate for bleeding was 4.8% in the aspirin group and 1% in the placebo group.

Other Antithrombotic Inhibitor Therapies

Ticlopidine

In a study of 173 patients, ticlopidine 250 mg twice daily or placebo was administered starting 2 days after operation. Over 90% of patients were restudied by digital angiography at 10, 180, and 360 days after operation. The proportion of distal anastomoses occluded in the placebo and treated groups, respectively, was reduced at 10 days 13.4% and 7.1% ($p < 0.05$), at 180 days 24.0% and 15% ($p < 0.02$), and at 360 days 26.1% and 15.9% ($p < 0.01$) (52). This single study needs confirmation. Ticlopidine has a delayed onset of action of 1 to 2 days and reaches a maximal effect at 3 to 5 days.

Low-Dose Aspirin

In other studies, aspirin dosage was reduced to 100 to 150 mg/day with significant reductions in vein graft occlusion in both studies (48,61).

Oral Anticoagulation

Oral anticoagulation also has successfully reduced aortocoronary vein graft occlusion when heparin and dipyridamole were administered three times daily for 7 days before starting oral anticoagulation versus no further therapy (36). A recent large study showed that oral anticoagulation is no better than aspirin alone in reducing vein graft occlusion 1 year after operation (15% of distal anastomoses occluded with aspirin 50 mg/day and 13% occluded with oral anticoagulation) (39). Unfortunately, an initial loading dose of at least 160 mg was not given. Patients with INRs of 1.8 to 3.8 had vein graft patency comparable with that of patients with INRs of 2.8–4.8 (40).

Low-dose warfarin plus aspirin 81 mg (INR 1.4) was no better than aspirin 81 mg alone in preserving vein graft patency at 4–5 years after coronary artery bypass graft surgery (62).

The following study confirms the efficacy of oral anticoagulation and the need for antithrombotic therapy for at least 1 year after operation. In a well-executed study comparing aspirin 50 mg (started the night before operation) plus dipyridamole 400 mg (started 2 days before operation) in two divided doses per day compared with oral anticoagulation (international normalized ratio 2.5 to 5.0) started on the first day after operation, graft angiography was obtained in 99% of patients 2 weeks after operation and 95% of patients 1 year after operation (63). Early graft occlusion occurred in 7% of both groups (16% and 19% of patients, respectively), and late graft occlusion occurred in 16% of distal anastomoses when therapy was continued for 1 year and in 23% of distal anastomoses if patients were switched to placebo at 3 months after operation.

Indobufen

Indobufen (200 mg twice daily) is a reversible inhibitor of platelet cyclooxygenase that was compared with aspirin 300 mg three times daily plus dipyridamole 75 mg three times daily in preventing occlusion of saphenous vein coronary artery bypass grafts. Of 803 patients randomized in this double-blind study, 552 (69%) had follow-up angiography 1 year after operation. All anastomoses were patent in 56% of indobufen-treated patients and 59% of aspirin-dipyridamole patients. The percentage of all anastomoses patent was also similar: 82% in the indobufen group and 83% in the aspirin-dipyridamole group. Mean postoperative blood loss was significantly less in the indobufen group (p = 0.04). Indobufen was as effective as aspirin plus dipyridamole in preventing aortocoronary saphenous vein graft occlusion (41).

CURRENT RECOMMENDATIONS

Aspirin reduces infarction and death in patients with unstable angina (see Chapter 13).

In addition, more than half of the patients presenting to the hospital with acute coronary syndromes are on aspirin, which probably reduces the severity of their syndrome from myocardial infarction to unstable angina. These benefits of reduced arterial thrombosis in these patients appear to outweigh the risks of a slightly greater need for reoperation for bleeding after bypass operation. Early withdrawal of antithrombotic therapy in patients with unstable angina increases the risk of recurrent ischemia and myocardial infarction (see Chapter 13).

Thus, in patients presenting with unstable angina who are awaiting aortocoronary bypass graft operation, aspirin may be continued daily up to the time of operation. In patients with rest angina, a heparin infusion to maintain the activated partial thromboplastin time at approximately twice control is also advisable before operation. When used with heparin, aspirin should be reduced to 80 mg/day. A 160-mg loading dose of aspirin will acutely minimize thromboxane A2 production, and 80 mg/day will maintain this effect with the lowest risk of side effects (64).

If patients have not been on aspirin before operation, aspirin should be started 1 hour after operation down the nasogastric tube at a minimum dose of 160 mg/day for loading, and thereafter may be administered at 80 to 325 mg/day and continued indefinitely. Patients who are at high risk (see Chapter 23) with low vein graft blood flow (less than 40 mg/min) or a small coronary artery lumen at the point of vein graft insertion (smaller than 1.5 mm), or with associated endarterectomy of the bypassed coronary artery, may be considered for empiric combination therapy with ticlopidine 250 mg twice daily. This combination therapy is an empiric extrapolation from two studies of oral anticoagulation plus aspirin versus ticlopidine plus aspirin after placement of coronary artery stents where occlusion was reduced by over 75–80% by ticlopidine plus aspirin (0.6% to 0.8% at 15 to 30 days after stenting) (65,66).

It is also critical to reduce all coronary risk factors, including cessation of smoking, treatment of hypertension, control of diabetes, and correction of lipid abnormalities. Progression of both aortocoronary vein graft disease and native coronary artery disease has been shown to be significantly reduced in patients with reduced LDL cholesterol and increased HDL cholesterol (26,62,67–70). LDL cholesterol should be reduced to <100 mg/dl (62). The only studies that have shown a significant regression in vein graft or coronary artery disease have been those in which the HDL cholesterol has been increased with specific therapy, such as with niacin (69,70). Unless impossible from an anatomic or technical standpoint, at least one internal mammary bypass graft should be included, and this is usually to the largest and most significant vessel for myocardial supply, the left anterior descending coronary artery. Use of the internal mammary artery graft appears responsible for reducing graft occlusion in retrospective and prospective studies and improving survival in retrospective studies (42–45).

Prevention of Late Vein Graft Disease and Occlusion

Late vein graft disease begins to appear at 3 years after operation. Thus far the best treatment for reducing obstructive changes in saphenous vein coronary artery bypass grafts appears to be aggressive lipid lowering to an LDL cholesterol <100 mg/dl (62). Control of risk factors such as diabetes, cessation of smoking, reduction of LDL cholesterol, and increase of HDL cholesterol appear to be important in reducing the arteriosclerotic process and the incidence of plaque rupture, coronary events, and stroke (26,62,69–71).

In patients with incomplete correction of risk factors, consideration may be given to long-term anticoagulant therapy along with low-dose aspirin at 80 mg/day in order to prevent the disastrous consequences of plaque rupture in a vein graft. This leads not only to local occlusion, but also to occlusion of the entire graft proximal and often distal to the ruptured lesion because vein grafts have no branches and thus are prone to long segments of occlusion. Thus, large amounts of thrombus accumulate in vein grafts, which makes them risky for performing balloon angioplasty or atherectomy.

Prolonged selective urokinase infusion combined with heparin plus aspirin therapy may be beneficial for clearing thrombus and preparing the patient for subsequent angioplasty (72). A promising alternative for patients with recent occlusion causing angina at rest may be a 3- to 5-day infusion of recombinant hirudin, which in one study (73) recanalized five of 10 occluded aortocoronary vein grafts, all of which were further improved by successful angioplasty.

Thrombosis of Late Vein Graft Occlusion

In vein grafts with late occlusion after 0 to 6 months (penetrable with a guide wire) local infusion of urokinase 50,000 to 100,000 IU/hr for a mean of 24 hours has been used with successful recanalization in 79% of patients (Hartmann J, personal communication, 1996). An alternative may be direct and serial injection into the thrombus 1 to 2 cm at a time with a 5 French Sones catheter using urokinase 20,000 IU per centimeter of thrombus (Schneider E, personal communication, 1996). A simultaneous 5,000-U bolus of heparin to an activated partial thromboplastin time 2.0 to 2.5 times control, plus daily aspirin and ticlopidine 250 mg twice daily, may reduce simultaneous rethrombosis and may be followed by percutaneous transluminal coronary angioplasty, directional coronary atherectomy, or coronary vein graft stenting after thrombus is cleared (74,75). Long-term therapy starting at hospital dismissal based on pathogenesis and risk (see Chapter 23) would be oral anticoagulation (international normalized ratio 2.0 to 3.0) plus aspirin 80 mg/day or aspirin 80–160 mg/day plus ticlopidine 250 mg twice daily as empiric therapy (discussed above). The role of these empiric therapies administered chronically needs further study.

CONCLUSION

In summary, aortocoronary vein graft occlusion is a thrombo-proliferative process over the first year which evolves into an atherosclerotic process evident pathologically by the third year after operation. Occlusion over the first year is reduced by 30 to 70% with antiplatelet therapy started by administration down the nasogastric tube within one to seven hours of operation.

The current recommendation is to start aspirin 160 to 325 mg down the nasogastric tube 1 hour after operation and continuing with 80 to 100 mg/day thereafter for the lifetime of the patient.

Patients who have had aortocoronary vein graft occlusion with recanalization may be considered for chronic combined therapy with warfarin anticoagulation to an INR of 2.0 to 3.0 plus aspirin 80 to 100 mg/day. An empiric alternative may be ticlopidine 250 mg twice daily plus aspirin 80 to 100 mg/day; on this therapy, white blood counts every two weeks are needed for the first three months to rule out neutropenia.

All patients undergoing aortocoronary bypass graft operation should have coronary risk factors minimized with the LDL cholesterol reduced to less than 100 mg/day, consideration of niacin or gemfibrizol therapy for HDL cholesterols under 35 mg/day, control of diabetes mellitus and hypertension, and total cessation of smoking.

REFERENCES

1. Fuster V, Badimon L, Badimon JJ, Chesebro JH. The pathogenesis of coronary artery disease and the acute coronary syndromes (two parts). *N Engl J Med* 1992; 326:242–250, 310–318.
2. Grundfest WS, Litvack F, Sherman T, et al. Delineation of peripheral and coronary detail by intraoperative angioscopy. *Ann Surg* 1985;202:394–400.
3. Chesebro JH, Toschi V, Lettino M, et al. Evolving concepts in the pathogenesis and treatment of arterial thrombosis. *Mt Sinai J Med* 1995;62:275–286.
4. Josa M, Lie JT, Bianco RL, Kaye MP. Reduction of thrombosis in canine coronary bypass vein grafts with dipyridamole and aspirin. *Am J Cardiol* 1981;47:1248–1254.
5. Fuster V, Dewanjee MK, Kaye MP, Josa M, Metke MP, Chesebro JH. Noninvasive radioisotopic technique for detection platelet deposition in coronary artery bypass grafts in dogs and its reduction with platelet inhibitors. *Circulation* 1979;60:1508–1512.
6. Bulkley BH, Hutchins GM. Pathology of coronary artery bypass graft surgery. *Arch Pathol Lab Med* 1978;102:273–280.
7. Majestky MW, Reidy MA, Bowen-Pope DF, Hart CE, Wilcox JN, Schwartz SM. PDGF ligand and receptor gene expression during repair of arterial injury. *J Cell Biol* 1990;111:2149–2158.
8. Linder V, Lappi DA, Baird A, Majack RA, Reidy MA. Role of basic fibroblast growth factor in lesion formation. *Circ Res* 1991;68:106–113.
9. Toschi V, Gallo R, Lettino M, et al. Tissue factor modulates the thrombogenicity of human atherosclerotic plaques. *Circulation* 1997;95:594–599.
10. Gallo R, Fallon JT, Toschi V, et al. Biphasic increase of tissue factor activity after angioplasty in porcine coronary arteries. *Circulation* 1995;92(suppl I):354.
11. Webster MWI, Chesebro JH, Heras M, Mruk JS, Grill DE, Fuster V. Effect of balloon inflation on smooth muscle cell proliferation in the porcine carotid artery [Abstract]. *J Am Coll Cardiol* 1990;15:165.
12. Capron L, Bruneval P. Influence of applied stress on mitotic response of arteries to injury with a balloon catheter: quantitative study in rat thoracic aorta. *Cardiovasc Res* 1989;23:941–948.
13. Chesebro JH, Webster MWI, Zoldhelyi P, Roche PC, Badimon L, Badimon JJ. Antithrombotic therapy in the progression of coronary artery disease. *Circulation* 1992;89(suppl 6);III-100–III-110.
14. Uni KK, Kottke BA, Titus JL, Frye RL, Wallace RB, Brown AL. Pathologic changes in aortocoronary saphenous vein grafts. *Am J Cardiol* 1974;34:526–532.
15. Metke MP, Lie JT, Fuster V, Josa M, Kaye MP. Reduction of intimal thickening in canine coronary bypass vein grafts with dipyridamole and aspirin. *Am J Cardiol* 1979;43:1144–1148.
16. Lie LT, Lawrie GM, Morris GC. Aortocoronary bypass saphenous vein graft atherosclerosis. *Am J Cardiol* 1977;40:906–914.
17. Badimon L, Badimon JJ, Penny W, Webster MWI, Chesebro JH, Fuster V. Endothelium and atherosclerosis. *J Hypertens* 1992;10(suppl):43–50.
18. Fingerle J, Johnson R, Clowes AW, Majestky MW, Reidy MA. Role of platelets in smooth muscle cell proliferation and migration after vascular injury in rat carotid artery. *Proc Natl Acad Sci U S A* 1989;86: 8412–8416.
19. Fingerle J, Au WPT, Clowes AW, Reidy MA. Intimal lesion formation in rat carotid arteries after endothelial denudation in absence of medial injury. *Arteriosclerosis* 1990;10:1082–1087.
20. Berk BC, Taubman MB, Gragoe EJ, Fenton FW, Griendling KK. Thrombin signal transduction mechanisms in rat vascular smooth muscle cells. Calcium and protein kinase C-dependent and -independent pathways. *J Biol Chem* 1990;265:17334–17340.
21. Snow AD, Bolender RP, Wright TN, Clowes AW. Heparin modulates the composition of the extracellular matrix domain surrounding arterial smooth muscle cells. *Am J Pathol* 1990;137:313–330.
22. Gallo R, Gertz SD, Fallon JT, Chesebro JH, Fuster V, Badimon JJ. Fibromuscular hyperplasia and thrombosis are the predominant mechanisms for late luminal narrowing after balloon angioplasty in porcine coronary arteries [Abstract]. *J Am Coll Cardiol* 1996;27(suppl):289.
23. Gallo R, Toschi V, Fallon JT, Chesebro JH, Fuster V, Badimon JJ. Prolonged thrombin inhibition reduces restenosis after balloon angioplasty in porcine coronary

arteries [Abstract]. *J Am Coll Cardiol* 1996;27(suppl): 320.

24. Fuster V. Mechanisms leading to myocardial infarction: insights from studies of vascular biology. *Circulation* 1994;90:2126–2146.

25. Falk E, Shah PK, Fuster V. Coronary plaque disruption. *Circulation* 1995;92:657–671.

26. Sacks FM, Pfeffer MA, Moye LA, et al., for the Cholesterol and Recurrent Events Trial Investigators. The effect of pravastatin on coronary events after myocardial infarction in patients with average cholesterol levels. *N Engl J Med* 1996;335:1001–1009.

27. Campeau L, Enjalbert M, Lesperance J, Vaislic C, Grondin CM, Bourassa MG. Atherosclerosis and late closure of aortocoronary saphenous vein grafts: sequential angiographic studies at 2 weeks, 1 year, 5 to 7 years, and 10 to 12 years after surgery. *Circulation* 1983;68 (suppl II):1–7.

28. Paz MA, Lupon J, Bosch X, Pomar JL, Sanz G. Predictors of early saphenous vein aortocoronary bypass graft occlusion. The GESIC Study Group. *Ann Thorac Surg* 1993;56:1101–1106.

29. Goldman S, Zadina K, Krasnicka B, et al., for the Department of Veterans Affairs Cooperative Study Group No. 297. Predictors of graft patency 3 years after coronary artery bypass graft surgery. *J Am Coll Cardiol* 1997;29:1563–1568.

30. Neitzel GF, Barboriak JJ, Pintar K, Qureshi I. Atherosclerosis in aortocoronary bypass grafts: morphologic study and risk factor analysis 6 to 12 years after surgery. *Arteriosclerosis* 1986;6:594–600.

31. Slimes BC, Nadeau P, Millette D, Campeau L. Late thrombosis of saphenous vein coronary bypass grafts: morphologic study and risk factor analysis 6 to 12 years after surgery. *Arteriosclerosis* 1986;6:594–600.

32. Walts AE, Fishbein MC, Matloff JM. Thrombosed, ruptured atheromatous plaques in saphenous vein coronary artery bypass grafts: 10 years experience. *Am Heart J* 1987;114:718–723.

33. Hoff HF, Beck GJ, Skibinski CI, et al. Serum Lp(a) level as a predictor of vein graft stenosis after coronary artery bypass surgery in patients. *Circulation* 1988;77: 1238–1244.

34. Chesebro JH, Clements I, Fuster B, et al. A platelet-inhibitor-drug trial in coronary-artery bypass operations: benefit of perioperative dipyridamole and aspirin therapy on early postoperative vein-graft patency. *N Engl J Med* 1982;307:73–78.

35. Goldman S. Copeland J, Moritz T, et al. Improvement in early saphenous vein graft patency after coronary artery bypass surgery with antiplatelet therapy: results of a Veterans Administration Cooperative Study. *Circulation* 1988;77:1324–1332.

36. Gohlke H, Gohlke-Barwolf C, Sturzenhofecker P, et al. Improved graft patency with anticoagulant therapy after aortocoronary bypass surgery: a prospective randomized study. *Circulation* 1981;64(suppl II):22–27.

37. Chesebro JH, Fuster V, Elveback LR, et al. Effect of dipyridamole and aspirin on late vein-graft patency after coronary bypass operations. *N Engl J Med* 1984; 310:209–214.

38. Goldman S, Copeland J, Moritz T, et al. Saphenous vein graft patency 1 year after coronary artery bypass surgery and effects of antiplatelet therapy: results of a

39. van der Meer J, Hillege HL, Kootstra GJ, et al., for the CABADAS Research Group of the Interuniversity Cardiology Institute of the Netherlands. Prevention of one-year vein graft occlusion after aortocoronary-bypass surgery: a comparison of low-dose aspirin, low-dose aspirin plus dipyridamole, and oral anticoagulants. *Lancet* 1993;342:257–264.

40. van der Meer J, Hillege HL, Dunselman PHJM, et al., for the CABADAS Research Group of the Interuniversity Cardiology Institute of the Netherlands. Oral anticoagulation in the prevention of one-year vein graft occlusion after aortocoronary bypass surgery: optimal therapeutic range and practical limitations. *Thromb Haemost* 1994;72:676–681.

41. Rajah SM, Nair U, Rees M, et al. Effects of antiplatelet therapy with indobufen or aspirin-dipyridamole on graft patency one year after coronary artery bypass grafting. *J Thorac Cardiovasc Surg* 1994;107: 1146–1153.

42. Loop D, Lytle BW, Cosgrove DM, et al. Influence of the internal-mammary-artery graft on 10-year survival and other cardiac events. *N Engl J Med* 1986;314:1–6.

43. Spencer FC. The internal mammary artery: the ideal coronary bypass graft? *N Engl J Med* 1986;314:1–6.

44. Lylte BW, Loop FD, Cosgrove DM, Ratliff NB, Easley K, Taylor PC. Long-term (5–12 years) serial studies of internal mammary artery and saphenous vein coronary bypass grafts. *J Thorac Cardiovasc Surg* 1990;95: 15–20.

45. Grondin CM, Campeau L, Lesperance J, Engalbert M, Bourassa MG. Comparison of late changes in internal mammary artery and saphenous vein grafts in 2 consecutive series of patients 10 years after operation. *Circulation* 1984;710(suppl I):208–212.

46. Pantely GA, Goodnight SH Jr, Rahimtoola SH, et al. Failure of antiplatelet and anticoagulant therapy to improve patency of grafts after coronary-artery bypass. *N Engl J Med* 1979;301:962–966.

47. Rajah SM, Salter MC, Donaldson DR, et al. Acetylsalicylic acid and dipyridamole improve the early patency of aorta-coronary bypass grafts. A double-blind, placebo-controlled, randomized trial. *J Thorac Cardiovasc Surg* 1985;90:373–377.

48. Lorenz RL, Weber M, Kotzur J, et al. Improved aortocoronary bypass patency by low-dose aspirin (100 mg daily). *Lancet* 1984;1:1261–1264.

49. Brown BG, Cukingnan RA, DeRouen T, et al. Improved graft patency in patients treated with platelet-inhibiting therapy after coronary bypass surgery. *Circulation* 1985;72:138–146.

50. Brooks N, Wright J, Sturridge M, et al. Randomized placebo controlled trial of aspirin and dipyridamole in the prevention of coronary vein graft occlusion. *Br Heart J* 1985;53:201–207.

51. Sharma GVRK, Khuri SF, Josa M, Folland ED, Parisi AF. The effect of antiplatelet therapy on saphenous vein coronary artery bypass graft patency. *Circulation* 1983;68(suppl II):218–221.

52. Limet R, David JL, Margotteauz P, Larock MP, Riego P. Prevention of aortocoronary bypass graft occlusion: beneficial effect of ticlopidine on early and late patency rates of venous coronary bypass grafts: double-

blind study. *J Thorac Cardiovasc Surg* 1987;94:
773–783.

53. Pumphrey CW, Fuster V, Dewanjee MK, Chesebro JH, Vliestra RE, Kaye MP. Comparison of the antithrombotic action of calcium antagonist drugs with dipyridamole in dogs. *Am J Cardiol* 1983;51:591–595.

54. Ekestrom SA, Gunnes S, Brodin UB. Effect of dipyridamole (persantine) on blood flow and patency of aortocoronary vein bypass grafts. *Scand J Thorac Cardiovasc Surg* 1990;24:191–196.

55. Fuster V, Chesebro JH. Current concepts of thrombogenesis: role of platelets. *Mayo Clin Proc* 1981;56:102–112.

56. Harker LA, Ross R, Slichter SF, Scott CR. Homocystine-induced arteriosclerosis: the role of endothelial cell injury and platelet response in its genesis. *J Clin Invest* 1976;58:731–741.

57. Steele P, Rainwater J, Vogel. Platelet suppressant therapy in patients with prosthetic cardiac valves: relationship of clinical effectiveness to alteration of platelet survival time. *Circulation* 1979;60:910–913.

58. Donadio JV, Anderson CF, Mitchell JC, et al. Membranoproliferative glomerulonephritis: a prospective clinical trial of platelet-inhibitor therapy. *N Engl J Med* 1984;310:1421–1426.

59. Goldman S, Copeland J, Moritz T, et al. Starting aspirin before operation: effects on early graft patency. *Circulation* 1991;84:520–526.

60. Gavaghan TP, Gebski V, Baron DW. Immediate postoperative aspirin improves vein graft patency early and late after coronary artery bypass graft surgery. *Circulation* 1991;83:1526–1533.

61. Sanz G, Pajaron A, Alegria E, et al. Prevention of early aortocoronary bypass occlusion by low-dose aspirin and dipyridamole. *Circulation* 1990;82:765–773.

62. The Post Coronary Artery Bypass Graft Trial Investigators. The effect of aggressive lowering of low-density lipoprotein cholesterol levels and low-dose anticoagulation on obstructive changes in saphenous-vein coronary artery bypass grafts. *N Engl J Med* 1997;336:153–162.

63. Pfisterer M, Jockers G, Regenass, et al. Trial of low-dose aspirin plus dipyridamole versus anticoagulants for prevention of aortocoronary vein graft occlusion. *Lancet* 1989;2:1–7.

64. Clarke RJ, Mayo G, Price P, FitzGerald GA. Suppression of thromboxane A2 but not of systemic prostacyclin by controlled-release aspirin. *N Engl J Med* 1991;325:1137–1141.

65. Schomig A, Neumann FJ, Kastrati A, et al. A randomized comparison of antiplatelet and anticoagulant therapy after the placement of coronary artery stents. *N Engl J Med* 1996;334:1084–1089.

66. STARS Trial Investigators. Presented at American Heart Association Meeting, November 11–13, 1996, New Orleans, LA.

67. Brensike FJ, Levy PR, Kelsey SF, et al. Effects of therapy with cholestyramine on progression of coronary arteriosclerosis: results of the NJLBI Type II Coronary Intervention Study. *Circulation* 1984;69:313–324.

68. Artntzenius AC, Kromhout D, Barth JD, et al. Diet, lipoproteins, and the progression of coronary arteriosclerosis. The Leiden Intervention Trial. *N Engl J Med* 1985;312:805–811.

69. Blankenhorn DH, Nessim SA, Johnson RL, Sanmarco ME, Azen SP, Cahin-Hempil L. Beneficial effects of combined colestipol-niacin therapy on coronary atherosclerosis and coronary venous bypass graft. *JAMA* 1987;257:3233–3240.

70. Brown G, Albers JJ, Fisher LD, et al. Regression of coronary artery disease as a result of intensive lipid-lowering therapy in men with high levels of apolipoprotein B. *N Engl J Med* 1990;323:1289–1298.

71. Scandinavian Simvastatin Survival Study Group. Randomized trial of cholesterol lowering in 4444 patients with coronary heart disease: the Scandinavian Simvastatin Survival Study (4S). *Lancet* 1994;344:1383–1389.

72. Sharaf BL, Bier JD, Ledley GS, Williams DO. Prolonged selective urokinase infusion versus PTCA from totally occluded coronary saphenous vein bypass graft [Abstract]. *J Am Coll Cardiol* 1991;17:337.

73. Chesebro JH, Rao AK, Schwartz D, et al. Endogenous thrombolysis and recanalization of occluded aortocoronary vein grafts with recombinant hirudin in patients with unstable angina. *Circulation* 1994;90(suppl I):568.

74. Holmes DR Jr, Topol EJ, Califf RM, et al. A multicenter, randomized trial of coronary angioplasty versus directional atherectomy for patients with saphenous vein bypass graft lesions. CAVEAT-II Investigators. *Circulation* 1995;91:1966–1974.

75. Laham RJ, Carrozza JP, Berger C, Cohen DJ, Kuntz RE, Baim DS. Long-term (4- to 6-year) outcome of Palmaz-Schatz stenting: paucity of late clinical stent-related problems. *J Am Coll Cardiol* 1996;28:820–826.

76. Fuster V, Chesebro JH. Role of platelets and platelet inhibitors in aortocoronary artery vein-graft disease. *Circulation* 1986;73:227–232.

*Cardiovascular Thrombosis: Thrombocardiology
and Thromboneurology, Second Edition,*
edited by M. Verstraete, V. Fuster, and E. J. Topol,
Lippincott–Raven Publishers, Philadelphia © 1998.

33

Antithrombotic Treatment in Percutaneous Transluminal Coronary Angioplasty and Stenting

Michel E. Bertrand, Eugène P. McFadden, and Eric Van Belle

Division of Cardiology B, Hôpital Cardiologique, 59037 Lille, France

Over the past 15 years percutaneous transluminal coronary angioplasty (PTCA) has been shown to be a very effective method of myocardial revascularization in humans. Improvements in the design of the equipment and increased investigator experience have resulted in a high level of primary procedural success (90% to 95%).

The introduction of any device in a coronary artery can provoke thrombotic phenomena leading to abrupt closure. For that reason, it was recommended from the early use of PTCA to systematically administer antithrombotic drugs to minimize such complications. Nowadays, interventional cardiologists treat more complex coronary lesions, including intracoronary thrombi, particularly in patients with unstable angina or acute myocardial infarction. As a result of these expanded indications, the rate of early occlusion or abrupt closure is still a matter of serious concern, which fortunately has been almost eliminated by coronary stenting.

In this chapter, after a brief overview of abrupt closure, we first consider the use of antithrombotic treatment during coronary intervention, and subsequently address the specific problems encountered with coronary stenting.

INCIDENCE, MECHANISMS, AND PREDICTORS OF ABRUPT CLOSURE AFTER BALLOON ANGIOPLASTY

Lincoff et al. (1) in an unselected group of 1,300 patients undergoing PTCA in a single institution observed complete or partial occlusion during the procedure or the subsequent hospitalization in 8.3% of cases. The occlusion rate was 4.2% in the series of Kuntz (2) in 1992. In our institution, among 4,566 patients treated with angioplasty between January 1, 1993, and December 31, 1996, 270 (5.9%) developed an abrupt closure. Wolfe et al. (3), in a prospective study that included nine centers in the United States and Canada, found a 7.1% incidence of established abrupt closure with a 3.9% incidence of impending occlusion. Most of our knowledge concerning the mechanisms of abrupt closure is derived from imaging with angioscopy or with intravascular ultrasound. The primary mechanism is related to extensive disruption of the media leading to the formation of obstructive dissection and flaps with concomitant intramural haematoma. Exposure of subendothelial components can cause platelet deposition and activation with formation of thrombin.

It is relatively rare that thrombus formation alone induces abrupt closure, but thrombus occurring as a consequence of the marked aggression of the arterial wall during angioplasty may contribute to acute closure both by mechanical obstruction and by favoring vasospasm. Unstable angina and diabetes mellitus have been shown to be good clinical predictors of abrupt closure. Numerous angiographic correlates of abrupt closure have been proposed. In our experience of 201 cases of abrupt closure that occurred in 3,679 consecutively dilated stenoses, multivariate analysis of qualitative and quantitative angiographic parameters identified three angiographic predictors of occlusion: increasing stenosis severity ($p < 0.0001$), left coronary location ($p < 0.003$), and lesion location in an angulated segment ($p < 0.05$) (4,5). The presence of a thrombus (defined angiographically) before the procedure was not identified as a risk factor, but angiography is certainly not the best tool to identify intracoronary thrombi, which are best assessed via angioscopy. It should also be noted that the majority of abrupt closures occur in the catheterization laboratory.

ANTITHROMBOTIC MANAGEMENT AND BALLOON ANGIOPLASTY

The antithrombotic management before, during, and after balloon angioplasty includes blockade of platelet aggregation and thrombus formation at the angioplasty site.

Aspirin and Other Antiplatelet Agents

The efficacy of aspirin is now well established, and administration of this drug is mandatory before angioplasty.

The incidence of occlusive intracoronary thrombi detected by angiography 30 minutes after PTCA is significantly lower in patients pretreated with aspirin (1.8%) than in untreated patients (10.7%) (6). In a study of the effects of aspirin and dipyridamole in the prevention of restenosis, the group receiving aspirin in combination with dipyridamole had a significantly lower rate of periprocedural Q-wave myocardial infarction (1.6%) than did the untreated group (7). The dose of aspirin required is not clear; one study that compared 80 mg to 1,500 mg/day of aspirin did not show any difference in the incidence of postprocedural myocardial infarction or emergency bypass surgery (8).

Barragan et al. (9) showed that pretreatment with ticlopidine was also an effective strategy. In 1987, White et al. (10) demonstrated that ticlopidine reduced the incidence of ischemic complications to 1.8% from 13.6% in the placebo group. In the TACT study (11) which, was a trial designed to assess the effect of ticlopidine on restenosis, we observed a rate of abrupt closure of 5.1% in the ticlopidine group compared with 16.2% in the placebo group.

In summary, antiplatelet treatment has been demonstrated to be effective in reducing ischemic complications during and immediately after angioplasty and is an absolute prerequisite in all patients undergoing angioplasty. Currently, no protocol submitted to an ethical committee would be accepted if antiplatelet therapy were not given before the procedure.

Heparin

There is a universal consensus regarding the need for heparin during angioplasty. Traditionally, patients receive 10,000 U of heparin before the procedure, followed by 5,000 U for each additional hour of procedural time. However, despite the fact that most patients receive this standard regimen, it is recognized that individual responses to heparin vary widely. Various factors such as body size, previous treatment with heparin, or concurrent administration of nitroglycerin have been shown to affect the response to heparin. It has been shown that 10% to 20% of patients were inadequately anticoagulated during coronary angioplasty after receiving standard 10,000 IU boluses of heparin before dilatation (14). To our knowledge, there is no available randomized trial to determine the optimal degree of anticoagulation during coronary angioplasty. McGarry et al. (15) and Dougherty et al. (16) have studied the relationship between degree of anticoagulation and the risk of complications. They concluded that an activated clotting time (ACT) greater than 300 seconds or an activated partial thromboplastin time (APTT) greater than or equal to three times control were associated with a low rate of periprocedural complications. Thus, it appears preferable to carefully adapt the dose of heparin to optimize the level of anticoagulation rather than to administer empiric standard doses of heparin.

Several different management strategies have been suggested in the 12 to 24 hours after the procedure. Most investigators continue heparin in patients who have suboptimal results after PTCA or whose lesions are complex, particularly if intracoronary thrombus is suspected. To date, three randomized trials (17–19) have failed to demonstrate a significant decrease in the incidence of periprocedural complications in patients who received heparin for 12 to 24 hours in comparison with those who received no heparin after the procedure.

Even in the absence of complications, many patients dilated late in the afternoon continue heparin overnight because sheath removal during the night poses a logistic problem. However, as pointed out by Walford et al. (20), bleeding complications are more frequent in patients who continue heparin for 12–24 hours compared with those who do not receive heparin after the procedure.

Hirudin/Hirulog

The Helvetica trial (21) was designed to study whether hirudin, a specific inhibitor of thrombin, was able to reduce restenosis. For that purpose, 1,154 patients were randomized to heparin (intravenous [i.v.] bolus of 10,000 IU followed by a continuous infusion of 15 IU/kg/hr for 24 hours) or to hirudin at one of two dose regimens (i.v. bolus of 40 mg followed by a continuous i.v. infusion of 0.2 mg/kg/hr for 24 hours or the same regimen plus 40 mg of hirudin given subcutaneously [s.c.] twice daily for 3 consecutive days). The incidence of early events (i.e., occurring in the 96 hours after angioplasty) was carefully noted. Forty-two patients of the 382 assigned to heparin, 30 of the 381 assigned to i.v. hirudin, and 21 of the 378 patients assigned to i.v. and s.c. hirudin experienced such events. The relative risk in the combined hirudin groups was 0.61 (95% confidence interval [CI] 0.41 to 0.90; p = 0.023). In a subgroup analysis of patients with unstable angina, the event rate was 21.6% in the heparin group, 5.3% in the i.v. hirudin group, and 12.3% in patients receiving i.v. and s.c. hirudin (combined relative risk with hirudin 0.41; 95% CI 0.21 to 0.78; p = 0.006). Despite the lack of effect on restenosis, this trial showed that hirudin was associated with an impressive reduction in the rate of major cardiac events in the first 96 hours after angioplasty as compared with heparin. In addition, there were no differences with respect to major or minor bleeding among the three groups (6.2%, 5.5%, and 7.7%, respectively).

Bivalirubin (hirulog) was compared with heparin in a randomized trial conducted in 121 centers in North America and in Europe (22). The study included 4,098 patients who had unstable angina and who underwent a single angioplasty procedure. Heparin was given i.v. (bolus of 175 IU/kg plus 15 IU/kg/hr for 18 to 24 hours) in 2,039 patients. The patients randomized to bivalirudin (n = 2,059) received an i.v. bolus of 1 mg/kg followed by a 4-hour infusion at a rate of 2.5 mg/kg/hr and a 14-to-24 hour infusion at a rate of 0.2 mg/kg. The primary endpoints were death, myocardial infarction, abrupt closure, emergency coronary arterial bypass grafting (CABG), intra-aortic balloon pumping, or repeated coronary angioplasty. Bivalirudin therapy was not associated with a significant reduction in primary endpoints (11.4% versus 12.2%) but did result in a lower incidence of bleeding (3.8% versus 9.8%). The only positive effect was observed in a subgroup of 704 patients with postinfarction unstable angina where hirulog treatment was associated with a significant reduction in primary endpoints (9.1% versus 14.2%, p = 0.04). Measurement of activated clotting times showed that hirulog resulted in a lower level of systemic anticoagulation.

Thrombolytic Agents

The role of thrombolytic therapy in the prevention of abrupt closure is controversial. Zeiher (23), in a small double blind randomized trial, showed that routine intracoronary infusion of urokinase was not superior to intracoronary heparin during coronary angioplasty. As pointed out by Grill (24), substantial resolution of large intracoronary thrombi can be achieved during coronary angioplasty by intracoronary or i.v. injection of t-PA or with large doses of intracoronary urokinase. In patients with recent myocardial infarction, O'Neill has shown that pretreatment with thrombolytic agents followed by angioplasty has a deleterious effect with more immediate complications and a higher rate of bleeding.

The most convincing data were derived from the TAUSA study (25), which included 469 patients with ischemic rest pain with or without a recent myocardial infarction who underwent coronary angioplasty. All patients received aspirin and 10,000 IU of heparin. One group received 250,000 U of urokinase in phase I or 500,000 U of urokinase in phase II. The other group received placebo. Al-

though angiographic correlates of thrombus were not significantly decreased by urokinase (13.8%) compared with placebo (18.0%), acute closure was more frequent (p < 0.02) with urokinase (10.2%) compared with placebo. This deleterious effect of urokinase was more frequent with the higher dose of urokinase than with the lower dose. Similarly, major ischemic cardiac events (ischemia, infarction, or emergency bypass surgery) also were increased with urokinase (12.9%) versus placebo (6.3%). Angiographic and clinical endpoints were more frequent with urokinase in patients with unstable angina without recent myocardial infarction than in patients who were undergoing angioplasty after a recent infarction.

This study clearly demonstrates that prophylactic thrombolytic therapy should not be used routinely before percutaneous transluminal coronary angioplasty (26).

Management of High-Risk Patients with New Antiplatelet Drugs (27–32)

Abciximab (c7E3 Monoclonal Antibody)

A chimeric monoclonal antibody Fab fragment (c7E3 Fab) directed against the platelet glycoprotein (GP)IIb/IIIa receptor was used in patients undergoing angioplasty who were at high risk for ischemic complications. The integrin GPIIb/IIIa receptor on the surface of the platelet is the final common pathway of platelet aggregation: it binds circulating adhesive macromolecules, particularly the von Willebrand factor, which can then cross-link receptors on adjacent platelets leading to platelet aggregation. The EPIC study (12) was a randomized double-blind trial conducted in 2,099 patients. They were randomized in three groups: one received placebo, the second received a bolus of c7E3 and an infusion of placebo, and the third received a bolus and an infusion of c7E3. As compared with placebo, the c7E3 bolus and infusion resulted at 30 days in a 35% reduction of major cardiac events (death, nonfatal myocardial infarction, unplanned surgical or interventional revascularization, unplanned implantation of a stent, or insertion of an intra-aortic balloon pump). The rates of these events were 12.8% and 8.3% (p = 0.008) in the placebo group and c7E3 bolus plus infusion group, respectively. A 10% reduction was observed with c7E3 alone (12.8% versus 11.5%) (p = 0.43). Bleeding episodes and transfusions were more frequent in the c7E3 bolus and infusion groups than in the other group. Thus, this trial showed a beneficial effect of effective blockade of the GPIIb/IIIa receptor in patients undergoing high-risk procedures.

To study the effects of c7E3 in more stable patients, the EPILOG (Evaluation of PTCA to Improve Long-term Outcome by c7E3 GPIIb/IIIa receptor blockade) study was designed (33). In this trial, all patients undergoing urgent or elective percutaneous coronary revascularization, except for unstable angina and myocardial infarction patients, could be randomized. The trial was designed to determine whether decreasing the dose of heparin could reduce bleeding. One of two arms of c7E3 and the placebo group received 100 U/kg heparin, whereas the other c7E3 arm was treated with only 70 U/kg heparin. All patients received 325 mg of aspirin orally. Abciximab was given as a bolus of 0.25 mg/kg 10 to 60 minutes before inflation of the balloon, followed by an infusion of 0.125 µg/kg/min.

The trial, conducted in 69 centers, was terminated at the first interim analysis, with 2,792 of the planned 4,800 patients enrolled.

The primary efficacy endpoint was death from any cause, myocardial infarction, or urgent revascularization within 30 days of randomization.

At 30 days, the composite endpoint rate was 11.7% in the placebo group with standard-dose heparin, 5.2% in the group assigned to abciximab with low-dose heparin (hazard ratio 0.43; 95% CI 0.3 to 0.6; p < 0.001), and 5.4% in the group assigned to abciximab with standard-dose heparin (hazard ratio 0.45; 95% CI 0.32 to 0.63; p < 0.001) (Fig. 33-1). The risk of bleeding was significantly reduced by the low dose of heparin.

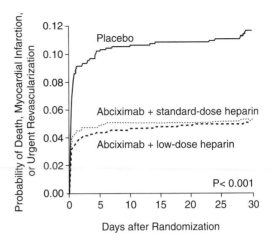

FIG. 33-1. EPILOG Study. Primary efficacy endpoint events (death, myocardial infarction, or urgent repeated revascularization) within 30 days after randomization, according to assigned treatment.

There were no significant differences among the groups in the risk of major bleeding, although minor bleeding was more frequent among patients receiving abciximab with standard-dose heparin. The CAPTURE (34) study was designed to enroll 1,400 patients with refractory unstable angina. This clinical presentation was defined as chest pain with significant electrocardiographic (ECG) changes and at least one episode of pain with ECG changes while treated for at least 2 hours with heparin and nitrates (oral or i.v.). The last episode of pain had to be within 48 hours of randomization, which was performed after diagnostic angiography if the patient had a lesion suitable for PTCA. The study medication was given 18 to 24 hours before PTCA until 1 hour after angioplasty. All patients received aspirin, heparin, and nitrates. Endpoints were assessed at day 30 and at 6 months. The primary endpoint at day 30 (death, myocardial infarction, or unplanned angiography) was reduced from 15.9% in the placebo group to 11.3% in the c7E3 group (p = 0.0072). Thus, it was decided to terminate the study prematurely. The number of myocardial infarctions was reduced by 50% (from 8.2% in the placebo group to 4.7% in the c7E3 group).

The need for urgent intervention was reduced from 10.9% to 7.8%. There was a modest increase of bleeding (major bleeding 3.8% with c7E3 versus 1.9% with placebo). These results are consistent with the EPIC and EPILOG trials and showed that 24-hour pretreatment with c7E3 reduces the complications of death, myocardial infarction, and reintervention with a modest increase in the risk of bleeding (27–35). However, contrary to what was observed in the EPIC trial, the initial benefit observed in the CAPTURE trial was lost at 6-month follow-up.

Tirofiban

Other antiplatelet agents have been used to reduce platelet-mediated thrombotic complications. Tirofiban is a synthetic, small-molecule, nonpeptide GPIIb/IIIa receptor blocker. It is a tyrosine derivative with a molecular weight of 495 and a highly selective inhibitor of fibrinogen binding to the platelet GPIIB/IIIa receptor. Preclinical and clinical studies have shown that tirofiban inhibits ex vivo aggregation in response to a variety of agonists, including adenosine diphosphate, collagen, epinephrine, and thrombin. The RESTORE trial (Randomized Efficacy Study of Tirofiban for Outcomes and Restenosis) was a randomized, double-blind, placebo-controlled trial of tirofiban in patients undergoing interventions (balloon angioplasty or atherectomy) within 72 hours of presentation with an acute ischemic coronary syndrome (unstable angina or acute myocardial infarction). Tirofiban was administered as a bolus of 10 µg/kg over 3 minutes followed by a 36-hour infusion of 0.15 µg/kg/min. Patients (n = 2,139) were randomized to placebo or tirofiban, and all received aspirin and heparin. The primary endpoint was a composite endpoint including the occurrence of death from any cause: myocardial infarction, CABG due to angioplasty failure or recurrent ischemia, repeat target vessel revascularization, or insertion of a stent for abrupt or threatened closure of the dilated segment. The tirofiban group had a 38% relative reduction in the composite endpoint at 2 days (p < 0.005) and a 27% relative reduction at 7 days (p = 0.022). This was mainly due to a reduction in nonfatal myocardial infarction and the need for repeat PTCA. However, at 30 days the reduction in adverse cardiac events was no longer statistically significant. The primary composite endpoint was reduced from 12.2% in the placebo group to 10.3% in the tirofiban group, a 16% relative reduction (p = 0.16). If only repeat PTCA or CABG performed on an emergency basis was included, the 30-day event rate in the composite endpoint decreased from 10.5% in the placebo group to 8.0% in the tirofiban group (relative reduction 24%; p = 0.052).

Major bleeding, including transfusion requirements, were not significantly different in the two groups (3.7% in the placebo versus 5.3% in the tirofiban group (p = 0.096). Thrombocytopenia was similar in the placebo and tirofiban group (0.9% and 1.1%, respectively).

Integrelin (IMPACT-II Study)

Eptifibatide (integrelin) is a cyclic heptapeptide in which the arginine component of the RGD sequence has been replaced by lysine (35). This modification results in more specific inhibition of the GPIIb/IIIA receptor. The benefit of eptifibatide as an adjunctive treatment during angioplasty was explored in a phase 3 randomized study, the IMPACT-II study (Integrelin to Manage Platelet Aggregation in Coronary Thrombosis) (31). This was a three-arm study with two doses of eptifibatide given over 24 hours after angioplasty in a large cohort of patients (n = 4,010). All patients randomized to eptifibatide received a 135 µg/kg bolus; the patients in one treatment group received an infusion of 0.5 µg/kg/min, whereas the patients in the second group received 0.75 µg/kg/min. The third group was a placebo group. All patients received aspirin and heparin. The primary efficacy endpoint was the composite of death, myocardial infarction, and the need for urgent/ emergency intervention (PTCA, CABG, or stent placement for abrupt closure by intention to treat during the procedure) within 30 days of enrollment.

A significant reduction in this endpoint was observed at 72 hours in the three groups (Fig. 33-2). By 30 days, the composite endpoint was observed in 11.4% of the patients of the placebo group compared with 9.2% in the 135/0.5 eptifibatide group (p = 0.063) and 9.9% in the 135/0.75 group (p = 0.022).

By treatment-received analysis, the 135/0.5 eptifibatide regimen induced a significant reduction in the composite endpoint (11.6 versus 9.1%, p = 0.035). However, the 135/0.75 regimen produced a less important reduction (11.6% versus 10.0%; p = 0.18). There was no difference in the rate of major bleeding between the eptifibatide and placebo groups.

The results of all these studies are consistent. During or immediately after angioplasty, these new antiplatelet agents are effective in decreasing the risk of death, myocardial infarction, or the need for urgent/emergency intervention in unstable or high-risk patients. However, the benefit is less obvious at 6 months' follow-up, but this is not completely unexpected because most of the critical events occur within hours after the procedure.

The data suggest that all patients benefit. The gradient between low- and high-risk patients in the EPILOG and IMPACT II trials showed no difference.

The use of platelet GPIIb/IIIA blockade also must be clearly defined in the era of new interventions, particularly coronary stenting, which is dramatically increasing. Even more, this technique has changed the concept of high-risk lesions and patients because a high-risk PTCA patient is one in whom it will be difficult for technical reasons to implant a coronary stent.

ANTITHROMBOTIC MANAGEMENT AFTER CORONARY STENTING

Puel and Sigwart performed the first stent implantation in 1986. There was immediately great excitement followed a few months later by disillusion. Acute and subacute stent thrombosis emerged as a major limitation to the use of intracoronary stents.

At that time, it was difficult to admit that despite full, even drastic anticoagulation, there was still an unacceptably high risk of subacute stent thrombosis. We have to remind ourselves that in the late 1980s it was recommended to treat patients with very high doses of heparin with additional dextran, aspirin, and dipyridamole followed by an intensive coumadin regimen with an INR between 3.5 and 4. As a result of this intensive anticoagulation, minor and major bleeding was frequent. Thus, in the early 1990s, stent implantation was reserved for bailout procedures after abrupt closure and in some centers for the treatment of saphenous vein graft lesions.

In 1993 and 1994, major advances were achieved in the management of patients after stent implantation. First, it was shown that optimal deployment of the stent was mandatory (36). Perfect apposition against the wall, with symmetrical stent expansion, can be confirmed with intravascular ultrasound guidance. However, this can be achieved more economically by increasing the inflation pressure (more than 14 atmospheres up to 22) during implantation of the prosthesis, which is thus well embedded into the vessel wall. Meanwhile, two landmark studies were performed and com-

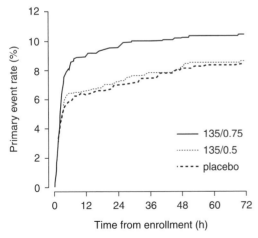

FIG. 33-2. IMPACT II trial. Composite primary endpoint events to 72 hours. Kaplan-Meier estimate.

pared the rate of restenosis after simple balloon angioplasty compared with stent implantation. The BENESTENT and STRESS studies clearly demonstrated that the rate of angiographic restenosis was significantly decreased in patients with stable angina and relatively large coronary vessels (>3 mm of diameter) by stent implantation (37,38). This was obtained at the expense of a greater risk of bleeding (13.5% versus 3.1%) due to full anticoagulation and a risk of subacute thrombosis, which was noted in 3.5% after stent implantation and 2.7% in the balloon group. The clinical restenosis rate was also better after stent implantation than after conventional balloon angioplasty.

Furthermore, different registries (TASTE registry, French registry) showed that the full anticoagulation regimen with heparin and coumadin that was the source of the high rate of vascular complications could be safely replaced by a two-pronged antiplatelet treatment combining ticlopidine with aspirin (39–45). Thanks to this new management, the risk of subacute thrombosis of the stent that was around 5% decreased to almost 0% in patients with elective stent placement. In addition, the risk of peripheral bleeding leading to transfusion or surgical repair (15% with the previous management) dramatically decreased to 0.5%. Thus, stent implantation to prevent abrupt closure became an accepted approach. However, this approach was only recognized after the presentation of three randomized trials. The first trial, called ISAR (Intracoronary Stenting and Antithrombotic Regimen) was a single-center, randomized comparison of antiplatelet and anticoagulant therapy after the placement of a Schatz Palmaz stent (46). The indications for stenting were extensive coronary artery dissection after PTCA, complete vessel closure, residual stenosis of 30% or more of the vessel diameter, and lesions in venous bypass grafts. Only patients in whom stenting was successful (i.e., in whom the stent was correctly placed at the desired position and there was less than 30% of residual narrowing) were randomized. The patients (n = 517) received ticlopidine (250 mg three times daily) plus as-

pirin (100 mg three times daily) (n = 257) or phenprocoumon (target INR 3.5 to 4.5). In patients assigned to antiplatelet treatment, heparin was discontinued 12 hours after stent placement; in those assigned to anticoagulation, heparin was continued for 5 to 10 days until adequate oral anticoagulation was achieved. Antiplatelet or oral anticoagulation was continued for 4 weeks.

Subacute occlusion of the stented vessel occurred in 0.8% of the ticlopidine aspirin group and in 5.4% of the anticoagulant therapy group (relative risk 0.14; 95% CI 0.02 to 0.62). Acute occlusions were not observed because they were excluded by protocol. With ticlopidine aspirin treatment, there was an 82% lower risk of myocardial infarction (0.8% in the ticlopidine group and 4.2% in the anticoagulation group; $p < 0.02$) and a 78% reduction in the need for repeat intervention (1.2% and 5.4%, respectively). The hemorrhagic events were significantly decreased with ticlopidine plus aspirin (0% versus 6.5%).

A second trial called FANTASTIC (Full Anticoagulation versus Aspirin Ticlopidine) was performed but had a different design (Table 33-1). This trial is a multicenter-randomized trial conducted with the Wiktor stent. Thirteen centers enrolled 473 patients. However, the protocol was slightly different from the ISAR trial because all patients after stent implantation were randomized, whatever the results of the stent placement (suboptimal results, distal dissection not completely by the stent, etc.). Coronary stenting was performed as an elective placement in 50.1% of patients and as a bailout procedure in 49.9% patients. The patients received ticlopidine 250 mg three times daily plus aspirin 100 to 325 mg at the discretion of the investigator for 6 weeks. After the procedure, heparin was discontinued 4 hours after stent implantation. Patients randomized to full conventional anticoagulation received heparin until stabilization of the oral anticoagulation plus aspirin at the same dose. Oral anticoagulation was continued for 6 weeks. The primary endpoint of the study was a composite of bleeding complications, including ecchymosis, hematomas, major bleed-

TABLE 33-1. *FANTASTIC Trial after Wiktor stent implantation*

	TAS	FAN	p	OR (95% CI)
Primary endpoint				
Ecchymosis >5 cm	16 (6.6%)	38 (16.5%)	0.006	0.36 (0.18–0.68)
Hematoma	25 (10.3%)	34 (14.8%)	0.13	0.66 (0.37–1.18)
Major bleeding	2 (0.8%)	7 (3.0%)	0.07	0.26 (0.04–1.4)
Transfusion	4 (1.6%)	6 (2.6%)	0.45	0.62 (0.14–2.51)
False aneurysm	2 (0.8%)	6 (2.6%)	0.13	0.31 (0.04–1.74)
Surgical repair	1 (0.4%)	2 (0.9%)	0.52	0.47 (0.01–9.04)
Composite endpoint	33 (13.5%)	48 (21%)	0.03	0.60 (0.36–0.99)
Secondary endpoint				
Acute thrombosis	6 (2.4%)	1 (0.4%)	0.06	0.17 (0.01–1.45)
Subacute thrombosis	1 (0.4%)	8 (3.5%)	0.01	0.12 (0.01–0.91)
Death	2 (0.8%)	5 (2.1%)	0.23	0.38 (0.05–2.25)
Nonfatal QWMI	3 (1.2%)	6 (2.6%)	0.27	0.47 (0.09–2.13)
Nonfatal NQWMI	9 (3.7%)	9 (3.9%)	0.9	0.94 (0.34–2.65)
Composite endpoint	14 (5.7%)	20 (8.6%)	0.221	0.64 (0.3–1.38)
Hospital stay	4.3 ± 3.6	6.4 ± 3.7	0.0001	

OR, odds ratio; QWMI, Q-wave myocardial infarction; NQWMI, non Q-wave myocardial infarction.

ings, blood transfusion, or surgical repair. The secondary endpoints were stent thrombosis and the length of in-hospital stay.

Subacute thrombosis was significantly lower in the ticlopidine plus aspirin group (0.4% versus 3.5%; p = 0.014). However, acute thrombosis still occurred (0.43% in the full anticoagulation group versus 2.4% in the ticlopidine plus aspirin group; p = 0.06), predominantly related to an initially suboptimal result after stent implantation or due to the delayed efficacy of ticlopidine. The stay in hospital was markedly reduced from 6.3 days (±3.6) with full anticoagulation to 4.3 (±3.4) days (p < 0.0001) with ticlopidine plus aspirin. Table 33-1 shows more details concerning the results of that study.

It is not clear whether the improved results obtained with the new antiplatelet regimen are solely related to the treatment after stent implantation or are also due to better deployment of the stents. Furthermore, one publication (47) suggested that with an optimal intravascular ultrasound-guided stent deployment strategy, aspirin alone was as effective as ticlopidine plus aspirin. In fact, the sample size of this study was too small to test that hypothesis. This was subsequently performed in the STARS trial, which compared three different strategies after a successful stent implantation: aspirin alone, aspirin plus war-

farin, and aspirin plus ticlopidine. The results were clear: the rate of subacute thrombosis was significantly lower in the ticlopidine plus aspirin group (0.6%) than in the other groups (aspirin plus warfarin, 2.4%). The group treated with aspirin alone had the highest rate of subacute thrombosis (3.6%).

Thus, nowadays the situation has been clarified. In the case of elective placement decided before the procedure, it is recommended to give ticlopidine plus aspirin 3 to 4 days before the procedure, then to proceed with stent implantation with standard heparinization (bolus of 10,000 U plus additional 5,000 U if the procedure lasts more than an hour). After successful implantation, the sheath is removed 4 hours later and the patient can be discharged the day after with a regimen of ticlopidine plus aspirin (100 to 325 mg) for 4 weeks.

If the stent was implanted in the context of a bailout situation or during an ad hoc PTCA, ticlopidine is started immediately. In the case of a long dissection not completely covered by stent and with a less than satisfactory result, it may be advisable to continue heparin for a few days but at the risk of serious bleeding complications.

It is recommended to control the hemogram at 2 weeks, 1 month, and 6 weeks after the procedure owing to the risk of neutropenia. This complication is not very frequent, observed in only 0.8% of patients receiving long-term treatment. Only one case of severe neutropenia (less than 1,500 white cells) was observed in the FANTASTIC study. The short duration of ticlopidine administration should preclude this complication, which is usually fully reversible after discontinuation of the treatment. In fact, rashes and gastrointestinal disturbances are more frequent and may require treatment cessation. In that case, if treatment is stopped after 3 weeks of therapy, one can leave the patient on aspirin alone. If treatment is stopped before 3 weeks, one may be obliged to start conventional anticoagulation therapy. In some particular cases, oral anticoagulation can be given in association with aspirin and ticlopidine when the patient has coexisting disease requiring oral anticoagulation, such as atrial fibrillation or deep vein thrombosis.

In conclusion, two-pronged antiplatelet treatment with ticlopidine and aspirin has dramatically decreased the risk of stent thrombosis. As a consequence, the number of stent implantations has markedly increased, and nowadays 50% to 75% of patients treated by angioplasty receive at least one stent. This practice has many important clinical consequences. The need for emergency bypass operation during PTCA is almost reduced to zero. This is not only the consequence of bailout stenting but also the result of a new strategy aiming to prevent abrupt closure by a systematic stent implantation in complex lesions. The rate of restenosis has decreased but is not completely abolished (48); the risk of mid-term occlusion or reocclusion in infarct-related vessels, chronic occlusion, and diabetics has almost disappeared; and lesions in saphenous vein grafts can be easily treated. Some problems are still not satisfactorily resolved, e.g., the problem of stenting in small vessels (<2.6 mm diameter).

CONCLUSION

Over the past 15 years, major advances have increased the safety of interventional procedures. Interventional cardiologists currently have an important armamentarium to prevent abrupt closure, which is a major contributor to the mortality and morbidity associated with angioplasty.

In summary, we make the following assertions:

1. All patients undergoing angioplasty must receive aspirin before the procedure.
2. The empiric standard dose of heparin (10,000 IU given before the procedure) should be replaced by a careful adaptation of the dose.
3. Hirudin is associated with a reduction in major cardiac events after angioplasty.
4. Prophylactic thrombolytic therapy, even in unstable angina, is not recommended.
5. New antiplatelet drugs (i.e., GPIIb/IIIa receptor blockers) are particularly effective and useful. A low-risk group of patients, as suggested in the EPILOG and IMPACT II trials, could benefit from these drugs, and under certain conditions it is possible that GPIIb/IIIA receptor blockers could be considered for routine, elective protection.
6. Management after coronary stenting is characterized by the superiority of the combination of ticlopidine and aspirin to prevent subacute thrombosis on all other treatment (and particularly full anticoagulation).
7. Besides these new pharmacologic approaches, which are undoubtedly useful, prophylactic stent implantation in patients who have suboptimal results has radically changed the problem of abrupt closure and early reocclusion. Most of the trials that were conducted 4 to 5 years ago comparing medical treatment or bypass surgery with coronary angioplasty have become completely obsolete. Undoubtedly, the stent is the "second wind" of coronary angioplasty.

REFERENCES

1. Lincoff AM, Popma JJ, Ellis SG, Hacker JA, Topol EJ. Abrupt vessel closure complicating coronary angio-

plasty: clinical, angiographic and therapeutic profile. *J Am Coll Cardiol* 1992;19:926–935.

2. Kuntz RE, Piana R, Pomerantz RM, et al. Changing incidence and management of abrupt closure following coronary intervention in the new device era. *Cathet Cardiovasc Diagn* 1992;27:183–190.

3. Wolfe M, Leya F, Bonan R, Ferguson J, Roubin GS. Predictors of outcome after balloon angioplasty: a prospective multicenter study [Abstract]. *Circulation* 1993;88:300.

4. Van Belle E, Bauters C, Lablanche J, McFadden E, Quandalle P, Bertrand M. Preprocedural stenosis severity is the most powerful determinant of acute outcome after coronary angioplasty [Abstract]. *Eur Heart J* 1994;25:3679.

5. Bauters C, Van Belle E, Lablanche JM, McFadden EP, Quandalle P, Bertrand ME. Predictive factors of primary success after coronary angioplasty. Qualitative and quantitative angiography of 3679 coronary stenosis before and after dilatation. *Arch Mal Coeur Vaiss* 1994;87:193–199.

6. Barnathan ES, Schwartz JS, Taylor L, et al. Aspirin and dipyridamole in the prevention of acute coronary thrombosis complicating coronary angioplasty. *Circulation* 1987;76:125–134.

7. Schwartz L, Bourassa MG, Lesperance J, et al. Aspirin and dipyridamole in the prevention of restenosis after percutaneous transluminal coronary angioplasty. *N Engl J Med* 1988;318:1714–1719.

8. Lembo NJ, Black AJ, Roubin GS, et al. Effect of pretreatment with aspirin versus aspirin plus dipyridamole on frequency and type of acute complications of percutaneous transluminal coronary angioplasty. *Am J Cardiol* 1990;65:422–426.

9. Barragan P, Sainsous J, Silvestri M, et al. Ticlopidine and subcutaneous heparin as an alternative regimen following coronary stenting. *Cathet Cardiovasc Diagn* 1994;32:133–138.

10. White CW, Chaitman B, Lassar TA. Antiplatelet agents are effective in reducing the immediate complications. TCA: results of the ticlopidine multicenter trial [Abstract]. *Circulation* 1987;76:IV-400.

11. Bertrand ME, Allain H, Lablanche JM. Results of a randomized trial of ticlopidine versus placebo for prevention of acute closure and restenosis after coronary angioplasty. The TACT study [Abstract]. *Circulation* 1990;82:III-90.

12. EPIC investigators. Use of a monoclonal antibody directed against the platelet glycoprotein IIb/IIIa receptor in high-risk coronary angioplasty. The epic investigation. *N Engl J Med* 1994;330:956–961.

13. Suzuki S, Sakamoto S, Adachi K, et al. Effect of argatroban on thrombus formation during acute coronary occlusion after balloon angioplasty. *Thromb Res* 1995;77:369–373.

14. Ferguson JJ, Dougherty KG, Gaos CM, Bush HS, Marsh KC, Leachman DR. Relation between procedural activated coagulation time and outcome after percutaneous transluminal coronary angioplasty. *J Am Coll Cardiol* 1994;23:1061–1065.

15. McGarry TF Jr, Gottlieb RS, Morganroth J, et al. The relationship of anticoagulation level and complications after successful percutaneous transluminal coronary angioplasty. *Am Heart J* 1992;123:1445–1451.

16. Dougherty KG, Gaos CM, Bush HS, Leachman DR,

Ferguson JJ. Activated clotting times and activated partial thromboplastin times in patients undergoing coronary angioplasty who receive bolus doses of heparin. *Cathet Cardiovasc Diagn* 1992;26:260–263.

17. Ellis SG, Roubin GS, Wilentz J, Douglas JS Jr, King SB 3d. Effect of 18- to 24-hour heparin administration for prevention of restenosis after uncomplicated coronary angioplasty. *Am Heart J* 1989;117:777–782.

18. Walford GD, Midei MM, Aversano TR. Heparin after PTCA: Increased early complications and no clinical benefit [Abstract]. *Circulation* 1991;84:II-591.

19. Reifart N, Schmidt A, Preusler W, Schwarz F. Is it necessary to heparinize for 24 hours after PTCA [Abstract]. *J Am Coll Cardiol* 1992;19:231.

20. Walford GD, Midei MM, Aversano TR, et al. Heparin after PTCA: increased early complications and no clinical benefit. *Circulation* 1991;84:II-592.

21. Serruys PW, Herrman JP, Simon R, et al. A comparison of hirudin with heparin in the prevention of restenosis after coronary angioplasty. Helvetica Investigators. *N Engl J Med* 1995;333:757–763.

22. Bittl J, Strony J, Brinker JA, Ahmed WH. Treatment with bivalirudin (hirulog) as compared with heparin during coronary angioplasty for unstable or post infarction angina. *N Engl J Med* 1995;333:764–769.

23. Zeiher AM, Kasper W, Gaissmaier C, Wolschlager Ch. Concomitant intracoronary treatment with urokinase during PTCA does not reduce acute complications: a double blind randomized study [Abstract]. *Circulation* 1990;82:III-189.

24. Grill HP, Brinker JA. Nonacute thrombolytic therapy: an adjunct to coronary angioplasty in patients with large intravascular thrombi. *Am Heart J* 1989;118:662–667.

25. Ambrose JA, Almeida OD, Sharma SK, et al. Adjunctive thrombolytic therapy during angioplasty for ischemic rest angina. Results of the tausa trial. Tausa investigators. Thrombolysis and angioplasty in unstable angina trial. *Circulation* 1994;90:69–77.

26. Neuhaus KL, Zeymer U. Prevention and management of thrombotic complications during coronary interventions. Combination therapy with antithrombins, antiplatelets, and/or thrombolytics: risks and benefits. *Eur Heart J* 1995;16(suppl L):63–67.

27. Simoons ML, de Boer MJ, van den Brand MJ, et al. Randomized trial of a GPIIb/IIIa platelet receptor blocker in refractory unstable angina. European Cooperative Study Group. *Circulation* 1994;89:596–603.

28. Tcheng JE. Glycoprotein IIb/IIIa receptor inhibitors: putting the EPIC, IMPACT II, RESTORE, and EPILOG trials into perspective. *Am J Cardiol* 1996;78:35–40.

29. Van de Werf F. More evidence for a beneficial effect of platelet glycoprotein IIb/IIIa-blockade during coronary interventions. Latest results from the EPILOG and CAPTURE trials. *Eur Heart J* 1996;17:325–326.

30. Ferguson JJ 3rd. EPILOG and CAPTURE trials halted because of positive interim results. *Circulation* 1996;93:637.

31. Schulman SP, Goldschmidt-Clermont PJ, Topol EJ, et al. Effects of integrelin, a platelet glycoprotein IIb/IIIa receptor antagonist, in unstable angina. A randomized multicenter trial. *Circulation* 1996;94:2083–2089.

32. de Feyter PJ, van den Brand MJ, Simoons ML, de Boer MJ, van Miltenburg A, van der Wieken LR. Antiplatelet therapy in therapy-resistant unstable angina. A pilot

study with REO PRO (c7E3). *Eur Heart J* 1995; 16(suppl L):36–42.

33. EPILOG investigators. Platelet glycoprotein IIB/IIIA receptor blockade and low-dose heparin during percutaneous coronary revascularization. *N Engl J Med* 1997;336:1689–1696.

34. CAPTURE Investigators. Randomized placebo-controlled trial of abciximab before and during coronary intervention in refractory unstable angina: the CAPTURE study. *Lancet* 1997;349:1429–1435.

35. IMPACT-II investigators. Randomized placebo-controlled trial of effect of eptifibatide on complications of percutaneous coronary intervention: IMPACT-II. *N Engl J Med* 1997;336:1689–1696.

36. Colombo A, Hall P, Nakamura S, et al. Intracoronary stenting without anticoagulation accomplished with intravascular ultrasound guidance. *Circulation* 1995;91: 1676–1688.

37. Serruys PW, de Jaegere P, Kiemenej F, Macaya C, Rutsch W. A comparison of balloon expandable stent implantation with balloon angioplasty in patients with coronary artery disease. *N Engl J Med* 1994;331: 489–495.

38. Fischman DL, Leon MB, Baim DS, et al. A randomized comparison of coronary stent placement and balloon angioplasty in the treatment of coronary artery disease. *N Engl J Med* 1994;331:496–501.

39. Barragan P, Sainsous J, Silvestri M, et al. Ticlopidine and subcutaneous heparin as an alternative regimen following coronary stenting. *Cathet Cardiovasc Diagn* 1994;32:133–138.

40. Van Belle E, McFadden EP, Lablanche JM, Bauters C, Hamon M, Bertrand ME. Two-pronged anplatelet therapy with aspirin and ticlopidine without systemic anticoagulation: an alternative therapeutic strategy after bailout stent implantation. *Coronary Artery Dis* 1995;6: 341–345.

41. Morice MC, Zemour G, Benveniste E, et al. Intracoronary stenting without coumadin: one month results of a French multicenter study. *Cathet Cardiovasc Diagn* 1995;35:1–7.

42. Lablanche JM, McFadden EP, Bonnet JL, et al. Combined antiplatelet therapy with ticlopidine and aspirin. A simplified approach to intracoronary stent management. *Eur Heart J* 1996;17:1373–1380.

43. Zemour G, Morice MC, Benveniste E, et al. Coronary artery stenting without antivitamin K. Results after a month. *Arch Mal Coeur Vaiss* 1996;89:291–297.

44. Goods CM, al Shaibi KF, Liu MW, et al. Comparison of aspirin alone versus aspirin plus ticlopidine after coronary artery stenting. *Am J Cardiol* 1996;78:1042–1044.

45. Karrillon GJ, Morice MC, Benveniste E, et al. Intracoronary stent implantation without ultrasound guidance and with replacement of conventional anticoagulation by antiplatelet therapy. 30 day clinical outcome of the French Multicenter Registry. *Circulation* 1996;94: 1519–1527.

46. Schomig A, Neumann FJ, Kastra A, et al. A randomized comparison of antiplatelet and anticoagulant therapy after the placement of coronary artery stents. *N Engl J Med* 1996;334:1084–1089.

47. Hall P, Nakamura S, Maiello L, et al. A randomized comparison of combined ticlopidine and aspirin therapy versus aspirin therapy alone after successful intravascular ultrasound guided stent implantation. *Circulation* 1996;93:215–222.

48. Serruys PW, Emanuelsson H, van der Giessen W, et al. Heparin coated Palmaz Schatz stents in human coronary arteries. Early outcome of the Benestent II Pilot Study. *Circulation* 1996;93:412–422.

Cardiovascular Thrombosis: Thrombocardiology and Thromboneurology, Second Edition,
edited by M. Verstraete, V. Fuster, and E. J. Topol,
Lippincott–Raven Publishers, Philadelphia © 1998.

34

Primary Prevention of Transient Ischemic Attack and Thromboembolic Stroke

Oscar Benavente, Robert G. Hart, and David G. Sherman

Department of Neurology, University of Texas Health Science Center, San Antonio, Texas 78284

Stroke is the third cause of death in the United States, and about 500,000 new cases occur every year. Worldwide, stroke is the number one cause of death due to the particularly high incidence of stroke in Asia. Stroke is a syndrome, caused by multiple etiologies (Fig. 34-1). Ischemic stroke is the most common form of stroke and is responsible for about 85% of all strokes (Fig. 34-2).

The incidence of ischemic and especially hemorrhagic stroke has declined over the past 20 years (1). This trend is attributed in part to changes in life-style and to a better control of hypertension over the past decade. However, due to the increasing mean age of the population in most Western nations, the absolute number of strokes continues to increase. Because there is an increasing number of U.S. citizens (about 36 million) over 65 years of age (the stroke-prone age group), the actual number of strokes is holding steady (2).

Because the brain is uniquely vulnerable to even brief ischemia and because it recovers poorly, primary prevention in ischemic stroke prevention offers the greatest potential for reducing the burden of this disease. In this chapter, we review clinical and epidemiologic data related to primary prevention in an attempt to provide "best estimates" of risk reduction. The management of hypertension, asymptomatic carotid stenosis, lipid-lowering intervention, and the use of aspirin in primary stroke prevention will be discussed.

Primary prevention begins with identification of risk factors for stroke and characterizing those at risk (Table 34-1). The toxicity and disutility of interventions must be considered in light of the stroke risk. For example, anticoagulation with warfarin is reasonable for selected patients with atrial fibrillation because the absolute reduction in stroke is 3% to 5% per year. On the other hand, for those with lower stroke risk who would have a smaller absolute reduction in stroke, interventions with less disutility would be sensible.

Although the efficacy of antithrombotic therapies is often expressed as the relative reduction, the absolute risk reduction is more important for individual patient management. Relative risk reduction is more generalizable,

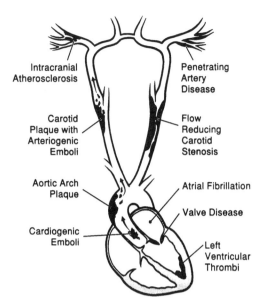

FIG. 34-1. Common cause of ischemic stroke and transient ischemic attack. Optimal management of the stroke syndrome requires proper diagnosis.

inasmuch as the absolute risk reduction is frequently difficult to accurately estimate in a specific patient subgroup because combinations of comorbid factors influence the absolute rate of events. The absolute risk reduction considers both the intrinsic rate of stroke

(Table 34-1) and the effect of therapy. For example, among survivors of myocardial infarction, chronic anticoagulation with warfarin reduces the stroke risk by 70%, but this impressive relative risk reduction is associated with an absolute reduction of only 1% per year (approximately 1.5% per year to approximately 0.5% per year, or 100 survivors of myocardial infarction would need to be given warfarin for 1 year to prevent one ischemic stroke). When expressed in terms of absolute risk reduction (or number needed to treat), the benefit of therapies often appears less impressive. Accurate estimates of the absolute risk reduction in stroke are important for primary prevention.

HYPERTENSION AND STROKE

Hypertension is the most powerful independent risk factor for ischemic stroke; it is a factor in almost 70% of strokes (3). The presence of hypertension increases the risk of stroke by six to seven times in both men and women (4). In borderline hypertension, the adjusted relative risk of stroke is about double (5).

The mechanisms by which hypertension causes ischemic stroke are several, and many of them coexist in the same patient. Hypertension promotes stroke by aggravating atherosclerosis in the aortic arch, carotid, and verte-

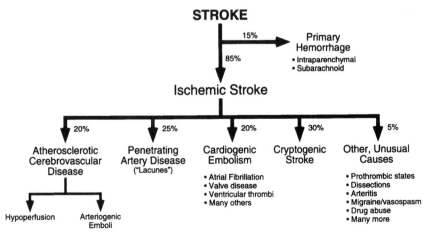

FIG. 34-2. Frequency of etiologies of ischemic stroke. Numbers represent aggregate estimates from stroke registries.

TABLE 34-1. *Absolute stroke rates in stroke-prone patients*

	Ischemic stroke rates
General population, age 70 yr	0.6%/yr
Asymptomatic bruit	1.5%/yr
Prior myocardial infarction	1.5%/yr
Asymptomatic carotid stenosis	2.0%/yr
Nonvalvular atrial fibrillation	5%/yr
TIA	6%/yr
Prior ischemic stroke	10%/yr

TIA, transient ischemic attack.
Vertebrobasilar TIA = 4%/yr vs. carotid TIA = 6%/yr. The risk in the first 12 months is about 10%, declining to 5%/yr thereafter. TIA with ipsilateral carotid stenosis of >70% carries a 15%/yr stroke risk. Transient monocular blindness carries a lower stroke risk than hemispheric TIA.

bral arteries. It also affects small-diameter penetrating arteries with arteriolosclerosis and lipohyalinosis formation, and contributes to ischemic heart disease, which can be complicated by stroke (6).

For both sexes and all ages, systolic and diastolic hypertension have been associated with an excess risk of ischemic and hemorrhagic stroke (7–9). Pooled data from a meta-analysis showed a 10- to 12-fold increase in the risk of stroke for people with a mean diastolic blood pressure of 105 mmHg (10). Although the value of treating severe hypertension has been known for a long time, only recently has the treatment of mild to moderate hypertension been extensively studied (11). A meta-analysis of 14 controlled clinical trials examined the association between treatment of hypertension (using diuretics or β-blockers) and the incidence of stroke (12). Data from this analysis, demonstrated a 45% reduction (95% confidence interval [CI] 33 to 50) in the incidence of stroke. This was achieved by decreasing the diastolic blood pressure by 6 mmHg. In individuals older than 65 years, antihypertensive therapy also was associated with a reduction in the incidence of stroke between 25% and 47%. The different therapeutic interventions have not been compared directly in randomized trials.

Isolated systolic hypertension (systolic pressure above 160 mmHg, and diastolic pressure below 90 mmHg), is frequently present after 55 years of age. It is more prevalent in women and affects about 30% of individuals between 65 and 74 years of age (13). Before the 1990s it was generally believed that isolated systolic hypertension in most elderly people should not be treated. The Systolic Hypertension in the Elderly Program (SHEP) was the first study to demonstrate that modest reduction in systolic hypertension induced a decreased incidence of stroke. Average follow-up was 4.5 years, and 4,736 hypertensive patients (systolic blood pressure >160 mmHg) over 60 years of age were entered into the trial. The interventions were chlorthalidone 12.5 mg/day (dose 1), 25 mg/day (dose 2) or/and atenolol 25 mg/day (dose 1), and 50 mg/day (dose 2). If patients were not controlled (systolic blood pressure >160 mmHg) at the end of each 4-week treatment period, the dose of the drug was increased or the low dose of a second drug (atenolol) was added to the first drug. Reductions of 11 mmHg in mean sytolic pressure and 3.4 mmHg in mean diastolic pressure in the treatment group led to a 36% reduction in the risk of stroke, fatal and nonfatal, compared with those receiving placebo. This was noticed in patients of all ages and both sexes (Fig. 34-3) (14).

In summary, sufficient convincing evidence supports the use of early antihyperten-

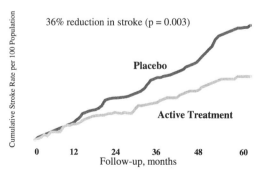

FIG. 34-3. Reduction in stroke in Systolic Hypertension in the Elderly Program (SHEP).

sive therapy to reduce the risk of stroke in all categories of hypertensive patients of all ages.

CAROTID ENDARTERECTOMY FOR PATIENTS WITH ASYMPTOMATIC CAROTID STENOSIS

Asymptomatic carotid stenosis is a common condition, often detected incidentally or in a patient with carotid bruit. Its prevalence ranges from 0.5% in people under 60, increasing to 10% in those over age 80 (an estimated 2 million North Americans) (15–17). Patients with asymptomatic carotid stenosis are at higher risk for ischemic stroke when compared with those without carotid disease, but the risk for stroke is relatively low compared with that in symptomatic patients with carotid stenosis (1–5). In addition, these patients have an excess risk of myocardial infarction and vascular death (15–19).

Carotid endarterectomy is a surgical procedure to remove atherosclerotic stenosis from the cervical carotid artery. The operation has been performed for more than 40 years on patients with signs or symptoms of cerebrovascular disease in an attempt to prevent strokes and restore cerebral blood flow. Carotid en-

darterectomy is efficacious for reducing ipsilateral stroke in patients with symptomatic carotid disease who have carotid stenosis ≥70%, the benefit becoming more evident with greater degrees of stenosis (20,21). Extrapolating these results, the assumption that carotid endarterectomy could usefully reduce ipsilateral strokes in asymptomatic patients has been made.

Six randomized clinical trials in asymptomatic patients with carotid stenosis have been conducted (the trial of Lagneau et al. was conducted in France and completed in 1989; it is still unpublished) (Table 34-2) (22–27). Interpretation of these trials is controversial. Two of the trials had a small sample size with very few outcomes, and no ipsilateral stroke occurred (22–25). The CASANOVA study had numerous crossovers, with results that were difficult to interpret (23). All trials entered patients with carotid stenosis of ≥50%; however, measurement of the degree of stenosis was not done using the same method or imaging studies, and direct comparison is thus confounded. Despite these methodologic differences, the data are consistent and convincingly suggest that carotid endarterectomy reduces the risk of stroke ipsilateral to asymptomatic carotid stenosis. However, the magnitude of reduction

TABLE 34-2. *Randomized clinical trials of endarterectomy for asymptomatic carotid stenosis*

Trials	Total patients	Mean age (yr)	Follow-up (mean yr)	Stenosis (%)	Antithrombotic therapy	
					Surgical group	Medical group
Southern Association for Vascular Surgery (1984)	29	63–64	3	72%[a]	None	ASA 1,300 mg/day
Mayo Asymptomatic Carotid Endarterectomy (1992)	71	NR	2	≥50%	None	ASA 80 mg/day
Veterans Trial (1993)	444	64–65	4	≥50%	ASA 1,300 mg/day	ASA 1,300 mg/day
ACAS (1995)	1,662	67	2.7	≥60%	ASA 325 mg/day	ASA 325 mg/day
L'AURC[b]	237	64	5	>70%	ASA 1,000 mg/day	ASA 1,000 mg/day
CASANOVA (1991)	410	65	3	50–90%	ASA 975 mg/day, dipyridamol 225 mg/day	ASA 975 mg/day, dipyridamol 225 mg/day

NR, not reported.
[a]Mean stenosis.
[b]Trial completed but not published.

TABLE 34-3. *Pooled analysis (five trials):*
Ipsilateral stroke: relative and absolute risk reduction

	Surgical group	Medical group	Relative risk reduction by CEA	CI	p	Absolute risk reduction[a]	NNT[a]
Ipsilateral stroke	3.5%	7.5%	51%	0.30–0.62	0.00001	4%	25

Data from Benavente et al., ref. 28.
NNT, number needed to treat; CEA, carotid endarterectomy.
[a]During a mean follow-up of 4.6 years.

is not large in unselected patients with asymptomatic carotid stenosis ≥50%.

A meta-analysis of all randomized trials, excluding the CASANOVA study (Table 34-3), showed a rate of ipsilateral stroke in the non-surgical group of 1.7% per year (Table 34-3) (28). The relative risk reduction for ipsilateral stroke of 51% was observed with an absolute risk reduction of 4% over a 4.6-year follow-up (Table 34-3). This translates to a reduction of less than 1% per year. Simply put, 100 patients would need to undergo carotid endarterectomy to prevent about one disabling or nondisabling stroke per year, or if the patients survive for longer than 4 years, one can argue that operating on approximately 25 patients might prevent one stroke. Patients who underwent surgical treatment had an increased incidence of early stroke as well as of vascular death (Table 34-4). The frequency of stroke (any vascular territory) within 30 days of entry was five times higher in the surgically treated group (odds ratio [OR] = 4.9; 95% confidence interval [CI] 2.5 to 10; p < 0.00001). The incidence of vascular deaths during the perioperative period was three times higher than in the medically treated patients (OR = 3.04, 95% CI 1 to 10; p < 0.065). A major limitation in the current analysis is the lack of uniformity in the measurement of carotid stenosis. This could result in subgroups of patients at markedly different risk for stroke being pooled. It is conceivable that particularly high-risk subgroups of patients with asymptomatic carotid stenosis exist who would substantially benefit from surgery. At present, such a subgroup has not been identified.

Accordingly, surgery cannot be routinely recommended for unselected patients with asymptomatic carotid stenosis eligible for these trials. The incidence of ipsilateral stroke was relatively low in the medically treated group. Consequently, carotid endarterectomy offered a small absolute stroke reduction that only became evident after the first year postsurgery. Performing 100 endarterectomies to prevent one stroke per year may be dubiously cost effective compared with other interventions. Massive screening programs in search of carotid disease are not justified at the present time, for the reasons described above.

Unquestionably, the prognosis and consequently the surgical benefit of carotid endarterectomy is different between patients with symptomatic and asymptomatic carotid stenosis. The magnitude of the benefit is definitively larger in symptomatic patients (Fig. 34-4).

TABLE 34-4. *Stroke and vascular death within 30 days postrandomization*

	Stroke (%)				Vascular death (%)			
	Medical group/n	Surgical group/n	Odds ratio	95% CI	Medical group/n	Surgical group/n	Odds ratio	95% CI
Pooled analysis (five trials)	3 (0.25) /1.225	28 (2.5) /1.215	4.94	2.5–10	1 (0.09) /1.225	7 (6) /1.215	3.04	1–10

Data from Benavente et al., ref. 28.

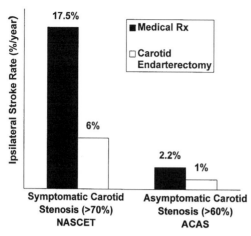

FIG. 34-4. Effect of carotid endarterectomy in carotid stenosis: symptomatic versus asymptomatic. NASCET, North American Symptomatic Carotid Endarterectomy Trial. Absolute risk reduction: 11.5% per year. Number needed to treat: nine patients would need to undergo carotid endarterectomy to prevent one stroke per year. ACAS, Asymptomatic Carotid Atherosclerosis Study. Absolute risk reduction: 1.2% per year. Number needed to treat: 83 patients would need to undergo carotid endarterectomy to prevent one stroke per year.

It is possible that patients at higher risk of stroke (i.e., higher degree of stenosis, rapidly progressive disease, silent cerebral infarcts, or ulcerated plaque) would benefit from carotid endarterectomy. However, until a risk stratification is validated and the results of the ongoing European Asymptomatic Carotid Surgery Trial are available, the management of patients with asymptomatic carotid disease continues to be controversial, influenced by individual patient preferences.

LIPID LOWERING FOR PRIMARY STROKE PREVENTION

Although hyperlipidemia is a well-established risk factor for coronary artery disease, its role as an independent risk factor for ischemic stroke was controversial until recently (29). The possible mechanisms by which hyperlipidemia increases the incidence of ischemic stroke are dependent on the development of atherosclerosis in the extracranial/intracranial vascular system and coronary arteries.

The value of lipid-lowering therapies for stroke prevention has been controversial, and only a few randomized trials have tested those agents for stroke prevention. A meta-analysis showed a decrease in the risk of non-fatal stroke (OR 0.88; 95% CI 0.70 to 1.11) and an excess of fatal stroke (OR 1.32; 95% CI 0.94 to 1.86) among men allocated to lipid-lowering agents. The excess of fatal strokes was attributed to a high incidence of intracerebral hemorrhage. A subgroup analysis of patients randomized to clofibrate showed a statistically significant reduction in the incidence of ischemic stroke (30). The trials included in this meta-analysis preceded the more recent studies that used 3-hydroxy-3-methylglutaryl coenzyme A (HMG-CoA) reductase inhibitors (statins).

In the Scandinavian Simvastatin Survival Study (known as 4S), patients with angina or prior myocardial infarction who had a total serum cholesterol level of ≥212 mg% (more than 5.5 mmol/L) were assigned to placebo or to simvastatin (HMG-CoA reductase inhibitor) and followed for an average of 5 years. A 35% decrease in low-density lipoprotein (LDL) cholesterol in the treated group was associated with a significant reduction of all causes of mortality, coronary events, and ischemic stroke. A post hoc analysis documented 98 strokes in 2,223 patients in the placebo group, as compared with 70 such events in 2,221 patients receiving simvastatin, corresponding to a risk reduction of 30% (p = 0.024). A subgroup analysis of nonembolic strokes showed a greater risk reduction (50%) (31).

Recent data from the multicenter Asymptomatic Carotid Progression Study (ACAPAS) has shown that lovastatin reverses the progression of intimal–medial thickening in carotid arteries. Patients with mild carotid stenosis and LDL cholesterol of 130–189 mg% were enrolled in the study and randomized to lovastatin or placebo (mean follow-up 36 months). A reduction in LDL cholesterol of 28% was associated with signicantly reversed progression of plaque thickness (p = 0.001). In addition, lovastatin appeared to reduce the incidence of stroke; five strokes occurred in the placebo arm and none in the treatment group; however, this trend was not statistically significant (32).

Due to the suspected relationship of increased cholesterol and increased risk of stroke; treatment recommendations at this time include aggressive hyperlipidemia management for those patients considered to be at risk for cerebrovascular disease. Patients with LDL cholesterol of more than 130 mg% with clinical coronary disease or mild asymptomatic carotid plaques should be considered candidates for dietary modification and therapy with HMG-CoA reductase inhibitors (statins). Although the value of statins for stroke prevention has not been tested specifically in higher risk patients with asymptomatic carotid stenosis, such treatment seems reasonable for those with mild to moderate carotid stenosis and LDL cholesterol of more than 130 mg%. Such treatment also may benefit the associated coronary artery disease so often coexistent in these patients.

CIGARETTE SMOKING AND THE RISK OF STROKE

Cigarette smoking is a major risk factor for ischemic stroke. Smoking may contribute to stroke by several mechanisms: i.e., increasing blood levels of fibrinogen and hematocrit, augmenting platelet aggregability, reducing high-density lipoprotein cholesterol levels, and damaging the vascular endothelium, which may promote atherosclerosis (33–37). Pooled data from a meta-analysis showed that the relative risk of stroke for smokers, as compared with nonsmokers, was 1.51 (95% CI 1.45 to 1.58). The stroke risk increased with the number of cigarettes smoked per day (38). Data from the Physician's Health Study showed that the age-adjusted relative risk of stroke was increased by 2.7 in heavy smokers, 2.0 in moderate smokers, and 1.3 in former smokers (not significant) compared with that seen in men who had never smoked. Accordingly, cigarette smoking is related to ischemic stroke, and there is a graded dose-response relationship.

Prospective studies have shown a significant reduction in the incidence of stroke after cigarette smoking cessation. In the Framingham study, the risk of stroke in former smokers, after 5 years of cessation, was not greater than those who never smoked. This trend also was observed in elderly smokers and in people who have been long-term smokers (39). The Nurses Health Study also confirmed a dramatic reduction in the risk of stroke after smoking cessation. The relative risk of stroke decreased from 1.0 in smokers to 0.4 in former smokers within 5 years after quitting (40).

Smoking cessation should be routinely urged because it is clearly a beneficial measure that substantially reduces the incidence of stroke and other vascular disease.

ASPIRIN FOR PRIMARY STROKE PREVENTION

Aspirin use has been convincingly demonstrated to reduce the risks of myocardial infarction, ischemic stroke, and vascular death for many patients when used for secondary stroke prevention (41). A meta-analysis of

TABLE 34-5. *Aspirin effect on stroke in low-risk patients*

Trials	N	Aspirin dose	Stroke[a]	
			Rate	% change
USPHS (42)	22,071	325 mg every other day	0.2%/yr	(+) 21%
British doctors (43)	5,139	500 mg/day	0.4%/yr	(+) 27%
ETDRS (44)	3,711	650 mg/day	0.8%/yr	(+) 17%
AGGREGATE				22% (p = 0.007)

[a]Includes both ischemic and hemorrhagic stroke; about 15% of strokes were hemorrhagic.

over 100 randomized clinical trials involving about 70,000 participants with vascular disease concluded that aspirin reduces these vascular events by about 25%, regardless of the aspirin dose (41).

In contrast, three randomized clinical trials assessing aspirin for primary prevention in low-risk people have shown an increased risk of stroke (Table 34-5). Myocardial infarction was reduced by aspirin in these trials, but stroke was consistently increased (aggregate estimate of 22%, p = 0.007) (42–44). These randomized trials of primary prevention included mostly men and middle-aged people.

At least part of the increased risk of stroke associated with aspirin use is due to a higher rate of hemorrhagic stroke. Aspirin increases hemorrhagic stroke both for people with and without manifest vascular disease (Table 34-6) (45). There is no apparent relationship between the aspirin dose and accentuation of hemorrhagic stroke based on indirect comparisons from randomized trials (Table 34-6) (45), although direct comparisons are limited to a handful of hemorrhagic events (46,47).

In most clinical series, 10% to 20% of strokes are hemorrhagic (41,42,48). Hence, a 1.75-fold increase in hemorrhagic stroke by aspirin would increase the overall stroke rate by about 12%, theoretically accounting for

about half of the "extra" strokes occurring in low-risk people who regularly use aspirin. However, uncertainties in these estimates are large, and it is possible that the entire increment of aspirin-induced stroke is accounted for by brain hemorrhages.

Although it is clear that aspirin use increases overall stroke rates and hemorrhagic stroke in low-risk patients, it is uncertain whether aspirin augments ischemic stroke in this population. The most reliable data are from the U.S. Physicians' Health Study (USPHS) (42), in which most strokes were categorized as ischemic or hemorrhagic based on neuroimaging or autopsy (49). There was an 11% excess of ischemic strokes in this randomized trial (91 on aspirin versus 82 on placebo). Although this difference was not statistically significant, it is not compatible with the overall reduction in ischemic stroke afforded by aspirin in high-risk patients, as defined by a meta-analysis of all available clinical trials (risk reduction 28 ± 5%) (41). Based on these results, it is plausible that the effects of aspirin on ischemic stroke in low-risk versus high-risk patients are importantly different.

The potential mechanisms by which aspirin increases ischemic stroke are not well defined. Aspirin has been variably reported to increase

TABLE 34-6. *Randomized trials relating aspirin to hemorrhagic stroke*

| | | No. of intracranial hemorrhages | | |
	Aspirin dose	Placebo	Aspirin	Relative risk
TIA/stroke patients				
UK-TIA (46)	300 mg/day	2	7	
UK-TIA (46)	1,200 mg/day	2	7	
SALT (60)	75 mg/day	3	8	
Pooled others (41)	Various	5	7	
Aggregate		10	22	2.2
Primary prevention				
USPHS (42)	325 mg/day	12	23	(p = 0.06)
British doctors (43)	500 mg/day	12	21	
Aggregate		24	44	1.8
Others				
Pooled prosthetic valves (61)	100–1,000 mg/day	7	15	
Stable angina	75 mg	2	5	
Aggregate		9	20	2.2
Antiplatelet Trialists (41)				
High-risk without TIA/stroke	Various	27	34	1.3

systemic blood pressure (especially if measured supine) and to antagonize the effect of certain antihypertensive drugs (50); hypertension is a strong, prevalent risk factor for stroke (51,52). In the UK-TIA study, blood pressure tended to be slightly higher in those receiving 1,200 mg versus 300 mg of aspirin daily (46). Thrombogenic effects of aspirin have been demonstrated experimentally, particularly at high doses, possibly relating to inhibition of endothelial-derived prostacyclin synthesis (53–55). In the absence of atherosclerotic vascular disease, for which the antiplatelet effect of aspirin reduces stroke, inhibition of prostacyclin may predispose to thrombosis (the "aspirin dilemma") (56). Hence, the low doses of aspirin that reduce myocardial infarction and enhance hemorrhagic stroke by virtue of the antiplatelet effect may be less likely to potentiate a separate competing prothrombotic effect based on prostacyclin inhibition (57). The clinical relevance of the effect of aspirin on prostacyclin remains unclear, however (56). Hypothetically, in patients with manifest vascular disease, the antiplatelet effect may dominate, causing a reduction in ischemic stroke, but potentially less so in low-risk populations. Paradoxically increased platelet adhesiveness has been reported in some patients taking aspirin (aspirin nonresponders), but the clinical consequences of these observations are unclear (58,59).

It remains unclear whether aspirin is beneficial in the primary prevention of ischemic stroke. Despite the existing data that show that aspirin produces an excess of hemorrhagic and ischemic stroke in low-risk patients, this cannot yet be considered conclusive due to the low event rate. Based on this evidence, aspirin cannot routinely be recommended for patients without manifest cardiovascular disease.

CONCLUSION

Because irreversible injury occurs so quickly after occlusion of an artery supplying the brain, stroke prevention rather than acute stroke treatment must be the focus in decreasing the devastation resulting from stroke. The decline in stroke incidence seen in the past two decades is likely due to risk factor management. Recent studies have critically examined primary prevention for subsets of high-risk patients (e.g., asymptomatic carotid stenosis, atrial fibrillation). Extrapolating the benefits for secondary prevention to primary prevention must be done with caution, as the data presented on aspirin and endarterectomy illustrate.

REFERENCES

1. Soltero L, Liu K, Cooper R, Stamler J, Garside D. Trends in mortality from cerebrovascular disease in the United States, 1960 to 1975. *Stroke* 1978;9:549–558.
2. American Heart Association. *Heart and Stroke Facts.* Dallas: American Heart Association, 1994.
3. Dunbabin DW, Sandercock PAG. Preventing stroke by the modification of risk factors. *Stroke* 1990;21(suppl IV):36–39.
4. Castelli WP, Anderson K. A population at risk. Prevalence of high cholesterol levels in hypertensive patients in the Framingham Study. *Am J Med* 1986;80:23–32.
5. Wolf PA. Epidemiology and Risk Factors Management. In: Welch KMA, Caplan LR, Reis DJ, Siesjo BK, Weir B (eds). *Primer on Cerebrovascular Diseases.* San Diego: Academic, 1997;751–757.
6. Phillips SJ, Whisnant JP. Hypertension and the brain the National High Blood Pressure Education Program. *Arch Intern Med* 1992;152:938–945.
7. Wolf PA, Cobb JL, D'Agostino RB. Epidemiology of stroke. In: Barnett HJM, Mohr JP, Stein BM, Yatsu FM (eds). *Stroke: Pathophysiology, Diagnosis, and Management.* 2nd ed. New York: Churchill Livingstone, 1992;3–27.
8. Sacco RL, Wolf PA, Bharucha NE, et al. Subarachnoid and intracerebral hemorrhage: natural history, prognosis and precursive factors in the Framingham Study. *Neurology* 1984;34:847–854.
9. Fiebach NH, Hebert PR, Stampfer MJ, et al. A prospective study of high blood pressure and cardiovascular disease in women. *Am J Epidemiol* 1989;130:646–654.
10. MacMahon SW, Peto R, Cutler JA, et al. Blood pressure, stroke, and coronary heart disease. I. Prolonged differences in blood pressure: prospective observational studies corrected for the regression dilution bias. *Lancet* 1990;335:765–774.
11. MacMahon SW, Cutler JA, Furberg CD, Payne GH. The effects of drug treatment for hypertension on morbidity and mortality from cardiovascular disease: a review of randomized controlled trials. *Prog Cardiovasc Dis* 1986;29(suppl 1):99–118.
12. Collins R, Peto R, MacMahon S, et al. Blood pressure, stroke and coronary heart disease. 2. Short-term reductions in blood pressure: overview of randomized drug trials in their epidemiological context. *Lancet* 1990;335:827–838.
13. Working Group on Hypertension in the Elderly. Statement on hypertension in the elderly. *JAMA* 1986;256:70–74.

14. SHEP Cooperative Research Group Prevention of stroke by antihypertensive drug treatment in older persons with isolated systolic hypertension: final results of the Systolic Hypertension in the Elderly Program (SHEP). *JAMA* 1991;265:3255–3264.

15. Ricci S, Flamini OF, Celani MG, Marini M, Antonini D, Bartolini E. Prevalence of internal carotid artery stenosis in subjects older than 49 years: a population study. *Cerebrovas Dis* 1991;23:1752–1760.

16. Prati P, Vanuzzo D, Casaroli M, et al. Prevalence and determinants of carotid atherosclerosis in a general population. *Stroke* 1992;23:1705–1711.

17. Meissner I, Wiebers DO, Whisnant JP, O'Fallon M. The natural history of asymptomatic carotid artery occlusive lesions. *JAMA* 1987;258:2704–2707.

18. Norris JW, Zhu CZ, Bornstein NM, Chambers BR. Vascular risk of asymptomatic carotid stenosis. *Stroke* 1991;22:1485–1490.

19. European Carotid Surgery Trialists' Collaborative Group. Risk of stroke in the distribution of an asymptomatic carotid artery. *Lancet* 1995;345:209–212.

20. North American Symptomatic Carotid Endarterectomy Trial Collaborators. Beneficial effect of carotid endarterectomy in symptomatic patients with high-grade carotid stenosis. *N Engl J Med* 1991;325:445–453.

21. European Carotid Surgery Trialists' Collaborative Group. MRC European Carotid Surgery Trial: interim results for symptomatic patients with severe (70–99%) or with mild (0–29%) carotid stenosis. *Lancet* 1991; 337:1235–1243.

22. Clagett GP, Youkey JR, Brigham RA, et al. Southern Association for Vascular Surgery. Asymptomatic cervical bruit and abnormal ocular pneumoplethysmography: a prospective study comparing two approaches to management. *Surgery* 1984;96:823–830.

23. The CASANOVA Study Group. Carotid surgery versus medical therapy in asymptomatic carotid stenosis. *Stroke* 1991;22:1229–1235.

24. Hobson RW II, Weiss DG, Fields WS, et al., and the Veterans Affairs Cooperative Study Group. Efficacy of carotid surgery for asymptomatic carotid stenosis. *N Engl J Med* 1993;328:221–227.

25. Mayo Asymptomatic Carotid Endarterectomy Study Group. Results of a randomized controlled trial of carotid endarterectomy for asymptomatic carotid stenosis. *Mayo Clin Proc* 1992;67:513–518.

26. Asymptomatic Carotid Atherosclerosis Study. Endarterectomy for asymptomatic carotid artery stenosis. *JAMA* 1995;273:1421–1428.

27. Lagneau P. Stenoses carotidiennes asymptomatics. *J Mal Vasc* 1993;18:209–212.

28. Benavente O, Moher D. Carotid endarterectomy for asymptomatic carotid stenosis: a meta-analysis of randomized controlled trials. (Submitted for publication.)

29. Tell GS, Crouse JR, Furberg CD. Relation between blood lipids, lipoproteins, and cerebrovascular atherosclerosis: a review. *Stroke* 1988;19:423–430.

30. Atkins D, Psaty BM, Koepsell TD, Longstreth WT Jr, Larson EB. Cholesterol reduction and the risk for stroke in men: a meta-analysis of randomized, controlled trials. *Ann Intern Med* 1993;119:136–145.

31. Randomized trial of cholesterol lowering in 4444 patients with coronary heart disease: the Scandinavian Simvastatin Survival Study (4S). *Lancet* 1994;344:1383–1389.

32. Furberg CD, Adams HP Jr, Applegate WB, et al. Effect of lovastatin on early carotid atherosclerosis and cardiovascular events. *Circulation* 1994;90:1679–1687.

33. Wihelmsen L, Svardsudd K, Korsan-Bengtsen K, Welin L, Tibblin G. Fibrinogen as a risk factor for stroke and myocardial infarction. *N Engl J Med* 1984; 311:501–505.

34. Renaud S, Blache D, Dumont E, Thevenon C, Wissendanger T. Platelet function after cigarette smoking in relation to nicotine and carbon monoxide. *Clin Pharmacol Ther* 1984;36:389–395.

35. Criqui MH, Wallace RB, Heiss G, et al. Cigarette smoking and plasma high-density lipoprotein cholesterol: the Lipid Research Clinics Program Prevalence Study. *Circulation* 1980;62(suppl IV):70–76.

36. Smith JR, Landaw SA. Smokers' polycythemia. *N Engl J Med* 1978;298:6–10.

37. Sieffert GF, Keown K, Moore WS. Pathologic effect of tobacco smoke inhalation on arterial intima. *Surg Forum* 1981;32:333–335.

38. Shinton R, Beevers G. Meta-analysis of relation between cigarette smoking and stroke. *Br Med J* 1989; 298:789–794.

39. Wolf PA, D'Agostino RB, Kannel WB, et al. Cigarette smoking as a risk factor for stroke: the Framingham Study. *JAMA* 1988;259:1025–1029.

40. Kawachi I, Colditz GA, Stampfer MJ, et al. Smoking cessation and decreased risk of stroke in women. *JAMA* 1993;269:232–236.

41. Antiplatelet Trialists Collaboration. Collaborative overview of randomized trials of antiplatelet therapy (part I). *Br Med J* 1994;308:81–106.

42. Steering Committee of the Physicians' Health Study Research Group. Final report on the aspirin component of the ongoing Physicians' Health Study. *N Engl J Med* 1989;321:129–135.

43. Peto R, Gray R, Collins R, et al. A randomized trial of prophylactic daily aspirin in British male doctors. *Br Med J* 1988;296:313–317.

44. Early Treatment of Diabetic Retinopathy Study Investigators. Aspirin effects in diabetes mellitus. *JAMA* 1992; 268:1292–1300.

45. Hart RG, Pearce LA. In vivo antithrombotic effect of aspirin dose versus nongastrointestinal bleeding [Letter]. *Stroke* 1993;24:138–139.

46. UK-TIA Study Group. The United Kingdom Transient Ischemic Attack (UK-TIA) Aspirin Trial. Final results. *J Neurol Neurosurg Psychiatry* 1991;54:1044–1054.

47. The Dutch TIA Study Group. A comparison of two doses of aspirin (30 mg vs. 283 mg a day) in patients after a transient ischemic attack or minor ischemic stroke. *N Engl J Med* 1991;325:1261–1266.

48. Kronmal RA, Hart RG, Manolio TA, et al. Aspirin use and incident stroke in the Cardiovascular Health Study. (Submitted for publication).

49. Berger K, Kase CS, Buring JE. Interobserver agreement in the classification of stroke in the Physicians' Health Study. *Stroke* 1996;27:238.

50. Johnson AG, Nguyen TV, Day RO. Do nonsteroidal anti-inflammatory drugs affect blood pressure? A meta-analysis. *Ann Intern Med* 1994;121:289–300.

51. Verhoef P, Hennekens CH, Malinow R, et al. A prospective study of plasma homocyst(e)ine and risk of stroke. *Stroke* 1994;25:1924.

52. Manolio TA, Kronmal RA, Burke GL, et al. Short-term predictors of incident stroke in older adults: the Cardiovascular Health Study. *Stroke* 1996;27:1479–1486.

53. Lekstrom JA, Bell WR. Aspirin in the prevention of thrombosis. *Medicine* 1991;70:161–178.

54. Zimmermann R, Thiessen M, Walter E, Morl H. Paradoxical effect of high-mid-low-dose aspirin in experimental arterial thrombosis. *Artery* 1980;8:422–425.

55. Kelton JG, Hirsh J, Carter CJ, Buchanan MR. Thrombogenic effect of high-dose aspirin in rabbits. *J Clin Invest* 1978;62:892–895.

56. Marcus AJ. Aspirin as an antithrombotic medication. *N Engl J Med* 1983;309:1515–1516.

57. Masotti G, Galanti G, Poggesi L, et al. Differential inhibition of protacyclin production and platelet aggregation by aspirin. *Lancet* 1979;2:1213–1216.

58. Buchanan MR, DeJana E, Gent M, Mustard JF, Hirsh J. Enhanced platelet accumulation onto injured carotid arteries in rabbits following aspirin treatment. *J Clin Invest* 1981;67:503–508.

59. Buchanan MR, Brister SJ. Individual variation in the effects of aspirin on platelet function: implications for the use of aspirin clinically. *Clin J Cardiol* 1995;11:221–227.

60. SALT Collaborative Group. Swedish Aspirin Low-Dose Trial (SALT) of 75 mg aspirin as secondary prophylaxis after cerebrovascular ischaemic events. *Lancet* 1991;338:1345–1349.

61. Hart RG, Boop BS, Anderson DC. Oral anticoagulants and intracerebral hemorrhage. Facts and hypotheses. *Stroke* 1995;26:1471–1477.

62. Juul-Moller S, Edvardsson N, Jahnmatz B, Rosen A, Sorensen S, Omblus R. Double-blind trial of aspirin in primary prevention of myocardial infarction in patients with stable chronic angina pectoris. *Lancet* 1992;340:1421–1425.

Cardiovascular Thrombosis: Thrombocardiology and Thromboneurology, Second Edition,
edited by M. Verstraete, V. Fuster, and E. J. Topol,
Lippincott–Raven Publishers, Philadelphia © 1998.

35

Thrombolytic Treatment of Thrombotic Stroke

Gregory J. del Zoppo and *Werner Hacke

*Department of Molecular and Experimental Medicine, The Scripps Research Institute,
La Jolla, California 92037; and *Department of Neurology, University of Heidelberg,
Heidelberg D69120, Germany*

Stroke, a group of heterogeneous cerebrovascular disorders that produce focal neurologic deficits, is the third leading cause of death and the most common cause of permanent disability in the Western hemisphere. Fixed or transient neurologic deficits of ischemic cerebrovascular disease result from in situ thrombosis (40% to 57%), atherothromboembolism (16% to 23%), subarachnoid hemorrhage (10% to 19%), intracerebral hemorrhage (4% to 18%), lacunae (14%), or other causes (1–3). Atherothromboembolic and thrombotic stroke are of particular importance because of their frequency, connection to clinically demonstrable cerebral arterial occlusions, and their clear impact on cerebral tissue integrity.

The association of thrombosis with cerebrovascular ischemia has been the basis for trials of plasminogen activators in ischemic stroke. Angiography-based studies of symptomatic carotid arterial territory thrombosis have demonstrated that arterial patency increases spontaneously with time from stroke onset, in a manner analogous to coronary artery patency in evolving acute myocardial infarction (4). Occlusion of symptomatic carotid arteries has been documented in 76% to 81% of patients within 6 hours (5,6), 58.7% at 24 hours (7), 57% at 3 days (8), and somewhat lower frequencies later (9). Yamaguchi et al. suggested that spontaneous recanalization is a relatively frequent occurrence after cerebral thromboembolism (10). Mori indicated that spontaneous recanalization may occur in 16.7% patients over 120 minutes in whom angiography was performed within a mean of 3.6 hours from symptom onset (11), whereas Yamaguchi reported a 4.4% frequency of spontaneous recanalization in a similar clinical setting (12). On this basis, efficacy studies of plasminogen activators in focal cerebral ischemia have been directed at two goals: (a) facilitation of cerebral arterial recanalization, considered necessary for neurologic recovery, and (b) enhancement of neurologic or clinical recovery alone, irrespective of vascular effects. Studies of the latter type are based on the presumption that the plasminogen activator does mediate recanalization, without independent verification of the site or extent of cerebral arterial occlusion. Initial studies of this genre were conducted in the late 1950s in which direct intra-arterial delivery (13) appeared to produce a superior recanalization to intravenous delivery (14), although the experiences were limited and not directly compared.

A significant change in the approach to stroke was realized in the early 1980s, when plasminogen activators were experimentally applied in the acute period (6 to 8 hours from symptom onset) (15). Acute intervention in patients selected by strict computed tomography (CT) scan and clinical criteria have been associated with evidence of benefit (11,16, 18). To study the efficacy of plasminogen activator delivery, two trial design approaches have been followed: (a) angiography-based studies that allow one to relate vascular outcome and clinical benefits, and (b) symptom-based studies that assess clinical outcome only without corroboration of vascular outcome. Experimental and clinical work suggest that plasminogen activators must be used within a short interval from symptom onset to limit hemorrhagic complications and enhance favorable outcome. The ramifications and limitations of both approaches rest on an understanding of the pathophysiology of focal cerebral ischemia.

PATHOPHYSIOLOGY OF FOCAL CEREBRAL ISCHEMIA

Thromboembolism Versus In Situ Thrombosis

Thromboembolism is responsible for approximately 75% of ischemic events (3).

However, embolic events may originate from thrombi in various locations: cardiac sources (e.g., atrial fibrillation, patent foramen ovale, intramural thrombus on hyperkinetic segments, valvular disease), atherosclerosis of the aorta and aortic arch, and atherosclerosis of the common and internal carotid arteries. Predilection sites for atheroma formation (Fig. 35-1) also serve as sources of atherothromboembolism. Thromboemboli may vary in composition and organization. Some thrombi contain calcifications, whereas others may be fresh and easily dissolvable. On the other hand, in contrast to one popular hypothesis, cardiac emboli are not always fresh or easily amenable to dissolution because some may be old and calcified. Unfortunately, little solid information exists concerning thrombus composition complicating the brain circulation (19). The volume and location of emboli probably influence the clinical signs and symptoms of the stroke syndrome and its

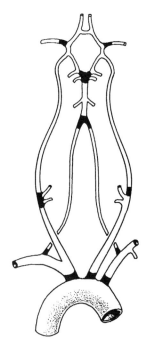

FIG. 35-1. Predilection sites for atheroma formation. These arterial sites provide foci for in situ thrombus formation and the origin of atherothromboemboli.

appearance on CT scans: large emboli from atheromas at the carotid bifurcation, for example, may lodge in proximal vessels, especially in the carotid T or the proximal middle cerebral artery (MCA) (20) (Fig. 35-2).

In situ thrombosis occurs in both the large, extracerebral brain-supplying vessels including the basal circle of Willis and its main arterial branches. Thrombotic occlusion of the brain microcirculation occurs during ischemia. The frequency of in situ thrombosis of large intracranial vessels leading to local arterial occlusion is low in white populations, but is more frequent among Asiatic groups and populations of African descent (21).

Neuronal Responses to Ischemia

Experimental studies of focal ischemia suggest a finite interval after cessation of blood flow beyond which significant irreversible ischemic neuronal damage and sustained neurologic deficit occurs (22–24). Clinical factors important to outcomes in acute ischemic stroke include the integrity of collateral anastomoses, time from symptom onset to evaluation, occlusion location, cellu-

lar vulnerability, and local flow characteristics. One angiography-based reperfusion study using a plasminogen activator suggested that clinical outcome may be enhanced by the presence of patent collateral anastomoses (25). The patency of the collateral circuit may bear on the potential for tissue functional recovery after cerebral ischemia. Astrup et al. postulated a zone of neuronal tissue peripheral to an irreversibly ischemic core that is metabolically injured, but functionally recoverable if sufficient blood flow could be restored within a short time (23). The existence of a penumbra has been implied by human positron emission tomography (PET) studies (26) and experimental preparations (27), although exact cellular/vascular correlates are not yet known. Also implied is a finite interval after cessation of blood flow beyond which irreversible ischemic neuronal damage occurs (22–24). Experimental preparations have suggested that certain regions of limited vascular flow and certain neuron populations are particularly sensitive to ischemia. Such regional or cellular "selective vulnerabilities" may place unknown, but strict limits on tissue recoverability. In addition, local

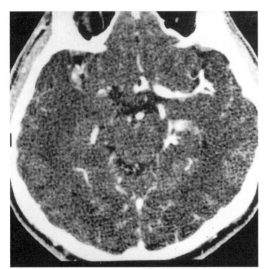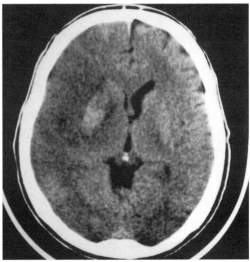

FIG. 35-2. Spiral CT angiography of a right carotid T M1 occlusion **(left panel)**. This occlusion resulted in an extended MCA infarction **(right panel)**. The CT scan was performed 36 hours after stroke onset. Note the hemorrhagic transformation of the external pallidum.

flow conditions may contribute to variation in the tissue distribution of nutrients or plasminogen activators. In an individual patient, these considerations may combine to define an individual limited interval of tolerated ischemia (28). For clinical trial design, a practical limit to treatment has taken this interval in humans as 3 to 6 hours.

Neuronal vulnerabilities are responsible for the neurologic findings that accompany cerebral arterial occlusion. However, neurologic status is a relatively poor predictor of cerebral arterial occlusion location (5,29). Saito et al. suggested that in the MCA territory clinical outcome is directly related to occlusion site (29). Specifically, five of 16 patients (31.3%) with distal M1 segment (MCA trunk) and M2 segment occlusions, and five of 17 (29.4%) with proximal M1 segment occlusions had fatal outcomes at 3 months, whereas only one of seven (14.3%) with M3 segment (branch) occlusions succumbed in the same time frame. M1 segment occlusions are generally associated with a very poor outcome typified by persistent disabling defects in 87.5% of untreated patients (30).

Mortality, however, is a rather weak indicator of occlusion location and has had limited utility as an outcome measure in acute stroke trials. To date, large-scale mortality outcome trials (e.g., International Stroke Trial [IST] [31]) have not been developed for thrombolysis. Stroke-related death and cardiac death have been reported to occur in 28% and 37%, respectively, of patients who have had transient ischemic attacks, indicating that cardiovascular mortality is a significant contributor to stroke outcome (32). More recent evaluations including data from placebo groups of large antithrombotic efficacy trials suggest a lower mortality rate. For instance, the combined outcome events of stroke, myocardial infarction, and death occurred in 14% of placebo patients over 2 years in the UK-TIA Study Group Trial (33). One-year mortality rates generally do not exceed 15%, most of which are due to cardiovascular causes (34). In a population of stroke patients not selected by vascular diagnostic techniques, expected differences in outcome based on occlusion location (e.g., M1 segment occlusions) or vascular pathology (e.g., lacunae) would not be readily apparent.

In general, patients with milder fixed deficits are more likely to fare better than are those with severe deficits. Substantial neurologic improvements in patients with carotid territory infarction and baseline Canadian Neurological Scale scores of ≥6.5 (normal = 10.0) were noted by Fieschi et al. (5,35). Stroke patients may display progressive improvement in the absence of treatment according to scoring instruments based on the neurologic examination (e.g., Scandinavian Stroke Scale [34]) (36).

Disability outcomes are reasonable targets as outcome measures for treatment trials in acute ischemic stroke. Although still in evolution, the use of measures of disability including the Rankin scale (37) modified for mortality and the Barthel index (38) provide convenient means of describing patient status. Their use in recent clinical trials (18,39) underscores the ability to describe large population responses to therapy.

Microvascular Responses to Ischemia

Limitations to the ability of plasminogen activators to enhance reperfusion (6,11, 40–42) and to improve clinical outcome (11, 17,18) draw attention to the relative contributions of early ischemic injury (18), individualization of the window for treatment (28), edema formation, and mechanisms of hemorrhagic transformation to poor outcome. These elements of focal cerebral ischemic injury underscore the central role that microvascular processes may play in clinical outcome (Table 35-1). Ultimate disability is the sum of the beneficial attributes of recanalization, inflammation, and preservation of collateral flow, and the negative effects of inflammation, plasmin generation, and hemorrhage within the ischemic microvascular bed. Approaches that limit the latter effects are likely to enhance beneficial outcome.

TABLE 35-1. *Microvascular processes and tissue injury*

Microvascular obstruction
  No-reflow phenomenon
  Platelet-fibrin deposition (in situ thrombosis)
  PMN leukocyte obstruction/adherence
  Compression
Free-radical generation
Cytokine synthesis
Increased endothelial cell permeability and edema
    formation
  Alterations in blood–brain barrier
  Leukocyte-enhanced permeability of
    postcapillary venules
Alterations in endothelial cell and astrocyte end-feet
    integrin expression
Alterations in basal lamina integrity
Hemorrhagic transformation

Although thrombotic occlusion of a major brain-supplying artery has nearly immediate consequences for neuron function, the downstream microvasculature also has distinct vulnerabilities to ischemic injury. In focal cerebral ischemia (and reperfusion) cytokine expression, upregulation of cellular adhesion receptors, and activation of leukocytes, platelets, and coagulation occur in the early moments after MCA occlusion. Hallenbeck et al. demonstrated accumulation of leukocytes in regions of low cerebral blood flow in a novel model of arterial embolism (43). del Zoppo et al. suggested that the microvascular perfusion defects that occur after focal cerebral ischemia in reperfusion may reflect polymorphonuclear (PMN) leukocyte adherence in the ischemic microvasculature via active adhesion receptor–counter-receptor interactions (44–47). Discrete studies have demonstrated that transmigration across postcapillary venules begins 4 to 6 hours after MCA occlusion, with maximal numbers of intravascular PMN leukocytes detected at 12 hours and maximal emigration by 24 hours in the anesthetized Wistar rat (48,49).

Adherence of PMN leukocytes to vascular endothelium initiates and augments local tissue injury via potent enzyme release and superoxide free-radical formation (50–56). Leukocyte transmigration requires sequential expression of the endothelial cell adhesion receptors P-selectin (45), intercellular adhesion molecule-1 (45), and E-selectin (47), and leukocyte and platelet counter-receptors that differentially mediate PMN leukocyte "rolling," and firm adherence to the endothelium. Mori et al. demonstrated that PMN leukocytes, upon activation, express the surface adhesion β_2-integrin counter-receptor CD18 during experimental focal cerebral ischemia (46). Prereperfusion blockade of CD18 has been shown to preserve microvascular patency (46). The strict temporal and spatial appearance of these adhesion receptors in focal cerebral ischemia supports the transition from immediate ischemic injury to inflammatory response.

Okada et al. demonstrated progressive accumulation by platelets by 24-hour reperfusion in the central ischemic zone (57). It is likely that platelets become activated as part of the ischemic process by thrombin, platelet-activating factor, and other stimuli and may be recruited by collaterals through patent microvessels to the ischemic core where they become activated.

Focal cerebral ischemia also affects the microvascular endothelium, astrocyte end-feet, and the basal lamina by initiating proteolytic events that affect the microvascular structure. Hamann et al. and Wagner et al. described significant reductions in antigens of collagen (type IV), laminin-1, laminin-5, and fibronectin of cellular origin, which comprise the microvascular extracellular matrix and basal lamina after MCA:O (58,59). Hemorrhage, together with loss of microvascular integrity, occurs in regions in which the extracellular matrix and basal lamina antigens are most affected (60). Profound and rapid disruptions in the interactions of endothelial cells and astrocytes with their matrix contacts occur pari passu. Tagaya and others have shown that the number of microvessels displaying integrin subunit $\alpha_1\beta_1$, responsible for the interaction of endothelial cells to laminin-1 and collagen (IV), decrease significantly within 2 hours of MCA:O (47,61), as does the microvascular expression of integrin $\alpha_6\beta_4$, a putative receptor for the adhesion of the astrocyte end-feet to laminin-5 (59). These events occur at the same time as neuron injury (62). It is apparent that the microvasculature undergoes rapid dynamic changes in the ischemic territory very soon after MCA occlusion.

CLINICAL MANIFESTATIONS OF FOCAL CEREBRAL ISCHEMIA

Stroke Subtypes

The efficacy of plasminogen activator exposure appears to vary among the subtypes of ischemic stroke. The identification of each stroke subtype can be made on clinical grounds, as well as with additional diagnostic studies such as angiography, Doppler ultrasonography, CT, magnetic resonance imaging (MRI), and cardiac assessment. Identification of a stroke subtype is not achieved in about 20% of the patients despite these efforts.

There is a difference in the incidence of intracranial in situ thrombosis between the anterior and the posterior circulations (63,64). In the anterior circulation, local thrombosis is rare, whereas embolic events are more frequent. In the posterior circulation, atherosclerotic occlusion is more frequently found in the distal vertebral arteries and the basilar artery, where it constitutes the single most important reason for basilar artery occlusion (65). This is also important with respect to reocclusion frequency. Reocclusion, a prominent problem after thrombolytic therapy in acute myocardial infarction, rarely, if ever, occurs in the carotid territory (25). However, it has been reported after the use of plasminogen activators for basilar artery occlusion (66).

Small vessel disease of the brain parenchyma leading to multiple, small ischemic areas in the basal ganglia and the white matter is usually the result of a local atherosclerotic process of the small perforators, so-called lipohyalinosis. In general, this condition has not been considered amenable to thrombolysis because disease of the small vessels not only leads to microvascular fibrin-containing occlusions, but also may lead to microaneur-

ysms with spontaneous hemorrhages. However, in one recent study, beneficial effects of tissue plasminogen activator (t-PA) were attributed to patients with small arterial disease as well as large arterial disease (39).

Hemorrhagic Transformation

Secondary hemorrhagic infarction and secondary parenchymal hematoma, as well as space-occupying edema, can be detected reliably using CT (Figs. 35-3 and 35-4). MRI has a higher sensitivity for small hemorrhages; however, their clinical relevance may be minimal. Characteristics of distinct secondary hemorrhagic events, which may occur either spontaneously or in consequence of acute treatment after antithrombotic substances, are given in Table 35-2 (6). Clinical deterioration due to secondary hemorrhage is the most important concern of the use of plasminogen activators in this setting. In unselected popula-

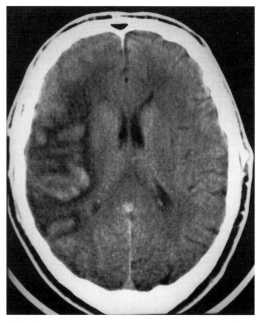

FIG. 35-3. Hemorrhagic infarction (6) of the HI2 type (18). Regions of this MCA infarction display high attenuation signals consistent with hemorrhage. No space-occupying effect is evident (see Table 35-2).

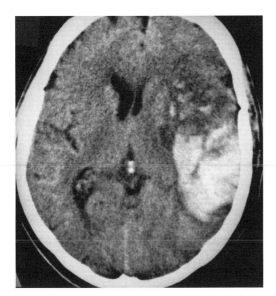

FIG. 35-4. Parenchymal hemorrhage (6) of the PH2 type (18). There is gross, parenchymal hemorrhage in more than 50% of the territory of this MCA territory infarct. A significant space-occupying effect is visible, which is due in part to brain edema but mainly caused by the additional volume of the parenchymal hemorrhage (see Table 35-3).

acute plasminogen activator intervention in ischemic stroke. In one placebo-controlled trial, symptomatic hemorrhage of any degree was seen in 52% of treated patients and 41% of placebo patients (11). A relationship between successful recanalization and the occurrence of hemorrhagic transformation has not definitively been established. Hemorrhagic infarction is restricted to the ischemic zone, whereas approximately 10% of parenchymal hematomas develop in brain areas outside the ischemic zone (6). In one study, clinical deterioration occurred in 54.5% of patients (six of 11) with parenchymal hematoma, but in only 19.1% of patients (four of 21) with hemorrhagic infarction (6). The frequency of hemorrhagic events appears to increase with delayed plasminogen activator administration, that is, 4 to 6 hours and more after treatment onset.

DIAGNOSTIC APPROACHES TO ACUTE ISCHEMIC STROKE

Imaging Techniques in Acute Ischemic Stroke

Primary diagnostic methods for delineating the degree and type of cerebral tissue injury include CT, MRI, and magnetic resonance angiography (MRA). Expertise in the assessment of subtle early infarctions may be essential not only for identification of patients who may be treated with thrombolytic agents, but also in patients with poor prognosis and the risk of hemorrhagic events and herniation.

CT is required to establish the differential diagnosis between a primary intracerebral he-

tions of ischemic stroke patients, a 2% to 4% frequency of spontaneous parenchymal hematoma with clinical deterioration in the development of embolic infarction has been described. In open trials of selected plasminogen activators, the incidence of intracranial hemorrhage with event-related clinical deterioration has varied between 0% and 18% (67). There is no clear correlation between t-PA dose or recanalization and hemorrhagic transformation among the majority of studies of

TABLE 35-2. *Characteristics of hemorrhagic transformation*

	CT scan features	Clinical features
Hemorrhagic Infarction	Patchy areas of high attenuation Indistinct margins Speckled or mottled appearance within region of infarction	Generally clinically silent
Parenchymatous hematoma	Homogeneous area of high attenuation, most often confined to region of infarction May have ventricular extension May have mass effect	More often contributing to clinical deterioration

morrhage and acute ischemic stroke. Other intracranial pathologies, including abscesses, apoplectic gliomas, encephalitis, sinus venous thrombosis, meningiomas and other tumors, and unexpected subarachnoid hemorrhage, may be identified using CT. CT will show evidence of intracerebral hemorrhage as early as 15 to 20 minutes after onset in volumes exceeding 0.5 ml. However, the definite size of the primary hemorrhage will only be assessable when CT is repeated after 6 to 12 hours, because its size is usually underestimated in the initial scan.

CT is required for documentation and assessment of the course of tissue injury. The initial CT scan may show early signs of infarct after hemispheric stroke as early as 2 hours from apparent symptom onset in some patients (68). Approximately 64% of patients with transient ischemic attacks show evidence of an infarction on the initial CT scan (69). Early hemispheric "infarct signs" include (a) focal effacement of the cortical sulci, (b) compression of the insular cistern, (c) focal loss of white/gray matter contrast and loss of internal capsule definition, and (d) slight compression of the lateral ventricles. Early infarct signs do not accurately reflect the final extent of the infarct—most infarcts will prove to be larger. In rare cases the infarct signs are in part reversible and may not represent infarcted tissue, but rather edema. In clinical trials, a second CT scan is required within 24 hours for assessment of hemorrhagic transformation. For final assessment of infarct volume, a repeat CT scan after 4 to 6 days is also recommended. CT is less helpful in detecting early infarct signs in brain stem or cerebellar stroke, although extensive infarcts of the cerebellar hemispheres can be detected. Early focal swelling may compress the fourth ventricle or the aqueduct leading to occlusive hydrocephalus, a sign that will not occur earlier than 24 hours after stroke.

Vascular alterations may be shown by CT. The hyperdense middle cerebral artery (HMCA) sign is present in 30% to 50% of acute internal cerebral artery (ICA)/MCA occlusions if studied within 6 hours of symptom onset (70–72) (Fig. 35-5). It does not always signify poor prognosis, although about 50% of the patients will develop a space-occupying hemispheric infarction. Recently, spiral CT scan technology has allowed CT angiography with some relative assessment of perfusion and collateral integrity, and only minor additional time (Fig. 35-6). However, its value in acute interventions remains to be established.

Magnetic resonance techniques, performed within minutes of ictus, may give information on (a) tissue morphology and early infarct signs, (b) brain perfusion (73,74), (c) arterial patency (by MRA), (d) cellular events (diffusion-weighted imaging [DWI]) (75), and (e) metabolic changes (spectroscopy). MRI and MRA cannot be performed in all acute stroke patients because of (a) the complexity of the examination and (b) problems in monitoring the patients within the magnet bore (76). For patients with slowly developing symptoms, clinical signs of organic brain syndrome, seizures, sinus venous thrombosis, and suspected arterial dissection, MRI and MRA

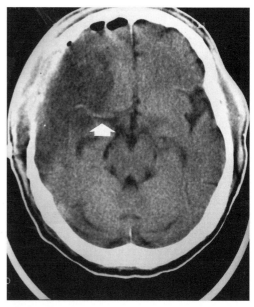

FIG. 35-5. Hyperdense middle cerebral artery (HMCA) sign (*arrow*) and resultant MCA territory infarct.

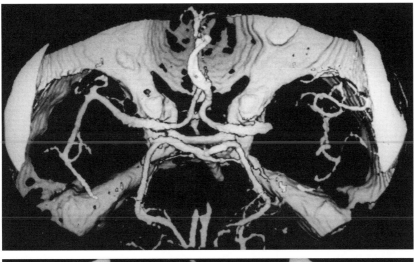

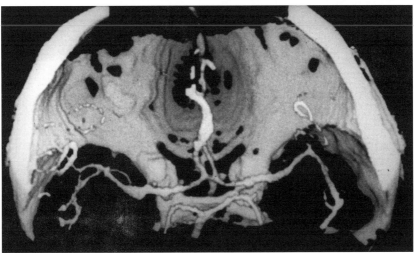

FIG. 35-6. Spiral CT scan definition of arterial events in acute thromboembolic stroke. Occlusion of proximal MCA **(top panel)** before thrombolysis. After intravenous t-PA, near complete reconstitution of MCA patency may be seen **(bottom panel).**

have become the imaging modalities of choice. In the latter condition, intramural hemorrhage can be easily demonstrated. MRA does not depict the vessel anatomy, but rather provides information on flow. Flow voids at regions of high-grade stenoses or pseudo-occlusion may cause overestimates of the degree of stenosis, and the resolution of the technique limits the utility of MRA. Although new and more rapid MR techniques will allow acute studies in severe stroke patients, little experience has been reported so far.

The Relationship of Imaging to Vascular/Tissue Responses

With the exception of obvious correlations between CT-detectable hemorrhagic transformation and the appearance of hemorrhage by gross and microscopic examination, little experimental or clinical correlative work has been reported which demonstrate cellular signatures of injury detectable by CT or MRI modalities at current resolutions. Nonetheless, alterations in DWI detectable by MRI early during experimental focal ischemia may reflect shifts of water in the extravascular compartment, which result from ischemic injury (75). DWI may allow visualization of intracellular disturbances (77). The nature of those shifts remains unclear, however.

MR spectroscopy and MR perfusion imaging may provide information on the physiologic state of the tissue and the ultimate risk of infarction. Fast T2*-weighted techniques combined with bolus application of a paramagnetic contrast agent allow an estimate of "capillary perfusion." In combination with echo-planar imaging techniques, which allow imaging of the whole brain within 200 to 500 milliseconds, absolute quantification of cerebral blood flow will be possible. These techniques have been used to monitor the pathophysiologic changes in experimental acute cerebral ischemia.

General Management of Acute Ischemic Stroke

Given the limited time frame for intervention, the acute stroke patient, even the one with milder symptoms, must be recognized as an urgently ill medical patient (78–80). Rapid evaluation and management of the patient who is a potential candidate for thrombolysis includes neurologic examination, emergency CT to exclude intracerebral hemorrhage and to assess early infarct signs, blood samples for routine laboratory (glucose, electrolytes, coagulation, hematology), Doppler ultrasonography of the carotid and vertebral arteries, and coordination of the critical care unit and angiographic facilities (81).

General treatment strategies to optimize blood oxygenation, pulmonary function, and cardiac output are required. Blood pressure should not be lowered unless systolic pressure exceeds 220 mmHg. Bleeding complications may be more frequent if uncontrolled hypertension is present. Use of plasminogen activators is discouraged if systolic blood pressure exceeds 180 mmHg after oral or parenteral nifedipine (10 mg) or parenteral clonidine (0.15 mg) (in Europe), or intravenous la-

betalol (2 mg/min) (in North America). The actions of nifedipine and clonidine may be rapid and excessive, and often difficult to predict, but subject to ready titration, whereas bradycardia and reduced cardiac output are unusual side effects of labetalol. Sodium nitroprusside may sometimes become necessary despite major side effects, including reflex tachycardia and coronary artery ischemia. For isolated elevation of diastolic blood pressure, nitroglycerine (in Europe) (82) and sodium nitroprusside (in North America) (83) are frequently used. Sodium nitroprusside, hydralazine, and calcium channel blockers have cerebral vasodilating effects and may increase intracerebral pressure (76,83).

The roles of temperature and serum glucose have been underestimated in clinical stroke management, although experimental data clearly show the negative effects of hyperthermia and hyperglycemia on infarct size and outcome (84–86). Normothermia is achieved by (a) simple physical methods including cooling of the legs and thighs, (b) antipyretic agents such as paracetamol or acetaminophen, and (c) early use of antibiotics in infection (e.g., aspiration pneumonia or urinary tract infection). Almost 25% of stroke patients have a pre-existing infection.

Prophylactic use of subcutaneous unfractionated heparin to prevent deep venous thrombosis (DVT) and consequent pulmonary embolism are standard approaches. One recent study suggests that subcutaneous low-dose heparin applied within 48 hours of symptom onset may significantly reduce mortality and disability from the initial stroke by 6 months (87).

ACUTE INTERVENTIONS WITH PLASMINOGEN ACTIVATORS

General Considerations

Evaluations of the safety and efficacy of plasminogen activators in focal cerebral ischemia require quantifiable clinical assessment techniques. Arterial recanalization frequency, regional cerebral blood flow (rCBF), and measures of neurologic function and disability have been applied. None of the neurologic scoring instruments (including the NIH stroke scale [NIHSS] [88–90], the Hemispheric Stroke Scale [HSS] [11], or modifications of specific scales [42]) used in acute ischemic stroke trials have been prospectively validated for long-term outcome (91), although interobserver correlations for some scales have been published (92). Disability outcome measures, including the Rankin scale modified for mortality (37) and the Barthel index (38,93), which have superseded such scoring instruments, also have not yet been prospectively validated as functional outcome measures in acute stroke efficacy trials. The applicability of the statistical methods for evaluation of disability outcome remain open to discussion. However, thrombolysis trials using disability outcome measures have provided a database to validate their utility and appropriateness for acute stroke outcome assessment (17,18).

Occlusion location is important to the facility with which recanalization occurs. Three prospective thrombolytic intervention trials indicate that proximal ICA and carotid T occlusions have a much lower recanalization incidence than do MCA branch lesions to either intravenous or regional thrombolytic infusion (6,11,94). The outcomes of several studies are consistent with the view that thrombus location and volume adversely influence their dissolution by endogenous or therapeutic thrombolysis (15,29,40,41,94–96). SPECT scan investigations have displayed restitution of rCBF in individual patients after plasminogen activator exposure; however, a correlation with outcome has not been consistently obtained (97,98). Ueda et al. have demonstrated that a threshold of rCBF reduction may be determined that correlates with the frequency of hemorrhagic transformation (99). That observation implies that a measure of baseline rCBF during the acute phase of stroke may allow selective withholding of plasminogen activators and potentially improved safety. As noted earlier, disability outcome at 3 months

has become a practical measure of stroke outcome, which lacks the limitations of mortality alone. Early stroke-related mortality has been used as an outcome in a number of acute stroke trials (100–103). Silver and colleagues demonstrated that cerebral edema from large hemispheric ischemic lesions led to transtentorial herniation and death in 36 of 46 patients (78%) who died in the first 7 days after the onset of stroke symptoms (104). This is consistent with the large number of fatal events (82%) in one retrospective pathology study (105).

Requirements for Treatment

Clinical Requirements

Elements relevant to treatment of focal cerebral ischemia with plasminogen activators include (a) time from symptom onset to treatment, (b) symptom severity, (c) stroke subtype, (d) age, and (e) otherwise formal contraindications to the treatment with plasminogen activators. Time from symptom onset to possible treatment is probably the most important qualifying clinical feature. Onset–treatment intervals range from almost 3 hours to 6 hours (6). Another important aspect is stroke severity because very mild stroke syndromes may improve completely with or without therapy. This supports the current exclusion of very mild stroke symptoms from thrombolytic intervention by a majority of investigators. More problematic is the margin between mild and moderate ischemic symptoms. Clearly, there is no role for thrombolytic intervention in completed stroke (18), that is, conditions characterized by a dense, complete hemiplegia, forced eye deviation, early somnolence and drowsiness, and, if the dominant hemisphere is involved, global aphasia. These patients frequently present with extended early infarct signs on CT scan (106). In addition to little if any benefit from thrombolytic intervention, they are at substantially increased risk for secondary hemorrhagic complications. Recent plasminogen activator studies exclude patients with the most severe stroke subtype from the trial (6,11,17,18). No prospective study has examined the effects of age on outcome. In some studies, treatment has been restricted to those under 80 years of age (18,101). Post hoc analyses have suggested age-related poor outcomes for thresholds at 75 years. Otherwise, known contraindications (e.g., recent trauma, intracranial neoplasms) to the use of plasminogen activators in cardiovascular disease apply (107).

Imaging Modalities

Pretreatment CT is mandatory to exclude intracranial hemorrhage as the underlying pathology of the stroke syndrome. Severe stroke with proximal vessel occlusion and scarce collaterals frequently appear as regions of low attenuation or early space occupying edema on the initial CT scan. Individuals showing large areas of hypodensity (more than 33% of the affected territory) early should not be treated with thrombolytic substances because such lesions correlate significantly with the extent of the infarct on follow-up CT scans. Recent analyses suggest that both secondary space-occupying lesions and hemorrhagic transformation might be associated with extended early infarct signs (18).

Modern spiral CT technology and MR techniques have not yet been featured in acute patient assessment because standard CT examinations can be performed more rapidly and less expensively. In few instances, perfusion and diffusion MR studies and MRA have been applied in acute stroke, but none have been tested prospectively in the setting of acute stroke therapy. PET studies have been used in the follow-up of patients receiving plasminogen activators.

Focal Cerebral Ischemia

Completed Stroke

There is no role for the use of plasminogen activators in completed stroke or "stroke in evolution." Although a small group of angiography-based studies demonstrated recanal-

ization after plasminogen activator application, clinical benefit was not formally tested (13,14,108–111). The frequency of symptomatic intracerebral hemorrhages in those trials supported the viewpoint that the use of fibrinolytic agents for stroke was unsafe and not clinically efficacious. A general contraindication of their use in stroke patients ensued (107). Since that time, a number of weaknesses of those studies have been addressed (15): (a) treatment is now initiated less than 6 hours from symptom onset; (b) stringent selection of patients with symptoms referable to arterial occlusions is recommended; (c) patients with completed stroke are excluded; (d) CT scanning techniques to rule out intracerebral hemorrhage as a cause of stroke are routinely applied; (e) there is a growing appreciation of the vascular natural history of each stroke subtype; and (f) the dose-rate/duration of plasminogen activator infusion has been applied in acceptable study design format.

Acute Thrombotic/Thromboembolic Stroke

With the appreciation from experimental focal ischemia studies that a finite interval after cessation of blood flow beyond which significant irreversible ischemic neuronal damage and sustained neurologic deficit occurs (22-24), and early experience in acute myocardial infarction management, the potential use of plasminogen activators in thrombotic and thromboembolic stroke received a practical basis. A practical clinical limit to treatment takes this interval in humans as 3 to 6 hours for clinical trial design.

Trials with Angiographic Selection and Intra-arterial Delivery

Intra-arterial studies have established the feasibility of cerebral arterial recanalization in acute thrombotic stroke patients (13,112–117). Larger prospective open trials of regional or local infusion of urokinase plasminogen activator (u-PA) or streptokinase (SK) have documented recanalization of acute carotid artery territory or vertebrobasilar artery territory occlusions (40,41,94,112,118–121).

Arterial recanalization has been reported in 46% to 100% of acutely treated patients with carotid territory focal ischemia. For instance, among 125 patients treated locally with u-PA, SK, or t-PA from four prospective open studies, 90 (72.0%) displayed arterial recanalization (Table 35-3) (40,41,118,119). Zeumer et al., del Zoppo et al., and Mori et al. demonstrated the feasibility of recanalization in carotid artery territory occlusions (40,94,113), the safety of angiographic techniques applied in the acute phase, the benign outcome of hemorrhagic infarction occurring during the period of thrombolysis (40), and that recanalization was associated with significant reduction in the infarction volume by CT (94). ICA occlusions were more resistant to recanalization than were distal MCA obstructions (41,94). Zeumer et al. indicated recanalization efficacy in the carotid artery with u-PA (40) and t-PA (alteplase) (112,122), in the vertebrobasilar artery (122), and in ophthalmic artery circulation (123). Ohtaki et al. and many others in Japan have demonstrated the feasibility of recanalization of symptomatic occlusions of the carotid and vertebrobasilar artery with either u-PA or t-PA by direct superselective intraarterial delivery in the acute setting (124).

Hemorrhagic transformation occurred in 20.0% to 32.5% of treated patients in four studies (40,41,118,119), excluding the report by Zeumer et al. (122). This frequency is consistent with that observed in other trials of proximal MCA occlusion. Ohtaki et al. experienced one hemorrhage in an M1 MCA occlusion (3.9%), whereas hemorrhagic transformation occurred in five of 26 MCA patients (19.2%) and two of 13 ICA patients (15.2%) by 24 hours (124–127). Overall, the incidence of parenchymal hematoma (mostly symptomatic) has not exceeded 11% in a single study.

Whether the frequency of hemorrhage might be different from the natural history requires placebo-controlled phase III prospective trials. The PROACT (Prolyse for Acute Cerebral Thromboembolism) trial compared recombinant pro-urikinase (rpro-UK) with placebo in a two-part, double-blinded, prospective dose-rate phase I/II study format. The trial was terminated after the 6-mg dose tier by the sponsor to review the data. An increase in 2-hour recanalization was associated with rpro-UK over placebo when the mode of delivery was controlled. Both recanalization frequency and hemorrhagic transformation were directly dependent on heparin dose (128).

TABLE 35-3. *Trials of acute carotid territory ischemia with angiographic selection*

	Agent	Patients	Recanalization		Hemorrhage with deterioration			
			N	%	Nil	HI	PH	%
Intra-arterial delivery								
del Zoppo (40)	SK/u-PA	20	18	90.0	16	4	0	0.0
Mori (41)	u-PA	22	10	45.5	18	1	3	13.6
Theron (118)	SK/u-PA	12	12	100.0	9	1	2	16.6
Matsumoto (119)	u-PA	40	24	60.0	27	9	4	—
Zeumer (122)	t-PA[a]/u-PA	31	29	93.5	25	6	0	0.0
Intravenous delivery								
del Zoppo (6)	t-PA[b]	93 (104)	32	34.4	72	21	11	9.6
Mori (11)	t-PA[b]	19	9	47.4	9	8	2	10.5
	C	12	2	16.7	7	4	1	0.0
von Kummer (25)	t-PA[a]	22	13	59.1	14	6	2	11.1
Yamaguchi (42)	t-PA[b]	47 (51)	10	21.3	27	20	4	7.8
	C	46 (47)	2	4.4	25	17	5	10.6

Numbers in parentheses, patients receiving any t-PA—intention to treat; C, control (placebo); HI, hemorrhagic infarction; PH, parenchymatous hematoma.
[a]Alteplase.
[b]Duteplase.

Trials with Angiographic Selection and Intravenous Delivery

Recanalization frequencies of 21.3% to 59.1%, of a total of 181 patients receiving t-PA, have been reported among five prospective angiography-based trials of intravenous t-PA (Table 35-3) (6,11,25,42,129). In an open prospective multicenter dose-escalation study of t-PA (duteplase) (6), recanalization at 60 minutes occurred in 34.4% of 93 patients across nine dose rates from 0.12 MIU/kg to 0.75 MIU/kg. Mori et al. in a three-arm, placebo-controlled, double-blind pilot trial demonstrated that immediate recanalization and clinical outcome at 30 days (inverted HSS) were significantly better in 19 subjects receiving 30 MIU (0.5 MIU/kg/60 min) than in 12 treated with placebo or 20 MIU (25). Interestingly, no significant change in outcome at 24 to 48 hours was observed. Yamaguchi et al. reported similar results in a multicenter placebo-controlled trial comparing 20 MIU t-PA (duteplase) in 47 patients with matched placebo in 46 patients (42). A prospective blinded comparison of the efficacy of 20 MIU versus 30 MIU per patient demonstrated equal neurologic recovery (16).

The frequency of hemorrhagic transformation was not different from that reported for intra-arterial infusion in the carotid territory (6,11,25,42,129). In the dose-rate escalation study, hemorrhagic infarction occurred in 20.2% and parenchymal hematoma in 10.6% of 104 treated patients (6,12). Parenchymal hematoma was typically lobar in distribution and usually (90.9%) confined to the region of ischemia (6,12). There was no relationship between hemorrhagic transformation and 60-minute recanalization, rt-PA dose rate, pretreatment exposure to antiplatelet agents, or pretreatment blood pressure (6). In the placebo-controlled trial of Mori et al., one parenchymal hematoma was observed in each of the t-PA/placebo groups although neurologic deterioration occurred only in the rt-PA groups (25). Yamaguchi et al. noted massive hemorrhage in 7.8% and 10.6% of patients in the t-PA group and placebo group, respec-

tively (42). The frequency of hemorrhagic transformation with neurologic deterioration ranged from 9.6% to 11.1% of a total of 196 patients (6,11,25), and overall among all angiography-based trials was about 10%.

Acute Ischemic Stroke

In the absence of angiographic evidence of cerebral arterial occlusion, stroke patients have been selected for treatment with thrombolytic substances on the basis of symptoms (and CT evidence) consistent with focal cerebral ischemia in the absence of cerebral hemorrhage.

Symptom-Based Clinical Trials with Intravenous Delivery

Three symptom-based, randomized, placebo-controlled trials of SK in acute ischemic stroke have exposed important concerns about risks of intracerebral hemorrhage (Table 35-4). Each study used a single intravenous infusion of 1.5×10^6 IU SK in the active arm. Hommel et al. described early termination of the Multicenter Acute Stroke Trial-Europe (MAST-E), a comparison of intravenous SK with placebo within 6 hours of the onset of MCA territory symptoms, when 10-day (p < 0.001) and 6-month (p < 0.01) mortality in the SK group significantly exceeded that of the placebo group (101). The incidence of symptomatic intracranial hemorrhage (24 of 135 [18.5%] versus 4 of 133 [3.0%]; p < 0.001) also was significantly higher in the SK group. Both findings were probably due to the increased severity of stroke patients entered into this trial. This was suggested by the high short-term mortality in the placebo group (18.1%). Interim analysis of adverse outcome after 300 patients entered within 4 hours of acute ischemic stroke in the Australia Streptokinase (ASK) trial, prompted the safety monitoring committee to advise termination of the >3-hour arm because of significant increased mortality or disability among patients in that arm (102). No apparent safety concern was

TABLE 35-4. *Randomized controlled trials of thrombolysis in acute ischemic stroke without angiographic selection*

	Agent	Patients	Treatment, Δ (T-0) hr	Clinical improvement (%)	Hemorrhage			
					Nil	HI	PH	%
MAST-E (136)	SK	156	<6.0	35.0	88	25	24	17.5
	C	154		18.1	116	13	4	0.3
ASK (137)	SK	106	<4.0	43.4				
	C	122		22.1				
MAST-I (100)	SK	313	<6.0	26.5	232	60	21	6.7
	C	309		11.7	280	27	2	0.7
ECASS (18)	t-PA	313	<6.0	35.9	179	72	62	19.8
	C	307		29.3	184	93	30	6.5
NINDS 1 (138)	t-PA	144	≤1.5, ≤3.0	1.2[a]	—		13	5.6
	C	147			—		3	0.0
NINDS 2	t-PA	168	≤1.5, ≤3.0	50[b], 31[c]	—		21	7.1
	C	165		38[b], 20[c]	—		8	2.1

Δ(T-0), time from symptom onset to treatment; HI, hemorrhagic infarction; PH, parenchymatous hematoma; SK, streptokinase; t-PA, tissue plasminogen activator (alteplase); C, control.
[a] Relative risk reduction.
[b] Barthel index.
[c] NIHSS.

observed for patients treated in the 0- to 3-hour window. Those findings are reminiscent of the earlier findings of Meyer et al. regarding the safety of SK in stroke (108). The Multicentre Acute Stroke Trial-Italy (MAST-I) terminated their trial of acute intravenous SK ± aspirin (ASA) within 6 hours of symptom onset after only 622 patients were entered (100,130). An excess 10-day case fatality frequency was associated with SK ± ASA ($2p < 0.00001$), most particularly when SK was given with ASA ($2p < 0.00001$) (100). A proper dose-finding study to arrive at a safe SK dose was not performed before any of those trials. The dose used reflected the dose for acute myocardial infarction (131,132).

A prospective two-part, four-armed, placebo-controlled disability outcome trial of t-PA (0.9 mg/kg) in acute ischemic stroke sponsored by the National Institutes of Neurological Diseases and Stroke (NINDS) with entry stratification of ≤90 minutes and 91 to 180 minutes from symptom onset reported an 11% to 13% increase in the number of patients with normal neurologic status at 3 months (133). In part 1, among 291 patients randomized to t-PA or placebo, no difference in NIHSS status at 24 hours was observed. In part 2, rt-PA recipients displayed a significant 11% to 13% absolute improvement over placebo in minimal or no disability (neurologic deficit) according to the Barthel index, modified Rankin scale score, Glasgow outcome scale score, and NIHSS at 3 months follow-up. No difference in mortality was observed. The observed benefit was seen in patients with the presumed stroke subtypes of small arterial disease, large arterial disease, or cardioembolic origin (17).

The frequency of cerebral hemorrhage with neurologic symptoms, however, was significantly greater among those patients treated with t-PA than with placebo (6.4% versus 0.6%, $2p < 0.001$). Symptomatic hemorrhage contributed significantly to mortality within the t-PA group at 3 months. Although the reasons for the lower frequency of symptomatic hemorrhage in the placebo group (0.6%) compared with literature reports (6,11,12) are not clear, they cannot be attributed to earlier arrival to the hospital setting or CT evaluation, or to more severe initial neurologic status. In any event, one possible common theme is the contribution of collateral patency during early focal ischemia to maintain perfusion of the ischemic vascular bed.

The European Cooperative Acute Stroke Study (ECASS), a prospective phase III, symptom-based, randomized study, compared 3-month disability outcomes and mortality in patients treated within 6 hours of symptom onset with intravenous infusion t-PA (1.1 mg/kg, maximum 100 mg) or placebo over 1 hour (18). Prospectively applied rules sought to exclude patients with evidence of large regions of hemispheric injury (early signs of ischemia) by neuroradiographic criteria. Intention-to-treat analysis demonstrated no apparent difference between the rt-PA and placebo-treated groups in neurologic status at 24 hours, with regard to median (or best outcome) Barthel index and modified Rankin scale scores at 90 days, or cumulative 90-day mortality. A mandated post hoc assessment of baseline CT scans in all patients defined a population with hemispheric injury not apparent to investigators on admission. Among 109 patients who were to be excluded, 66 (60.6%) had CT scan changes including the presence of major early infarct signs. These contributed to the substantial reduction in efficacy in this trial. When that group was eliminated from the analysis, a significant increase in median (or best outcome) Barthel index and modified Rankin scale score was derived. A significantly higher proportion of patients with intracerebral hemorrhage causing neurologic deterioration or death occurred with rt-PA (19 of 313) compared with placebo (seven of 307). A singular interpretation of these data is that the lack of benefit in functional outcome and neurologic recovery was "driven" by a subgroup of patients with clinically significant early cerebral injury at increased risk for hemorrhage or further deterioration after intravenous thrombolysis. The overall analysis suggested that when a subgroup of patients (e.g., with early infarct signs) at high risk for poor outcome or hemorrhage would be excluded, 90-day disability outcome would be favorably affected. Defining the subgroup or subgroups represented by the excluded patients is of major importance to the application of this approach within 6 hours from symptom onset.

Summary

The feasibility and efficacy of plasminogen activators, applied within the early hours of ischemic stroke, to improve 90-day outcome follows on a substantial body of experimental and clinical work that has demonstrated the relevance and safety of this approach. Taken together, the ECASS and NINDS studies indicate the enormous importance of patient selection to reduce the hemorrhagic risk attendant to the use of plasminogen activators in stroke (17,18). Both studies suggest that at the current state, CT scans and neurologic scores at study entry do not completely identify those at risk for hemorrhage, although proper attention to the presence and extent of ischemic injury on initial CT scan is likely to address hemorrhagic risk in part. However, it is currently not possible to separate benefit from hemorrhagic risk in a given patient based on simple clinical criteria. The experience of those studies suggests that poor neurologic status at outset and reduced rCBF may reflect cerebral tissue injury, which contributes to significant neuroparenchymal hemorrhage with deterioration upon exposure to plasminogen activators. ECASS-2, a follow-up study in progress, uses t-PA at 0.9 mg/kg/60 min and will test the hypothesis that increased clinical acumen at detecting early ischemic signs by CT can enhance favorable outcome. Criteria for patient treatment (in the experimental setting) require a short interval from symptom onset to treatment and the absence of apparent tissue injury on initial CT scan.

ACUTE INTERVENTION WITH DEFIBRINATING AGENTS

One report has appeared supporting the safety of the defibrinating agent ancrod in acute ischemic stroke when a reduction in fibrinogen of 100 mg/dl was maintained (134). A phase III study in acute stroke is in progress.

CONCLUSION

The experimental and clinical use of plasminogen activators in acute ischemic stroke has exposed the importance of vascular integrity to functional recovery.

1. Recanalization of carotid and vertebrobasilar arterial territory occlusion has been shown to be technically feasible within 3 to 6 hours of symptom onset.
2. However, the optimal plasminogen activator, its dose rate, and delivery system have yet to be defined in either arterial territory.
3. Complete thrombotic occlusions of the cervical ICA appear more resistant to thrombolysis than occlusions of the stem and major branches of the MCA. Early clinical studies suggested that recanalization was associated with a decrease in infarct volume by CT assessment. Two prospective phase III trials, the ECASS and the NINDS studies, indicate the range of clinical outcomes achievable and central risks to the use of plasminogen activators in acute focal cerebral ischemia.
4. Any potential benefit with t-PA in a stroke population was nullified by the treatment of patients with subtle signs of ischemic injury on CT scan (ECASS).
5. Treatment of acute ischemic stroke patients within 3 hours of symptom onset was associated with improvement in outcome (NINDS) and has led to recommendations for use (135).
6. Phase III trials of intravenous SK in carotid territory stroke demonstrated increased mortality in some patients consistent with increased stroke severity and/or excessive SK dosage. Hemorrhagic transformation accompanies the use of fibrinolytic agents.
7. The frequency of hemorrhagic infarction and parenchymal hematoma formation is significantly increased by delayed intervention, diastolic hypertension, dose, and the presence of severe ischemia on baseline CT scan.
8. In one group of selected ischemic stroke patients, although t-PA was shown to significantly increase the number of patients with minimal to no neurologic residua

treated within 3 hours of symptom onset (NINDS), the hemorrhagic risk also contributed significantly to mortality.
9. Future efforts must be directed to the reduction of this risk.

ACKNOWLEDGMENT

This work was supported in part by grant NS 26945 of the National Institutes of Neurological Diseases and Stroke.

REFERENCES

1. Mohr JP, Caplan LR, Melski JW, et al. The Harvard Cooperative Stroke Registry: a prospective registry of patients hospitalized with stroke. *Neurology* 1978;28: 754–762.
2. Sacco RL, Wolf PA, Kannel WB, McNamara PM. Survival and recurrence following stroke: the Framingham Study. *Stroke* 1982;13:290–295.
3. Mohr JP, Barnett HJM. Classification of ischemic strokes. In: Barnett HJM, Stein BM, Mohr JP, Yatsu FM (eds). *Stroke: Pathophysiology, Diagnosis and Management.* Vol. 1. New York: Churchill Livingstone, 1986;281–291.
4. DeWood MA, Spores J, Notske R, et al. Prevalence of total coronary occlusion during the early hours of transmural myocardial infarction. *N Engl J Med* 1980; 303:897–902.
5. Fieschi C, Argentino C, Lenzi GL, Sacchetti ML, Toni D, Bozzao L. Clinical and instrumental evaluation of patients with ischemic stroke within the first six hours. *J Neurol Sci* 1989;91:311–321.
6. del Zoppo GJ, Poeck K, Pessin MS, et al. Recombinant tissue plasminogen activator in acute thrombotic and embolic stroke. *Ann Neurol* 1992;32:78–86.
7. Solis OJ, Roberson GR, Taveras JM, Mohr J, Pessin MS. Cerebral angiography in acute cerebral infarction. *Rev Interam Radiol* 1977;2:19–25.
8. Fieschi C, Bozzao L. Transient embolic occlusion of the middle cerebral and internal carotid arteries in cerebral apoplexy. *J Neurol Neurosurg Psychiatry* 1969;32:236–240.
9. Irino T, Taneda M, Minami T. Angiographic manifestations in post-recanalized cerebral infarction. *Neurology* 1977;27:471–475.
10. Yamaguchi T, Minematsu K, Choki J, Ikeda M. Clinical and neuroradiological analysis of thrombotic and embolic cerebral infarction. *Jpn Circ J* 1984;48: 50–58.
11. Mori E, Yoneda Y, Tabuchi M, et al. Intravenous recombinant tissue plasminogen activator in acute carotid artery territory stroke. *Neurology* 1992;42: 976–982.
12. Yamaguchi T, Hayakawa T, Kikuchi H. Intravenous tissue plasminogen activator ameliorates the outcome of hyperacute embolic stroke. *Cerebrovasc Dis* 1993;3: 269–272.
13. Clarke RL, Cliffton EE. The treatment of cerebrovas-

cular thrombosis and embolism with fibrinolytic agents. *Am J Cardiol* 1960;30:546–551.

14. Sussman BJ, Fitch TSP. Thrombolysis with fibrinolysin in cerebral arterial occlusion. *JAMA* 1958;167:1705–1709.

15. del Zoppo GJ, Zeumer H, Harker LA. Thrombolytic therapy in acute stroke: possibilities and hazards. *Stroke* 1986;17:595–607.

16. Yamaguchi T, Kikuchi H, Hayakawa T, for the Japanese Thrombolysis Study Group. Clinical efficacy and safety of intravenous tissue plasminogen activator in acute embolic stroke: a randomized, double-blind, dose-comparison study of duteplase. In: Yamaguchi T, Mori E, Minematsu K, del Zoppo GJ (eds). *Thrombolysis in Acute Ischemic Stroke III.* Tokyo: Springer-Verlag, 1995;223–229.

17. The National Institute of Neurological Disorders and Stroke rt-PA Stroke Study Group. Tissue plasminogen activator for acute ischemic stroke. *N Engl J Med* 1995;333:1581–1587.

18. Hacke W, Kaste M, Fieschi C, et al. Intravenous thrombolysis with recombinant tissue plasminogen activator for acute hemispheric stroke. The European Cooperative Acute Stroke Study (ECASS). *JAMA* 1995;274:1017–1025.

19. Pilz P, Ladurner G, Griebnitz E. Neuropathological findings after thrombolytic therapy in acute ischemic stroke. In: Hacke W, del Zoppo GJ, Hirschberg M (eds). Thrombolytic Therapy in Acute Ischemic Stroke. Heidelberg: Springer-Verlag, 1991;224–227.

20. Hacke W. Thrombolysis, stroke subtypes and embolus type. In: del Zoppo GJ, Hacke W (eds). *Thrombolytic Therapy in Acute Stroke II.* Heidelberg: Springer-Verlag, 1993;151–159.

21. Schoenberg BS, Schulte BPM. Cerebrovascular disease: epidemiology and geopathology. In: Vinken PJ, Bruyn GW, Klawans HL, Toole JF (eds). *Handbook of Clinical Neurology, Vascular Diseases Part 1.* Amsterdam: Elsevier, 1988;1–26.

22. Astrup J, Symon L, Branston NM, Lassen N. Cortical evoked potential and extracellular K- and H- at critical levels of brain ischemia. *Stroke* 1977;8:51–57.

23. Astrup J, Siesjö BK, Symon L. Thresholds in cerebral ischemia—the ischemic penumbra. *Stroke* 1981;12:723–725.

24. Skyhoj-Olsen T, Larsen B, Herring M, Skawer EB, Lassen NA. Blood flow and vascular reactivity in collateral perfused brain tissue: evidence of an ischemic penumbra. *Stroke* 1983;14:332–341.

25. von Kummer R, Hacke W. Safety and efficacy of intravenous tissue plasminogen activator and heparin in acute middle cerebral artery. *Stroke* 1992;23:646–652.

26. Powers WJ. The ischemic penumbra: usefulness of PET. In: del Zoppo GJ, Mori E, Hacke W (eds). *Thrombolytic Therapy in Acute Ischemic Stroke II.* Heidelberg: Springer-Verlag, 1993;17–21.

27. Garcia JH, Yoshida Y, Chen H, et al. Progression from ischemic injury to infarct following middle cerebral artery occlusion in the rat. *Am J Pathol* 1993;142:623–635.

28. Baron JC, von Kummer R, del Zoppo GJ. Treatment of acute ischemic stroke. Challenging the concept of a rigid and universal time window [Editorial]. *Stroke* 1995;26:2219–2221.

29. Saito I, Segawa H, Shiokawa Y, Taniguchi M, Tsutsumi

K. Middle cerebral artery occlusion: correlation of computed tomography and angiography with clinical outcome. *Stroke* 1987;18:863–868.

30. Fisher CM. The natural history of middle cerebral artery trunk occlusion. In: Austin GM (ed). *Microneurosurgical Anastomoses for Cerebral Ischemia.* Springfield: Charles C Thomas, 1976;146–154.

31. The International Stroke Trial Collaborative Group. The International Stroke Trial. Preliminary results. Part II: effects of heparin [Abstract]. *Stroke* 1997;28:231.

32. Whisnant JP, Matsumoto N, Elveback LR. Transient cerebral ischemic attacks in a community, Rochester, Minnesota, 1955 through 1969. *Mayo Clin Proc* 1973;48:194–198.

33. The UK-TIA Study Group. United Kingdom transient ischaemic attack (UK-TIA) aspirin trial: interim results. *Br Med J* 1988;1:316–320.

34. Scandinavian Stroke Study Group. Multicenter trial of hemodilution in ischemic stroke—background and study protocol. *Stroke* 1985;16:885–890.

35. Coté R, Hachinski VC, Shurtell BL, Norris JW, Wolfson C. The Canadian Neurological Scale: a preliminary study in acute stroke. *Stroke* 1986;17:731–737.

36. Wityk RJ, Pessin MS, Kaplan RF, Caplan LR. Serial assessment of acute stroke using the NIH stroke scale. *Stroke* 1994;25:362–365.

37. Rankin J. Cerebral vascular accidents in patients over the age of 60. II. Prognosis. *Scott Med J* 1957;2:200–215.

38. Loewen SC, Anderson BA. Reliability of the modified motor assessment scale and the Barthel index. *Phys Ther* 1988;68:1077–1081.

39. The NINDS rt-PA Stroke Study Group. Tissue plasminogen activator for acute ischemic stroke. *N Engl J Med* 1995;333:1581–1587.

40. del Zoppo GJ, Ferbert A, Otis S, et al. Local intra-arterial fibrinolytic therapy in acute carotid territory stroke: a pilot study. *Stroke* 1988;19:307–313.

41. Mori E, Tabuchi M, Yoshida T, Yamadori A. Intracarotid urokinase with thromboembolic occlusion of the middle cerebral artery. *Stroke* 1988;19:802–812.

42. Yamaguchi T. Intravenous tissue plasminogen activator in acute thromboembolic stroke: a placebo-controlled, double-blind trial. In: del Zoppo GJ, Mori E, Hacke W (eds). *Thrombolytic Therapy in Acute Ischemic Stroke II.* Heidelberg: Springer-Verlag, 1993;59–65.

43. Hallenbeck JM, Dutka AJ, Tanishima T, et al. Polymorphonuclear leukocyte accumulation in brain regions with low blood flow during the early postischemic period. *Stroke* 1986;17:246–253.

44. del Zoppo GJ, Schmid-Schönbein GW, Mori E, Copeland BR, Chang C-M. Polymorphonuclear leukocytes occlude capillaries following middle cerebral artery occlusion and reperfusion in baboons. *Stroke* 1991;22:1276–1283.

45. Okada Y, Copeland BR, Mori E, Tung MM, Thomas WS, del Zoppo GJ. P-selectin and intercellular adhesion molecule-1 expression after focal brain ischemia and reperfusion. *Stroke* 1994;25:202–211.

46. Mori E, Chambers JD, Copeland BR, Arfors KE, del Zoppo GJ. Inhibition of polymorphonuclear leukocyte adherence suppresses non-reflow after focal cerebral ischemia. *Stroke* 1992;23:712–718.

47. Haring HP, Berg EL, Tsurushita N, Tagaya M, del

Zoppo GJ. E-selectin appears in non-ischemic tissue during experimental focal cerebral ischemia. *Stroke* 1996;27:1386–1392.

48. Dereski MO, Chopp M, Knight RA, Chen H, Garcia JH. Focal cerebral ischemia in the rat: temporal profile of neutrophil responses. *Neurosci Res Commun* 1992; 11:179–186.

49. Garcia JH, Liu KF, Yoshida Y, Lian J, Chen S, del Zoppo GJ. Influx of leukocytes and platelets in an evolving brain infarct (Wistar rat). *Am J Pathol* 1994; 144:188–199.

50. Babior BM, Curnutte JT, McMurrich BJ. The particulate superoxide-forming system from human neutrophils: properties of the system and further evidence supporting its participation in the respiratory burst. *J Clin Invest* 1976;58:989–996.

51. McIntyre TM, Patel KD, Zimmerman GA, Prescott SM. Oxygen radical-mediated leukocyte adherence. In: Granger DN, Schmid-Schönbein GW (eds). *Physiology and Pathophysiology of Leukocyte Adhesion.* New York: Oxford University Press, 1995;261–277.

52. Suematsu M, Schmid-Schönbein GW, Chavez-Chavez RH, et al. In vivo visualization of oxidative changes in microvessels during neutrophil activation. *Am J Physiol* 1993;264:H881–H891.

53. Grisham MB, Gaginella TS, Von Ritter C, Tamai H, Be RM, Granger DN. Effects of neutrophil-derived oxidants on intestinal permeability, electrolyte transport, and epithelial cell viability. *Inflammation* 1990;14: 531–542.

54. Whatley RE, Nelson P, Zimmerman GA, et al. The regulation of platelet-activating factor production in endothelial cells—the role of calcium and protein kinase C. *J Biol Chem* 1989;264:6325–6333.

55. Patel KD, Zimmerman GA, Prescott SM, McEver RP, McIntyre TM. Oxygen radicals induce human endothelial cells to express GMP-140 and bind neutrophils. *J Cell Biol* 1991;112:749–759.

56. Zimmerman GA, McIntyre TM, Mehra M, Prescott SM. Endothelial cell-associated platelet-activating factor: a novel mechanism for signaling intercellular adhesion. *J Cell Biol* 1990;110:529–540.

57. Okada Y, Copeland BR, Fitridge R, Koziol JA, del Zoppo GJ. Fibrin contributes to microvascular obstructions and parenchymal changes during early focal cerebral ischemia and reperfusion. *Stroke* 1994;25: 1847–1854.

58. Hamann CF, Okada Y, Fitridge R, del Zoppo GJ. Microvascular basal lamina antigens disappear during cerebral ischemia and reperfusion. *Stroke* 1995;26: 2120–2126.

59. Wagner S, Tagaya M, Koziol JA, Quaranta V, del Zoppo GJ. Rapid disruption of an astrocyte interaction with the extracellular matrix mediated by $\alpha_6\beta_4$ during focal cerebral ischemia/reperfusion. *Stroke* 1997;28: 858–865.

60. Hamann GF, Okada Y, del Zoppo GJ. Hemorrhagic transformation and microvascular integrity during focal cerebral ischemia/reperfusion. *J Cereb Blood Flow Metab* 1996;16:1373–1378.

61. del Zoppo GJ, Haring HP, Tagaya M, Wagner S, Akamine P, Hamann GF. Loss of $\alpha_1\beta_1$ integrin immunoreactivity on cerebral microvessels and astrocytes following focal cerebral ischemia/reperfusion [Abstract]. *Cerebrovasc Dis* 1996;6:9.

62. Tagaya M, Liu KF, Copeland B, et al. DNA scission following focal brain ischemia: temporal differences in two species. *Stroke* 1997;28:1245–1254.

63. Caplan LR. Vertebrobasilar occlusive disease. In: Barnett HS, Mohr J, Stein B, Yatsu F (eds). *Stroke. Pathophysiology, Diagnosis and Management.* New York: Churchill Livingstone, 1986;549–619.

64. Brückmann H, Ferbert A, del Zoppo GJ, Hacke W, Zeumer H. Acute vertebral basilar thrombosis: Angiologic-clinical comparison and therapeutic implications. *Acta Radiol* 1986;369:28–42.

65. Brückmann H, Ferbert A, del Zoppo GJ, Hacke W, Zeumer H. Acute vertebral-basilar thrombosis: angiologic-clinical comparison and therapeutic implications. *Acta Radiol* 1987;369(suppl):3842.

66. Brandt T, von Kummer R, Müller-Kuppers M, Hacke W. Thrombolytic therapy of acute basilar artery occlusion: variables affecting recanalization and outcome. *Stroke* 1996;27:875–881.

67. del Zoppo GJ, Pessin MS, Mori E, Hacke W. Thrombolytic intervention in acute thrombotic and embolic stroke. *Semin Neurol* 1991;11:368–384.

68. von Kummer R, Meyding-Lamade U, Forsting M, et al. Sensitivity and prognostic value of early CT in occlusion of the middle cerebral artery trunk. *AJNR* 1994;15:9–15.

69. Caplan LR. Are terms such as completed stroke or RIND of continued usefulness? *Stroke* 1983;14: 431–433.

70. Gacs G, Fox AJ, Barnett HJ, Vinuela F. CT visualization of intracranial arterial thromboembolism. *Stroke* 1983;14:756–762.

71. Tomsick T, Brott T, Barsan W, Broderick J, Haley ECJ, Spiller J. Thrombus localization with emergency cerebral CT. *AJNR* 1992;13:257–263.

72. Wolpert SM, Bruckmann H, Greenlee R, Wechsler L, Pessin MS, del Zoppo GJ, and the rt-PA Acute Stroke Study Group. The neuroradiologic evaluation of patients with acute stroke treated with recombinant tissue plasminogen activator. *AJNR* 1993;14:313.

73. Moseley ME, Wedland MF, Kuchorczyk J. Magnetic resonance imaging of diffusion and perfusion. *Top Magn Reson Imaging* 1991;3:50–67.

74. Forsting M, Reith W, Dörfler A, von Kummer R, Hacke W, Sartor K. MRI in acute cerebral ischaemia: perfusion imaging with superparamagnetic iron oxide in a rat model. *Neuroradiology* 1994;36:23–26.

75. Minematsu K, Li L, Fisher M, et al. Diffusion weighted magnetic resonance imaging: rapid and quantitative detection of focal brain ischemia. *Neurology* 1992;42:235–240.

76. Kanal E, Shellock FG. Policies, guidelines and recommendations for MR-imaging safety and patient management. *J Magn Reson Imaging* 1992;2: 247–248.

77. Warach S, Gaa J, Siewert B, Wielopolski P, Edelman RR. Acute human stroke studied by whole brain echo planar diffusion-weighted magnetic resonance imaging. *Ann Neurol* 1995;37:231–241.

78. Brott T, Fieschi C, Hacke W. Ischemic stroke: general therapy. In: Hacke W (ed). *NeuroCritical Care.* New York: Springer-Verlag, 1994;553–577.

79. Hacke W, Krieger D, Hirschberg M. General principles in the treatment of acute ischemic stroke. *Cerebrovasc Dis* 1991;1:93–99.

80. Grotta J. Medical and surgical therapy for cerebrovascular disease. *N Engl J Med* 1987;315:1505–1516.
81. Hacke W, Bogousslavsky J, Brott T, et al. European strategies for early intervention in stroke. *Cerebrovasc Dis* 1996;6:315–324.
82. Hacke W, Stingele R, Steiner T, Schuchardt V, Schwab S. Critical care of acute ischemic stroke. *Intens Care Med* 1995;21:856–862.
83. Brott T, McCarthy C. Antihypertensive therapy in stroke. In: Fisher M (ed). *Medical Therapy of Acute Stroke.* New York: Dekker, 1989;117–141.
84. Dietrich WD, Busto R, Alonso O, Globus MY, Ginsberg MD. Intraischemic but not postischemic brain hypothermia protects chronically following global forebrain ischemia in rats. *J Cereb Blood Flow Metab* 1993;13:541–549.
85. Dietrich WD, Alonso O, Busto R. Moderate hyperglycemia worsens acute blood-brain barrier injury after forebrain ischemia in rats. *Stroke* 1993;24:111–116.
86. Pulsinelli W, Levy D, Sigsbee B, Scherer P, Plum F. Increased damage after ischemic stroke in patients with hyperglycemia with or without established diabetes mellitus. *Am J Med* 1983;74:540–544.
87. Kay R, Wong KA, Yu YL, et al. Low-molecular weight heparin in the treatment of acute ischemic stroke. *N Engl J Med* 1995;333:1588–1593.
88. Brott T, Adams HP, Olinger CP, et al. Measurements of acute cerebral infarction: a clinical examination scale. *Stroke* 1989;20:864–870.
89. Brott TG, Haley EC Jr, Levy DE, et al. Urgent therapy for stroke. Part I. Pilot study of tissue plaminogen activator administered within 90 minutes. *Stroke* 1992;23:632–640.
90. Haley EC Jr, Levy DE, Brott TG, et al. Urgent therapy for stroke. Part II. Pilot study of tissue plasminogen activator administered 91–180 minutes from onset. *Stroke* 1992;23:641–645.
91. Hantson L, De Weerdt W, De Keyser J, et al. The European Stroke Scale. *Stroke* 1994;25:2215–2219.
92. Lyden P, Brott T, Tilley B, et al. Improved reliability of the NIH Stroke Scale using video training. *Stroke* 1994;25:2220–2226.
93. Mahoney FJ, Barthel DW. Functional evaluation. The Barthel index. *Md Med J* 1965;14:61–65.
94. Mori E. Fibrinolytic recanalization therapy in acute cerebrovascular thromboembolism. In: Hacke W, del Zoppo GJ, Hirschberg M (eds). *Thrombolytic Therapy in Acute Ischemic Stroke.* Heidelberg: Springer-Verlag, 1991;137–146.
95. Moulin D, Lo R, Chiang J, Barnett H. Prognosis in middle cerebral artery occlusion. *Stroke* 1985;16:282–288.
96. Hacke W, Schwab S, Horn M, Spranger M, DeGeorgia M, von Kummer R. Malignant middle cerebral artery territory infarction. *Arch Neurol* 1996;53:309–315.
97. Overgaard K, Sperling B, Boysen G, et al. Thrombolytic therapy in acute ischemic stroke. A Danish pilot study. *Stroke* 1993;24:1439–1446.
98. Baird AE, Donnan GA, Austin MC, Fitt GJ, Davis SM, McKay WJ. Reperfusion after thrombolytic therapy in ischemic stroke measured by single-photon emission computed tomography. *Stroke* 1994;25:79–85.
99. Ueda T, Hatakeyama T, Kumon Y, Sakaki S, Uraoka T. Evaluation of risk of hemorrhagic transformation in local intra-arterial thrombolysis in acute ischemic stroke by initial SPECT. *Stroke* 1994;25:298–303.
100. Multicentre Acute Stroke Trial-Italy (MAST-I) Group. Randomised controlled trial of streptokinase, aspirin, and combination of both in treatment of acute ischaemic stroke. Lancet 1995;346:1509–1514.
101. The Multicenter Acute Stroke Trial—Europe Study Group. Thrombolytic therapy with streptokinase in acute ischemic stroke. *N Engl J Med* 1996;335:145–150.
102. Donnan GA, Davis SM, Chambers BR, et al. Streptokinase for acute ischemic stroke with relationship to time of administration. *JAMA* 1996;276:961–966.
103. Diener H, Hacke W, Hennerici M, Rädberg J, Hantson L, De Keyser J, for the Lubeluzole International Study Group. Lubeluzole in acute ischemic stroke. A double-blind, placebo-controlled phase II trial. *Stroke* 1996;27:76–81.
104. Silver FL, Norris JLO, Lewis AJ, Hachinski VC. Early mortality following stroke: a prospective review. *Stroke* 1984;15:492–496.
105. Shaw CM, Alvord EC Jr, Berry RG. Swelling of the brain following ischemic infarction with arterial occlusion. *Arch Neurol* 1959;1:161–177.
106. von Kummer R, Bozzao L, Manelfe C. *CT Diagnosis of Hemispheric Brain Infarction.* Heidelberg: Springer-Verlag, 1995.
107. NIH Consensus Conference. Thrombolytic therapy in treatment. *Br Med J* 1980;280:1585–1587.
108. Meyer JS, Gilroy J, Barnhart MI, Johnson JF. Anticoagulants plus streptokinase therapy in progressive stroke. *JAMA* 1964;189:373.
109. Araki G, Minakami K, Mihara H. Therapeutic effect of urokinase on cerebral infarction. *Rinsho Kenkyu* 1973;50:3317–3326.
110. Fletcher AP, Alkjaersig N, Lewis M, et al. A pilot study of urokinase therapy in cerebral infarction. *Stroke* 1976;7:135–142.
111. Hanaway J, Torack R, Fletcher AP, Landau WM. Intracranial bleeding associated with urokinase therapy for acute ischemic hemispheral stroke. *Stroke* 1976;7:143–146.
112. Zeumer H, Freitag HJ, Grzyka U, Neunzig HP. Local intra-arterial fibrinolysis in acute vertebrobasilar occlusion. Technical developments and recent results. *Neuroradiology* 1989;31:336–340.
113. Zeumer H. Survey of progress: vascular recanalizing techniques in interventional neuroradiology. *J Neurol* 1985;231:287–294.
114. Atkin N, Nitzberg S, Dorsey J. Lysis of intracerebral thromboembolism with fibrinolysin. Report of a case. *Angiology* 1964;15:346–439.
115. Meyer JS, Herndon RM, Gotoh F, Tazaki Y, Nelson JN, Johnson JF. Therapeutic thrombolysis. In: Millikan CH, Siekert RG, Whisnant JP (eds). *Cerebral Vascular Diseases, Third Princeton Conference.* New York: Grune & Stratton, 1961;160–177.
116. Nenci GG, Gresele P, Taramelli M, Agnelli G, Signorini E. Thrombolytic therapy for thromboembolism of vertebrobasilar artery. *Angiology* 1983;34:561–571.
117. Miyakawa T. The cerebral vessels and thrombosis. *Rinsho Ketsueki* 1984;25:1018–1026.
118. Theron J, Courtheoux P, Casaseo A, et al. Local intra-arterial fibrinolysis in the carotid territory. *AJNR* 1989;10:753–765.

119. Matsumoto K, Satoh K. Topical intraarterial urokinase infusion for acute stroke. In: Hacke W, del Zoppo GJ, Hirschberg M (eds). *Thrombolytic Therapy in Acute Ischemic Stroke.* Heidelberg: Springer-Verlag, 1991; 207–212.

120. Hacke W, Zeumer H, Ferbert A, Brückmann H, del Zoppo GJ. Intra-arterial thrombolytic therapy improves outcome in patients with acute vertebrobasilar occlusive disease. *Stroke* 1988;19:1216–1222.

121. Möbius E, Berg-Dammer E, Kühne D, Nahser HC. Local thrombolytic therapy in acute basilar artery occlusion: experience with 18 patients. In: Hacke W, del Zoppo GJ, Hirschberg M (eds). *Thrombolytic Therapy in Acute Ischemic Stroke.* Heidelberg: Springer-Verlag, 1991;213–215.

122. Zeumer H, Freitag HJ, Zarella F, Thie A, Arnig C. Local intra-arterial fibrinolytic therapy in patients with stroke: urokinase vs. recombinant tissue plasminogen activator (rt-PA). *Neuroradiology* 1993;35:159–162.

123. Freitag HJ, Zeumer H, Knospe V. Acute central retinal artery occlusion and the role of thrombolysis. In: del Zoppo GJ, Mori E, Hacke W (eds). *Thrombolytic Therapy in Acute Ischemic Stroke II.* Heidelberg: Springer-Verlag, 1993;103–105.

124. Ohtaki M, Shinya T, Yamamura A, Minamida Y, et al. Local fibrinolytic therapy using superselective catheterization for patients with acute cerebral embolism within 10 hours. In: Tomita M, Mchedlishvili A, Rosenblum W, Heiss WD, Fukuuchi Y (eds). *Microcirculatory Stasis in the Brain.* Amsterdam: Elsevier Science, 1993;539–545.

125. Higashida RT, Halbach VV, Barnwell SL, Dowd CF, Hieshima GB. Thrombolytic therapy in acute stroke. *J Endovasc Surg* 1994;1:415.

126. Barnwell SL, Clark WM, Nguyen TT, O'Neill OR, Wynn ML, Coull BM. Safety and efficacy of delayed intraarterial urokinase therapy with mechanical clot disruption for thromboembolic stroke. *AJNR* 1994;15: 1817–1822.

127. Jansen O, von Kummer R, Forsting M, Hacke W, Sartor K. Thrombolytic therapy in acute occlusion of the intracranial internal carotid artery bifurcation. *AJNR* 1995;16:1977–1986.

128. del Zoppo GJ, Higashida RT, Furlan AJ, et al. PROACT: a phase II randomized trial of recombinant pro urokinase by direct arterial delivery in acute middle cerebral artery stroke. *Stroke* 1998 (in press).

129. Yamaguchi T. Intravenous rt-PA in acute embolic stroke. In: Hacke W, del Zoppo GJ, Hirschberg M (eds). *Thrombolytic Therapy in Acute Ischemic Stroke.* Heidelberg: Springer-Verlag, 1991;168–174.

130. Tognoni G, Roncaglioni MC. Dissent: an alternative interpretation of MAST-I. *Lancet* 1995;346:1504–1515.

131. Gruppo Italiano Per Lo Studio Della Streptochinasi Nell'Infarto Miocardico (GISSI). Effectiveness of intravenous thrombolytic treatment in acute myocardial infarction. *Lancet* 1986;1:397–401.

132. Gruppo Italiano Per Lo Studio Della Streptochinasi Nell'Infarto Miocardico (GISSI). GISSI-2: a factorial randomized trial of alteplase versus streptokinase and heparin versus no heparin among 12,490 patients with acute myocardial infarction. *Lancet* 1990;336: 65–71.

133. Madison EL, Goldsmith EJ, Gerard RD, Gething MJ, Sambrook JF. Serpin-resistant mutants of human tissue-type plasminogen activator. *Nature* 1989;339:721–724.

134. Ancrod for the treatment of acute ischemic brain infarction. The Ancrod Stroke Study Investigators. *Stroke* 1994;25:1755–1759.

135. Adams HP Jr, Brott TG, Furlan AJ, et al. Guidelines for thrombolytic therapy for acute stroke: a supplement to the guidelines for the management of patients with acute ischemic stroke. A statement for healthcare professionals from a special writing group of the Stroke Council, American Heart Association. *Circulation* 1996;94:1167–1174.

136. Hommel M, Boissel JP, Cornu C, et al. Termination of trial of streptokinase in severe acute ischemic stroke [Letter]. *Lancet* 1995;345:578–579.

137. Donnan GA, Davis SM, Chambers BR, et al. Trials of streptokinase in severe acute ischaemic stroke. *Lancet* 1995;345:578–579.

138. The National Institutes of Neurological Disorders and Stroke rt-PA Stroke Study Group. Tissue plasminogen activator for acute ischemic stroke. *N Engl J Med* 1995;333:1581–1587.

Cardiovascular Thrombosis: Thrombocardiology and Thromboneurology, Second Edition,
edited by M. Verstraete, V. Fuster, and E. J. Topol,
Lippincott–Raven Publishers, Philadelphia © 1998.

36

Secondary Prevention of Thromboembolic Stroke

Jan van Gijn and *Ale Algra

*University Department of Neurology, University Hospital Utrecht, 3508 GA Utrecht, The Netherlands;
and *Department of Neurology, The Julius Center for Patient-Oriented Research, Utrecht University,
3584 CG Utrecht, The Netherlands*

DIAGNOSIS OF TRANSIENT ISCHEMIC ATTACK AND MINOR ISCHEMIC STROKE

It would be improper to discuss treatment without saying at least a few words about diagnosis. Precisely because the symptoms are transient, the diagnosis is difficult. Many other disorders can resemble a transient ischemic attack (TIA), the most common of which are migraine, syncope, overbreathing, postural vertigo, hypoglycemia, and epilepsy (1,2). The criteria that have been adopted to define true TIAs are phrased in rather abstract terms (3), which may result in a disappointing interobserver reliability (4). Structured checklists in plain language help to improve this (5).

The arbitrary time limits of 24 hours and 6 weeks that have been devised to separate TIAs, reversible ischemic neurologic deficits (RINDs), and minor strokes have little value in terms of management. Most attacks that resolve within 1 day do so within 60 minutes (6), but even with these short-lived deficits the computed tomography (CT) scan later may show a relevant infarct. In a large series, the proportion of patients with an infarct on CT scanning that was appropriate to the symptoms gradually increased with the duration of the (longest) attack: 10% with symptoms of less than 30 minutes, 20% if these lasted 5 to 24 hours, 40% if recovery took 1 to 6 weeks, and 50% with deficits persisting beyond 6 weeks (7). Hence, the differences between TIAs, RINDs, and minor strokes are quantitative rather than qualitative.

A distinction should be made with regard to stroke subtype (8). Treatment and prognosis are fairly different for strokes originating from cardiac emboli and those due to presumed arterial disease. Within the latter group, the site and degree of narrowing of extracerebral arteries determines whether surgical or medical therapy should be the first choice in secondary prevention.

PREVENTION AFTER CEREBRAL ISCHEMIA OF PRESUMED ARTERIAL ORIGIN

The annual combined risk of death from all vascular causes, nonfatal stroke, or nonfatal myocardial infarction in patients who have a TIA or nondisabling ischemic stroke of presumed arterial origin ranges between 4% and 11% in clinical trials (9,10). The corresponding estimate for population-based studies is 9% per year (11). Two main options of secondary prevention are available: one medical, the other surgical. These approaches have overlapping indications.

Medical Treatment

Aspirin

The Antiplatelet Trialists' Collaboration published an overview of all controlled clinical trials on antiplatelet drugs in the prevention of major vascular events available by March 1990 (9). The main measure of outcome chosen for the analysis was the composite event "vascular death, nonfatal stroke, or nonfatal myocardial infarction" (whichever occurred first), because this combination was considered to be the most relevant from the patient's point of view. Moreover, the composite measure provides the largest number of events for analysis that are likely to be influenced by antiplatelet treatment. TIA and minor ischemic stroke were studied in 18 trials, totalling 11,707 patients. The relative odds reduction for the combined vascular outcome was 22%, the corresponding relative risk reduction 18%, with a 95% confidence interval (CI) of 12% to 24%. It might be argued that the potential degree of protection is somewhat greater than this, because the compliance in these trials averaged 80% or less at 1 year after randomization, and also because some of the controls probably took antiplatelet drugs, for whatever reason. Another reason why the true degree of protection might be higher is that a variety of antiplatelet drugs were considered in this analysis, including suloctidyl, which has only a weak effect on platelets and has disappeared from the market.

Meta-analysis is not without disadvantages. Such analyses are mainly based on published trials only, and negative trials may remain undiscovered; the overall appreciation thus may be hampered by this publication bias. Also, in some respects the interpretation of the data of the antiplatelet meta-analysis is problematic because all antiplatelet agents have been included in the analysis. This probably does not affect the main conclusions of the overview because aspirin was by far the most common drug, and no antiplatelet agent was found more or less effective than others. However, most of the comparisons between antiplatelet agents were indirect (between trials and not within trials). Moreover, the CIs are wide enough, even though trials in other cardiovascular diseases were included, to be consistent with the possibility that the effects of aspirin have been diluted with those of some inactive drugs. This egalitarian approach of the overview analysts is most obvious in the representation of the pioneering Canadian Cooperative trial, which involved almost 600 patients (12). There were four groups in this trial: aspirin, sulfinpyrazone, both, or neither (double placebo). A dosage of 1,300 mg of aspirin per day, with or without sulfinpyrazone being simultaneously given, reduced the incidence of vascular events by 30%. However, if the analysis was restricted to the patients who did not receive sulfinpyrazone, the results for aspirin only were not favorable: the relative risk reduction was -3% (95% CI -66% to 34%) (10), but the investigators themselves concluded from their trial that aspirin worked and sulfinpyrazone did not.

To disentangle the confusion that some felt because of the combined analyses of different antiplatelet drugs, we reanalyzed the data provided in an appendix of the report on the second cycle of the Antiplatelet Trialists' Collaboration (10). Moreover, we wanted to determine whether the efficacy of low, medium, and high doses of aspirin were different because this was another contentious issue (13). We identified 10 randomized trials of aspirin only versus control treatment in 6,171 patients after a TIA or nondisabling stroke (12,14–22). Figure 36-1 shows the relative risks and corresponding relative risk reductions with their 95% CIs for all aspirin trials separately. There was virtually no difference between the risk reduction for a low dose (13%), medium dose (9%), and high dose (14%), allowing the calculation of an overall estimate that was 13% (95% CI 4% to 21%). There were two direct comparisons about the dose of aspirin. The UK-TIA trial showed no difference between the results of 300 and 1,200 mg aspirin daily (16). The Dutch TIA Trial evaluated the effect of two doses of a water-soluble preparation of aspirin (30 and 283 mg/day) in 3,131 patients during a mean follow-up of 2.6 years (23); the age- and sex-adjusted hazard ratio for the

group receiving the lower dose was 0.91 (95% CI 0.76 to 1.09), indicating no difference between the results of 30- and 283-mg doses.

Recently, the results of the second European Stroke Prevention Study (ESPS-2) were published (see below) (24). One of its comparisons was between 50 mg aspirin daily and placebo in patients after cerebral ischemia; the relative risk reduction (13%, 95% CI -1% to 25%) was exactly the same as that of the cumulative evidence so far. In conclusion, aspirin in any daily dose of 30 mg or higher reduces the risk of major vascular events by 20% at most.

Side Effects

It was known before its second life as an antithrombotic agent that the incidence of hemorrhagic complications and gastrointestinal symptoms with aspirin was dose dependent. However, it is difficult to compare the incidence of these side effects between different studies because criteria tend to be less precise and the auditing procedures less rigid than for the main outcome events. A comparison of bleeding complications or gastrointestinal symptoms between different groups within one study gives at least some idea of the relative frequency of side effects because these have been recorded without knowledge of treatment allocation.

In placebo-controlled trials with 1,000 to 1,300 mg of aspirin, the incidence of side effects was two to three times as high as in patients on placebo (12,16,20,25). The most detailed report is from the UK-TIA study: gastrointestinal bleeding occurred in 1% of the patients on placebo, 3% on 300 mg of aspirin, and 5% on 1,200 mg; approximately half of the patients in each group required admission to hospital. Indigestion, nausea, heartburn or vomiting was reported by 26% of the patients on placebo, 31% of those on 300 mg of aspirin, and 41% of those on 1,200 mg (16).

With low-dose aspirin, the incidence of hemorrhagic complications can be decreased even further. In the 30-mg group of the

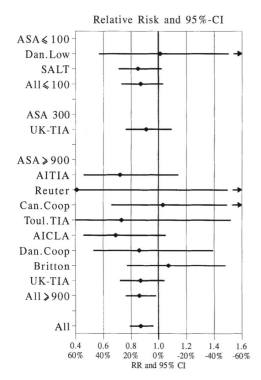

FIG. 36-1. Relative risks and corresponding relative risk reductions with 95% CIs for all aspirin trials separately, two low-dose (<100 mg/day) trials combined, one medium-dose trial, all high-dose (>>900 mg/day) trials combined, and all aspirin trials combined. ASA, acetylsalicylic acid (aspirin). (Adapted from Algra and van Gijn, ref. 9, with permission.)

Dutch TIA trial, major bleeding complications (requiring hospital attendance) were slightly less common than in the 300-mg group (relative risk 0.80; 95% CI 0.53 to 1.21), and significantly fewer minor bleeds occurred (relative risk 0.61, 95% CI 0.43 to 0.86). Even gastric discomfort or unspecified side effects were reported significantly less often with 30 mg than with 300 mg (16% versus 19%, relative risk 0.83) (23). In the Swedish trial with 75 mg of aspirin, bleeding complications occurred in 7.2% of the patients treated with aspirin versus 3.2% in the placebo group (for severe bleeding the proportions were 1.6% and 0.6%, respectively) (15).

Other Antiplatelet Drugs

Ticlopidine

Ticlopidine hydrochloride does not inhibit the cyclooxygenase pathway, like aspirin, but the adenosine diphosphate pathway of platelet aggregation. Two major trials with this drug have been completed in patients with cerebrovascular disease (26,27).

In the Canadian American Ticlopidine Study (CATS), 1,072 patients with stroke were randomized between ticlopidine (250 mg twice daily) and placebo. The qualifying stroke had occurred 1 week to 4 months before and had not left the patients bedridden, although 70% required some assistance with activities of daily living. Analysis of all randomized patients (except 19 ineligible cases) for the same composite vascular outcome used by the Antiplatelet Trialists showed a relative risk reduction with ticlopidine of 23% (95% CI 0% to 40%) (26). In other words, the benefits are similar to those of aspirin only (Fig. 36-1) (10).

A direct comparison with aspirin was made in the Ticlopidine Aspirin Stroke Study (TASS) (27). A total of 3,069 patients with transient or nondisabling focal ischemia of the brain or retina was randomized between ticlopidine (250 mg twice daily) or aspirin (650 mg twice daily). The occurrence of nonfatal myocardial infarction was not re-ported in the original report (27), but data on the composite event of vascular death, nonfatal stroke, or nonfatal myocardial infarction were reported in the appendix of the report of the second cycle of the Antiplatelet Trialists' Collaboration (9). The relative risk difference was a 6% advantage in favor of ticlopidine, but the 95% CI was compatible with no difference at all: -7% to 17% (28).

Thus, according to present evidence, ticlopidine is about equally effective as aspirin. Unfortunately, ticlopidine is definitively more toxic. Diarrhea and skin rashes were reported in up to 20% and 14%, respectively (27), and neutropenia in about 1% (26,27). The rate of noncompliance because of side effects was higher than that for high-dose aspirin (21% versus 14.5%) (27). The neutropenia is reversible, as are the other side effects, provided ticlopidine administration is stopped in time; if it occurs it does so within 3 months, during which period a blood count should be done every 2 weeks. A final consideration is that ticlopidine is much more expensive than aspirin and that it has not been approved in several countries.

Clopidogrel

Clopidogrel is a new thienopyridine derivative, chemically related to ticlopidine; it also blocks the adenosine diphosphate pathway of platelet aggregation. CAPRIE was a randomized, blinded, international trial designed to assess the relative efficacy of clopidogrel (75 mg daily) and aspirin (325 mg daily) in reducing the risk of the composite outcome event vascular death, nonfatal stroke, or nonfatal myocardial infarction (29). Patients were enrolled in three diagnostic strata: ischemic stroke (6431 patients), myocardial infarction (6302 patients), and peripheral arterial disease (6452 patients). The overall relative risk reduction by clopidogrel was 8.7% (95% CI 0.3 to 16.5). The relative risk reductions differed in a statistically significant fashion ($p = 0.042$) between the strata: 7.3% for ischemic stroke, -3.7% for myocardial infarction, and 23.8% for peripheral arterial disease (Fig. 36-2). The notion that not all vascular disease is the same is further underlined by the differential efficacy of antiplatelet drugs in the analyses of the Antiplatelets Trialists' Collaboration, which show a relative risk reduction of 35% in unstable angina, 26% in acute myocardial infarction, 21% in previous myocardial infarction, and 17% after cerebral ischemia. Thus, assessment of the separate strata in CAPRIE is warranted. For the patients who entered the trial with an ischemic stroke, the 95% CI of the relative risk reduction of clopidogrel versus aspirin was -5.7% to 18.7%. Because of the small, statistically nonsignificant advantage, and low cost of aspirin, clopidogrel is not attractive as a drug of first choice for patients after cerebral ischemia. Moreover, the CAPRIE study group has plans to launch another trial with clopidogrel in the stroke stratum.

Sulfinpyrazone

Sulfinpyrazone is a uricosuric drug that inhibits platelet aggregation by reversible inactivation of cyclooxygenase via its metabolites. The drug has fallen into disrepute with neurologists because it offered no demonstrable pro-

tection against stroke in small trials (9) or in subgroups of medium-sized trials (12). It may have fallen victim to the play of chance, however, because the results were much better in large trials of patients with myocardial infarction. Taken together, all trials with sulfinpyrazone in patients with vascular disease indicate a relative risk reduction of 17% (95% CI 4% to 27%) for the composite event stroke, myocardial infarction, or vascular death (9). Therefore, some clinicians advocate not only ticlopidine but also sulfinpyrazone as an alternative for patients who cannot tolerate aspirin (30). Certain allergic phenomena are shared with aspirin, however: peptic ulcer, bronchospasm, and skin rashes. Additional side effects may include renal failure by deposits of urate in the tubuli and—rarely—aplastic anemia.

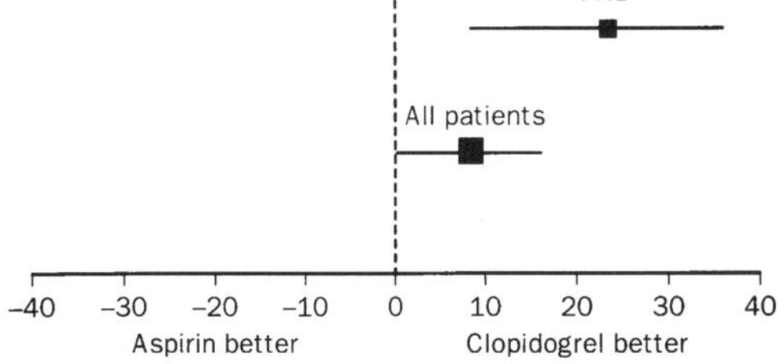

Dipyridamole

This drug seems to have an antithrombotic effect in certain animal models, but it has long remained unclear whether strokes were actually prevented by this drug or any other vascular complication (31). In patients with cerebrovascular disease, good results were initially achieved only on the coat-tails of aspirin (9,20,25).

Recently the results of the second European Stroke Prevention Study (ESPS-2) were published (24). ESPS-2 was a randomized, placebo-controlled, double-blind trial comparing the effects of low-dose aspirin (50 mg daily), dipyridamole (400 mg daily), or the combination of both drugs with placebo treatment in 6,602 patients with a prior ischemic stroke or TIA. In the analysis of all major vascular events (vascular death, nonfatal stroke or nonfatal myocardial infarction), combination therapy yielded the best results in comparison with aspirin only, the relative risk being 0.78 (95% CI 0.67 to 0.91) (Diener HC, personal communication). However, the applicability of these results in clinical practice is difficult for several reasons. First, four earlier studies compared the combination therapy and aspirin only (19,20,32,33); data on these studies have been listed in an appendix

FIG. 36-2. Relative risk reductions and 95% CIs by disease group in the CAPRIE trial. MI, myocardial infarction; PAD, peripheral arterial disease. (From the CAPRIE Steering Committee, ref. 29, with permission.)

of the report on the second cycle of the Antiplatelet Trialists' Collaboration (9). The combined evidence from these four studies for the same composite outcome event yields a Mantel-Haenszel relative risk of 0.97 (95% CI 0.78 to 1.22). This is rather different from the result obtained in ESPS-2. Poisson regression analysis shows that this difference approaches statistical significance (p = 0.13). This trial should be interpreted with caution also because of ethical problems with the use of placebo and allegations of scientific fraud (34), although the data in question have been excluded from the analysis. In short, doubt continues to exist on the effectiveness of dipyridamole as an adjuvant to aspirin.

Anticoagulant Drugs

Oral anticoagulant drugs might be more effective than aspirin in preventing vascular complications after cerebral ischemia. Secondary prevention trials after myocardial infarction indicate that treatment with oral anticoagulant drugs is associated with a risk reduction approximately twice that of treatment with aspirin or other antiplatelet drugs (9,35–38). Few data are available on the efficacy and safety of oral anticoagulant treatment in patients with cerebral ischemia (39), except in those with atrial fibrillation (40).

The aim of SPIRIT (Stroke Prevention In Reversible Ischemia Trial) was to compare the efficacy and safety of oral anticoagulants (international normalized ratio [INR] 3.0 to 4.5) and 30 mg aspirin daily. Patients referred to a neurologist in one of 58 collaborating centers because of a transient ischemic attack or minor ischemic stroke (Rankin grade ≤3) were eligible. Randomization was concealed, treatment assignment was open, and assessment of outcome events was masked; recruitment of 3,000 patients was planned with an average follow-up of 2.9 years. The primary measure of outcome was the composite event "death from all vascular causes, stroke, myocardial infarction, or major bleeding complication" (i.e., the usual threefold outcome event was expanded by the inclusion of major bleeding complications).

The trial was stopped after the first interim analysis. A total of 1,316 patients participated; the mean follow-up was 14 months. There was an excess of the primary outcome event in the anticoagulant group (81 of 651), versus 36 of 665 in the aspirin group (hazard ratio 2.3, 95% CI 1.6 to 3.5) (41). This excess could be attributed to 53 major bleeding complications (27 intracranial; 17 fatal) during anticoagulant therapy versus six on aspirin (three intracranial, one fatal). Calculation of INR-specific incidence rates (42) showed that the bleeding incidence increased by a factor of 1.45 (95% CI 1.33 to 1.58) for each 0.5-U increase of the achieved INR. The most important other risk factors for intracerebral hemorrhages were age over 65 years (relative risk 2.5; 95% CI 1.1 to 5.7) and leukoaraiosis (bilateral patchy or diffuse areas of hypodensity on CT or hyperintensity on T2-weighted MRI corresponding with the cerebral white matter) (43,44), centrally recorded for the baseline CT scan (relative risk 7.5, 95% CI 3.4% to 16%). The numbers of ischemic outcome events (ischemic stroke, myocardial infarction, and nonhemorrhagic vascular death) were so small because of the early termination of the study (anticoagulants 27 versus aspirin 27; hazard ratio 1.03), that the results are entirely consistent with the initial assumption that there would be an approximately 20% further reduction of ischemic events with anticoagulants (95% CI of the hazard ratio 0.60 to 1.75). We therefore concluded that (a) anticoagulant therapy with an INR range of 3.0 to 4.5 in patients after cerebral ischemia of presumed arterial origin is not safe; and (b) anticoagulant therapy with an intensity of INR 2.0 to 3.0 might be both safe and efficacious in patients after cerebral ischemia, and the efficacy and safety of such an anticoagulation regimen deserves further study.

Surgical Treatment

Carotid Endarterectomy

There used to be two great problems with the surgical treatment of carotid atheroma.

One was, and still is, that it can be applied to only a small proportion of patients with TIAs: the attacks have to be in the carotid territory, the clinical features should indicate dysfunction of the cortex and not of the internal capsule (in the latter case lacunar infarcts due to small-vessel disease should be suspected) (45,46), the patients should be fit and willing to undergo the operation, and the angiogram should show an accessible lesion in the carotid bifurcation—in that order. This leaves less than one third of all TIA patients (47).

The biggest problem, until the early 1990s, was the uncertainty about the risk/benefit ratio with carotid endarterectomy. In some patients the operation causes the very stroke that it should prevent, usually as a result of thromboembolism (48). The rate of stroke or death varies widely between series, from 2.5% to 25% (47), but the most common estimate was between 6% and 8%, half of which are deaths or disabling strokes (49). The crucial question is—assuming that carotid endarterectomy per se reduces the risk of stroke—how long it takes before the break-even point is reached.

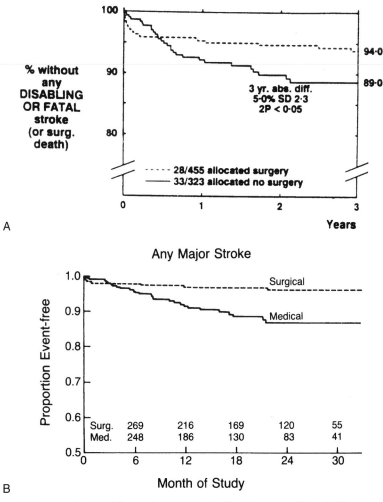

FIG. 36-3. Survival curves for disabling or fatal stroke in the European Carotid Surgery Trial **(A)** and the North American Symptomatic Carotid Endarterectomy Trial **(B)**. (From the European Carotid Surgery Trialists' Collaborative Group, ref. 50 [A]; and the North American Symptomatic Carotid Endarterectomy Trial Collaborators, ref. 51 [B]; with permission.)

Not until the 1980s were two randomized surgical trials performed: the European Carotid Surgery Trial (ECST) and the North American Symptomatic Carotid Endarterectomy Trial (NASCET); both studies published an interim report in 1991 (50,51). It is an admirable demonstration of scientific integrity on the part of the collaborating surgeons that they were willing to put carotid endarterectomy to the test. In patients with severe carotid stenosis (70% to 99% diameter reduction), the risk of disabling or fatal stroke decreased dramatically, from 11% to 6% after 3 years in the ECST (Fig. 36-3A) and from 13% to 4% after 2 years in the NASCET (Fig. 36-3B). These numbers include surgical risks; the break-even point occurred after about 6 months. The small proportion of strokes after initially successful surgery were mainly infarcts in another territory or hemorrhages. For patients with mild carotid stenosis (0% to 29% diameter reduction; included only in the ECST), the risk of stroke without surgery was so low that after more than 3 years the surgical complications still outweighed the benefits. According to an interim report from the ECST, patients with mild carotid stenosis (30% to 69%) have little to gain from the operation (52). The NASCET trial is still continuing follow-up for this intermediate group, but the method of measuring carotid stenosis differs between the two trials (53); by ECST standards the degree of stenosis in this intermediate group of the NASCET trial would not be 30% to 69%, but 58% to 82%.

Extracranial–Intracranial Bypass Surgery

In the 1970s, neurosurgeons developed a technique of anastomosing the superficial temporal branch of the external carotid artery to a cortical branch of the middle cerebral artery. This bypass constituted a potential treatment modality for the secondary prevention of stroke in patients with symptoms of cerebral ischemia in whom the arterial lesion was not amenable to endarterectomy, that is, patients with occlusion or inaccessible stenosis of the internal carotid artery, or with stenosis of the stem of the middle cerebral artery. The rationale was that in most of these patients the cerebral circulation might be hemodynamically compromised.

Fortunately, a well-designed clinical trial undertook to assess the benefits of the operation before it had prematurely established itself in clinical practice. In a world-wide effort, 1,377 patients were randomized to undergo the operation (plus best medical care) or to receive only the best medical care (54). The result was disappointing in that bypass surgery was safe in skilled hands but did not protect against ipsilateral stroke or against stroke in general, despite a patency rate of 97% (55). Even subgroup analysis, according to clinical or radiologic criteria, failed to identify subgroups of patients for whom the operation might still be beneficial. There were contorted criticisms by disappointed surgeons to the effect that patients who had undergone surgery outside the trial would have been the very patients who stood to benefit (56,57).

Yet the hope is still alive that sophisticated metabolic and hemodynamic assessments can identify a subgroup of patients with a low-flow state in whom an increased risk of stroke might be averted by means of an artificial bypass (58), although according to some reports the stroke rate in such hemodynamically compromised groups is rather low (59). Technical advances in bypass surgery are still being made, such as constructing a high-flow bypass with the distal anastomosis at the intracranial portion of the internal carotid artery or the proximal part of the middle cerebral artery, by means of Excimer laser; this technique does not necessitate temporary clamping of the internal carotid artery (60,61). However, appropriate or even plausible indications for extracranial–intracranial bypass surgery remain to be defined.

Carotid Angioplasty

Percutaneous transluminal balloon angioplasty is a common procedure in the treatment of atherosclerotic narrowing in coronary arteries or arteries supplying the legs, but its application in arteries supplying the brain has been delayed by concerns about the risk of distal embolization. Perhaps the most rational indications, at least in theory, are (a) postendarterectomy restenosis (62); (b) severe narrowing of the internal carotid artery in combination with hemodynamic symptoms and perceived hazards of surgery (63); and (c) surgically inaccessible lesions such as in the middle cerebral artery (64) or in the posterior circulation (65,66). Some surgeons consider performing angioplasty even in patients with severe, symptomatic stenosis of the internal carotid artery, given the undeniable risk of carotid endarterectomy (7% to 8% perioperative strokes, half of which are disabling) (50,51). Up to now, observational series of such patients seem to indicate that the complication rate is of the same order of magnitude as surgery (67–69). Angioplasty may be safer with protective measures against embolization or with stenting. Only controlled trials of angioplasty in these different situations can resolve the questions about its efficacy, but this needs to be an international effort because a formidable number of patients is required to attain useful results. At least one such trial is ongoing (70).

PREVENTION AFTER CEREBRAL ISCHEMIA OF CARDIAC ORIGIN

In the European Atrial Fibrillation Trial (EAFT) 1,007 patients with nonrheumatic atrial fibrillation were enrolled who had had a TIA or minor ischemic stroke (40). Patients were randomized between open oral anticoagulation (INR target range 2.5 to 4.0), aspirin 300 mg daily, or aspirin matching placebo (group 1, n = 669). If patients had a contraindication against anticoagulation, they were randomized between aspirin and placebo only (group 2, n = 338). Primary outcome after a mean follow-up of 2.3 years was the composite event "death from all vascular causes, nonfatal stroke, nonfatal myocardial infarction or systemic embolism," whichever occurred first.

The annual rate of the primary outcome was 15% among the aspirin-treated patients (groups 1 and 2), against 19% in those allocated to placebo (hazard ratio 0.83, 95% CI 0.65 to 1.05). In patients allocated to anticoagulants, the yearly rate of the composite outcome event was 8%, whereas this rate was 17% in the placebo group of group 1 (hazard ratio 0.53; 95% CI 0.36 to 0.79; Fig. 36-4). In a direct comparison, anticoagulants proved to be more effective than aspirin (95% CI 0.41 to 0.87). The incidence of major bleeding complications was 0.9% per year on aspirin and 2.8% in the anticoagulant group. A detailed on-treatment analysis of the anticoagulant therapy showed that the optimal achieved INR was between 2.0 and 4.0; the target should be set at 3.0 (71). Most major bleeding complications were observed at anticoagulant intensities with INRs of 5.0 or higher; no intracranial bleeds were identified.

In a subgroup of the VA-SPINAF study, 46 patients with atrial fibrillation and cerebral ischemia were randomized between anticoagulation (INR 1.4 to 2.8) and placebo (72). Two ischemic strokes occurred in the anticoagulation group and 4 with placebo; the resulting relative risk was 0.66 (95% CI 0.12 to 3.60).

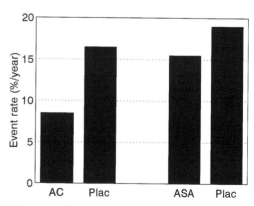

FIG. 36-4. Annual event rates for the primary composite outcome "death from all vascular causes, nonfatal stroke, nonfatal myocardial infarction or systemic embolism" in the European Atrial Fibrillation Trial, ref. 40. The left two bars originate from group 1 (no contraindications for anticoagulants), and the right two bars are from group 2 (contraindication for anticoagulants).

SPAF-3 was a randomized clinical trial in 1,044 patients with atrial fibrillation and at least one thromboembolic risk factor; 36% had had a previous stroke or TIA (73). Patients were allocated to either adjusted-dose warfarin (INR target 2.0 to 3.0) or fixed-dose warfarin (INR 1.2 to 1.5) together with aspirin (325 mg daily). The trial was stopped early after a follow-up of 1.1 years. There were 11 ischemic strokes in the adjusted-dose warfarin group and 43 plus one systemic embolus in the combination therapy group. The corresponding relative risk reduction was 75% (95% CI 52% to 87%). The rates of major bleeding were similar in both treatment groups.

In conclusion, anticoagulation with a target value of INR 3.0 is the preferred therapy for prevention in patients with nonrheumatic atrial fibrillation and cerebral ischemia. If a contraindication exists against anticoagulation, aspirin in a daily dose of 300 mg is a safe, but less effective, alternative.

CONCLUSION

Certainties

The importance of risk factor modification (especially hypertension) goes without saying. Carotid endarterectomy is indicated in patients with cortical symptoms or signs and severe carotid stenosis (70% to 99% diameter reduction). Aspirin is still the mainstay of medical treatment; any dose over 30 mg is as effective as higher doses, yet the rate of reduction of vascular outcome events by aspirin is only in the order of 15% and leaves much room for improvement. Anticoagulation therapy with an INR range of 3.0 to 4.5 in patients after cerebral ischemia of presumed arterial origin is not safe. In patients with nonrheumatic atrial fibrillation and cerebral ischemia, anticoagulation with a target value of INR 3.0 is the preferred therapy.

Uncertainties

Because of the small, statistically nonsignificant, advantage and the low cost of aspirin,

clopidogrel is not attractive as drug of first choice in patients after cerebral ischemia. However, clopidogrel may be considered when there is allergy to aspirin, when aspirin has failed to prevent arterial thrombosis, or in patients with extensive peripheral arterial disease. Doubt exists on the effectiveness of dipyridamole as an adjuvant to aspirin. Current evidence does not yet justify performing extracranial–intracranial bypass surgery or carotid angioplasty for the purpose of secondary prevention of cerebral ischemia, except in the context of a clinical trial.

Open Questions

Currently available data are consistent with the assumption that anticoagulant therapy with an intensity of INR 2.0 to 3.0 might be both safe and efficacious in patients after cerebral ischemia. Atherosclerotic disease in different organs responds differently to antithrombotic treatment, and perhaps even medical treatment for the prevention of ischemic stroke should be fine-tuned according to pathogenesis (e.g., large versus small vessel disease).

REFERENCES

1. Dennis MS, Bamford JM, Sandercock PAG, Warlow CP. Incidence of transient ischemic attacks in Oxfordshire, England. *Stroke* 1989;20:333–339.
2. Landi G. Clinical diagnosis of transient ischaemic attacks. *Lancet* 1992;339:402–405.
3. The Ad Hoc Committee on the classification and outline of cerebrovascular disease. II. *Stroke* 1975;6:566–616.
4. Kraayeveld CL, van Gijn J, Schouten HJA, Staal A. Interobserver agreement for the diagnosis of transient ischemic attacks. *Stroke* 1984;15:723–725.
5. Koudstaal PJ, van Gijn J, Staal A, Duivenvoorden HJ, Gerritsma JGM, Kraayeveld CL. Diagnosis of transient ischemic attacks: improvement of interobserver agreement by a check-list in ordinary language. *Stroke* 1986;17:723–728.
6. Levy DE. How transient are transient ischemic attacks? *Neurology* 1988;38:674–677.
7. Koudstaal PJ, van Gijn J, Frenken CWGM, et al. TIA, RIND, minor stroke: a continuum or different subgroups? *J Neurol Neurosurg Psychiatry* 1992;55:95–97.
8. Bamford J. Clinical examination in diagnosis and subclassification of stroke. *Lancet* 1992;339:400–402.
9. Antiplatelet Trialists' Collaboration. Collaborative overview of randomised trials of antiplatelet therapy—I: Prevention of death, myocardial infarction, and stroke by prolonged antiplatelet therapy in various categories of patients. *Br Med J* 1994;308:81–106.

10. Algra A, van Gijn J. Aspirin at any dose above 30 mg offers only modest protection after cerebral ischaemia. *J Neurol Neurosurg Psychiatry* 1996;60:197–199.
11. Warlow C. Secondary prevention of stroke. *Lancet* 1992;339:724–727.
12. Canadian Cooperative Study group. A randomized trial of aspirin and sulfinpyrazone in threatened stroke. *N Engl J Med* 1978;299:53–59.
13. Dyken ML, Barnett HJM, Easton JD, et al. Low-dose aspirin and stroke—"It ain't necessarily so." *Stroke* 1992;23:1395–1399.
14. Boysen G, Sorensen PS, Juhler M, Andersen AR, Boas J, Olsen JS, et al. Danish very-low-dose aspirin after carotid endarterectomy trial. *Stroke* 1988;19: 1211–1215.
15. The SALT Collaborative Group. Swedish Aspirin Low-dose Trial (SALT); 75 mg aspirin as secondary prophylaxis after cerebrovascular ischaemic events. *Lancet* 1991;338:1345–1349.
16. UK-TIA Study Group. The United Kingdom transient ischaemic attack (UK-TIA) aspirin trial: final results. *J Neurol Neurosurg Psychiatry* 1991;54:1044–1054.
17. Fields WS, Lemak NA, Frankowski RF, Hardy RJ. Controlled trial of aspirin in cerebral ischemia. *Stroke* 1977; 8:301–316.
18. Reuther R, Dorndorf W, Loew D. Behandlung transitorisch-ischämischer Attacken mit Azetylsalizylsäure. *Munch Med Wochenschr* 1980;122:795–798.
19. Guiraud-Chaumeil B, Rascol A, David J, Boneu B, Clanet M, Bierme R. Prévention des récidives des accidents vasculaires cérébraux ischémiques par les anti-agrégants plaquettaires. Résultats d'un essai thérapeutique controlé de 3 ans. *Rev Neurol (Paris)* 1982;138: 367–385.
20. Bousser MG, Eschwege E, Haguenau M, et al. "AICLA" controlled trial of aspirin and dipyridamole in the secondary prevention of atherothrombotic cerebral ischemia. *Stroke* 1983;14:5–14.
21. Sorensen PS, Pedersen H, Marquardsen J, et al. Acetylsalicylic acid in the prevention of stroke in patients with reversible cerebral ischemic attacks. A Danish cooperative study. *Stroke* 1983;14:15–22.
22. Swedish Cooperative Study. High-dose acetylsalicylic acid after cerebral infarction. Stroke 1987;18:325–334.
23. The Dutch TIA Trial Study Group. A comparison of two doses of aspirin (30 mg vs. 283 mg a day) in patients after a transient ischemic attack or minor ischemic stroke. *N Engl J Med* 1991;325:1261–1266.
24. Diener HC, Cunha L, Forbes C, Sivenius J, Smets P, Lowenthal A. European Stroke Prevention Study 2. Dipyridamole and acetylsalicylic acid in the secondary prevention of stroke. *J Neurol Sci* 1996;143:1–13.
25. European Stroke Prevention Study Group. European stroke prevention study: principal endpoints. *Lancet* 1987;2:1351–1354.
26. Gent M, Blakely JA, Easton JD, et al. The Canadian American Ticlopidine Study (CATS) in thromboembolic stroke. *Lancet* 1989;1:1215–1220.
27. Hass WK, Easton JD, Adams HP, et al. A randomized trial comparing ticlopidine hydrochloride with aspirin for the prevention of stroke in high-risk patients. *N Engl J Med* 1989;321:501–507.
28. Van Gijn J, Algra A. Ticlopidine, trials, and torture. *Stroke* 1994;25:1097–1098.
29. CAPRIE Steering Committee. A randomised, blinded, trial of clopidogrel versus aspirin in patients at risk of ischaemic events (CAPRIE). *Lancet* 1996;348: 1329–1339.
30. Warlow C. Ticlopidine, a new antithrombotic drug: but is it better than aspirin for longterm use? *J Neurol Neurosurg Psychiatry* 1990;53:185–187.
31. FitzGerald GA. Dipyridamole. *N Engl J Med* 1987;316: 1247–1257.
32. American-Canadian Co-operative Study Group. Persantin aspirin trial in cerebral ischemia. Part II: endpoint results. *Stroke* 1983;16:406–415.
33. Kaye J. A trial to evaluate the relative roles of dipyridamole and aspirin in the prevention of deep vein thrombosis in stroke patients. (Boehringer Ingelheim internal report.) Bracknell, Berkshire: Boehringer Ingelheim, 1990.
34. Enserink M. Fraud and ethics charges hit stroke drug trial. *Science* 1996;274:2004–2005.
35. The Sixty Plus Reinfarction Study Research Group. A double-blind trial to assess long-term oral anticoagulant therapy in elderly patients after myocardial infarction. *Lancet* 1980;2:989–994.
36. Smith P, Arnesen H, Holme I. The effect of warfarin on mortality and reinfarction after myocardial infarction. *N Engl J Med* 1990;323:147–152.
37. Anticoagulants in the Secondary Prevention of Events in Coronary Thrombosis (ASPECT) Research Group. Effect of long-term oral anticoagulant treatment on mortality and cardiovascular morbidity after myocardial infarction. *Lancet* 1994;343:499–503.
38. The EPSIM Research Group. A controlled comparison of aspirin and oral anticoagulants in prevention of death after myocardial infarction. *N Engl J Med* 1982;307: 701–708.
39. Jonas S. Anticoagulant therapy in cerebrovascular disease: a review and meta-analysis. *Stroke* 1988;19:1043–1048.
40. EAFT (European Atrial Fibrillation Trial) Study Group. Secondary prevention in non-rheumatic atrial fibrillation after transient ischaemic attack or minor stroke. *Lancet* 1993;342:1255–1262.
41. The Stroke Prevention in Reversible Ischemia Trial (SPIRIT) Study Group. Comparison of anticoagulant drugs (INR 3.0–4.5) and aspirin (30 mg per day) for secondary prevention after cerebral ischaemia of presumed arterial origin: a randomised clinical trial stopped for safety reasons. *Ann Neurol* 1997;42:57–65.
42. Rosendaal FR, Cannegieter SC, van der Meer FJM, Briët E. A method to determine the optimal intensity of oral anticoagulant therapy. *Thromb Haemost* 1993;69: 236–239.
43. van Swieten JC, Hijdra A, Koudstaal PJ, van Gijn J. Grading white matter lesions on CT and MRI: a simple scale. *J Neurol Neurosurg Psychiatry* 1990;53: 1080–1083.
44. Pantoni L, Garcia JH. Pathogenesis of leukoaraiosis. A review. *Stroke* 1997;28:652–659.
45. Kappelle LJ, van Latum JC, Koudstaal PJ, van Gijn J for the Dutch TIA Study Group: Transient ischemic attacks and small-vessel disease. *Lancet* 1991;337:339–341.
46. Hankey GJ, Warlow CP. Lacunar transient ischaemic attacks: a clinically useful concept. *Lancet* 1991;337: 335–338.
47. Warlow C. Carotid endarterectomy: does it work? *Stroke* 1984;15:1068–1076.
48. Krul JMJ, van Gijn J, Ackerstaff RGA, Eikelboom BC,

Theodorides T, Vermeulen FFE. Site and pathogenesis of infarcts associated with carotid endarterectomy. *Stroke* 1989;20:324–328.

49. North American Symptomatic Carotid Endarterectomy Study Group. Carotid endarterectomy: three clinical evaluations. *Stroke* 1987;18:987–989.

50. European Carotid Surgery Trialists' Collaborative Group. MRC European Carotid Surgery Trial: interim results for symptomatic patients with severe (70–99%) or with mild (0–29%) carotid stenosis. *Lancet* 1991;337:1235–1243.

51. North American Symptomatic Carotid Endarterectomy Trial Collaborators. Beneficial effect of carotid endarterectomy in symptomatic patients with high-grade carotid stenosis. *N Engl J Med* 1991;325:445–453.

52. European Carotid Surgery Trialists' Collaborative Group. Endarterectomy for moderate symptomatic carotid stenosis: interim results from the MRC European Carotid Surgery Trial. *Lancet* 1996;347:1591–1593.

53. Rothwell PM, Gibson RJ, Slattery J, Sellar RJ, Warlow CP. Equivalence of measurements of carotid stenosis. A comparison of three methods on 1001 angiograms. European Carotid Surgery Trialists' Collaborative Group. *Stroke* 1994;25:2435–2439.

54. EC/IC Bypass Study Group. The international cooperative study of extracranial/intracranial arterial anastomosis (EC/IC Bypass Study): methodology and entry characteristics. *Stroke* 1985;16:397–405.

55. EC-IC Bypass Study Group. Failure of extracranial-intracranial arterial bypass to reduce the risk of ischemic stroke. Results of an international randomised trial. *N Engl J Med* 1985;313:1191–1200.

56. Sundt TM. Was the international trial of extracranial-intracranial arterial bypass representative of the population at risk? *N Engl J Med* 1987;316:814–816.

57. Barnett HJM, Sackett D, Taylor DW, et al. Are the results of the extracranial-intracranial bypass trial generalizable? *N Engl J Med* 1987;316:820–824.

58. Vorstrup S, Paulson OB. Extracranial-intracranial bypass revisited. *Cerebrovasc Dis* 1992;2:61–62.

59. Powers WJ, Tempel LW, Grubb RL. Influence of cerebral hemodynamics on stroke risk: one-year follow-up of 30 medically treated patients. *Ann Neurol* 1989;25:325–330.

60. Tulleken CAF, van Dieren A, Verdaasdonk RM, Berendsen W. End-to-side anastomosis of small vessels using an Nd:YAG laser with a hemispherical contact probe. *J Neurosurg* 1992;76:546–549.

61. Tulleken CAF, Verdaasdonk RM, Berendsen W, Mali WPThM. Use of the excimer laser in high-flow bypass surgery of the brain. *J Neurosurg* 1993;78:477–480.

62. Yadav JS, Roubin GS, King P, Iyer S, Vitek J. Angioplasty and stenting for restenosis after carotid endarterectomy—initial experience. *Stroke* 1996;27: 2075–2079.

63. Brown MM, Butler P, Gibbs J, Swash M, Waterston J. Feasibility of percutaneous transluminal angioplasty for carotid artery stenosis. *J Neurol Neurosurg Psychiatry* 1990;53:238–243.

64. Clark WM, Barnwell SL, Nesbit G, O'Neill OR, Wynn ML, Coull BM. Safety and efficacy of percutaneous transluminal angioplasty for intracranial atherosclerotic stenosis. *Stroke* 1995;26:1200–1204.

65. Terada T, Higashida RT, Halbach VV, et al. Transluminal angioplasty for arteriosclerotic disease of the distal vertebral and basilar arteries. *J Neurol Neurosurg Psychiatry* 1996;60:377–381.

66. Nakatsuka H, Ueda T, Ohta S, Sakaki S. Successful percutaneous transluminal angioplasty for basilar artery stenosis: technical case report. *Neurosurgery* 1996;39: 161–164.

67. Gil-Peralta A, Mayol A, Marcos JRG, et al. Percutaneous transluminal angioplasty of the symptomatic atherosclerotic carotid arteries—results, complications, and follow-up. *Stroke* 1996;27:2271–2273.

68. Eckert B, Zanella FE, Thie A, Steinmetz J, Zeumer H. Angioplasty of the internal carotid artery: results, complications and follow-up in 61 cases. *Cerebrovasc Dis* 1996;6:97–105.

69. Theron JG, Payelle GG, Coskun O, Huet HF, Guimaraens L. Carotid artery stenosis: treatment with protected balloon angioplasty and stent placement. *Radiology* 1996;201:627–636.

70. Major ongoing trials. Carotid and Vertebral Artery Transluminal Angioplasty Study (CAVATAS). *Stroke* 1996;27:358.

71. The European Atrial Fibrillation Trial Study Group. Optimal oral anticoagulant therapy in patients with non-rheumatic atrial fibrillation and recent cerebral ischemia. *N Engl J Med* 1995;333:5–10.

72. Ezekowitz MD, Bridgers SL, James KE, et al. Warfarin in the prevention of stroke associated with non-rheumatic atrial fibrillation. *N Engl J Med* 1992;327: 1406–1412.

73. Stroke Prevention in Atrial Fibrillation Investigators. Adjusted-dose warfarin versus low-intensity, fixed-dose warfarin plus aspirin for high-risk patients with atrial fibrillation: stroke Prevention in Atrial Fibrillation III randomised clinical trial. *Lancet* 1996;348: 633–638.

Cardiovascular Thrombosis: Thrombocardiology and Thromboneurology, Second Edition, edited by M. Verstraete, V. Fuster, and E. J. Topol, Lippincott–Raven Publishers, Philadelphia © 1998.

37

Peripheral Arterial Occlusion: Thromboembolism and Antithrombotic Therapy

Raymond Verhaeghe and *Henri Bounameaux

*The Center for Molecular and Vascular Biology, University of Leuven, B-3000 Leuven, Belgium; and *Division of Angiology and Hemostasis, University Hospital of Geneva, CH-1211 Geneva 14, Switzerland*

This chapter addresses atherosclerotic peripheral arterial disease, the most common cause of obstruction of blood flow to the lower limbs. Other degenerative or inflammatory arterial disorders (Table 37-1) that also result in a reduction of blood flow are rare in comparison with atherosclerosis. We particularly focus on the thromboembolic complications of peripheral atherosclerosis and on antithrombotic and thrombolytic therapy. Other therapeutic principles and general management are discussed only in the general context of thromboembolism and their prevention.

ATHEROSCLEROSIS AND THROMBOSIS IN PERIPHERAL ARTERIAL DISEASE: PRIMARY PREVENTION

Atherosclerosis is a multi-organ disorder characterized by localized plaque formation in selected sites of the arterial tree. Coronary arteries and the carotid bifurcation are particularily prone to plaque formation, as are the leg arteries, which are more often affected than arteries of similar size in the arms, perhaps because of a difference in hydrostatic pressure and in exercise-related variation of blood flow.

TABLE 37-1. *Etiology of peripheral arterial occlusive disease in the legs*

Degenerative arterial disease
  Atherosclerosis
  Mönckeberg's medial sclerosis
  Medial cystic degeneration
  Fibromuscular dysplasia
Inflammatory arterial disease
  Thromboangiitis obliterans (Buerger's disease)
  Systemic giant cell arteritis (Horton)
  Takayasu's disease
  Arteritis associated with connective tissue disease
Arterial thrombosis
  Idiopathic
  Associated with thrombophilia (causal relationship frequently uncertain)
  Immunologic (e.g., associated with lupuslike anticoagulant or induced by heparin)
Miscellaneous
  Peripheral arterial embolism
  Arterial trauma
  Arterial spasm (drug-induced or spontaneous)

Clinical manifestations of atherosclerosis in the legs include acute (thrombotic or embolic) occlusion of a leg artery and chronic arterial insufficiency resulting in intermittent claudication or rest pain and gangrene. The management of these two clinical conditions is discussed at the end of this chapter. In fact, the risk of a leg amputation is relatively low (5% or less), but the patients with symptomatic leg ischemia have a much reduced life expectancy due to arterial disease in vital organs. Their overall mortality rates at 5, 10, and 15 years are about 30%, 50%, and 70%, respectively, due to cardiovascular causes (myocardial infarction, stroke) in two thirds of the cases and to noncardiovascular causes (e.g., lung cancer) for the remaining third (1). Thus, the therapeutic approach of these patients should achieve two complementary goals: it should eliminate ischemic symptoms in the leg and, secondly, it should prevent progression of atherosclerosis and reduce the incidence of its thrombotic complications in other vascular beds as well as in the legs (secondary prevention).

Primary prevention of peripheral arterial disease mainly rests on control of the well-known risk factors of atherosclerosis. Atherosclerotic disease of the lower extremities is strongly related to cigarette smoking, hypercholesterolemia (particularily low-density lipoprotein and very low density lipoprotein hypercholesterolemia), diabetes mellitus, and hypertension. Smoking has an independent effect greater than other risk factors. Almost all patients younger than 70 years of age who attend vascular clinics or require peripheral arterial intervention are current or recent smokers. Increasing evidence that risk factors influence the early preclinical stages of atherosclerosis strengthens the belief that risk factor modification early in life will contribute to primary prevention of peripheral arterial disease. Campaigns against smoking set up by health authorities and by the antitobacco movement were reinforced by reports on the health risk of ambient smoke (2) and resulted in a gradual decline of tobacco consumption in developed countries. Prevalence estimates of adult regular smokers vary now between 25% and 30%, down from a peak of over 40% in the 1960s. At the same time, improved detection and treatment of hypertension, reduction of blood cholesterol due to changes in dietary habits, and treatment with cholesterol-lowering drugs and an improved level of fitness in the population may have contributed to the decline of mortality from coronary heart disease over the past 25 years. A recent report of the U.S. Physicians' Health Study concludes that moderate alcohol intake appears to decrease the risk of leg arterial disease in apparently healthy men, but the effect is easily overwhelmed by smoking (3).

Most data on risk factor control in leg arterial disease are from secondary prevention studies. Cessation of smoking was associated with an improvement of 86% of the maximum treadmill walking distance compared with only 24% in the subjects who continued smoking (4). Lowering of plasma cholesterol slowed the arteriographic progression of femoral atherosclerosis (5), and a similar effect has been obtained with antiplatelet drugs in a placebo-controlled trial (6). In the U.S. Physicians' Health Study, a primary prevention study, the relative risk of peripheral arteral surgery was lower (0.54, p = 0.03) in the aspirin group than in the control group

(7). The question of whether antiplatelet drugs are worthwhile in primary prevention of leg arterial disease merits further study.

THERAPEUTIC PRINCIPLES TO RELIEVE ARTERIAL OCCLUSION

Vascular Surgery

Circulation to the legs can be reestablished by two basic techniques: thrombendarterectomy and bypass grafting (Fig. 37-1). The former technique is less frequently performed in recent years. Thrombendarterectomy of the proximal part of the deep femoral artery (profundaplasty) is a well-tolerated operation to improve the collateral blood supply to the limb when the superficial femoral artery is occluded. The implantation of an aortofemoral Dacron graft is the common surgical technique to treat extensive aortoiliac disease. The graft starts with a terminoterminal (end-to-end) or terminolateral (end-to-side) anastomosis close to the origin of the renal arteries and ends on the femoral arteries. A proximal end-to-end anastomosis saves the normal pelvic circulation and decreases the risk of postoperative impairment of erection. For infrainguinal reconstruction, the saphenous vein bypass graft remains the preferred material. The saphenous vein is totally removed, reversed because of its valves, and sewn proximally on the common femoral and distally on the popliteal or tibial artery. In most patients, the distal anastomosis descends below the knee joint. A prosthetic graft is a second choice alternative at this level because of poorer long-term results. An elegant but delicate technique for long reconstructions is the venous bypass in situ. The proximal saphenous vein is slightly moved and anastomosed on the femoral artery in the groin, whereas the smaller distal end is mobilized and fixed on the popliteal or tibial artery. Side branches have to be ligated and the valves destroyed with a suitable instrument. Many patients who undergo vascular surgery have multisegmental arterial occlusive disease. This is almost certainly the case if they have critical ischemia. The proximal lesion is repaired first, usually by aortofemoral bypass grafting.

The decision to operate on a patient with arterial disease of the legs depends on several factors: the severity of the patient's symptoms, the level of the main arterial obstruction (aortoiliac or infrainguinal), the risk of the operation, the expected late result of the procedure balanced against the natural history of the disease, the general prognosis of the patient, and the best available alternative treatment. Some surgeons feel that surgical intervention should be reserved for patients with

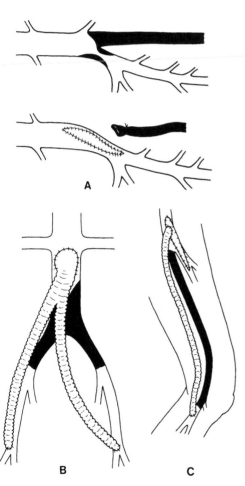

FIG. 37-1. Schematic presentation of common surgical procedures. **A:** Profundaplasty with ligation of the occluded superficial femoral artery. **B:** Aortofemoral bypass graft. **C:** Femoropopliteal bypass graft.

critical leg ischemia that endangers the limb (so-called limb salvage surgery), but others propose surgery to patients with disabling claudication as well. The severity of the symptoms has to be evaluated in conjunction with the level of the main obstructive lesion: aortoiliac reconstruction produces better late results than infrainguinal bypass surgery. Age, life expectancy, and physical condition are important determinants to select a patient for surgery and may influence the choice of the procedure. For instance, in an elderly person with a high cardiac risk for major abdominal surgery, alternative techniques may be considered, such as an axillofemoral graft. Infrainguinal reconstruction in patients in whom the distal circulation is impaired should be reserved for true limb salvage because long-term patency decreases in the presence of a poor run-off.

Results of arterial surgery are reported in terms of survival, limb salvage, and patency of the reconstruction. The operative mortality of aortoiliac surgery is low (1% to 2%), but it increases in patients with critical ischemia (4% to 5%). The long-term patency rate of aortofemoral bypass grafting is fairly high (85% to 90% at 5 years and 70% to 75% at 10 years), but a considerable proportion of patients need a reintervention to achieve this result. For patients with intermittent claudication, the late results are better than for those with critical ischemia who often have multilevel disease. Early complications occur in 5% of the patients who undergo surgery: renal failure, severe bleeding, acute thrombosis, and intestinal ischemia are the most common. Late complications include graft thrombosis, graft infection, anastomotic false aneurysm, and aortoenteric erosion or fistula. The long-term results of infrainguinal bypass surgery depend largely on the particular selection of the patients considered. Factors that affect the late result are the extent of the distal disease, the site of the terminal anastomosis, and the type of graft material used. In general, autologous vein grafts carry better patency rates than prosthetic grafts, and the difference is magnified with more distal terminal anasto-

mosis. Approximate 1-year patency rates in patients with critical leg ischemia vary from 75% for femoropopliteal vein grafts with above-knee distal anastomosis to 40% for femorotibial prosthetic grafts (8).

Percutaneous Revascularization Procedures

Introduced by Dotter and Judkins in 1964, the transluminal treatment of atherosclerotic obstructive lesions of the leg arteries became accepted worldwide only after the development by Grüntzig of a double-lumen polyvinyl balloon catheter in 1974. Later, the technique became popular to treat lesions in other regions as well, particularly in the coronary arteries. We will focus here on the use of percutaneous transluminal angioplasty (PTA) and on stenting of the leg arteries and briefly comment on other developments of the transluminal technique.

Percutaneous Transluminal Angioplasty of the Leg Arteries

The PTA procedure is devided into three phases: (a) an artery is punctured using the classical Seldinger technique, (b) the obstructive lesion is crossed with a guide wire, and (c) the ballon catheter is passed over the guide wire and inflated until adequate enlargement of the arterial lumen is obtained. PTA stretches the wall, ruptures the atherosclerotic plaque, and causes a localized tear of the intima and media. In the healing phase, the tear retracts and the arterial lumen is enlarged. The ankle pressure, measured before and after the procedure, confirms the hemodynamic improvement.

PTA is technically feasible for lesions listed in Table 37-2. As for surgery, the procedure is only justified if symptoms are disabling the patient or endanger the limb. The initial technical result as demonstrated on a control angiography at the end of the procedure determines the primary success rate (Fig. 37-2). Patency rate is defined as the percentage of patients in whom the artery is still open

TABLE 37-2. *Indications for percutaneous transluminal angioplasty and for iliac stents*

Percutaneous angioplasty
  Optimal lesions
    Short stenosis of the common or external iliac artery
    Isolated stenosis of the superficial femoral or popliteal artery
    Isolated short obstruction (<3 cm) of the superficial femoral artery
  Possibly treatable
    Stenosis at surgical anastomosis
    Multiple stenoses of the superficial femoral artery
    Longer obstruction (3–10 cm) of the superficial femoral artery
    Short obstruction of distal popliteal artery
    Stenosis of the proximal deep femoral artery
    Stenosis of the abdominal aorta
  For limb salvage only
    Longer obstruction (>10 cm) of the femoropopliteal axis (?)
    Stenosis of the calf arteries
Iliac stents
  Failure of angioplasty
  Recurrent lesion (after angioplasty)
  Complicated lesions (long, eccentic, ulcerated, calcified)
  Occlusion of iliac artery

Data directly comparing PTA with surgery are limited and the significance of such a comparison can be questioned. Nonetheless, in two randomized trials, clinical outcome was similar after a mean follow-up of 1 and 4 years, respectively (14,15). In one study, patients treated initially with PTA needed additional vascular procedures more frequently to maintain patency during the study period (15). On the other hand, a randomized trial compared PTA with conservative management in patients with claudication due to short obstructive lesions: at 6 months improvement

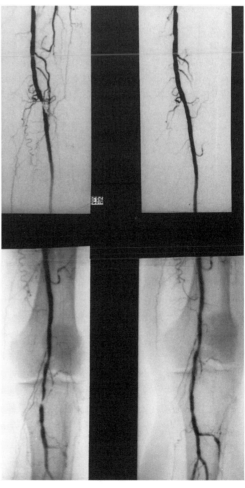

FIG. 37-2. Stenosis of the superficial femoral artery relieved with angioplasty **(top, left and right)**. Recurrent claudication 4 years later due to popliteal artery stenosis again treated with angioplasty **(bottom, left and right)**.

for a given period of observation after initial technical success of the procedure and is calculated by means of the life table method. Average primary success and patency rates for iliac and femoropopliteal PTA are listed in Table 37-3. In a prospective series of 984 PTAs, Johnston et al. (9–11) identified the following factors as important for the long-term prognosis: (a) clinical stage (claudication versus limb salvage), (b) site (common iliac artery versus other), (c) extent of disease (stenosis versus occlusion), (d) distal runoff (good versus poor). These factors together with differences in threshold to define success most probably explain the variation in early and late results reported in the literature.

Few patients are candidates for infrapopliteal PTA; if they are, results of PTA appear comparable with what is achieved with distal bypass surgery. In a series of 145 lesions treated in 114 endangered limbs, the cumulative 2-year limb salvage rate was 83%, similar to that obtained in 320 patients treated surgically in the same institution over the same time period (12,13).

TABLE 37-3. *Approximate immediate and long-term results after PTA (ideal lesions)*

	Technical success rate (%)	Patency rate at 3–5 years (%)
Iliac artery	>90	80–85
Femoropopliteal artery	80–85	60–65

Technical success: excellent result on control angiography at end of procedure. Patency rate: percentage of open angioplasty sites after initial technical success (life table method).

in walking and quality of life was significantly better and progression of atherosclerosis slower in patients treated with PTA (16). Starting from a literature review on 26 studies with data on mortality, morbidity, patency, and cost, Hunink et al. evaluated the relative benefits and cost-effectiveness of femoropopliteal revascularization with PTA versus bypass surgery (17). They used a multistate transition simulation model (Markov process) for decision analysis and concluded that PTA was the preferred treatment for claudication if they had a treatable lesion, whereas in those with critical limb ischemia, bypass surgery is preferred for an occlusion and PTA for a stenosis.

The complications of PTA are listed in Table 37-4. Surgical intervention for bleeding, false aneurysm, or acute ischemia is required in 1% to 2%. Thrombosis and/or distal embolization leading to amputation is rare (0.2%). Other rare complications are renal

TABLE 37-4. *Local complications of PTA*

	Mahler (18) (%)	AHA (19) (%)
Puncture site		
Hematoma	4.7	3.4
False aneurysm	0.2	0.5
AV fistula		0.1
Angioplasty site		
Dissection	0.4	0.4
Thrombosis		3.2
Wall rupture	Very rare	0.3
Peripheral embolization (thrombus, plaque material)	0.4	2.3

failure (0.2%), (fatal) myocardial infarction (0.1% to 0.2%), or stroke (18,19).

Stents in Leg Arteries

Among the novel techniques introduced over the past 10 years to improve the results of PTA, the insertion of intravascular metallic stents under fluoroscopic control has gained widespread acceptance. Various self-expandable stents (e.g., Gianturco stents or Wall stents) and balloon-expandable stents (e.g., Palmaz stents or Strecker stents) have been developed; they act as a scaffold to hold open a vessel segment. Within 4 to 6 weeks after their implantation, they become covered with a true endothelium (20). Initially reserved to rescue failed PTA (because of intima dissection or acute occlusion due to elastic recoil) and to remedy recurrent disease after an initial PTA, their use has expanded to primary stenting of complicated lesions (Fig. 37-3). Stents are inherently thrombogenic, and neointimal hyperplasia develops in stented arteries; both problems are more common in infrainguinal as compared with iliac vessels.

Stenting of iliac arteries was first used as an adjunct to PTA in the presence of a suboptimal result of simple dilatation (confirmed by hemodynamic measurements), as well as in occlusion, restenosis, or extensive intima dissection, which compromise the outcome. Because they provide rigid support of the arterial lumen after PTA, stents also facilitate the percutaneous treatment of iliac artery lesions, which would hardly be accessible for simple PTA such as long-segment stenosis and occlusion (Table 37-2). Several investigators have published primary success rates over 90% with iliac stents, and the first follow-up studies report a 4-year patency of 85% (21–24). In centers with a liberal use of iliac stenting, the demand for surgical reconstruction in obstructive aortoiliac disesase decreases markedly.

In the femoropopliteal region, restenosis and reocclusion remain significant problems after PTA, and with stent insertion a better

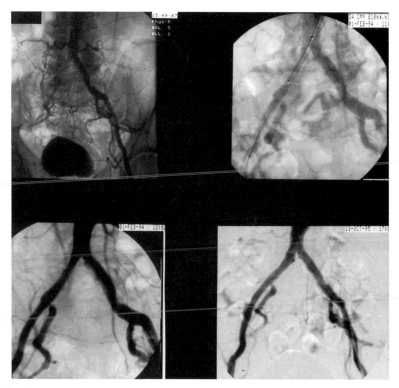

FIG. 37-3. Occlusion of the right common iliac artery causing incapacitating claudication for 8 months **(top left)**. Primary recanalization and insertion of a Wall stent **(top right and bottom left)**. Normal patency is maintained 20 months later **(bottom right)**.

outcome was expected. The stent most widely used so far for infrainguinal disease is the Wall stent, with a patency rate of approximately 70% at 6 months and 50% at 1 year (25,26). Thus, the initial expectation does not appear to be fulfilled, and the exact role of stenting in femoropopliteal disease is not definitively established.

Areas of research and future development are new (e.g., biodegradable) materials and coating of stents with drugs to inhibit and prevent thrombosis and to modify the vessel wall response to injury. A mechanical solution to the problem of ingrowth of scar tissue within the stent is the concept of endovascular stented grafts or stents with a thin polyester covering. Promising early results were reported in patients with obstructive aortoiliac disease, but long-term results and femoropopliteal use are still awaited (27,28).

Other Developments in Percutaneous Revascularization

Of all other auxiliary methods purported to complement classical balloon PTA that were introduced and too rapidly promoted under commercial pressure over the past 10 to 15 years (directional atherectomy, rotational angioplasty, laser-assisted angioplasty, and ultrasonic angioplasty), none ultimately withstood critical evaluation and gained uncontested acceptance for clinical use. However, some centers keep using directional atherectomy or rotational angioplasty for particular indications.

Thrombolytic Therapy

Intravenous administration of a thrombolytic agent through a peripheral vein as currently used in acute myocardial infarction or pulmonary embolism was investigated some 25 to 30 years ago but has been replaced almost completely by intra-arterial catheter-directed infusion.

Procedure

The procedure usually starts with a diagnostic angiography. The most appropriate vascular access—ipsilaterally or contralaterally—is chosen on the basis of physical examination (arterial pulses in the groin) and duplex ultrasound localization of the occlusion. In practice, ipsilateral anterograde common femoral puncture is preferred if the occlusion starts at a distance below the inguinal ligament and the femoral pulse is normal; the contralateral femoral artery is taken if the femoral pulse on the affected side is weak or absent.

A guide wire is passed through the thrombus; successful lysis is much more likely with a positive guide wire traversal test suggesting a soft recent clot (29). A catheter is then imbedded within the thrombus for local infusion of the thrombolytic agent. Several types of catheters (usually 4F or 5F caliber) are suitable (e.g., standard endhole catheters, catheters with multiple sideholes or with sideslits that open only when a threshold intraluminal pressure is reached). Several infusion techniques can be used. Stepwise infiltration means repeated injection of a small fixed dose of lytic agent into the thrombus (e.g., every 5 to 15 minutes), while advancing the catheter progressively until the open distal lumen is reached. Continuous infusion using a steady-flow pump is less laborious and thus more popular; it is frequently combined with initial "bolusing" or "lacing" of the thrombus with thrombolytic agent. This is achieved by retracting the catheter from distally in the thrombus to proximally while infiltrating it over its entire length with lytic agent. Initial bolusing shortens the duration of lytic therapy for peripheral arterial occlusion (30,31). Accelerating lysis and shortening treatment time is also the aim of the "pulse spray" infusion

technique, in which the agent is forcefully injected through a catheter with multiple side slits and endhole occlusion (32). Superiority of any catheter system or infusion technique remains to be established. The duration of the lytic procedure also can be reduced with the use of adjunctive techniques, which intend to debulk the thrombus mass. Examples are the simple catheter aspiration thromboembolectomy or the still experimental mechanical thromboembolectomy with the hydrolyser (33) or with the clotbuster (a high-speed rotating impeller) (34).

Progression of lysis is followed by clinical evaluation and noninvasive testing, as well as by repeated injection of contrast fluid at intervals of 4 to 12 hours or earlier if rapid clearance is anticipated (Fig. 37-4). Between two controls, the catheter is advanced into the remaining clot and the infusion is continued. Thrombolytic treatment is considered to have failed, and normally stopped, if after 12 to 24 hours no lysis is observed. In the large majority of patients, the postlysis angiography identifies a causative arterial lesion that can usually be corrected by a complementary endovascular procedure, although occasionally a surgical intervention is required to improve the circulation to the limb and to prevent early rethrombosis. Opinions differ on the value of simultaneous heparinization during thrombolysis to prevent catheter-related thromboembolism. Heparin can be infused through a peripheral vein or through a proximal sheath around the arterial catheter. Dosages vary from 200 to 1,000 IU/hr. After a successful procedure, most patients receive antithrombotic prophylaxis with aspirin or a similar drug. Others prefer systemic heparin followed by coumarinic drugs.

Choice of Lytic Agent

In the early days of catheter thrombolysis, streptokinase was the most widely used agent, but in recent years urokinase and alteplase (rt-PA) largely superseded streptokinase in clinical practice. For urokinase, dosage schemes varied initially, but the low-dose concept was

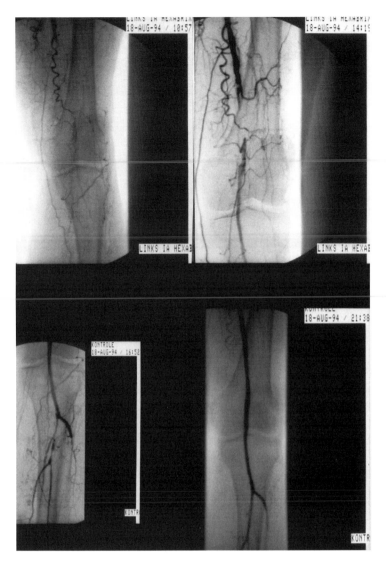

FIG. 37-4. Acute ischemia with a viable limb due to a recent occlusion of the left distal superficial femoral artery **(top left),** for which an intrathrombotic infusion of rt-PA is started with progressive lysis **(top right and bottom left).** Lysis restores normal patency of the superficial femoral, popliteal, and fibular artery, but flow in the anterior tibial remains slow **(bottom right).**

gradually abandoned in favor of higher dosages with progressive tapering (35,36). With rt-PA, an opposite move occurred with higher doses (10 or 5 mg/hr or 0.1 mg/kg/hr) being replaced by lower ones (1 or 0.5 mg/hr) because no obvious benefit from using the higher doses was observed. Acceptable dosage schemes for the three thrombolytic agents are summarized in Table 37-5. With

delivery systems that pursue accelerated lysis, initial bolus injections may be used as described above.

From retrospective pooled analysis of published reports, rt-PA is frequently claimed to achieve the speediest and most efficacious thrombolysis, whereas urokinase has the reputation of highest safety. Prospective randomized studies that compare different agents di-

TABLE 37-5. *Agents and therapeutic schemes in local thrombolysis for peripheral arterial disease*

Stepwise infusion	
Streptokinase	1,000–3,000 IU every 3–5 min
Urokinase	3,000–4,000 IU every 3–5 min
Continuous infusion	
Streptokinase	5,000 (or 10,000) IU per hour (eventually with loading dose of up to 40,000 IU)
Urokinase	Low dose: variable schemes up to 100,000 IU/hr (eventually with variable loading dose)
	High dose: 4,000 IU/min up to antegrade flow
	1,000 IU/min up to complete lysis (modifications possible)
rt-PA	Low dose: 0.5 or 1 mg/hr
	High dose: 3, 5, or 10 mg/hr
	0.05 or 0.1 mg/kg/hr
Intrathrombus bolusing or lacing	
Urokinase	120,000–250,000 IU lacing dose (or 2,500 IU/cm) followed by continuous infusion
rt-PA	3×5 mg (5–10 min interval) followed by 0.05 mg/kg/hr
Forced periodic (pulse spray) infusion:	
Urokinase	25,000 IU/ml: 0.2 ml every 30 sec for 20 min and every 60 sec thereafter
	20,000 IU/cm occlusion length (microhole balloon catheter)
rt-PA	0.5 mg/ml: 0.2 ml every 30 sec for 20 min, every 60 sec thereafter
	0.5–1 mg/cm occlusion length (microhole balloon catheter)
Intraoperative thrombolysis	
Streptokinase	50,000–150,000 IU slow bolus or infusion over 30 min
Urokinase	250,000–500,000 IU bolus or infusion over 30 min
	1,000–2,000 IU/min into distal thrombus
rt-PA	3×5 mg bolus over 30 min

rectly are few. One open trial compared intra-arterial streptokinase (SK) to intra-arterial and intravenous rt-PA in 60 patients with recent onset or deterioration of limb ischemia (37): initial angiographic success was significantly greater with intra-arterial rt-PA (100%) than with intra-arterial SK (80%; p < 0.04) or intravenous rt-PA (45% p < 0.01), the 30-day limb salvage rate being 80%, 60%, and 45%, respectively. In another open randomized trial on 32 patients, rt-PA initially produced significantly faster lysis than urokinase, but the 24-hour and 30-day success rate did not achieve statistical significance (38). In the STILE trial (Surgery versus Thrombolysis for Ischemia of the Lower Extremity), there was no difference in efficacy or bleeding complications in patients receiving rt-PA compared with urokinase in a randomized but open fashion (39). Thus, there is at present no definite scientific proof of superiority of any agent for peripheral thrombolysis in terms of efficacy or safety.

New thrombolytic agents being developed for clinical use include recombinant human urokinase (40), recombinant pro-urokinase (41), and recombinant staphylokinase (42–44).

Clinical Application

Clinical experience with intra-arterial catheter-directed thrombolysis in acute limb ischemia started in the late 1970s. Many descriptive series are relatively small and contain a mixed population of patients with arterial occlusions of different origin, location, and extent, and with a variable degree of ischemia. The therapeutic success rate thus varies largely (from 25% to 85%). Four studies compared thrombolysis to surgical intervention. A small randomized trial tested the intra-arterial continuous infusion of 30 mg alteplase over 3 hours versus surgical thrombectomy in 20 patients with recent (less than 14 days) occlusion and severe leg ischemia. Considerable lysis was obtained in 60% of patients treated with alteplase, and half of them subsequently had angioplasty but two early reocclusions occurred. Thrombectomy restored blood flow immediately in 65% of cases (45). Ouriel et al. (36) compared initial thrombolysis with adjunctive angioplasty or surgery versus immediate surgery in 114 patients with limb-threatening ischemia of less than 7 days' duration.

Successful thrombolysis was obtained in 70% of the patients. Limb salvage was similar in the two groups (82% at 1 year), but cumulative survival was significantly improved in patients randomized to thrombolysis due to fewer cardiopulmonary complications in hospital (84% versus 58% at 1 year, p = 0.01). The large multicenter STILE trial selected patients with non-embolic worsening of limb ischemia within the preceding 6 months to evaluate thrombolysis as part of a treatment strategy. The study was terminated at 393 patients because surgical revascularization appeared a more effective treatment at the first interim analysis, primarily because of a reduction in ongoing/recurrent ischemia. Failure of catheter placement occurred in 28% of patients randomized to lysis, and they were counted as treatment failures. A post hoc analysis according to duration of ischemia indicated that patients with recent (less than 14 days) deterioration had shorter hospital stays, lower amputation rates at 1 month, and improved amputation-free survival at 6 months if initially treated with thrombolysis (39). At 1-year follow-up, only recently thrombosed bypass grafts but not native arteries had benefited from thrombolysis (46,47). Phase I of the TOPAS trial was designed as a dose-ranging trial to evaluate three doses of recombinant urokinase in comparison with surgery. The amputation-free survival rate at 1 year was 75% in 52 patients treated initially with 4,000 IU/min of urokinase (the best group) and 65% in 58 surgically treated patients, this difference not reaching statistical significance (40).

In chronic arterial obstruction leading to limb-threatening ischemia, surgery or angioplasty is the treatment of choice for most patients. Descriptive series frequently included patients with occlusion of up to 6 months' duration and reported variable lysis rates. The STILE trial only evaluated such patients versus surgery prospectively: results obtained from a post hoc analysis indicate that surgical revascularization was superior (39).

The therapeutic options in patients with an occluded bypass graft leading to severe ischemia are either surgical revision and thrombectomy, catheter directed thrombolysis, or insertion of a new graft. Thrombolysis appears attractive in patients with poor filling of distal vessels on the pretreatment angiography: lysing the thrombus may show a correctible causative lesion and eventually clear the thrombosed outflow vessels. In descriptive reports, success rates of thrombolysis have varied as much for occluded grafts (25% to 75%) as for native arteries, and long-term outcome is still debated. In a secondary analysis of the STILE trial, patients with a recently occluded bypass graft (less than 14 days) had a lower major amputation rate at 1 year follow-up (20% versus 48%; p = 0.026), whereas those with graft occlusion of more than 14 days had a better outcome when treated surgically (46). Proper catheter positioning within the thrombus is an occasional problem with occluded grafts; in STILE, positioning failed in 39% of the occluded grafts, an inexplicably high rate. Experts agree that grafts that occlude within the first few days after their insertion need surgical revision rather than thrombolytic treatment (48).

Recent operation is generally considered to be a contraindication to thrombolytic therapy, but intraoperative thrombolysis has paradoxically emerged as a frequently successful adjuvant to permit surgical thromboembolectomy in patients with extensive distal thrombosis in whom complete thrombectomy is difficult. A thrombolytic drug is then infused over a short period into the distal artery containing the thrombus. Urokinase has become the most frequently used agent for this application. In a prospective, randomized, blinded, and placebo-controlled trial, three doses of urokinase were investigated (125,000, 250,000, and 500,000 IU). Bolus infusions of these doses were safe and associated with breakdown of complexed fibrin (elevated D-dimer) but not with depletion of fibrinogen. Patients receiving urokinase had a significantly lower mortality rate compared with that of placebo controls (49).

Complications

Complications of peripheral thrombolysis are summarized in Table 37-6. Intracranial bleeding or severe systemic bleeding is the most significant risk associated with any thrombolytic therapy. It also occurs with fibrin-specific thrombolytic agents due to lysis of pre-existing hemostatic plug or to depletion of coagulation factors; it also may be a consequence of concomitant or continued anticoagulation.

In a review of 19 prospectively followed series of patients undergoing peripheral thrombolysis published from 1974 to 1988, the overall incidence of hemorrhagic stroke was 1%, and the incidence of major and minor hemorrhage was 5.1 and 14.8%, respectively (50). There were no control groups in these series. The British Thrombolysis Study group reported recently an incidence of hemorrhagic and ischemic stroke of 2.3%, half of which occurred during the thrombolytic session (51). By contrast, McNamara et al. (52), reviewing the American experience, calculated a lower risk of intracranial hemorrhage with peripheral intra-arterial thrombolysis than with systemic thrombolytic infusions for myocardial infarction (0.1% to 0.5% versus 0.3% to 0.5%), but two recent American prospective randomized trials comparing surgery to thrombolysis recorded intracranial bleeding rates of 1.2% and 2.1%, respectively (39,40).

Overt or occult gastrointestinal bleeding is rare; early bleeding usually results from an undiagnosed peptic ulcer. Retroperitoneal bleeding may occur spontaneously in elderly patients but more frequently results from inadvertent posterior wall puncture. Unexpected back pain, the sudden development of hypotension, or anemia without obvious blood loss should prompt a search for a retroperitoneal hematoma using ultrasound. Pericatheter bleeding (or bleeding at other arterial or venous puncture sites) is common,

typically delayed in onset, usually minor, and controlled with local pressure.

Major bleeding should prompt interruption of infusion of thrombolytic agent and heparin. Administration of fresh frozen plasma or blood may be considered depending on the clinical need.

Episodes of distal embolization by fragments of the lysing clot are observed in 10% to 15% of the patients undergoing peripheral thrombolysis. Small emboli in tiny arteries are usually lysed during the course of continued thrombolysis. Emboli that occlude larger distal arteries are potentially more harmful. Although some subsequently dissolve by additional fibrinolytic agent, additional measures such as thrombus aspiration or surgical intervention may be required if profound leg ischemia develops and the clinical condition does not improve quickly with continued lysis.

Catheter manipulation in the arterial lumen entails a definite risk of thrombosis, wall dissection, or vessel spasm. Several measures have been proposed to prevent pericatheter thrombosis—the use of thin catheters or catheters with side holes, an increase in flow rate, or simultaneous infusion of heparin—but it is uncertain whether these measures are effective. In the event of pericatheter thrombosis, further thrombolytic therapy is required. Undetected pericatheter thrombosis may lead to immediate reocclusion of the reopened vessel upon withdrawal of the catheter; in this event, urgent surgical intervention may be needed.

ANTITHROMBOTIC THERAPY IN SECONDARY PREVENTION

Antithrombotic Therapy and Natural History of Peripheral Arterial Disease

Effect on General Prognosis

Most clinicians are not convinced that long-term oral anticoagulation is needed in patients with peripheral arterial obstructive

TABLE 37-6. *Complications of thrombolysis*

Major bleeding	5%
Intracranial bleeding	1%
Minor bleeding	10–15%
Distal embolization	10–15%
Catheter complications	5–10%

disease. Two Dutch prospective trials suggest a lower incidence of vascular events in patients on oral anticoagulants (53,54). More recently, Kretschmer et al. (55) selected patients who had vascular surgery in the femoropopliteal region to study the influence of oral anticoagulants on long-term mortality: they report a longer survival in the anticoagulated group (120 months versus 73 months in the control group).

In general, patients with peripheral arterial disease receive aspirin or (in some countries) ticlopidine to decrease the incidence of thromboembolic vascular events. The collaborative overview of randomized trials of antiplatelet therapy, the meta-analysis of the Antiplatelet Trialists' Collaboration, calculated that the vascular risk was reduced to a similar extent (odds reduction of $27 \pm 2\%$) in a category of high-risk patients of mixed origin as in patients with prior myocardial infarction ($25 \pm 4\%$), with acute myocardial infarction ($29 \pm 4\%$), or with prior stroke/transient ischemic accident (TIA) ($22 \pm 4\%$). This mixed category was subdivided, and peripheral vascular disease was one of the major subgroups. The meta-analysis showed that there was no significant evidence of heterogeneity between the results of the subgroups: almost all of the subgroup results appear to favor treatment, even though the risk reductions are not conventionally significant for all subgroups. The authors state that "the most likely conclusion may well be that antiplatelet therapy is likely to be protective for any high risk patients with clinically evident occlusive vascular disease unless there is some special contra-indication" (56). Although the meta-analysis is referred to as "the aspirin papers," a closer look at the individual results of unconfounded randomized comparisons (4) shows that in the subcategory of intermittent claudication the number of patients included in placebo-controlled ticlopidine trials far exceeds that of aspirin trials. Further evidence for a beneficial effect of ticlopidine comes from another double-blind multicenter study that enrolled 615 patients; 304 were assigned to ticlopidine

treatment and 311 to placebo for 24 weeks. Four patients in the ticlopidine group and 12 in the placebo group experienced a vascular event (sudden death, myocardial infarction, or stroke) during the follow-up period (relative risk 2.93 with 95% confidence interval [CI] 0.96 to 8.99; risk reduction 68%; p = 0.04; intention-to-treat analysis). The risk reduction was consistent when subgroups (diabetic and nondiabetic patients) were analyzed separately (57). Clopidogrel (75 mg daily), a novel thienopyridine derivative like ticlopidine, was compared with aspirin (325 mg daily) in a randomized, blinded, international megatrial. In the subgroup of 6,452 patients with peripheral arterial disease followed for 1 to 3 years, the relative risk reduction for the occurrence of a vascular event was 24% (p = 0.0028) for clopidogrel as compared with aspirin (58).

Effect on Local Evolution

Aspirin and ticlopidine are the only platelet drugs that have been shown to retard the progression of atheroslerosis and the occurrence of thrombotic complications in legs of patients with arterial disease. Three trials had an angiographic endpoint. In one it was progression to total occlusion, but in the other two angiographic changes were quantified into a score, which represents a rather crude way of evaluating the progression of atherosclerotic lesions, and doubt remains about the clinical significance of the observed changes (6,59, 60) (Table 37-7). Two other reports, one with aspirin and one with ticlopidine, point to a lower need of vascular surgery in patients who receive antithrombotic drugs, thus suggesting slower progression to advanced stages of ischemia (7,57).

Data on the functional clinical evolution are available for several trials with ticlopidine. A meta-analysis on four placebo-controlled trials (61,62) and a fifth controlled study (63) all showed a significantly better evolution of walking capacity with ticlopidine, although the beneficial functional effect of the com-

TABLE 37-7. *Effect of antiplatelet therapy on local progression of leg arterial disease*

Aspirin (-dipyridamole)	
Schoop et al. (59)[a]	
Placebo	58%
Aspirin (1 g)	20[b]
Aspirin-dipyridamole (1 g to 225 mg)	34[b]
Hess et al. (6)[c]	
Placebo	+6.2 points
Aspirin (1 g)	+4.4 points
Aspirin-dipyridamole (1 g to 225 mg)	+2.2[b]
Ticlopidine	
Stiegler et al. (60)[d]	
Placebo	+4.2 points
Ticlopidine (500 mg)	+0.1[b]

[a]Occlusion rate in femoral artery stenosis (n = 300; follow-up 4.5 yr).
[b]Significantly different from placebo.
[c]Angiographic progression in leg arteries (n = 199; follow-up 2 yr).
[d]Angiographic progression in leg arteries (n = 43; follow-up 1 yr).

pound may be related to hemorheologic improvement rather than to its antiplatelet action (64). By contrast, walking distance improved in the two treatment groups in a multicenter study, but no significant difference was reached between ticlopidine and placebo. The number of patients with at least 50% improvement was slightly greater in the ticlopidine-treated group (57).

Because thrombosis is only the final step in a long atherosclerotic evolution of the leg arteries, long-term anticoagulation is unlikely to represent a major advance in the pharmacologic prevention of local progression of peripheral arterial occlusive disease. From a slower deterioration of the ankle pressure index in patients treated with anticoagulants, de Smit and van Urk concluded that this was a delayed progression (54).

Antithrombotic Therapy in Arterial Surgery

Several problems may arise after implantation of a graft or after a thrombendarterectomy of which early thrombosis, restenosis, and late occlusion are relevant to antithrombotic prevention. Early thrombosis may be fa-

vored by the nonthromboresistant nature of prosthetic materials or endarterectomized surfaces but is frequently related to poor surgical indication or to technical errors. Myointimal hyperplasia is the main cause of restenosis, particularly at the anastomotic sutures, but occasionally diffuse and late graft occlusion results from progression of the atherosclerotic disease with decreasing inflow and increasing outflow obstruction. Development of new atherosclerotic lesions in the bypass graft frequently aggravates the situation, whereas embolic complications originating from surgical sites are less common—they occur when hemodynamic forces that favor disruption and fragmentation surpass adhesive forces.

The daily concern is how to maintain patency of the arterial reconstruction. Although few problems arise with aortofemoral reconstruction, the situation is particularly delicate for bypasses that extend below the groin, and the main problems arise when the diameter of the graft decreases below 6 mm. For identical conditions, autologous vein grafts produce better late patency rates than prosthetic grafts, and this explains the popularity of the saphenous vein as first-choice graft material in infrainguinal reconstruction. Apart from a correct application of surgical techniques, adjunctive measures, and methods of surveillance of grafts as outlined in Chapter 20, many vascular surgeons prescribe antiplatelet drugs to their patients postoperatively for a prolonged period of time with the hope of improving patency rates. Clinical trials to substantiate their practice are not numerous and are usually small. The fourth American College of Chest Physicians (ACCP) Consensus Conference on Antithrombotic Therapy analyzed five published randomized prospective trials (Table 37-8) (65). The study population in these trials is a mixture of patients with vein grafts and prosthetic grafts. Three studies reported a significant advantage of antiplatelet treatment, usually aspirin associated with dipyridamole, started before surgery and continued for a variable period, over placebo to maintain patency of infrainguinal arterial bypass (66–68). One trial suggests that the ef-

TABLE 37-8. *Antiplatelet therapy in infrainguinal grafts*

Authors (ref.)	Patients (n)	Type of graft	Follow-up	Patency (%)	Comment
Green et al. (66)	49	Prosthetic	1 yr	Aspirin 88 Aspirin-dip 62.5 Placebo 25	
Goldman and McCollum (67)	53	Prosthetic	1 yr	Aspirin-dip 67 Placebo 36	$p < 0.05$
Clyne et al. (68)	111	Vein (93) Prosthetic (55)	1 yr Life table	Aspirin-dip 84 Placebo 65	$p = 0.012$ Benefit entirely in prosthetic grafts within first month
Kohler et al. (69)	100	Vein (51) Prosthetic (51)	2 yr Life table	Aspirin-dip 67 Placebo 57	Not significant Treatment started postsurgery
McCollum et al. (70)	549	Vein	3 years	Aspirin-dip 61 Placebo 60	More myocardial infarction and stroke with placebo

Dip, dipyridamole.

fect is limited to prosthetic grafts and that it is confined to the first postoperative month. The fourth trial followed 100 patients with distal reconstruction, one third of whom received a prosthetic graft, and found no difference in the results between active drug and placebo, but the treatment was started after surgery only (69). In the fifth study on more than 500 patients undergoing saphenous vein femoro-popliteal bypass surgery followed over 2 years, patients treated with antiplatelet therapy had fewer myocardial infarctions and strokes but no better graft patency (70). Antiplatelet drugs were started before surgery, and this may have caused more wound hematomas and greater transfusion requirements. The Consensus Conference therefore recommends aspirin 325 mg daily (with or without dipyridamole, 75 mg three times daily) for prosthetic infrainguinal arterial bypass grafts as a useful adjunct to maintain patency. An optimal protection requires aspirin to be started before surgery (65). The ACCP recommendation is supported by a recent meta-analysis made by the Antiplatelet Trialists' Collaboration on 11 randomized trials including over 2,000 patients with peripheral arterial grafts: antiplatelet drugs reduce the incidence of graft occlusion by one third (from 24% to 16%) (71).

Some clinicians advocate the use of oral anticoagulants for the first few months after implantation of a vascular graft or eventually for lifelong use if the graft is at high risk of thrombosis. They base their decision on personal experience rather than on controlled clinical trials, although the data obtained by Kretschmer et al. (55,72) in patients with autologous vein grafts lend some support to their practice. In this study, anticoagulants appeared to favorably influence long-term graft patency and limb salvage as well as to prolong life expectancy, even though some patients had to discontinue coumarin therapy because of bleeding complications. Two recent trials evaluated the effect of low molecular weight heparin in infrainguinal bypass graft surgery: enoxaparin reduced early (10 days) graft thrombosis compared with unfractionated heparin (73), and dalteparin (given for 3 months) was superior to conventional antiplatelet therapy in maintaining patency at 1 year in patients with critical limb ischemia (74).

Antithrombotic Therapy in Percutaneous Revascularization Procedures

The published results of peripheral angioplasty are obtained with many patients taking antithrombotic drugs, at least for a while after the procedure. In fact, the tradition to pre-scribe antithrombotic agents to patients who undergo percutaneous transluminal angio-plasty appears logical. Platelets rapidly ad-here on sites of intimal injury and disruption induced by indwelling catheters and other in-struments. Most centers advise using aspirin, and many start the day before the procedure. During the catheter procedure, heparin is rou-tinely used to inhibit platelet stimulation and subsequent thrombus formation (and is occa-sionally continued for the first hours after the procedure). The fourth ACCP Consensus Conference on Antithrombotic Therapy (65) issued the following recommendation to re-duce the incidence of periprocedural throm-boembolic events (largely based on data from studies in patients undergoing coronary an-gioplasty): use (a) aspirin before angioplasty and (b) heparin during angioplasty, and (c) continue with aspirin after angioplasty.

Historically, the use of antithrombotic agents to prevent (re)thrombosis in the early phase of balloon angioplasty appears to be based on the observation by Zeitler et al. (75) that the incidence of early rethrombosis (less than 2 weeks) with aspirin alone was similar to that with the combination aspirin and he-parin (four of 87 and six of 90, respectively) and much lower than with heparin alone (four of 19), whereas the bleeding risk at the punc-ture site was lowest with aspirin alone (six versus 11). Although the data were obtained in a nonrandomized fashion, they were appar-ently accepted widely as evidence for the effi-cacy of periprocedural aspirin in percuta-neous revascularization. A second German study from the pioneers' period found much higher early recurrence rates with aspirin: 30% after 2 weeks but 16% with aspirin com-bined with dipyridamole (76).

Properly controlled clinical trials that ad-dress the need for antithrombotic prevention after peripheral angioplasty are not numerous and rarely distinguish early reocclusion from late restenosis. Four trials were published in the German and Swiss literature in the 1980s (77–80). Their interpretation is not made easy by the fact that they all compare two regimens

of antithrombotic therapy and only two include a placebo group. Recurrence rates at 6 months to 1 year varied between 21% and 36%. The overall impression from these studies is that the use of antiplatelet agents may have little impact on the rate of late recurrence of stenosis, but a definite conclusion is not possible.

In the 1990s two properly designed studies that included a placebo group were published. In the first, 199 patients were randomized into three treatment groups: placebo and 100 mg and 330 mg aspirin (both combined with 75 mg dipyridamole) three times daily. The study treatment was started within 2 hours after a successful femoropopliteal angioplasty. The endpoint was clinical and/or angiographic de-terioration after 6 months. Deterioration oc-curred in 63%, 51%, and 39% of the patients in the three treatment groups when clinical and angiographic data were combined and in 60%, 53%, and 38%, respectively, when an-giographic data were analyzed separately. The difference between placebo and the highest dose of aspirin was statistically significant in both analyses ($p = 0.01$ and 0.04, respec-tively) (81). How deterioration has to be translated into terms of reocclusion and/or restenosis is not detailed. The second study compared 50 mg of aspirin combined with 400 mg of dipyridamole daily for 3 months to placebo in 223 patients. Treatment was started 1 day before angioplasty, and the endpoint was an overall statement of whether the an-gioplasty site was patent, restenosed, or oc-cluded. This conclusion was reached by the vascular surgeon on the basis of clinical signs and symptoms in combination with pressure measurements and ultrasonographic or angio-graphic findings. Cumulative patency rates at 1, 3, 6, and 12 months of follow-up were sim-ilar in the two treatment groups (82). The main differences with the first study are the very low daily dose of aspirin and the inclu-sion of iliac angioplasty (more than 40% of the patients), which is expected to have a higher late patency rate.

The issue of low- versus high-dose aspirin was specifically addressed in two recent tri-als. A German study randomized 359 patients to 50 or 900 mg aspirin daily for 12 months after aortoiliac or femoropopliteal angioplasty. All patients received an unblinded loading dose of 1 g aspirin before the procedure. Event-free survival after 1 year was 84% and 85% for the low- and the high-dose aspirin group, respectively. The only independent predictor of reocclusion/restenosis in a multivariate analysis was a long (more than 3 cm) femoral artery occlusion (83). An Austrian study randomized 216 patients to 100 or 1,000 mg aspirin daily for 24 months after femoropopliteal angioplasty. Treatment was started only 3 days after a succesful procedure because all patients received periprocedural intravenous aspirin and heparin. By intention-to-treat analysis the cumulative patency rate at 2 years of follow-up was 62.6% and 62.5% in the low- and high-dose aspirin group, respectively (84). These two studies reported fewer serious gastrointestinal side effects with the lower dose of aspirin. A third study compared low-dose aspirin (50 mg daily) combined with dipyridamole (400 mg) versus oral anticoagulants for 12 months after successful femoropopliteal angioplasty in 160 patients. All patients received aspirin before angioplasty and randomization occurred 24 hours after the procedure. The endpoint of the study was the angiographically verified patency rate of the dilated arterial segment at 1 year: it was 69% with aspirin and dipyridamole and 53% with oral anticoagulants (p = 0.18) (85).

The current practice of periprocedural heparin and aspirin is not seriously challenged, even if it is not strictly followed in all centers. The data from recent studies on early reocclusion (6% reocclusion rate at 30 days in the Swedish trial [82] and 5% at 3 days in the Austrian trial [84]) confirm previously published rates. Better antithrombotic prophylaxis would not prevent mechanical obstruction by an intimal flap. The consequences of early reocclusion—if limited to the angioplasty site—are often not dramatic: the patient returns to its prior status, and a second recanalization attempt can be planned or an alternative endovascular or conventional surgical procedure considered. On the other hand, the overall result of the studies on the effect of aspirin on late restenosis (and reocclusion) is meager and rather disappointing. To conclude that a low dose of aspirin is as effective as a high dose has little significance (except for the lower complication rate) as long as we do not know whether aspirin has any effect at all on late events (which many experts doubt).

The debate on the value of antithrombotic drugs in peripheral angioplasty is admittedly rather academic. As discussed earlier, practitioners have two good reasons to prescribe aspirin to their patients with arterial disease in the lower limbs: their general outlook and the local progression of the disease.

The whole discussion on the use of antithrombotic therapy in percutaneous transluminal angioplasty may be repeated *mutatis mutandis* for all other forms of percutaneous revascularization, but up to now there are few data to discuss. In the early days of stent insertion, it was common to prescribe anticoagulant drugs to avoid stent thrombosis. This recommendation was soon abandoned for the iliac region, where long-term patency appears satisfactory with the commonly used antiplatelet therapy. However, in the femoropopliteal region, maintenance of stent patency is as great a problem as it is with infrainguinal bypass surgery and angioplasty. A recent study evaluated the immediate and mid-term outcomes of vascular stents implanted in the femoral and popliteal arteries in 32 patients who received daily low-dose aspirin only. The primary patency rate was 75% at 18 months, and this result was interpreted as proof that long-term anticoagulation was not needed. The role of aspirin was not questioned in this study (86).

For coronary stents, ticlopidine combined with aspirin appears to offer superior antithrombotic prophylaxis, but no study has reported on the results of this combination with peripheral stents (87). Clinical studies with inhibitors of angiotensin-converting enzyme were disappointing. Failure of current therapies prompts research into alternative forms of intervention, including new gene therapy approaches such as antisense strategies (oligonucleotides targeted to inhibit the expression of genes believed to be critical for the pathogenesis of restenosis) or local overexpression of genes encoding vasodilatory, antithrombotic, or antiproliferative proteins (88,89).

MANAGEMENT OF ACUTE LEG ISCHEMIA

The functional integrity of an extremity depends to a large extent on an adequate blood supply through the main arteries. Sudden arterial occlusion with almost instantaneous and complete interruption of blood flow rapidly jeopardizes the limb's viability and is almost invariably due to arterial thrombosis or arterial embolism. Thrombosis is frequently the end-stage of advanced atherosclerosis; the severity of ischemia is inversely related to the degree of pre-existing and developed collateral circulation. Thrombosis also occurs with other degenerative or inflammatory diseases, with trauma, and in venous or synthetic grafts. Transsection, laceration, and external compression (e.g., by bone fragments) lead to occlusive events with trauma, but thrombosis occurs from blunt trauma as well. The daily use of intra-arterial catheters for diagnostic or therapeutic procedures and for monitoring purposes accounts for an increasing number of acute arterial occlusions. Hypovolemia, hyperviscosity, and hypercoagulability as observed in shock, thrombocytosis, polycythemia, and malignant disorders frequently predispose to this complication. More than 80% of arterial emboli arise from the heart. Causes include atrial fibrillation associated with valvular disease, prosthetic valves, and mural thrombi in an infarcted or cardiomyopathic dilated left ventricle. Noncardiac causes are arterial aneurysms, ulcerated atherosclerotic lesions, and percutaneous or surgical arterial procedures. Most noncerebral emboli occlude arteries to the lower limbs, whereas the upper extremity is far less frequently affected. The frequency of embolism is equal in the iliofemoral segment and in the popliteal and tibial area. Rare causes of acute leg ischemia are severe arterial spasm and aortic dissection without distal re-entry.

Irrespective of whether an acute arterial occlusion is due to thrombosis or embolism, a number of urgent measures are to be taken. The ischemic leg is placed in a position of about 15 degrees dependency to avoid further impairment to capillary perfusion. Direct heating of the cold leg and mechanical trauma are avoided. Heparin treatment is initiated at a therapeutic dosage to prevent extension of thrombosis or recurrent embolism. Further therapeutic measures will depend on whether the acute occlusion is caused by embolism in a healthy artery or by thromboembolism in an atheromatous artery.

Embolism in Healthy Arteries

In patients with a clinical diagnosis of acute ischemia due to a proximal embolism as evidenced by the sudden onset of the symptoms, the presence of an embolic source, absence of previous claudication, and normal physical findings in the unaffected leg, emergency thromboembolectomy for prompt removal of the emboli and of secondary stagnation thrombi is the treatment of choice in nearly all patients. Percutaneous clot aspiration or thrombolysis also may be used for distal emboli. Postintervention imaging is advised to ascertain completeness of clot removal.

Thromboembolism in Atheromatous Arteries

Most of the arterial thromboses and many of the emboli are superimposed on atheromatous plaques in an already impaired arterial circulation. Many patients have had longstanding stenotic lesions of the occluded vessel with development of sufficient collaterals to retain viability of the extremity. Final occlusion in these patients is frequently not a dramatic event, and emergency treatment may not be needed. Elective vascular repair at a later stage offers better perspectives on optimal results in such patients. In addition, a better visualization of run-off vessels is obtained if angiography can be delayed until further collateral circulation has developed, whereas contrast injection in the acute stage correctly localizes the occlusion but frequently fails to show distal vessels. If expectant treatment is preferred, close monitoring of the condition of the limb is required, and continued heparin administration is advised.

Although surgical management remains the first choice for patients with acute limb-threatening ischemia in many centers, catheter thrombolysis combined with angioplasty of the causative lesion is a valuable alternative. Primary amputation should be performed for irreversible ischemia.

Trauma

In most cases of occlusion caused by trauma, early surgery with appropriate repair of the injured vessel is the preferred treatment. With trauma, the prognosis of the limb is mainly determined by the duration of ischemia. Early thrombectomy is indicated in iatrogenic acute arterial occlusion; thrombolysis is an alternative treatment in selected patients.

"Blue Toe" Syndrome

A number of patients present with acute and often recurrent pain and ischemia in the toes and fingers, even though the blood supply through the larger arteries appears intact as shown by normal peripheral pulses and systolic pressures. This so-called blue toe (or blue finger) syndrome may be due to obstruction of the microcirculation in patients with essential or secondary thrombocythemia. The platelets of these patients aggregate spontaneously in vitro. Usually, the symptoms respond to symptomatic treatment with aspirin and skin perfusion improves quickly. The underlying cause of the thrombocytosis needs investigation and proper treatment. Similar but more lasting symptoms of distal ischemia are occasionally caused by peripheral microembolization of atherosclerotic debris or cholesterol emboli originating from ulcerated lesions in proximal arteries. Here, eradication of the source of atheroembolism without further delay is usually indicated. Anticoagulants do not help to prevent cholesterol emboli and may even produce deleterious effects, possibly by preventing the cementing of cholesterol plaque by fibrin. The important role of fibrin in stabilizing plaques is underlined by the occurence of peripheral cholesterol emboli during thrombolytic treatment, e.g., for myocardial infarction.

Prevention of Recurrent Thromboembolism

Heparin administration started before or during intervention for acute embolic ischemia is continued and relayed with oral anticoagulants to prevent new embolic episodes. If the source of embolism can be corrected or eradicated, e.g., atrial fibrillation secondary to hyperthyroidism or an aneurysm, anticoagulation will be temporary only.

Prevention of recurrent thromboembolism in diseased arteries is a much more complicated and disputed problem. First, a clear distinction between a thrombotic and an embolic occlusion is frequently difficult in the individual patient, especially the elderly with pre-existing atherosclerosis in the limbs. Furthermore, the benefits of antithrombotic therapy have not been definitively and unequivocally established in this clinical condition. Most centers advise the temporary use of oral anticoagulants or antiplatelet agents after thrombembolectomy or thrombolysis in order to prevent early recurrent thromboembolism. Short-term prophylaxis suffices when thrombosis was initiated by a unique incident, a puncture, or catheter manipulation. Long-term use of these agents is mainly a question of secondary prevention.

MANAGEMENT OF CHRONIC ISCHEMIA OF THE LEG

Treatment of Intermittent Claudication

Prevention

Secondary prevention of progression of atherosclerosis in patients with peripheral arterial occlusive disease of the leg arteries is not restricted to the use of antithrombotic drugs. Reducing the risk factors is probably at least as important. Thus, patients with intermittent claudication should stop smoking, and they should seek treatment to control their hypertension, diabetes, and hyperlipidemia. Abstaining from smoking can even result in an increase of the walking distance.

Vascular Surgery and PTA

Vascular surgery and PTA relieve symptoms of ischemia; therefore, their application should depend in the first place on the severity of the symptoms. Thus, careful evaluation of the handicap for the individual patient is a crucial issue: a walking distance of only 40 m may be sufficient for an 80-year-old institutionalized patient, whereas a younger, active person may feel very disabled by a walking distance of 300 m or even more.

Walking Training

Daily physical exercise has been shown in several studies to markedly increase the walking distance in patients with intermittent claudication. Weitz et al. (90) reviewed all trials on exercise training: the improvement in pain-free walking time and distance ranged from 44% to 290%, with an average increase of 134%. Maximum walking time and distance increased from 25% to 183%, with an average increase of 96%. Proposed mechanisms for the effects of training on walking distance include an increase of muscle blood flow during exercise due to development of collateral vessels, redistribution of blood flow within the leg, improved metabolism of muscle cells in trained skeletal muscle, improved rheologic properties of blood, and increased pain tolerance. Up to now, there is little evidence to definitely favor any of these hypotheses.

Methods of exercise therapy include simple walking regimens, dynamic and static leg exercise, and individual training programs on treadmill. A recent meta-analysis emphasizes the need for a program using three weekly 30-minute sessions of walking to near-maximal pain over a period of at least 6 months (91).

Drug Treatment

How might drugs improve the symptoms of effort ischemia in patients with arterial disease? Vasodilatation was the initial remedy for all the symptoms of arterial obstruction, but because this concept has been completely abandoned, other characteristics of the same drugs are emphasized. For instance, they improve various factors that disturb blood rheology and correct perfusion in the microcirculation. The problem is that the clinical use of drugs in arterial disease of the legs depends on the results of therapeutic efficacy trials with clinical end-points that are relatively crude and soft. The demonstration of a pharmacodynamic effect under well-controlled conditions is not necessarily relevant for the clinical situation.

Cameron et al. (92) analyzed all trials of drug therapy in claudicants that were published during the period 1965 to 1985 and found a total of 75 trials that had studied 33 different pharmacologic agents. They found that (a) treadmill exercise, the most relevant method of evaluating symptoms in this condition, was used in only half of the trials; (b) a significant negative relation existed between sample size and therapeutic response, suggesting that improvement in walking distance was likely to have been biased by nonpublication of small trials with negative results; (c) one fourth of all trials were uncontrolled, most of them (84%) reporting benefit from drug treatment, compared with only 32% of placebo-controlled trials; and (d) one fourth of the trials reported data from fewer than 20 patients. Thus, the vast majority of published trials on drug treatment of intermittent claudication were unlikely to have made a satisfactory assessment of drug efficacy.

This critical assessment should be kept in mind when positive results on claudication distance are reported with new compounds, as was recently the case for pentoxifylline, for ticlopidine (an antiplatelet drug), and for Lcarnitine (a substance claimed to improve pyruvate utilization and oxidative phosphorylation efficiency in ischemic skeletal muscle). Despite an increasing number of positive randomized placebo-controlled and double-blind trials, most authorities would still dispute the efficacy of drug treatment in intermittent claudication.

Treatment of Critical Limb Ischemia

Definition

A strict definition of chronic critical limb ischemia as a condition that endangers the limb is not easy because of its capricious natural history and because of the placebo effect of many therapeutic measures proposed to patients who face an amputation. In the early 1980s, critical ischemia was thought to be present if ischemic pain at rest persisted for at least 4 weeks and the ankle pressure was below 40 mmHg, or below 60 mmHg if skin necrosis already developed (93,94). This definition did not extend to diabetic patients. A prospective study in Great Britain on 428 ischemic legs in 409 patients reported an overall mortality at 1 year of 18% and a 26% amputation rate in survivors (95). Thus, only 56% of the patients were alive with their two legs 1 year after their initial presentation with limb ischemia. The study further showed that patients with pain at rest and ankle pressure below 40 mmHg had a poorer outcome than those with a pressure above 40 mmHg; in patients with gangrene this difference was not upheld. A slightly different terminology was therefore proposed to define critical ischemia: (a) rest pain and an ankle pressure lower than 40 mmHg or (b) rest pain with ulceration. Diabetics represent a different subset of patients both with regard to clinical presentation and to prognosis after revascularization procedures. Differences may be accounted for by the presence of neuropathy, the increased risk of infection, and the impaired healing response in diabetics. With this background, a European Working Group on Critical Limb Ischemia tried to reach a consensus and adopted the following definition of critical ischemia: persistently recurring rest pain requiring regular analgesia for more than 2 weeks and/or ulceration or gangrene of the foot and toes, plus ankle pressure below 50 mmHg and/or toe pressure below 30 mmHg. For the definition of critical ischemia in diabetics and in patients with calcified arteries, a toe systolic pressure below 30 mmHg is needed (96).

Assessment of Critical Ischemia

Careful clinical assessment should be complemented by noninvasive measurement of ankle systolic pressure using the Doppler probe. Segmental measurements (at thigh, calf, and ankle levels) may help to define the location of the main obstructive lesions. This method is achievable with little training. More sophisticated techniques include the measurement of systolic pressure at the great toe level using strain-gauge plethysmography, laser Doppler, and the measurement of transcutaneous oxygen tension using a polarographic probe.

Great toe systolic pressure is of particular interest in patients (mostly diabetics) with calcified ankle arteries in whom systolic pressures measured at the ankle with the sphygmomanometer are overestimated. Toe pressures lower than 30 mmHg indicate permanent foot ischemia. Values between 30 and 40 mmHg are compatible with viability of the limb but usually do not permit healing of ischemic lesions. If digital ulcers or gangrene is present, transcutaneous oxygen tension may help assess the severity of arterial insufficiency, especially in diabetics. Values that are lower than 10 mmHg on the dorsum of the foot generally indicate critical ischemia of the foot. The response to postural changes or to oxygen breathing has a prognostic value in patients with critical limb ischemia: if the transcutaneous oxygen pressure does not increase above 10 mmHg, the outlook for the foot appears particularly poor. The method also has been proposed as a useful tool to adequately determine the amputation level, the critical value being around 20 mmHg (97).

Therapeutic Approach

Ideally, there should be an interdisciplinary approach to the treatment of patients with critical limb ischemia. Apart from investigations outlined above, optimal therapeutic decision making requires an angiographic evaluation of the macrocirculation in most patients. Restoration of the blood supply through the main arteries is the primary therapeutic approach if practicable. Because the majority of patients have multilevel disease, surgical reconstruction is the first option in most of them. However, some patients are aided by angioplasty of a single lesion, e.g., a stenotic lesion in the femoropopliteal region.

Surgical or chemical (with phenol or absolute alcohol) sympathectomy has been used for decades as a last resort in patients with critical limb ischemia. The procedure usually leads to some warming of the foot and subjective improvement by alleviation of rest pain. Vascular reconstruction is sometimes combined with lumbar sympathectomy in order to improve the run-off in critical ischemia. Unequivocal evidence that sympathectomy is effective as a limb salvage procedure is almost nonexistent. Spinal cord stimulation has been proposed to relieve rest pain and to increase skin blood flow, but published data are uncontrolled.

There is no evidence for the efficacy of primary drug treatment to relieve critical limb ischemia. Anticoagulation, antiplatelet therapy, vasoactive drugs, or fibrinogen-lowering drugs have been proposed, but their efficacy has never been proven in properly designed studies. Prostacyclin, prostacyclin analogues, as well as prostaglandin E_1 act favorably on activated platelets and leukocytes and may improve microcirculation. The stable analogue iloprost has been investigated in the largest number of patients. In clinical trials, those who received the drug had a significantly greater probability of completing the follow-up period alive without amputation than did those who received placebo (98).

CONCLUSION

Vascular surgery, although a fairly young discipline, sets the standard in peripheral revascularization. Percutaneous techniques initially regarded with skepticism have now become accepted complementary practice for selected patients. The main challenge is not how to reopen a vessel but rather how to keep a reopened vessel patent.

Patients with peripheral arterial disease should be prescribed aspirin (or possibly ticlopidine). This recommendation is based on the evidence that antiplatelet therapy reduces the risk of vascular events in these patients. By contrast, their usefulness to improve late results of angioplasty, stenting, or grafting of obstructed arteries is doubtful, and their presumed effect on early rethrombosis is poorly documented.

Few defend the long-term use of oral anticoagulants unless for specific aims such as prevention of recurrent embolism or perhaps improving the patency rate of infrainguinal venous bypass grafts.

Contrary to new risky techniques, promising drugs (e.g., the glycoprotein IIb/IIIa antagonists) are usually first tested in coronary disease. Unexpected findings such as the recently reported differential effect of clopidogrel in peripheral as compared with cardiac disease argue against extrapolation of data and general conclusions and may stimulate further research into specific aspects of the peripheral vascular bed.

REFERENCES

1. Dormandy J, Mahir M, Ascady G, et al. Fate of the patient with chronic leg ischemia. A review article. *J Cardiovasc Surg* 1989;30:50–57.
2. Kritz H, Schmid P, Sinzinger H. Passive smoking and cardiovascular risk. *Arch Intern Med* 1995;155:1942–1948.
3. Camargo CA Jr, Stampfer MJ, Glynn RJ, et al. Prospective study of moderate alcohol consumption and risk of peripheral arterial disease in US male physicians. *Circulation* 1997;95:577–580.
4. Quick CRG, Cotton LT. The measured effect of stop-

ping smoking on intermittent claudication. *Br J Surg* 1982;69(suppl):24–26.

5. Duffield RGM, Lewis B, Miller NE, Jamieson CW, Brunt JNH, Colchester ACF. Treatment of hyperlipidaemia retards progression of symptomatic femoral atherosclerosis. *Lancet* 1983;2:639–642.

6. Hess H, Mietaschk A, Deichsel G. Drug-induced inhibition of platelet function delays progression of peripheral occlusive arterial disease. A prospective double-blind arteriographically controlled trial. *Lancet* 1985;1:415–419.

7. Goldhaber SZ, Manson JE, Stampfer MJ et al. Low-dose aspirin and subsequent peripheral arterial surgery in the Physicians' Health Study. *Lancet* 1992;340:143–145.

8. European Working Group on Critical Leg Ischaemia. Second European consensus document on chronic critical leg ischemia. *Circulation* 1991;84(suppl IV):1–26.

9. Johnston KW, Rae M, Hogg-Johnston SA, et al. 5-year results of a prospective study of percutaneous transluminal angioplasty. *Ann Surg* 1987;206:403–413.

10. Johnston KW. Femoral and popliteal arteries: reanalysis of results of balloon angioplasty. *Radiology* 1992;183:767–771.

11. Johnston KW. Iliac arteries: reanalysis of results of balloon angioplasty. *Radiology* 1993;186:207–212.

12. Schwarten DE, Cutcliff WB. Arterial occlusive disease below the knee. Treatment with percutaneous transluminal angioplasty performed with low-profile catheters and steerable guide wires. *Radiology* 1989;169:71–74.

13. Schwarten DE. Clinical and anatomical considerations for non-operative therapy in tibial disease and results of angioplasty. *Circulation* 1991;83(suppl I):86–90.

14. Holm Jan, Arfvidsson B, Jivegard L, et al. Chronic lower limb ischemia. A prospective randomized controlled study comparing the 1-year results of vascular surgery and percutaneous transluminal angioplasty (PTA). *Eur J Vasc Surg* 1991;5:517–522.

15. Wolf GL, Wilson SE, Cross AP, Deupree RH, Stason WB, for the principal investigators and their associates of Veterans Administration Cooperative Study Number 199. Surgery or balloon angioplasty for peripheral vascular disease: a randomized clinical trial. *J Vasc Intervent Radiol* 1993;4:639–648.

16. Whyman MR, Fowkes FG, Kerracher EM, et al. Randomised controlled trial of percutaneous transluminal angioplasty for intermittent claudication. *Eur J Vasc Endovasc Surg* 1996;12:167–172.

17. Hunink MGM, Wong JB, Donaldson MC, Meyerovitz MF, de Vries J, Harrington DP. Revascularization for femoropopliteal disease. A decision and cost-effectiveness analysis. *JAMA* 1995;274:165–171.

18. Mahler F. *Katheterinterventionen in der Angiologie*. New York: Georg Thieme Verlag, 1990;1–202.

19. Pentecost MJ, Criqui MH, Dorros G, et al. Guidelines for peripheral percutaneous transluminal angioplasty of the abdominal aorta and lower extremity vessels. *Circulation* 1994;89:511–531.

20. Palmaz JC, Tio FO, Schatz RA et al. Early endothelisation of balloon-expandable stents: experimental observations. *J Intervent Radiol* 1988;3:119–124.

21. Palmaz JC, Garcia O, Schatz RA, et al. Placement of balloon-expandable stents in iliac arteries: first 171 patients. *Radiology* 1990;174:969–975.

22. Günther RW, Vorwerk D, Antonucci F, et al. Iliac artery stenosis or obstruction after unsuccessful balloon angioplasty. Treatment with a self-expandable stent. *Am J Radiol* 1991;156:389–393

23. Murphy KD, Encarnacion CE, Le VA, Palmaz JC. Iliac artery stent placement with the Palmaz stent: follow-up study. *J Vasc Intervent Radiol* 1995;6:321–329.

24. Henry M, Amor M, Ethevenot G, et al. Palmaz stent placement in iliac and femoropopliteal arteries: primary and secondary patency in 310 patients with 2–4 year follow-up. *Radiology* 1995;197:167–174.

25. Zollikofer CL, Antonucci F, Pfyffer M, et al. Arterial stent placement with use of the Wallstent: mid-term results of clinical experience. *Radiology* 1991;179:449–456.

26. Sapoval MR, Long AL, Raynaud AC, Beyssen BM, Fiessinger JN, Gaux JC. Femoropopliteal stent placement: long-term results. *Radiology* 1992;184:833–839.

27. Pernes JM, Auguste MA, Hovasse D, Gignier P, Lasry B, Lasry JL. Long iliac stenosis: initial clinical experience with the Cragg endoluminal graft. *Radiology* 1995;196:67–71.

28. Marin ML, Veith FJ, Sanchez LA, et al. Endovascular repair of aortoiliac disease. *World J Surg* 1996;20:679–686.

29. Ouriel K, Shortell CK, Azodo MW, Guitterrez OH, Marder VJ. Acute peripheral arterial occlusion: predictors of success in catheter-directed thrombolytic therapy. *Radiology* 1994;93:561–566.

30. Sullivan KL, Gardiner GA, Shapiro MJ, Bonn J, Levin DC. Acceleration of thrombolysis with a high-dose transthrombus bolus technique. *Radiology* 1989;173:805–808.

31. Braithwaite BD, Buckenham TM, Galland RB, Heather BP, Earnshaw JJ. A prospective randomised trial of high dose versus low dose tissue plasminogen activator infusion in the management of acute limb ischaemia. *Br J Surg* 1997;84:646–650.

32. Bookstein JJ, Fillmeth B, Roberts A, Valji K, Davis G, Machado T. Pulsed spray pharmacomechanical thrombolysis: preliminary clinical results. *Am J Roentgenol* 1989;152:1097–1100.

33. Reekers JA, Kromhout JH, van der Waal K. Catheter for percutaneous thrombectomy: first clinical experience. *Radiology* 1993;188:871–874.

34. Coleman CC, Krenzel C, Dietz CA, Nazarion GK, Amplatz K. Mechanical thrombectomy: results of early experience. *Radiology* 1993;189:803–805.

35. McNamara TO, Fischer JR. Thrombolysis of peripheral arterial and graft occlusions: improved results using high-dose urokinase. *Am J Roentgenol* 1985;144:769–775.

36. Ouriel K, Shortell CK, De Weese JA, et al. A comparison of thrombolytic therapy with operative vascularization in the initial treatment of acute peripheral arterial ischemia. *J Vasc Surg* 1994;19:1021–1030.

37. Berridge DC, Gregson RHS, Hopkinson BR, Makin GS. Randomized trial of intra-arterial recombinant tissue plasminogen activator, intravenous plasminogen activator and intra-arterial streptokinase in peripheral arterial thrombolysis. *Br J Surg* 1991;78:988–995.

38. Meyerovitz MF, Goldhaber SZ, Reagan K, et al. Recombinant tissue-type plasminogen activator versus urokinase in peripheral arterial and graft occlusions: a randomized trial. *Radiology* 1990;175:75–78.

39. The STILE investigators. Results of a prospective randomised trial evaluating surgery versus thrombolysis for ischaemia of the lower extremity. The STILE trial. *Ann Surg* 1994;220:251–268.
40. Ouriel K, Veith FJ, Sasahara AA, for the TOPAS Investigators. Thrombolysis or peripheral arterial surgery (TOPAS): phase I results. *J Vasc Surg* 1996;23: 64–75.
41. Hartmann JR, Enger EL, Villiard EM, Sasahara AA. Dose ranging trial of intraarterial r-prourokinase (A-74187) for thrombolysis of total peripheral arterial occlusions [Abstract 869–865]. *J Am Coll Cardiol* 1994; 23(suppl):95.
42. Vanderschueren S, Stockx L, Wilms G, et al. Thrombolytic therapy of peripheral arterial occlusion with recombinant staphylokinase. *Circulation* 1995;92: 2050–2057.
43. Collen D, Moreau H, Stockx L, Vanderschueren S. Recombinant staphylokinase variants with altered reactivity. II. Thrombolytic properties and antibody induction. *Circulation* 1996;84:1216–1234.
44. Collen D, Stockx L, Lacroix H, Suy R, Vanderschueren S. Recombinant staphylokinase variants with altered reactivity. IV. Identification of variants with reduced antibody induction but intact potency. *Circulation* 1997;95: 463–472.
45. Nilsson L, Albrechtsson U, Jonung T, et al. Surgical treatment versus thrombolysis in acute arterial occlusion: a randomized controlled study. *Eur J Vasc Surg* 1992;6:189–193.
46. Comerota AJ, Weaver FA, Hosking JD, et al. Results of prospective, randomized trial of surgery versus thrombolysis for occluded lower extremity bypass grafts. *Am J Surg* 1996;172:105–112.
47. Weaver FA, Comerota AJ, Youngblood M, Froehlich J, Hosking JD, Papanicolaou G, and the STILE investigators. Surgical revascularization versus thrombolysis for nonembolic lower extremity native artery occlusions: results of a prospective randomized trial. *J Vasc Surg* 1996;24:513–523.
48. Working Party on thrombolysis in the management of limb ischaemia. Thrombolysis in the management of limb arterial occlusion. Towards a consensus interim report. *J Intern Med* 1996;240:343–355.
49. Comerota AJ, Rao KA, Throm RC, et al. A prospective, randomized, blinded, and placebo controlled trial of intra-operative intra-arterial urokinase infusion during lower extremity revascularization: regional and systemic effects. *Ann Surg* 1993;218:534–543.
50. Berridge DC, Niakin GS, Hopkinson BR. Local low-dose intra-arterial thrombolytic therapy, the risk of major stroke and haemorrhage. *Br J Surg* 1989;76: 1230–1233.
51. Dawson K, Armon A, Braithwaite B, et al. Stroke during intra-arterial thrombolysis: a survey of experience in the UK [Abstract]. *Br J Surg* 1996;83:568.
52. McNamara TO, Goodwin SC, Kandarpa K. Complications of thrombolysis. *Semin Intervent Radiol* 1994;11: 134–144.
53. Hamming JJ, Hensen A, Loeliger EA. The value of long-term coumarin treatment in peripheral sclerosis. Clinical trial [Abstract]. *Thromb Haemost* 1965;21:405.
54. de Smit P, van Urk H. The effect of long-term treatment with oral anticoagulants in patients with peripheral vascular disease. In: Tilsner V, Matthias FR (eds). *Arterielle*

Verschlusskrankheit und Blutgerinnung. Basel, Switzerland: Editiones Roche, 1987;211–217.
55. Kretschmer G, Herbst F, Prager M, et al. A decade of oral anticoagulant treatment to maintain autologous vein grafts for femoropopliteal atherosclerosis. *Arch Surg* 1992;127:1112–1115.
56. Antiplatelet Trialists' Collaboration. Collaborative overview of randomized trials of antiplatelet therapy. I. Prevention of death, myocardial infarction and stroke by prolonged antiplatelet therapy in various categories of patients. *Br Med J* 1994;308:81–101.
57. Blanchard J, Carreras LO, Kindermans M, and the EMATAP-group. Results of EMATAP: a double-blind placebo-controlled multicentre trial of ticlopidine in patients with peripheral arterial disease. *Nouv Rev Fr Hematol* 1993;35:523–528.
58. CAPRIE Steering Committee. A randomised, blinded, trial of clopidogrel versus aspirin in patients at risk of ischaemic events (CAPRIE). *Lancet* 1996;348: 1329–1339.
59. Schoop W, Levy H, Schoop B, Gaentsch A. Experimentelle und klinische Studien zu der sekundären Prävention der peripheren Arteriosklerose. In: Bollinger A, Rhyner K (eds). *Thrombozytenfunktionshemmer.* Stuttgart: Georg Thieme Verlag, 1983;49–58.
60. Stiegler H, Hess H, Mietaschk A, Trampisch HJ, Ingrisch H. Einfluss von Ticlopidine auf die perifere obliterierende Arteriopathie. *Dtsch Med Wochenschr* 1984; 109:1240–1243.
61. Boissel JP, Peyrieux JC, Destors JM. Is it possible to reduce the risk of cardiovascular events in subjects suffering from intermittent claudication of the lower limbs? *Thromb Haemost* 1989;62:681–685.
62. Arcan JC, Panak E. Ticlopidine in the treatment of peripheral occlusive arterial disease. *Semin Thromb Haemost* 1989;15:167–170.
63. Balsano F, Coccheri S, Libretti A, et al. Ticlopidine in the treatment of intermittent claudication: a 21-month double blind trial. *J Lab Clin Med* 1989;114:84–91.
64. Palareti G, Poggi M, Torricelli P, et al. Long-term effects of ticlopidine on fibrinogen and haemorheology in patients with peripheral arterial disease. *Thromb Res* 1988;52:621–629.
65. Clagett GP, Krupski WC. Antithrombotic therapy in peripheral arterial occlusive disease. *Chest* 1995;108 (suppl):431–443.
66. Green RM, Roederscheimer R, DeWeese JA. Effects of aspirin and dipyridamole on expanded polytetrafluoroethylene graft patency. *Surgery* 1982;82:1016–1026.
67. Goldman M, McCollum C. A prospective study to examine the effect of aspirin plus dipyridamole on the patency of prosthetic femoro-popliteal grafts. *Vasc Surg* 1984;18:217–221.
68. Clyne CAC, Archer TJ, Atahura LK, et al. Random control trial of a short course of aspirin and dipyridamole (Persantin) for femorodistal grafts. *Br J Surg* 1987;74: 246–248.
69. Kohler TR, Kaufman JL, Kacoyanis G, et al. Effect of aspirin and dipyridamole on the patency of lower extremity bypass grafts. *Surgery* 1984;96:462–466.
70. McCollum C, Alexander C, Kenchington G, et al. Antiplatelet drugs in femoro-popliteal vein bypasses: a multicenter trial. *J Vasc Surg* 1991;13:150–162.
71. Antiplatelet Trialists' Collaboration. Collaborative overview of randomized trials of antiplatelet treatment. Part

II: Maintenance of vascular graft or arterial patency by antiplatelet therapy. *Br Med J* 1994;309:159–168.

72. Kretschmer G, Wenzl E, Piza F, et al. The influence of anticoagulant treatment on the probability of function in femoropopliteal vein bypass surgery: analysis of a clinical series (1970–1985) and interim evaluation of a controlled clinical trial. *Surgery* 1987;102:453–459.

73. Samama CM, Gigou F, Ill P, for the Enoxart study group. Low-molecular-weight heparin vs. unfractionated heparin in femorodistal reconstructive surgery: a multicenter open randomized study. *Ann Vasc Surg* 1995;9(suppl):45–53.

74. Edmonson RA, Cohen AT, Das SK, Wagner MB, Kakkar VJ. Low-molecular weight heparin versus aspirin and dipyridamole after femoropopliteal bypass grafting. *Lancet* 1994;344:914–918.

75. Zeitler E, Reichold J, Schoop W, Loew D. Einfluss von Acetylsalicylsäure auf das Frühergebnis nach perkutaner Rekanalisation arterieller Obliterationen nach Dotter. *Dtsch Med Wochenschr* 1973;98:1285–1288.

76. Hess H, Müller-Fassbender H, Ingrisch H, Mietaschk A. Verhütung von Wiederverschlüssen nach Rekanalisation obliterierter Arterien mit der Katheter-methode. *Dtsch Med Wochenschr* 1978;103:1994–1997.

77. Staiger J, Mathias K, Friederich M, Heiss HW, Konrad S, Spillner G. Perkutane Katheterrekanalisation (Dotter-Technik) bei peripherer arterieller Verschluss-krankheit. *Herz Kreislauf* 1980;12:383–386.

78. Heiss HW, Mathias K, Beck AH, König K, Betzner M, Just H. Rezidivprophylaxe mit Acetylsalicylsäure und Dipyridamol nach perkutaner transluminaler Angioplastie der Beinarterien bei obliterierender Arteriosklerose. *Cor Vas* 1987;1:25–34.

79. Mahler F, Schneider E, Gallino A, Bollinger A. Combination of suloctidil and anticoagulation in the prevention of reocclusion after femoro-popliteal PTA. *Vasa* 1987;16:381–385.

80. Schneider E, Mahler F, Do DD, Biland L. Zur Rezidivprophylaxe nach perkutaner transluminaler Angioplastie (PTA): Antikoagulation versus Ticlopidin. *Vasa* 1988;17(suppl 20):355–356.

81. Heiss HW, Just H, Middleton D, Deichsel G. Reocclusion prophylaxis with dipyridamole combined with acetylsalicylic acid following PTA. *Angiology* 1990;41:263–269.

82. Study group on pharmacological treatment after PTA. Platelet inhibition with ASA/dipyridamole after percutaneous balloon angioplasty in patients with symptomatic lower limb arterial disease. A prospective double-blind trial. *Eur J Vasc Surg* 1994;8:83–88.

83. Ranke C, Creutzig A, Luska G, et al. Controlled trial of high-versus low-dose aspirin treatment after percutaneoustransluminal angioplasty in patients with peripheral vascular disease. *Clin Invest* 1994;72:673–680.

84. Minar E, Ahmadi A, Koppensteiner R, et al. Comparison of effects of high-dose and low-dose aspirin on restenosis after femoropopliteal percutaneous transluminal angioplasty. *Circulation* 1995;91:2167–2173.

85. Do DD, Mahler F. Low-dose aspirin combined with dipyridamole versus anticoagulants after femoropopliteal percutaneous transluminal angioplasty. *Radiology* 1994;193:567–571.

86. White GH, Liew SC, Waugh RC. Early outcome and intermediate follow-up of vascular stents in the femoral and popliteal arteries without long-term anticoagulation. *J Vasc Surg* 1995;21:270–279.

87. Schömig A, Neumann FJ, Kastrati A, et al. A randomized comparison of antiplatelet and anticoagulant therapy after the placement of coronary stents. *N Engl J Med* 1996;334:1084–1089.

88. Bennett MR, Schwartz SM. Antisense therapy for angioplasty restenosis. Some critical considerations. *Circulation* 1995;92:1981–1993.

89. Gibbons GH, Dzau VJ. Molecular therapies for vascular diseases. *Science* 1996;272:689–693.

90. Weitz JI, Byrne J, Clagett GP, et al. Diagnosis and treatment of chronic arterial insufficiency of the lower extremities: a critical review. *Circulation* 1996;94:3026–3049.

91. Gardner AW, Poehlman ET. Exercise rehabilitation programs for the treatment of claudication pain. A meta-analysis. *JAMA* 1995;274:975–980.

92. Cameron HA, Waller PC, Ramsay LE. Drug treatment of intermittent claudication: a critical analysis of the methods and findings of published clinical trials, 1965–1985. *Br J Clin Pharmacol* 1988;26:569–576.

93. Bell PRF, Challesworth D, DePalma RG, Jamieson C. The definition of critical ischaemia of a limb. *Br J Surg* 1982;69:52.

94. Ad Hoc Committee on Reporting Standards. Suggested standards for reports dealing with lower extremity ischemia. *J Vasc Surg* 1986;4:80–94.

95. Wolfe JHN. The definition of critical ischemia—Is this a concept of value? In: Greenhalgh RM, Jamieson CW, Nicolaides AN (eds). *Limb Salvage and Amputation for Vascular Disease.* Philadelphia: WB Saunders, 1988:3–10.

96. European Working Group on Critical Leg Ischaemia. Second European consensus document on chronic critical leg ischemia. *Circulation* 1991;84(suppl IV):1–26.

97. Wütschert R, Bounameaux H. Determination of amputation level in ischemic limbs: re-appraisal of the measurement of transcutaneous oxygen tension. *Diabetes Care* 1997;20:1315–1319.

98. Dormandy JA, Loh A. Critical limb ischaemia. In: Tooke JE, Lowe GDO. *A Textbook of Vascular Medicine.* London: Arnold, 1996;221–236.

Cardiovascular Thrombosis: Thrombocardiology and Thromboneurology, Second Edition,
edited by M. Verstraete, V. Fuster, and E. J. Topol,
Lippincott–Raven Publishers, Philadelphia © 1998.

38

Primary Prevention of Venous Thrombosis and Pulmonary Embolism

Russell D. Hull, Graham F. Pineo, *Gary E. Raskob, and †Vijay V. Kakkar

*Departments of General Internal Medicine and Medicine, University of Calgary/Foothills Hospital, Calgary, Alberta T2N 4N1, Canada; *Department of Biostatistics, Epidemiology, and Medicine, University of Oklahoma Health Sciences Center, Oklahoma City, Oklahoma 73190; and †Thrombosis Research Institute, London SW3 6LR, United Kingdom*

Pulmonary embolism is responsible for approximately 150,000 to 200,000 deaths per year in the United States (1,2). Despite significant advances in the prevention and treatment of venous thromboembolism (venous thrombosis and pulmonary embolism), pulmonary embolism remains the most common preventable cause of hospital death (3). Venous thromboembolism usually occurs as a complication in patients who are sick and hospitalized, but it may also affect ambulant and otherwise healthy individuals. Many patients who die from pulmonary embolism succumb suddenly or within 2 hours after the acute event, i.e., before therapy can be initiated or take effect (4). Therefore, prevention is the key to reducing death and morbidity from venous thromboembolism. Effective and safe prophylactic measures against venous thromboembolism are now available for most high-risk patients (5–8). This chapter highlights practical approaches to the prevention of venous thromboembolism.

PATHOGENESIS OF VENOUS THROMBOEMBOLISM

Deep vein thrombosis (DVT) most commonly arises in the deep veins of the calf muscles or, less commonly, in the proximal deep veins of the leg. Deep venous thrombosis confined to the calf veins is associated with a low risk of clinically important pulmonary embolism (9–12). However, without treatment, approximately 20% of calf-vein thrombi extend into the proximal venous system (13,14) where they pose a serious and potentially life-threatening disorder. Untreated proximal venous thrombosis is associated with a 10% risk of fatal pulmonary embolism and at least a 50% risk of pulmonary embolism or recurrent venous thrombosis (11,12,15). Furthermore, the postphlebitic syndrome is associated with extensive proximal venous thrombosis and carries its own long-term morbidity.

It is now well established that clinically important pulmonary emboli arise from thrombi in the proximal deep veins of the legs (16–20). Other less common sources of pulmonary embolism include the deep pelvic veins, renal veins, inferior vena cava, right heart, and occasionally axillary veins. The clinical significance of pulmonary embolism depends on the size of the embolus and the cardiorespiratory reserve of the patient.

RISK FACTORS FOR VENOUS THROMBOEMBOLISM

Factors predisposing to the development of venous thromboembolism are shown in Table 38-1 (see also Chapter 6). Patients undergoing surgical procedures should be assessed for thromboembolic risks prior to surgery, as this determines the prophylactic approach. For example, the incidence of thromboembolism in patients in the low-risk

TABLE 38-1. *Factors predisposing to the development of venous thromboembolism*

Clinical risk factors
  Surgical and nonsurgical trauma
  Previous venous thromboembolism
  Immobilization
  Malignant disease
  Heart disease
  Leg paralysis
  Age (>40)
  Obesity
  Estrogens
  Parturition
Inherited or acquired abnormalities
  Activated protein C resistance
  Protein C deficiency
  Protein S deficiency
  Antithrombin III deficiency
  Anticardiolipin syndrome
  Heparin-induced thrombocytopenia

group undergoing minor surgical procedures is such that the potential complications and expense of prophylaxis may not be warranted. However, others, determined by the type of surgery, may be at risk of deep vein thrombosis if they have one or more risk factors.

The risk of calf vein thrombosis, proximal vein thrombosis, and fatal pulmonary embolism has been assessed by objective tests for patients undergoing a variety of surgical procedures (Table 38-2). The risk of postoperative deep vein thrombosis can be identified as low, moderate, or high, depending on the surgical procedure and the presence or absence of additional risk factors (21).

PREVENTION OF VENOUS THROMBOEMBOLISM

Without prophylaxis, the frequency of fatal pulmonary embolism ranges from 0.1% to 0.8% in patients undergoing elective general surgery (22–24), 2% to 3% in patients undergoing elective hip replacement (25), and 4% to 7% in patients undergoing surgery for a fractured hip (26). It is surprising that not all physicians and surgeons comply with the recommendations for prophylaxis of venous thromboembolism despite the fact that there is convincing evidence for the efficacy and safety of a number of agents (26,27). In a retrospective audit of hospitals in Massachusetts, it was shown that prophylaxis of venous thromboembolism even in high-risk patients was grossly underutilized, particularly in non-teaching hospitals (28). In orthopedic surgery, as shown in surveys conducted in England and Sweden, some form of prophylaxis, usually in the form of drugs, is used in the majority of cases (29,30).

There are two approaches to the prevention of fatal pulmonary embolism: (a) secondary prevention involves the early detection and treatment of subclinical venous thrombosis by screening postoperative patients with objective tests that are sensitive for venous thrombosis; and (b) primary prophylaxis is carried out using either drugs, physical methods or a combination of both methods that are effec-

TABLE 38-2. *Risk of venous thromboembolism assessed by objective test*

Risk category	Calf vein thrombosis	Proximal vein thrombosis	Fatal pulmonary embolism
High Risk	40–80%	10–30%	1–5%
Major orthopedic surgery of lower limbs			
General urologic surgery in patients older than 40 years with recent history of DVT or PE			
Extensive pelvic or abdominal surgery for malignant disease			
Moderate Risk	10–40%	2–10%	0.1–0.8%
General surgery in patients older than 40 years that lasts 30 minutes or more, in patients younger than 40 years on oral contraceptives, and women over 35 years having emergency cesarean section			
Low Risk	<10%	<1%	<0.01%
Minor surgery, i.e., <30 min, in patients older than 40 years without additional risk factors			
Uncomplicated surgery in patients younger than 40 years without additional risk factors			

From Nicolaides et al., ref. 8, with permission.

tive in preventing deep vein thrombosis. The latter approach, primary prophylaxis, is preferred in most clinical circumstances. Furthermore, prevention of deep venous thrombosis and pulmonary embolism is more cost-effective than treatment of the complications when they occur (31–35). Secondary prevention by case-finding studies should never replace primary prophylaxis. It should be reserved for patients in whom primary prophylaxis is either contraindicated or relatively ineffective.

Thromboprophylaxis can be directed toward three components of Virchow's triad, namely, blood flow, factors within the blood itself, and the vascular endothelium. Some methods act on all three, resulting in a reduction of venous stasis, prevention of the hypercoagulable state induced by tissue trauma and other factors, and protection of the endothelium. Whichever method is used, thromboprophylaxis should probably be initiated prior to induction of anesthesia, as it has been demonstrated that the thrombotic process commences intraoperatively (13) The ideal thromboprophylactic agent would prevent all DVTs, be free from side effects, be simple to apply or administer (e.g., oral administration), need no laboratory monitoring, and be cost-effective.

None of the available approaches meets all of these criteria. The selection of a particular thromboprophylactic method therefore depends on the type of surgery, the overall risk category into which the patient falls, and the preference of the responsible clinician. For example, it may not be appropriate to treat with anticoagulants patients at very high risk of bleeding or at risk of complications secondary to bleeding, or to use mechanical devices on patients who have peripheral ischemia. For all surgical patients it is important to reduce tissue trauma, shorten the anesthetic time, and promote early postoperative mobilization.

The prophylactic measures most commonly used are low-dose or adjusted dose unfractionated heparin, low molecular weight heparin, oral anticoagulants (International Normalized Ratio [INR] of 2 to 3; see "Specific Prophylactic Measures," below), intermittent pneumatic leg compression, and graduated compression stockings. More recently, studies on the prevention of venous thrombosis following orthopedic surgery have been performed with specific antithrombin agents, i.e., hirudin and hirulog. Other less common measures include the use of aspirin and intravenous dextran.

It has become standard practice to commence prophylaxis, for example, with low-dose heparin, prior to anesthesia in patients undergoing thoracoabdominal surgery, and in Europe prophylaxis is started the night before surgery in patients undergoing total hip or total knee replacement surgery. In North America, because of the concern about postoperative bleeding, prophylaxis for patients having total knee or total hip replacement has been started postoperatively (36). This difference in the patterns of practice may account for the differences in the rates of postoperative venous thrombosis in Europe and North America (37). In a pooled analysis of level 1 trials comparing preoperative enoxaparin in Europe with postoperative enoxaparin in North America, the respective total deep vein thrombosis rates following total hip replacement were 8.8% (95% CI 6.5 to 11.7) and 15.6% (95% CI 13.0 to 18.7), a difference favoring preoperative enoxaparin of 6.83% (95% CI 2.9 to 10.7). Clinical trials are currently underway to compare the efficacy and safety of preoperative prophylaxis with postoperative commencement of prophylaxis within the same trial.

The duration of prophylaxis required after high-risk procedures such as total joint replacement is currently under intensive study. There is evidence that thrombin can be generated after the discontinuation of prophylaxis 1 week after total hip replacement and these laboratory abnormalities can be demonstrated up to 35 days postoperatively (38). Studies from Europe have demonstrated the presence of venous thrombosis at day 28 to 35 (39–42). In three of these studies, negative venograms were required at discharge before patients could continue on either low molecular weight heparin or placebo (38–40). Thrombosis rates were lower in patients who continued on low molecular weight heparin as compared to those on placebo. Similar studies are underway in North America. These studies support the need for extended prophylaxis after such procedures for 28 to 35 days.

Patterns of clinical practice with respect to the prevention of venous thromboembolism and the appropriate use of anticoagulants for the treatment of thrombotic disease have been influenced very strongly by recent consensus conferences. The American College of Chest Physicians has held four consensus conferences on antithrombotic therapy (43). Recommendations from the Fourth American College of Chest Physicians Consensus Conference on Antithrombotic Therapy have recently been published. Rules of evidence for assessing the literature were applied to all recommendations regarding prevention and treatment of thrombotic disease, thereby indicating which recommendations were based on solid clinical evidence, which were based on extrapolation of evidence from related clinical disorders, and which were based only on nonrandomized clinical trials or case series (44). Data from the European Consensus Conference on the Prevention of Venous Thromboembolism were published in International Angiology in 1992 (21). A more recent International Consensus Statement is in press. In both reports a number of unanswered questions relating to the prevention of venous thrombosis were identified.

SPECIFIC PROPHYLACTIC MEASURES

Low-Dose Heparin

The effectiveness of low-dose unfractionated heparin for preventing deep vein thrombosis has been established by multiple randomized clinical trials. Low-dose subcutaneous heparin is usually given in a dose of 5,000 U 2 hours preoperatively, and then postoperatively every 8 or 12 hours. Most of the patients in these trials underwent abdominothoracic surgery, particularly for gastrointestinal disease, but patients having gynecologic and urologic surgery as well as mastectomies or vascular procedures were also included. Pooled data from meta-analyses confirm that low-dose heparin significantly reduces the incidence of all deep vein thrombosis, proximal deep vein thrombosis, and all pulmonary emboli including fatal pulmonary emboli (5–8).

The International Multicentre Trial also established the effectiveness of low-dose heparin for preventing fatal pulmonary embolism, a clinically and significantly striking reduction from 0.7% to 0.1% (p < 0.005) (24).

The incidence of major bleeding complications is not increased by low-dose heparin, but there is an increase in minor wound hematomas. The platelet count should be monitored regularly in all patients on low-dose heparin to detect the rare but significant development of heparin-induced thrombocytopenia. Low-dose heparin has the advantage of being relatively inexpensive, easy to administer, and it does not require anticoagulant monitoring.

Adjusted Dose Heparin

The use of adjusted dose subcutaneous heparin was shown to be an effective approach for prophylaxis compared with low-dose heparin in patients undergoing total hip replacement (45). Adjusted dose heparin therapy decreased the incidence of deep vein thrombosis significantly (13% versus 39%) without any increase in the frequency of bleeding complications. Adjusted dose heparin has not become popular because of the time and expense required for laboratory monitoring.

Low Molecular Weight Heparin

A number of low molecular weight heparin fractions have been evaluated by randomized clinical trials in moderate-risk general surgical patients (46–54). The low molecular weight heparins that have been most extensively evaluated include dalteparin, nadroparin, enoxaparin, and tinzaparin. In randomized clinical trials comparing low molecular weight heparin with unfractionated heparin, the low molecular weight heparins given once or twice daily have been shown to be as effective or more effective in preventing thrombosis (46–54). In most of the trials, similarly low frequencies of bleeding for low molecular weight heparin and low-dose unfractionated heparin were documented, although the incidence of bleeding was significantly lower in the group as evidenced by a reduction in the incidence of wound hematoma, severe bleeding, and the number of patients requiring reoperation for bleeding (46).

A number of randomized control trials have been performed with low molecular weight heparin comparing it with either placebo, intravenous dextran, unfractionated heparin, or warfarin for the prevention of venous thrombosis following total hip replacement (55–64) (Table 38-3). The drugs under investigation and their dosage schedules vary from one clinical trial to another, making comparisons across trials difficult. Furthermore, it has been shown that even within the same clinical trial there can be considerable intercenter variability (63). Low molecular weight heparin is usually started the night before surgery in the European trials, in contrast to North American trials where it is started 12 to 24 hours postoperatively. Total bleeding rates vary quite widely across trials as well, making comparisons difficult.

Although the number of patients undergoing total knee replacement now equals those undergoing total hip replacements, there have been fewer trials in this patient population (63–67). Recent clinical trials comparing low molecular weight heparin with either placebo or warfarin are shown in Table 38-4. Although the rates of DVT with low molecular weight heparin are significantly lower than those with warfarin, the rates continue to be high (63,64,66,67). Clinical trials using new antithrombin agents and a combination of low molecular weight heparin and intermittent pneumatic compression are currently underway.

A meta-analysis showed low molecular weight heparin to be more effective than unfractionated heparin in the prevention of venous thrombosis, but the risk of bleeding was slightly higher (68). It should be noted, however, that the findings of meta-analyses evaluating the low molecular weight heparins should be interpreted with caution because all of the low molecular weight heparins differ.

Two recent decision analyses compared the cost effectiveness of enoxaparin with warfarin

TABLE 38-3. *Randomized trials of low molecular weight heparin prophylaxis for deep vein thrombosis following hip replacement surgery: total deep vein thrombosis and bleeding*

Reference	Treatment	No. of patients	Total deep vein thrombosis (%)	Total bleeding (%)
Turpie et al. (55)	Enoxaparin	40	10.0	4.0
	Placebo	40	60.6	4.0
Torholm et al. (56)	Dalteparin	58	16.0	NA
	Placebo	54	35.0	NA
Lassen et al. (57)	Tinzaparin	93	31.0	9.5
	Placebo	97	45.0	12.6
Danish Enoxaparin Study Group (58)	Enoxaparin	108	6.5	13.9
	Dextran 70	111	21.6	23.4
Levine et al. (59)	Enoxaparin	258	19.4	5.1
	Unfractionated heparin	263	23.2	9.3
Leyvraz et al. (45)	Nadroparin (Fraxiparin)	198	12.6	0.5
	Unfractionated heparin	199	16.0	1.5
Eriksson et al. (60)	Dalteparin (Fragmin)	67	30.2	1.5
	Unfractionated heparin	68	42.4	7.4
Planes et al. (61)	Enoxaparin	120	12.5	2.4
	Heparin	108	25.0	1.8
Colwell et al. (62)	Enoxaparin	136	21.0	10.0
	Enoxaparin	136	6.0	12.0
	Heparin	142	1.5	12.0
Hull et al. (63)	Tinzaparin (Logiparin)	332	21.0	4.1
	Warfarin	340	23.0	3.8
Hamulyak et al. (64)	Nadroparin	195	13.8	2.4[a]
	Warfarin	196	13.8	5.2

NA, not available.
[a]Clinically important plus minor bleeding for combined hip and knee replacement patients.

in patients undergoing hip replacement (69,70). Although enoxaparin was more expensive than low-dose warfarin, its cost effectiveness compared favorably with other medical interventions. A recent economic evaluation of low molecular weight heparin versus warfarin prophylaxis after total hip or knee replacement indicated that low molecular weight heparin was cost-effective (71).

Recent studies have shown that low molecular weight heparin is superior to low-dose unfractionated heparin in patients suffering

TABLE 38-4. *Randomized control trials of low molecular weight heparin prophylaxis for deep vein thrombosis bleeding following total knee replacement: total deep vein thrombosis and bleeding*

Reference	Treatment	No. of patients	Total deep vein thrombosis (%)	Total bleeding (%)
Leclerc et al. (65)	Enoxaparin	41	20.0	6.1
	Placebo	54	65.0	6.2
Hull et al. (63)	Tinzaparin	317	45.0	4.4
	Warfarin	324	54.0	2.4
Leclerc et al. (66)	Enoxaparin	206	37.0	33.0
	Warfarin	211	52.0	30.0
Heit et al. (67)	Ardeparin	232	27.0[a]	7.9
	Warfarin	222	38.0	4.4
Hamulyak et al. (64)	Nadroparin	65	24.6	2.4[b]
	Warfarin	61	37.7	5.2

[a]Venogram on operated leg only.
[b]Clinically important and minor bleeding for combined hip and knee replacement patients.

multiple trauma (72) and equally effective in medical patients (73,74).

The low molecular weight heparinoid danaparoid (Organon) has been evaluated in patients undergoing surgery for cancer (75), hip fractures (76,77), and total hip replacement (78). The thrombosis rates were similar with danaparoid and unfractionated heparin in patients undergoing cancer surgery (75). In patients undergoing surgery for hip fracture, the deep vein thrombosis rates were significantly lower compared with intravenous dextran (76) (13% versus 35%) and with low-intensity warfarin (7% versus 21%) (77). More blood transfusions were required in the dextran group. Compared with placebo, the rates of deep vein thrombosis following total hip replacement were significantly lower (15.5% versus 56.6%) (78).

Oral Anticoagulants

For prophylaxis, oral anticoagulants (coumarin derivatives) can be commenced preoperatively, at the time of surgery, or in the early postoperative period. Oral anticoagulants commenced at the time of surgery or in the early postoperative period may not prevent small venous thrombi from forming during surgery, or soon after surgery, because the antithrombotic effect is not achieved until the third or fourth postoperative day. However, oral anticoagulants are effective in inhibiting the extension of these thrombi, thereby preventing clinically important venous thromboembolism.

The postoperative use of warfarin following total hip or total knee replacement surgery has been compared with low molecular weight heparin (63,64,66,67) or intermittent pneumatic compression with little or no difference in the incidence of postoperative venous thrombosis or bleeding (79–81). When warfarin was initiated in small doses 7 to 10 days preoperatively to prolong the prothrombin time (PT) 1.5 to 3.0 seconds and then less intense warfarin was started the night of surgery, the results were similar to those when warfarin was started postoperatively (81).

In patients with hip fractures, warfarin was compared with aspirin and placebo: The rates of deep vein thrombosis were 20% for warfarin, 40.9% for aspirin, and 46% for placebo (82). Compared with placebo, very low doses of oral anticoagulants (warfarin 1 mg per day) decreased the postoperative thrombosis rate in patients undergoing gynecologic surgery or major general surgery (83) and decreased the thrombosis rate in indwelling central line catheters (84). There was no increase in bleeding rates. Very-low-dose warfarin, however, did not provide protection against deep vein thrombosis following hip or knee replacement (85).

Intermittent Leg Compression

The use of intermittent pneumatic leg compression prevents venous thrombosis by enhancing blood flow in the deep veins of the legs, thereby preventing venous stasis. It also increases blood fibrinolytic activity, which may contribute to its antithrombotic properties. Intermittent pneumatic leg compression is effective for preventing venous thrombosis in moderate-risk general surgical patients (86) following cardiac surgery (87) and in patients undergoing neurosurgery (88–90). In patients undergoing hip surgery, intermittent pneumatic compression of the calf is effective for preventing calf vein thrombosis, but it is relatively ineffective against proximal vein thrombosis (91).

Intermittent pneumatic compression of the calf decreased distal venous thrombosis following knee replacement, but proximal thrombosis rates remained high (92). Studies with calf and thigh compression significantly decreased the incidence of both distal and proximal thrombosis rates (93).

Intermittent pneumatic compression is virtually free of clinically important side effects and offers a valuable alternative in patients who have a high risk of bleeding. It may produce discomfort in the occasional patient and should not be used in patients with overt evidence of leg ischemia caused by peripheral vascular disease. A variety of well-accepted, comfortable, and effective intermittent pneumatic devices are currently available which may be applied preoperatively, at the time of operation, or in the early postoperative period. These devices should be used for the entire period until the patient is fully ambulatory with only temporary removal for nursing care or physiotherapy.

Graduated Compression Stockings

Graduated compression stockings (GCSs) are a simple, safe, and moderate effective form of thromboprophylaxis. It is by no means clear how GCS achieve a thromboprophylactic effect. It has been shown that they increase the velocity of venous blood flow (94–96) and thus GCS are recommended in low-risk patients and as an adjunct in those with medium and high risk. The only major contraindication is peripheral vascular disease. The majority of studies in patients undergoing general abdominal and gynecologic procedures have shown a reduction in the incidence of DVT. A comprehensive meta-analysis concluded that in studies using sound methods there was a highly significant risk reduction of 68% in patients at moderate risk of postoperative thromboembolism (97). However, there is no conclusive evidence that GCS are effective in reducing the incidence of fatal and nonfatal PE. It is not known as to whether wearing GCS following discharge from hospital is efficacious.

Other Agents

Although meta-analyses indicate that aspirin decreases the frequency of venous thrombosis following general or orthopedic surgery, this reduction is significantly less than that obtained using other agents. Aspirin, therefore, cannot be recommended for the prevention of venous thrombosis in high-risk patients (98). Also, although intravenous dextran has been shown to be effective in the prevention of venous thrombosis following major orthopedic surgery, it is cumbersome, expensive, and associated with significant side effects (see also Chapter 13). It has therefore been replaced by other agents.

Studies using specific antithrombin agents (hirudin or hirulog) have been performed in patients undergoing total hip replacement (99,100). Hirudin, started preoperatively, was superior to unfractionated heparin in preventing venous thrombosis following total hip replacement (99,100).

ANESTHESIA AND THROMBOEMBOLISM

Lumbar epidural anesthesia results in higher flow velocity in the femoral vein than general anesthesia (GA) (101). The same is not true for thoracic epidural anesthesia (102). The incidence of postoperative DVT may be lower in those undergoing lumbar epidurals. In open prostatectomy, epidural anesthesia was compared to GA and less DVT occurred in those having epidurals (103). Studies comparing the incidence of DVT following general anesthesia or thoracic extradural anesthesia in general abdominal surgery have now shown significant differences (104,105). A randomized study of patients undergoing elective abdominal surgery compared morphine for analgesia and low-dose heparin with epidural analgesia with no prophylactic antithrombotic treatment (106). The incidence of deep venous thrombosis (^{125}I-fibrinogen scan) was 32% after general anesthesia and low-dose heparin and 34% after epidural analgesia with no prophylactic antithrombotic treatment (p < 0.9).

Regional anesthesia combined with unfractionated heparin or low molecular weight heparin raises another issue. Spinal hematoma is a recognized complication of epidural and spinal anesthesia and there are obvious concerns regarding the safety of combining these invasive techniques with anticoagulant thromboprophylactic agents. However, intraspinal hemorrhages may occur spontaneously or in conjunction with coexisting pathology, such as bleeding disorders, spinal neoplasia, and vascular abnormalities lying in close proximity to the spinal cord. They are well documented in association with therapeutic anticoagulation. The complications of regional anesthesia have been investigated in three studies with a total of 164,701 patients. There were no reported cases of spinal hematomas. A review of surgical patients in clinical trials using heparin thrombo-prophylaxis where the type of anesthesia was defined showed no intraspinal hematomas in 9,013 patients receiving low molecular weight heparin in combination with epidural or spinal anesthesia (107). There is one case report of a spinal hematoma in a patient receiving prophy-lactic unfractionated heparin in combination with epidural anesthesia and two case reports of spinal bleeding in patients receiving low molecular weight heparin prophylaxis. How-ever, only one of these patients had epidural catheterization. These data suggest that there is little or no increased risk associated with com-bination of regional anesthesia and heparin thromboprophylaxis. In patients undergoing major surgery, particularly those at high risk of thromboembolic disease, the risks of deep vein thrombosis and fatal pulmonary embolism far outweigh the risks of spinal hemorrhage.

SPECIFIC RECOMMENDATIONS

The recommended primary prophylactic approach depends on the patient's risk cate-gory and the type of surgery. In assessing the literature relating to the prevention of venous thromboembolism, the rules of evidence as defined by Cook et al. have been used (43). They are summarized as follows:

Level I—Randomized trials with low false-positive (α) and low false-negative (β) er-rors.
Level II—Randomized trials with high false-positive (α) and high false-negative (β) er-rors.
Level III—Nonrandomized concurrent cohort studies.
Level IV—Nonrandomized historical cohort studies.
Level V—Case series.

Unless indicated, all recommendations in the following section are based on level I evi-dence.

Low-Risk Patients

Apart from early ambulation, specific pro-phylaxis is usually not recommended (44).

However, prophylaxis for low-risk patients is recommended in certain circumstances. It is the clinical custom in some countries to use graduated compression stockings but this is not based on evidence from clinical trials.

Moderate-Risk Patients

General Abdominal, Thoracic, or Gynecologic Surgery

In moderate-risk patients the use of subcu-taneous low-dose unfractionated heparin (5,000 U every 8 or 12 hours) or subcuta-neous low molecular weight heparin is rec-ommended (5,8,44). Subcutaneous low mole-cular weight heparin is as effective as subcutaneous heparin prophylaxis and has the advantage of a once-daily injection. An alter-native recommendation is the use of intermit-tent pneumatic compression until the patient is ambulatory. This method is indicated in pa-tients at high risk for bleeding. Pharmacologic methods may be combined with graduated compression stockings in selected patients.

Neurosurgery

These patients should receive intermittent pneumatic compression. This approach may be used in conjunction with graduated com-pression stockings (8,44). Low-dose heparin is an acceptable alternative.

High-Risk Patients

Elective Hip Replacement

Several approaches are effective. Subcuta-neous low molecular weight heparin given once or twice daily is effective and safe. Sev-eral such agents are approved for use in Eu-rope and North America. At present in North America, these agents are approved for post-operative use only. Prophylaxis with oral anti-coagulants adjusted to maintain an INR of 2.0 to 3.0 is effective and is associated with a low risk of bleeding (8,44). Other effective ap-proaches include adjusted dose subcutaneous unfractionated heparin and intermittent pneumatic compression. However, rates of proximal venous thrombosis are higher with intermittent pneumatic compression than with the other approaches.

Elective Knee Replacement

Although intermittent pneumatic compression was shown in earlier studies to be effective and to be a still-useful alternative, the current prophylaxis of choice is low molecular weight heparin given once or twice daily postoperatively (44,68). Oral anticoagulants are less effective than low molecular weight heparin and cannot be recommended.

Hip Fractures

Two approaches to prophylaxis are available: oral anticoagulation (82) (INR = 2.0 to 3.0) or fixed-dose subcutaneous low molecular weight heparin started preoperatively (44). The combined use of intermittent pneumatic compression with low molecular weight heparin or warfarin may provide additional benefit in certain patients (not level I).

Multiple Trauma

Multiple trauma represents a high risk for thrombosis (44). Low molecular weight heparin is the prophylaxis of choice (72). Intermittent pneumatic compression has been recommended, where feasible, because it eliminates any risk for bleeding. Other alternatives include low-dose unfractionated heparin or warfarin based on extrapolation from other high-risk situations such as hip fracture and hip replacement surgery. Insertion of an inferior vena cava filter has been recommended for very-high-risk situations where anticoagulants may be contraindicated, but this recommendation is based on level V data.

Acute Spinal Cord Injury Associated with Paralysis

Low molecular weight heparin is the most effective prophylaxis (44). Adjusted dose heparin has also been shown to be effective.

Low-dose heparin and intermittent pneumatic compression are less effective. Combining intermittent pneumatic compression with low molecular weight heparin or adjusted dose heparin may provide additional benefit, but this is not supported by data.

OTHER CONDITIONS

Medical Patients

These patients should be classified as low, moderate, or high risk for venous thromboembolism depending on their underlying medical condition and other comorbid factors, such as immobility, previous deep vein thrombosis, cancer, and the like. Low-risk patients should be considered for graduated compression stockings. For patients following myocardial infarction who have no other significant risk factors, anticoagulant with heparin/warfarin is recommended (108). In the presence of congestive heart failure and/or pulmonary infections, either low-dose heparin or low molecular weight heparin is recommended (73). For patients with ischemic strokes and lower limb paralysis, low-dose heparin or low molecular weight heparin is recommended (109). Intermittent pneumatic compression may be used for high-risk patients who are at high risk for bleeding, although this is not based on clinical trial data.

Pregnancy

The use of subcutaneous low-dose heparin is the prophylaxis of choice for pregnant patients who are at high risk for deep vein thrombosis and pulmonary embolism, although data on efficacy from controlled trials are lacking (8). The benefits of prophylaxis are uncertain in patients undergoing cesarean section, particularly if they have no additional risk factors (8). For patients having an emergency cesarean section, prophylaxis with low-dose unfractionated heparin or low molecular weight heparin is recommended. Low molecular weight heparin has been studied in case series for the prevention of venous thrombosis in high-risk pregnancies (110), but there have been no prospective clinical trials to date. In most countries, low molecular weight heparin has not been approved for use in pregnancy.

CONCLUSION

Based on a large number of level I clinical trials and a smaller number of meta-analyses, evidence-based recommendations for the prevention of venous thrombosis in a number of clinical situations can be made: medical patients, general surgery, hip fracture, elective total joint replacement, and multiple trauma. Furthermore, evidence from level I clinical trials supports the use of a number of prophylactic approaches: low-dose heparin, low molecular weight heparin, oral anticoagulants, intermittent pneumatic compression, and graduated compression stockings.

There are numerous clinical situations where further level I clinical trials are required before specific recommendations can be made. These include a number of orthopedic problems, including pelvic fractures and back surgery, and minimally invasive procedures such as arthroscopic surgery or laparoscopic surgery. Although venous thrombosis following total knee replacement can be reduced with the use of low molecular weight heparin when compared with warfarin or low-dose heparin, the thrombosis rates remain high, and better prophylactic measures are required. Uncertainties regarding the most effective use of prophylactic agents continue to stimulate further work in this field. These questions include the safety of anticoagulants used in conjunction with spinal anesthesia, whether low molecular weight heparin is more effective started preoperatively as opposed to postoperatively, and whether once-daily or twice-daily administration of low molecular weight heparin is more effective.

There are a number of interesting topics that have not as yet been addressed. These include the large number of newer antithrombotic agents which are under development, and with the exception of the use of hirudin

following total hip replacement their effectiveness and safety remains unexplored. No level I studies have been carried out in pregnancy, either for the prevention of venous thromboembolism in high-risk patients or for the treatment of proximal venous thrombosis when it occurs. The venogram remains the gold standard for the detection of asymptomatic venous thrombosis following surgery, but this procedure has its drawbacks. Further work on the use of newer investigative modalities, including ultrasound, computed tomographic scanning, and magnetic resonance imaging, may provide more practical and acceptable alternatives to the venogram. Finally, the ultimate goal of prophylaxis should be the elimination of fatal pulmonary embolism in medical and surgical patients, and that at the present time is an unfulfilled goal.

REFERENCES

1. Dismuke SE, Wagner EH. Pulmonary embolism as a cause of death. The changing mortality in hospitalized patients. *JAMA* 1986;255:2039–2042.
2. Dalen JE, Alpert JS. Natural history of pulmonary embolism. *Prog Cardiovasc Dis* 1975;17:257–270.
3. Anderson FA, Wheeler HB, Goldberg RJ, et al. A population-based perspective of the hospital incidence and case-fatality rates of deep vein thrombosis and pulmonary embolism. *Arch Intern Med* 1991;151: 933–938.
4. Donaldson GA, Williams C, Scanell J, et al. A reappraisal of the application of the Trendelenburg operation to massive fatal embolism. *N Engl J Med* 1963;268: 171–174.
5. Clagett GP, Reisch JS. Prevention of venous thromboembolism in general surgical patients. Results of meta-analysis. *Ann Surg* 1988;208:227–240.
6. Collins R, Scrimgeour A, Yusef S, et al. Reduction in fatal pulmonary embolism and venous thrombosis by perioperative administration of subcutaneous heparin. *N Engl J Med* 1988;318:1162–1173.
7. Colditz GA, Tuden RL, Oster G. Rates of venous thrombosis after general surgery: combined results of randomized clinical trials. *Lancet* 1986;19:143–146.
8. Nicolaides AN, Bergqvist D, Hull R. Prevention of Venous Thromboembolism. International Consensus Statement. *Int Angiol* 1997;16:3–38.
9. Hull RD, Hirsh J, Carter CJ, et al. Diagnostic efficacy of impedance plethysmography for clinically suspected deep-vein thrombosis: a randomized trial. *Ann Intern Med* 1985;102:21–28.
10. Huisman MV, Buller HE, ten Cate JW, et al. Serial impedance plethysmography for suspected deep venous thrombosis in outpatients. The Amsterdam General Practitioner Study. *N Engl J Med* 1986;314:823–828.

11. Moser KM, Le Moine JR. Is embolic risk conditioned by location of deep venous thrombosis? *Ann Intern Med* 1981;94:439–444.

12. Huisman MV, Buller HR, ten Cate JW, et al. Management of clinically suspected acute venous thrombosis in outpatients with serial impedance plethysmography in a community hospital setting. *Arch Intern Med* 1989;149:511–513.

13. Kakkar VV, Flanc C, Howe CT, et al. Natural history of post-operative deep-vein thrombosis. *Lancet* 1969; 2:230–233.

14. Lagerstedt CI, Fagher BO, Olsson CG, et al. Need for long-term anticoagulant treatment in symptomatic calf-vein thrombosis. *Lancet* 1985;2:515–518.

15. Hull RD, Delmore T, Genton E, et al. Warfarin sodium versus low-dose heparin in the long-term treatment of venous thrombosis. *N Engl J Med* 1979;301:855–858.

16. Huisman MV, Buller HR, ten Cate JW, et al. Unexpected high prevalence of silent pulmonary embolism in patients with deep venous thrombosis. *Chest* 1989; 95:498–502.

17. Sevitt S, Gallagher N. Venous thrombosis and pulmonary embolism. A clinico-pathological study in injured and burned patients. *Br J Surg* 1961;48: 475–489.

18. Mavor GE, Galloway JMD. The iliofemoral venous segment as a source of pulmonary emboli. *Lancet* 1967;1:871–874.

19. Hull RD, Hirsh J, Carter CJ, et al. Diagnostic value of ventilation-perfusion lung scanning in patients with suspected pulmonary embolism. *Chest* 1985;88: 819–828.

20. A collaborative study by the PIOPED Investigators. Value of the ventilation/perfusion scan in acute pulmonary embolism: results of the Prospective Investigation of Pulmonary Embolism Diagnosis (PIOPED). *JAMA* 1990;263:2753–2769.

21. Kakkar VV, Adams PC. Preventive and therapeutic approach to venous thromboembolism. Can death from pulmonary embolism be prevented? *J Am Coll Cardiol* 1986;8:146B–158B.

22. Skinner DB, Salzman EW. Anticoagulant prophylaxis in surgical patients. *Surg Gynecol Obstet* 1967;125: 741–746.

23. Shephard RM, White HA, Shirkey AL. Anticoagulant prophylaxis of thromboembolism in post-surgical patients. *Am J Surg* 1966;112:698–702.

24. International Multicentre Trial: prevention of fatal postoperative pulmonary embolism by low doses of heparin. *Lancet* 1975;2:45–64.

25. Coventry MB, Nolan DR, Beckenbaugh RD. "Delayed" prophylactic anticoagulation: a study of results and complications in 2,012 total hip arthroplasties. *J Bone Joint Surg [Am]* 1973;55:1487–1492.

26. Eskeland G, Solheim K, Skhorten F. Anticoagulant prophylaxis, thromboembolism and mortality in elderly patients with hip fracture: a controlled clinical trial. *Acta Chir Scand* 1986;131:16–29.

27. Kakkar V, Stamatakis JD, Bentley PG, et al. Prophylaxis for post-operative deep-vein thrombosis. *JAMA* 1979;241:39–42.

28. Anderson FA, Wheeler HB, Goldberg RJ, et al. Physician practices in the prevention of venous thromboembolism. *Ann Intern Med* 1991;115:581–595.

29. Bergqvist D. Prevention of postoperative deep vein thrombosis in Sweden: results of a survey. *World J Surg* 1980;4:489–495.

30. Laverick MD, Croak SA, Mollan RA. Orthopedic surgeons and thromboprophylaxis. *Br Med J* 1991;303: 549–550.

31. Salzman EW, Davies GC. Prophylaxis of venous thromboembolism. Analysis of cost-effectiveness. *Ann Surg* 1980;191:207–218.

32. Hull R, Hirsh J, Sackett DL, et al. Cost-effectiveness of primary and secondary prevention of fatal pulmonary embolism in high-risk surgical patients. *Can Med Assoc J* 1982;127:990–995.

33. Oster G, Tuden RL, Colditz GA. A cost-effectiveness analysis of prophylaxis against deep vein thrombosis in major orthopedic surgery. *JAMA* 1987;257: 203–208.

34. Bergqvist D, Matzsch T, Jendteg S, et al. The cost-effectiveness of prevention of post-operative thromboembolism. *Acta Chir Scand* 1990;556(suppl): 36–41.

35. Hauch O, Kyattar SC, Jorensen LN. Cost-benefit analysis of prophylaxis against deep vein thrombosis in surgery. *Semin Thromb Hemost* 1991;3(suppl 17): 280–283.

36. Kearon C, Hirsh J. Starting prophylaxis for venous thromboembolism postoperatively. *Arch Intern Med* 1995;155:366–372.

37. Hull RD, Pineo GF, Valentine KA, Stagg V, Brant RF. Preoperative low molecular weight heparin (LMWH) is more effective than postoperative LMWH in the prevention of deep vein thrombosis (DVT) in patients undergoing total hip replacement (THR): a pooled analysis. *Blood* 1996;88(suppl):660(A).

38. Dahl OE, Aspelin T, Arnesen H, et al. Increased activation of coagulation and formation of late deep venous thrombosis following discontinuation of thromboprophylaxis after hip replacement surgery. *Thromb Res* 1995;80:299–306.

39. Bergqvist D, Benoni G, Bjorgell O, et al. Low molecular weight heparin (Enoxaparin) as prophylaxis against venous thromboembolism after total hip replacement. *N Engl J Med* 1996;335:696–700.

40. Planes A, Vochelle N, Darmon JY, et al. Risk of deep-venous thrombosis after hospital discharge in patients having undergone total hip replacement: double-blind randomized comparison of enoxaparin versus placebo. *Lancet* 1996;348:224–228.

41. Dahl OE, Andreassen G, Aspelin T, et al. Prolonged thromboprophylaxis following hip replacement surgery—results of a double-blind prospective, randomized, placebo-controlled study with Dalteparin (fragmin). *Thromb Haemost* 1997;77:26–31.

42. Lassen M, Borris L. Prolonged thromboprophylaxis with low molecular weight heparin (Fragmin) after elective total hip arthroplasty—a placebo controlled study. *Thromb Haemost* 1995;73:1104.

43. Cook DJ, Guyatt GH, Laupacis A, Sackett DL, Goldberg J. Rules of evidence and clinical recommendations on the use of antithrombotic agents. *Chest* 1995; 108(4):227S–230S.

44. Clagett GP, Anderson FA, Heit J, Levine M, Wheeler HB. Prevention of venous thromboembolism. *Chest* 1995;108:312S–334S.

45. Leyvraz PF, Richard J, Bachmann F, et al. Adjusted versus fixed dose subcutaneous heparin in the preven-

tion of deep–vein thrombosis after total hip replacement. *N Engl J Med* 1983;309:954–958.

46. Kakkar VV, Cohen AT, Edmonson RA, et al. Low molecular weight versus standard heparin for prevention of venous thromboembolism after major abdominal surgery. *Lancet* 1993;341:259–265.

47. Kakkar VV, Murray WJG. Efficacy and safety of low-molecular-weight heparin (CY216) in preventing postoperative venous thromboembolism: a co-operative study. *Br J Surg* 1985;72:786–791.

48. Bergqvist D, Matzsch T, Brumark U, et al. Low-molecular-weight heparin given the evening before surgery compared with conventional low-dose heparin in prevention of thrombosis. *Br J Surg* 1988;75:888–891.

49. Samama M, Bernard P, Bonnardot JP, et al. Low-molecular-weight heparin compared with unfractionated heparin in prevention of postoperative thrombosis. *Br J Surg* 1988;75:128–131.

50. The European Fraxiparin Study Group. Comparison of a low-molecular-weight heparin and unfractionated heparin for the prevention of deep vein thrombosis in patients undergoing abdominal surgery. *Br J Surg* 1988;75:1058–1063.

51. Caen JP. A randomized double-blind study between a low-molecular-weight heparin Kabi 2165 and standard heparin in the prevention of deep-vein thrombosis in general surgery. A French multicentre trial. *Thromb Haemost* 1988;59:216–220.

52. Leizorovicz A, Picolet H, Peyrieux JC, et al. Prevention of perioperative deep vein thrombosis in general surgery: a multicentre double-blind study comparing two doses of logiparin and standard heparin. *Br J Surg* 1991;78:412–416.

53. Nurmohamed MT, Verhaeghe R, Haas S, et al. A comparative trial of a low molecular weight heparin (Enoxaparin) versus standard heparin for the prophylaxis of postoperative deep vein thrombosis in general surgery. *Am J Surg* 1995;169:567–571.

54. Bergqvist D, Burmark US, Flordal PA, et al. Low molecular weight heparin started before surgery as prophylaxis against deep vein thrombosis: 2500 versus 500 XaI units in 2070 patients. *Br J Surg* 1995;82:496–501.

55. Turpie AGG, Levine MN, Hirsh J, et al. A randomized controlled trial of low-molecular-weight heparin (enoxaparin) to prevent deep-vein thrombosis in patients undergoing elective hip surgery. *N Engl J Med* 1986;315:925–929.

56. Torholm C, Broeng L, Jorgensen PS, et al. Thromboprophylaxis by low-molecular-weight heparin in elective hip surgery: a placebo controlled study. *J Bone Joint Surg [Br]* 1991;73:434–438.

57. Lassen MR, Borris LC, Christiansen HM, et al. Prevention of thromboembolism in 190 hip arthroplasties. *Acta Orthop Scand* 1991;62:33–38.

58. The Danish Enoxaparin Study Group. Low-molecular weight heparin (Enoxaparin) vs. Dextran 70. *Arch Intern Med* 1991;151:1621–1624.

59. Levine MN, Hirsh J, Gent M, et al. Prevention of deep vein thrombosis after elective hip surgery: a randomized trial comparing low molecular weight heparin with standard unfractionated heparin. *Ann Intern Med* 1991;114:545–551.

60. Eriksson BI, Kälebo P, Anthmyr BA, et al. Prevention of deep vein thrombosis and pulmonary embolism after total hip replacement. *J Bone Joint Surg [Am]* 1991;73:484–493.

61. Planes A, Vochelle N, Fagola M, et al. Prevention of deep vein thrombosis after total hip replacement: the effect of low-molecular-weight heparin with spinal and general anaesthesia. *J Bone Joint Surg [Br]* 1991; 73:418–423.

62. Colwell CW, Spiro TE, Trowbridge AA, et al. Use of Enoxaparin, a low-molecular-weight heparin, and unfractionated heparin for the prevention of deep venous thrombosis after elective hip replacement. *J Bone Joint Surg* 1994;76:3–14.

63. Hull RD, Raskob GE, Pineo GF, et al. A comparison of subcutaneous low-molecular-weight heparin with warfarin sodium for prophylaxis against deep-vein thrombosis after hip or knee implantation. *N Engl J Med* 1993;329:1370–1376.

64. Hamulyak K, Lensing AWA, van der Meer J, et al. Subcutaneous low molecular weight heparin or oral anticoagulants for the prevention of deep vein thrombosis in elective hip and knee replacement? *Thromb Haemost* 1995;74:1428–1431.

65. Leclerc JR, Geerts WH, Desjardins L, et al. Prevention of deep vein thrombosis after major knee surgery—a randomized, double-blind trial comparing a low-molecular-weight heparin fragment (Enoxaparin) to placebo. *Thromb Haemost* 1992;67:417–423.

66. Leclerc JR, Geerts WH, Desjardins L, et al. Prevention of venous thromboembolism after knee arthroplasty—a randomized, double-blind trial comparing a low molecular weight heparin fragment (Enoxparin) to warfarin [Abstract]. *Thromb Haemost* 1995;73:1103.

67. Heit J, Berkowitz S, Bona R, et al. Efficacy and safety of Normiflow (a LMWH) compared to warfarin for prevention of venous thromboembolism following total knee replacement: a double-blind, dose-ranging study [Abstract]. *Thromb Haemost* 1995;73:A739.

68. Nurmohamed MT, Rosendaal FR, Büller HR, et al. Low molecular weight heparin in the prophylaxis of venous thrombosis: a meta-analysis. *Lancet* 1992; 340:152–156.

69. O'Brien BJ, Anderson DR, Goeree R. Cost-effectiveness of enoxparin versus warfarin prophylaxis against deep-vein thrombosis after total hip replacement. *Can Med Assoc J* 1994;150:1083–1089.

70. Menzin J, Colditz GA, Regan MM, Richner RE, Oster G. Cost-effectiveness of Enoxaparin vs. low dose warfarin in the prevention of deep-vein thrombosis after total hip replacement surgery. *Arch Intern Med* 1995; 155:757–764.

71. Hull RD, Raskob GE, Rosenbloom D, et al. Treatment of proximal vein thrombosis with subcutaneous low molecular weight heparin vs. intravenous heparin. *Arch Intern Med* 1997;159:289–294.

72. Geerts WH, Jay RM, Code KI, et al. A comparison of low-dose heparin with low-molecular-weight heparin as prophylaxis against venous thromboembolism after major trauma. *N Engl J Med* 1996;335:701–707.

73. Harenberg J, Roebruck P, Heene DL, on behalf of the Heparin Study in Internal Medicine Group. Subcutaneous low molecular weight heparin versus standard heparin and the prevention of thromboembolism in medical inpatients. *Haemostasis* 1996;26:127–139.

74. Bergmann JF, Neuhart E. A multicenter randomized double-blind study of Enoxaparin compared with un-

fractionated heparin in the prevention of venous thromboembolic disease in elderly inpatients bedridden for an acute medical illness. *Thromb Haemost* 1996;7:529–534.

75. Gallus A, Cade J, Ockelford P, et al. Orgaran (Org 10172) or heparin for preventing venous thromboembolism after elective surgery for malignant disease? A double-blind, randomized multicentre comparison. *Thromb Haemost* 1993;70:562–567.

76. Bergqvist D, Kettunen K, Fredin H, et al. Thromboprophylaxis in hip fracture patients—a prospective randomized comparative study between ORG 10172 and dextran. *Surgery* 1991;109:617–622.

77. Gerhart TN, Yett HS, Robertson LK, et al. Low-molecular-weight heparinoid compared with warfarin for prophylaxis of deep vein thrombosis in patients who are operated on for fracture of the hip. A prospective, randomized trial. *J Bone Joint Surg* 1991;73(4):494–502.

78. Hoek J, Nurmohamed MT, ten Cate H, et al. Prevention of deep vein thrombosis following total hip replacement by a low-molecular-weight heparinoid. *Thromb Haemost* 1989;62(suppl):1637.

79. Francis CW, Pellegrini VD, Marder VJ, et al. Comparison of warfarin and external pneumatic compression in prevention of venous thrombosis after total hip replacement. *JAMA* 1992;267:2911–2915.

80. Paiement GD, Wessinger SJ, Waltman WC, et al. Low-dose warfarin versus external pneumatic compression. *Ann Intern Med* 1990;112:423–428.

81. Francis CW, Pellegrini Jr VD, Leibert KM. Comparison of two warfarin regimens in the prevention of venous thrombosis following total knee replacement. *Thromb Haemost* 1996;75:706–711.

82. Power PJ, Gent M, Jay R, et al. A randomized trial of less intense postoperative warfarin or aspirin therapy in the prevention of venous thromboembolism after surgery for fractured hip. *Arch Intern Med* 1989;149:771–774.

83. Poller L, McKernan A, Thomson JM, et al. Fixed minidose warfarin: a new approach to prophylaxis against venous thrombosis after major surgery. *Br Med J* 1987;285:1309–1312.

84. Bern MM, Lokich JJ, Wallach SR, et al. Very low doses of warfarin can prevent thrombosis in central venous catheters. *Ann Intern Med* 1990;112:423–428.

85. Dale C, Gallus A, Wycherley A, et al. Prevention of venous thrombosis with minidose warfarin after joint replacement. *Br Med J* 1991;303:224.

86. Roberts VC, Sabri S, Beely AH, et al. The effect of intermittently applied external pressure on the hemodynamics of the lower limb in man. *Br J Surg* 1972;59:233–236.

87. Ramos R, Salem BI, Pawlikowski MP, et al. The efficacy of pneumatic compression stockings in the prevention of pulmonary embolism after cardiac surgery. *Chest* 1996;109:82–85.

88. Turpie AGG, Gallus A, Beattie WS, et al. Prevention of venous thrombosis in patients with intracranial disease by intermittent pneumatic compression of the calf. *Neurology* 1977;27:435–438.

89. Turpie AGG, Delmore T, Hirsh J, et al. Prevention of venous thrombosis by intermittent sequential calf compression in patients with intracranial disease. *Thromb Res* 1979;16:611–616.

90. Skillman JJ, Collins RR, Coe NP, et al. Prevention of deep vein thrombosis in neurosurgical patients: a controlled, randomized trial of external pneumatic compression boots. *Surgery* 1978;83:354–358.

91. Hull RD, Raskob G, Gent M, et al. Effectiveness of intermittent pneumatic leg compression for preventing deep vein thrombosis after total hip replacement. *JAMA* 1990;263:2313–2317.

92. Hull RD, Delmore TJ, Hirsh J, et al. Effectiveness of intermittent pulsatile elastic stockings for the prevention of calf and thigh vein thrombosis in patients undergoing elective knee surgery. *Thromb Res* 1979;16:37–45.

93. Mckenna R, Galante J, Bachmann F, et al. Prevention of venous thromboembolism after total knee replacement by high-dose aspirin or intermittent calf and thigh compression. *Br Med J* 1980;1:514–517.

94. Meyerowitz BR, Nelson R. Measurement of the velocity of blood in lower limb veins with and without compression surgery. *Surgery* 1964;56:481–486.

95. Sigel B, Edelstein AL, Felix WR. Compression of the deep venous system of the lower leg during inactive recumbency. *Arch Surg* 1973;106:38–43.

96. Lawrence D, Kakkar VV. Graduated, static, external compression of the lower limb: a physiological assessment. *Br J Surg* 1980;67:119–121.

97. Wells PS, Lensing AWA, Hirsh J. Graduated compression stockings in the prevention of postoperative venous thromboembolism. A meta-analysis. *Arch Intern Med* 1994;154:67–72.

98. Antiplatelet Trialists' Collaboration. Collaborative overview of randomized trials of antiplatelet therapy—III: Reduction in venous thrombosis and pulmonary embolism by antiplatelet prophylaxis among surgical and medical patients. *Br Med J* 1994;308:235–246.

99. Eriksson BI, Ekman S, Kalebo P, et al. Prevention of deep-vein thrombosis after total hip replacement: direct thrombin inhibition with recombinant hirudin, CGP 39393. *Lancet* 1996;347:635–639.

100. Eriksson BI, Goteborg SE, Lindbratt S, et al. Prevention of Thromboembolism with use of recombinant hirudin. *J Bone Joint Surg* 1997;79:326–333.

101. Polkolainen E, Hendolin H. Effects of lumbar epidural analgesia and general anesthesia on flow velocity in the femoral vein and postoperative deep vein thrombosis. *Acta Chir Scand* 1983;149:361–364.

102. Otton PE, Wilson EJ. The cardiocirculatory effects of upper thoracic epidural analgesia. *Can Anaesth Soc J* 1966;13:541–549.

103. Hendolin H, Mattila MAK, Poikolainen E. The effect of lumbar epidural analgesia on the development of deep vein thrombosis of the legs after open prostatectomy. *Acta Chir Scand* 1981;147:425–429.

104. Hendolin H, Tuppurainen T, Lahtinen J. Thoracic epidural analgesia and deep vein thrombosis in cholecystectomized patients. *Acta Chir Scand* 1982;148:405–409.

105. Mellbring G, Dahlgren S, Reiz S, et al. Thromboembolic complications after major abdominal surgery. Effect of thoracic epidural analgesia. *Acta Chir Scand* 1983;149:263–268.

106. Hjortso NC, Neumann P, Frosig F, et al. A controlled study on the effect of epidural analgesia with local anesthetics and morphine on morbidity after abdominal surgery. *Acta Anaesthesiol Scand* 1985;29:790–796.

107. Bergqvist D, Lindblad B, Matzsch T. Low molecular weight heparin for thromboprophylaxis and epidural/spinal anesthesia—is there a risk? *Acta Anaesth Scand* 1992;36:605–609.

108. Cairns JA, Lewis HD, Meade TW, Sutton GC, Theroux P. Antithrombotic agents in coronary artery disease. *Chest* 1995;108:380S–400S.

109. Sherman DG, Dyken ML, Gent M, et al. Antithrombotic therapy for cerebrovascular disorders. *Chest* 1995;108:444S–455S.

110. Hunt BJ, Dought HA, Majumdar G, et al. Thrombo prophylaxis with low molecular weight heparin (Fragmin) in high risk pregnancies. *Thromb Haemost* 1997; 77:39–43.

*Cardiovascular Thrombosis: Thrombocardiology
and Thromboneurology, Second Edition,*
edited by M. Verstraete, V. Fuster, and E. J. Topol,
Lippincott–Raven Publishers, Philadelphia © 1998.

39

Treatment of Deep Venous Thrombosis and Pulmonary Embolism

Jan W. ten Cate, *Hervé Sors, and †Samuel Z. Goldhaber

*Centre of Haemostasis, Thrombosis, and Atherosclerosis Research,
Academic Medical Centre, 1105 AZ Amsterdam, The Netherlands;
*Department of Pneumology and Intensive Care, Hôpital Laennec, 75007 Paris, France; and
†Cardiovascular Division, Brigham and Women's Hospital, Boston, Massachusetts 02115*

The annual incidence of venous thromboembolism (VTE) in the general population of the Western world is about 1 per 1,000 (1,2). Prevention of recurrence and of a fatal outcome constitutes the principal rationale for anticoagulant treatment. Additional goals are prevention of venous insufficiency (due to post-thrombotic syndrome) and of pulmonary hypertension. Despite improved management strategies, VTE still heralds a fatal outcome in a substantial proportion of patients, with 1-year all-cause mortality rates of 24% for pulmonary embolisms (PEs) (3) and 10% to 14% for DVT patients at 3 to 6 months follow-up, respectively (4,5). Although fatal outcomes are mostly due to concomitant serious disorders, such as cancer, cardiovascular and infectious diseases, recurrent PE still accounts for the morbidity and mortality of some patients.

ANTICOAGULATION

With the introduction of heparin in 1937 (6) and of dicumarol in 1941 (7), medical treatment of VTE became feasible. Treatment is usually started with an initial course of adjusted dose heparin to achieve immediate optimal anticoagulation. Coumarin treatment is begun concurrently and requires several days to reach sufficient therapeutic anticoagulation. The need for heparinization has been unequivocally demonstrated. In a randomized double-blind study (8), patients with confirmed proximal deep vein thrombosis receiving only oral anticoagulants had 20% recurrent thromboembolic events at follow-up for 6 months versus 6.7% in patients conventionally treated with adjusted dose heparin and oral anticoagulants started concurrently. Initial heparinization and long-term treatment with oral anticoagulants are therefore considered the standard therapeutic approach.

The development of low molecular weight heparins and their evaluation versus standard unfractionated heparin in the initial treatment of VTE has changed the outlook for VTE treatment considerably. Standard unfractionated heparin is a heterogeneous mixture of highly sulfated polysaccharide chains with molecular weights ranging from 5,000 to 30,000 daltons and an average molecular weight of approximately 15,000 daltons (see Chapter 11). Heparin evokes its anticoagulant activity by binding to a unique pentasaccharide sequence of the natural anticoagulant antithrombin (9), thereby inducing a conformational change and greatly enhancing the activity of this inhibitor toward thrombin, factor Xa, and other activated clotting factors. The inhibition of thrombin requires that heparin bind antithrombin and thrombin simultaneously, requiring a heparin chain length of at least 18 monosaccharide units of approximately 4,800 daltons (10). In addition to its effect on coagulation via antithrombin, heparin (particularly the high molecular weight chains of heparin) interacts with platelets, thereby impairing hemostasis and in part explaining bleeding as its major side effect (11) (Fig. 39-1).

To circumvent this problem, heparin has been fractionated into low molecular weight heparins (LMWHs) ranging from 4,000 to 8,000 daltons. Heparins containing at least the

pentasaccharide antithrombin binding sequence suffice to accelerate the inhibition of activated factor X, without requiring a "direct" interaction between heparin and the activated clotting factors (12). These preparations yielded more short chains of 18 or fewer saccharide units with increased anti-Xa to anti-IIa ratios (2:1 to 4:1) and reduced antiplatelet activity (13).

Hence it was postulated that due to these characteristics LMWH would have an improved balance of benefit to risk compared with heparin. Experimental animal studies indeed showed less bleeding with LMWH, despite the same antithrombotic efficacy, compared with unfractionated heparin (14,15). These encouraging observations plus the longer elimination half-lives and much greater bioavailability of LMWHs following subcutaneous injections compared to unfractionated heparin have greatly stimulated their evaluation in clinical studies.

Unfractionated Heparin

Unfractionated heparin is adjusted according to the activated partial thromboplastin time (APTT) method, using a sensitive thromboplastin, to obtain values of 1.5 to 2.5 times the control, which correspond to a heparin level of 0.2 to 0.4 IU/ml by protamine titration assay (16). Use of a nomogram may assist in achieving an adequate therapeutic anticoagulant response soon after the initiation of heparin (17). The importance of exceeding the lower limit of the target APTT range within 24 to 48 hours has been emphasized in view of a higher risk of recurrent VTE at suboptimal heparinization (18,19).

Hence, a bolus dose of 5,000 IU heparin followed by continuous intravenous infusion starting at 30,000 to 35,000 IU per 24 hours combined with laboratory monitoring of the APTT once per day appears a reasonable recommendation for clinical practice. If required, heparin may be administered by the subcutaneous route as well and seems effective, provided that the heparin dosage is APTT-adjusted and that adequate APTTs (target APTT

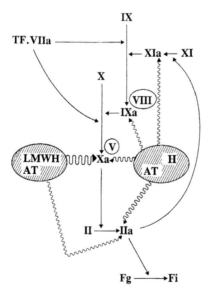

FIG. 39-1. Low molecular weight heparin (LMWH) and standard heparin (H) complex with antithrombin (AT) to inhibit activated clotting factors.

1.5 to 2.5 times control using a sensitive thromboplastin) are obtained as early as possible (20,21).

A 5-day heparin treatment course is currently regarded as the standard regimen provided that heparinization is only discontinued at a therapeutic International Normalized Ratio (INR) on two measurements at least 24 hours apart following concurrently started oral anticoagulant treatment.

Low Molecular Weight Heparin

The efficacy and safety of LMWH have been directly compared with unfractionated heparin in the initial treatment of DVT. LMWHs were administered in a fixed dose on a weight-adjusted basis, by subcutaneous injection, and without laboratory monitoring. In contrast, unfractionated heparin was administered with laboratory monitoring and subsequent dose adjustment.

Two recent studies in large cohorts of patients (22,23) evaluated the use of LMWH in the out-of-hospital setting, whereas conventional heparin treatment intravenously was provided in hospital (Table 39-1). Of those patients randomized to LMWH, more than half were able to be treated at home, either immediately or after a brief stay in hospital. Efficacy and safety was similar in both heparin groups. However, the measurements of quality of life indicated that patients treated with LMWH performed better, in terms of social and physical function, without any detrimental effect of home treatment on their sense of well-being and ability to cope. The potential economic consequence of home treatment is obvious because a 60% to 70% reduction in the number of hospital days was achieved in patients receiving LMWH.

In a recent multicenter study (24a), 1,021 patients with symptomatic DVT (750 patients) or PE (271 patients) were randomized to fixed dose subcutaneous LMWH (510 patients) or adjusted dose continuous intravenous unfractionated heparin (511 patients). Oral anticoagulant treatment was commenced concurrently and continued for 12 weeks. Efficacy and safety outcome events recorded over this period were blindly adjudicated. Twenty-seven (5.3%) of the 510 LMWH-treated patients had proven recurrent VTE versus 25 patients (4.9%) of the 511 patients treated with unfractionated heparin, which met the a priori criteria established for equivalence. Sixteen (3.1%) patients treated with LMWH and 12 (2.3%) patients receiving unfractionated heparin experienced a major bleeding episode. Overall, mortality was 7.4% and similar in the two groups. These findings suggest that fixed dose LMWH is as effective and safe as adjusted dose unfractionated heparin intravenously and can be recommended as initial treatment across the full spectrum of patients with venous thromboembolism. Furthermore, LMWH administered subcutaneously is an attractive alternative to intravenous heparin due to the advantage of simplicity of administration and the potential for home treatment.

In another recent study (24b), 612 patients with symptomatic PE were randomized to either a fixed dose LMWH (304 patients) or intravenous unfractionated heparin in an adjusted fashion. Oral anticoagulant treatment was started concurrently and continued for at least three months.

The primary end point was a combined outcome event defined as death, symptomatic recurrent VTE, or major bleeding within the first eight days of the study. This combined end point was also assessed at day 90.

TABLE 39-1. *Thromboembolic complications during initial treatment and long-term follow-up*

Source (no. patients)	VTE complications		Relative risk reduction (95% CI)	P	Duration of follow-up
	LMWH	Heparin			
Koopman et al. (22)	14/202	17/198	20%	>0.2	6 months
Levine et al. (23)	13/247	17/253	22%	>0.2	3 months

In the first eight days of treatment, 9 patients in each treatment group reached one of the end points (2.9 percent in the unfractionated heparin group, 3.0 percent in the LMWH treated group; 95 percent confidence interval, −2.7 to 2.6). By day 90, 22 patients in the unfractionated heparin group (7.1 percent) and 18 patients assigned to LMWH (5.9 percent) had reached at least one endpoint (95 percent confidence interval, −2.7 to 5.1). The risk of major bleeding was similar throughout the study.

These findings suggest equivalence for efficacy and safety of both treatment regimens in patients with PE who did not require thrombolytic therapy or embolectomy.

Coumarins

The duration of oral anticoagulant therapy is usually limited to 3 months in patients with a first deep venous thrombosis, a practice that is mainly based on the retrospective study of Coon and Willis (25). In this case-control study, a sharp decline in the recurrence rate was observed in patients receiving at least 3 months of anticoagulant treatment. Whether this is indeed the optimal treatment period cannot be concluded from this study.

Two small (26,27) and one larger, more recent randomized trial (28) addressed the effect of different duration of oral anticoagulant therapy in patients with VTE. The first study (26) compared a 1-month course of oral anticoagulant therapy with 6 months treatment, whereas the other investigation randomized (27) patients to either 3 to 12 months or 1.5 to 6 months. As the incidence of recurrence was not clearly different between the two groups in both studies, no definite conclusions can be drawn because the number of enrolled patients was small and the strategy of diagnosing recurrent episodes of DVT was inconsistent.

In the third study, patients with a first episode of VTE (790 DVT patients and 107 PE patients) were randomized to either 6 weeks of oral anticoagulant therapy (443 patients) or 6 months (454 patients) at a target INR of 2.0 to 2.85 (28). Initial treatment consisted of either adjusted dose unfractionated heparin or LMWH administered subcutaneously for at least 5 days prior to randomization. Objective and adequate diagnostic techniques were used to assess the recurrent events, i.e., contrast venography for recurrent DVT and pulmonary scintigraphy and angiography for recurrent PE. The incidence of recurrence at 2-year follow-up for all patients was 14.0%. Among the 6-weeks-treated patients, the incidence was 18.1% (95% CI 14.5 to 21.6), and 9.5% (95% CI 6.8 to 12.2) for the 6-month-treated patients, which is a clinically important difference. No differences were found for the rates of major hemorrhage or mortality. In fact, the rate of fatal PE was low, i.e., 0.6% for all patients. Interestingly, the increased rate of recurrences in the 6-week treatment group occurred mainly after treatment cessation within a period of 4.5 months. Thereafter, the incidences in both groups increased gradually, linearly, and in parallel during the remaining follow-up of 2 years. Overall, the incidences over 2 years in the 6-month treatment group were approximately half of those in the 6-week treatment group, regardless of risk factors and regardless of whether the initial diagnosis was proximal DVT, isolated calf DVT, or PE.

Two studies have demonstrated that factor V Leiden is associated with an increased risk of recurrent PE or DVT at long-term follow-up after anticoagulation is discontinued (29,30). In the more recent study, among 251 unselected patients with a first episode of symptomatic DVT, 16% had the factor V Leiden genetic mutation (29). Patients were followed for an average of 4 years, after an initial 3-month period of oral anticoagulation. With up to 8 years of follow-up, those with factor V Leiden had a 40% recurrence rate, and those without the mutation had an 18% recurrence rate (p < 0.01). Of the recurrent events, 51% were in the leg involved with the initial DVT, 35% were in the contralateral leg, and 14% had PE.

In an additional trial, patients with two separate episodes of venous thromboembolism were randomized after the recurrent episode to 6 months versus indefinite anticoagulation (31). After an average of 4 years of follow-up, 21% of those in the 6-month group suffered recurrent DVT or PE compared with 3% in the group with indefinite anticoagulation. No cases of fatal recurrent PE could be confirmed, although one was suspected in the 6-month group. However, the major hemorrhage rate was 3% in the 6-month group and 9% in the indefinite anticoagulation group.

In conclusion, in view of the high risk for recurrence in patients with permanent risk, at present 6 months of anticoagulation therapy seems advisable. Indefinite anticoagulation therapy should be considered in patients with VTE and active cancer, particularly in those receiving chemotherapy (32). Indefinite anticoagulation therapy should also be considered in patients with inherited thrombophilia such as factor V Leiden or following a recurrent episode of unprovoked VTE (33).

THROMBOLYTIC THERAPY

Pulmonary Embolism

Anticoagulation, the cornerstone of PE management, is called "treatment" but also constitutes secondary prevention of recurrent PE. PEs differ markedly in size and physiologic effect. Therefore, risk stratification is crucial to determine which patients should receive anticoagulation alone and which patients should be considered candidates for thrombolysis or embolectomy.

Thrombolysis appears to be lifesaving in patients with massive PE who present with systemic arterial hypotension as a manifestation of cardiogenic shock (34). Over the past decade, the protocol for giving thrombolytics to pulmonary embolism patients has been streamlined so that it is safer, less expensive, and less time consuming (35). If thrombolysis is contraindicated or fails, suction catheter embolectomy or open surgical embolectomy may be considered (36). The likelihood of success can be optimized by proceeding with these primary therapeutic interventions without delay. Waiting for the development of

pressor-dependent cardiogenic shock leads to an unfavorable metabolic state and poor prognosis, with increased catecholamine release and decreased perfusion of vital organs.

Thrombolysis may also reduce the rate of recurrent PE in patients with preserved blood pressure but worsening right ventricular dysfunction, which can often only be detected on echocardiogram. In a trial of 101 PE patients randomized to rt-PA 100 mg/2 hours followed by heparin or to heparin alone (37), all presented with normal systemic arterial pressure, and slightly less than half had right ventricular dysfunction on echocardiogram. Among patients assigned to rt-PA followed by heparin, none died or had recurrent PE. In contrast, among the 55 patients who received heparin alone, 5 had recurrent PE, despite therapeutic levels of anticoagulation, and 2 of these were fatal (p = 0.06). All 5 were heparin-alone-treated patients who presented with the combination of normal systemic arterial pressure plus echocardiographic evidence of right ventricular hypokinesis.

In our current paradigm, we often consider patients to be potentially "hemodynamically unstable" if they have moderate or severe right ventricular dysfunction, even in the presence of normal systemic arterial pressure. However, the risks of major bleeding must first be carefully considered. In an overview of five PE thrombolysis trials conducted by the Venous Thromboembolism Research Group over the past decade, 4 of 312 patients suffered intracranial hemorrhage within 24 hours of receiving rt-PA or urokinase. Two of these four patients died from hemorrhagic stroke. One of the two survivors had a history of seizures and received thrombolysis in violation of the protocol. Overall, systemic arterial diastolic hypertension at the time of hospital admission increased the risk of intracranial hemorrhage. Notably, no patient under age 57 years suffered hemorrhagic stroke (38).

Patients with normal systemic arterial pressure and normal right ventricular function generally have a good prognosis following

PE. For such individuals, anticoagulation alone is usually adequate; an inferior vena caval filter can be placed if major bleeding from anticoagulation is likely.

Deep Venous Thrombosis

The occasional patient with massive iliofemoral venous thrombosis should be considered for thrombolytic therapy if there are no contraindications. Patients and their physicians must weigh the risk of worse venous insufficiency without thrombolysis versus the increased risk of intracranial or other major hemorrhage with thrombolysis (39). In the presence of a venous bed that is completely obstructed by thrombus (40), systemically given thrombolysis usually fails, probably because the lytic agent cannot physically gain contact with the clot. Under such circumstances, catheter-directed thrombolysis is preferable. However, only about 1 in 20 patients with DVT is an appropriate candidate for any thrombolysis (41,42).

PULMONARY EMBOLECTOMY

Surgical Approach

The surgical approach to pulmonary embolectomy has evolved considerably since Trendelenburg's original description in 1908 (43). Currently, the most commonly used procedure involves normothermic cardiopulmonary bypass (CPB) with or without aortic cross-clamping (36). In severely compromised patients, preoperative circulatory support with partial femoral bypass has been advocated to allow time for diagnostic procedures, surgical preparation, and institution of CPB (44). This approach should be reserved for patients who cannot immediately undergo operation. Temporary venous inflow occlusion or unilateral embolectomy might be considered when CPB is not available or is contraindicated (45), although these procedures have largely been abandoned because of high mortality (36). In such cases, a transvenous embolectomy is usually the procedure of

choice. Whatever the procedure, the role of emergent pulmonary embolectomy remains controversial. The decision to proceed with surgical embolectomy must therefore be highly individualized on a case-by-case basis.

There is a general consensus that pulmonary embolectomy should be considered for hemodynamically compromised patients (shock) if thrombolytic therapy is contraindicated and for those with a deteriorating hemodynamic condition despite intensive medical treatment, including the use of thrombolytics (36,46). Indications for surgery also largely depend on the training and availability of the surgical team.

Mortality in patients referred for pulmonary embolectomy with an erroneous diagnosis approaches 100%, highlighting the need for an unquestionable diagnostic method before surgery is considered, even if this requires partial CPB while diagnostic procedures are performed. Although direct evidence of PE is best provided by pulmonary angiography, alternative imaging modalities may ultimately replace pulmonary angiography, especially transesophageal echocardiography and spiral CT angiography, which both allow direct visualization of proximal clots (48,49). Although a high-probability lung scan is also considered as a valuable diagnostic tool, it cannot specifically diagnose proximal emboli suitable for operation and therefore cannot provide the sole basis for such an important therapeutic decision. Even in the modern settings of CPB and surgical techniques, operative mortality of pulmonary embolectomy for acute PE has ranged from 8% to 56% (36). More recent estimates of mortality in large series average 20% to 40% (50–52), a figure close to mortality with medical therapy in comparable patients (53).

In a series of 96 patients, multivariate analysis identified cardiac arrest and underlying cardiopulmonary disease as predictors of mortality (51). Among patients who have had cardiac arrest, mortality has been reported between 50% and 94% (54). Reported postoperative complications include right heart failure, adult respiratory distress syndrome, pulmonary hemorrhage, mediastinitis, acute renal failure, and severe neurologic sequelae resulting from brain damage. The risk of subsequent fatal PE during the postoperative course is the major rationale for perioperative vena cava filter insertion, although the clinical validity of caval interruption in this setting remains questioned.

Most long-term survivors of surgical pulmonary embolectomy had no or minimal clinical symptoms. Late mortality is mainly due to unrelated conditions rather than recurrent embolization or postembolic pulmonary hypertension (51,52).

Transvenous Approach

Transvenous catheter embolectomy of the pulmonary artery was first described by Greenfield and colleagues in 1971 (55). The embolectomy device (10-Fr steerable catheter) is inserted through the femoral or jugular vein by surgical venotomy and guided under fluoroscopy into the pulmonary artery. Clots are then removed by means of a suction cup. The procedure may have to be repeated several times in order to obtain a significant clot extraction. To date, Greenfield's group has reported 46 patients with a 76% success rate and a 69% overall survival (56). Timsit et al., using the same procedure in 18 patients, reported a 72% survival rate (57). The procedure resulted in immediate improvement in 11 patients (61%) and was unsuccessful in 7. Good results were associated with minimizing the duration of hemodynamic impairment.

An alternative to catheter embolectomy is catheter fragmentation of proximal clots with distal dispersion (58), thereby decreasing the extent of pulmonary vascular obstruction. Other transvenous procedures have been proposed, including ultrasound-assisted aspiration, laser- assisted embolectomy, and clot fragmentation using several devices (Kensey catheter, Amplatz thrombectomy device) (36). Although most of these procedures have been successfully evaluated in vitro or in animal experiments, there are only limited clinical data.

At present, the transvenous techniques are not available in most hospitals. In those where the equipment and expertise for transvenous catheter embolectomy exist, this procedure is an alternative to surgical embolectomy if surgery is contraindicated or not readily available. Any extension of indications of transvenous embolectomy to other patients with massive PE warrants appropriate clinical trials. However, catheter extraction does appear to be technically feasible with a low mortality rate in properly selected patients.

INFERIOR VENA CAVAL PROCEDURES

Inferior vena cava interruption (IVCI) to prevent PE has undergone major evolution over the past three decades. Direct surgical approaches (ligation and external clipping) have given way to transvenous devices placed under fluoroscopic control and introduced through the jugular or femoral vein.

The Mobin-Uddin umbrella filter was first released for general clinical use in 1970 (59). The higher rate of caval patency of the Kimray-Greenfield filter, which became available soon after, made it for a long time the favored device for IVCI (60). Since the 1980s, a number of newer transvenous devices designed for percutaneous insertion have been developed. Now the most widely used in United States and Europe are the Vena Tech, Bird's Nest, Titanium Greenfield, and Simon-Nitinol filters (61). At this time, definitive conclusions on the comparative merits of the available filters cannot be drawn firmly. Important parameters include the ability to retain major clots, high IVC patency, and minimal access site complications. Long-term retrievable filters are now emerging and will probably supplant existing devices, at least in patients for whom IVCI is only needed for a limited time (62).

With most devices and increasing skill, perioperative complications of filter insertion (tilting, malposition, migration, fracture, complications at puncture site) are now infrequent. New or increased lower extremity DVT, filter occlusion, and, to a lesser extent, recurrent PE remain the more frequent long-term filter-related complications (63).

Available data suggest that the risk of filter placement for prevention of recurrent PE is fully justified in the following circumstances: (a) PE or extensive DVT and absolute contraindication for anticoagulation, (b) major bleeding on anticoagulation for embolism or venous thrombosis, (c) failure of adequate anticoagulation to prevent recurrent PE (54,61).

Vena cava interruption may be considered for patients with cor pulmonale resulting from chronic embolization and after surgical or transvenous embolectomy. Prophylactic indications for IVCI warrant further clinical evaluation, although the low complication rates of the new filters should widen the indications for their use in some particularly vulnerable patients, including those with extensive trauma, visceral cancer, or undergoing hip or knee replacement.

CONCLUSION

We have learned that anticoagulation is the cornerstone of management for PE and DVT and that low molecular weight heparin (LMWH) provides a promising approach to therapy. Recent studies have demonstrated that LMWH is effective and that among carefully selected patients LMWH can help shorten (or even eliminate) hospitalization for uncomplicated venous thromboembolism. For patients with massive PE, thrombolysis or embolectomy can be life saving. It is uncertain whether thrombolysis should be administered to patients with the combination of normal systemic arterial pressure and right ventricular dysfunction on echocardiogram. However, evidence is accumulating to support this viewpoint, and a definitive clinical trial will contribute pivotal results. In the future, development of optimal devices to remove PE and DVT and improvements in inferior vena caval filters can be expected.

The "take-home" points are summarized as follows:

1. The initial anticoagulant treatment of patients with a confirmed first episode of DVT or PE consists of either unfraction-
ated heparin intravenously in a dose adjusted to rapidly achieve APTT values of 1.5 to 2.5 times the control, or LMWH in a fixed (body-weight-adjusted) dose subcutaneously. The initial treatment should continue until the INR values of concurrently started coumarin treatment are within the therapeutic range of 2.0 to 3.0 at repeated measurements within two subsequent days.

2. The duration of coumarin treatment in patients with a first DVT or PE may be defined by the presence of temporary (e.g., post-surgery) risk factors or persistence thereof. For the first category, three months of oral anticoagulant treatment may be considered adequate. Prolonged and even indefinite anticoagulation should be considered in patients with active cancer, particularly in those receiving chemotherapy, in patients with inherited thrombophilia (e.g., factor V Leiden), or following recurrent episodes of unprovoked venous thromboembolism.

3. Thrombolysis should be considered for patients with massive iliofemoral vein thrombosis or massive PE. For patients in cardiogenic shock, thrombolysis or embolectomy can be life saving. Embolectomy is especially worthwhile when thrombolysis has failed or is contraindicated.

4. Inferior vena cava interruption should be considered in patients with PE or extensive DVT and absolute contraindication for anticoagulation, those who experienced major bleeding on anticoagulation, and those in whom adequate anticoagulation failed to prevent recurrent PE.

REFERENCES

1. Kierkegaard A. Incidence of acute deep venous thrombosis in two districts. A phlebographic study. *Acta Chir Scand* 1980;146:267–269.
2. Anderson FA, Wheeler HB, Goldberg RJ. A population-based perspective of the hospital incidence and case-fatality rates of deep vein thrombosis and pulmonary embolism. The Worcester DVT study. *Arch Intern Med* 1991;151:933–938.
3. Carson JL, Kelley MA, Duff A, et al. The clinical

course of pulmonary embolism. *N Engl J Med* 1992;
326:1240–1245.

4. Prandoni P, Lensing AWA, Büller HR, et al. Comparison of subcutaneous low-molecular-weight heparin with intravenous standard heparin in proximal deep-vein thrombosis. *Lancet* 1992;339:441–445.

5. Hull RD, Raskob GE, Pineo GF, et al. Subcutaneously low-molecular-weight heparin compared with continuous intravenous heparin in the treatment of proximal-vein thrombosis. *N Engl J Med* 1992;326:975–981.

6. Murray DWG, Jacques LB, Perrett TS, Best Ch. Heparin and the thrombosis of veins following injury. *Surgery* 1937;2:163–187.

7. Stahman MA, Hübner CF, Link KP. Studies on the hemorrhagic sweet clover disease V. Identification and synthesis of the hemorrhagic agent. *J Biol Chem* 1941; 138:513–527.

8. Brandjes DPM, Heyboer H, Büller HR, et al. Acenocoumarol and heparin compared with acenocoumarol alone in the initial treatment of proximal-vein thrombosis. *N Engl J Med* 1992;327:1485–1489.

9. Choay J, Petitou M, Lormean JC, et al. Structure activity relationship in heparin:a synthetic pentasaccharide with high affinity for antithrombin III and eliciting high antifactor Xa activity. *Biochem Biophys Res Commun* 1983;116:492–499.

10. Casu B, Oreste P, Torri G, et al. The structure of heparin oligosaccharide fragments with high anti-factor Xa activity containing the minimal antithrombin III-binding sequence. *Biochem J* 1981;197:599–609.

11. Salzman EW, Rosenberg RD, Smith MH, et al. Effect of heparin and heparin fractions on platelet aggregation. *J Clin Invest* 1980;65:64–73.

12. Lindahl U, Thunberg L, Bäckström G, et al. Extension and structural variability of the antithrombin-binding sequence in heparin. *J Biol Chem* 1984;259: 12368–12376.

13. Messmore HL, Griffin Jr B, Fareed J, et al. In vitro studies of the interaction of heparin, low molecular weight heparin and heparinoids with platelets. *Ann NY Acad Science* 1989;556:217–233.

14. Carter CJ, Kelton JG, Hirsh J, et al. The relationship between the hemorrhagic and antithrombotic properties of low molecular weight heparin in rabbits. *Blood* 1982;59:1239–1245.

15. Ockelford PA, Carter CJ, Cerskus A, et al. Comparison of the in vivo hemorrhagic and antithrombotic effects of a low antithrombin III affinity heparin fraction. *Thromb Res* 1982;27:679–690.

16. Hirsh J. Heparin. *N Engl J Med* 1991;324:1565–1574.

17. Cruickshank MK, Levine MN, Hirsh J, et al. A standard heparin nonogram for the management of heparin therapy. *Arch Intern Med* 1991;151:333–337.

18. Hull RD, Raskob GE, Hirsh J, et al. Continuous intravenous heparin compared with intermittent subcutaneous heparin in the initial treatment of proximal vein thrombosis. *N Engl J Med* 1986;315:1109–1114.

19. Hull RD, Raskob GE, Rosenbloom D, et al. Heparin for 5 days compared with 10 days in the initial treatment of proximal venous thrombosis. *N Engl J Med* 1990;322:1260–1264.

20. ten Cate JW, Koopman MMW, Prins MH, Büller HR. Treatment of venous thromboembolism. *Thromb Haemost* 1995;74:197–203.

21. Hirsch DR, Lee TH, Morrison RB, Carlson W, Gold-

haber SZ. Shortened hospitalization by means of adjusted-dose subcutaneous heparin for deep venous thrombosis. *Am Heart J* 1996;131:276–280.

22. Koopman MMW, Prandoni P, Piovella F, et al. Treatment of venous thrombosis with intravenous unfractionated heparin administered in the hospital as compared to subcutaneous low-molecular-weight heparin administered at home. *N Engl J Med* 1996;334: 682–687.

23. Levine MN, Gent M, Hirsh J, et al. A comparison of low-molecular-weight heparin administered primarily at home with unfractionated heparin administered in the hospital for proximal deep-vein thrombosis. *N Engl J Med* 1996;334:677–668.

24a. The Columbus Investigators. Low molecular weight heparin in the treatment of patients with venous thromboembolism. *N Engl J Med* 1997;337:657–662.

24b. Simonneau G, Sors H, Charbonnier B, et al. A comparison of low-molecular-weight heparin with unfractionated heparin for acute pulmonary embolism. *N Engl J Med* 1997;337:663–669.

25. Coon WW, Willis PW. Recurrence of venous thromboembolism. *Surgery* 1973;73:823–827.

26. Holmgren K, Andersson G, Fagrell B, et al. One month versus six month therapy with oral anticoagulants after symptomatic deep vein thrombosis. *Acta Med Scand* 1985;218:279–284.

27. Schulman S, Lockner D, Juhlin-Danfelt A. The duration of oral anticoagulant treatment after deep vein thrombosis. *Acta Med Scand* 1985;217:547–552.

28. Schulman S, Rhedin AS, Lindmarker P, et al. A comparison of six weeks with six months of oral anticoagulant therapy after a first episode of venous thromboembolism. *N Engl J Med* 1995;332:1661–1665.

29. Simioni P, Prandoni P, Lensing AWA, et al. The risk of Recurrent venous thromboembolism in patients with an Arg506 Gln mutation in the gene for factor V (factor V Leiden). *N Engl J Med* 1997;336:399–403.

30. Ridker PM, Miletich JP, Stampfer MJ, Goldhaber SZ, Lindpaintner K, Hennekens CH. Factor V Leiden and risks of recurrent idiopathic venous thromboembolism. *Circulation* 1995;92:2800–2802.

31. Schulman S, Granqvist S, Holmström M, et al., and the Duration of Anticoagulation Trial Study Group. The duration of oral anticoagulant therapy after a second episode of venous thromboembolism. *N Engl J Med* 1997;336:393–398.

32. Levine MN, Gent M, Hirsh J, et al. The thrombogenic effect of anticancer drug therapy in women with stage II breast cancer. *N Engl J Med* 1988;318:404–407.

33. Hirsh J. The optimal duration of anticoagulant therapy for venous thrombosis. *N Engl J Med* 1995;332: 1710–1711.

34. Jerjes-Sanchez C, Ramirez-Rivera A, Garcia M de L, et al. Streptokinase and heparin versus heparin alone in massive pulmonary embolism: a randomized controlled trial. *J Thrombosis Thrombolysis* 1995;2:227–229.

35. Goldhaber SZ. Contemporary pulmonary embolism thrombolysis. *Chest* 1995;107:45S–51S.

36. Meyer G, Tamiser D, Reynaud P, Sors H. Acute pulmonary embolectomy. In: Goldhaber SZ (ed). *Cardiopulmonary Diseases and Cardiac Tumors*. Volume III in Braunwald E (series ed). *Atlas of Heart Diseases*. Philadelphia: Current Medicine, 1995;6.1–6.12.

37. Goldhaber SZ, Haire WD, Feldstein ML, et al. Al-

teplase versus heparin in acute pulmonary embolism: randomised trial assessing right ventricular function and pulmonary perfusion. *Lancet* 1993;341:507–511.

38. Kanter DS, Mikkola KM, Patel SR, Parker JA, Goldhaber SZ. Thrombolytic therapy for pulmonary embolism. Frequency of intracranial hemorrhage and associated risk factors. *Chest* 1997;111:1241–1245.

39. O'Meara JJ III, McNutt RA, Evans AT, Moore SW, Downs SM. A decision analysis of streptokinase plus heparin as compared with heparin alone for deep-vein thrombosis. *N Engl J Med* 1994;330:1864–1869.

40. Meyerovitz MF, Polak JF, Goldhaber SZ. Short-term response to thrombolytic therapy in deep venous thrombosis: Predictive value of venographic appearance. *Radiology* 1992;184:345–348.

41. Brown WD, Goldhaber SZ. How to select patients with deep vein thrombosis for tPA therapy. *Chest* 1989;95: 276S–278S.

42. Markel A, Manzo RA, Strandness DE Jr. The potential role of thrombolytic therapy in venous thrombosis. *Arch Intern Med* 1992;152:1265–1267.

43. Trendelenburg F. Ueber die operative behandlung der embolie der lungenarterie. *Arch Klin Chir* 1908;86: 686–700.

44. Gray HH, Miller GAH, Paneth M. Pulmonary embolectomy: its place in the management of pulmonary embolism. *Lancet* 1988;1:1441–1445.

45. Clarke DB, Abrams LD. Pulmonary embolectomy: a 25 year experience. *J Thorac Cardiovasc Surg* 1986; 92:442–445.

46. Beall AC. Pulmonary embolectomy. *Ann Thorac Surg* 1991;51:179.

47. Hudson ER, Smith TP, McDermott VG, et al. Pulmonary angiography performed with iopamidol: complications in 1,434 patients. *Radiology* 1996;198: 61–65.

48. Torbicki A. Echocardiography in pulmonary embolism. In: Morpurgo M (ed). *Pulmonary Embolism.* New York: Marcel Dekker, 1994;153–178.

49. Van Rossum AB, Pattynama PMT, Tjin A, et al. Pulmonary embolism: validation of spiral CT angiography in 149 patients. *Radiology* 1996;201:467–470.

50. Gray HH, Morgan JM, Paneth M, Miller GAH. Pulmonary embolectomy: indications and results. *Br Heart J* 1987;57:572.

51. Meyer G, Tamisier D, Sors H, et al. Pulmonary embolectomy: a 20-year experience at one center. *Ann Thorac Surg* 1991;51:232–236.

52. Schmid C, Zietlow S, Wagner TOF, Laas J, Borst HG. Fulminant pulmonary embolism: symptoms, diagnostics, operative technique, and results. *Ann Thorac Surg* 1991;52:1102–1107.

53. Gulba DC, Schmid C, Borst HG, Lichtlen P, Dietz R, Luft FC. Medical compared with surgical treatment for massive pulmonary embolism. *Lancet* 1994;343: 576–577.

54. Hyers TM, Hull RD, Weg JG. Antithrombotic therapy for venous thromboembolic disease. *Chest* 1995;108: 335S–351S.

55. Greenfield LJ, Bruce TA, Nichols NB. Transvenous pulmonary embolectomy by catheter device. *Ann Thorac Surg* 1971;174:881–886.

56. Greenfield LJ, Proctor MC, Williams DM, et al. Long-term experience with transvenous catheter pulmonary embolectomy. *J Vasc Surg* 1993;18:450–458.

57. Timsit JF, Reynaud P, Meyer G, et al. Pulmonary embolectomy by catheter device in massive pulmonary embolism. *Chest* 1991;100:655–658.

58. Brady AJB, Crake T, Oakley CM. Percutaneous catheter fragmentation and distal dispersion of proximal pulmonary embolus. *Lancet* 1991;338:1186–1189.

59. Mobin-Uddin K, Callard GM, Bolooki H, Rubinson R, Michie D, Jude JR. Transvenous caval interruption with umbrella filter. *N Engl J Med* 1972;286:55–58.

60. Greenfield LJ, Peyton R, Crute S, Barnes R. Greenfield vena caval filter experience. Late results in 156 patients. *Arch Surg* 1981;116:1451–1456.

61. Bergqvist D. The role of vena caval interruption in patients with venous thromboembolism. *Prog Cardiovasc Dis* 1994;37:25–37.

62. Yune HY. Inferior vena cava filter: search for an ideal device. *Radiology* 1989;172:15–16.

63. Ferris EJ, McCowan TC, Carver DK, McFarland DR. Percutaneous inferior vena caval filters: follow-up of seven designs in 320 patients. *Radiology* 1993;188: 851–856.

Cardiovascular Thrombosis: Thrombocardiology
and Thromboneurology, Second Edition,
edited by M. Verstraete, V. Fuster, and E. J. Topol,
Lippincott–Raven Publishers, Philadelphia © 1998.

40

Secondary Prevention of Deep Vein Thrombosis and Pulmonary Embolism

Alexander G. G. Turpie

Department of Medicine, McMaster University, Hamilton, Ontario L8L 2X2, Canada

Recent studies have put the clinical management of venous thromboembolism on a firm scientific basis. Antithrombotic therapy is mandatory in the management of acute deep vein thrombosis (DVT) and pulmonary embolism because the frequency of thromboembolic complications in untreated patients is high (1). Heparin is standard in the initial management of most patients with venous thrombosis and is effective in the relief of symptoms and in the prevention of extension. In addition, heparin is effective in preventing fatal and nonfatal pulmonary embolism in patients with major vein thrombosis and in recurrence in patients whose initial presentation was pulmonary embolism (2). Randomized trials have established that, following an initial period of treatment with heparin, long-term anticoagulant therapy is necessary for optimal management of deep vein thrombosis or pulmonary embolism. Secondary prophylaxis with oral anticoagulants or subcutaneous heparin in therapeutic doses are the current methods of choice, but recent studies suggest that low molecular weight heparin may be used as an alternative.

ANTICOAGULANT MANAGEMENT OF VENOUS THROMBOEMBOLISM

Heparin followed by warfarin is standard treatment for those patients with venous thromboembolism (Table 40-1). The recommendation that patients be treated initially with heparin is based on the results of a clinical trial that compared oral anticoagulants in combination with heparin versus oral anticoagulants alone, which was stopped early because of a high incidence of recurrent venous thromboembolism in the group of patients treated with oral anticoagulants alone (3).

A retrospective study and a series of prospective trials have established the requirement for secondary prophylaxis in the management of venous thromboembolism. Treatment options available for secondary prophylaxis of deep vein thrombosis are oral anticoagulants, subcutaneous unfractionated heparin, and low molecular weight heparin. Good data on low molecular weight heparins for secondary prophylaxis are still lacking, but the evidence on the efficacy and safety of oral anticoagulants or adjusted dose subcutaneous heparin is solid.

TABLE 40-1. *Anticoagulant treatment of venous thromboembolism*

Suspected DVT
- Heparin 5,000 U IV or low molecular weight heparin SC
- Imaging study

Confirmed DVT
- Rebolus heparin 5,000–10,000 U IV or low molecular weight heparin q12h SC
- IV infusion 1,300 U/hour
- APTT 1.5–2.5 times control
- Daily platelet count
- Oral anticoagulants begun on day 1
- Discontinue heparin after 5–7 days
- Warfarin for 3 months at INR 2.0–3.0.

Adapted from Hyers et al., ref. 8.

The initial recommendations for long-term use of oral anticoagulants came from a retrospective study (4) that showed fewer episodes of recurrent thromboembolism among patients discharged home on long-term anticoagulant therapy compared with patients not receiving anticoagulants. A series of prospective randomized clinical trials, the results of which are summarized in Table 40-2, have put this recommendation on a firm scientific basis (5–7). In each study, the recurrence rate of venous thromboembolism and the rate of bleeding over a 3-month period was compared among different anticoagulant regimens. In the first study, warfarin monitored to give an INR 3.0 to 4.5 was compared with low-dose subcutaneous unfractionated heparin in a dose of 5,000 units q12h (5). The same oral anticoagulant regimen was then compared with

TABLE 40-2. *Treatment of deep vein thrombosis outcomes in randomized trials of secondary prophylaxis*

	Recurrence	Bleeding
Low-dose heparin	25.7%	0.0%
Hull et al. (5)		
Adjusted dose heparin	3.8%	1.9%
Hull et al. (6)		
Warfarin INR 2.0–3.0	2.1%	4.3%
Hull et al. (7)		
Warfarin INR 3.0–4.5		
Hull et al. (5)	0.0%	21.2%
Hull et al. (6)	1.9%	17.0%
Hull et al. (7)	2.0%	22.4%

fixed adjusted dose heparin administered subcutaneously to give a mid-interval activated partial thromboplastin time (APTT) of 1.5 to 2.0 times control (6). Finally, two intensities of warfarin anticoagulation monitored to achieve either a less intense INR of 2.0 to 3.0 or a standard intensity of 3.0 to 4.5 were directly compared (7). The comparison of warfarin with low-dose heparin was the first demonstration in a prospective trial (5) that patients who received oral anticoagulant therapy had a reduced risk of recurrent venous thromboembolism, thus establishing the requirement for secondary prophylaxis. In this study, of the 33 patients who received standard warfarin none had recurrences compared with 9 of 35 patients (25%) on low-dose subcutaneous heparin who had recurrent thromboembolism over a 3-month period. However, five of the patients receiving warfarin with a target INR of 3.0 to 4.5 had an overt bleeding complication, whereas none of the patients on low-dose heparin had a bleeding complication. In the second study (6), in which the dose of subcutaneous heparin was adjusted to prolong the APTT to 1.5 to 2.0 times control, there was no difference in the recurrence rates between the heparin- and warfarin-treated patients that were low in both groups (2 of 53 and 2 of 52, respectively), but there was a substantially lower incidence of hemorrhage in those patients who had the adjusted dose of subcutaneous heparin (1 of 53) compared with standard warfarin treatment (9 of 53). In the third study (7), in which low-intensity warfarin (INR 2.0) was compared with the standard target for warfarin (INR 3.0 to 4.5), both levels of anticoagulation were found to be effective in reducing the risk of recurrence, but the risk of bleeding was markedly lower in those patients with the less intensive level of anticoagulation in whom 2 of 47 (4.3%) treated at the less intense level had a bleeding episode, compared with 11 of 49 (22%) in the patients treated at the higher level of anticoagulation ($p = 0.015$).

Thus, it was demonstrated that oral anticoagulation with warfarin at a target INR of 2.0 to 3.0 was effective and safe for secondary prophylaxis of deep vein thrombosis and is now recommended as the treatment of choice in this clinical setting (8). An alternative is the use of adjusted dose subcutaneous unfractionated heparin to prolong the mid-interval APTT to 1.5 to 2.0 times control. This adjusted dose regimen of heparin is the treatment of choice in pregnant patients who require anticoagulant therapy. Two recent studies (9,10) have demonstrated the efficacy and safety of low molecular weight heparin for secondary prophylaxis and offer a practical alternative to oral anticoagulants or adjusted dose heparin but more data are required before this regimen can be recommended for routine use.

DURATION OF ANTICOAGULATION THERAPY

The optimal duration of anticoagulant therapy for deep vein thrombosis remains controversial. The retrospective study (4) suggested that in the absence of anticoagulants the risk of recurrence remained significant for about 3 months after the initial event but was substantially less in patients who remained on anticoagulants. Based on this observation, 12 weeks of anticoagulation therapy was usually recommended.

The recent prospective studies have shown that 3 months of treatment is associated with a low risk of recurrence in most patients after initial treatment with heparin (5–7). A number of prospective studies have recently addressed the duration of anticoagulant therapy specifically and have clarified the issue. The duration of anticoagulation therapy for venous thromboembolism was studied in a prospective trial (11) in 712 patients with venous thromboembolic disease who were randomized to anticoagulant therapy for 4 weeks or for 12 weeks and the frequency of death and recurrence of deep vein thrombosis and pulmonary embolism during follow-up was compared. The group receiving 4 weeks of therapy had twice as many bad outcomes as compared to those who received 12 weeks of therapy. The frequency of fatal events was approximately the same for the two groups. Al-

though there are some methodologic limitations to the study, the evidence strongly suggested that optimum duration of anticoagulation therapy for deep venous thromboembolism should be at least 3 months. In this study, patients who had a transient risk factor for venous thromboembolism (e.g., patients with postoperative deep vein thrombosis) had a low risk of recurrence during the period of follow-up, whereas patients without readily identifiable risk factors were at a higher risk for recurrence of venous thrombosis. This difference in recurrence among different patient groups was also noted in a study of 260 symptomatic patients with proven DVT who were followed for 2 years in a management study (12). In this study, DVT was secondary to a known risk factor in half of the patients. These patients had a very low risk of recurrence in the follow-up period. On the other hand, one in four of the remaining patients who had idiopathic thromboembolic disease had recurrent venous thromboembolism over the 2-year period after the anticoagulant treatment was discontinued at 3 months. In addition, 17% of patients in whom cancer was not diagnosed at the time of their initial DVT developed overt cancer during the 2-year follow-up period.

The largest prospective study evaluating the duration of anticoagulant therapy was recently published (13) in which 6 weeks of oral anticoagulant therapy was compared with 6 months of therapy in 887 patients with a first episode of venous thromboembolism that was initially treated with heparin or low molecular weight heparin. After 2 years of follow-up, there were 123 recurrences of venous thromboembolism in total; 80 recurrences occurred in 443 patients who were treated for 6 weeks (18.1%; 95% confidence interval [CI], 14.5 to 21.6) and 43 in the 452 patients who were treated for 6 months (9.5%; 95% CI, 6.8 to 12.2). The odds ratio for recurrent venous thromboembolism in the group treated for 6 weeks only was 2.1 (95% CI, 1.4 to 3.1). There was no difference in mortality or in the rate of major hemorrhagic complications between the 6-week- and 6-month-treated patients. However, there was no difference in the incidence of recurrent events in the two groups at follow-up 6 to 24 months after the initial episode, with a linear increase in the cumulative risk, corresponding to 5% to 6% annually. These observations suggest that longer term anticoagulation may be necessary in some patients, particularly those with idiopathic thrombosis. In a recent study (14), it was shown that patients with recurrent venous thrombosis may require even longer secondary prophylaxis. In this study with a mean follow-up of 3.9 years, patients with recurrent venous thrombosis treated for 6 months had a greater risk (20.7%) of recurrent thromboembolism compared with the patients treated indefinitely in whom the recurrence rate was significant lower at 2.6% (p < 0.001). The rate of major bleeding complications was greater in the patients treated indefinitely (8.6%) compared with the patients treated for 6 months (2.7%). This difference, however, was not statistically significant (p = 0.084).

CALF VEIN THROMBOSIS

The requirement for initial anticoagulant therapy with heparin and long-term treatment in patients with calf vein thrombosis is less certain than for proximal vein thrombosis. Calf vein thrombosis is considered by many authorities to be benign with a low risk of complications including recurrence acutely and long-term complications such as chronic venous insufficiency or the postphlebitic syndrome. Also, it is commonly held that pulmonary embolism is uncommon in patients with isolated calf vein thrombosis. Based on the uncertainty regarding the significance of calf vein thrombosis, recommendations for its management vary from no treatment, surveillance only, short-term anticoagulants, or full anticoagulant therapy with heparin followed by warfarin.

Calf vein thrombosis may occur in outpatients who are symptomatic or may occur in hospitalized patients as a complication of other medical conditions or surgical procedures. In the latter, calf vein thrombosis is usually asymptomatic and often remains undetected. Management strategies for both clinical settings have been developed based on the results of natural history studies, management studies in symptomatic patients with negative noninvasive tests, and from prospective trials evaluating anticoagulant therapy in patients with symptomatic calf vein thrombosis confirmed by objective tests.

Information on the clinical course of calf vein thrombosis in the hospital setting has been obtained from control of placebo-treated patients in studies evaluating thrombosis prophylaxis in high-risk medical or surgical patients. Early studies on thrombosis prevention in patients undergoing general surgical procedures using fibrinogen leg scanning to detect venous thrombosis demonstrated that without prophylaxis 20% of calf vein thrombi propagated into the proximal segments (15). In addition, 20% of these proximal thrombi embolized to the lungs. A recent study using venous duplex scanning reported an extension rate of 28% in symptomatic and asymptomatic patients with isolated calf vein thrombosis (16). Based on these data, it has been suggested that when calf vein thrombosis is diagnosed in patients at risk of extension such as postoperative and medically ill patients, treatment with anticoagulants should be instituted followed by secondary prophylaxis. Whether low-dose unfractionated heparin is sufficient to prevent extension or embolization in such patients has not been conclusively demonstrated; thus, treatment with therapeutic dose unfractionated heparin followed by warfarin, as recommended for proximal vein thrombosis (2), should probably be administered. However, since the majority of calf vein thrombi remain undetected in these patients, the most efficient way to reduce the risk of venous thromboembolism and its complication is to ensure that all patients at risk receive primary prophylaxis (17).

Perhaps the confusion regarding the requirement for anticoagulant treatment of calf vein thrombosis is based partly on different interpretations of the studies evaluating noninvasive diagnostic tests in the management of suspected venous thromboembolism using long-term clinical outcomes to assess efficacy. Most authorities recommend that patients with suspected venous thrombosis who are symptomatic but have negative noninvasive tests, a proportion of whom will have calf vein thrombosis, do not require anticoagulant therapy based on good outcomes at follow-up (18,19). This recommendation has been erroneously interpreted as being evidence that patients with calf vein thrombosis do not require acute or long-term treatment. These studies determined the clinical utility of noninvasive diagnostic tests including impedance plethysmography (IPG) and venous Doppler ultrasound in the management of suspected deep vein thrombosis in symptomatic patients. Both techniques will reliably detect symptomatic proximal thrombi but are relatively insensitive for the detection of calf vein thrombosis (20,21). Management studies using IPG or venous Doppler ultrasound to determine the safety of withholding anticoagulants in symptomatic patients with normal tests have demonstrated that patients with serial tests that remain negative, which excludes calf vein thrombi that extend into the proximal segments, do not require anticoagulants based on the absence of recurrent disease during long-term follow-up (19). Thus management of symptomatic patients without anticoagulants who have negative serial tests has been widely adopted. However, it has to be emphasized that this strategy is based on serial testing and not on a single negative test, and therefore applies to patients who have calf vein thrombi that do not extend into the proximal segments. The utility of such an approach may be improved by taking into account prior clinical probability of venous thromboembolism (22) and may be further improved by the use of ancillary blood tests such as the D-dimer test, which may reliably exclude venous thrombosis if it is negative and may ultimately allow a treatment decision to be made based on the results of the first noninvasive test (23).

Evidence to support the use of long-term anticoagulants in symptomatic calf vein thrombosis confirmed by objective tests comes from small randomized trials that have demonstrated a higher rate of recurrence in untreated patients compared with treated patients. In one study (24), patients with symptomatic calf vein thrombosis initially treated with intravenous heparin were randomized to receive secondary prophylaxis with warfarin at a target INR of 2.5 to 4.2 or no antithrombotic treatment. During 3 months follow-up, 8 (29%) of 28 patients who did not receive warfarin had recurrent venous thromboembolism compared with none in the warfarin-treated group (p = 0.01). Furthermore, at 1 year, 19% of the 28 patients in the untreated group had recurrent venous thrombosis compared with only one of the patients treated with warfarin. These data suggest that patients with symptomatic calf vein thrombosis, like patients with proximal vein thrombosis, require anticoagulant treatment for a minimum of 3 months.

However, there are no studies that have specifically addressed the optimal antithrombotic regimen or duration of treatment of patients with calf vein thrombosis. One study suggested that less intense anticoagulation may be required in the treatment of symptomatic calf vein thrombosis compared with proximal vein thrombosis (5). In this study in which warfarin was compared with low-dose heparin for 3 months after initial therapeutic dose intravenous heparin therapy, there were no recurrences in patients with isolated calf vein thrombosis with either treatment; on the other hand, patients with proximal vein thrombosis treated with low-dose heparin had a high rate of recurrence (9 of 19; 47%) in comparison to those treated with warfarin, suggesting that recurrence or extension of calf vein thrombosis may be adequately treated by low-dose heparin. However, the use of low-dose heparin in the treatment of calf vein thrombosis will have to be tested prospectively before it is adopted for clinical use in this setting.

In the study evaluating the optimal duration of secondary prophylaxis with oral anticoagulants in the treatment of deep vein thrombosis, the relative risk of recurrence with calf vein thrombosis was the same as that for proximal

TABLE 40-3. *Treatment of deep venous thrombosis with low molecular weight heparins:*
a meta-analysis

	LMWH	Heparin	RR (95% CI)	P
Recurrent venous thromboembolism	17/540 (3.1%)	38/546 (6.6%)	53% (18%–73%)	<0.01
Major bleeding	6/753 (0.8%)	21/759 (2.8%)	71% (31%– 85%)	<0.005
Mortality	21/540 (3.9%)	39/546 (7.1%)	45% (10%– 69%)	<0.04

Data from Lensing et al., ref. 25.

vein thrombosis during follow-up (13). In this study, similar to patients with proximal thrombosis, patients with calf vein thrombosis who were treated for 6 months had a recurrence rate that was >50% lower than that observed in patients treated for only 6 weeks. These data suggest that treatment of calf vein thrombosis with anticoagulants may be necessary for an extended period to prevent recurrence of disease or extension and provides additional support for the routine use of long-term oral anticoagulants in patients with calf vein thrombosis. Because there are no good data on optimal anticoagulant regimen for patients with calf vein thrombosis, the treatment shown to be effective in patients with proximal vein thrombosis should be used (8).

The new data demonstrating the feasibility of the outpatient management of patients with deep vein thrombosis with low molecular weight heparin is likely to facilitate the management of patients with calf vein thrombosis. Several studies have demonstrated the safety and efficacy of low molecular weight heparin in the treatment of proximal vein thrombosis (25). A pooled analysis of the comparative trials is shown in Table 40-3. Two large trials recently demonstrated that it is safe and effective to treat many patients with proximal deep vein thrombosis with fixed dose weight-adjusted low molecular weight heparin given subcutaneously at home (26,27). Thus, patients with calf vein thrombosis who are likely to be less symptomatic and are less likely to suffer thromboembolic complications than patients with proximal vein thrombosis will be particularly suited to outpatient treatment.

CONCLUSION

Randomized trials have established the requirement for continued anticoagulant therapy following initial treatment with heparin for patients with venous thromboembolism. Recent studies have demonstrated that patients with recurrent thrombosis require long-term anticoagulants and those with idiopathic thrombosis require treatment for a minimum of one year.

The target INR for oral anticoagulant therapy for patients with venous thromboembolism is 2.0 to 3.0. Adjusted dose subcutaneous heparin or fixed dose low molecular weight heparin are alternatives in patients in whom oral anticoagulants are contraindicated or impractical.

REFERENCES

1. Dalen JE, Alpert JS. Natural history of pulmonary embolism. *Prog Cardiovasc Dis* 1975;17:257–270.
2. Barritt DW, Jordan SC. Anticoagulant drugs in the treatment of pulmonary embolism. A controlled trial. *Lancet* 1960; 1:1309–1312.
3. Brandjes DPM, Heijboer H, Buller HR, de Rijk, M Jagt, ten Cate JW. Acenocoumarol and heparin compared with acenocoumarol alone in the initial treatment of proximal vein thrombosis. *N Engl J Med* 1992;327:1485–1489.
4. Coon WW, Willis PW. Recurrence of venous thromboembolism. *Surgery* 1973;73:823–827.
5. Hull RD, Delmore T, Genton E, et al. Warfarin sodium versus low-dose heparin in the long-term treatment of venous thrombosis. *N Engl J Med* 1979;301:855–859.
6. Hull RD, Delmore T, Carter C, et al. Adjusted subcutaneous heparin versus warfarin sodium in the long-term treatment of venous thrombosis. *N Engl J Med* 1982;306:189–194.
7. Hull RD, Hirsh J, Jay R, et al. Different intensities of oral anticoagulant therapy in the treatment of proximal vein thrombosis. *N Engl J Med* 1982;307:1676–1681.
8. Hyers TM, Hull RD, Weg JG. Antithrombotic therapy for venous thromboembolic disease. *Chest* 1995;108:335S–352S.

9. Pini M, Pattacini C, Quintavalla R, et al. Subcutaneous vs. intravenous heparin in the treatment of deep venous thrombosis: a randomized clinical trial. *Thromb Haemost* 1990;64:222–226.

10. Monreal M, Lafoz E, Olive A, delRio L, Vedia C. Comparison of subcutaneous unfractionated heparin with a low molecular weight heparin (Fragmin) in patients with venous thromboembolism and contraindications to coumarin. *Thromb Haemost* 1994;71:7–11.

11. Research Committee of the British Thoracic Society. Optimal duration of anticoagulation for deep vein thrombosis and pulmonary embolism. *Lancet* 1992; 340:873–876.

12. Prandoni P, Lensing AWA, Buller HR, et al. Deep vein thrombosis and the incidence of subsequent symptomatic cancer. *N Engl J Med* 1993;327:1128–1133.

13. Schulman S, Rhedin AS, Lindmarker P, et al. A comparison of six weeks with six months of oral anticoagulant therapy after a first episode of venous thromboembolism. *N Engl J Med* 1995;332:1661–1665.

14. Schulman S, Granqvist S, Holmstrom M, et al. The duration of oral anticoagulant therapy after a second episode of venous thromboembolism. *N Engl J Med* 1997;336:393–398.

15. Kakkar VV, Howe CT, Flanc C, Clarke MB. Natural history of postoperative deep vein thrombosis. *Lancet* 1969;2:230–233.

16. Lohr JM, James KV, Desmukh RM, Hasselfeld KA. Calf vein thrombi are not a benign finding. *Am J Surg* 1995;170:86–90.

17. Clagett GP, Anderson FA, Heit J, Levine MN, Wheeler HB. Prevention of venous thromboembolism. *Chest* 1995;1:312S–334S.

18. Hull R, Hirsh J, Carter C, et al. Diagnostic efficacy of impedance plethysmography for clinically suspected deep vein thrombosis: a randomized trial. *Ann Intern Med* 1985;102:18–21.

19. Huisman MV, Buller HR, ten Cate JW, et al. Management of clinically suspected acute venous thrombosis in outpatients with serial impedance plethysmography in a community hospital setting. *Arch Intern Med* 1989;149: 511–513.

20. Heijboer H, Buller HR, Lensing AWA, et al. A comparison of real-time compression ultrasonography with impedance plethysmography for the diagnosis of deep vein thrombosis in symptomatic outpatients. *N Engl J Med* 1993;329:1365–1369.

21. Hull R, Hirsh J, Sackett DL, et al. Replacement of venography in suspected venous thrombosis by impedance plethysmography and 125 I-fibrinogen leg scanning. A less invasive approach. *Ann Intern Med* 1981;94:12–15.

22. Wells P, Hirsh J, Anderson DR, et al. Accuracy of clinical assessment of deep vein thrombosis. *Lancet* 1995; 345:1326–1330.

23. Wells PS, Brill-Edwards P, Stevens P, et al. A novel and rapid whole-blood assay for D-dimer in patients with clinically suspected deep vein thrombosis. *Circulation* 1995;91:2184–2187.

24. Lagerstedt CI, Olsson CG, Fagher BO, et al. Need for long-term anticoagulant treatment in symptomatic calf vein thrombosis. *Lancet* 1985;2:515–518.

25. Lensing AWA, Prins MH, Davidson BL, Hirsh J. Treatment of deep venous thrombosis with low molecular weight heparins. A meta-analysis. *Arch Intern Med* 1995;155:601–607.

26. Levine M, Gent M, Hirsh J, et al. A comparison of low molecular weight heparin administered primarily at home with unfractionated heparin administered in the hospital for proximal deep vein thrombosis. *N Engl J Med* 1996;334:677–681.

27. Koopman MWM, Prandoni P, Piovella F, et al., for the TASMAN Study Group. Treatment of venous thrombosis with intravenous unfractionated heparin administered in the hospital as compared with subcutaneous low molecular weight heparin administered at home. *N Engl J Med* 1996;334:682–687.

Cardiovascular Thrombosis: Thrombocardiology and Thromboneurology, Second Edition,
edited by M. Verstraete, V. Fuster, and E. J. Topol,
Lippincott–Raven Publishers, Philadelphia © 1998.

41

Perinatal Thromboembolic Disease: Risk to the Fetus and Newborn

Anton Heinz Sutor, *Maureen Andrew, *Lu Ann C. Brooker, and †Sara J. Israels

*Department of Pediatric Hematology, University of Freiburg, D-79117 Freiburg, Germany;
*Department of Pediatrics, McMaster University, Hamilton, Ontario L8V 1C3, Canada; and
†Department of Pediatrics and Child Health, Univeristy of Manitoba, Winnipeg,
Manitoba R3E 0V9, Canada*

Thromboembolic events (TEs) in newborns are increasing in frequency and are predominantly secondary to the presence of central venous lines (CVLs) and arterial catheters (1,2). Recent registries have outlined the epidemiology of TEs in newborns and brought recognition to the seriousness of the problem (1–7). Despite the frequency and seriousness of TEs in newborns, there is a paucity of controlled trials assessing treatment and prophylaxis in the perinatal period. Currently, guidelines for newborns are modified recommendations for adults (8,9). However, information from both clinical and basic studies suggests that the optimal administration of antithrombotic therapy in newborns will differ significantly from adults. The objective of the following review is to discuss the relevance of hemostasis to the incidence, pathogenesis, clinical presentation, diagnosis, laboratory testing, and treatment of newborns with thrombotic complications. The influence of detection and treatment of maternal thromboembolic disease on the fetus is also considered.

DEVELOPMENTAL HEMOSTASIS

The Coagulation System

Coagulation proteins do not cross the placental barrier but are synthesized by fetuses

TABLE 41-1. *Reference values for components of the coagulation system in healthy fetuses (19–27 weeks GA) and premature infants at birth (28–31 weeks GA)*

| Coagulation tests | Gestational age (weeks) | |
	19–27 M SD	28–31 M B
PT(sec)	—	15.4(14.6–16.9)†
APTT (sec)	—	108(80.0–168)†
Fibrinogen (g/l)	1.0(±0.43)∞	2.56(1.60–5.50)†
II (U/ml)	0.12(±0.02)	0.31(0.19–0.54)†
V (U/ml)	0.41(±0.10)~	0.65(0.43–0.80)†
VII (U/ml)	0.28(±0.04)	0.37(0.24–0.76)†
VIII (U/ml)	0.39(±0.14)~	0.79(0.37–1.26)†
vWF (U/ml)	0.64(±0.13)~	1.41(0.83–2.23)†
IX (U/ml)	0.10(±0.01)	0.18(0.17–0.20)†
X (U/ml)	0.21(±0.03)	0.36(0.25–0.64)†
XI (U/ml)	—	0.23(0.11–0.33)†
XII (U/ml)	0.22(±0.03)	0.25(0.05–0.35)†
PK (U/ml)	—	0.26(0.15–0.32)†
HMWK (U/ml)	—	0.32(0.19–0.52)†
AT (U/ml)	0.24(±0.03)°	0.28(0.20–0.38)†
HCII (U/ml)	0.27(±0.05)°	—
Protein C (U/ml)	0.11(±0.03)	—

From Andrew et al., ref. 23, with permission.

GA, gestational age; PT, prothrombin time; APTT, active partial thromboplastin time; VIII, factor VIII procoagulant; vWF, von Willebrand factor; PK, prekallikrein; HK, high molecular weight kininogen; III, antithrombin III; HCIII, heparin cofactor II; SD, standard deviation.

All factors except fibrinogen are expressed as units per milliliter (U/ml) where pooled plasma contains 1.0 U/ml. Values are extrapolated from designated references: 13 (∞), 16 (~); 18 ( ); 20 (°); (178) †. Results for the age group 19–27 weeks gestational age are expressed as a mean (M) ± SD. The age group 28–31 weeks gestational age is expressed as mean followed by the lower and upper boundary (B).

as early as 10 weeks gestational age (GA) (Table 41-1) (10–22). Tables 41-2 to 41-5 provide reference ranges for coagulation proteins for premature (30 to 36 weeks gestational age) and full-term infants during the first 6 months of life (23).

Coagulant Proteins

Plasma concentrations of the vitamin K (VK)–dependent coagulant proteins (factors [F] II, VII, IX, and X) are decreased at birth and during the first months of life (23–29). The prolonged prothrombin time (PT) at birth reflects the low levels of three VK-dependent factors. Similarly, plasma concentrations of the four contact factors (FXI, FXII, prekallikrein, and high molecular weight kininogen) are decreased at birth and gradually increase to values approaching those in adults by 6 months of life (23–25,30). The prolonged activated partial thromboplastin time (APTT) during the first months of life primarily reflects the low levels of the four contact factors (31). Plasma levels of other coagulant proteins including fibrinogen, FVIII, von Willebrand factor (vWF), FV, and FXIII are not decreased at birth (see Tables 41-2 and 41-3) (23–25,30,32–41). Both vWF levels and high molecular weight multimers are increased at birth and for the first 3 months of life (42). Fibrinogen is present in a fetal form and is characterized by increased sialic acid content compared to adult fibrinogen (43–45). However, the physiologic significance of this is unknown.

Inhibitors of Coagulation

Plasma concentrations of antithrombin (AT), protein C, protein S, and heparin cofactor II (HCII) are decreased during the first weeks of life, with levels similar to levels in adults with heterozygous deficiency of one of

TABLE 41-2. *Reference values for coagulation tests in healthy full-term infants during the first 6 months of life*

Coagulation Tests	Day 1 M B	Day 5 M B	Day 30 M B	Day 90 M B	Day 180 M B	Adult M B
PT (sec)	13.0(10.1–15.9)*	12.4(10.0–15.3)*	11.8(10.0–14.3)*	11.9(10.0–14.2)*	12.3(10.7–13.9)*	12.4(10.8–13.9)
INR 1.00	(0.53–1.62)	0.89(0.53–1.48)	0.79(0.53–1.26)	0.81(0.53–1.26)	0.88(0.61–1.17)	0.89(0.64–1.17)
APTT (sec)	42.9(31.3–54.5)	42.6(25.4–59.8)	40.4(32.0–55.2)	37.1(29.0–50.1)*	35.5(28.1–42.9)*	33.5(26.6–40.3)
TCT (sec)	23.5(19.0–28.3)*	23.1(18.0–29.2)	24.3(19.4–29.2)	25.1(20.5–29.7)*	25.5(19.8–31.2)*	25.0(19.7–30.3)
Fibrinogen (g/L)	2.83(1.67–3.99)*	3.12(1.62–4.62)*	2.70(1.62–3.78)*	2.43(1.50–3.79)*	2.51(1.50–3.87)*	2.78(1.56–4.00)
II (U/ml)	0.48(0.26–0.70)	0.63(0.33–0.93)	0.68(0.34–1.02)	0.75(0.45–1.05)	0.88(0.60–1.16)	1.08(0.70–1.46)
V (U/ml)	0.72(0.34–1.08)	0.95(0.45–1.45)	0.98(0.62–1.34)	0.90(0.45–1.32)	0.91(0.55–1.27)	1.06(0.62–1.50)
VII (U/ml)	0.66(0.28–1.04)	0.89(0.35–1.43)	0.90(0.42–1.38)	0.91(0.39–1.43)	0.87(0.47–1.27)	1.05(0.67–1.43)
VIII (U/ml)	1.00(0.50–1.78)*	0.88(0.50–1.54)*	0.91(0.50–1.57)	0.79(0.50–1.25)*	0.73(0.50–1.09)	0.99(0.50–1.49)
vWF (U/ml)	1.53(0.50–2.87)	1.40(0.50–2.54)	1.28(0.50–2.46)	1.18(0.50–2.06)	1.07(0.50–1.97)	0.92(0.50–1.58)
IX (U/ml)	0.53(0.15–0.91)	0.53(0.15–0.91)	0.51(0.21–0.81)	0.67(0.21–1.13)	0.86(0.36–1.36)	1.09(0.55–1.63)
X (U/ml)	0.40(0.12–0.68)	0.49(0.19–0.79)	0.59(0.31–0.87)	0.71(0.35–1.07)	0.78(0.38–1.18)	1.06(0.70–1.52)
XI (U/ml)	0.38(0.10–0.66)	0.55(0.23–0.87)	0.53(0.27–0.79)	0.69(0.41–0.97)	0.86(0.49–1.34)	0.97(0.67–1.27)
XII (U/ml)	0.53(0.13–0.93)	0.47(0.11–0.83)	0.49(0.17–0.81)	0.67(0.25–1.09)	0.77(0.39–1.15)	1.08(0.52–1.64)
PK (U/ml)	0.37(0.18–0.69)	0.48(0.20–0.76)	0.57(0.23–0.91)	0.73(0.41–1.05)	0.86(0.56–1.16)	1.12(0.62–1.62)
HK (U/ml)	0.54(0.06–1.02)	0.74(0.16–1.32)	0.77(0.33–1.21)	0.82(0.30–1.46)*	0.82(0.36–1.28)*	0.92(0.50–1.36)
XIIIa (U/ml)	0.79(0.27–1.31)	0.94(0.44–1.44)*	0.93(0.39–1.47)*	1.04(0.36–1.72)*	1.04(0.46–1.62)*	1.05(0.55–1.55)
XIIIb (U/ml)	0.76(0.30–1.22)	1.06(0.32–1.80)	1.11(0.39–1.73)*	1.16(0.48–1.84)*	1.10(0.50–1.70)	0.97(0.57–1.37)

From Andrew et al., ref. 24, with permission.

PT, prothrombin time; APTT, activated partial thromboplastin time; TCT, thrombin clotting time; VIII, factor VIII procoagulant; vWF, von Willebrand factor; PK, prekallikrein; HK, high molecular weight kininogen; INR, International Normalized Ratio.

All factors except fibrinogen are expressed as units per milliliter (U/ml) where pooled plasma contains 1.0 U/ml. All values are expressed as mean (M) followed by the lower and upper boundary encompassing 95% of the population (B). Between 40 to 77 samples were assayed for each value for the population has been given.

*Values that are indistinguishable from those of the adult.

TABLE 41-3. *Reference values for coagulation tests in healthy premature infants (30–36 weeks gestation) during the first 6 months of life*

Coagulation Tests	Day 1 M B	Day 5 M B	Day 30 M B	Day 90 M B	Day 180 M B	Adult M B
XPT (sec)	13.0(10.6–16.2)*	12.5(10.0–15.3)*	11.8(10.0–13.6)*	12.3(10.0–14.6)	12.5(10.0–15.0)*	12.4(10.8–13.9)
INR 1.0	(0.61–1.70)	0.91(0.53–1.48)	0.79(0.53–1.11)	0.88(0.53–1.32)	0.91(0.53–1.48)	0.89(0.64–1.17)
APTT (sec)	53.6(27.5–79.4)†	50.5(26.9–74.1)	44.7(26.9–62.5)	39.5(28.3–50.7)	37.5(27.2–53.3)	33.5(26.6–40.3)
TCT (sec)	24.8(19.2–30.4)	24.1(18.8–29.4)*	24.4(18.8–29.9)	25.1(19.4–30.8)	25.2(18.9–31.5)	25.0(19.7–30.3)
Fibrinogen (g/L)	2.43(1.50–3.73)*†	2.80(1.60–4.18)*†	2.54(1.50–4.14)	2.46(1.50–3.52)	2.28(1.50–3.60)	2.78(1.56–4.00)
II (U/ml)	0.45(0.20–0.77)	0.57(0.29–0.85)†	0.57(0.36–0.95)	0.68(0.30–1.06)	0.87(0.51–1.23)	1.08(0.70–1.46)
V (U/ml)	0.88(0.41–1.44)*†	1.00(0.46–1.54)*	1.02(0.48–1.56)*	0.99(0.59–1.39)	1.02(0.58–1.46)*	1.06(0.62–1.50)
VII (U/ml)	0.67(0.21–1.13)	0.84(0.30–1.38)	0.83(0.21–1.45)	0.87(0.31–1.43)	0.99(0.47–1.51)*	1.05(0.67–1.43)
VIII (U/ml)	1.11(0.50–2.13)	1.15(0.53–2.05)*†	1.11(0.50–1.99)	1.06(0.58–1.88)*†	0.99(0.50–1.87)*†	0.99(0.50–1.49)
vWF (U/ml)	1.36(0.78–2.10)	1.33(0.72–2.19)	1.36(0.66–2.16)	1.12(0.75–1.84)*†	0.98(0.54–1.58)*	0.92(0.50–1.58)
IX (U/ml)	0.35(0.19–0.65)†	0.42(0.14–0.74)†	0.44(0.13–0.80)	0.59(0.25–0.93)	0.81(0.50–1.20)	1.09(0.55–1.63)
X (U/ml)	0.41(0.11–0.71)	0.51(0.19–0.83)	0.56(0.20–0.92)	0.67(0.35–0.99)	0.77(0.35–1.19)	1.06(0.70–1.52)
XI (U/ml)	0.30(0.08–0.52)†	0.41(0.13–0.69)†	0.43(0.15–0.71)†	0.59(0.25–0.93)*	0.78(0.46–1.10)	0.97(0.67–1.27)
XII (U/ml)	0.38(0.10–0.66)†	0.39(0.09–0.69)†	0.43(0.11–0.75)	0.61(0.15–1.07)	0.82(0.22–1.42)	1.08(0.52–1.64)
PK (U/ml)	0.33(0.09–0.57)	0.45(0.25–0.75)	0.59(0.31–0.87)	0.79(0.37–1.21)	0.78(0.40–1.16)	1.12(0.62–1.62)
HK (U/ml)	0.49(0.09–0.89)	0.62(0.24–1.00)†	0.64(0.16–1.12)*†	0.78(0.32–1.24)	0.83(0.41–1.25)*	0.92(0.50–1.36)
XIIIa (U/ml)	0.70(0.32–1.08)	1.01(0.57–1.45)*	0.99(0.51–1.47)*	1.13(0.71–1.55)*	1.13(0.65–1.61)*	1.05(0.55–1.55)
XIIIb (U/ml)	0.81(0.35–1.27)	1.10(0.68–1.58)*	1.07(0.57–1.57)*	1.21(0.75–1.67)	1.15(0.67–1.63)	0.97(0.57–1.37)

From Andrew et al., ref. 25, with permission.

PT, prothrombin time; APTT, activated partial thromboplastin time; TCT, thrombin clotting time; VIII, factor VIII procoagulant; vWF, von Willebrand factor; PK, prekallikrein; HK, high molecular weight kininogen; INR, International Normalized Ratio.

All factors except fibrinogen are expressed as units per milliliter (U/ml) where pooled plasma contains 1.0 U/ml. All values are given as a mean (M) followed by the lower and upper boundary encompassing 95% of the population (B). Between 40 to 96 samples were assayed for each value for the newborn. Some measurements were skewed due to a disproportionate number of high values. The lower limits which excludes the lower 2.5% of the population has been given (B).

*Values that are indistinguishable from those of the adult.

†Measurements are skewed owing to a disproportionate number of high values.

TABLE 41-4. *Reference values for the inhibitors of coagulation in healthy full-term infants during the first 6 months of life*

Inhibitor Levels	Day 1 M B	Day 5 M B	Day 30 M B	Day 90 M B	Day 180 M B	Adult M B
AT (U/ml)	0.63(0.39–0.87)	0.67(0.41–0.93)	0.78(0.48–1.08)	0.97(0.73–1.21)*	1.04(0.84–1.24)*	1.05(0.79–1.31)
α2M (U/ml)	1.39(0.95–1.83)	1.48(0.98–1.98)	1.50(1.06–1.94)	1.76(1.26–2.26)	1.91(1.49–2.33)	0.86(0.52–1.20)
C1E-INH (U/ml)	0.72(0.36–1.08)	0.90(0.60–1.20)*	0.89(0.47–1.31)	1.15(0.71–1.59)	1.41(0.89–1.93)	1.01(0.71–1.31)
α1AT (U/ml)	0.93(0.49–1.37)*	0.89(0.49–1.29)*	0.62(0.36–0.88)	0.72(0.42–1.02)	0.77(0.47–1.07)	0.93(0.55–1.31)
HCII (U/ml)	0.43(0.10–0.93)	0.48(0.00–0.96)	0.47(0.10–0.87)	0.72(0.10–1.46)	1.20(0.50–1.90)	0.96(0.66–1.26)
Protein C (U/ml)	0.35(0.17–0.53)	0.42(0.20–0.64)	0.43(0.21–0.65)	0.54(0.28–0.80)	0.59(0.37–0.81)	0.96(0.64–1.28)
Protein S (U/ml)	0.36(0.12–0.60)	0.50(0.22–0.78)	0.63(0.33–0.93)	0.86(0.54–1.18)*	0.87(0.55–1.19)*	0.92(0.60–1.24)
TM (AU) (179)	10.55(4.84–16.25)				7.26(3.96–10.56)	4.60(2.9–6.3)
TFPI (U/ml)**	0.7331*					0.8270

Reference values for the inhibitors of coagulation in healthy premature infants (30–36 weeks gestation) during the first six months of life

Inhibitor Levels	Day 1 M B	Day 5 M B	Day 30 M B	Day 90 M B	Day 180 M B	Adult M B
AT (U/ml)	0.38(0.14–0.62)†	0.56(0.30–0.82)	0.59(0.37–0.81)†	0.83(0.45–1.21)†	0.90(0.52–1.28)†	1.05(0.79–1.31)
α2M (U/ml)	1.10(0.56–1.82)†	1.25(0.71–1.77)	1.38(0.72–2.04)	1.80(1.20–2.66)	2.09(1.10–3.21)	0.86(0.52–1.20)
C1E-INH (U/ml)	0.65(0.31–0.99)	0.83(0.45–1.21)	0.74(0.40–1.24)†	1.14(0.60–1.68)*	1.40(0.96–2.04)	1.01(0.71–1.31)
α1AT (U/ml)	0.90(0.36–1.44)*	0.94(0.42–1.46)*	0.76(0.38–1.12)†	0.81(0.49–1.13)*†	0.82(0.48–1.16)*	0.93(0.55–1.31)
HCII (U/ml)	0.32(0.10–0.60)†	0.34(0.10–0.69)	0.43(0.15–0.71)	0.61(0.20–1.11)	0.89(0.45–1.40)*†	0.96(0.66–1.26)
Protein C (U/ml)	0.28(0.12–0.44)†	0.31(0.11–0.51)	0.37(0.15–0.59)†	0.45(0.23–0.67)†	0.57(0.31–0.83)†	0.96(0.64–1.28)
Protein S (U/ml)	0.26(0.14–0.38)†	0.37(0.13–0.61)	0.56(0.22–0.90)	0.76(0.40–1.12)†	0.82(0.44–1.20)	0.92(0.60–1.24)

From Andrew et al., ref. 24, with permission.

AT, antithrombin III; α2-M, α2-macroglobulin; C1E-INH, C1esterase inhibitor; α1–AT, α1-antitrypsin; HCII, heparin cofactor II; TM, thrombomodulin (179). All values are expressed in units per milliliter (U/ml) where pooled plasma contains 1.0 U/ml. All values are given as a mean (M) followed by the lower and upper boundary encompassing 95% of the population (B). Between 40 and 75 samples were assayed for each value for the newborn. Some measurements were skewed due to a disproportionate number of high values. The lower limits, which exclude the lower 2.5% of the population, have been given (B).

*Values that are indistinguishable from those of the adult.

†Values different from those of full-term infants.

**Cord blood (51).

TABLE 41-5. *Reference values for the components of the fibrinolytic system in healthy full-term infants during the first 6 months of life*

Fibrinolytic System	Day 1 M B	Day 5 M B	Day 30 M B	Day 90 M B	Day 180 M B	Adult M B
Plasminogen (U/ml)	1.95(1.25–2.65)	2.17(1.41–2.93)	1.98(1.26–2.70)	2.48(1.74–3.22)	3.01(2.21–3.81)	3.36(2.48–4.24)
t-PA (ng/ml)	9.60(5.00–18.9)	5.60(4.00–10.0)*	4.10(1.00–6.00)*	2.10(1.00–5.00)*	2.80(1.00–6.00)*	4.90(1.40–8.40)
α2AP (U/ml)	0.85(0.55–1.15)	1.00(0.70–1.30)*	1.00(0.76–1.24)*	1.08(0.76–1.40)*	1.11(0.83–1.39)*	1.02(0.68–1.36)
PAI (U/ml)	6.40(2.00–15.1)	2.30(0.00–8.10)*	3.4(0.00–8.80)*	7.20(1.00–15.3)	8.10(6.00–13.0)	3.6(0.00–11.0)

Reference values for the components of the fibrinolytic system in healthy premature infants during the first 6 months of life

Fibrinolytic System	Day 1 M B	Day 5 M B	Day 30 M B	Day 90 M B	Day 180 M B	Adult M B
Plasminogen (U/ml)	1.70(1.12–2.48)†	1.91(1.21–2.61)†	1.81(1.09–2.53)	2.38(1.58–3.18)	2.75(1.91–3.59)†	3.36(2.48–4.24)
t-PA (ng/ml)	8.48(3.00–16.70)	3.97(2.00–6.93)*	4.13(2.00–7.79)*	3.31(2.00–5.07)*	3.48(2.00–5.85)*	4.96(1.46–8.46)
α2AP (U/ml)	0.78(0.40–1.16)	0.81(0.49–1.13)†	0.89(0.55–1.23)†	1.06(0.64–1.48)*	1.15(0.77–1.53)	1.02(0.68–1.36)
PAI (U/ml)	5.40(0.00–12.2)*†	2.50(0.00–7.10)*	4.30(0.00–11.8)*	4.80(1.00–10.2)*†	4.90(1.00–10.2)*†	3.60(0.00–11.0)
uPA (ng/ml)	0.18(0.08–0.28)^**		0.32(0.18–0.46)^			
PAI–2 (ng/ml)	<1.6**					<1.6

From Andrew et al., ref. 24; and Reverdiau-Moalic et al., ref. 58, with permission.

t-PA, tissue plasminogen activator; α2AP, α2-antiplasmin; PAI, plasminogen activator inhibitor; uPA, urokinase plasminogen inhibitor.

For α2AP, values are expressed as units per milliliter (U/ml) where pooled plasma contains 1.0 U/ml. Plasminogen units are those recommended by the Committee on Thrombolytic Agents. Values for t-PA are given as nanograms per milliliter. Values for PAI are given as units per milliliter where one unit of PAI–1 activity is defined as the amount of PAI–1 that inhibits 1 IU of human single-chain t-PA. All values are given as a mean (M) followed by the lower and upper boundary encompassing 95% of the population (B).

*Values that are indistinguishable from those of the adult.

†Values that are different from those of the full-term infant.

**Cord blood.

these inhibitors. Only protein C levels remain low at 6 months of age and do not reach adult values until early childhood (46). A "fetal" form of protein C differs from the adult form by a twofold increase in single-chain protein C (47). Total amounts of protein S are decreased at birth due to the absence of C4B-binding protein (48,49). However, functional protein S activity is similar to adult values because protein S is completely present in the free active form. In contrast, levels of C1-esterase inhibitor and α_2-macroglobulin (α_2M) are in the adult range at birth and increase to values surpassing adult levels by 6 months of age (see Table 41-4) (23) A third coagulation inhibitor is tissue factor pathway inhibitor (TFPI). Cord plasma concentrations of TFPI are decreased to 64% of adult values (50,51).

Regulation of Thrombin

Regulation of thrombin is a key step in hemostasis. The generation of thrombin is delayed and decreased in newborn plasma reflecting decreased plasma concentrations of coagulant proteins, particularly prothrombin, and increased plasma concentrations of α_2M (23). The capacity of newborn plasma to generate thrombin is similar to adults receiving therapeutic amounts of warfarin or heparin (52).

The Fibrinolytic System

Components of the Fibrinolytic System

Plasma concentrations of plasminogen are only 50% of adult values whereas levels of α_2-antiplasmin (α_2AP), the main inhibitor of plasmin, are 80% of adult values (see Table 41-5). Plasma concentrations of tissue plasminogen activator (t-PA), the main physiologic activator of plasminogen, and plasminogen activator inhibitor (PAI-1), the main inhibitor of t-PA, are significantly increased over adult values (23–25,29,53,54). Increased levels of t-PA and PAI-1 on day 1 of life are in marked contrast to values from cord blood

where levels of these proteins are decreased (53–55). The latter discrepancies are likely explained by enhanced release of t-PA and PAI-1 from the endothelium shortly after birth. PAI-2 levels are detectable in cord blood but at significantly lower concentrations than for pregnant women (56). Plasminogen, like fibrinogen, has a fetal form that may have decreased activity as well as binding to cellular receptors for plasminogen (57). Cord levels of urokinase plasminogen activator (u-PA) are decreased to 56% to 74% of adult values (58).

Regulation of Fibrinolysis

Short whole-blood clotting times, short euglobulin lysis times, and increased plasma concentrations of the Bβ15-42 fibrin-related peptides are consistent with activation of the fibrinolytic system at birth (24,54,59). However, the capacity of the fetal fibrinolytic system to generate plasmin in response to thrombolytic agents is decreased compared to adults (60), reflecting decreased plasma concentrations of plasminogen (42).

Platelet Function

In vitro studies of cord blood platelets show decreased activation to a variety of physiologic agonists (61,62), reduced synthesis and response to thromboxane (42), and impaired mobilization of intracellular calcium (63). Despite reduced platelet function, the bleeding time in newborns is shorter than in adults (27,64,65). Several mechanisms contribute to this enhanced platelet–vessel wall interaction. These mechanisms include increased plasma concentrations of vWF; enhanced function of vWF due to a disproportional increase in the high molecular weight multimers; large red cells; and increased hematocrits (23–25).

Blood Vessel Wall

The vessel wall plays a complex role in hemostasis, preventing thrombotic complications under physiologic conditions and promoting fibrin formation when injured. One of the anticoagulant properties of endothelial cell surfaces is mediated by lipoxygenase and cyclooxygenase metabolites of unsaturated fatty acids. Prostacyclin (PGI_2) production from cord vessels exceeds that of vessels from adults (66). A second endothelial cell–mediated antithrombotic property is promotion of AT neutralization of thrombin by cell surface proteoglycans. Structurally, there is evidence that vessel wall glycosaminoglycans (GAGs) are increased by mass and antithrombotic activity in the prepubertal animal compared to adults (67,68). Nitric oxide (NO), or endothelium-derived relaxing factor, is a labile humeral agent that modulates vascular tone in the fetal and postnatal lung and contributes to the normal decline in pulmonary vascular resistance at birth. Like PGI_2, NO is a potent inhibitor of platelet activation and adhesion to the damaged vessel wall. When measured directly, thrombin generation in cord plasma is decreased in the presence of human umbilical endothelial cells compared to plastic by cell surface promotion of AT inhibition of thrombin (69).

VENOUS THROMBOEMBOLIC DISORDERS IN NEWBORNS

Congenital Prethrombotic Disorders

Homozygous Prethrombotic Disorders

Patients who are homozygotes or double heterozygotes for congenital prethrombotic disorders usually present in the early postnatal period or as newborns or young children (70–73). Approximately 40 patients with homozygous protein C or S deficiency are reported in the literature. All patients presenting as newborns had undetectable levels of protein C (or protein S) whereas children with delayed presentation had detectable levels ranging between 0.05 to 0.20 U/ml. Clinically, newborns usually presented with cerebral and/or ophthalmic damage that occurred in utero and purpura fulminans within hours of birth (71,73–78). Purpura fulminans is an acute, lethal syndrome with rapidly progressive hemorrhagic necrosis of the skin due to dermal vascular thrombosis (79–81). Small ecchymotic lesions increase in size and become purplish black with bullae, necrosis, and, ultimately, gangrene (80,81). The lesions occur mainly on the extremities but can occur on the buttocks, abdomen, scrotum, scalp, pressure points, and sites of previous punctures.

The diagnosis of homozygous protein C/S deficiency is made by a combination of an undetectable protein C/S level, a heterozygous state in the parents, and, ideally, identification of the molecular defect. The presence of very low levels of protein C in the absence of clinical manifestations cannot be considered diagnostic because physiologic plasma levels can be as low as 0.12 U/ml at birth. Homozygous forms of AT, or HCII, deficiency have not been confirmed in newborns but would likely present with life-threatening thromboembolic complications.

Until the specific disorder is identified, initial therapy usually consists of 10 to 20 ml/kg of fresh frozen plasma (FFP) (82). With these doses plasma levels of protein C and, similarly, protein S vary from peak values of 15% to 32% and trough levels that are low but measurable (73,83). Doses of protein C concentrate have ranged from 20 to 60 U/kg per dose (70,71). Replacement therapy should be continued until all of the clinical lesions resolve, which is usually 6 to 8 weeks. Subsequent therapeutic options consist of oral anticoagulation therapy, replacement therapy with either FFP or protein C concentrate, and liver transplantation (84).

Heterozygote Prethrombotic Disorders

Patients with single-gene defects for recognized inherited prethrombotic disorders rarely present with their first thromboembolic complication during childhood, unless there is an acquired pathologic event that unmasks the problem (85–87). Clinical presentations reflect the site of the thrombus and purpura fulminans does not occur.

Activated protein C resistance (APCR) is the most common congenital prethrombotic disorder, occurring in 3% to 5% of the Caucasian population (88). APCR was discovered in 1993 by Dahlback and is a point mutation in factor V (R506Q), called factor V Leiden, which confers resistance of FVa to degradation by APC (89). Deficiencies or dysfunction of protein C, protein S, and AT are less common than APCR and reflect a variety of molecular defects (90). The diagnosis of congenital prethrombotic disorders based on activity assays must be made using age related normal values (23,24,26). The contribution of prethrombotic disorders to thrombotic disease in newborns is unknown. However, individual cases and case series implicate prethrombotic disorders as contributing to thrombotic disease in sick newborns (78,91,92). The risk of thrombosis during childhood from the heterozygous state of other congenital risk factors (such as APC resistance, plasminogen deficiency, HCII deficiency, dysfibrinogenemia) is unknown at this time. Although there is general agreement on the initial treatment of TEs with anticoagulants, there is a paucity of information on the benefits and safety for long-term prophylaxis versus careful monitoring with intermittent prophylaxis. Therapies are similar to those in the absence of a congenital prethrombotic disorder except that specific factor replacement may be helpful (93–95). AT concentrates administered as boluses (125 U and 250 U) (95) increase AT levels from 0.10 U/ml to 0.75 and 1.48 U/ml, respectively, at 1 hour (95). Alternatively, continuous infusions of AT at a rate of 2 U/kg/hour maintains a plasma level of 0.40 to 0.50 U/ml (95).

Acquired Prethrombotic Disorders

Incidence

Symptomatic thromboembolic complications secondary to illness or the presence of a catheter occur more frequently in sick newborns than at any other age during childhood, with an incidence of approximately 2.4 per 1,000 hospital admissions (2). Catheters provide many of the requirements that initiate thrombus formation and are responsible for the majority of venous thrombotic complications in newborns (2,96,97). Renal vein thrombosis (RVT) is the most common non-catheter-related thrombosis (2). The following section discusses the most common acquired thrombotic complications in newborns.

Venous Catheter-Related Thrombosis

Umbilical venous catheters and other forms of CVLs are responsible for >80% of all venous thrombi in newborns (1,3,98–104). Based on autopsy studies, 20% to 65% of infants who die with an umbilical venous catheter in place have an associated thrombus (105,106). Long-term complications of umbilical venous catheters, which include portal hypertension, splenomegaly, gastric and oesophageal varices, and hypertension, have not been rigorously studied. Short-term complications such as PE are rarely diagnosed in sick newborns because the clinical symptoms are similar to those of respiratory distress syndrome (RDS). The use of ventilation lung scintigram in newborns has facilitated the diagnosis of PE (107).

Renal Vein Thrombosis

Of all childhood age groups, newborns <1 month of age are most often affected with renal vein thrombosis (RVT) (79%). Some infants develop RVT in utero. The incidence in males and females is similar and the left and right side are equally affected. Presenting symptoms in newborns, which are influenced by the extent and rapidity of thrombus formation, consist of a flank mass, hematuria, proteinuria, thrombocytopenia, and a nonfunctioning kidney. Symptoms of thrombus extension into the inferior vena cava can include cold, cyanotic, and edematous lower extremities. Pathologic states characterized by reduced renal blood flow, increased blood viscosity, hyperosmolality, or hypercoagulability are the main causes of RVT. Coagulation disorders associated with RVT include mild thrombocytopenia (which may reflect consumption), mildly prolonged coagulation screening tests, and increased fibrinogen/fibrin degradation products. Newborns with RVT should be evaluated for an underlying congenital prethrombotic disorder (108). Ultrasound is the radiographic test of choice for diagnosis because of the ease of testing and its sensitivity to an enlarged kidney.

Supportive care alone for unilateral RVT in the absence of uraemia, or extension into the inferior vena cava (IVC) has been suggested. Heparin therapy should be considered for bilateral RVT or RVT that extends into the IVC to prevent PE or complete renal failure. Thrombolytic therapy should be considered in the presence of bilateral RVT and pending renal failure. Eighty-five percent of newborns survive their RVT; however, studies assessing long-term morbidity such as hypertension and renal atrophy are needed.

Sinovenous Thrombosis

Sinovenous thrombosis in newborns is characterized by thrombosis of the intracranial venous system and frequently presents with seizures, lethargy, and/or intermittent hyperexcitability. Heparin therapy is currently recommended for adults based on positive results in one randomized controlled trial (109). Although there are no controlled studies in newborns, the common pathophysiology and relatively poor prognosis (109–114) suggest that therapy with heparin or low molecular weight heparin (LMWH) should be considered (115).

Other

Spontaneous venous thrombosis is very rare but may occur in adrenal veins, the IVC, portal vein, and hepatic veins (75,116–118). Other causes of thrombotic complications include the presence of antiphospholipid antibodies (119–122) and maternal diabetes.

Diagnosis

Although contrast angiography using nonionic contrast media is the diagnostic tool of choice for most venous thrombosis outside the central nervous system (CNS), it is not feasible for many newborns. Other less invasive tests, such as duplex ultrasound and color Doppler, are frequently helpful, but their precision and accuracy in neonatal thrombotic disease is still uncertain (123,124).

ARTERIAL THROMBOEMBOLISM IN NEWBORNS

Arterial Catheter–Related Thrombosis

Arterial catheters are a necessity in the management of critically ill newborns. However, arterial catheters are responsible for >80% of all arterial thrombi in newborns (1). Patients may present with loss of catheter patency or, less commonly, with severe symptomatic vessel obstruction (125–128). Acute symptoms of arterial thrombi reflect the location of the catheter and include renal hypertension, intestinal necrosis, and peripheral gangrene (117). Asymptomatic catheter-related thrombi occur more frequently, as evidenced by both postmortem (116,129) and angiographic studies (130–133). Long-term side effects of symptomatic and asymptomatic thrombosis are not clear but may be significant (117).

Diagnosis

Contrast angiography remains the diagnostic test of choice but is frequently not feasible. Duplex ultrasound and color Doppler offer advantages but their sensitivity and specificity are unknown. A review of 20 neonates with aortic thrombosis treated in one institution revealed that ultrasonography failed to identify thrombosis in four patients, three of whom had complete aortic obstruction (134).

Prophylaxis with Heparin

The effectiveness of low-dose heparin infusions (3 to 5 U per hour) was assessed in seven studies using three outcomes: patency, local thrombus, and intracranial hemorrhage (ICH)

(135–140). Reduced patency, which is likely linked to the presence of local thrombus, is prolonged by low-dose heparin (136–140). Local thrombosis (which may occur within hours) was assessed by ultrasound in two studies that were too small to be inclusive (135, 138). The evidence linking heparin to ICH in newborns is similarly weak (139,141). Based on current evidence, prophylactic heparin in small doses through the catheter can be recommended to prolong arterial catheter patency in newborns (117).

TREATMENT OF VENOUS AND ARTERIAL THROMBOEMBOLISM IN NEWBORNS

There is a lack of consensus for the treatment of TEs in newborns, which reflects a lack of controlled trials. Recommendations for adults are extrapolated to newborns but in all likelihood do not reflect optimal therapy. Current therapeutic options include supportive care alone, heparin/LMWH therapy, thrombolytic therapy, and thrombectomy. For most infants who develop a thrombotic complication, it is a catheter-related thrombus and clinically silent. In most nurseries, catheters are not routinely screened for associated thrombosis, so by exclusion most infants with clinically silent thrombi receive supportive care alone.

Heparin/Low Molecular Weight Heparin Therapy

Heparin's anticoagulant activities are mediated by catalysis of AT inhibition of thrombin and factor Xa as well as other coagulant enzymes. Newborns have been described as both sensitive and resistant to heparin compared to adults. Observations suggesting that newborns are sensitive to heparin are (a) thrombin generation by newborn plasma is both delayed and decreased compared to adults (and similar to plasma from adults receiving therapeutic amounts of heparin) (52,142); (b) in the presence of low heparin

concentrations, the capacity of newborn plasmas to generate thrombin is barely measurable (143); and (c) clot bound thrombin is decreased in newborns reflecting low levels of prothrombin (144). Observations suggesting that newborns are resistant to heparin are as follows: (a) heparin clearance is accelerated (145,146); (b) plasma concentrations of AT are decreased to levels frequently less than 0.40 U/ml, which may limit heparin's antithrombotic activities (23–25); and (c) studies in newborn piglets show that low AT levels limit the antithrombotic effectiveness of heparin (95,147).

Indications for heparin therapy in newborns remain unclear because the risk/benefit ratio is unknown and the relative risk of major bleeding is likely increased compared to that of adults. Heparin therapy should be considered for infants with extending thrombotic complications or with threatened organ or limb viability. One approach is to use heparin in doses that achieve the lower therapeutic range for adults (Table 41-6). Monitoring of the thrombus with objective tests such as ultrasonography can be helpful.

Optimal duration of therapy with heparin is uncertain. One approach is to treat with heparin for 10 to 14 days and then discontinue therapy. Ultrasound can be used to determine if there is extension of the thrombus. If there is subsequent extension of the thrombus, 3 months of anticoagulation therapy should be considered. When possible, oral anticoagulants should be avoided in newborns because of the risk of bleeding and difficulties in monitoring. There are clear exceptions to this approach such as homozygous protein C/S deficiency or recurrent thrombosis.

Two adverse effects of heparin are serious bleeding, particularly an ICH and heparin-induced thrombocytopenia (HIT) (149–151). In the absence of an alternative etiology, thrombocytopenic patients should be evaluated for HIT and alternative anticoagulant therapy instituted if required. Long-term heparin should be avoided because of the risk of osteopenia. Optimal heparin requirements in newborns can only be determined in controlled clinical trials.

TABLE 41-6. *Protocol for systemic heparin administration and adjustment for newborns*

I. Loading dose: Heparin 75 U/kg IV over 10 minutes.
II. Initial maintenance dose: 28 U/kg/hour for infants <1 year.
III. Adjust heparin to maintain APTT 60–85 seconds (assuming this reflects an anti-factor Xa level of 0.35 to 0.70):

APTT (sec)	Bolus (U/kg)	Hold (min)	% Rate change	Repeat APTT
<50	50	0	+10%	4 hr
50–59	0	0	+10%	4 hr
60–85	0	0	0	Next day
86–95	0	0	-10%	4 hr
96–120	0	30	-10%	4 hr
>120	0	60	-15%	4 hr

IV. Obtain blood for APTT 4 hours after administration of the heparin loading dose and 4 hours after every change in the infusion rate.
V. When APTT values are therapeutic, a daily CBC, and APTT.

From Michelson et al., ref. 180, with permission.
CBC, complete blood count; APTT, activated partial thromboplastin time.

In the future, new anticoagulant drugs, such as LMWH, potentially offer significant therapeutic advantages over heparin for newborns (117,152). The advantages of LMWH include predictable bioavailability, minimal monitoring, ease of administration, less bleeding, and equal or increased efficacy. LMWHs are particularly helpful in patients, such as sick premature infants, who are vulnerable to bleeding complications. Dose finding studies are available for two LMWHs in small infants (153,154).

Oral Anticoagulant Therapy in Newborns

Coumarins function by reducing plasma concentrations of the VK- dependent proteins. In newborns, levels of the VK-dependent proteins are similar to those found in adults receiving therapeutic amounts of oral anticoagulants for DVT/PE (23–25,143,155–157). In addition, newborn stores of VK are low and, if the newborns are breast-fed, VK intake is marginal (158). These features increase the sensitivity of newborns to oral anticoagulants and, potentially, their risk of bleeding. Formula-fed newborns may develop a resistance to oral anticoagulants due to VK supplementation of formulas. Oral anticoagulant therapy should be avoided when possible during the first month of life (124,158). Unfortunately, a small number of infants require long-term anticoagulation therapy and heparin cannot be used for extended periods of time because of the risk of osteopenia. LMWH is an option to be considered; however, studies in newborns are limited (154).

The optimal therapeutic INR range is unknown for newborns and almost certainly differs from that of adults. Recommendations for oral anticoagulation therapy in adults can be used as a guideline with the goal of using the lowest effective dose, which can be individualized to some extent (Table 41-7). Mechanisms responsible for the age dependency of dosing with oral anticoagulants are not completely clear. One reason could be that oral anticoagulants act in the extracellular space which is larger in infants. If the dose is calculated according to body weight in kilograms, an infant requires approximately double the quantity of a drug compared to adults or older children. Dosing of drugs in newborns can be calculated per square meter of body surface (159). For phenprocoumon, the average maintenance dose is 1.4 mg per m^2 per day with wide variations (160).

Maintenance doses for therapeutic amounts of oral anticoagulants are age-dependent, with infants having the highest (0.32 mg per kg) requirements. Once a stable response has been established, weekly or biweekly measurements

TABLE 41-7. *Protocol for oral anticoagulation therapy to maintain an INR between 2 and 3 for newborns*

I. Day 1: If the baseline INR is 1.0 to 1.3:
Dose = 0.2 mg/kg orally

II. Loading days 2 to 4: If the INR is:

INR	Action
1.1–1.4	repeat loading dose
1.5–1.9	50% of loading dose
2.0–3.0	50% of loading dose
3.0–3.5	25% of loading dose
>3.5	hold until INR <3.5 then restart at 50% less than the previous dose.

III. Long-term oral anticoagulation dose guidelines:

INR	Action
1.1–1.4	increase by 20% of dose
1.5–1.9	increase by 10% of dose
2.0–3.0	no change
3.1–3.5	decrease by 20% of dose
>3.5	hold dose, check INR daily until INR <3.5, then restart at 20% less than the previous dose.

From Michelson et al., ref. 180, with permission.
INR, International Normalized Ratio.

of the INR are required with frequent dose adjustments (8,161) due to alterations in diet, medications, and intercurrent illnesses. Daily supplementation of breast-fed infants with small amounts of commercial formulas reduces their sensitivity to oral anticoagulants and the risk of sudden increases in INR values.

Antiplatelet Agents in Newborns

Antiplatelet agents are rarely used in newborns for the purpose of antithrombotic therapy. The hyporeactivity of neonatal platelets and paradoxically short bleeding time suggest that optimal use of antiplatelet agents will differ in newborns compared to adults. Aspirin is the most commonly used antiplatelet agent. Empiric low doses of 1 to 5 mg/kg/day have been proposed as adjuvant therapy for Blalock-Taussig shunts, some endovascular stents and some cerebrovascular events (162).

Thrombolytic Therapy in Newborns

Thrombolytic therapy is frequently administered in low doses to restore catheter patency (Table 41-8). Less frequently, thrombolytic therapy is administered in systemic doses (Table 41-8), usually to newborns with threatening organ or limb loss. The activities of thrombolytic agents are reduced in newborns because of physiologically decreased plasminogen levels that result in an impaired capacity to thrombolyse fibrin clots (60, 123,163–165). Increasing plasma concentrations of plasminogen, along with thrombolytic therapy, can increase fibrin clot lyses. If an infant does not respond to thrombolytic therapy, replacement of plasminogen should be considered. Embolectomy can be curative,

TABLE 41-8. *Thrombolytic therapy for newborns*

I. Low dose for blocked catheters

	Regimen	Monitoring
Instillation	UK (5,000 U/ml) 1.5–3.0 ml/lumen 2–4 hr	None
Infusion	UK (150 U/kg/hr) per lumen 12–48 hr	Fibrinogen, TCT, PT, APTT

II. Systemic thrombolytic therapy[a]

	Load	Maintenance	Monitoring
UK	4,400 U/kg	4,400 U/kg/hr, 6–12 hr	Fibrinogen, TCT, PT, APTT
SK	2,000 U/kg	2,000 U/kg/hr, 6–12 hr	Same
t-PA	None	0.1–0.6 mg/kg/hr for 6 hr	Same

From Michelson et al., ref. 180, with permission.
UK, urokinase; SK, streptokinase; t-PA, tissue plasminogen activator; TCT, thrombin clotting time; PT, prothrombin time; APTT, activated partial thromboplastin time.
[a]Start heparin therapy either during or immediately upon completion of thrombolytic therapy. A loading dose of heparin may be omitted. The length of time for optimal maintenance is uncertain.
Note: Values provided are starting suggestions; some patients may respond to longer or shorter courses of therapy.

but it is technically difficult and the thrombus may reoccur even when anticoagulant therapy is used.

RISKS OF MATERNAL THROMBOSIS FOR THE INFANT

Diagnostic Procedures

The diagnosis of DVT/PE in pregnant women is problematic because of potential risk of irradiation to the fetus. A small increase in the relative risk of childhood cancer is suggested by a literature review following low-dose (<5 rads) in utero radiation exposure (166). With careful use of diagnostic procedures, it is possible to keep the fetal exposure to radiation at <0.50 rads for diagnosing DVT and PE (166).

ANTICOAGULANT AND THROMBOLYTIC DRUGS DURING PREGNANCY AND LACTATION

Heparin

Neither heparin or LMWH crosses the placenta and therefore either one can be used during pregnancy (167). When compared to uncomplicated pregnancies, there is no difference (168) in the outcome of pregnancies in mothers treated with heparin for venous thromboembolism or prosthetic heart valves in terms of prematurity, spontaneous abortions, stillbirths, neonatal deaths, or congenital malformations (169). Heparin is not excreted into breast milk and can be given in the puerperium.

Oral Anticoagulants

Oral anticoagulants taken during the first trimester of pregnancy can induce an embryopathy characterized by intrauterine growth retardation, microcephaly, optic atrophy, nasal hypoplasia, and/or stippled epiphyses (170). CNS defects may be induced during any trimester and may be related to bleeding with subsequent impaired growth of brain

tissue. In the third-trimester oral anticoagulants may cause an anticoagulant effect in the fetus, particularly at the time of delivery (170). In general, heparin or LMWH is substituted for oral anticoagulants during pregnancy (170).

Breast Feeding

There are two convincing studies that show that oral anticoagulants are not excreted into breast milk and that breast-fed newborns are not at risk for a coumadin-induced coagulopathy (171,172).

Aspirin

Fetal Risk

Maternal use of low-dose aspirin (<60 mg) has not been shown to increase hemorrhagic complications in newborns and has less inhibitory effect on fetal than maternal thromboxane production (173,174). Aspirin and other salicylates may be excreted into breast milk in low concentrations. It is recommended that aspirin be used cautiously by the mother during lactation because of potential adverse effects in the breast-fed infant (175,176).

CONCLUSION

The use of anticoagulation therapy in the treatment of newborns with DVT, PE, or arterial thrombosis continues to be highly individualized. Further clinical investigation is needed before more definite recommendations can be made.

If short-term anticoagulation therapy is not used, the thrombus should be closely monitored with objective tests and, if extending, anticoagulation therapy reinstituted.

If anticoagulation is used, a short course (10 to 14 days) of intravenous heparin should be sufficient to prolong the APTT to the therapeutic range that corresponds to an antifactor Xa level of 0.3 to 0.7 U/ml. The thrombus should be closely monitored with objective tests for evidence of extension or recurrent disease. This grade C recommendation is based on unpublished data (124). If the thrombus extends following discontinuation of heparin therapy, oral anticoagulation therapy should be considered.

If LMWHs are used, they must be monitored with an antifactor Xa assay and not an APTT. Newborns have increased dose requirements with an average of 1.69 U/kg SC BID (enoxaparin) to achieve therapeutic heparin levels (153). For older children an initial dose of 1.0 mg/kg SC BID is usually sufficient to achieve therapeutic heparin levels (180).

The use of thrombolytic agents in the treatment of venous thromboembolism continues to be highly individualized. Further clinical investigation is needed before more definitive recommendations can be made. Supplementation with plasminogen (FFP) may be helpful (60,124).

REFERENCES

1. Schmidt B, Andrew A. A prospective international registry of neonatal thrombotic diseases [Abstract]. *Pediatr Res* 1994;35(part 2):170a.
2. Schmidt B, Andrew M. Neonatal thrombosis: report of a prospective Canadian and International registry. *Pediatrics* 1995;96:939–943.
3. Andrew M, David M, Adams M, et al. Venous thromboembolic complications (VTE) in children: first analyses of the Canadian Registry of VTE. *Blood* 1994;83:1251–1257.
4. Schmidt B, Andrew M. Neonatal thrombosis: a critical appraisal of the available evidence on prevention, diagnosis and treatment. In: Suzuki S, Hathaway WE, Bonnar J, Sutor AH (eds). *Perinatal Thrombosis and Hemostasis.* Tokyo: Springer, 1991;137–144.
5. Sutor AH. Vitamin K deficiency bleeding in infancy. *Semin Thromb Haemost* 1995;22:317–329.
6. Sutor A, Engelhardt W, Mehraein S, Uhl M, Zurborn KH. Anticoagulation in thrombosis of childhood: present state. In: Sutor AH (ed). *Antikoagulation bei Thrombosen im Kindesalter.* Stuttgart: Schattauer, 1997;293–335.
7. Sutor AH. Thrombocytosis in childhood. *Semin Thromb Haemost* 1995;21:330–339.
8. Andrew M, Marzinotto V, Brooker L, et al. Oral anticoagulant therapy in pediatric patients: a prospective study. *Thromb Haemost* 1994;71:265–269.
9. Andrew M, Marzinotto V, Blanchette V, et al. Heparin therapy in pediatric patients: a prospective cohort study. *Pediatr Res* 1994;35:78–83.
10. Cade J, Hirsh J, Martin M. Placental barrier to coagulation factors: its relevance to the coagulation defect at birth and to haemorrhage in the newborn. *Br Med J* 1969;2:281–283.
11. Kisker C, Robillard J, Clarke W. Development of blood coagulation—a fetal lamb model. *Pediatr Res* 1981; 15:1045–1050.
12. Andrew M, O'Brodovich H, Mitchell L. The fetal lamb coagulation system during normal birth. *Am J Hematol* 1988;28:116–118.
13. Holmberg L, Henriksson P, Ekelund H, Astedt B. Coagulation in the human fetus, comparison with term newborn infants. *J Pediatrics* 1974;85:860–864.
14. Jensen A, Josso S, Zamet P, Monset-Couchard M, Minkowski A. Evolution of blood clotting factors in premature infants during the first ten days of life: a study of 96 cases with comparison between clinical status and blood clotting factor levels. *Pediatr Res* 1973;7:638–644.
15. Mibashan R, Rodeck C, Thumpson J, Edwards R, Singer J, White J. Plasma assay of fetal factors VIIIc and IX for prenatal diagnosis of haemophilia. *Lancet* 1979;1:1309–1311.
16. Forestier F, Daffos F, Galacteros F, Bardakjian J, Rainaut M, Berezard Y. Hematological values of 163 normal fetuses between 18 and 30 weeks of gestation. *Pediatr Res* 1986;20:342–346.
17. Forestier F, Cox WL, Daffos F, et al. The assessment of fetal blood samples [Abstract]. *Am J Obstet Gynecol* 1988;158:1184.
18. Forestier F, Daffos F, Rainaut M, Sole Y, Amiral J. Vitamin K dependent proteins in fetal hemostasis at mid trimester pregnancy. *Thromb Haemost* 1985;53: 401–403.
19. Forestier F, Daffos E, Sole Y, et al. Prenatal diagnosis of hemophilia by fetal blood sampling under ultrasound guidance [Abstract]. *Haemostasis* 1986;16:346.
20. Toulon P, Rainaut M, Aiach M, Roncato M, Daffos F, Forestier F, et al. Antithrombin III (ATIII) and heparin cofactor II (HCII) in normal human fetuses (21st–27th week) [Letter]. *Thromb Haemost* 1986;56:237.
21. Barnard DR, Simmons MA, Hathaway WE. Coagulation studies in extremely premature infants. *Pediatr Res* 1979;13:1330–1335.
22. Nossel HL, Lanzkowsky P, Levy S, Mibashan RS, Hansen JDL. A study of coagulation factor levels in women during labour and in their newborn infants. *Thromb Diath Haemorrh* 1966;16:185.
23. Andrew M, Paes B, Milner R, et al. Development of the human coagulation system in the full-term infant. *Blood* 1987;70:165–172.
24. Andrew M, Paes B, Johnston M. Development of the hemostatic system in the neonate and young infant. *Am J Pediatr Hematol Oncol* 1990;12:95–104.
25. Andrew M, Paes B, Milner R, et al. Development of the human coagulation system in the healthy premature infant. *Blood* 1988;72:1651–1657.
26. Andrew M, Vegh P, Johnston M, Bowker J, Ofosu F, Mitchell L. Maturation of the hemostatic system during childhood. *Blood* 1992;80:1998–2005.
27. Künzer W, Niederhoff H, Sutor AH. Haemostase der Neugeborenen. *Hämostaseologie* 1990;10:104–115.
28. Andrew MD. Developmental hemostasis: Relevance to hemostatic problems during childhood. *Semin Thromb Haemost* 1995;21:341–356.
29. Ries M. Besonderheiten der Gerinnung und Fibrinolyse im Neugeborenenalter. In: Sutor AH (ed). *Antikoagulation bei Thrombosen im Kindesalter.* Stuttgart: Schattauer, 1997;87–97.

30. Aballi A, de Lamerens S. Coagulation changes in the neonatal period and in early infancy. *Pediatr Clin North Am* 1962;9:785–817.

31. Andrew M, Karpatkin M. A simple screening test for evaluating prolonged partial thromboplastin times in newborn infants. *J Pediatrics* 1982;101:610–612.

32. Bleyer W, Hakami N, Shepard T. The development of hemostasis in the human fetus and newborn infant. *J Pediatrics* 1971;79:838–853.

33. Hathaway WE, Bonnar J. Bleeding disorders in the newborn infant. In: Oliver TKJ (ed). *Perinatal Coagulation. Monographs in Neonatology.* New York: Grune and Stratton, 1978;115–169.

34. Gross S, Melhorn D. Exchange transfusion with citrated whole blood for disseminated intravascular coagulation. *J Pediatrics* 1971;78:415–419.

35. Buchanan G. Coagulation disorders in the neonate. *Pediatr Clin North Am* 1986;33:203–220.

36. Montgomery R, Marlar R, Gill J. Newborn haemostasis. *Clin Hematol* 1985;14:443–460.

37. Gibson B. Neonatal haemostasis. *Arch Dis Child* 1989;64:503–506.

38. Göbel U, Voss HC, Petrich C, Jürgens H, Oliver A. Etiopathology and classification of acquired coagulation disorders in the newborn infant. *Klinische Wochenschrift* 1979;57:81–86.

39. McDonald M, Hathaway W. Neonatal haemorrhage and thrombosis. *Semin Perinatol* 1983;7:213–225.

40. Strothers J, Boulton F, Wild R, Ibbotson R, Millar P, Lloyd M, Snodgrass H. Neonatal coagulation [Letter]. *Lancet* 1975;1:408–409.

41. Bahakim H, Gader A, Galil A, Babbar FA, Gaafar TH, Edrees YB. Coagulation parameters in maternal and cord blood at delivery. *Ann Saudi Med* 1990;10:149–155.

42. Stuart M, Dusse J, Clark A, Walenga R. Differences in thromboxane production between neonatal and adult platelets in response to arachidonic acid and epinephrine. *Pediatr Res* 1984;18:823–826.

43. Witt I, Muller H, Kunter LJ. Evidence for the existence of fetal fibrinogen. *Thromb Diath Haemorrh* 1969;22:101–109.

44. Hamulyak K, Nieuwenhuizen W, Devillee PP, Hemker HC. Re-evaluation of some properties of fibrinogen purified from cord blood of normal newborns. *Thromb Res* 1983;32:301–320.

45. Galanakis DK, Mosesson MW. Evaluation of the role of in vivo proteolysis (fibrinogenolysis) in prolonging the thrombin time of human umbilical cord fibrinogen. *Blood* 1976;48:109–118.

46. Karpatkin M, Manucci PM, Mannuccio Manniuci P, Bhogal M, Vigano S, Nardi M. Low protein C in the neonatal period. *Br J Haematol* 1986;62:137–142.

47. Manco-Johnson MJ, Marlar R, Hathaway WE. Neonatal protein C: evidence for a dysfunctional protein and for the predisposition to thrombosis [Abstract]. *Thromb Haemost* 1985;54:838.

48. Moalic P, Gruel Y, Body G, Foloppe P, Dalahousse B, Leroy J. Levels and plasma distribution of free and c4b-BP-bound protein S in human fetuses and fullterm newborns. *Thromb Res* 1988;49:471.

49. Schwarz HP, Muntean W, Watzke H, Richter B, Griffin JH. Low total protein S antigen but high protein S activity due to decreased c4b-binding protein in neonates. *Blood* 1988;71:562.

50. Buckell M. The effect of citrate on euglobin methods of estimating fibrinolytic activity. *J Clin Pathol* 1958;11:403.

51. Weissbach G, Harenberg J, Wendisch J, Pargac N, Thomas K. Tissue factor pathway inhibitor in infants and children. *Thromb Res* 1994;73:441–446.

52. Schmidt B, Ofosu F, Mitchell L, Brooker L, Andrew M. Anticoagulant effects of heparin in neonatal plasma. *Pediatr Res* 1989;25:405–408.

53. Corrigan J. Neonatal thrombosis and the thrombolytic system. Pathophysiology and therapy. *Am J Pediatr Hematol Oncol* 1988;10:83–91.

54. Corrigan J, Sluth J, Jeter M, Lox C. Newborn's fibrinolytic mechanism: Components and plasmin generation. *Am J Hematol* 1989;32:273–278.

55. Kolindewala JK, Das BK, Dube B, Bhargava B. Blood fibrinolytic activity in neonates: effect of period of gestation, birth weight, anoxia and sepsis. *Ind Pediatrics* 1987;24:1029.

56. Lecander I, Astedt B. Specific plasminogen activator inhibitor of placental type PAI 2 occurring in amniotic fluid and cord blood. *J Lab Clin Med* 1987;110:602–605.

57. Edelberg JM, Enghild JJ, Pizzo SV, Gonzalez-Gronow M. Neonatal plasminogen displays altered cell surface binding and activation kinetics. Correlation with increased glycosylation of the protein. *J Clin Invest* 1990;86:107–112.

58. Reverdiau-Moalic P, Gruel Y, Delahousse B, et al. Comparative study of the fibrinolytic system in human fetuses and in pregnant women. *Thromb Res* 1991;61:489–499.

59. Muntean W, Zenz W, Finding K. Acquired thrombin inhibitor in a 9-year-old child after total correction of univentricular heart with pulmonary atresia and administration of fibrin glue. *Wien Klin Wochenschr* 1992;104:101–104.

60. Andrew M, Brooker L, Paes B, Weitz J. Fibrin clot lysis by thrombolytic agents is impaired in newborns due to a low plasminogen concentration. *Thromb Haemost* 1992;68:325–330.

61. Mull MM, Hathaway WE. Altered platelet function in newborns. *Pediatr Res* 1970;4:229–237.

62. Israels S, Daniels M, McMillan E. Deficient collagen-induced activation in the newborn platelet. *Pediatr Res* 1990;27:337–343.

63. Gelman B, Setty BN, Chen D, Amin-Hanjani S, Stuart MJ. Impaired mobilization of intracellular calcium in neonatal platelets. *Pediatr Res* 1996;39:692–696.

64. Sutor AH, Heidmann M, Künzer W. Die Blutungszeitbestimmung im Sauglingsalter und Kindesalter und ihre klinische Anwendung. *Med Welt (NF)* 1974;25:401–404.

65. Andrew M, Castle V, Mitchell L, Paes B. A modified bleeding time in the infant. *Am J Hematol* 1989;30:190–191.

66. Jacqz EM, Barrow SE, Dollery CT. Prostacyclin concentrations in cord blood and in the newborn. *Pediatrics* 1985;76:954–957.

67. Kumar V, Berenson G, Ruiz H, Dalferes E, Strong J. Acid mucopolysaccharides of human aorta. Part 1. Variations with maturation. *J Atheroscler Res* 1967;7:573.

68. Andrew M, Mitchell L, Paes B, et al. An anticoagulant dermatan sulphate proteoglycan circulates in the preg-

nant woman and her fetus. *J Clin Invest* 1992;89: 321–326.

69. Xu L, Delorme M, Berry L, et al. Thrombin generation in newborn and adult plasma in the presence of an endothelial surface [Abstract]. *Thromb Haemost* 1991; 65:1230.

70. Dreyfus M, Magny J, Bridey F, et al. Treatment of homozygous protein C deficiency and neonatal purpura fulminans with a purified protein C concentrate. *N Engl J Med* 1991;325:1565–1568.

71. Dreyfus M, Masterson M, David M, et al. Replacement therapy with a monoclonal antibody purified protein C concentrate in newborns with severe congenital protein C deficiency. *Semin Thromb Hemost* 1995;21:371–381.

72. Wehinger H. Therapie des genetisch bedingten protein-C-Mangels. In: Sutor AH (ed). *Thrombosen im Kindersalter.* Basel: Roche, 1992;S311–S314.

73. Mahasandana C, Suvatte V, Chuansumvita A, et al. Homozygous protein S deficiency in an infant with purpura fulminans. *J Pediatrics* 1990;117:750–753.

74. Hartman KR, Manco-Johnson M, Rawlings JS, Bower DJ, Marlar RA. Homozygous protein C deficiency: early treatment with warfarin. *Am J Pediatr Hematol Oncol* 1989;11:395–340.

75. Jochmans K, Lissens W, Vervoort R, Peeters S, De Waele M, Liebaers I. Antithrombin-Gly 424 Arg: a novel point mutation responsible for type 1 antithrombin deficiency and neonatal thrombosis. *Blood* 1994; 83:146–151.

76. Hartman R, Manco-Johnson M, Rawlings J, Bower D, Marlar R. Homozygous protein C deficiency: early treatment with Warfarin. *Am J Pediatr Hematol Oncol* 1989;11:395–401.

77. Nowak-Göttl U, Auberger K, Göbel U, et al. Inherited defects of the protein C anticoagulant system in childhood thrombo-embolism. *Eur J Pediatrics* 1996;155: 921–927.

78. Pipe SW, Schmaier A, Nichols WC, Ginsburg D, Bozynski MEA, Castle VP. Neonatal purpura fulminans in assicoation with factor V R506Q mutation. *J Pediatrics* 1996;128:706–709.

79. Auletta M, Headington J. Purpura fulminans: a cutaneous manifestation of severe protein C deficiency. *Arch Dermatol* 1988;124:1387–1391.

80. Adcock D, Brozna J, Marlar R. Proposed classification and pathologic mechanisms of purpura fulminans and skin necrosis. *Semin Thromb Haemost* 1990;16: 333–340.

81. Adcock D, Hicks M. Dermatopathology of skin necrosis associated with purpura fulminans. *Semin Thromb Haemost* 1990;16:283–292.

82. Estelles A, Garcia-Plaza I, Dasi A, et al. Severe inherited protein C deficiency in a newborn infant. *Thromb Haemost* 1984;52:53–56.

83. Marlar R, Montgomery R, Broekmans A. Report on the diagnosis and treatment of homozygous protein C deficiency. Report of the working party on homozygous protein C deficiency of the ISTH Subcommittee on protein C and protein S. *Thromb Haemost* 1989; 61:529–531.

84. Marlar R, Montgomery R, Broekmans A, and the working party. Diagnosis and treatment of homozygous protein C deficiency. *J Pediatrics* 1989;114:528–534.

85. Aschka I, Aumann V, Bergmann F, et al. Prevalence of factor V Leiden in children with thromboembolism. *Eur J Pediatrics* 1996;155:1009–1014.

86. Tabbutt S, Griswold WR, Ogino MT. Multiple thromboses in a premature infant associated with maternal phospholipid antibody syndrome. *J Perinatol* 1994;14: 66–70.

87. Sperling MA, Menon RK. Infant of the diabetic mother. *Curr Ther Endocrinol Metab* 1994;5:372–376.

88. Dahlback B, Hildebrand B. Inherited resistance to activated protein C is corrected by anticoagulant cofactor activity found to be a property of factor V. *Proc Natl Acad Sci USA* 1994;91:1396–1400.

89. Sun X, Evatt B, Griffin JH. Blood coagulation Factor Va abnormality associated with resistance to activated protein C in venous thrombophilia. *Blood* 1994;83: 3120–3125.

90. Koeleman BPC, van Rumpt D, Hamulyak K, Reitsma PH, Bertina RM. Factor V Leiden: an additional risk factor for thrombosis in protein S deficient families. *Thromb Haemstas* 1995;74:580–583.

91. Kodish E, Potter C, Kirschbaum NE, Foster PA. Activated protein C resistance in a neonate with venous thrombosis. *J Pediatrics* 1995;127:645–648.

92. Uttenreuther-Fisher MM, Ziemer S, Gaedicke G. Resistance to activated protein C (APCR): reference values of APC-ratios for children. *Thromb Haemost* 1996; 76:813–821.

93. Schander K, Niesen M, Rehm A, Budde U, Muller N. Diagnose und therapie eines kongenitalen antithrombin III Mangel in der neonatalen Periode. *Blut* 1980;40:68.

94. Soutar R, Burrows P, Marzinotto V, Doyle J, Andrew M. Overtight diaper precipitating iliac vein thrombosis in antithrombin III deficient neonate. *Arch Dis Child* 1993;69:599.

95. Shiozaki A, Arai T, Izumi R, Niiya K, Sakuragawa N. Congenital antithrombin III deficient neonate treated with antithrombin III concentrates. *Thromb Res* 1993; 70:211–216.

96. Krafte-Jacobs B, Sivit C, Majia R, Pollack M. Catheter-related thrombosis in critically ill children: comparison of catheters with and without heparin bonding. *J Pediatrics* 1995;126:50–54.

97. Rand T, Kohlhauser C, Popow C. Sonographic detection of internal jugular vein thrombosis after central venous catheterization in the newborn period. *Pediatr Radiol* 1994;24:577–580.

98. David M, Andrew M. Venous thromboembolism complications in children: a critical review of the literature. *J Pediatrics* 1993;123:337-346.

99. Sutor AH, Weissbach G, Schreiber R, Bruhn HD, Seifried E. Thrombosen im Kindesalter. *Hämostaseologie* 1992;12:82–93.

100. Guenthard J, Wyler F, Nars PW. Neonatal aortic thrombosis mimicking coarctation of the aorta. *Eur J Pediatrics* 1995;154:163–164.

101. Suri M, Ramji S, Thirupuram S, Sharma BK. Spontaneous aortic thrombosis in a neonate. *Ind Pediatrics* 1994;31:846–849.

102. Kawahira Y, Kishimoto H, Lio M. Spontaneous aortic thrombosis in a neonate with multiple thrombi in the main branches of the abdominal aorta. *Cardiovasc Surg* 1995;3:291–321.

103. Martin JE, Moran JF, Cook LS, Goertz KK, Mattioli L. Neonatal aortic thrombosis complicating umbilical artery catheterization: successful treatment with

retroperitoneal aortic thrombectomy. *Surgery* 1989; 105:793–796.

104. Uva MS, Serraf A, Lacour-Gayat F. Aortic arch thrombosis in the neonate. *Ann Thorac Surg* 1993;55: 990–992.

105. Khilnani P, Goldstein B, Todres ID. Double lumen umbilical venous catheters in critically ill neonates: a randomized prospective study. *Crit Care Med* 1991;19: 1348–1351.

106. Wigger HJ, Bransilver BR, Blanc WA. Thromboses due to catheterization in infants and children. *J Pediatrics* 1970;76:1.

107. O'Brodovich H, Coates J. Quantitative ventilation perfusion lung scans in infants and children: utility of a submicronic radiolabelled aerosol to assess ventilation. *J Pediatrics* 1984;105:377–383.

108. Rogers P, Silva M, Carter J, Wadsworth L. Renal vein thrombosis and response to therapy in a newborn due to protein C deficiency. *Eur J Pediatrics* 1989;149: 124–125.

109. Einhaupl KM, Villringer A, Meister W, et al. Heparin treatment in sinus venous thrombosis. *Lancet* 1991; 338:597–600.

110. Barron TF, Gusnard DA, Zimmerman RA, Clancy RR. Cerebral venous thrombosis in neonates and children. *Pediatr Neurol* 1992;8:112–116.

111. Govaert P, Achten E, Vanhaesebrouck P. Deep cerebral venous thrombosis in thalamo-ventricular hemorrhage of the term newborn. *Pediatr Radiol* 1992;22:123–127.

112. Klowat B, Fahnenstich H, Hansmann M, Keller E, Bartmann P. Konnatale sinusthrombose. *Monatsschr Kinderheilkd* 1996;144:609–12.

113. Lee WT, Wang PJ, Young C, Shen YZ. Cerebral venous thrombosis in children. *Acta Paediatr Scand* 1995;36: 425–430.

114. Einhaupl KM, Masuhr F. Zerebralsinus und Venenthrombosen. *Therapeutische Umshau* 1996;53:552–558.

115. deVeber G, Andrew M, Adams M, et al. Treatment of pediatric sinovenous thrombosis with low molecular weight heparin [Abstract]. *Ann Neurol* 1995;38(3):S32.

116. Schmidt B, Zipursky A. Thrombotic disease in newborn infants. *Clin Perinatol* 1984;11:461–488.

117. Schmidt B, Andrew M. Neonatal thrombotic disease: prevention, diagnosis and therapy. *J Pediatrics* 1988; 113:407–410.

118. Andrew M, Berube C, Adams M, Vegh P. The relationship between non-specific inhibitors in children with systemic lupus erythematosus and thromboembolic complications: a cross-sectional study. *J Pediatrics* 1996. Submitted.

119. Contractor S, Hiatt M, Kasmin M, Kim HC. Neonatal thrombosis with anticardiolipin antibody in baby and mother. *Am J Perinatol* 1992;9:409–410.

120. Israels SJ, Seshia SS. Childhood Stroke associated with protein C or S deficiency. *J Pediatrics* 1987;111: 562–564.

121. Kodish E, Potter C, Kirschbaum N, Foster P. Activated protein C resistance in a neonate with venous thrombosis. *J Pediatrics* 1995;127:645–648.

122. Zenz W, Muntean W, Gallistl S, Leschnik B, Beitzke A. Inherited resistance to activated protein C in a boy with multiple thromboses in early infancy. *Eur J Pediatrics* 1995;154:285–288.

123. Leititis JU. Die Behandlung von Obstruktionen und Thrombosen bei zentralvenosen Kathetern. In: Sutor AH (ed). *Thrombosen im Kindesalter.* Basel: Roche, 1992;S153–164.

124. Schmidt B, Andrew M. Report of scientific and standardization subcommittee on neonatal hemostasis diagnosis and treatment of neonatal thrombosis. *Thromb Haemost* 1992;67:381–382.

125. Burrows P, Benson L, Williams W, et al. Iliofemoral arterial complications of balloon angioplasty for systemic obstructions in infants and children. *Circulation* 1990;82:1697–1704.

126. Mortensson W, Hallbook T, Lundstrom N. Percutaneous catheterization of the femoral vessels in children. II. Thrombotic occlusion of the catheterized artery: frequency and causes. *Pediatr Radiol* 1975;4:1–9.

127. Mortensson W. Angiography of the femoral artery following percutaneous catheterization in infants and children. *Acta Radiol (Diagn)* 1976;17:581–593.

128. Freed M, Keane J, Rosenthal A. The use of heparinization to prevent arterial thrombosis after percutaneous cardiac catheterization in children. *Circulation* 1974; 50:565–569.

129. O'Neill JA, Neblett WWI, Born ML. Management of major thromboembolic complications of umbilical artery catheters. *J Pediatr Surg* 1981;16:972–978.

130. Neal WA, Reynolds JW, Jarvis CW, Williams HJ. Umbilical artery catheterization: demonstration of arterial thrombosis by aortography. *Pediatrics* 1972; 50:6–13.

131. Goetzman BW, Stadalnik RC, Bogren HG, Blankenship WJ, Ikeda RM, Thayer J. Thrombotic complications of umbilical artery catheters: a clinical and radiographic study. *Pediatrics* 1975;56:374.

132. Olinsky A, Aitken FG, Isdale JM. Thrombus formation after umbilical arterial catheterization: an angiographic study. *S Afr Med J* 1975;49:1467–1470.

133. Mokrohisky ST, Levine R, Blumhagen JB, Wesenberg RL, Simmons SA. Low positioning of umbilical artery catheters increases associated complications in newborn infants. *N Engl J Med* 1978;299:561.

134. Vailas G, Brouillette R, Scott J, Shkolnik A, Conway J, Wiringa K. Neonatal aortic thrombosis: recent experience. *J Pediatrics* 1986;109:101–108.

135. Jackson J, Truog W, Watchko J, Mack L, Cyr D, Van Belle G. Efficacy of thromboresistant umbilical artery catheters in reducing aortic thrombosis and related complications. *J Pediatrics* 1987;110:102–105.

136. David R, Merten D, Anderson J, Gross S. Prevention of umbilical artery catheter clots with heparinized infusates. *Dev Pharm Therapeut* 1981;2:117–126.

137. Bosque E, Weaver L. Continuous versus intermittent heparin infusion of umbilical artery catheters in the newborn infant. *J Pediatrics* 1986;108:141–143.

138. Horgan M, Bartoletti A, Polonsky S, Peters J, Manning T, Lamont B. Effect of heparin infusates in umbilical arterial catheters on frequency of thrombotic complications. *J Pediatrics* 1987;111:774–778.

139. Ankola P, Atakent Y. Effect of adding heparin in very low concentration to the infusate to prolong the patency of umbilical artery catheters. *Am J Perinatol* 1993;10:229–232.

140. Rajani K, Goetzman B, Wennberg R, Turner E,

Abildgaard C. Effect of heparinization of fluids infused through an umbilical artery catheter on catheter patency and frequency of complications. *Pediatrics* 1979;63:552–556.

141. Lesko S, Mitchell A, Epstein M, Louik C, Gracoia G, Shapiro S. Heparin use a risk factor for intraventricular hemorrhage in low birth weight infants. *N Engl J Med* 1986;314:1156–1160.

142. Andrew M, Schmidt B, Mitchell L, Paes B, Ofosu F. Thrombin generation in newborn plasma is critically dependent on the concentration of prothrombin. *Thromb Haemost* 1990;63:27–30.

143. Andrew M, Mitchell L, Vegh P, Ofosu F. Thrombin regulation in children differs from adults in the absence and presence of heparin. *Thromb Haemost* 1994; 72:836–842.

144. Patel P, Weitz J, Brooker L, Paes B, Andrew M. Decreased thrombin activity of fibrin clots prepared in cord plasma compared to adult plasma. *Pediatr Res* 1996;39:826–830.

145. Andrew M, Ofosu F, Schmidt B, Brooker L, Hirsh J, Buchanan M. Heparin clearance and ex vivo recovery in newborn piglets and adult pigs. *Thromb Res* 1988; 52:517–527.

146. McDonald MM, Jacobson LJ, Hay WW, Hathaway WE. Heparin clearance in the newborn. *Pediatr Res* 1981;15:1015–1018.

147. Schmidt B, Buchanan M, Ofosu F, Brooker L, Hirsh J, Andrew M. Antithrombotic properties of heparin in a neonatal piglet model of thrombin induced thrombosis. *Thromb Haemost* 1988;60:289–292.

148. Sutor AH. Blutgerinnungsstörung und Infektion in der padiatrie. In: Tilsner V, Matthias FR (eds). *Entzundung und Blutgerinnung.* Basel: Roche, 1990;135–150.

149. Murdoch I, Beattie R, Silver D. Heparin–induced thrombocytopenia in children. *Acta Paediatr* 1993;82: 495–497.

150. Spadone D, Clark F, James E, Laster J, Hoch J, Silver D. Heparin-induced thrombocytopenia in the newborn. *J Vasc Surg* 1992;15:306–311.

151. Mocan H, Beattie T, Murphy A. Renal venous thrombosis in infancy: long-term follow-up. *Pediatr Nephrol* 1991;5:45–49.

152. Hirsh J, Levine M. Low molecular weight heparin. *Blood* 1992;79:1–17.

153. Massicotte P, Adams M, Marzinotto, V, Brooker L, Andrew M. Low molecular weight heparin in pediatric patients with thrombotic disease: a dose finding study. *J Pediatrics* 1996;128:313–318.

154. Massicotte MP, Adams M, Leaker M, et al. A nomogram to establish therapeutic levels of the low molecular weight heparin (LMWH), clivarine in children requiring treatment for venous thromboembolism (VTE) [Abstract]. *Thromb Haemost* 1997:June (suppl PS–1154):282.

155. Hathaway W, Corrigan J. Report of scientific and standardization subcommittee on neonatal hemostasis. *Thromb Haemost* 1991;65:323–325.

156. Corrigan J. Normal hemostasis in fetus and newborn: coagulation. In: Polin R, Fox W (eds). *Fetal and Neonatal Physiology.* Philadelphia: Saunders, 1992; 1368–1371.

157. Hathaway WE, Bonnar J (eds). *Hemostatic Disorders of the Pregnant Woman and Newborn Infant.* New York: Elsevier, 1987.

158. Bovill E, Soll R, Lynch M, et al. Vitamin K1 metabolism and the production of des-carboxy prothrombin and protein C in the term and premature neonate. *Blood* 1993;81:77–83.

159. Sutor AH. Präanalytische Fehlerquellen bei der diagnose von Thromboembolien im Kindesalter. In: Sutor AH (ed). *Thrombosen im Kindesalter. Risikofaktoren, Diagnose, Prophylaxe, Therapie.* Basel: Roche, 1992; 217–219.

160. Sutor AH. Thrombosen im Kindesalter. Riskofaktoren, Diagnose, Therapie, Prophyaxe (zusammenfassung). In: Sutor AH (ed). *Thrombosen im Kindesalter.* Basel: Roche, 1992;471–501.

161. Litin SC, Gastineau DA. Current concepts in anticoagulant therapy. *Mayo Clin Proc* 1995;70:266–272.

162. Hathaway WE. Use of antiplatelet agents in pediatric hypercoagulable states. *Am J Dis Child* 1984;138: 301–304.

163. Leaker M, Brooker L, Mitchell L, Weitz J, Superina R, Andrew M. Fibrin clot lysis by tissue plasminogen activator (tPA) is impaired in plasma from pediatric patients undergoing orthotopic liver transplantation. *Transplantation* 1995;60:144–147.

164. Levy M, Benson LN, Burrows PE, et al. Tissue plasminogen activator for the treatment of thromboembolism in infants and children. *J Pediatrics* 1991;118: 467–472.

165. Muntean W, Beitzke A, Riccabona M, et al. Fibrinolytische therapie arterieller verschlusse mit rT-PA nach herzkatheteruntersuchung. In: Sutor AH (ed). *Thrombosen im Kindesalter.* Basel: Roche, 1992; S387–S392.

166. Ginsberg JS, Hirsh J, Rainbow AJ, Coates G. Risks to the fetus of radiologic procedures used in the diagnosis of maternal venous thromboembolic disease. *Thromb Haemost* 1989;61:189–196.

167. Astedt B. Thrombotische probleme wahrend schwangerschaft und geburt und ihre bedeutiung fur den fetus und neugeborenen. In Sutor AH (ed). *Thrombosen im Kindesalter.* Basel: Roche, 1992;173–178.

168. Ginsberg JS, Hirsh J, Turner DC. Risks to the fetus of anticoagulant therapy during pregnancy. *Thromb Haemost* 1989;61:197–203.

169. Briggs GG, Freeman RK, Sumner JY. *Drugs in Pregnancy and Lactation: A Reference Guide to Fetal and Neonatal Risk.* Baltimore: Williams and Wilkins, 1991; 40–48a, 158–163c, 292–294h.

170. Ginsberg JS, Hirsh J. Use of antithrombotic agents during pregnancy. *Chest* 1995;184(suppl 4):305S–311S.

171. Orme ME, Lewis PJ, De Swiet M. May mothers given warfarin breast-feed their infants? *Br Med J* 1977;1: 1564–1565.

172. McKenna R, Cole ER, Vasan U. Is warfarin sodium contraindicated in the lactating mother? *J Pediatrics* 1983;103:325–327.

173. Benigni A, Gregorini G, Frusca T, et al. Effect of low-dose aspirin on fetal and maternal generation of thromboxane by platelets in women at risk for pregnancy-induced hypertension. *N Engl J Med* 1989;321: 357–362.

174. Louden KA, Broughton Pipkin F, Heptinstall S, et al.

Neonatal platelet reactivity and serum thromboxane B2 production in whole blood: the effect of maternal low dose aspirin. *Br J Obstet Gynaecol* 1994;101: 203–208.

175. Chaplin S, Sanders GL, Smith JM. Drug excretion in human breastmilk. *Adv Drug React Ac Pois Rev* 1982;1:255–287.

176. Unsworth J, d'Assis-Fonseca, Beswick DT. Serum salicylate levels in a breast fed infant. *Ann Rheum* 1987;46:638–639.

177. Pfeiffer O, Dabrowski U, Dabrowski J, Stein S, Strube K, Geyer R. Carbohydrate structure of a thrombin like serine protease from agkistrodon rhodostroma. *Eur J Biochem* 1992;205:961.

178. Barnard D, Simmons M, Hathaway W. Coagulation studies in extremely premature infants. *Pediatr Res* 1979;13:1330–1335.

179. Aurousseau M, Amiral J, Boffa M. Level of plasma thrombomodulin in neonates and children [Abstract]. *Thromb Haemost* 1991;65:1232.

180. Michelson AD, Bovill E, Andrew M. Antithrombotic therapy in children. *Chest* 1995;108:506S–522S.

Cardiovascular Thrombosis: Thrombocardiology and Thromboneurology, Second Edition,
edited by M. Verstraete, V. Fuster, and E. J. Topol,
Lippincott–Raven Publishers, Philadelphia © 1998.

42

Venous and Arterial Thromboembolism in Users of Oral Contraceptives and Hormone Replacement Therapy

Kathelijne Peerlinck and *Frits R. Rosendaal

*The Center for Molecular and Vascular Biology, University of Leuven, B-3000 Leuven, Belgium; and
*Departments of Clinical Epidemiology and Haematology, Leiden University Medical Center,
2300 RC Leiden, The Netherlands*

The association between the use of oral contraceptives with an increased thromboembolic risk has first been described in the early 1960s when case reports were published on pulmonary embolism (1) and ischemic stroke (2) in women using these drugs. The magnitude of the thromboembolic risk was thought to be related to the estrogen content; however, recent reports have shown relative risks of 4 to 6 for deep vein thrombosis with recent low-estrogen-containing anti-contraceptives, which is not substantially different from older reports. Furthermore, hormonal replacement therapy, which has an extremely low estrogen content compared to anticonceptives, still increases the risk for venous thromboembolism by 2.1- to 3.6-fold. Several recent studies have shown that it is not just the estrogen component of anticonceptives that is responsible for the risk of venous thrombosis since preparations containing a third-generation progestin (desogestrel, gestodene) lead to a twofold higher risk than products containing a second-generation progestin (mostly levonorgestrel).

Studies published in the 1970s showed an increased risk of thrombotic stroke and an increased risk of acute myocardial infarction in current users of oral contraceptive agents. Recently published case-control studies no longer find an increased risk of ischemic stroke with the current use of low-dose anticonceptives (<50 μg estrogen), with the exception of hypertensive or smoking women. Current users of postmenopausal hormone substitution have a relative risk of 0.50 of coronary heart disease as compared to nonusers. The association of progestin to estrogen does not seem to attenuate the cardioprotective effects of postmenopausal estrogen therapy.

ORAL CONTRACEPTIVES AND RISK OF VENOUS THROMBOEMBOLISM

The association of the use of oral contraceptives and an increased risk of venous thromboembolic disease has been well established in a series of epidemiologic studies (3–5). Several studies have suggested a dose-response relation between the estrogen component of oral contraceptives and the magnitude of the thrombotic risk (6–8), which extends from 50 to 30 µg of estrogen (9). In the latter study the relative risk of venous thromboembolism in users of oral contraceptives containing >50 µg of estrogen as compared to those taking <50 µg of estrogen was 1.7. In the WHO Collaborative Study of Cardiovascular Disease and Steroid Hormone Contraception (10), the odds ratios for venous thromboembolic disease tended to be lower when first- and second-generation progestagens were used in combination with low (<50 µg estrogen) rather than higher estrogen doses; in the Leiden thrombophilia study (11) the risk conferred by oral contraceptives containing 30 or 50 µg ethinylestradiol was the same. The risk reduction that has occurred by lowering the estrogen content of oral contraceptives, if any, has certainly not been a dramatic one. The early case-control studies in the 1960s reported relative risks for idiopathic deep vein thrombosis ranging from 4 to 8 (12–14), whereas in the most recent studies oral contraceptives still are found to be associated with a four- to sixfold increased risk (10,15,16). No other lifestyle or environmental risk factor influenced in a consistent way the risk for venous thromboembolism with the exception of body mass index, which was a weak independent risk factor; the odds ratios associated with venous thromboembolism were higher among those with a body mass index (BMI) above 25 kg/m^2 than among those with smaller BMIs (10).

Several studies published in 1995–1996 came with an unexpected result: The risk for venous thromboembolism is not only influenced by estrogen content but also by type of progestagen used. So-called third-generation oral contraceptives, containing desogestrel or gestodene as a progestagen, were associated with a twofold higher risk for venous thromboembolism than those containing a second-generation progestagen such as levonorgestrel. The published studies were a subanalysis of women exposed to third-generation oral contraceptive pills of the WHO Collaborative Study of Cardiovascular Disease and Steroid Hormone Contraception (17); a case-control study of current users of the oral contraceptive pill from the British general practice research database (18); a reanalysis of the Leiden thrombophilia study (11); and a multinational case-control study (15). All studies indicated a doubling of the adjusted odds ratio for venous thromboembolism in patients taking third- rather than second- generation oral contraceptive pills.

Venous thromboembolism is quite rare in the age group of women taking oral contraceptives. Most recent studies report incidences of around 1 per 10 000 women years; this figure increases to 4 per 10,000 women years in women using second-generation contraceptives and around 6 to 10 per 10,000 with the use of third-generation contraceptives.

Low-dose oral contraceptives containing third-generation progestagens seem to be less androgenic and have less impact on carbohydrate and lipoprotein metabolism than other low-dose preparations (19); recent reviews have concluded that these third-generation preparations do not differ from earlier low-dose contraceptives in their impact on hemostatic variables. The changes in hemostatic parameters, at least for those that can be measured, in women using oral contraceptives are minor and generally remain within the normal range. Furthermore, it has been suggested that the use of oral contraceptives induces changes in the procoagulant and anticoagulant pathways that may counterbalance each other (19–21). Recently it was shown, using a method measuring endogenous thrombin potential of plasma, that the sensitivity to activated protein C (APC) was decreased in women using oral contraceptives, independent of the kind of contraceptive used. Women who used third-generation oral contraceptives were less sensitive to APC than women using second-generation oral contraceptives and became comparable to female carriers of the factor V Leiden mutation which causes inherited APC resistance and is the most common cause of inherited thrombophilia (22). Joining their data on impaired APC sensitivity with epidemiologic data, these authors suggest that the increased incidence of venous thrombosis in women using oral contraceptives, especially in those using third-generation contraceptives, might be explained by acquired APC resistance. The exact molecular mechanism behind the thrombogenic potential of oral contraceptives remains to be elucidated (23).

The increased risk of venous thromboembolism appears to be related to current use of anticonceptives. In the WHO study (10) the increased odds ratios were fully realized within 4 months of starting oral contraceptives and had resolved within 3 months of stopping. These findings are in keeping with previous publications (4,24,25) and suggest that disturbance of coagulation balances induced by the anticonceptive are involved.

RISK OF VENOUS THROMBOSIS WITH POSTMENOPAUSAL HORMONE REPLACEMENT THERAPY

Until recently the risk of venous thromboembolism associated with postmenopausal hormone replacement therapy was thought to be probably nonexistent or at most very small; however, few epidemiologic studies had assessed the relation between postmenopausal hormones and thrombotic disease and most of them were too small to provide reliable estimates (26–28). The risk of venous thromboembolism associated with oral anticonceptives is to a large extent attributable to its estrogen content and the hemostatic alterations induced by postmenopausal replacement therapy on hemostatic parameters have been shown to be similar though less pro-

nounced than with oral contraceptives; the paradoxical absence of increased venous thromboembolic risk was explained by the significantly lower estrogen content of postmenopausal hormones and different type of estrogen used. The results of three large studies studying the effect of postmenopausal hormone replacement therapy on venous thromboembolism (29,30) or pulmonary embolism (31) resolved the apparent paradox. In each of these studies a twofold to fourfold increased risk of venous thromboembolism was shown with estrogen-only as well as with combined estrogen-progestagen hormone replacement therapy. The risk seems to be higher shortly after the start of therapy (29,30). In these studies, women suffering from thromboembolic disease who had other risk factors for thrombosis, such as recent trauma or surgery, previous thromboembolism, cardiac disease, diabetes, or cancer, were excluded. Further research will be needed to establish the safety of postmenopausal hormone therapy when other risk factors for venous thromboembolism, including obesity, recent surgery, immobilization, or thrombophilic conditions, are present.

RISK OF VENOUS THROMBOEMBOLISM IN WOMEN WITH INHERITED THROMBOPHILIA TAKING EXOGENOUS HORMONES

Hereditary defects in the natural anticoagulant pathways, the antithrombin pathway (including antithrombin deficiency), and the protein C pathway (including deficiencies of protein C and protein S and resistance to activated protein C) predispose patients to the development of venous thromboembolism. Data on the thrombotic risk of women with antithrombin (AT), protein C (PC), and protein S (PS) deficiencies taking oral contraceptives are anecdotal due to the low prevalence of these defects. In a retrospective study of 96 women with proven deficiencies of either AT, PC, or PS, Pabinger et al. (32) found that the probability for thrombosis was significantly higher in AT deficient patients taking oral contraceptives as compared to AT deficient patients not taking contraceptives. In patients with protein C or protein S deficiency there was no clear difference between users or non-users of oral contraceptives. Due to the higher prevalence of resistance to activated protein C, generally explained by the factor V Leiden mutation, more data are available concerning the risk of venous thrombosis associated with the use of oral contraceptives in this group. Data from the Leiden Thrombophilia Study (16) showed a fourfold increased risk for thrombosis among users of oral contraceptives, an eightfold increased risk of thrombosis among carriers of the factor V Leiden mutation compared with noncarriers, and a >30-fold increased risk for women who both were carriers of the mutation and used oral contraceptives. In this study the incidence of first venous thrombosis in women aged 15 to 49 years not using oral contraceptives was 0.8 per 10,000 person-years in noncarriers of factor V Leiden and 5.7 per 10,000 person-years in carriers of the mutation; in users of contraceptives the incidences rose to 3.0 per 10,000 person-years and 28.5 per 10,000 person-years, respectively. The absolute increase in thrombosis risk due to oral contraceptives is much larger in women who carry the factor V Leiden mutation than in women who do not. In a study of 29 patients homozygous for the factor V Leiden mutation oral contraceptives were found to enhance the risk of clinical manifestation of venous thrombosis at a young age (33). The factor V Leiden mutation was also shown to enhance the risk of deep vein thrombosis associated with oral contraceptives containing a third-generation progestagen (11). The risk of factor V Leiden carriers using a desogestrel containing anticonceptive is almost 50-fold increased as compared with noncarrier nonusers.

Although an enhancement of the risk of venous thromboembolism associated with the use of postmenopausal hormone replacement therapy by these hereditary thrombophilic conditions might be anticipated no data on this subject are currently available.

ORAL CONTRACEPTIVES AND RISK OF STROKE AND MYOCARDIAL INFARCTION

The issue of an increased risk of stroke associated with the use of oral contraceptives has been addressed in several, mostly retrospective studies (34,35). Relative risks among users of contraceptives in these studies were found between 3.7 and 4.8. Since most of these studies were conducted during a period when pills with a high estrogen and progestagen content were widely used, several recent studies were undertaken to address the question of whether recent contraceptives with low hormone contents still carry an increased risk of stroke. In a Danish retrospective case-control study of women aged 15 to 44 years who had suffered a thromboembolic attack without known predisposing factor, a crude odds ratio of 3 was found (36). After correcting for confounders such as age, smoking, and years of schooling, pills containing 50 μg estrogen were associated with an odds ratio for cerebral thromboembolic attack of 2.9 and those containing 30 to 40 μg estrogen with an odds ratio of 1.8. Progesterone-only pills did not increase the risk of a cerebral thromboembolic attack. Cigarette smoking increased the risk of cerebral thromboembolic attacks by 50% independent of oral contraceptive use or age. In the report of the WHO Collaborative Study of Cardiovascular Disease and Steroid Hormone Contraception (37) the overall odds ratio of ischemic stroke in women aged 20 to 44 taking combined oral contraceptives was 2.99 in Europe and 2.93 in non-European countries. Odds ratios associated with contraceptives containing <50 μg of estrogen were 1.53 and substantially higher (5.30) for preparations containing >50 μg of estrogen. In this study odds ratios were lower in younger women and those who did not smoke, but among current users of oral contraceptives with a history of hypertension the odds ratio was 10.7.

The same study group (38) reported no increased risk of hemorrhagic stroke associated with contraceptives in women younger than

35 years. Odds ratios were >2 for women older than 35 years and >3 for those who also smoked cigarettes. Current users of oral contraceptives with a history of hypertension (with the exception of pregnancy-related hypertension) had a 10- to 15-fold increased risk of hemorrhagic stroke as compared with nonusers without history of hypertension.

Another recent study of the risk of stroke in users of low-dose oral contraceptives (containing <50 μg of estrogen) did not show an increased risk for ischemic stroke or for hemorrhagic stroke (39). A positive interaction between the current use of oral contraceptives and smoking was found with respect to the risk of hemorrhagic stroke. Considering the width of their confidence interval and the results of the Danish study (36), Pettiti and colleagues conclude that the true relative risk of stroke among users of oral contraceptives, as compared with nonusers, is <2.5. Since the absolute incidence of ischemic stroke in young healthy women is small (5.4/100,000 women-years according to Pettiti), the absolute increase in incidence of stroke in current users of oral contraceptives will also be small.

Shortly after their introduction oral contraceptives were associated with acute myocardial infarction in a case report (40). This association was thereafter confirmed in several case-control and cohort studies (41–44). More recent studies conducted in the 1990s and dealing mainly with newer contraceptives, which have low estrogen content and are used by younger women who do not have other risk factors for cardiovascular disease, could no longer demonstrate increases in risk of acute myocardial infarction associated with oral contraceptives (45–47). In the WHO Collaborative Study of Cardiovascular Disease and Steroid Hormone Contraception, 368 women aged 20 to 44 with a definite or possible acute myocardial infarction who were admitted to hospital were studied (48). Women from Africa, Asia, Europe, and Latin America were included. The overall odds ratio for acute myocardial infarction was 5.0 in Europe and 4.8 in the developing countries. However,

odds ratios associated with the use of oral contraceptives were not increased in women without other cardiovascular risk factors such as smoking or hypertension. The estimated excess risk in such women in the European centers was about 3 per 106. Among oral contraceptive users who smoke 10 or more cigarettes per day, the odds ratios were >20 and the degree of excess risk associated with oral contraceptives is substantial only in older women who smoke (about 400 per 106 women-years). Whereas a risk reduction for cardiovascular events associated with third-generation as compared with second-generation progestagens has been anticipated based on less androgenic activity with an advantageous effect on lipid profile and possibly carbohydrate mechanism (49), it has yet to be clarified as to whether the risk of arterial diseases during treatment with the newer formulations differs from that of the older preparations (50). Two studies have failed to show a difference in the risk of ischemic stroke for users of third-generation contraceptives compared to second-generation contraceptives (37,51). Initial results of an international case-control study suggest a reduced risk of myocardial infarction associated with third-generation oral contraceptives as compared with second-generation preparations, but are based on a small number of cases (n = 6) and controls (n = 34) (odds ratio of 0.45 with wide confidence intervals) (52). This study confirms that the greatest risk for health comes from smoking while taking the pill, rather than from the type of pill being used; young women smokers who use the pill are 10 times more likely to suffer myocardial infarction than users who don't smoke (53).

While consistent reports show an increased risk of venous thrombotic disease with third-generation oral contraceptives, it is not yet clear if and how they differ from second-generation contraceptives in their risk on myocardial infarction. If the latter will prove to be the case, decision analysis models will have to be set up that take into account the differences in age-dependent baseline risks for venous and arterial thrombotic disease. Such model may lead to preferential use of second-generation contraceptives in younger women and third-generation contraceptives in older women (54).

As for the risk of venous thromboembolism, the increased risk for myocardial infarction is associated with current use of anticonceptives. No increase in odds ratio was apparent with increasing duration of use among current users, and odds ratios were not increased in women who had stopped using oral contraceptives, even after long exposure (48). This again suggests that the effects are due to disturbances in coagulation rather than to, for instance, an atherogenic effect.

POSTMENOPAUSAL HORMONE REPLACEMENT THERAPY AND CARDIOVASCULAR RISK REDUCTION

In a meta-analysis of many observational studies (55) an overall risk reduction of approximately 36% was found when estrogen users were compared with those who had never used estrogen. Furthermore, the data suggest that most of this apparent protection is among the current hormone users who had a relative risk of 0.49. An even greater benefit was found in women with coronary heart disease: A summary relative risk from angiographic studies comparing women with occlusion to those without was 0.39. In several studies a reduction of all-cause mortality was documented (56,57). In a recent study of mortality associated with long-term postmenopausal hormone therapy (58), the age-adjusted relative risk of death from any cause was 0.54 in estrogen users and was largely due to reductions in coronary heart disease. However, currently much debate is ongoing whether the protective effect seen in these studies may be due, at least in part, to selection bias. Different authors observed that women who use estrogen replacement therapy are healthier and have a better cardiovascular risk profile prior to estrogen replacement therapy than women who do not take hormones (59–61). However, adjustment for known cardiac risk factors in many of the large studies did not have a major impact on the results (56,57,62).

The proposed mechanisms of cardiovascular protection are a reduction of low-density lipoprotein, an increase of high-density lipoprotein, and an increase of triglycerides that results in an overall improvement of the lipid profile (63). Estrogen replacement therapy has been found to reduce lipoprotein(a) levels toward premenopausal values (64) and to impede the oxidation of low-density lipoprotein (LDL) cholesterol (65). The effects of estrogen replacement therapy on the coagulation system are inconsistent: it lowers fibrinogen and plasminogen activator inhibitor but it also lowers antithrombin and protein C, which have an anticoagulant function (66). Estrogen replacement therapy also favorably influences endothelium function and vascular tone (67,68).

Currently, to avoid abnormal endometrial proliferation and endometrial cancer, a progestin is associated with the estrogen. However, progestins tend to raise LDL and lower HDL levels (69) and to oppose the effects of estrogen on vascular tone (70). In three recent studies an almost identical reduction in cardiovascular risk was found when women receiving estrogens plus progestin were compared with women receiving estrogen only (71–73). In addition, the decrease of plasminogen activator inhibitor I induced by estrogen or estrogen combined with medroxyprogesterone acetate was not different in a recent randomized crossover study (74).

CONCLUSION

Currently used combined oral anticonceptives with low estrogen content still hold an increased risk of venous thromboembolism. The risk of thromboembolism is not confined to the estrogen component but is also dependent on the type of progesterone.

Postmenopausal hormone replacement therapy carries a two- to fourfold risk of venous thromboembolism.

Inherited thrombophilia and oral contraceptives have a synergistic effect on the risk of venous thromboembolism.

The risk of stroke and myocardial infarction associated with the use of oral contraceptives is very small in young women without other cardiovascular risk factors. When other risk factors such as smoking or hypertension are present, the risk increases substantially.

Postmenopausal hormone replacement therapy reduces cardiovascular risk regardless whether estrogen only or combined estrogen-progestin treatment are used. However the magnitude of this reduction still is matter of debate; many authors argue that selection towards healthier women with less preexisting cardiovascular risk factors for treatment with estrogen replacement may bias the results.

REFERENCES

1. Jordan WM. Pulmonary embolism. *Lancet* 1961;2: 1146–1147.
2. Lorentz IT. Parietal lesion and "Enovid." *Br Med J* 1962;2:1191.
3. Stadel BV. Oral contraceptives and cardiovascular disease (first of two parts). *N Engl J Med* 1981;305:612–618.
4. Vessey MP. Female hormones and vascular disease—an epidemiological overview. *Br J Fam Plann* 1980 (suppl):1–12.
5. Sartwell PE, Stolley PD. Oral contraceptives and vascular disease. *Epidemiol Rev* 1982;4:95–109.
6. Inman WH, Vessey MP, Westerholm B, Engelund A. Thromboembolic disease and the steroidal content of oral contraceptives. A report to the Committee on Safety of Drugs. *Br Med J* 1970;2:203–209.
7. Stolley PD, Tonascia JA, Tockman MS, Sartwell PE, Rutledge AH, Jacobs MP. Thrombosis with low-estrogen oral contraceptives. *Am J Epidemiol* 1975;102:197–208.
8. Bottinger LE, Bowan G, Eklund G. Oral contraceptives and thromboembolic disease: effects of lowering oestrogen content. *Lancet* 1980;1:1097–1101.
9. Gerstman BB, Piper JM, Tomita DK, Ferguson WJ, Stadel BV, Lundin FE. Oral contraceptive estrogen dose and the risk of deep venous thromboembolic disease. *Am J Epidemiol* 1991;133:32–37.
10. Venous thromboembolic disease and combined oral contraceptives. Results of international multicentre case-control study. World Health Organization Collaborative Study of Cardiovascular Disease and Steroid Hormone Contraception. *Lancet* 1995;346:1575–1582.
11. Bloemenkamp KW, Rosendaal FR, Helmerhorst FM, Buller HR, Vandenbroucke JP. Enhancement by factor V Leiden mutation of risk of deep-vein thrombosis associated with oral contraceptives containing a third-generation progestagen. *Lancet* 1995;346:1593–1596.
12. Inman WH, Vessey MP. Investigation of deaths from pulmonary, coronary, and cerebral thrombosis and embolism in women of child-bearing age. *Br Med J* 1968; 2:193–199.
13. Vessey MP, Doll R. Investigation of relation between use of oral contraceptives and thromboembolic disease. *Br Med J* 1968;2:199–205.
14. Sartwell PE, Masi AT, Arthes FG, Greene GR, Smith HE. Thromboembolism and oral contraceptives: an epidemiologic case-control study. *Am J Epidemiol* 1969; 90:365–380.
15. Spitzer WO, Lewis MA, Heinemann LA, Thorogood M, MacRae KD. Third generation oral contraceptives and risk of venous thromboembolic disorders: an international case-control study. Transnational Research Group on Oral Contraceptives and the Health of Young Women. *Br Med J* 1996;312:83–88.
16. Vandenbroucke JP, Koster T, Briët E, Reitsma PH, Bertina RM, Rosendaal FR. Increased risk of venous thrombosis in oral-contraceptive users who are carriers of factor V Leiden mutation. *Lancet* 1994;344:1453–1457.
17. Effect of different progestagens in low oestrogen oral contraceptives on venous thromboembolic disease. World Health Organization Collaborative Study of Cardiovascular Disease and Steroid Hormone Contraception. *Lancet* 1995;346:1582–1588.
18. Jick H, Jick SS, Gurewich V, Myers MW, Vasilakis C. Risk of idiopathic cardiovascular death and nonfatal venous thromboembolism in women using oral contraceptives with differing progestagen components. *Lancet* 1995;346:1589–1593.
19. Speroff L, DeCherney A. Evaluation of a new generation of oral contraceptives. The Advisory Board for the New Progestins. *Obstet Gynecol* 1993;81:1034–1047.
20. Stubblefield PG. The effects on hemostasis of oral contraceptives containing desogestrel. *Am J Obstet Gynecol* 1993;168:1047–1052.
21. Newton JR. Classification and comparison of oral contraceptives containing new generation progestogens. *Hum Reprod Update* 1995:1:231–263.
22. Rosing J, Tans G, Nicolae GAF, et al. Oral contraceptives and venous thrombosis: different sensitivities to activated protein C in women using second- and third-generation oral contraceptives. *Br J Haematol* 1997;97: 233–238.
23. Vandenbroucke JP, Rosendaal FR. End of the line for "third-generation-pill" controversy? *Lancet* 1997;349: 1113–1114.
24. Helmrich SP, Rosenberg L, Kaufman DW, Strom B, Shapiro S. Venous thromboembolism in relation to oral contraceptive use. *Obstet Gynecol* 1987;69:91–95.
25. Stadel BV. Oral contraceptives and cardiovascular disease (second of two parts). *N Engl J Med* 1981;305: 672–677.
26. Surgically confirmed gallbladder disease, venous thromboembolism, and breast tumors in relation to postmenopausal estrogen therapy. A report from the Boston Collaborative Drug Surveillance Program, Boston University Medical Center. *N Engl J Med* 1974; 290:15–19.
27. Pettiti DB, Wingerd J, Pellegrin F, Ramcharan S. Risk of vascular disease in women: smoking, oral contraceptives, noncontraceptive estrogens, and other factors. *JAMA* 1979;242:1150–1154.
28. Devor M, Barrett Connor E, Renvall M, Feigal D Jr,

Ramsdell J. Estrogen replacement therapy and the risk of venous thrombosis. *Am J Med* 1992;92:275–282.

29. Daly E, Vessey MP, Hawkins MM, Carson JL, Gough P, Marsh S. Risk of venous thromboembolism in users of hormone replacement therapy. *Lancet* 1996;348: 977–980.

30. Jick H, Derby LE, Myers MW, Vasilakis C, Newton KM. Risk of hospital admission for idiopathic venous thromboembolism among users of postmenopausal oestrogens. *Lancet* 1996;348:981–983.

31. Grodstein F, Stampfer MJ, Goldhaber SZ, et al. Prospective study of exogenous hormones and risk of pulmonary embolism in women. *Lancet* 1996;348: 983–987.

32. Pabinger I, Schneider B. Thrombotic risk of women with hereditary antithrombin III-, protein C- and protein S-deficiency taking oral contraceptive medication. The GTH Study Group on Natural Inhibitors. *Thromb Haemost* 1994;71:548–552.

33. Rintelen C, Mannhalter C, Ireland H, et al. Oral contraceptives enhance the risk of clinical manifestation of venous thrombosis at a young age in females homozygous for factor V Leiden. *Br J Haematol* 1996;93:487–490.

34. Thorogood M, Mann J, Murphy M, Vessey M. Fatal stroke and use of oral contraceptives: findings from a case-control study. *Am J Epidemiol* 1992:136:35–45.

35. Mettinger KL, Soderstrom CE, Neiman J. Stroke before 55 years of age at Karolinska Hospital 1973-77. A study of 399 well-defined cases. Risk indicators and etiological considerations. *Acta Neurol Scand* 1984;70: 415–422.

36. Lidegaard O. Oral contraception and risk of a cerebral thromboembolic attack: results of a case-control study. *Br Med J* 1993;306:956–963.

37. Ischaemic stroke and combined oral contraceptives: results of an international, multicentre, case-control study. WHO Collaborative, Study of Cardiovascular Disease and Steroid Hormone Contraception. *Lancet* 1996; 348:498–505.

38. WHO Collaborative Study of Cardiovascular Disease and Steroid Hormone Contraception. Haemorrhagic stroke, overall stroke risk, and combined oral contraceptives: results of an international, multicentre, case-control study. *Lancet* 1996;348:505–510.

39. Petitti DB, Sidney S, Bernstein A, Wolf S, Quesenberry C, Ziel HK. Stroke in users of low-dose oral contraceptives. *N Engl J Med* 1996;335:8–15.

40. Boyce J, Fawcett JW, Nall EWP. Coronary thrombosis and Conovid. *Lancet* 1963;1:111.

41. Mann JI, Thorogood M, Waters WE, Powell C. Oral contraceptives and myocardial infarction in young women: a further report. *Br Med J* 1975;3:631–632.

42. Jick H, Dinan B, Rothman KJ. Oral contraceptives and nonfatal myocardial infarction. *JAMA* 1978;239: 1403–1406.

43. Shapiro S, Slone D, Rosenberg L, Kaufman DW, Stolley PD, Miettinen OS. Oral-contraceptive use in relation to myocardial infarction. *Lancet* 1979:1:743–747.

44. Slone D, Shapiro S, Kaufman DW, Rosenberg L, Miettinen OS, Stolley PD. Risk of myocardial infarction in relation to current and discontinued use of oral contraceptives. *N Engl J Med* 1981;305:420–424.

45. Thorogood M, Mann J, Murphy M, Vessey M. Is oral contraceptive use still associated with an increased risk of fatal myocardial infarction? Report of a case-control study. *Br J Obstet Gynaecol* 1991;98:1245–1253.

46. Rosenberg L, Palmer JR, Lesko SM, Shapiro S. Oral contraceptive use and the risk of myocardial infarction. *Am J Epidemiol* 1990:131:1009–1016.

47. Sidney S, Petitti DB, Quesenberry CP Jr, Klatsky AL, Ziel HK, Wolf S. Myocardial infarction in users of low–dose oral contraceptives. *Obstet Gynecol* 1996;88: 939-944.

48. Acute myocardial infarction and combined oral contraceptives: results of an international multicentre case-control study. WHO Collaborative Study of Cardiovascular Disease and Steroid Hormone Contraception. *Lancet* 1997;349:1202–1209.

49. Wilde MI, Balfour JA. Gestodene. A review of its pharmacology, efficacy and tolerability in combined contraceptive preparations. *Drugs* 1995;50:364–395.

50. Kuhl H. Comparative pharmacology of newer progestogens. *Drugs* 1996;51:188–215.

51. Lidegaard O, Milsom I. Oral contraceptives and thrombotic diseases: impact of new epidemiological studies. *Contraception* 1996;53:135–139.

52. Lewis MA, Spitzer WO, Heinemann LA, MacRae KD, Bruppacher R, Thorogood M. Third generation oral contraceptives and risk of myocardial infarction: an international case-control study. Transnational Research Group on Oral Contraceptives and the Health of Young Women. *Br Med J* 1996;312:88–90.

53. McPherson K. Third generation oral contraception and venous thromboembolism. *Br Med J* 1996;312:68–69.

54. Schwringl PJ, Shelton J. Modeled estimates of myocardial infarction and venous thromboembolic disease in users of second and third generation oral contraceptives. *Contraception* 1997;55:125–129.

55. Grodstein F, Stampfer M. The epidemiology of coronary heart disease and estrogen replacement in postmenopausal women. *Prog Cardiovasc Dis* 1995;38: 199–210.

56. Bush TL, Barrett Connor E, Cowan LD, et al. Cardiovascular mortality and noncontraceptive use of estrogen in women: results from the Lipid Research Clinics Program Follow-up Study. *Circulation* 1987;75:1102–1109.

57. Henderson BE, Paganini Hill A, Ross RK. Decreased mortality in users of estrogen replacement therapy. *Arch Intern Med* 1991:151:75–78.

58. Ettinger B, Friedman GD, Bush T, Quesenberry CP Jr. Reduced mortality associated with long-term postmenopausal estrogen therapy. *Obstet Gynecol* 1996;87: 6–12.

59. Posthuma WF, Westendorp RG, Vandenbroucke JP. Cardioprotective effect of hormone replacement therapy in postmenopausal women: is the evidence biased? *Br Med J* 1994;308:1268–1269.

60. Sturgeon SR, Schairer C, Brinton LA, Pearson T, Hoover RN. Evidence of a healthy estrogen user survivor effect. *Epidemiology* 1995;6:227–231.

61. Matthews KA, Kuller LH, Wing RR, Meilahn EN, Plantinga P. Prior to use of estrogen replacement therapy, are users healthier than nonusers? *Am J Epidemiol* 1996:143:971–978.

62. Stampfer MJ, Colditz GA, Willett WC, et al. Postmenopausal estrogen therapy and cardiovascular disease. Ten-year follow-up from the nurses' health study. *N Engl J Med* 1991;325:756–762.

63. Walsh BW, Schiff I, Rosner B, Greenberg L, Ravnikar V, Sacks FM. Effects of postmenopausal estrogen replacement on the concentrations and metabolism of plasma lipoproteins. *N Engl J Med* 1991;325:1196–1204.

64. Sacks FM, McPherson R, Walsh BW. Effect of post-menopausal estrogen replacement on plasma Lp(a) lipoprotein concentrations. *Arch Intern Med* 1994:154: 1106–1110.

65. Sacks MN, Rader DJ, Cannon RO. Oestrogen and inhibition of oxidation of low-density lipoproteins in postmenopausal women. *Lancet* 1994;343:269–270.

66. Nabulsi AA, Folsom AR, White A, et al. Association of hormone-replacement therapy with various cardiovascular risk factors in postmenopausal women. The Atherosclerosis Risk in Communities Study Investigators. *N Engl J Med* 1993;328:1069–1075.

67. Herrington DM, Braden GA, Williams JK, Morgan TM. Endothelial-dependent coronary vasomotor responsiveness in postmenopausal women with and without estrogen replacement therapy. *Am J Cardiol* 1994;73: 951–952.

68. Reis SE, Gloth ST, Blumenthal RS, et al. Ethinyl estradiol acutely attenuates abnormal coronary vasomotor responses to acetylcholine in postmenopausal women. *Circulation* 1994;89:52–60.

69. Miller VT, Muesing RA, LaRosa JC, Stoy DB, Phillips EA, Stillman RJ. Effects of conjugated equine estrogen with and without three different progestogens on lipoproteins, high-density lipoprotein subfractions, and apolipoprotein A-I. *Obstet Gynecol* 1991;77:235–240.

70. Sarrel PM. *Blood Flow: Treatment of the Post-menopausal Woman—Basic and Clinical Aspects.* New York: Raven Press, 1994;251–252.

71. Falkeborn M, Persson I, Adami HO, et al. The risk of acute myocardial infarction after oestrogen and oestrogen-progestogen replacement. *Br J Obstet Gynaecol* 1992;99:821–828.

72. Psaty BM, Heckbert SR, Atkins D, et al. The risk of myocardial infarction associated with the combined use of estrogens and progestins in postmenopausal women. *Arch Intern Med* 1994:154:1333–1339.

73. Grodstein F, Stampfer MJ, Manson JE, et al. Postmenopausal estrogen and progestin use and the risk of cardiovascular disease. *N Engl J Med* 1996;335: 453–461.

74. Kon Koh K, Mincemoyer R, Bui MN, et al. Effects of hormone-replacement therapy on fibrinolysis in postmenopausal women. *N Engl J Med* 1997;336:683–690.

Cardiovascular Thrombosis: Thrombocardiology and Thromboneurology, Second Edition,
edited by M. Verstraete, V. Fuster, and E. J. Topol,
Lippincott–Raven Publishers, Philadelphia © 1998.

43

Anticoagulants During Pregnancy

Jeffrey S. Ginsberg and Jack Hirsh

Department of Medicine, McMaster University, Hamilton, Ontario L8N 3Z5, Canada

Antithrombotic therapy during pregnancy is used for the treatment and prophylaxis of venous thromboembolic disease, for the prevention and treatment of systemic arterial embolism associated with valvular heart disease and/or prosthetic heart valves, and for the prevention of fetal growth retardation and pregnancy loss in patients with antiphospholipid antibodies as well as patients with pregnancy-induced hypertension. Because antithrombotic agents can produce complications in both the mother and fetus, their use during pregnancy raises concerns. It is difficult to establish definitive guidelines because the evidence on which recommendations can be based is derived primarily from retrospective studies in pregnant patients. In this chapter, we review the fetal and maternal effects of antithrombotic agents including oral anticoagu-

lants, unfractionated heparin, low molecular weight heparins (LMWHs), and aspirin, and provide recommendations for their use during pregnancy.

EPIDEMIOLOGY OF VENOUS THROMBOEMBOLISM

Pregnancy and the postpartum state are considered to be high-risk situations for venous thromboembolism (VTE), but the absolute risks are probably small. There are two recent observations that have the potential to affect the management of pregnant women with venous thrombosis: (a) In the absence of a clinical or laboratory risk factor, patients who present with idiopathic deep vein thrombosis (DVT) have a much higher recurrence rate than patients who develop DVT in association with a transient risk factor (1–3), and (b) there is hereditary resistance to activated protein C that predisposes affected individuals to VTE (4,5).

Randomized trials and a cohort study have shown that patients who develop "secondary" DVT in the presence of a transient risk factor, such as major orthopedic or abdominal surgery, have a much lower incidence of recurrent VTE than patients who develop idiopathic DVT or DVT in association with an ongoing risk factor (e.g., patients with metastatic cancer) (1–3). This has an impact on the prognosis of DVT and has the potential to influence the risk of recurrent venous thrombosis in pregnant women with previous VTE. Although accurate estimates of the true incidence of recurrent VTE are not available in such women, it is reasonable to assume that women whose original DVT occurred secondary to a transient risk factor have a lower overall risk of recurrent VTE in association with pregnancy than women whose original DVT was idiopathic or associated with an ongoing risk factor. Consequently, it seems reasonable to follow low-risk women by surveillance and to use active prophylaxis in high-risk women.

Activated protein C resistance is caused by a mutation in the factor V gene that alters a binding site of factor V for activated protein C, factor V Leiden (5). The abnormality can be detected using an activated partial thromboplastin time (APTT)–based assay or by identification of the specific genetic mutation (5). Activated protein C resistance has been reported to occur in approximately 5% of the "normal" population and in 20% to 40% of unselected patients with DVT (5), and therefore might be the most common hereditary cause of VTE. To date, there are few published studies on the incidence of activated protein C resistance in pregnant women with previous VTE, but until further information becomes available women with activated protein C resistance (both with and without a history of previous VTE) should be considered to have an increased risk for VTE.

It is likely that women with congenital deficiencies of antithrombin III, protein C, or protein S, or the persistent presence of antiphospholipid antibodies have an increased risk of VTE during pregnancy and the puerperium (6–8). Women with previous VTE might also have an increased risk of recurrent VTE during pregnancy and the puerperium, but the results are conflicting (9–12). Retrospective studies have reported the incidence of recurrent VTE to be as high as 15% during pregnancy in women with previous DVT (12,13). In contrast, the results of one randomized trial reported that 1 of 20 untreated patients (5%) with previous VTE developed recurrent antepartum VTE (10) and a cohort study (published in letter form) reported that none of 59 pregnant patients with previous VTE developed antepartum recurrence (9). Conclusions from these studies are limited by the relatively small numbers and lack of description of the inception cohorts. Clinical trials are required to establish the true incidence of recurrent VTE in pregnant women as well as the safety and efficacy of anticoagulant therapy in preventing recurrent VTE.

ANTICOAGULANT THERAPY DURING PREGNANCY

The agents currently available for the prevention and treatment of VTE include heparin and heparin-like compounds (unfractionated heparin, LMWH, and heparinoids) and coumarin derivatives.

Fetal Complications of Anticoagulant Therapy During Pregnancy

There are two potential fetal complications of maternal anticoagulant therapy: teratogenicity and bleeding. Heparin does not cross the placenta and therefore cannot cause fetal bleeding or teratogenicity, although bleeding at the uteroplacental junction is possible (13). Two recent studies strongly suggest that heparin therapy is safe for the fetus (14,15).

In contrast to heparin, coumarin derivatives cross the placenta and can cause both bleeding in the fetus and teratogenicity (16,17). Coumarin derivatives can cause an embryopathy, consisting of nasal hypoplasia and/or stippled epiphyses after in utero exposure to oral anticoagulants during the first trimester of pregnancy (Fig. 43-1), and central nervous system abnormalities that can occur after exposure to such drugs during any trimester (16). It is possible that coumarin derivatives are safe during the first 6 weeks of gestation, but there is a risk of embryopathy if they are taken between 6 and 12 weeks gestation (18). In addition, these oral anticoagulants have an anticoagulant effect in the fetus that is a concern, particularly at the time of delivery when the combination of the anticoagulant effect and trauma of delivery can lead to neonatal bleeding.

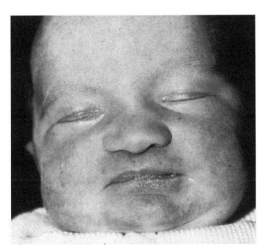

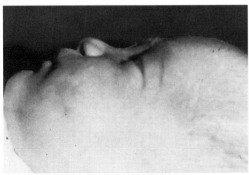

FIG. 43-1. A newborn with warfarin embryopathy who exhibits nasal hypoplasia. There are no signs of epiphyseal stippling.

Maternal Complications of Anticoagulant Therapy During Pregnancy

In a recent cohort study, the rate of major bleeding in pregnant patients treated with heparin therapy was 2% (15), which is consistent with the reported rates of bleeding associated with heparin therapy in nonpregnant patients (19) and with warfarin therapy (20) when used for the treatment of DVT. Adjusted dose, subcutaneous heparin can cause a persistent anticoagulant effect at the time of delivery, which can complicate its use prior to labor (21). In a recent study, an anticoagulant effect persisted for up to 28 hours after the last injection of adjusted dose subcutaneous heparin, frequently resulting in deliveries that were complicated by a prolonged APTT (21). The mechanism for this phenomenon is unclear; however, to avoid an unwanted anticoagulant effect during delivery in women receiving adjusted dose subcutaneous heparin, heparin can be discontinued 24 hours prior to elective induction of labor. If spontaneous labor occurs in women receiving adjusted dose subcutaneous heparin, careful monitoring of the APTT is required; if the APTT is prolonged near delivery, protamine sulfate may be required to reduce the risk of bleeding.

Long-term heparin therapy causes osteoporosis; the mechanism is unknown. Five recent studies provide estimates of the risk of heparin-induced osteoporosis with long-term heparin (22–26). The results of these studies show that although the risk of symptomatic fractures is low (2% or less), an asymptomatic reduction in bone density, detected radiographically, occurs in up to one third of women receiving long-term (>1 month) heparin therapy. The radiologic effects of heparin are at least partly reversible. Women with reduced bone density due to heparin might be predisposed to future fractures. Although none of the five studies showed that the risk of osteoporosis is dependent on the dose of heparin used and the duration of heparin therapy, none was sufficiently large to exclude such relationships.

In some women, there can be considerable discomfort associated with twice-daily self-administered heparin injections. An indwelling subcutaneous Teflon catheter (Insuflon), which must be replaced weekly, is a useful approach in pregnant women who require long-term heparin (27).

Use of Anticoagulants in the Nursing Mother

Heparin is not secreted into breast milk and can be administered safely to nursing mothers (28). There are two reports that warfarin does not induce an anticoagulant effect in the breast-fed infant when the drug is administrated to a nursing mother (29,30). Therefore, the use of warfarin in women who require anticoagulant therapy post partum is reasonable; these women should be encouraged to breast-feed.

Low Molecular Weight Heparins and Heparinoids

There is accumulating experience with the use of these agents both in pregnant and nonpregnant patients for the prevention and treatment of DVT (29–34). Based on the results of large clinical trials in nonpregnant patients, LMWH and heparinoids are at least as effective and safe as unfractionated heparin for the treatment of patients with acute proximal DVT (32,33) and for the prevention of DVT in patients undergoing surgery (35). They have the advantage of a longer plasma half-life and a more predictable dose response than unfractionated heparin.

There is also evidence that LMWH and heparinoids do not cross the placenta (37–40). These agents have potential advantages over unfractionated heparin during pregnancy because they cause less heparin-induced thrombocytopenia (HIT) (41), have the potential for once-daily administration, and may have a lower risk of heparin-induced osteoporosis (35,36,42). In pregnant women who develop HIT and require ongoing anticoagulant therapy, use of the heparinoid danaparoid sodium is recommended because it is an effective antithrombotic agent and has much less cross-reactivity with unfractionated heparin than

LMWH and therefore less potential to produce recurrent HIT (43). These agents are more expensive than unfractionated heparin but are suitable substitutes for unfractionated heparin in the prevention and treatment of VTE in pregnant women. Anecdotal experience suggests that LMWH should be considered in patients with intractable painful skin reactions to unfractionated heparin.

EFFICACY OF ANTICOAGULANTS FOR THE PREVENTION AND TREATMENT OF VTE DURING PREGNANCY

There is a lack of data about the efficacy of anticoagulants for the prevention and treatment of VTE during pregnancy. Accordingly, the recommendations about their use during pregnancy is based largely on extrapolations from data in nonpregnant patients and case reports and case series of pregnant patients. Based on the safety data, heparin is the drug of choice for the prevention and treatment of VTE during pregnancy.

The results of a large randomized trial in nonpregnant patients have shown that full-dose intravenous (IV) heparin, followed by 3 months of twice daily subcutaneous (SC) heparin therapy, in doses adjusted to prolong a midinterval APTT into the therapeutic range (adjusted dose SC heparin) is safe and effective (19). Therefore, it seems reasonable to extrapolate these results to pregnant patients with DVT and PE and use IV heparin followed by at least 3 months of adjusted dose SC heparin.

Pregnant women with previous VTE probably have an increased risk for recurrent VTE, but the magnitude of the risk is unknown. It is likely that the risk of recurrence is higher in women with previous idiopathic VTE than in women who developed VTE in association with a transient risk factor (1–3). It is unclear as to whether women who developed VTE in association with previous pregnancy have a relatively greater risk of recurrence. Based on the current state of knowledge, there are two reasonable approaches to pregnant patients with previous VTE: (a) active prophylaxis with heparin and (b) clinical surveillance with or without regular noninvasive tests such as venous compression ultrasonography (CUS) or impedance plethysmography (IPG). Subcutaneous (SC) heparin, 5000 IU twice daily, is effective and safe for the prevention of VTE in high-risk nonpregnant patients (44) and its use has been recommended in pregnant patients. However, there is a concern that a dose of heparin 5,000 U SC every 12 hours may be insufficient in high-risk situations because it does not reliably produce detectable heparin levels. There are also published data indicating that more intense heparin therapy, in doses that produce plasma heparin levels (measured as anti-factor Xa activity) of 0.1 to 0.2 IU/ml, is associated with low recurrence rates (25). The advantage of this latter approach is that it is more likely to produce a consistent anticoagulant effect throughout pregnancy, but its use is likely to increase the risks of bleeding and osteoporosis and requires lab monitoring. Until comparative clinical trials are performed, it is our belief that either approach is reasonable.

In pregnant women with previous VTE who cannot use or refuse to use heparin, an alternative is clinical surveillance with or without regular IPG or CUS. We have an ongoing trial that is testing the safety of this approach, which is dependent on detection and treatment of VTE before the development of major PE. When using a surveillance approach, it is important that the clinician recognize the relative insensitivity of IPG and CUS to asymptomatic proximal DVT (45). This approach is certainly reasonable in women who developed previous VTE in association with a previous risk factor (e.g., leg fracture), in whom the risk of recurrence is likely to be low and might be reasonable in all women with previous VTE.

MANAGEMENT OF PREGNANT WOMEN WITH PROSTHETIC HEART VALVES

Women of childbearing age with valvular heart disease pose problems because of the lack of reliable data on the efficacy and safety of antithrombotic therapy during pregnancy and the concern that bioprosthetic heart valves deteriorate at an accelerated rate dur-

ing pregnancy (46). In a recent retrospective survey describing outcomes in pregnant women with mechanical heart valves, it was concluded that (a) warfarin was safe and not associated with embryopathy and (b) unfractionated heparin was associated with more thromboembolic and bleeding complications than warfarin (46). The concern about thromboembolic complications has been reported in other studies (47). However, the reported high rates of thromboembolism might also be explained by inadequate heparin dosing and/or the use of an inappropriate target therapeutic range. Nevertheless, these recent publications do raise the concern that patients with mechanical heart valves are resistant to moderate doses of heparin and draw attention to the need to use adequate heparin doses in such patients. Insufficient heparin dosing is associated with treatment failure, emphasizing the need for adequate initial heparinization and stringent monitoring (48). Contemporary APTT reagents are more sensitive to the anticoagulant effect of heparin and, therefore, a minimum target APTT ratio of 1.5 times control is likely to be inadequate and a target APTT ratio of at least twice that of the control should be attained (49). The higher rate of thromboembolic events reported in heparin-treated compared to warfarin-treated women is based on retrospective studies and is difficult to interpret because the adequacy of heparin dosing was usually not reported in these studies and a minimum target APTT ratio of 1.5 times control was often used. Long-term twice daily subcutaneous heparin, in doses adjusted to prolong a midinterval APTT into the therapeutic range, has been shown to be as effective and safe as long-term warfarin (International Normalized Ratio [INR] of 2.5 to 4.9) for the treatment of acute venous thrombosis (19). Such doses of heparin might be less effective than warfarin in preventing arterial thromboembolism in patients with mechanical heart valves but there are no data available to support or refute this conclusion.

At present, there are insufficient grounds to make definitive recommendations about optimal antithrombotic therapy in pregnant patients with mechanical heart valves because properly designed studies have not been performed. Substantial concern remains about the fetal safety of warfarin, the efficacy of subcutaneous heparin in preventing thromboembolic complications, and the risks of maternal bleeding with various regimens. Extrapolating from the results of a recent randomized trial of nonpregnant patients with mechanical prosthetic heart valves or bioprosthetic heart valves and either chronic atrial fibrillation or previous thromboembolic events, it is reasonable to add low-dose (80 to 100 mg per day) aspirin throughout pregnancy to the anticoagulant regimen (50). This recommendation is limited by the lack of safety and efficacy data on the combination of heparin and aspirin. Warfarin should probably be avoided between 6 and 12 weeks gestation (to avoid embryopathy) and close to term (to avoid delivery of an anticoagulated fetus) but is reasonable at other times; in many European countries, warfarin throughout pregnancy has been used with success and with a very low incidence of warfarin embryopathy (46). We believe that it is reasonable to use subcutaneous heparin either during these periods only, with warfarin, target INR of 2.5 to 3.5, at other times, or to use heparin throughout pregnancy. Subcutaneous heparin should be initiated in doses of 17,500 to 20,000 U every 12 hours and adjusted to prolong a 6-hour postinjection APTT into the therapeutic range; strong efforts should be made to ensure an adequate anticoagulant effect because inadequate doses of heparin are ineffective. LMWH or heparinoids are probably reasonable substitutes for unfractionated heparin because they appear to reduce the risk of bleeding and osteoporosis and do not cross the placenta. However, before they are recommended for routine use, additional information is required about dosing.

ANTIPHOSPHOLIPID ANTIBODIES

Antiphospholipid antibodies (APLA) can be detected using clotting assays (lupus anticoagulant) or immunoassays (anticardiolipin antibodies) (51), and have been reported to occur in systemic lupus erythematosus, with certain drugs and in apparently healthy individuals (see Chapter 47). There is convincing evidence that the presence of APLA is associated with an increased risk of thrombosis (7,51) and pregnancy loss (52). Thus, pregnant individuals with APLA should be considered at risk for both pregnancy loss and thrombosis. The management of these patients is problematic because very few large clinical trials evaluating therapy have been performed. Regimens that have been evaluated include aspirin (ASA) alone (53) or in combination with prednisone (53,54), unfractionated heparin (55,56) or LMWH (57), and intravenous gammaglobulin (58). Two recent randomized trials provide guidelines for the prevention of pregnancy loss in women with APLA. In the first, 202 women with an antibody (APLA or others) were randomly allocated to receive ASA and prednisone or placebo (57), and there was no significant improvement in pregnancy outcome with ASA and prednisone, either in the entire group or in the subgroup with APLA. In the second trial, 90 patients were randomly allocated to ASA or ASA plus heparin (56); there was a significant improvement in the live birth rate in ASA plus heparin–treated patients. Studies evaluating LMWH for prevention of pregnancy loss are ongoing (57).

Based on current evidence, any recommendations on management must be tentative. Women with APLA and a history of multiple pregnancy losses are considered candidates for heparin plus ASA, but the supporting evidence is based on one randomized trial. Whether the patient with APLA and either no or one pregnancy loss should be treated with such therapy is unclear. Pregnant women with APLA and previous venous thrombosis should also be considered to be candidates for heparin therapy. Women with APLA and no previous venous thrombosis should be managed either with low-dose heparin therapy or a combination of clinical surveillance combined with IPG or CUS throughout pregnancy.

SAFETY OF ASPIRIN DURING PREGNANCY

Potential complications of aspirin during pregnancy include birth defects and bleeding in the neonate and in the mother. The results of a recent meta-analysis (59) and a large (>9,000 patients) randomized trial (60) reported that low-dose (60 to 150 mg per day) aspirin therapy administered during the second and third trimesters of pregnancy in women at risk for pregnancy-induced hypertension or intrauterine growth retardation was safe for the mother and fetus because no increase in maternal or neonatal adverse effects occurred in aspirin-treated individuals. Thus, low-dose (<150 mg per day) aspirin during the second and third trimesters appears to be safe, but the safety of higher doses of aspirin and/or aspirin ingestion during the first trimester remains a subject of debate.

CONCLUSION

The relatively poor quality of evidence from the published studies makes it difficult to provide clear-cut recommendations (Table 43-1). Because it is safe for the fetus, heparin is the anticoagulant of choice during pregnancy for situations in which its efficacy is established. The evidence for the efficacy of heparin for the prevention and treatment of venous thromboembolic disorders during pregnancy is based on nonrandomized studies. Although it is likely that full doses of heparin are effective for the prevention of systemic embolism in patients with mechanical heart valves, studies demonstrating the efficacy of heparin in such patients have not been published. Low doses of heparin or poorly controlled heparin therapy appear not to be effective in preventing systemic embolism in patients with mechanical heart valves (18).

TABLE 43-1. *Summary of recommendations*

Clinical problem	Treatment
Previous venous thrombosis or pulmonary embolism prior to current pregnancy	Heparin (5,000 U q12h adjusted to produce a heparin level of 0.1–0.2 U/ml) throughout pregnancy followed by warfarin post partum for 4 to 6 weeks
	or
	Clinical surveillance combined with periodic IPG or compression ultrasound followed by warfarin post partum for 4 to 6 weeks
Venous thrombosis or pulmonary embolism during current pregnancy	Unfractionated heparin in full intravenous doses for 5–10 days, followed by q12h subcutaneous injections to prolong 6-hour postinjection APTT into the therapeutic range until delivery. Warfarin can then be used post partum. LMWH are a suitable substitute for unfractionated heparin.
Planning pregnancy in patients who are being treated with long- term oral anticoagulants	Either unfractionated heparin q12h subcutaneously to prolong 6-hour postinjection APTT into the therapeutic range
	or
	Frequent pregnancy tests and substitute heparin (as above) for warfarin when pregnancy achieved
Mechanical heart valve	Either unfractionated heparin q12h valves subcutaneously to prolong 6-hour postinjection APTT into the therapeutic range
	or
	Adjusted dose subcutaneous heparin until the 13th week, warfarin (target INR 2.5–3.0) until the middle of the third trimester, then adjusted dose subcutaneous heparin until delivery
	The addition of aspirin 80–100 mg PO od to either regimen should be considered
APLA and >1 previous pregnancy loss	Aspirin plus heparin
APLA and previous venous thrombosis	Heparin q12h subcutaneously to prolong 6-hour postinjection APTT into the therapeutic range

Previous Venous Thromboembolism (Prophylaxis)

In pregnant women with a history of previous venous thromboembolic disease, the true risk of recurrence in untreated patients is unknown and estimates range from 0 to 15% (9–13). Consequently, some form of prophylaxis or surveillance should be considered. A recent cohort study reported that the incidence of symptomatic recurrence in pregnant women with previous thromboembolism who were treated with heparin was very low (15). Therefore, a reasonable approach to patients with previous venous thromboembolism is to use low-dose heparin (either 5,000 U every 12 hours SC or adjusted to produce a heparin level of 0.1 to 0.2 U/ml) throughout pregnancy. Alternatively, heparin could be withheld ante partum and the patient followed by clinical surveillance and periodic IPG or compression ultrasonography. With either option, heparin and warfarin should then be used post partum for 4 to 6 weeks.

Treatment of Venous Thromboembolism During Pregnancy

In patients who develop venous thrombosis during pregnancy, full doses of heparin should be given by intravenous infusion for 5 to 10 days and then by subcutaneous injection twice daily in full doses, until term. Subcutaneous low molecular weight heparin is a reasonable substitute for unfractionated heparin. Heparin should be discontinued immediately before delivery and then both heparin and warfarin can be started post partum. Once a therapeutic INR is obtained, heparin can be discontinued and warfarin administered for a further 4 to 6 weeks.

Unexpected Pregnancy or Planned Pregnancy In Patients Who Are Being Treated with Long-Term Anticoagulants

Patients on long-term oral anticoagulant therapy for venous thromboembolism or patients with mechanical heart valves present problems when planning pregnancy of if pregnancy occurs unexpectedly. It is possible that oral anticoagulants are safe during the first 6 weeks of gestation, but there is a risk of warfarin embryopathy if warfarin is taken between 6 and 12 weeks of gestation. Ideally, such women should be counseled before pregnancy occurs. If anticoagulant therapy is indicated during pregnancy the risks should be explained before conception. If pregnancy is still desired two options can be considered. The first is to perform frequent pregnancy tests and to substitute heparin for warfarin when pregnancy is achieved. The second is to replace warfarin with heparin before conception is attempted. Both approaches have limitations; the first assumes that warfarin is safe during the first 4 to 6 weeks of gestation and the second increases the duration of exposure to heparin and therefore to a higher risk of osteoporosis.

Prophylaxis in Patients with Mechanical Heart Valves

The management of pregnant patients with mechanical heart valves is problematic because the efficacy of heparin is not established. Nevertheless, it is highly likely that full doses of heparin are effective in preventing systemic embolism. Two approaches have been recommended: the first is to use heparin therapy throughout pregnancy administered twice daily by subcutaneous injection in doses adjusted to keep the midinterval APTT in the therapeutic range (at least twice that of the control). The second approach is to use heparin until the thirteenth week, change to warfarin until the middle of the third trimester, and restart heparin therapy until delivery. Although the latter approach might avoid warfarin embryopathy, other fetopathic effects (e.g., central nervous system abnormalities) are still possible. Therefore, before this approach is recommended the potential risks should be explained to the patients. A further potential problem with the use of oral anticoagulants during pregnancy arises from the clear statement in the manufacturer's package insert that coumarin is contraindicated during pregnancy. This statement carries with it medicolegal implications that would also have to be discussed with the patient if a choice is made to use oral anticoagulants during pregnancy. In view of recent concerns about the efficacy of heparin and the recent demonstration that aspirin is useful in combination with warfarin in nonpregnant patients, we believe that low-dose aspirin (80 to 100 mg per day) should be considered in combination with anticoagulants in patients with mechanical heart valves.

Pregnancy and APLA

Pregnant patients with APLA and a history of multiple pregnancy losses are candidates for aspirin plus heparin. For pregnant patients with APLA and a history of no or one pregnancy loss, low-dose ASA alone during the second and third trimester seems reasonable because it is relatively safe and may be effective. Patients with APLA and a history of venous thrombosis are candidates for long-term anticoagulant therapy. During pregnancy, adjusted dose subcutaneous heparin therapy seems reasonable. In the absence of previous venous thrombosis, pregnant patients with APLA should be considered to be at risk for the development of venous thrombosis and either followed with a combination of clinical surveillance and noninvasive tests (IPG or compression ultrasonography) or treated with low-dose subcutaneous heparin.

REFERENCES

1. Prandoni P, Lensing AWA, Buller HR, et al. Deep-vein thrombosis and the incidence of subsequent symptomatic cancer. N Engl J Med 1992;327:1128–1133.
2. Research Committee of the British Thoracic Society. Optimum duration of anticoagulation for deep-vein thrombosis and pulmonary embolism. Lancet 1992; 340:873–876.
3. Levine MN, Hirsh J, Gent M, et al. Optimal duration of oral anticoagulant therapy: A randoized trial comparing four weeks with three months of warfarin in patients with proximal deep vein thrombosis. Thromb Haemost 1995;74:606–611.
4. Svensson PJ, Dahlback B. Resistance to activated protein C as a basis for venous thrombosis. N Engl J Med 1994;330:517–522.
5. Dahlback B. Inherited thrombophilia: resistance to activated protein C as a pathogenic factor of venous thromboembolism. Blood 1995;85:607–614.
6. Conard J, Horellou MH, Van Dreden P, Lecompte T, Samama M. Thrombosis and pregnancy in congenital deficiencies in ATIII, protein C or protein S: study of 78 women. Thromb Haemost 1990;63:319–320.
7. Long AA, Ginsberg JS, Brill-Edwards P, et al. The relationship of antiphospholipid antibodies to thromboembolic disease in systemic lupus erythematosus: a cross-sectional study. Thromb Haemost 991;66:520–524.
8. Friederich PW, Sanson B, Simioni P, et al. Frequency of pregnancy-related venous thromboembolism in anticoagulant factor-deficient women: implications for prophylaxis. Ann Intern Med 1996;125:955–960.
9. De Swiet M, Floyd E, Letsky E. Low risk of recurrent thromboembolism in pregnancy. Br J Hosp Med 1987;38:264.
10. Howell R, Fidler J, Letsky E, De Swiet M. The risk of antenatal subcutaneous heparin prophylaxis: a controlled trial. Br J Obstet Gynecol 1983;90:1124–1128.
11. Badaracco MA, Vessey M. Recurrent venous thromboembolic disease and use of oral contraceptives. Br Med J 1974;1:215–217.
12. Tengborn L. Recurrent thromboembolism in pregnancy and puerperium. Is there a need for thromboprophylaxis? Am J Obstet Gynecol 1989;160:90–94.
13. Flessa HC, Klapstrom AB, Glueck MJ, Will JJ. Placental transport of heparin. Am J Obstet Gynecol 1965;93: 570–573.
14. Ginsberg JS, Hirsh J, Turner DC, Levine MN, Burrows R. Risks to the fetus of anticoagulant therapy during pregnancy. Thromb Haemost 1989;61:197–203.
15. Ginsberg JS, Kowalchuk G, Hirsh J, Brill-Edwards, Burrows R. Heparin therapy during pregnancy: Risks to the fetus and mother. Arch Intern Med 1989;149: 2233–2236.
16. Hall JAG, Paul RM, Wilson KM. Maternal and fetal sequelae of anticoagulation during pregnancy. Am J Med 1980;68:122–140.
17. Becker MH, Genieser NB, Finegold M, Miranda D, Spackman T. Chondrodysplasia punctata: Is maternal warfarin a factor? Am J Dis Child 1975;129:356–359.
18. Iturbe-Alessio I, Fonseca MC, Mutchnik O, Santos MA, Zajarias A, Salazar E. Risks of anticoagulant therapy in pregnant women with artificial heart valves. N Engl J Med 1986;315:1390–1393.
19. Hull RD, Delmore TJ, Carter CJ, et al. Adjusted subcutaneous heparin versus warfarin sodium in the long-term treatment of venous thrombosis. N Engl J Med 1982;306:189–194.
20. Hull R, Hirsh J, Jay R, et al. Different intensities of oral anticoagulant therapy in the treatment of proximal-vein thrombosis. N Engl J Med 1982;307:1676–1681.
21. Anderson DR, Ginsberg JS, Burrows R, Brill-Edwards P. Subcutaneous heparin therapy during pregnancy: A need for concern at the time of delivery. Thromb Haemost 1991;63:248–250.
22. Ginsberg JS, Kowalchuk G, Hirsh J, et al. Heparin effect on bone density. Thromb Haemost 1990;64:286–289.
23. Dahlman T, Lindvall N, Hellgren M. Osteopenia in pregnancy during long-term heparin treatment: a radiological study post-partum. Br J Obstet Gynecol 1990;97:221–228.
24. Barbour LA, Kick SD, Steiner JF, et al. A prospective

study of heparin-induced osteoporosis using bone densitometry. *Am J Obstet Gynecol* 1994;170:862–869.

25. Dahlman TC. Osteoporotic fractures and the recurrence of thromboembolism during pregnancy and the puerperium in 184 women undergoing thromboprophylaxis with heparin. *Am J Obstet Gynecol* 1993;168: 1265–1278.

26. Douketis JD, Ginsberg JS, Burrows RF, Duku EK, Webber CE, Brill-Edwards P. The effects of long-term heparin therapy during pregnancy on bone density. *Thromb Haemost* 1996;75:254–257.

27. Anderson DR, Ginsberg JS, Brill-Edwards P, Demers C, Burrows RF, Hirsh J. The use of an indwelling teflon catheter for subcutaneous heparin administration during pregnancy. *Arch Intern Med* 1993;153:841–844.

28. O'Reilly R. Anticoagulant, antithrombotic and thrombolytic drugs. In: Gilman AG, et al (eds). *The Pharmacologic Basis of Therapeutics.* New York: Macmillan, 1980;1347–1366.

29. Orme ML'e, Lewis PJ, De Swiet M, Serlin MJ, Sibeon R, Baty JD. May mothers given warfarin breast-feed their infants? *Br Med J* 1977;1:1564–65.

30. McKenna R, Cale ER, Vasan U. Is warfarin sodium contraindicated in the lactating mother? *J Pediatrics* 1983;103:325–27.

31. Gillis S, Shushan A, Eldor A. Use of low molecular weight heparin for prophylaxis and treatment of thromboembolism in pregnancy. *Int J Gynecol Obstet* 1992; 39:297–301.

32. Melissari E, Parker CJ, Wilson NV, et al. Use of low molecular weight heparin in pregnancy. *Thromb Haemost* 1992;68:652–656.

33. Hull RD, Raskob GE, Pineo GF, et al. Subcutaneous low-molecular-weight heparin compared with continuous intravenous heparin in the treatment of proximal-vein thrombosis. *N Engl J Med* 1992;326:975–982.

34. Prandoni P, Lensing AWA, Buller HR, et al. Comparison of subcutaneous low-molecular-weight heparin with intravenous standard heparin in proximal deep-vein thrombosis. *Lancet* 1992;339:441–445.

35. Hull R, Raskob G, Pineo G, et al. A comparison of subcutaneous low-molecular-weight heparin with warfarin sodium for prophylaxis against deep-vein thrombosis after hip or knee implantation. *N Engl J Med* 1993;329:1370–1376.

36. Monreal M, Lafoz E, Olive A, del Rio L, Vedia C. Comparison of subcutaneous unfractionated heparin with a low molecular weight heparin (Fragmin) in patients with venous thromboembolism and contraindications for coumarin. *Thromb Haemost* 1994;71:7–11.

37. Hunt BJ, Doughty G, Majumdar G, et al. Thromboprophylaxis with low molecular weight heparin (Fragmin) in high risk pregnancies. *Thromb Haemost* 1997;77: 39–43.

38. Forestier F, Daffos F, Capella-Pavlovsky M. Low molecular weight heparin (PK 10169) does not cross the placenta during the second trimester of pregnancy: study by direct fetal blood sampling under ultrasound. *Thromb Res* 1984;34:557–560.

39. Forestier F, Daffos F, Rainaut M, Toulemonde F. Low molecular weight heparin (CY 216) does not cross the placenta during the third trimester of pregnancy. *Thromb Haemost* 1987;57:234.

40. Omri A, Delaloye JF, Anderson H, Bachmann F. Low molecular weight heparin NOVO (LHN-1) does not cross the placenta during the second trimester of pregnancy. *Thromb Haemost* 1989;61:55–56.

41. Warkentin TE, Levine MN, Hirsh J, et al. Heparin-induced thrombocytopenia in patients treated with low-molecular-weight heparin or unfractionated heparin. *N Engl J Med* 1995;332:1330–1335.

42. Shaughnessy SG, Young E, Deschamps P, Hirsh J. The effects of low molecular-weight and standard heparin on calcium loss from fetal rat calvaria. *Blood* 1995;86: 1368–1373.

43. Magnani HN. Heparin-induced thrombocytopenia (HIT): an overview of 230 patients treated with Orgaran (Org 10172). *Thromb Haemost* 1993;70:554–561.

44. Collins R, Scrimgeour A, Yusuf S, Phil D, Peto R. Reduction in fatal pulmonary embolism and venous thrombosis by perioperative administration of subcutaneous heparin. Overview of results of randomized trials in general, orthopedic, and urologic surgery. *N Engl J Med* 1988;318:1162–1173.

45. Ginsberg JS, Caco CC, Brill-Edwards PA, Panju AA, Bona R, Demers CM. Venous thrombosis in patients who have undergone major hip or knee surgery: detection with compression US and impedance plethysmography. *Radiology* 1991;181:651–654.

46. Sbarouni E, Oakley CM. Outcome of pregnancy in women with valve prostheses. *Br Heart J* 1994;71: 196–201.

47. Salazar E, Izaguirre R, Verdejo J, Mutchinick O. Failure of adjusted doses of subcutaneous heparin to prevent thromboemoblic phenomena in pregnant patients with mechanical cardiac valve prostheses. *J Am Coll Cardiol* 1996;27:1698–1703.

48. Hirsh J. Heparin. *N Engl J Med* 1991;324:1565–1574.

49. Brill-Edwards P, Ginsberg JS, Johnston M, Hirsh J. Establishing a therapeutic range for heparin. *Ann Intern Med* 1993;119:104–109.

50. Turpie AGG, Gent M, Laupacis A, et al. A comparison of aspirin with placebo in patients treated with warfarin after heart-valve replacement. *N Engl J Med* 1993;329: 524–529.

51. Love PE, Santoro SA. Antiphospholipid antibodies: anticardiolipin and the lupus anticoagulant in systemic lupus erythematosus (SLE) and in non-SLE disorders. *Ann Intern Med* 1990;112:682–698.

52. Ginsberg JS, Brill-Edwards P, Johnston M, et al. Relationship of antiphospholipid antibodies to pregnancy loss in patients with systemic lupus erythematosus: a cross-sectional study. *Blood* 1992;80:975–980.

53. Silver RK, MacGregor SN, Sholl JS, Hobart JM, Neerhof MG, Ragin A. Comparative trial of prednisone plus aspirin versus aspirin alone in the treatment of anticardiolipin antibody positive obstetric patients. *Am J Obstet Gynecol* 1993;169:1411–1417.

54. Laskin C, Bombardier C, Mandel F, Ritchie K, Hannah M, Farine D. A randomized controlled trial of prednisone and ASA in women with autoantibodies and unexplained recurrent fetal loss. Society of Perinatal Obstetricians 1996 Annual Meeting, Hawaii. *N Engl J Med* 1997;337:148–153.

55. Cowchock FS, Reece EA, Balaban D, Branch DW, Plouffe L. Repeated fetal losses associated with antiphospholipid antibodies: A collaborative randomized trial comparing prednisone with low-dose heparin treatment. *Am J Obstet Gynecol* 1992;166:1318–1323.

56. Rai RS, Regan L, Dave M, Cohen H. Randomised trial

of aspirin versus aspirin and heparin in pregnant women with the antiphospholipid syndrome [Abstract]. *Lupus* 1996;5:578.

57. Laskin C, Ginsberg J, Farine D, et al. Low molecular weight heparin and ASA therapy in women with autoantibodies and unexplained recurrent fetal loss. Society of Perinatal Obstetricians 1997 Annual Meeting, California.

58. Foley-Nolan D, Buchan PC, Gooi HC. Intravenous immunoglobulin treatment of the antiphospholipid antibody syndrome in pregnancy [Abstract]. *Br J Rheumatol* 1994;33:34.

59. Imperiale TF, Stollenwerk PA. A meta-analysis of low-dose aspirin for the prevention of pregnancy-induced hypertensive disease. *JAMA* 1991;266:260.

60. CLASP Collaborative Group. CLASP: A randomised trial of low dose aspirin for the prevention and treatment of pre-eclampsia among 9364 pregnant women. *Lancet* 1994;343:619–29.

*Cardiovascular Thrombosis: Thrombocardiology
and Thromboneurology, Second Edition,*
edited by M. Verstraete, V. Fuster, and E. J. Topol,
Lippincott–Raven Publishers, Philadelphia © 1998.

44

Thrombosis in Cancer Patients

Kenneth B. Hymes and Simon Karpatkin

*Departments of Hematology and Medicine,
New York University Medical Center, New York, New York 10016*

Patients with malignancies have an increased incidence of thrombotic and thromboembolic disorders, an observation that has been confirmed innumerable times since the original description of Trousseau (1). This chapter will attempt to describe the clinical syndromes of hypercoagulability and neoplasia, to characterize the laboratory abnormalities seen in these syndromes, and to discuss the biological events that may underlie these associations.

Coagulation disorders in patients with malignancies are major complications of these diseases. As many as 15% of patients with tumors have either thrombotic or hemorrhagic events (2). As many as 30% have clinically asymptomatic coagulation disorders (3). The clinical presentations of hypercoagulability include classic Trousseau's syndrome, disseminated intravascular coagulation (DIC), nonbacterial thrombotic endocarditis, and thrombotic thrombocytopenic purpura. These entities may

either complicate the course of patients with known malignant diseases or serve as the presenting symptoms of these disorders.

TROUSSEAU'S SYNDROME AND PULMONARY EMBOLIZATION

The original description of hypercoagulability in malignancy by Trousseau was recurrent superficial venous thromboses, typically involving the upper extremities (1). This entity has been expanded to include both deep and superficial thrombosis of any vessels including the superior or inferior vena cava, the jugular, axillary, femoral veins, and the dorsal veins of the penis (3). Clots in superficial veins may coexist with deep venous thrombi and lead to pulmonary embolization. Thromboemboli are common occurrences in 7% to 9% of hospitalized cancer patients; in autopsy studies the incidence of thrombosis or thromboembolism is as high as 28% of cancer patients (4). Cancer-related in situ thromboses or thromboemboli respond more slowly to heparin anticoagulation than thromboses occurring in other settings. Following cessation of heparin or conversion to warfarin anticoagulation thrombosis may commonly reoccur in the same site or at new sites (3,5).

Recurrent or recalcitrant thromboses in patients not known to have a malignancy may represent the presence of an occult tumor. Prandoni et al. studied 250 patients with first presentation of lower extremity deep venous thrombosis (DVT) in a prospective study of the association of venous thrombosis and cancer (6). Patients were stratified into those with and without identifiable predisposing factors for thrombosis (such as lower extremity trauma, prolonged immobilization, antithrombin III deficiency). The incidence of malignancy in patients without an identifiable predisposition was 10.5% compared to 1.9% with a known predisposing factor. All of the patients with occult malignancies were diagnosed within 2 years of the thrombosis with the majority of patients (11/15) diagnosed within 6 months of their presentation with DVT. This information is similar to that reported by Monreal (7) and Aderka (8) who independently found a cancer incidence of 23% within the 2 years of presentation with idiopathic DVT.

Adenocarcinomas are typically reported as the most common neoplasms found in this setting with pancreatic, bronchogenic, prostatic, gastric, and colonic malignancies presenting in decreasing order of frequency in one large series (3). Myeloid malignancies (most often acute promyelocytic leukemia) are present in 9% of patients with Trousseau's syndrome (3). This information suggests that patients presenting with idiopathic DVT should be screened for an occult malignancy.

The natural history of Trousseau's syndrome is modulated by the underlying malignancy; however, some observations on its behavior are noteworthy. Treatment of the underlying malignancy rarely results in a complete remission; consequently, the prothrombotic tendency does not disappear. Anti-platelet therapy with aspirin or dipyridamole as well as anticoagulation with warfarin usually has no effect on the frequency of thrombotic events (5). Heparin anticoagulation has been demonstrated to reduce the levels of fibrin split products, circulating fibrin monomer, and to decrease the severity of thromboses (5). Regulation of the level of anticoagulation is more difficult in patients with the hypercoagulability of malignancy and is associated with an increased risk of hemorrhage (9).

Treatment of malignant diseases may be associated with a paradoxically increased risk of venous thrombosis. In studies of patients receiving adjuvant chemotherapy for stage II breast carcinoma, there was a 6.8% incidence of deep venous thromboses in patients receiving cytotoxic chemotherapy (cyclophosphamide, methotrexate, vincristine, 5-fluorouracil, doxorubicin) and with hormonal therapy (tamoxifen) (10). No DVTs were noted after conclusion of the chemotherapy, implicating the treatment as the cause of the events (10). Serial evaluations of coagulation function showed a decrease in the vitamin K–dependent coagulation factors II and VII and the anticoagulant proteins C and S (11). It is not clear if these abnormalities were the result of decreased vitamin K intake (due to chemotherapy-induced anorexia), reduced hepatic protein synthesis of coagulation factors as a result of the chemotherapy, reduced generation of activated protein C due to chemotherapy-induced endothelial damage with resultant reduction in levels of functional thrombomodulin (required to activate protein C), or a combination of these disorders. Of note is that a comparison of chemotherapy regimens with and without tamoxifen revealed a 10-fold increase in the incidence of DVTs (12.7 versus 1.2%) in postmenopausal women (12). The weak estrogenic effect of tamoxifen may contribute to the thrombotic events observed in these patients by reducing plasma levels of antithrombin III or affecting unknown procoagulant events. Although no study has demonstrated reduction in antithrombin III by tamoxifen to <70% of baseline value, the possibility remains that a lesser reduction of the level of this protein coupled with the defects mentioned previously might contribute to thrombosis.

DISSEMINATED INTRAVASCULAR COAGULATION

Routine and specialized laboratory studies give evidence of activation of both the thrombotic and fibrinolytic pathways in patients with cancer (13,14). Coagulation factors V, VIII, and XI, fibrin/fibrinogen degradation products, and D dimers are all elevated in patients with malignancy. Platelet counts may be elevated or decreased in patients with malignancies. More specific and sophisticated measurements of intravascular thrombosis and fibrinolysis including fibrinopeptide A (the product of the cleavage of fibrinogen by thrombin), F1+2 (the peptide produced by the cleavage of prothrombin by factor Xa), thrombin–antithrombin III complexes, or plasminogen are abnormal in patients with malignancies. Unfortunately, none of these laboratory assays are characteristic of the hypercoagulabilty of malignancy because they can be influenced by impairment of hepatic function, availability of nutrients (vitamin K), alterations in efficiency of their clearance (due to shock and hypoperfusion), increase in their synthetic rate (as acute phase reactants), or the presence of other activators of coagulation such as endotoxin.

EFFECTS OF MALIGNANCY ON THROMBOREGULATORY PROTEINS

The vitamin K–dependent anticoagulant proteins, protein C and its cofactor protein S, confer protection against pathologic venous thrombosis by enzymatic inactivation of factors Va and VIIIa. Forty percent of plasma protein S is in an unbound biologically active state, whereas the remaining 60% circulates bound to a carrier protein C4bp. Plasma levels of C-4bp are increased as acute phase proteins in both inflammatory diseases and malignancy leading to a decrease in concentration of functional protein S and an increase in the risk of thrombosis.

Protein C is converted to its active form (PCa) by thrombin in the presence of the endothelial-associated protein thrombomodulin. TNF-α and other cytokines decrease endothelial synthesis of thrombomodulin and cause this protein to be shed from the endothelial cell (15); the reduction in thrombomodulin-bound thrombin reduces generation of PCa and increases the thrombotic tendency in patients with malignancies.

A recently discovered mutation at amino acid 506 of factor V renders this protein resistant to inactivation by proteins C and S. The mutated factor V (factor V Leiden) has been identified in as many as 50% of patients with unexplained venous thrombosis. It is not known if this mutation contributes to hypercoagulable events seen in association with malignant disease. In one study (16) the incidences of thrombosis in cancer patients with and without this mutation were similar. Nonetheless, resistance to PCa should be part of the screening studies of all patients with recurrent or atypical venous thrombosis.

NONBACTERIAL THROMBOTIC ENDOCARDITIS

Nonbacterial thrombotic endocarditis (NBTE), or marantic endocarditis, is the arterial equivalent of Trousseau's syndrome. Its clinical presentation as showers of arterial thrombi to brain, gut, spleen, or extremities is an infrequent but spectacular preterminal event in patients with cancers. This diagnosis was seldom made ante mortem; however, with the advent of Doppler and transesophageal echocardiography the diagnosis can be made. In a large antemortem study Edoute et al. used transesophageal echocardiography to discover mitral or aortic thrombi in 19% of 200 patients with known malignancies (17). (A control group of 100 patients without malignancies had an incidence of valvular thrombi of 2%.) Management of this problem once discovered is limited to an attempt to treat the underlying malignancy and suppress intravascular thrombosis and embolization with heparin. As in the case of

Trousseau's syndrome, the prognosis of the disease depends on the availability of effective antineoplastic treatment.

THROMBOTIC MICROANGIOPATHY IN CANCER

Sporadic cases of thrombotic microangiopathies (TM) [either identified as the hemolytic uremic syndrome (HUS) or thrombotic thrombocytopenic purpura (TTP)] have been observed in association with malignant diseases for many years. With the recent advent of aggressive multidrug chemotherapeutic regimens and the use of high-dose chemotherapy, total body irradiation (TBI) therapy, and bone marrow transplantation, the incidence of these disorders has increased. In a review of 168 patients undergoing autologous or allogeneic bone marrow transplantation following treatment with TBI and cyclophosphamide, 16 (9.5%) developed HUS within the first year (18). In other studies using different myeloablative regimens similar rates of TTP and or HUS occurred (19). When rates of this complication for allogeneic and autologous transplants were compared, a slightly higher incidence of TM was noted in patients receiving allogeneic bone marrow. One possible explanation for this observation is the frequent use of cyclosporin A (CSA) as an immunosuppressant in the allograft recipients (20).

The etiology of this disorder may reside in the endothelial damage caused by the pretransplant conditioning regimens. Increased levels of high molecular weight von Willebrand factor (vWF) have been found in the plasma of patients receiving these treatments indicative of perturbation of the endothelium, simulating derangements of vWF multimer distribution seen in other forms of TM (21). CSA has a similar effect on vWF multimer composition (22) and has been shown to increase platelet aggregation, enhance platelet generation of thromboxane A_2, and reduce prostacyclin I_2 synthesis by cultured endothelial cells (23,24).

VENO-OCCLUSIVE DISEASE OF THE LIVER

The hypercoagulable syndrome, venous-occlusive disease of the liver (VOD), seen in association with allogeneic bone marrow transplantation, needs to be distinguished from TM. This major cause of morbidity and mortality in patients in the transplant setting is characterized by painful hepatomegaly, jaundice, weight gain, ascites, and occlusion of the hepatic or portal veins usually appearing 2 to 3 weeks after the initiation of high-dose chemotherapy (24). The small intrahepatic branches of the hepatic vein show subendothelial thickening, thrombosis, and obliteration of the lumen (25). The subendothelial location of the characteristic histopathologic lesion is reminiscent of TM; however, no classic hyalin thrombi are noted, and microangiopathic hemolytic anemia is absent. Prospective studies of coagulation function in patients undergoing allogeneic BMT have identified a low protein C level as an independent risk factor for developing VOD (26); however, these studies have not stratified their patients by severity of preexisting liver disease. Thus it is possible that the depressed protein C level is a marker for a hepatic lesion predisposing to VOD.

PATHOPHYSIOLOGIC MECHANISMS LEADING TO HYPERCOAGULABILITY

Tissue Factor

Tissue factor (TF) is a 44-kDa transmembrane glycoprotein located within the adventitia which comes into contact with blood after vascular injury (Fig. 44-1). TF then complexes with coagulation factor VII in the blood and converts it to its active form, VIIa. The vascular endothelium, which has no TF on its surface, can be induced to express TF by several agents: hypoxia, endotoxin, tumor necrosis factor (TNF)–α, interleukin-1 (IL-1), interferon (IFN)–γ, immune complexes, CSA, and thrombin (27,28). Similar observations

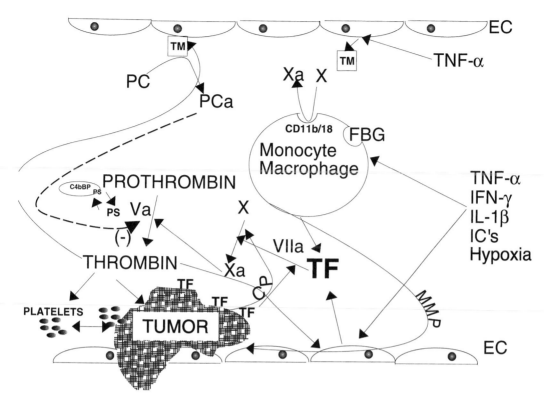

FIG. 44-1. Endothelial cells (EC) and monocyte/macrophages are stimulated by TNF-α, IFN-γ, IL-1β, immune complexes (ICs), or hypoxia to express tissue factor (TF). TF drives the generation of thrombin, which activates protein C (PCa) in the presence of thrombomodulin (TM). Thrombin stimulation of platelets and tumor cells increases their binding to each other. Tumor cells constitutively express TF and the tumor-associated cysteine proteinase (CP), which activates factor X independently of TF and factor VIIa. Procoagulant functions of the monocyte integrin CD11b/18 include activation of factor X and binding of fibrinogen (FBG). Activated monocytes secrete matrix metalloproteinases (MMP), which digest the subendothelial matrix and promote tumor invasiveness. TNF-α mediates the release of TM, thus reducing activation of protein C. The anticoagulant function of PCa on Va is also inhibited by sequestration of its cofactor, protein S (PS), by C4b-binding protein. (C4bBP is an acute phase protein that is increased in malignancy and inflammation.)

have been made with monocytes (29). This event initiates the "extrinsic" coagulation pathway by proteolytic cleavage of factor X to Xa, which in turn converts prothrombin to thrombin. TF is constitutively expressed on a broad range of benign tissues, tumor biopsies (30), and myelomonocytic cell lines (31) as measured by immunologic techniques (32,33) and by binding of peptides bearing sequences derived from factor VII (32).

In vivo evidence of the role of TF in the hypercoagulable state in cancer includes increased levels of TF in the serum and urine of patients with advanced malignancies (27, 34–36). Akasura et al. (34) measured the plasma concentration of TF in patients with DIC resulting from hepatic failure, sepsis, lymphoid or myeloid malignancies, and solid tumors. Plasma TF levels were only elevated in patients with solid tumors and correlated with the severity of the DIC. The biological activity of TF in these patients is supported by the observation of increased levels of factor VIIa and fibrinogen fragment 1+2 indicating activation of the extrinsic pathway, generation of thrombin, and cleavage of fibrinogen. Because DIC is frequently seen in patients with acute promyelocytic leukemia it is reasonable to expect that TF will be expressed on cells of myelomonocytic lineage although normal peripheral blood polymorphonuclear cells have undetectable levels.

Other sources of TF may also participate in the hypercoagulability of cancer. TNF treatment of mice bearing methylcholanthrene A–induced sarcomas induced TF expression in endothelial cells, monocytes, and macrophages; this expression was independent of the tumor cell TF and could be inhibited by transfection of antisense TF cDNA (37). Thus, the source of increased levels of TF found in patients with malignancies may be derived from constitutive tumor expression as well as an inducible host expression. Therapeutic suppression of host sources of TF by either modulating cytokine secretion or function or by molecular techniques inhibiting translation of active TF might provide avenues for controlling pathologic thrombosis in cancer patients.

Tumor-Associated Coagulation Protein

Gordon et al. (38) described the procoagulant activity of extracts of a variety of solid tumors. These extracts accelerated the clotting of plasma and appeared to function independently of factors VII, VIII, and IX (39). These investigators concluded that the activity directly activated factor X, bypassing both the intrinsic and extrinsic pathways. Further purification of this activity (40) identified a proteolytic procoagulant cysteine proteinase enzyme with a molecular mass of 68 kDa. The protein has been identified in a variety of tumor types including colon, breast, lung, kidney, and melanoma (39). The biosynthesis of the protein may be vitamin K– dependent since warfarin has been observed to decrease both procoagulant and metastatic activity of coagulation protein (CP) bearing experimental tumor cell lines (41). Extracts from corresponding benign tissues do not contain this activity. Increased levels of CP have correlated with the metastatic behavior of individual melanoma tumor samples (39).

Unlike TF, CP is expressed in acute myelocytic leukemia cells, and in some small studies plasma levels of CP correlate with response to treatment and subsequent relapse. Treatment of acute promyelocytic cell lines with all-trans retinoic acid results in granulocytic maturation and reduction in CP activity (42).

Specific Procoagulant Activity of Monocytes

Cells of the monocyte macrophage lineage can function as initiators of blood coagulation in addition to their role in host defense and antigen processing. Increases in monocyte procoagulant activity have been observed in patients with a variety of solid tumors (28,43,44) as well as in patients with infectious and inflammatory diseases (45). These cells have a distinct pathway leading to the activation of coagulation factors other than the TF pathway mentioned previously. Monocytes have an integrin receptor Mac-1 (CD11b/CD18), which can bind factor X/Xa as well as fibrinogen thus serving as an assembly point for coagulation factor Xa interaction with the prothrombinase complex with formation of thrombin and generation of fibrin (46).

The complexity of these events has been amplified by the discovery of the colocalization of the urokinase receptor (CD87) with the CD11b–CD18 complex as well (47). These receptors, when engaged with their respective ligands, provide sites for both the generation of fibrin and its degradation. These receptors also function as sites for cellular adhesion to the connective tissue matrix with CD11b/CD18 binding to fibrin and CD87 binding to vitronectin. Activated monocytes also secrete matrix metalloproteinases (MMPs), which digest the extracellular matrix (48–51). Secretion of these enzymes (including collagenases, gelatinases, and stromelysins) by tumor cells increase tissue invasion and metastasis (52) and is associated with a malignant phenotype in tumor cell lines (53). Expression of mRNAs for MMP-9 (a 92-kDa gelatinase), MMP-11 (stromelysin-3), and TIMP-1 was found in malignant but not benign tumors of the lung, colon, and breast (53). Cytokines secreted by monocytes modulate the expression of MMPs by other tissues including vascular smooth muscle cells, thus amplifying the degradation of the extracellular matrix at sites of unstable atheromatous plaques (54). The contribution of this latter source of MMPs to tumor invasiveness has yet to be documented. The coordination of fibrin generation, fibrin(ogen)olysis, and localization of inflammatory cells suggests a mechanism whereby local activation of coagulation might participate in tumor growth, adhesion, and/or invasion.

Endothelial Cells

The vascular endothelium actively regulates thrombosis by secretion or expression of TF, prostaglandins, platelet-activating factor (PAF), vWF, selectins, nitric oxide, thrombomodulin, thrombospondin, plasminogen activator inhibitor (PAI-1), and endothelin (ET). The balance of procoagulant versus anticoagulant activity can be influenced by thrombin, TNF-α, IL-1β, and IFN-γ, which are increased in patients with malignancies. Thrombin increases secretion of the procoagulant molecules PAF (55), TF (27), and vWF (56), whereas the same agonist induces anticoagulants PGI$_2$ (55) and activated protein C (57). TNF-α increases the expression of E-selectin and intercellular adhesion molecule–1 leading to increased adhesion of leukocytes and accelerated generation of monocyte TF (58,59). In addition, TNF-α and IL-1β increase TF expression on the abluminal surface of endothelial cells (59), enhance release of thrombomodulin (15) and PAI (60) from the endothelial cell surface (reducing the function of these proteins at the endothelial surface), and induce secretion of platelet-activating factor (61). However, these same cytokines induce synthesis of the antithrombotic prostaglandin PGI$_2$ (55). In addition the presence of other cytokines, including IL-4, can inhibit the TNF effect on TF and PAI (60).

Levels of the vasospastic agent ET or the vasodilatory agent nitric oxide may be af-

fected by the same mediators discussed above. It is noteworthy that high levels of plasma ET-1 has been observed in patients with DIC and malignancy (62). The authors suggest that this peptide might cause vasospasm and aggravate the DIC process by facilitating the formation of intravascular microthrombi, ultimately leading to ischemic end-organ dysfunction. Whether the elevation of plasma ET-1 is a cause of malignancy induced DIC or a consequence of endothelial damage remains to be elucidated. These observations suggest that an intricate regulatory mechanism exists that modulates the thrombogenic actions of cytokines and thrombin at the level of the endothelial cell.

ROLE OF PLATELETS IN TUMOR CELL METASTASIS AND GROWTH

Alterations in platelet number and function are well described in patients with neoplastic diseases. More significantly, these derangements may influence the local growth and metastatic spread of the tumor. Platelet counts are increased in 30% to 60% of patients with malignancies (14), although the absolute platelet count does not correlate with an increased risk for thrombotic events. In vitro studies, however, indicate that platelets may directly interact with the malignant cells.

Platelet–Tumor Cell Adhesion

Gasic et al. observed that tumor cells were able to aggregate platelets in vitro and that a reduction in platelet number reduced the efficiency of pulmonary metastases in a murine system (63); this was confirmed and extended by Pearlstein et al. (64). Human and xenogeneic tumor cell lines preferentially adhere to platelet monolayers and this adhesion is inhibited by the murine monoclonal antibody 10E5 or the peptide RGDS, reagents that interfere with the binding of von Willebrand factor (vWF), fibronectin, or fibrinogen to the platelet integrin GPIIb-IIIa receptor (65). In vivo experiments showed that the antimetastatic effect of thrombocytopenia induced by a murine antiplatelet antibody was transient (6 hours) and that it could be abrogated by infusion of human platelets (64). Thus the platelet requirement appears to be an early event on platelet–tumor–endothelial cell adhesion resulting in the retention of tumor cells within the vasculature via platelet–tumor thrombus formation. The prometastatic effect of these platelet transfusions could be reduced by 10E5 (65), and metastases could be inhibited by RGDS (66), the same reagents that reduced in vitro platelet–tumor adhesion. In addition, monospecific antimurine vWF inhibited experimental pulmonary metastases in the absence of thrombocytopenia (65). These experiments indicate that the GPIIb-IIIa receptor and its ligands on platelets interact with tumor cells and support their metastatic ability. Tumor cells may also possess GPIIb-IIIa-like integrins on their membranes, which permit binding to subendothelial adhesive ligands such as fibronectin, fibrin, or vWF (67–70). Indeed, both melanoma cell lines and melanoma biopsies (but not benign pigmented skin lesions) contained immunoreactive GPIIb-IIIa (69). This integrin was not detected on other tumor specimens, but it is likely that other integrin receptors for vitronectin or laminin may participate in tumor adhesion to the subendothelium or to platelets.

Role of Thrombin in Platelet–Tumor Cell Adhesion, Metastasis, and Tumor Growth

In addition to its participation in fibrin formation and protein C anticoagulant activation, thrombin can interact with its receptor on cell membranes and function as a platelet aggregation agonist or as a growth factor for fibroblasts, smooth muscle, endothelial and tumor cells (71–77). A cellular thrombin receptor has been cloned and identified as a member of the G-protein-coupled seven-transmembrane- spanning family of receptors. This receptor is unique because thrombin cleavage of its N-terminal portion between the amino acids arginine-serine at position 41–42 is required for receptor activation. This generates a tethered ligand that interacts with

the extracellular second loop of the receptor and initiates intracellular signaling. Peptides containing the sequences of the tethered ligand (thrombin receptor activation peptides, or TRAPs) have thrombin-like activity on platelets, smooth muscle cells, endothelial cells, and tumor cells (78–82).

Thrombin treatment of platelets activates GPIIb-IIIa avidity for ligands, induces the release of platelet fibronectin and vWF, and enhances platelet–tumor adhesion two- to fourfold (83). Thrombin treatment of tumor cells also increases their adhesion to platelets, endothelial cells, fibronectin, and vWF two- to threefold indicating the presence of a thrombin receptor on tumor cells (77). Thrombin treatment of tumor cells enhances the formation of pulmonary metastases following their intravenous injection into syngeneic mice 10- to 160-fold (77). These observations suggest that thrombin can function as a tumor growth promotor, either via enhanced adhesion to platelets and endothelial cells or by some other mechanism, e.g., the activation of tumor growth. This latter suggestion is supported by the observation that thrombin-treated murine CT26 and B16F10 cells enhance their in vivo metastatic growth despite absence of increased adhesion to platelets or fibronectin (77).

Binding of ^{125}I thrombin to tumor cell lines HM29 and SK-Mel-28 melanoma, and HeLa cervical CA, occurs in a saturation-dependent manner that is inhibitable with nonradiolabeled thrombin. These data indicate the presence of a thrombin receptor(s) on the human tumor cell lines (84). Treatment of human tumor cells with TRAP also stimulates their adhesion to platelets and fibronectin in vitro suggesting that the tumor cell thrombin receptor is of the seven- transmembrane-spanning family. This has been confirmed by reverse transcriptase–polymerase chain reaction (RT-PCR) analysis of thrombin receptor mRNA of six human tumors (82). TRAP (and by inference thrombin) may influence tumor cell growth by stimulation of tyrosine kinases. TRAP treatment of tumor cell lines induced changes in tyrosine phosphorylation in four of six tumor lines studied (82). In other cell lines thrombin treatment activates a variety of genes including urokinase-type plasminogen activator in PC-3 prostate cancer cells (85), platelet-derived growth factor and E-selectin in human umbilical endothelial cells (86), monocyte chemotactic factor in monocytic cells (87,88), atrial natriuretic factor in myocardium (89), tissue factor in endothelial cells (90), and the oncogene c-fos in endothelial cells (91) and the megakaryocytic cell line CHRF-288 (92).

These observations suggest that thrombin can regulate the growth of malignancies and that the aggressive growth of tumors associated with intravascular coagulation is an effect of the DIC and not its cause.

CONCLUSION

Thus, low-grade thrombin formation induced by TF activation of tumor cells (93–100) may be harmful to some patients with malignancies because it may predispose to metastatic progression of the lesion by enhancing tumor cell adhesion and/or tumor cell growth. This creates a vicious cycle in which greater tumor burden induces greater thrombin generation, which in turn enhances tumor adhesion, growth, and/or metastasis. Of interest is the observation that low-grade intravascular coagulation (thrombin generation) has been observed in most patients with solid tumors (101–103), with increasing severity with progression of disease. Persistent elevation was associated with a poor prognosis.

The thrombotic events seen in patients with malignant diseases are the result of multiple alterations in the physiologic mechanisms which regulate thrombosis and fibrinolysis. The intersection of many of these pathways on thrombin both as a product of multiple proteolytic pathways and an initiator of cell regulatory events gives support to the concept of its seminal importance in thrombosis associated with cancer as well as the induction of a metastatic phenotype. This understanding may lead to pharmacologic means of modulating thrombin activity not only as a procoagulant but as a mediator of tumor spread and growth.

REFERENCES

1. Trousseau A. *Phlegmasia alba dolens. Clinique Medicale de l'Hotel-Dieu de Paris*, vol 3. London: New Sydenham Society, 1865;94–105.
2. Edwards RL, Rickles FR, Moritz TE, et al. Abnormalities of blood coagulation tests in patients with cancer. *Am J Clin Pathol* 1987;88:596–602.
3. Stack GJ, Levin J, Bell WR. Trousseau's syndrome and other manifestations of chronic disseminated coagulopathy in patients with neoplasms: clinical, pathophysiologic, and therapuetic features. *Medicine* 1977;56:1–37.
4. Saeger W, Genzkow M. Venous thrombosis and pulmonary embolism in post-mortem series: probable cause by correlations of clinical data and basic diseases. *Pathol Res Pract* 1994. 190:394–9.
5. Bell WR, Starksen NF, Tong S, Porterfield JK. Trousseau's syndrome. Devastating coagulopathy in the absence of heparin. *Am J Med* 1985;79:423–430.
6. Prandoni P, Lensing AW, Buller HR, et al. Deep-vein thrombosis and the incidence of subsequent symptomatic cancer (see comments). *N Engl J Med* 1992;327:1128–1133.
7. Monreal M, Lafoz E, Casals A, et al. Occult cancer in patients with deep venous thrombosis. A systematic approach. *Cancer* 1991;67:541–545.
8. Aderka D, Brown A, Zelikovski A, Pinkhas J. Idiopathic deep vein thrombosis in an apparently healthy patient as a premonitory sign of occult cancer. *Cancer* 1986;57:1846–1849.
9. Schwartz RE, Marrero AM, Conlon KC, Burt M. Inferior vena cava filters in cancer patients: indications and outcome. *J Clin Oncol* 1996;4:652–657.
10. Levine M, Gent M, Hirsch J, et al. The thrombogenic effect of anticancer drug therapy in women with stage II breast cancer. *N Engl J Med* 1988;318:404–408.
11. Rogers JS, Murgo AJ, Fontana JA, Raich PC. Chemotherapy for breast cancer decreases plasma protein C and protein S. *J Clin Oncol* 1988;6:276–281.
12. Pritchard KI, Pater J, Paul N, et al. Thromboembolic complications related to chemotherapy in postmenopausal women with axillary node positive receptor positive breast cancer [Abstract]. *Proc ASCO* 1989;8:25.
13. Falanga A, Barburi T, Rickles FR, et al. Guidelines for clotting studies in caner patients. For the Scientific and Standardization Committee of the Subcommittee on Hemostasis and Malignancy International Society of Thrombosis and Hemostasis. *Thromb Haemost* 1993;70:540.
14. Rickles FR, Edwards RL. Activation of blood coagulation in cancer: Trousseau's syndrome revisited. *Blood* 1983;62:14.
15. Boehme MW, Deng Y, Raeth U, et al. Release of thrombomodulin from endothelial cells by concerted action of TNF-alpha and neutrophils: in vivo and in vitro studies. *Immunology* 1996;87:134–140.
16. Otterson GA, Monahan BP, Harold N, Steinberg SM, Frame JN, Kaye FJ. Clinical significance of the FV:Q506 mutation in unselected oncology patients. *Am J Med* 1996;01:406–412.
17. Edoute Y, Haim N, Rinkevich D, Brenner B, Reisner SA. Cardiac valvular vegetations in cancer patients: a prospective echocardiographic study of 200 patients. *Am J Med* 1997;102:252–258.

18. Rabinowe SN, Soiffer RJ, Tarbell NJ, et al. Hemolytic-uremic syndrome following bone marrow transplantation in adults for hematologic malignancies. *Blood* 1991;77:1837–1844.

19. Juckett M, Perry EH, Daniels BS, Weisdorf DJ. Hemolytic uremic syndrome following bone marrow transplantation. *Bone Marrow Transplant* 1991;7:405–409.

20. Zeigler ZR, Shadduck RK, Nemunaitis J, Andrews DF, Rosenfeld CS. Bone marrow transplant-associated thrombotic microangiopathy: a case series. *Bone Marrow Transplant* 1995;15:247–253.

21. Zeigler ZR, Rosenfeld CS, Andrews DF, et al. Plasma von Willebrand Factor Antigen (vWF:AG) and thrombomodulin (TM) levels in Adult Thrombotic Thrombocytopenic Purpura/Hemolytic Uremic Syndromes (TTP/HUS) and bone marrow transplant-associated thrombotic microangiopathy (BMT-TM). *Am J Hematol* 1996;53:213–220.

22. Charba D, Moake JL, Harris MA, Hester JP. Abnormalities of von Willebrand factor multimers in drug-associated thrombotic microangiopathies. *Am J Hematol* 1993;42:268–277.

23. Grace AA, Barradas MA, Mikhailidis DP, et al. Cyclosporine A enhances platelet aggregation. *Kidney Int* 1987;32:889–895.

24. Brown Z, Neild GH, Lewis GP. Mechanism of inhibition of prostacyclin synthesis by cyclosporine in cultured human umbilical vein endothelial cells. *Transplant Proc* 1988;20:654–657.

25. Shulman HM, Hinterberger W. Hepatic veno-occlusive disease—liver toxicity syndrome after bone marrow transplantation. *Bone Marrow Transplant* 1992;10:197–214.

26. Catani L, Gugliotta L, Mattioli Belmonte M, et al. Hypercoagulability in patients undergoing autologous or allogeneic BMT for hematological malignancies. *Bone Marrow Transplant* 1993;12:253–259.

27. Camerer E, Kolsto AB, Prydz H. Cell biology of tissue factor, the principal initiator of blood coagulation. *Thromb Res* 1996;81:1–41.

28. Rao LV. Tissue factor as a tumor procoagulant. *Cancer Metastasis Rev* 1992;11:249–266.

29. Schwager I, Jungi TW. Effect of human recombinant cytokines on the induction of macrophage procoagulant activity. *Blood* 1994;83:152–160.

30. Rickles FR, Hair GA, Zeff RA, Lee E, Bona RD. Tissue factor expression in human leukocytes and tumor cells. *Thromb Haemost* 1995;74:391–395.

31. Hair GA, Padula S, Zeff R, et al. Tissue factor expression in human leukemic cells (see comments). *Leukemia Res* 1996;20:1–11.

32. Contrino J, Hair GA, Schmeizl MA, Rickles FR, Kreutzer DL. In situ characterization of antigenic and functional tissue factor expression in human tumors utilizing monoclonal antibodies and recombinant factor VIIa as probes. *Am J Pathol* 1994;145:1315–1322.

33. Callander NS, Varki N, Rao LV. Immunohistochemical identification of tissue factor in solid tumors. *Cancer* 1992;70:1194–1201.

34. Asakura H, Kamikubo Y, Goto A, et al. Role of tissue factor in disseminated intravascular coagulation. *Thromb Res* 1995;80:217–224.

35. Carty N, Taylor I, Roath OS, el-Baruni K, Francis JL. Urinary tissue factor activity in malignancy. *Thromb Res* 1990;57:473–478.

36. Kakkar AK, DeRuvo N, Chinswangwatanakul V, Tebbutt S, Williamson RC. Extrinsic-pathway activation in cancer with high factor VIIa and tissue factor. *Lancet* 1995;346:1004–1005.

37. Zhang Y, Deng Y, Wendt T, et al. Intravenous somatic gene transfer with antisense tissue factor restores blood flow by reducing tumor necrosis factor–induced tissue factor expression and fibrin deposition in mouse meth-A sarcoma. *J Clin Invest* 1996;97:2213–2224.

38. Gordon SG, Franks JJ, Lewis B. Cancer procoagulant: a factor X activating procoagulant from malignant tissue. *Thromb Res* 1975;6:127–137.

39. Donati MB, Gambacorti-Passerini C, Casali B, et al. Cancer procoagulant in human tumor cells: evidence from melanoma patients. *Cancer Res* 1986;46:6471–6474.

40. Falanga A, Gordon SG. Isolation and characterization of cancer procoagulant: a cysteine proteinase from malignant tissue. *Biochemistry* 1985;24:5558–5567.

41. Colucci M, Delaini F, De Bellis Vitti G, Locati D, Poggi A. Warfarin inhibits both procoagulant activity and metastatic capacity of Lewis lung carcinoma cells. *Biochem Pharmacol* 1983;32:1689–1691.

42. Falanga A, Consonni R, Marchetti M, et al. Cancer procoagulant in the human promyelocytic cell line NB4 and its modulation by all-trans-retinoic acid. *Leukemia* 1994;8:156–159.

43. Dasmahapatra KS, Cheung NK, Spillert C, Lazaro E. An assessment of monocyte procoagulant activity in patients with solid tumors. *J Surg Res* 1987;43:158–163.

44. Morgan D, Edwards RL, Rickles FR. Monocyte procoagulant activity as a peripheral marker of clotting activation in cancer patients. *Haemostasis* 1988;18:55–65.

45. Cermak J, Key NS, Bach RR, Balla J, Jacob HS, Vercellotti GM. C-reactive protein induces human peripheral blood monocytes to synthesize tissue factor. *Blood* 1993;82:513–520.

46. Plescia J, Altieri DC. Activation of Mac-1 (CD11b/CD18)-bound factor X by released cathepsin G defines an alternative pathway of leucocyte initiation of coagulation. *Biochem J* 1996;319:873–879.

47. Simon DI, Rao NK, Xu H, et al. Mac-1 (CD11b/CD18) and the urokinase receptor (CD87) form a functional unit on monocytic cells. *Blood* 1996;88:3185–3194.

48. Lacraz S, Isler P, Vey E, Welgus HG, Dayer JM. Direct contact between T lymphocytes and monocytes is a major pathway for induction of metalloproteinase expression. *J Biol Chem* 1994;269:22027–22033.

49. Malik N, Greenfield BW, Wahl AF, Kiener PA. Activation of human monocytes through CD40 induces matrix metalloproteinases. *J Immunol* 1996;156:3952–3960.

50. McGeehan GM, Becherer JD, Bast RC Jr, et al. Regulation of tumour necrosis factor-alpha processing by a metalloproteinase inhibitor. *Nature* 1994;370:558–561.

51. Zhang Y, DeWitt DL, McNeely TB, Wahl SM, Wahl LM. Secretory leukocyte protease inhibitor suppresses the production of monocyte prostaglandin H synthase-2, prostaglandin E2, and matrix metalloproteinases. *J Clin Invest* 1997;99:894–900.

52. Swallow CJ, Murray MP, Guillem JG. Metastatic colorectal cancer cells induce matrix metalloproteinase release by human monocytes. *Clin Exp Metast* 1996;14:3–11.

53. Kossakowska AE, Huchcroft SA, Urbanski SJ, Edwards DR. Comparative analysis of the expression patterns of metalloproteinases and their inhibitors in breast neoplasia, sporadic colorectal neoplasia, pulmonary carcinomas and malignant non-Hodgkin's lymphomas in humans. *Br J Cancer* 1996;73:1401–1408.

54. Lee E, Grodzinsky AJ, Libby P, Clinton SK, Lark MW, Lee RT. Human vascular smooth muscle cell-monocyte interactions and metalloproteinase secretion in culture. *Arterioscl Thromb Vasc Biol* 1995;15:2284–2289.

55. Cabre F, Tost D, Suesa N, et al. Synthesis and release of platelet-activating factor and eicosanoids in human endothelial cells induced by different agonists. *Agents and Actions* 1993;38:212–219.

56. Sporn LA, Marder VJ, Wagner DD. Inducible secretion of large, biologically potent von Willebrand factor multimers. *Cell* 1986;46:185–193.

57. Esmon CT. The role of protein C and thrombomodulin in the regulation of blood coagulation. *J Biol Chem* 1989;264:4347–4350.

58. Sterner-Kock A, Braun RK, Schrenzel MD, Hyde DM. Recombinant tumour necrosis factor-alpha and platelet-activating factor synergistically increase intercellular adhesion molecule-1 and E-selectin dependent neutrophil adherence to endothelium in vitro. *Immunology* 1996;87:454–460.

59. Lo SK, Cheung A, Zheng Q, Silverstein RL. Induction of tissue factor on monocytes by adhesion to endothelial cells. *J Immunol* 1995;154:4768–4777.

60. Martin NB, Jamieson A, Tuffin DP. The effect of interleukin-4 on tumour necrosis factor-alpha induced expression of tissue factor and plasminogen activator inhibitor-1 in human umbilical vein endothelial cells. *Thromb Haemost* 1993;70:296–301.

61. Schmid E, Muller TH, Budzinski RM, Binder K, Pfizenmaier K. Signalling by E-selectin and ICAM-1 induces endothelial tissue factor production via autocrine secretion of platelet-activating factor and tumor necrosis factor alpha. *J Interferon Cytokine Res* 1995;15:819–25.

62. Ishibashi M, Ito N, Fujita M, Furue H, Yamaji T. Endothelin-1 as an aggravating factor of disseminated intravascular coagulation associated with malignant neoplasms. *Cancer* 1994;73:191–195.

63. Gasic GJ, Gasic TF, Stewart CC. Antimetastatic effects associated with platelet reduction. *Proc Natl Acad Sci USA* 1968;61:46–52.

64. Pearlstein E, Ambrogio C, Karpatkin S. Effect of antiplatelet antibody on the development of pulmonary metastases following injection of CT26 colon adenocarcinoma, Lewis lung carcinoma, and B16 amelanotic melanoma tumor cells into mice. *Cancer Res* 1984;44:3884–3887.

65. Karpatkin S, Pearlstein E, Ambrogio C, Coller BS. Role of adhesive proteins in platelet tumor interaction in vitro and metastasis formation in vivo. *J Clin Invest* 1988;81:1012–1019.

66. Humphries MJ, Olden K, Yamada KM. A synthetic peptide from fibronectin inhibits experimental metastases of murine melanoma cells. *Science* 1986;467:467–470.

67. Boukerche H, Berthier-Vergnes O, Tabone E, et al. Platelet melanoma cell interaction is mediated by the glycoprotein IIb-IIIa complex. *Blood* 1989;74:658–663.

68. Grossi IM, Hatfield JS, Fitzgerald LA, et al. Role of tumor cell glycoproteins immunologically related to glycoproteins Ib and IIb/IIIa in tumor cell-platelet and tumor cell-matrix interactions. *FASEB J* 1988;2:2385–2395.

69. McGregor BC, McGregor JL, Weiss LM. Presence of cytoadhesions (IIb-IIIa-like glycoproteins) on human metastatic melanomas but not on benign melanocytes. *Am J Clin Pathol* 1989;92:495–499.

70. Boukerche H, Berthier-Vergues O, Bailly JF. A monoclonal antibody against the blood platelet glycoprotein IIb/IIIa complex inhibits human melanoma growth in vivo. *Blood* 1989;74:909–912.

71. Chen LB, Buchanan JM. Mitogenic activity of blood components. I. Thrombin and prothrombin. *Proc Natl Acad Sci USA* 1975;72:131–135.

72. Carney DH, Glenn KC, Cunningham DD. Conditions which affect initiation of animal cell division by trypsin and thrombin. *J Cell Physiol* 1978;95:13–22.

73. Carney DH, Stiemberg J, Fenton JW. Initiation of proliferative events by human a-thrombin requires both receptor binding and enzymic activity. *J Cellular Biochem* 1984;26:181–195.

74. Glenn KC, Carney DH, Fenton JW, et al. Thrombin active site regions required for fibroblast receptor binding and initiation of cell division. *J Biol Chem* 1980;255:6609–6616.

75. Morris DL, Ward JB, Carney DH. Thrombin promotes cell transformation in Balb 3T3/A31-1-13 cells. *Carcinogenesis (Lond.)* 1992;13:67–73.

76. McNamara CA, Sarembok IJ, Gimple LW. Thrombin stimulation of smooth muscle cell proliferation is mediated by a proteolytic, receptor-mediated mechanism. *J Clin Invest* 1992;91:94–98.

77. Nierodzik ML, Kajumo F, Karpatkin S. Effect of thrombin treatment of tumor cells on adhesion of tumor cells to platelets in vitro and tumor metastasis in vivo. *Cancer Res* 1992;52:3267–3272.

78. Vu T-KH, Hung DT, Wheaton VI, Coughlin SR. Molecular cloning of a functional thrombin receptor reveals a novel proteolytic mechanism of receptor activation. *Cell* 1991;64:1057–1068.

79. Ngaiza JR, Jaffe EA. A 14 amino acid peptide derived from the amino terminus of the cleaved thrombin receptor elevates intracellular calcium and stimulates prostacyclin production in human endothelial cells. *Biochem Biophys Res Commun* 1991;179:1656–1661.

80. Vassallo RR, Kieber-Emmons T, Chichowski K, Brass LF. Structure–function relationships in the activation of platelet thrombin receptors by receptor-derived peptides. *J Biol Chem* 1992;27:6081–6085.

81. Zhong C, Hayzer DJ, Corson M, Runge MS. Molecular cloning of the rat smooth muscle thrombin receptor:evidence for in vitro regulation by basic fibroblast growth factor. *J Biol Chem* 1992;267:16975–16979.

82. Nierodzik ML, Bain RM, Liu L-X, Shivji M, Takeshita K, Karpatkin S. Presence of the seven transmembrane thrombin receptor on human tumour cells: effect of activation on tumour adhesion to platelets and tumor tyrosine phosphorylation. *Br J Haematol* 1996;92:452–457.

83. Nierodzik ML, Plotkin A, Kajumo F, et al. Thrombin stimulates tumor-platelet adhesion in vitro and metastasis in vivo. *J Clin Invest* 1991;87:229–236.

84. Klepfish A, Greco MA, Karpatkin S. Thrombin stimulates melanoma tumor-cell binding to endothelial cells and subendothelial matrix. *Int J Cancer* 1993; 53:978–982.

85. Yoshida E, Verrusio EN, Mihara H, Oh D, Kwann HC. Enhancement of the expression of urokinase-type plasminogen activator from PC-3 human prostate cancer cells by thrombin. *Cancer Res* 1994;54:3300–3306.

86. Shankar R, de la Motte CA, Poptic EJ, DiCorleto PE. Thrombin receptor-activating peptides differentially stimulate platelet-derived growth factor production, monocytic cell adhesion, and E.-selectin expression in human umbilical vein endothelial cells. *J Biol Chem* 1994;269:13936–13942.

87. Colotta F, Sciacca FL, Sironi M, Liuni W, Rabiet MJ, Mantovani A. Expression of monocyte chemotactic protein-1 by monocytes and endothelial cells exposed to thrombin. *Am J Pathol* 1994;144:975–981.

88. Grandaliano G, Valente AJ, Abboud HE. A novel biologic activity of thrombin: stimulation of monocyte chemotactic protein production. *J Exp Med* 1994;179: 1737–1746.

89. Glembotski CC, Irons CE, Krown KA, Murray SF, Sprenkle AB, Sei CA. Myocardial alpha-thrombin receptor activation induces hypertrophy and increases atrial natriuretic factor gene expression. *J Biol Chem* 1993;268:20646–20652.

90. Bartha K, Brisson C, Archipoff G, et al. Thrombin regulates tissue factor and thrombomodulin mRNA levels and activities in human saphenous vein endothelial cells by distinct mechanisms. *J Biol Chem* 1993;268:421–427.

91. Lampugnani MG, Lolotta F, Polentarutti N, et al. Thrombin induces c-fos expression in cultured human endothelial cells by a Ca++ dependent mechanism. *Blood* 1990;76:1173–1180.

92. Dorn GW, Davis MG. Thrombin, but not thromboxane, stimulates megakaryocytic differentiation in human megakaryoblastic leukemia cells. *J Pharmacol Exp Ther* 1992;262:1242–1247.

93. Lerner WA, Pearlstein E, Ambrogio C, et al. A new mechanism for tumor-induced platelet aggregation: comparison with mechanism shared by other tumors with possible pharmacologic strategy toward prevention of metastases. *Int J Cancer* 1983;31:463–469.

94. Bastida E, Ordinas A, Escolar G, et al. Tissue factor in microvesicles shed from U87 MG human glioblastoma cells induces coagulation, platelet aggregation and thrombogenesis. *Blood* 1984;64:177–184.

95. Dvorak HF, Van deWater L, Bitzer AM, et al. Procoagulant activity associated with plasma membrane vesicles shed by cultured tumor cells. *Cancer Res* 1983; 43:4334–4342.

96. Gordon SG, Cross BA. A factor X-activating cysteine protease from malignant tissue. *J Clin Invest* 1981;67: 1665–1671.

97. Honn KV, Sloane BF, Cavanaugh PG. Role of the coagulation system in tumor-cell-induced platelet aggregation and metastasis. *Haemostasis* 1988;18:37–46.

98. Kadish JL, Wenc KM, Dvorak HF. Tissue factor activity of normal and neoplastic cells: quantitation and species specificity. *JNCI* 1983;70:551–557.

99. Pearlstein E, Ambrogio C, Gasic G. Inhibition of the platelet aggregating activity of two human adenocarcinomas of the colon and an anaplastic murine tumor with a specific thrombin inhibitor: dansylarginine N(3-ethyl-1,5-pentanediyl)amide. *Cancer Res* 1981;41:4535–4539.

100. Curatolo L, Colucci M, Cambini AL, et al. Evidence that cells from experimental tumors can activate coagulation factor X. *Br J Cancer* 1979;40:228–233.

101. Merskey C, Johnson AJ, Harris JU, et al. Isolation of fibrinogen-fibrin related antigen from human plasma by immune-affinity chromatography: its characterization in normal sujects and in defibrinating patients wtih abruptio placentae and disseminated cancer. *Br J Haematol* 1980;44:655–670.

102. Peuscher FW, Cleton FJ, Amstrong L, et al. Significance of plasma fibrinopeptide A (FPA) in patients with malignancy. *J Lab Clin Med* 1980;96:5–14.

103. Rickles FR, Edwards RC, Barb C, et al. Abnormalities of blood coagulation in patients with cancer: fibrinopeptide A generation and tumor growth. *Cancer* 1983; 51:301–307.

*Cardiovascular Thrombosis: Thrombocardiology
and Thromboneurology, Second Edition,*
edited by M. Verstraete, V. Fuster, and E. J. Topol,
Lippincott–Raven Publishers, Philadelphia © 1998.

45

Hemostasis and Solid Organ Transplantation

Beverley J. Hunt, *Sudhir S. Kushwaha, and †Magdi H. Yacoub

*Department of Cardiothoracic Surgery, National Heart and Lung Institute,
Imperial College School of Medicine, London SE1 7EH, United Kingdom;
*Department of Cardiology, Mount Sinai Medical Center, New York, New York 10029; and
†Department of Cardiothoracic Surgery, National Heart and Lung Institute, Harefield Hospital,
Harefield, Middlesex UB9 6JH, United Kingdom*

Transplantation is one of the major medical successes of the end of the twentieth century. It is widely accepted as effective management of end-stage organ failure for the liver, kidney, heart, and lungs. Today the overall 1-year survival of cardiac transplant recipients is nearly 90% and 5-year survival of 50% with a return to near-normal quality of life (1). However, the scarcity of donor organs means that only about 300 heart transplants are performed annually in Britain. In the United States approximately 17,000 persons per year under the age of 55 could benefit from cardiac transplantation, but no more than 2,200 viable donor hearts are available per year (2). The worldwide shortage in donor organs has led to a scientific interest in xenotransplantation.

There are residual problems in transplantation. If transplantation is to realize its potential in the third millennium, then it is essential that these problems be addressed. Many of the early and late problems are partly or entirely due to hemostatic abnormalities. In this chapter the hemostatic aspects of solid organ transplantation will be discussed.

PERIOPERATIVE BLEEDING

Kidney transplantation does not appear to involve any excessive morbidity and mortality above that of operating on any patient with end-stage renal failure. The use of liver transplantation, however, produces a unique bleeding diathesis (3).

Liver Transplantation

Preexisting liver disease alters the hemostatic balance by reduced production of hemostatic proteins and impaired clearance of activated hemostatic factors. Other abnormalities secondary to cirrhosis exist, including thrombocytopenia with decreased platelet function and functionally abnormal fibrinogen. During orthotopic liver transplantation a further complication ensues: hyperfibrinolysis. This is caused by the presence of excessive tissue plasminogen activator (t-PA) and urokinase (4). Usually t-PA is inhibited by complex formation with plasminogen activator inhibitor-1 (PAI-1) with subnormal levels of antiplasmin. The t-PA and t-PA/PAI-1 complexes are rapidly cleared from the blood by a normal liver with a plasma half-life of 3 to 5 minutes. Thus high levels of t-PA and u-PA are found in liver failure and notably during the anhepatic phase of liver transplantation, with extremely high levels at the time of reperfusion of the donor liver (4). This may relate to plasminogen activator release from the perturbed donor liver endothelial cells caused by hypoxia and acidosis. The contact system can also contribute to activation of fibrinolysis but there is little activation of this during orthotopic liver transplantation (5). There is evidence to suggest that the cause of liver failure will alter the patients hemostatic response during orthotopic liver transplantation; for in primary biliary cirrhosis there is better preservation of coagulation proteins (6). Perioperatively during liver transplantation in patients with primary biliary cirrhosis there is greater thrombin generation and less fibrinolysis, again suggesting that these patients are more prothrombotic than others (6).

Aprotinin (Trasylol), a powerful antifibrinolytic with possible platelet preservative effects, is widely prescribed perioperatively in liver transplantation in a high-dose regimen to ameliorate hyperfibrinolysis and reduce bleeding (7,8). The major antifibrinolytic effects of aprotinin during orthotopic liver transplantation are as an antiplasmin agent. Aprotinin may also inhibit t-PA release but has no effect on urokinase release (4). High concentrations of plasmin-generated fibrinogen degradation products (FDPs) have been shown to inhibit platelet function (9). By inhibiting plasmin and therefore reducing FDP levels, aprotinin may thus prevent inhibition of platelet function and thereby have a platelet preservative effect.

Heart and/or Lung Transplantation

Heart transplantation (HT), heart and lung transplantation (HLT), and lung transplantation (LH) necessitate the use of cardiopulmonary bypass and are associated with a hemorrhagic tendency. Cardiopulmonary bypass requires the use of heparin, induces hemodilution and activation of fibrinolysis, and produces thrombocytopenia and platelet function abnormalities (10). Whether during heart and/or lung transplantation there are additional or pronounced hemostatic changes above those normally seen during open cardiac surgery is not known and requires further study. Certainly the prolonged period of time on cardiopulmonary bypass required for some cases will exacerbate the hemostatic changes. Blood component usage during HT and HLT is greater than simpler open cardiac surgery (11). A retrospective study of 172 heart transplants at Harefield revealed the use of a median (interquartile range) of 12 (8 to 20) units of blood components of which 6 (4 to 8) constituted red cell components. In 1989 50 HLTs required a median of 18 (9 to 29) units of blood components of which 8 (5 to 11) were red cell components. As expected, those who have had previous cardiac surgery and/or previous transplantation required more blood. The highest risk of operative mortality occurred in patients with a previous thoracic operation and pleural adhesions (12). Perioperative bleeding from the posterior mediastinum, especially in Eisenmenger's syndrome, due to more prominent posterior mediastinal collaterals can leave large raw areas in which it is difficult to secure surgical hemostasis. The use of fibrin glue in combination with improved surgical techniques reduces blood loss (13). Aprotinin (Trasylol) used perioperatively whether in low-dose or high-dose regimen (2 million kIU given to the patient prior to cardiopulmonary bypass, 2 million kIU into the bypass equipment, and 500,000 kIU/hour) significantly reduces bleeding and the use of blood components (14–16). Even with the low-dose aprotinin 70% of patients treated with aprotinin underwent transplantation without the need of nonautologous blood compared with only 30% in the control group. Tranexamic acid given as an infusion perioperatively (17) also reduces bleeding during cardiopulmonary bypass, but there are as yet no published reports of its use during transplant operations.

HEMOSTASIS DURING ACUTE REJECTION

The main emphasis in transplantation research has been placed on immunologic mechanisms in graft rejection. There have been few studies of hemostasis until the recent explosion of interest in a special form of rejection, i.e., the hyperacute rejection seen in xenotransplantation. Hyperacute rejection is due to rejection mediated by preformed antibody, binding to antigen, activating complement, and initiating intravascular thrombosis. The classic example is the mistaken use of a donor organ that is blood group A in a group B recipient. The recipient's plasma contains anti-A antibodies that bind to endothelial A antigen, and the donor organ will be rejected within minutes. Histology of the donor organ shows generalized microvascular thrombosis. This is discussed below in the section on xenotransplantation.

Acute allograft rejection involves activation of cell-mediated response mainly through T lymphocytes. Early studies of coagulation during acute allograft rejection showed no significant changes in levels of fibrinogen, thrombin, factor V, or platelets (18).

A blood marker of acute rejection has remained elusive in solid organ transplantation and so histology of a biopsy of donor tissue remains the gold standard for diagnosing acute rejection. Many of the marker studied including levels of soluble leukocyte adhesion molecules fail to discriminate between rejection and infection, for they increase in both. This suggests that endothelial cell activation

and/or damage is occurring. We have therefore studied another product of endothelial cells in plasma—von Willebrand factor (vWF)—serially with C-reactive protein (CRP) levels during rejection episodes in heart transplant recipients (HTRs) (19). During moderate or severe rejection there was a significant increment in levels of vWF and CRP. However similar to other endothelial cell markers such as vascular-cellular adhesion molecules (VCAM), there was also an increment of vWF during systemic cytomegalovirus infections. A simultaneous increment of CRP suggested that part of the rise of vWF may be due to an acute phase response.

Decreased fibrinolytic potential has been described during acute rejection episodes in renal transplant recipients (20). Otherwise there are few recent studies of hemostatic changes during acute rejection; instead research has concentrated on accelerated coronary artery disease, which is probably an expression of chronic rejection.

CHRONIC GRAFT VASCULOPATHY

A chronic vasculopathy can occur after any solid organ transplant. It of most concern after heart transplantation where it limits long-term survival. Thus most research in this area has concentrated on the vasculopathy after heart transplantation which is also known as accelerated coronary artery disease (ACAD) within the donor heart, occurring as early as 3 months after transplantation (20). It affects 6% of the Harefield cardiac transplant recipients at 1 year and progresses to a prevalence of 17% after 3 years. Other centers have reported an incidence of 18% at 1 year and 44% at 3 years (21). It accounts for 40% of all deaths or retransplants in cardiac transplant recipients (21,22).

There are many similarities between naturally occurring atheroma and ACAD, although the latter tends to affect the coronary arteries concentrically rather than occurring as plaques only in medium and large vessels. There is diffuse, concentric intimal proliferation that may be present as early as 1 week after transplantation (23,24). In most cases the internal elastic lamina of the coronary vessels remains intact except for small breaks, whereas the asymmetric plaques of nontransplant atheroma usually contain calcium and disrupt the lamina. ACAD is confined to the allograft tissue and involves not only the great arteries but, unusually, the veins (23). The angiographic appearance usually reveals a mixture of focal atherosclerotic lesions, as well as diffuse and concentric narrowing of coronary vessels, with tapering and pruning are common in the secondary and tertiary branches. Complete obstruction of coronary arteries occurs in the advanced stages of the disease, and there is a striking lack of collateral blood vessel development. Serial angiograms remain the standard for detection of ACAD, although more recently intravascular echo has been used to diagnose ACAD through quantifying of the degree of intimal thickening (25).

Regular screening is important because the patients have denervated hearts and thus do not have angina. The first clinical event as a consequence of the disease may be sudden death.

There is a consensus that in ACAD, similar to Ross's hypothesis for nontransplant atherosclerosis (26), damage to the endothelium is the initial event and it is mediated by immune mechanisms. This is supported by the limitation of the lesions to the transplanted organ and the presence of peptide-specific antiendothelial antibodies in heart transplant recipients with ACAD (27), the presence of T cells in the atherosclerotic lesions (28), and improved survival with improved HLA matching (29).

Although these two types of atheroma are purported to have different initiating factors, the progression of atheroma may be influenced by some of the same factors, such as hyperlipidemia (30). Thus we hypothesized that prothrombotic changes may influence progression as occurs in nontransplant atheroma (31) because fibrin deposition occurs in ACAD (20). The deposition of fibrin in transplanted hearts has been associated with the loss of thrombomodulin and an-

tithrombin III from overlying endothelium. Loss of thrombomodulin alone was associated with cellular rejection. Endothelium is coated with antithrombin III bound to heparan sulfate proteoglycan molecules that bind and inactivate thrombin. This endothelial antithrombin III is lost during vascular rejection (32).

A proposed hypothesis of these interactions is shown in Fig. 45-1 (see below). As indicated in the diagram, the host-versus-graft immune response (by the production of acute phase response cytokines such as IL-6) will produce prothrombotic changes, as will the use of prednisolone and possibly cyclosporin.

We conducted a large cross-sectional study of coagulation and fibrinolysis in 115 clinically stable heart transplant recipients who were 1 year or more post transplantation. The majority were receiving cyclosporin and azathioprine immunosuppression alone. They were compared with an age-matched group of patients with stable ischemic heart disease (IHD) and healthy controls. The results are shown in Table 45-1.

Prothrombotic hemostatic changes including increases in acute phase proteins such as fibrinogen and antithrombin III and decreased fibrinolytic potential occur postoperatively and during acute rejection episodes, as described in renal transplant recipients (20). This study therefore excluded samples from immediate post-transplantation patients and

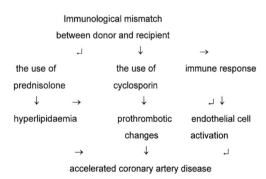

FIG. 45-1. A proposed pathogenesis of accelerated coronary artery disease in heart transplant recipients. (From Hunt et al., ref. 31, with permission.)

TABLE 45-1. *Levels of hemostatic proteins in heart transplant recipients as compared to healthy controls and those with stable ischemic heart disease*

Variables	Controls (n = 23)	Ischemic heart disease (n = 21)	Heart transplant recipients (n = 115)	Significance
Fibrinogen, Clauss (g/L)	3.03 (2.82–3.24)	3.17 (2.97–3.37)	3.70 (3.59–3.81)	p = 0.001
Fibrinogen, clot opacity (g/L)	3.47 (3.07–3.87)	4.00 (3.58–4.42)	4.50 (4.32–4.68)	p = 0.001
Prothrombin (IU/ml)	1.05 (1.00–1.11)	1.09 (1.03–1.15)	1.06 (1.04–1.09)	p = 0.66
Factor V (IU/ml)	0.96 (0.88–1.04)	0.97 (0.89–1.06)	0.95 (0.89–0.99)	p = 0.88
Factor VII (IU/ml)	0.99 (0.89–1.10)	1.03 (0.92–1.14)	1.16 (1.12–1.21)	p = 0.003
Factor VIII (IU/ml)	0.98 (0.81–1.16)	0.91 (0.72–1.09)	1.06 (0.98–1.13)	p = 0.29
Factor IX (IU/ml)	1.04 (0.92–1.16)	1.16 (1.04–1.28)	1.01 (0.95–1.06)	p = 0.07
Factor X (IU/ml)	1.03 (0.97–1.10)	1.06 (0.99–1.12)	1.11 (1.08–1.14)	p = 0.07
wWF antigen (IU/ml)	1.00 (0.80–1.26)	1.13 (0.92–1.41)	1.72 (1.58–1.88)	p = 0.001
C-reactive protein (U/ml)	6.54 (5.09–7.99)	15.9 (14.4–17.4)	7.67 (6.49–8.85)	p = 0.002
Interleukin-6 (pg/ml)	1.3 (0.02–0.67)	1.67 (0.37–2.97)	1.59 (0.44–2.74)	p = 0.44
Antithrombin III (IU/ml)	0.93 (0.82–1.05)	1.02 (0.90–1.15)	1.15 (1.10–1.20)	p = 0.002
Protein C activity (U/ml)	1.04 (0.91–1.17)	1.30 (1.14–1.46)	1.33 (1.23–1.43)	p = 0.002
Protein C antigen (U/ml)	0.99 (0.79–1.18)	1.57 (1.32–1.81)	1.15 (1.01–1.29)	p = 0.001
Protein S, free (U/ml)	1.01 (0.91–1.11)	0.99 (0.87–1.12)	0.97 (0.90–1.05)	p = 0.8
Protein S, total (U/ml)	1.09 (0.99–1.19)	0.86 (0.73–0.99)	0.82 (0.77–0.89)	p = 0.001
Euglobulin clot lysis time (min)	265 (56.2)	360 (86.2)	360 (83.6)	p = 0.008
t-PA antigen (ng/ml)	4.70 (3.50–5.90)	7.34 (6.13–8.55)	7.54 (6.42–8.66)	p = 0.001
PAI activity (IU/ml)	6.8 (5.4–8.2)	7.7 (6.3–9.2)	9.3 (8.1–10.5)	p = 0.076
Plasminogen (IU/ml)	1.1 (1.03–1.18)	1.03 (0.95–1.11)	1.10 (1.06–1.13)	p = 0.24
α_2-Antiplasmin (IU/ml)	1.1 (1.05–1.16)	1.17 (1.11–1.23)	1.12 (1.09–1.14)	p = 0.19

Results are expressed as means (95% confidence limits), except for euglobulin clot lysis time, for which medians (range) are shown.

those with an acute rejection episode within the previous three months.

Coagulation

Changes are characterized by significantly increased levels of fibrinogen, factor VII, and factor VIII. Stepwise discriminant analysis of the three groups (heart transplant recipients, those with ischemic heart disease, and controls) using the various hemostatic variables showed that fibrinogen was the best discriminator, correctly classifying 55.6% of HTRs, 40% of IHD, and 66.7% of controls. This increase in fibrinogen levels may not reflect an acute phase response in view of normal C-reactive protein and IL-6 levels. Epidemiologic studies have shown that fibrinogen levels are independent risk predictors for nontransplant coronary artery disease and that they correlate with the extent of atheromatous coronary artery disease (see Chapter 5). It is thus interesting to find that in transplant recipients fibrinogen levels are the best discriminators of accelerated coronary artery disease. Simi-

larly, factor VII levels and, to a lesser extent, the other vitamin K–dependent factors, II, IX, and X, are less strong predictors of the complications of primary atherosclerosis and accelerated coronary disease (see Chapter 5). Thus the pattern of changes in coagulation factors is similar in transplant and nontransplant atherosclerosis. Whether in this relationship the changes in coagulation factors are causal or reactive is not clear in transplant-related coronary artery disease (or, indeed, in non- transplant coronary artery disease).

Physiologic Anticoagulants

Antithrombin III and protein C levels are increased whereas protein S levels are reduced after heart transplantation. These proteins are altered by acute phase response but the normal levels of CRP and interleukin-6 levels suggest that these changes were not related to an inflammatory or acute phase response. Increased levels of antithrombin III and protein C activity have also been found in renal transplant recipients (33,34). Antithrombin III levels were increased in all heart transplant recipients, whereas protein C increases were confined to the group transplanted for ischemic heart disease, suggesting that the increases in antithrombin III were a posttransplant phenomenon related perhaps to the use of immunosuppressants. Increased plasma antithrombin III levels are surprisingly associated with the development of atheromatous heart disease (35), but the nature of this relationship is far from clear.

Fibrinolysis

Fibrinolytic activity was poor in those transplanted for ischemic heart disease compared with those transplanted for other causes, with increased levels of t-PA and non-significantly increased levels of PAI-1, suggesting that there was an increase in both t-PA and PAI-1 but with a net increase in PAI-1 production as associated with nontransplant atheroma (36,37). The increase in both t-PA antigen and PAI activity suggests that the decrease in fibrinolytic activity was probably due to a net increase in PAI-1 production as occurs in non-transplant atherosclerosis. Plasminogen and α_2-antiplasmin levels were not significantly different in either groups.

Decreased fibrinolysis as measured by the hemostatometer (38) has been seen in renal transplant recipients and attributed to the use of cyclosporin and prednisolone. The recent cloning of the PAI-1 gene has demonstrated a glucocorticoid sensitive enhancer element (39), suggesting that the poor fibrinolysis seen in renal transplant recipients was possibly related to prednisolone stimulating PAI-1 production and thus cyclosporin may have no detrimental effect on fibrinolysis.

In normal hearts and stable cardiac allografts t-PA is present in the vascular smooth muscle of arteries and arterioles. Biopsies of failing cardiac allografts have shown depletion of t-PA from these smooth muscle cells (40) and accelerated coronary artery disease develops in many of the grafts. A recent study examined the biopsies from HTRs to assess t-PA by immunocytochemistry (41) and correlated this with angiographic evidence of coronary artery disease. It showed that grafts with early depletion of t-PA showed subsequent angiographic evidence of accelerated coronary artery disease. Moreover, the depletion of t-PA was associated with earlier and more severe disease as well as decreased graft survival.

Patients with accelerated coronary artery disease show a tendency for all coagulation factor levels to be higher; this reached significance for factor IX. Factor IX has not been identified as a factor that has a firm relationship with the development with coronary artery disease. One possible explanation of the increased level of factor IX is that these patients have increased turnover of hemostasis and thus increased generation of thrombin and prothrombin activation peptides. In the rabbit, the prothrombin activation peptide has been shown to regulate the synthesis of vitamin K–dependent proteins (42), such as factor IX. It would be interesting to measure prothrombin fragment$_{1+2}$ levels in the transplant recipients.

Platelets

De Lorgil et al. have shown that platelets of heart transplant recipients exhibited a marked platelet hyperaggregability to adenosine diphosphate as compared to controls and that the secondary wave of ADP-mediated platelet aggregation was not significantly inhibited by the use of aspirin 250 mg daily unlike nontransplant patients (43). In multiple regression analysis, ADP-induced platelet aggregation was positively related to glucose and inversely related to *n*-3 fatty acids from platelet phospholipids (44). Similar changes have been described in renal transplant recipients (45,46). This supports the hypothesis that a generalized platelet disorder occurs after transplantation, regardless of the type of organ transplanted and whether cyclosporin is used. The same group found that in those patients who died or required retransplantation the majority had multiple thrombi in the coronary tree and these patients had previously shown enhanced ex vivo platelet aggregability (47).

Lipoprotein (a)

Lipoprotein (a) consists of one or two molecules of a glycoprotein called apolipoprotein (a) bound to a lipid -apoB100 by a disulfide bridge. Interest in lipoprotein (a) was stimulated by the discovery that there was a striking homology between the DNA sequence of apolipoprotein (a) and plasminogen (48). The apo(a) molecule is composed of an N-terminal variable repeat of the plasminogen kringle IV (a kringle is named after a Danish cake, the shape of which it resembles), a single kringle, and the plasminogen protease domain. This suggested that lipoprotein (a) might have a prothrombotic role by interfering with the numerous physiologic functions of plasminogen. In vitro lipoprotein (a) in physiologic concentrations can inhibit the binding of plasminogen to its endothelial receptor by 25%, thus reducing its activation (49). It can also bind directly to fibrin, blocking the thrombolytic effects of plasmin (48). Indeed, in a number of studies, Smith (50) has shown that Lp(a) colocalizes with fibrin(ogen) and may thus inhibit fibrinolysis. Moreover, induction by Lp(a) of plasminogen activator inhibitor–1 in endothelial cells could also contribute to thrombogenesis (51). Such effects are difficult to study in vivo, and firm evidence of an in vivo effect are still lacking.

We have found that lipoprotein (a) levels are increased after transplantation (Table 45-2) and also an increased concentration of serum Lp(a) is an important and independent risk factor for the development of accelerated coronary artery disease (52).

Although a cross-sectional study suggested that the use of cyclosporin may increase lipoprotein (a) levels (53), a longitudinal study by Farmer et al. (54) suggested that lipoprotein (a) concentrations can fall after transplantation. Our own observations from a prospective study in heart and/or lung transplant recipients suggest that cyclosporin does not affect lipoprotein (a) concentrations for up to 6 months after transplantation (Table 45- 3) (55).

Lipoprotein (a) is a risk factor for arterial atheromatous disease, including coronary artery disease and restenosis after angioplasty (56), and is a particularly strong risk factor in young patients with cardiovascular disease and in those who also have elevated low-density lipoprotein (LDL) levels (57,58). Thus, in populations with high total cholesterol and LDL levels such as the cardiac transplant recipients, Lp(a) levels are more critical than those with normal lipid levels. In a group of 115 patients with familial hypercholesterolemia selected from two London lipid clinics, Lp(a) was found to be the most important risk factor in multivariate analysis (59). Thus, the finding that lipoprotein (a) levels are increased in cardiac transplant recipients who tend to have increased levels of LDL, suggests that close attention to lipid lowering therapy is required in this group.

Effect of Indication for Transplantation

Many of transplant recipients were transplanted for IHD and therefore probably had preexisting prothrombotic changes, which may explain some of the changes seen. Those transplanted for IHD showed a trend of having higher levels of coagulation factors than those without, which reached significance for prothrombin and factor IXc. Those who were

TABLE 45-2. *Fasting serum lipid and lipoprotein values according to the presence or absence of ACAD*

Variable	No ACAD (n = 97)	ACAD (n = 33)	Significance
Total cholesterol (mmol/L)	63 (1.7)	7.1 (2)	p = 0.02
LDL cholesterol (mmol/L)	4.4 (1.0)	4.9 (1.6)	p = 0.03
Triglycerides (mmol/L)	2.0 (1.0)	2.3 (1.3)	p = 0.54
HDL cholesterol (mmol/L)	1.15 (1.0)	1.4 (0.9)	p = 0.68
Lipoprotein (a) (mg/dl)	22 (1-170)	71 (3-193)	p = 0.0006

TABLE 45-3. *A study of lipid levels including lipoprotein(a) after transplantation*

Type of transplant (no.)	Lipoprotein (a) Pretransplant levels (mg/L)	6 months	p value
Cardiac (33)	222 (7-702)	199 (3.7-700)	0.90
Lung (11)	355 (54-700)	353 (8.5-700)	0.44
TOTAL (4)	247 (7.2-700)	201 (3.7-700)	0.61

transplanted for IHD had greater prothrombotic changes than the controls with IHD, suggesting not unexpectedly that those transplanted for atheromatous disease had more extensive disease than their controls and/or that posttransplantation factors, such as the use of prednisolone and cyclosporin, exacerbated the changes.

Effect of Immunosuppression

Transplant recipients had significantly increased levels of fibrinogen, vWF antigen, and antithrombin III when compared with their pertinent control groups, suggesting that these changes may have been partially due to the use of immunosuppression. The use of cyclosporin has been associated with thromboembolic phenomena after renal transplantation (60), microangiopathic hemolysis (61), and hepatic veno-occlusive disease after bone marrow transplantation (62).

Vaziri et al. (63) conducted a cross-sectional study of hemostasis in renal transplant recipients, with eight receiving cyclosporin and prednisolone and five being maintained on prednisolone and azathioprine. They found that both groups had significant elevation of factor IX and vWF antigen, as in our study. Those receiving cyclosporin had the highest levels of vWF and also had elevations of protein C concentration. These studies, in conjunction with this and others, again suggest that cyclosporin may be responsible for the increased levels of vWF, factor IX, and protein C seen post transplantation.

Cyclosporin toxicity has been previously associated with elevated levels of vWF in renal transplant recipients (64). vWF is also an acute phase protein, and thus increased plasma vWF levels in the absence of increased levels of CRP or obvious thrombus formation suggest endothelial injury, perturbation, or activation (65). In vitro studies of the effect of cyclosporin on vWF release by the endothelium have shown that cyclosporin, and also its vehicle (for cyclosporin is not water-soluble), called cremophor EL, affect vWF production (66). When they were added separately or alone to cultured human endothelial cells in combination with physiologic agonists such as thrombin or histamine, there was a concentration-dependent increase in the amount of vWF released. How cyclosporin increases plasma levels of factor IX and C is uncertain.

Modulating Coagulation and Fibrinolysis After Transplantation

We conducted a study of the safety and efficacy and effect on lipid levels, coagulation, and fibrinolysis of bezafibrate and omega-3 marine triglycerides. Bezafibrate is a fibric acid derivative that in addition to its lipid-modulating effects (67) has been shown to enhance anticoagulation (68) and to reduce plasma viscosity and fibrinogen levels (69,70).

Bezafibrate reduced total cholesterol, triglyceride, LDL cholesterol, and apolipoprotein B, and increased HDL cholesterol and apolipoprotein A1. Maxepa induced a reduction only in triglyceride levels but had no significant effect on cholesterol or coagulation and fibrinolysis. Both drugs similarly caused an insignificant increase in lipoprotein (a) levels.

After bezafibrate treatment, as expected, there was a significant reduction in fibrinogen, and also factor X levels, but an increase in levels of factor II, VII, VIII, and IX. The reduction of mean fibrinogen levels by bezafibrate has also been described in nontransplant patients (70). This beneficial effect may be counteracted by the concomitant increased levels of vitamin K–dependent coagulation factors, which similarly, but less strongly than fibrinogen, are indicators of the risk of coronary artery disease.

Unfortunately, bezafibrate increased serum creatinine levels, as has been described in nontransplant patients, without any associated increase in urea, creatine phosphokinase, or cyclosporin blood level. Because cyclosporin nephrotoxicity is a major problem after transplantation, the use of another, nonessential, potentially nephrotoxic drug is of concern.

There are no studies of the long-term use of conventional anticoagulants in transplant recipients. Aziz et al. showed that the addition of daily low molecular weight heparin to cyclosporin reduced the severity of accelerated CAD and the extent of parenchymal rejection in rats with heterotopic heart transplants (72).

HEMOSTASIS AND XENOTRANSPLANTATION

The pig is currently being investigated as a prospective donor in xenotransplantation, but a pig-to-human transplant is a discordant combination that would result in a xenograft reaction: the donor organ is rejected with a rapidity typical of hyperacute rejection in allotransplantation. The endpoint of hyperacute rejection, whether it follows a major ABO mismatch or a discordant xenograft, is microvascular thrombosis (73), which causes organ dysfunction and death.

Hemostasis and Hyperacute Rejection

The current hypothesis of organ rejection in the pig-to-human xenograft reaction is that the recipient has preformed antipig antibodies that bind to xenoantigens on the porcine endothelium, activating complement and causing subsequent hemostatic activation and thrombosis.

Hemostatic activation is a consequence of antibody and complement deposition although the mechanisms are not fully understood. Platelets can be affected by components of the complement system. The assembly of C5-C (the final part of the complement pathway) potentiates thrombin-stimulated platelet aggregation (74). Complement-induced endothelial cell vesiculation results in the release of membrane microparticles expressing binding sites for factor Va and increased prothrombinase activity (75). Furthermore, xenoantibody and complement cause rapid cleavage of heparan sulfate proteoglycan from the endothelial cell surface (76).

Hemostasis and Endothelial Cell Activation

Endothelial cell activation plays a role in hemostatic activation, although this is not peculiar to xenotransplantation (77). Resting endothelial cells form a tight monolayer that presents an antithrombotic surface to blood cells and plasma proteins. In endothelial cell activation there are changes such that the endothelial cell surface becomes prothrombotic due to loss of heparin sulfate, thrombomodulin, increased production of PAI-1, the secretion of platelet-activating factor (PAF), and the expression of tissue factor. This is associated with a shape change allowing the efflux of protein through to the subendothelial space, is known as endothelial cell activation, and results in local platelet adhesion and aggregation, fibrin generation, and leukocyte traffic through the endothelium.

However, the speed of hyperacute rejection (within minutes) suggests that endothelial cell activation is not responsible for this, as the majority of the changes require gene transcription and protein synthesis, i.e., 2 to 6 hours.

Pathologic Activation of Hemostasis

Pathologic activation of hemostasis by definition bypasses physiologic hemostatic pathways. A major concern in xenotransplantation is that molecular incompatibilities between species will lead to adverse events, one of which may be pathologic activation of hemostasis. It has been shown that when a pig heart is perfused with human blood, despite complement depletion with cobra venom factor, hyperacute rejection was delayed but not prevented (78,79).

Moreover, there is the unacknowledged but well-recognized assumption that in situations when porcine organs are perfused with human blood the clotting process needs to be slowed down or inhibited to permit study of the immunologic aspects (15 U heparin/ml is required in the working pig heart and lung model; R. N. Pierson, personal communication). The ex vivo perfusion of a porcine liver with human blood and a pig-to-human liver xenograft have demonstrated prominent fibrin deposition on porcine endothelium associated with only weak binding of human IgM and IgG and absence of complement components (80).

Prior to the recent resurgence of interest in xenotransplantation, molecular discordances had been recognized between porcine and human hemostasis. It was noted that after hemophiliacs were treated with porcine factor VIII concentrates they developed thrombocytopenia. It was found that the factor VIII concentrates contained large amounts of porcine vWF, which can aggregate human platelets in vivo. Porcine vWF is structurally different from human vWF and can activate human platelets (81) by binding to the glycoprotein Ib receptor. vWF is produced from porcine endothelium; thus there is a potential for a porcine graft to produce a chronic thrombocytopenia due to platelet consumption.

More recently other incompatibilities have been found, including the inability of porcine tissue factor pathway inhibitor to inhibit human factor Xa (82) and the lack of potency of porcine tissue factor with human plasma (83).

Hunt et al. focused on the direct activation of human hemostasis by porcine endothelium (i.e., in the absence of xenoantibody and complement). Preliminary in vitro results suggested that, in addition to physiologic ac-

tivation of hemostasis, there may also be pathologic or nonphysiologic activation of the common pathway of coagulation (84). Direct activation of the common pathway was investigated by applying purified human prothrombin and factor X separately to porcine endothelium. Incubation of human prothrombin resulted in its activation (85). This did not occur when human prothrombin was added to human endothelial cells. Further studies suggested that the mechanism by which human prothrombin is activated by porcine endothelial cells is due to a conformational change in prothrombin upon binding to the porcine endothelial cells, exposing catalytic sites with subsequent autocatalytic cleavages. These observations have necessarily been made in vitro using a purified system in an attempt to dissect out the complex processes occurring in plasma. In vivo, continuous thrombin generation by porcine endothelial cells would overwhelm local anticoagulant mechanisms and local clot formation would occur. Moreover, the consumption of prothrombin and subsequent activation of platelets by thrombin may lead to a bleeding diathesis; this fulfills the criteria for disseminated intravascular coagulation.

Liver Xenotransplantation

As most of the hemostatic proteins are synthesized by the liver, if a liver is transplanted across species then the recipient will assume the hemostatic profile of the donor. In the case of the pig-to-human combination, it has been shown that the level of coagulation factors between the two species is markedly different, with high levels of factors V, VII, IX, XI, and XII, and lower levels of prothrombin in the pig (83). The long-term effects of this on the recipient are uncertain. It is interesting to note that the Galα1,3-Gal epitope occurs in carbohydrate chains of the porcine factor coagulation factors such as porcine fibrinogen (86) and factor VIII, which is not present in human factor VIII (87). Thus these molecules could be potential targets for the xenoantibody, but this has not been studied.

CONCLUSION

Hemostatic changes feature in many aspects of solid organ transplantation. There are unique changes during the orthotopic liver transplantation that require careful management. The fact that hemostasis is altered after transplantation may be partially due to the use of immunosuppressive drugs. The relationship of these changes to the development of chronic rejection is uncertain but may be similar to that between hemostasis and nontransplant atheroma. Hemostatic barriers will need to be overcome before pig-to-human xenotransplantation is a reality. Studies of the relationships between hemostasis and facets of transplantation are in their infancy but require exploration because they may reveal new potential avenues for managing problems in transplant recipients.

REFERENCES

1. Hosenpud JD, Novick RJ, Breen TJ, Daily OP. The Registry of the International Sociaety for Heart and Lung Transplantation: eleventh official report—1994. *J Heart Lung Transplant* 1994;13:561–570.
2. Evans RW, Orians CE, Ascher NL. The potential supply of organ donors. *JAMA* 1992;267:239–246.
3. McNichol PL, Liu G, Harley ID, et al. Blood loss and transfusion requirements in liver transplantation: experience with the first 75 cases. *Anaesth Intensive Care* 1994;22:666–671.
4. Segal HC, Hunt BJ, Cottam S, et al. Fibrinolytic activity during orthotopic liver transplantation with and without aprotinin. *Transplantation* 1994;58:1356–1360.
5. Segal H, Hunt BJ, Cottam S, et al. Changes in the contact system during orthotopic liver transplantation with and without aprotinin. *Transplantation* 1995;59:366–370.
6. Segal H, Cottam S, Potter D, Hunt BJ. Coagulation and fibrinolysis in primary biliary cirrhosis compared to other liver disease and during orthotopic liver transplantation. *Hepatology* 1997;25:683–688.
7. Scudamore CH, Randall TE, Jewesson PJ, et al. Aprotinin reduces the need for blood products during liver transplantation. *Am J Surg* 1996;169:546–549.
8. Patrassi GM, Viero M, Sartori MT, et al. Aprotinin efficacy on intraoperative bleeding and transfusion requirements in orthotopic liver transplantation. *Transfusion* 1994;34:507–511.
9. Gouin, I, Lecompte T, Morel MC, et al. In vitro effect of plasmin on human platelet function in plasma. *Circulation* 1992;85:935.
10. Hunt BJ. Modifying perioperative bleeding. *Blood Rev* 1991;5:168–176.
11. Hunt BJ, Sacks D, Amin S, Yacoub MH. The perioperative use of blood components during heart and heart-lung transplantation. *Transfusion* 1992;32:57–62.
12. Harjula A, Baldwin JC, Starnes VA, et al. Proper donor selection for heart-lung transplantation. The Stanford experience. *J Thorac Cardiovasc Surg* 1987;94:874–880.
13. Vouhe PR, Dartevelle PG. Heart-lung transplantation. Technical modifications that may improve the early outcome. *J Thorac Cardiovasc Surg* 1989;97:906–910.
14. Havel M, Owen AN, Simon P, et al. Decreased use of donated blood and reduction of bleeding after orthotopic heart transplantation by use of aprotinin. *J Heart Lung Transplant* 1992;11:348–349.
15. Kesten S, de Hoyas A, Chaparro C, Westney G, Winton T, Maurer JR. Aprotinin reduces blood losss in lung transplant recipients. *Ann Thorac Surg* 1995;59:877–879.
16. Prendergast W, Furukawa S, Beyer J, Eisen HJ, McClurken JB, Jeevanandam V. Defining the role of aprotinin in heart transplantation. *Ann Thorac Surg* 1996;62:670–674.
17. Shore-Lesserson L, Reich DL, Vela-Cantos F, Ammar T, Arisan Ergin M. Tranexamic acid reduces transfusions and mediastinal drainage in repeat cardiac surgery. *Anesth Analg* 1996;83:18–26.
18. Rodriguez-Erdmann F, Guttman RD. Coagulation in renal allograft rejection. *N Engl J Med* 1969;281:1428.
19. Hunt BJ, Funnell L, Segal H, Yacoub M. Plasma von Willebrand factor and C-reactive protein levels as markers of acute rejection after heart transplantation [Abstract]. *Am Coll Cardiology Meeting* 1991.
20. Faulk WP, Garguilo P, McIntyre JA, Bang NU. Hemostasis and fibrinolysis in renal transplantation. *Semin Thromb Haemost* 1989;15:88.
21. Gao SZ, Schoeder JS, Alderman EL, et al. Prevalence of coronary artery disease in heart transplant survivors. Comparison of cyclosporin and azathioprine regimens. *Circulation* 1989;8:100–105.
22. Uretsky BR, Kormos RL, Zerbe TR, et al. Cardiac events after heart transplantation: incidence and predictive value of coronary angiography. *J Heart Lung Transplant* 1992;11:45–51.
23. Billingham ME. Histopathology of graft coronary disease. *J Heart Lung Transplant* 1992;11:S38–44.
24. Hosenpud JD, Shipley GD, Wagner CR. Cardiac allograft vasculopathy: current concepts, recent developments and future directions. *J Heart Lung Transplant* 1992;11:9–23.
25. Tobis JM, Malley J, Mahon D, et al. Intravascular ultrasound imaging of human coronary arteries in vivo. *Circulation* 1991;83:913–926.
26. Ross R. The pathogenesis of atherosclerosis: an update. *N Engl J Med* 1986;314:488–500.
27. Dunn MJ, Crisp SJ, Rose ML, et al. Anti-endothelial antibodies and coronary artery disease after transplantation. *Lancet* 1992;339:1566–1570.
28. Salomon RN, Hughes CCW, Schoen Fl. Human coronary transplantation associated arteriosclerosis: evidence for a chronic immune reaction to activated graft endothelial cells. *Am J Pathol* 1991;138:791–798.
29. Smith JD, Rose ML, Pomerance A, Burke M, Yacoub MH. Reduction of cellular rejection and increase in longer term survival after heart transplantation after HLA-DR matching. *Lancet* 1995;346:1318–1322.
30. Johnson MR. Transplant coronary disease. Nonimmunological risk factors. *J Heart Lung Transplant* 1992;11:124–132.

31. Hunt BJ, Segal H, Yacoub M. Haemostasis in heart transplant recipients and the relationship with accelerated coronary sclerosis. *Transplantation* 1993;55: 309–315.

32. Labarrere CA, Pitts D, Halbrook H, Faulk WP. Natural anticoagulant pathways in normal and transplanted human hearts. *J Heart Lung Transplant* 1992;11:342–347.

33. Vanrenterghem Y, Lerut T, Roels L, et al. Thromboembolic complications and haemostatic changes in cyclosporin-treated cadaver kidney allograft recipients. *Lancet* 1985;1:999.

34. Cohen H, Neild GH, Mackie IJ, Machin SJ. Persistent decreased fibrinolytic activity in cyclosporin-treated renal allograft recipients. *Fibrinolysis* 1988;2:197.

35. Yue RH, Evtler MN, Starr T, et al. Alterations of plasma antithrombin II levels in ischaemic heart disease. *Thromb Haemost* 1976;35:598.

36. Hamsten A, Wiman B, de Faire U, et al. Increased plasma levels of a rapid inhibitor of tissue plasminogen activator in young survivors of myocardial infarction. *N Engl J Med* 1985;313:1557–63.

37. Hamsten A, de Faire U, Wallidius G, et al. Plasminogen activator inhibitor in plasma: risk factor for recurrent myocardial infarction. *Lancet* 1987;2:3–9.

38. Baker LRI, Tucker B, Kovacs IB. Enhanced on vitro haemostasis and reduced thrombolysis in cyclosporine-treated renal transplant recipients. *Transplantation* 1990;49:905.

39. Zonneveld AJ, Curndes SA, Loskntoft DJ. Type 1 plasminogen activator inhibitor gene, functional analysis and glucocorticoid regulation of its promoter. *Proc Natl Acad Sci USA* 1988;85:5525.

40. Labarrere CA, Pitts D, Halbrook H, Faulk WP. Tissue plasminogen activator, plasminogen activator inhibitor-1 and fibrin as indexes of clinical course in cardiac allograft recipients: an immunocytochemical study. *Circulation* 1994;89:1599–1608.

41. Labarrere CA, Pitts D, Nelson DR, Faulk WP. Vascular tissue plasminogen activator and the development of coronary artery disease in heart transplant recipients. *N Engl J Med* 1995;33:111–116.

42. Mitropoulos JA, Esnouf MP. The prothrombin activation peptide regulates synthesis of the vitamin -K-dependent proteins in the rabbit. *Thromb Res* 1990;57:541–549.

43. De Lorgeril M, Dureau G, Boissonnat P et al. Increased platelet aggregation after heart transplantation: influence of aspirin. *J Heart Lung Transplant* 1991;10: 600–603.

44. De Lorgeril M, Loire R, Guidollet J, et al. Accelerated coronary atherosclerosis after heart transplantation. The role of enhanced platelet aggregation and thrombosis. *J Intern Med* 1993;233:343–350.

45. Frampton G, Parbtani A, Marchesi D, et al. In vivo platelet activation with in vitro hyperaggregability to arachidonic acid in renla allograft recipients. *Kidney Int* 1987;23:506–513.

46. Grace AA, Barrados MA, Mikhailidis DP, et al. Cyclosporine A enhances platelet aggregation. *Kidney Int* 1987;32:889–895.

47. de Lorgeril M, Dureau G, Boissonnat P, et al. Platelet function and composition on heart transplant recipients compared with nontransplanted coronary patients. *Atheroscl Thromb* 1992;12:222–230.

48. Miles LA, Fless GM, Scanu AM, et al. A potential basis for the thrombotic risks associated with lipoprotein (a). *Nature* 1989;339:301–303.

49. Hajjar KA, Gavish D, Breslow JL, et al. Lipoprotein (a) modulation of endothelial cell surface fibrinolysis and its potential role in atherosclerosis. *Nature* 1989;339: 303–305.

50. Smith EB, Cochran S. Factors influencing the accumulation of lipid derived from low density lipoprotein. *Atherosclerosis* 1990;84:173–181.

51. Etingin OR, Hajjar DP, Hajjar KA, Harpel PC, Nachman RL. Lipoprotein (a) regulates plasminogen activator inhibitor type 1 expression in endothelial cells. *J Biol Chem* 1991;266:2459–2465.

52. Barbir M, Kushwaha S, Hunt BJ, et al. Lipoprotein(a) and accelerated coronary artery disease in cardiac transplant recipients. *Lancet* 1992;340:1500–1502.

53. Webb AT, Reavely DA, O Donnell M, O Connor B, Seed M, Brown EA. Does cyclosporin increase lipoprotein (a) concentrations in renal transplant recipients? *Lancet* 1993;341:268–270.

54. Farmer JA, Ballantyne CM, Frazier OH, et al. Lipoprotein (a) and apolipoprotein changes after cardiac transplantation. *J Am Coll Cardiol* 1991;18:926–930.

55. Hunt BJ, Parratt R, Rose M, Yacoub M. Does cyclosporin affect lipoprotein(a) concentrations. *Lancet* 1994;343:119–120.

56. Scott J. Lipoprotein (a) [Editorial]. *Br Med J* 1991; 303:663–664.

57. Durrington PN, Ishola N, Hunt L, et al. Apolipoproteins (a), A1 and B and parental history in men with early onset ischaemic heart disease. *Lancet* 1988;1:1070–1073.

58. Armstrong VW, Cremer P, Eberle E, et al. The association between serum Lp(a) concentrations and angiographically assessed coronary atherosclerosis: dependence on serum LDL levels. *Atherosclerosis* 1986;62: 249–257.

59. Seed M, Hoppichler F, Reaveley D, et al. Relation of serum lipoprotein (a) concentration and apolipoprotein (a) phenotype to coronary heart disease in patients with familial hypercholesterolaemia. *N Engl J Med* 1990; 322:1494–1499.

60. Vanrenterghem Y, Lerut T, Roels L, et al. Thromboembolic complications and haemostatic changes in cyclosporin-treated cadavar kidney allograft recipients. *Lancet* 1985;1:999.

61. Holler E, Kolb HJ, Hiller E, et al. Microangiopathy in patients on cyclosporin prophylaxis who developed acute graft versus host disease after HLA -identical bone marrow transplantation. *Blood* 1989;73:2018.

62. McDonald GB, Sharma P, Matthews DE, et al. Veno-occlusive disease of the liver after bone marrow transplantation. *Hepatology* 1984;4:116.

63. Vaziri ND, Ismail M, Martin DC, et al. Blood coagulation, fibrinolysis and inhibitory profiles in renal transplant recipients: comparison of cyclosporine and azathioprine. *Int J Artif Organs* 1992;15:365–369.

64. Brown Z, Neild GH, Willoughby JJ, et al. Increased factor VIII as an index of vascular injury in cyclosporin nephrotoxicity. *Transplantation* 1986;42:150.

65. Anonymous. Factor VIII related antigen and vasculitis [Editorial]. *Lancet* 1988;1:1203.

66. Collins P, Wilkie M, Razak K, et al. Cyclosporine and cremaphor modulate von Willebrand factor release from cultured human endothelial cells. *Transplantation* 1993; 56:1218–1223.

67. Olsson AG, Lang PD, Vollmar J. Effect of bezafibrate during 4.5 years of treatment of hyperlipoproteinemia. *Atherosclerosis* 1985;55:195–203.

68. Zimmerman R, Ehlers W, Walter E, et al. The effect of bezafibrate on the fibrinolytic enzyme system and the drug interaction with racemic phenprocoumon. *Atherosclerosis* 1978;29:477–485.

69. Arntz HR, Leonhardt H, Lang PD, Vollmar J. Effects of bezafibrate and Clofibrate on blood rheology and lipoproteins in primary hyperlipoproteinaemia. *J Clin Trials* 1981;18:280–286.

70. Almer LO, Kjellstrom T. The fibrinolytic system and coagulation during bezafibrate treatment of hypertriglyceridemia. *Atherosclerosis* 1986;61:81–85.

71. Dick TBS, Marples J, Ledermann HM, Whittington J. Comparative study of once and three times daily regimes of bezafibrate in patients with primary hyperlipoproteinaemia. *Curr Med Res Opin* 1981;7:489–502.

72. Verrier ED. A reduction in accelerated graft coronary artery disease and improvement in cardiac allograft survival using low molecular weight heparin in combination with cyclosporine. *J Heart Lung Transplant* 1993; 12:634–643.

73. Larsen S, Starklint H. Histopathology of kidney xenograph rejection. In: Cooper DKC, et al. (eds). *Xenotransplantation.* New York: Springer, 1997;17:228–254.

74. Polley MJ, Nachman RL. Human complement in thrombin-mediated platelet function. Uptake of the C5-C9 complex. *J Exp Med* 1979;150:633.

75. Weidmer T, Esmon CT, Sims PJ. Complement proteins C5b-9 stimulate procoagulant activity through platelet prothrombinase. *Blood* 1986;68:875.

76. Platt JL, Vercellotti GM, Lindman GJ, et al. Release of heparan sulphate from endothelial cells. *J Exp Med* 1990;171:1363.

77. Bach FH, Robson SC, Winkler H, et al. Barriers to xenotransplantation. *Nature Med* 1995;1:869–873.

78. Hunt BJ, Dunning J, Segal H, et al. Pig-to-human xenograft reaction: is haemostatic activation dependent on the presence of anti-pig antibodies or complement? *Transplant Proc* 1994;26:1156.

79. Jurd KM, Lee J, Ciarns T, Hunt BJ. Effect of Galα1,3Gal 1,4GlcNAc and complement depletion on haemostatic activation in an in vitro model of the pig to human xenograft reaction. *Transplant Proc* 1996;28:637–638.

80. Makowka L, Cramer DV, Hoffman A, Sher L, Podesta L. Pig liver xenografts as a temporary bridge for human allografting. *Xeno* 1993;1:17.

81. Paretti FI, Mazzucato M, Bottini E, Mannucci PM. Interaction of porcine von Willebrand factor with the platelet glycoproteins Ib and IIb/IIIa complex. *Br J Haematol* 1992;82:81.

82. Kopp CW, Siegel JB, Hancock WW, et al. Effect of porcine endothelial tissue factor pathway inhibitor on human coagulation factors. *Transplantation* 1997;63: 749–758.

83. Reverdiau-Moalic P, Watier H, Vallee I, et al. Comparative study of porcine and human blood coagulation systems: possible relevance in xenotransplantation. *Transplant Proc* 1996;28:643–644.

84. Jurd KM, Cairns T, Hunt BJ. Activation of haemostasis in an in vitro model of the pig-to-human xenograft reaction. *Transplant Proc* 1994;26:1159.

85. Jurd Km, Gibbs RV, Hunt BJ. Activation of human prothrombin by porcine endothelial cells—a potential barrier to xenotransplantation. *Blood Coag Fibrinol* 1996; 7:336.

86. Blanchard D, Thibandeau K, Soulillou JP. Porcine antigenic targets for human natural antibodies. *Xeno* 1995; 3:68.

87. Hironaka T, Furukawa K, Esmon CT, et al. Structural study of the sugar chains of porcine factor VIII-tissue and species-specific glycosylation of factor VIII. *Arch Biochem Biophys* 1993;307:316.

Cardiovascular Thrombosis: Thrombocardiology and Thromboneurology, Second Edition,
edited by M. Verstraete, V. Fuster, and E. J. Topol,
Lippincott–Raven Publishers, Philadelphia © 1998.

46

The Antiphospholipid Syndrome

Jef Arnout and *Luis Carreras

The Center for Molecular and Vascular Biology, University of Leuven, B-3000 Leuven, Belgium*; and Instituto de Cardiologia y Cirugia Cardiovascular, 1093 Buenos Aires, Argentina

INTRODUCTION

The antiphospholipid syndrome (APS) is defined as the association of antiphospholipid antibodies (aPL), i.e., lupus anticoagulant (LA) and/or anticardiolipin antibodies (aCL), with arterial or venous thrombosis, recurrent fetal loss, thrombocytopenia, or neurologic disorders (Table 46-1). This chapter summarizes the gradual development of the concept of this syndrome, the clinical features with which it is associated, the pathophysiology, laboratory diagnosis, and treatment of aPL.

HISTORICAL BACKGROUND

The gradual development of the notion "APS" started simultaneously in the 1950s from two medical disciplines. On the one hand, rheumatologists reported that a chronic biological false- positive test for syphilis identified a subset of patients with systemic lupus erythematosus (SLE) and other autoimmune diseases who had a high incidence of thrombosis, obstetric complications, and thrombocytopenia (1,2). On the other hand, hematologists described an aspecific coagulation inhibitor in patients with SLE manifested by prolongation of the whole-blood clotting time and the prothrombin time, without reduction of any specific clotting factor then measurable (3). This aspecific coagulation inhibitor, which appeared not to be associated with a bleeding tendency, was named the "lupus anticoagulant" (LA) by Feinstein and Rapaport (4) and was regarded as a laboratory curiosity until Bowie et al. (5) drew attention to the high prevalence of thrombotic complications in SLE patients with this "anticoagulant." The LA was later also found to be asso-

TABLE 46-1. *Definition of the antiphospholipid syndrome*

Laboratory finding
  Laboratory findings
    Persistently elevated aPL and/or lupus
      anticoagulant
    Lupus anticoagulant
    Anticardiolipin antibodies (IgG or IgM, moderate
      or high titer)
  Clinical findings
    Thrombosis: arterial and/or venous
    Recurrent fetal loss
    Thrombocytopenia
    Neurologic disorders

Note: Diagnosis is based on the persistence of at least one laboratory abnormality and/or at least once clinical manifestation.

ciated with obstetrical complications and thrombocytopenia (6,7). Only in the 1980s did it become clear that antibodies interacting with phospholipids are responsible for the chronic biological false- positive syphilis serology and the in vitro LA effect. Physico-chemical and immunologic analysis indicated that the LA consists of immunoglobulins of the IgG and/or the IgM isotype (7). The fact that the LA often delays both the intrinsic and extrinsic coagulation pathways without affecting the thrombin time pointed to the prothrombinase complex as the site of action. The following circumstantial evidence suggested that LAs impede clotting by competing with the coagulation factors for the available negatively charged phospholipid (PL) surface in the prothrombinase complex: (a) only PL-dependent clotting times were prolonged by LAs; (b) the effect of the LA was often more pronounced when reducing the PL content in the assay system; and (c) preincubation with lipids or tissue thromboplastin reduced the inhibitor effect. A more direct indication that LAs are antibodies directed against anionic PL came from Thiagarajan et al. who described a monoclonal IgM LA that formed precipitin lines with anionic PL (8). This finding also shed new light on the observation that patients with LA often have a false-positive syphilis serology because cardiolipin, a key component of the antigen used in the Venereal Disease Research Laboratory (VDRL) test, is

an anionic PL with which an aPL could react. Highly sensitive solid phase techniques for the detection of aCL were then introduced (9,10). With these sensitive assays the majority of SLE patients with an LA also had elevated aCL levels and a statistically significant relation between these two types of aPL was observed. aCL antibodies and LAs in patients with SLE appear to be associated with thrombosis, cerebral infarction, fetal loss, and thrombocytopenia. This association is now termed the APS (11). Some patients with these clinical symptoms and laboratory findings but not fulfilling the criteria for lupus are diagnosed as suffering from a "primary APS" (12).

ANTIPHOSPHOLIPID ANTIBODIES: CLINICAL ASSOCIATIONS

Association Between Antiphospholipid Antibodies and Thrombosis

Since Bowie et al. (1963) described the occurrence of thrombotic complications in patients with SLE and the LA, this intriguing phenomenon has provoked a great deal of interest (5). Excluding case reports, Carreras and Vermylen (1982) while reviewing the literature found that of 211 patients with LA, 61 (28.9%) had presented with arterial or venous thrombosis (13). Lechner and Pabinger-Fasching, reviewing the literature in 1985, observed that of 259 patients with LA, 85 (32.8%) had developed thrombosis (14). In many early studies, an unexplained thrombosis was one of the reasons to search for the LA. This obviously leads to an overestimation of the prevalence of thrombosis in patients with LA. To further delineate the association between LA, aCL, and thrombosis, it is useful to study the prevalence of such combinations within the same disease. In 1990, Love and Santoro published a meta-analysis of the thus far published reports on the APS (15). In their analysis only studies in which the laboratory diagnosis of aPL was based on minimal diagnostic criteria (16,17) were included. A history of thrombosis was noted in

42% of 340 SLE patients with an LA and only in 12% of 338 SLE patients without an LA (p < 0.001). When patients were stratified according to the presence of aCL, 40% of the 300 patients with aCL and 18% of the 364 patients without such antibody had suffered from thrombosis (p < 0.001). When only consecutive series were included in the analysis, similar highly significant differences were found. From these data the association between aPL and a history of thrombosis appears to be established, at least in SLE patients. The study by Love and Santoro did not permit firm conclusions to be drawn regarding an association between aPL and a history of thrombosis in patients without SLE. The available retrospective studies also could not answer the crucial question of whether aPL are associated with an increased risk for future, initial, or recurrent thromboembolic complications. A few recent prospective trials provide evidence that elevated aPL are indeed a real risk factor for thrombosis. A substudy of the Physician's Health Study found a relationship between the aCL titer at entry to the study and the subsequent risk for thrombosis and pulmonary embolism in healthy adult men (18). Another prospective cohort study of unselected patients with suspected deep venous thrombosis or pulmonary embolism showed a strong association between proven venous thromboembolism and the presence of an LA (19). There was no association between the presence of aCL and venous thromboembolism because of the high frequency of elevated aCL levels in patients without proven venous thromboembolism. The Italian Registry of aPL evaluated the natural history and the risk for thrombosis in a cohort of 360 unselected patients followed for 4 years (20). The annual incidence of both venous and arterial thromboses seemed to depend on either a history of thrombosis or a high titer of aCL. Asymptomatic patients with aPL have an incidence of thrombosis of 0.9% per patient-year. In patients with a positive history of thrombosis a high recurrency rate has been reported resulting in an annual incidence between 5% and 10% per patient-

year (20,21). Whether the thrombotic risk depends on the type, titer, and isotype of aPL is not yet entirely clear. Retrospective studies had shown that both LAs and aCL are associated with thrombosis. More recent studies give conflicting results. In the Italian registry study, only a correlation between high levels of aCL and thrombosis was found, whereas other investigators reported that the LA is a stronger risk factor for thrombosis than aCL (19,22).

The nature of the thrombotic episodes seen in patients with aPL deserves some further comment. Virtually all arterial or venous sites may be involved and approximately 70% of the thrombotic events are venous and 30% are arterial (23,24). Peripheral deep venous thrombosis and pulmonary embolism are the most common venous events. In addition, thrombosis of hepatic veins, inferior and superior vena cava, mesenteric veins, adrenal veins, cerebral veins, axillary veins, etc., have been reported. Among the common arterial locations are the cerebral, coronary, axillary, brachial, iliofemoral, aorta, mesenteric, carotid, and retinal arteries.

A few remarkable associations of aPL and thrombosis have been made. Asherson et al. reported the association between the LA and pulmonary hypertension in patients with SLE (25). They speculated that in these cases pulmonary hypertension may have been caused by intrapulmonary thrombosis. The LA appears to be the most common laboratory abnormality in patients with thromboembolic pulmonary hypertension (26). Hamsten et al. found aCL in 8 of 62 young survivors of a myocardial infarction; these patients with aCL were particularly prone to new thromboembolic complications (27). This finding has, however, been challenged by others (28). It should be noted that these studies were performed on survivors of myocardial infarction or in patients with established coronary heart disease. In a recent prospective study on a cohort of initially healthy middle-aged dyslipidemic men, high aCL levels were found to be an independent risk factor for myocardial infarction (29). In addition, a highly significant association between preoperative raised aCL levels and late graft occlusion has been reported in patients having coronary artery bypass graft surgery (30). An association has further been suggested between aPL and Degos's disease, a rare multisystemic vasculopathy characterized by widespread thrombosis, particularly of the vessels of the skin, the central nervous system, and gastrointestinal tract (31). Several reports in the pediatric and even neonatal literature have also noted the association of an LA with thrombosis, a very rare clinical event in childhood (32,33).

Antiphospholipid Antibodies and Pregnancy

The first report on the association of a circulating coagulation inhibitor, a chronically false-positive syphilis serology and recurrent abortion, came from Laurell and Nilsson in 1957 (6). One of the two patients described had five consecutive fetal losses in the third month of each pregnancy. In 1975, Nilsson et al. reported a case of a woman with a history of deep vein thrombosis and unexplained recurrent intrauterine death (34). The patient had no apparent autoimmune disease and in the placenta of one of the pregnancies microscopic necrosis and fibrin deposits were noted. In 1980, Soulier and Boffa described three women with recurrent abortions, thrombosis, and a circulating anticoagulant (35). This paper also proposed that the recurrent abortions could be linked with the thrombotic process that was observed in the placental vessels (see also below). In the beginning of the 1980s, the association of the LA with thrombosis or recurrent abortion became more generally recognized (36).

Love and Santoro, in their meta-analysis, evaluated the frequency of fetal loss in retrospective studies of patients with SLE or related autoimmune disorders (15). The percentage of patients who had had one or more fetal losses ranged from 13% to 68% in aPL-positive patients and from 3% to 42% in aPL-negative patients. However, since many of the studies included in this analysis did not report the number of fetal losses per patient, it was

impossible to distinguish whether there was a general tendency for fetal loss in all patients with aPL or multiple pregnancy failures in only a few patients. From their analysis the authors conclude that retrospective studies only suggest but do not firmly prove an association between aPL and a history of fetal loss in patients with SLE. A cross-sectional study on 42 SLE patients, however, found a significant relationship between aPL and pregnancy loss (37).

Whether aPL are independent risk factors for subsequent fetal loss can only be answered in prospective studies. In the limited number of such studies included in the meta-analysis by Love and Santoro, a significantly higher incidence of fetal loss (59%) was found in SLE patients with aCL than in patients without these antibodies (5%) (15). Similar differences were observed when patients were stratified according to the presence or absence of an LA. These studies show that patients with SLE who have aPL and a history of multiple pregnancy failures are at high risk for experiencing subsequent fetal loss.

The question of whether patients without SLE or lupus-like disorders but with elevated aPL have an increased risk for fetal loss is more difficult to answer. One way to approach this problem is to study the prevalence of aPL in patients with recurrent fetal loss in comparison with a control population. McNeil et al. summarized 16 such studies published between 1981 and 1989 (38). Of the 827 patients with recurrent idiopathic fetal loss, 238 (29%) were found to have aPL. Dividing the patients into LA and aCL subgroups, the average frequency of each was 25% and 37%, respectively. The prevalence of aPL in healthy pregnant women or women with explained fetal loss, used as control groups in these studies, was very low. Even if the proportion of SLE patients in a number of these studies is not precisely known, this analysis strongly suggests a more general relationship between aPL and recurrent fetal loss.

Prospective controlled studies on this matter are scarce but support the general belief that aPL are associated with an increased risk for subsequent fetal loss (39,40). Infante-Rivard et al. recently published a case-control study on aPL and fetal loss performed on 331 woman with spontaneous abortion or fetal death and 993 controls. This study could not show a relation between aPL and a first pregnancy loss (41). The search for aPL should only be part of the exploration of women with previous fetal death, recurrent idiopathic abortions, or a history of thromboembolic disease. Screening for aPL might also be useful in patients with SLE and in patients with a history of severe pre-eclampsia (42). Persistently positive results for aPL tests are found in approximately 15% of women with a history of recurrent miscarriage, defined as three or more consecutive pregnancy losses (43). Without specific treatment, these women have a rate of subsequent fetal loss of approximately 90% (43,44).

Clinical reports have suggested that thrombosis and fetal loss are more common in patients with high positive aCL titers (42,46) and that IgGs are more likely to be associated with thrombosis or fetal loss than IgM (46,47).

A frequent finding in case reports on the association of recurrent fetal loss with an LA is extensive infarction of the placenta (35,36,48). Extensive placental infarction indicates that there must be a widespread abnormality of the uteroplacental vasculature. Lesions of fibrinoid necrosis and intraluminal thrombosis in the spiral arteries of the basal plate of the grossly infarcted placenta have been reported (49). The decrease in maternal blood flow to the placenta as a consequence of these stenotic vascular lesions is considered to be the cause of fetal loss. These findings have more recently been confirmed in a histopathologic study of 47 placentas from women with intrauterine death with and without aPL (50). Extensive placental infarction has, however, not been found in all patients with aPL (51), but abnormal Doppler flow studies of the uteroplacental circulation (52) further support a pathogenetic role of vascular disturbances in fetal growth retardation and death associated with aPL.

Infants born of mothers with aPL are generally normal, except for complications associated with prematurity. However, in some neonates, thromboses of the renal vein, inferior vena cava, middle cerebral artery, and aorta have been found. Since IgG cross the placenta, the APS should be considered in the differential diagnosis of neonatal thrombosis (32,33).

Association Between Antiphospholipid Antibodies and Neurologic Disorders

Many authors have reported cerebral infarctions in association with aCL or the LA (53–56). Recurrent stroke and vascular dementia are feared consequences of aPL but other neurologic disorders such as amaurosis fugax (57), Sneddon's syndrome (58,59), Degos's disease (31), atypical migraine, encephalopathy, chorea, epilepsy, and myelopathy are also reported to be associated with these antibodies (60).

In the meta-analysis performed by Love and Santoro, nine studies were included evaluating the association between neurologic disorders and aPL in patients with SLE (15). Neurologic disorders were found in 38% of 135 patients with an LA compared to 21% of 180 patients without these antibodies (p < 0.001). When patients were stratified according to the presence of aCL, 49% of 57 patients with aCL had neurologic manifestations compared to only 12% of 108 patients without these antibodies (p < 0.001). A report by "the aPL in stroke" study group, on 255 consecutive first ischemic stroke patients without SLE and an equal number of age- and sex-matched nonstroke patients, showed a significantly increased frequency of aCL in these stroke patients (9.7% in stroke patients versus 4.3% in controls; p < 0.03) (61). The authors also concluded that the association of aCL and stroke was independent of other important stroke risk factors. Several recent prospective studies have confirmed these findings, but others have not (60). Cardiac emboli are probably a major cause of cerebrovascular symptoms in patients with the APS (see below).

Association Between Antiphospholipid Antibodies and Thrombocytopenia

Although in a few of the earliest described patients the LA was reported to be associated with some hemorrhagic manifestations, bleeding phenomena were rapidly found to be rare and usually could be ascribed to severe hypoprothrombinemia or severe thrombocytopenia. Lechner was probably the first to suggest that thrombocytopenia is more common in SLE patients with LA (7). Love and Santoro, in their meta-analysis, showed that patients with SLE or closely related disorders who tested positive for either the LA or aCL were on average three times more likely to have a history of moderate to severe thrombocytopenia than were aPL-negative patients (15). Approximately 25% of the patients with an APS have a mild thrombocytopenia. Severe thrombocytopenia is not a common finding and is only rarely associated with hemorrhagic complications. Two possible mechanisms to explain this thrombocytopenia have been proposed. aCL could be directly responsible because they can bind to activated platelets; for this interaction, a PL-binding protein, β_2-glycoprotein I (β_2GPI), is needed (62). Alternatively, specific antiplatelet antibodies directed against platelet membrane glycoproteins, often found in patients with aPL and thrombocytopenia, could be responsible (63). Of interest is that prednisone therapy normalizes platelet counts in such patients and reduces the levels of platelet-associated antibodies without affecting aPL titers (64).

Antiphospholipid Antibodies and Valvular Disease

The association of valve lesions with SLE was first described by Libman and Sacks in 1924 (65). Libman-Sacks vegetations have been reported in about one third of SLE patients. Several reports mention the presence of nonbacterial thrombotic endocarditis or mitral valve vegetation in patients with aPL and recurrent stroke (66,67). A few recent prospective studies confirm the association between

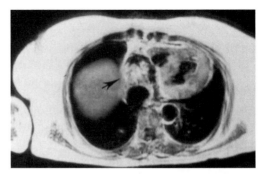

FIG. 46-1. CT scan of a 65-year-old patient with increasing dyspnea upon exertion, thrombocytopenia, positive antinuclear factor, positive lupus anticoagulant and anticardiolipin antibodies. Echocardiography and CT scan revealed a large pedunculated mass *(arrow)* in the right atrium, prolapsing through the tricuspid valve suggesting a myxoma. The partly granulomatous, partly gelatinous, partly fibrotic, and partly calcified mass was removed surgically. Pathologic examination showed old thrombus with calcification and fibrosis; no myxoma.

aPL and valvular heart disease in patients with and without SLE (61,68,69). In the study of Cervera et al., 65% of aPL-positive SLE patients had heart valve abnormalities (69). Heart valve abnormalities are slightly less common in patients with the primary APS (21). In most cases, the abnormalities are of minor hemodynamic significance and do not cause clinically overt valvular heart disease. Occasionally, severe valvular insufficiency can be the result of a massive intracavitary thrombus attached to the valve lesions (see Fig. 46-1). Several studies have highlighted a frequent concomitant occurrence of valve abnormalities and cerebrovascular ischemic events. These studies and limited pathologic findings suggest that not only in situ thrombosis of cerebral or carotid vessels but also a cardioembolic mechanism may be responsible for the development of stroke in patients with aPL (70).

The Catastrophic Antiphospholipid Syndrome

A minority of patients with aPL may develop an acute and catastrophic APS characterized by a sudden and explosive onset of multiple vascular occlusions affecting the central nervous, cardiac, renal, and pulmonary systems as well as intra-abdominal organs such as the adrenal gland, bowel, and pancreas (71). The clinical condition may mimic disseminated intravascular coagulation, thrombotic thrombocytopenic purpura, or the hemolytic uremic syndrome.

Cutaneous Manifestations Associated with Antiphospholipid Antibodies

Widespread skin necrosis was one of the first cutaneous complications reported in association with aPL. Since then many other clinical features such as livedo reticularis, leg ulcers, necrotizing purpura, Sneddon's syndrome, Degos's disease, distal cutaneous ischemia, widespread cutaneous necrosis, peripheral gangrene, and thrombophlebitis have been reported in association with aPL (72). Dermal vessel thrombosis, usually without vasculitis, may be considered characteristic of these skin lesions.

Primary Versus Secondary Antiphospholipid Syndrome

Whether the clinical features of the APS are in any way influenced by the presence or absence of SLE has recently been addressed in a multicenter trial on 114 patients who were followed during an average period of 2 years (21). Patients with primary and secondary APS have similar clinical profiles as they had similar frequencies of venous thrombosis, pulmonary embolism, arterial thrombosis, fetal loss, thrombocytopenia, livedo reticularis, pulmonary hypertension, and chorea at entry. Hemolytic anemia, neutropenia, and endocardial valve disease were more common in patients with SLE. The incidence of thrombosis, thrombocytopenia, and fetal loss during follow-up was similar in both patient groups. The primary APS (PAPS) should probably not be regarded as an early manifestation of the secondary APS because no patient with PAPS developed SLE in this series (21).

Antiphospholipid Antibodies and Infectious Disease

Elevated aPL levels are often found in association with infectious disease (for review, see 38). LAs have been described following mumps, hepatitis A, common childhood infections, and so forth. Elevated aCL, mainly IgM, are frequent in mycoplasma, chickenpox, hepatitis A, infectious mononucleosis, parvovirus, rubella, adenovirus, mumps, Lyme disease, and bacterial septicemia. In virtually all cases where follow-up samples were tested, aPL occurring in these infections were transient. In human immunodeficiency virus (HIV) infection, the occurrence of aPL was most common when opportunistic infections were present and tended to disappear upon resolution of the infection.

Drug-Induced Antiphospholipid Antibodies

APL have been found in association with the administration of various drugs (for review, see 38). Chlorpromazine and other drugs of the phenothiazine group are the most common cause of drug-induced aPL. About half of patients treated with chlorpromazine for a period longer than 1 year have elevated aPL levels, almost exclusively IgM. Other drugs, such as hydralazine, propranolol, procainamide, quinidine, amoxicillin, streptomycin, and so forth, also have been reported to induce aPL albeit much less frequently. Patients with drug-induced aPL do, however, not seem to develop the typical clinical complications associated with these antibodies.

PATHOGENIC MECHANISMS OF ANTIPHOSPHOLIPID ANTIBODIES

Interference with Natural Antithrombotic Pathways

The interest in aPL was kindled by early reports suggesting that these antibodies could be pathogenic. A causal relationship between these antibodies and thrombosis has been proposed via interference with several natural PL-dependent antithrombotic pathways.

Prostacyclin Production

Carreras et al. described a young woman with strong LA, arterial thromboses, and recurrent intrauterine death (73). They showed that the plasma of this patient impeded the production of prostacyclin by rat aorta rings, human myometrial tissue, and bovine aortic endothelial cells in culture. The hampered production could be restored by the addition of arachidonic acid. These authors suggested that the LA decreases the production of antithrombotic prostacyclin by interfering with the PL substrate from which arachidonic acid is released and hereby could be responsible for thrombosis in uteroplacental arteries. In a recent paper, Watson et al. (74). showed that the LA in a subset of thrombosis-prone patients decrease thrombin-mediated endothelial prostacyclin production. The same authors provided convincing evidence that these antibodies inhibit phospholipase A_2 activity in intact endothelial cells (75). These authors further confirmed that the inhibitory effect of the aPL on prostacyclin production is reversed by addition of exogenous arachidonic acid and showed that the enzymatic activity of various forms of phospholipase A_2 is inhibited by the aPL. It should, however, be noted that not all plasmas containing LA reduce prostacyclin formation (76,77).

The study of the effect of aPL on the production of PGI_2 by human umbilical vein endothelial cells has focused on the regulation of cyclooxygenase (Cox). It was demonstrated that patient IgGs stimulate the synthesis of newly described inducible Cox-2 without affecting the constitutive Cox-1 (78). This could reflect cell activation by these antibodies (see further). The "in vivo" significance of Cox-2 induction still is unknown.

The Protein C Pathway

Shortly after the description of the protein C pathway, Comp et al. (79) reported on an LA inhibiting protein C activation in the presence of thrombin, thrombomodulin, and PL. This finding was later described in more detail by two French groups (80,81). In addition, LAs have been found to prevent inactivation of factor Va by activated protein C on a PL surface (82). Finally, a reduction in protein S levels and function has been reported in patients with aPL (83). Inhibition of the protein C/protein S anticoagulant pathway has been confirmed by many groups but seems to depend on the type of PL used in the assay (84). However, again not all aPL impede the protein C anticoagulant pathway (85). Moreover, inhibition of the protein C system would not adequately explain the increased incidence of arterial thrombosis and fetal loss in patients with aPL because such complications are hardly observed in patients with protein C deficiency.

Effects on Other Antithrombotic Pathways

Cosgriff and Martin (1981) described a low-functional and high-antigenic antithrombin III level in a patient with the LA and recurrent thrombosis, implying interference with antithrombin III activity (86). More recently, aPL were also found to bind to heparin and thereby inhibit the formation of antithrombin–thrombin complexes (87).

Angles-Cano et al. (1979), using the venous occlusion test, found reduced or absent fibrinolytic capacity in 24 of 28 patients with SLE (88). Twelve of these patients had an LA and five had thrombotic episodes. More recent studies have evaluated the fibrinolytic capacity in patients with LAs but no consistent correlation between changes in the fibrinolytic potential and the presence of aPL could be found (89,90).

Another potential mechanism for aPL-induced thrombosis is the in vivo interference of these antibodies with the placental anticoagulant protein I, also named annexin V. Annexins are potent inhibitors of phospholipase A_2; they also inhibit coagulation reactions by preventing the assembly of activated coagulation factors on PL surfaces. In a recent study, Sammaritano et al. (91) showed that placental anticoagulant protein I and aCL compete for the binding to anionic PL, immobilized on microtiter wells. In clotting systems, aPL and placental anticoagulant protein I interacted additively.

Cellular Activation by Antiphospholipid Antibodies

Antiphospholipid Antibody Antigens

Two different groups almost simultaneously described that aCL are not directed against cardiolipin itself but against the complex that insolubilized cardiolipin forms with β_2GPI, a plasma protein with anticoagulant properties (92,93). Although the role of β_2GPI as cofactor for the binding of aCL to immobilized cardiolipin is still debated by some investigators (94), many groups have confirmed these findings. A number of studies demonstrated that the β_2GPI-dependent binding to PL can be used to discriminate between autoimmune aPL and those found in patients following infections (95,96). There also is evidence that β_2GPI undergoes a conformational change upon binding to anionic PL (97) and the resulting presentation of neo-epitopes is thought to be responsible for the aCL binding (98,99). The importance of β_2GPI was further stressed by the finding that some aCL can bind directly to this protein immobilized on irradiated microtiter plates in the absence of cardiolipin (100,101). Irradiation causes oxygenation of polystyrene plastic and increases its negative charge; β_2GPI bound to such a modified surface undergoes structural changes (101). In addition, several groups reported an excellent correlation between aCL titers and anti-β_2GPI (102–104), giving rise to the idea that autoimmune aCL and anti-β_2GPI are actually the same. Convincing experimental support for this has recently been provided by Roubey et al. (105). These authors showed that aCL are in fact anti-β_2GPI with an intrinsically low affinity toward fluid phase β_2GPI. Upon γ irradiation of microtiter plates, more β_2GPI is bound to the surface and this increased antigen density is responsible for low-affinity interactions to occur. Increased antigen density also could take place on anionic PL and therefore the

physiologic target of aCL is likely to be β_2GPI bound to membranes of activated cells.

The importance of β_2GPI for the binding of aPL is further underlined by the finding that a number of LAs exert their anticoagulant properties in a β_2GPI-dependent way and therefore appear to be directed against complexes of this protein with PL (106–108).

However, not all aPL are directed against β_2GPI bound to anionic PL. Bevers et al. showed that at least some LAs are directed against the complex formed by prothrombin and anionic PL rather than against PL itself (109). Antibodies binding to other protein–PL complexes such as protein C-PL and protein S-PL have also been found in plasma from patients with the APS (110). Not only complexes between proteins and anionic PL seem to be involved. Some patients have been described with antibodies binding to phosphatidylethanolamine, a neutral PL. Also for this binding, plasma proteins are required such as high and low molecular weight kininogen and sometimes prekallikrein and factor XI (111). One may hypothesize that aPL consist of a family of antibodies with varying affinities for protein–PL complexes (112,113) (Table 46-2).

Antibodies against β_2GPI–PL complexes are, however, the most frequently found aPL in patients with the APS and the importance of β_2GPI in the APS has been further emphasized by a series of findings. Monoclonal and polyclonal antibodies raised against β_2GPI bind to cardiolipin; some of them have LA activity (114). Passive and active immunization

TABLE 46-2. *Antigenic targets of antiphospholipid antibodies: phospholipid-binding proteins*

Major antigens:
  β_2-glycoprotein I
  Prothrombin
Others
  Protein C
  Protein S
  Thrombomodulin
  Annexin V
  High/low molecular weight kininogen
  Factor XI

of mice with such antibodies results in the induction of an experimental APS (115–117). In addition, several groups have demonstrated that an APS can be induced in animals upon immunization with β_2GPI alone (118–119). Pierangeli et al. recently reported on the thrombogenic effects of murine aCL, which suggests that these antibodies may be pathogenic in patients with APS (120).

Effect of Antiphospholipid Antibodies on Platelets

Sera of some patients with SLE and aPL increase thromboxane B_2 generation by platelet-rich plasma stimulated by collagen or arachidonic acid (77). In addition, purified IgG obtained from patients with the APS enhances thrombin-induced platelet activation and thromboxane formation (121). These findings are compatible with the increased urinary secretion of thromboxane B_2 metabolites observed in patients with the APS (122,123). That aPL are directly responsible for the observed effects is supported by the finding that affinity-purified aCL raised in rabbits induce a concentration-dependent activation of human platelets (124). The mechanism behind this was recently studied. Shi et al. showed that human aCL only bind to activated platelets and that this binding is β_2GPI-dependent (62). These authors also studied the influence of aCL on platelet aggregation and secretion but were unable to show any significant effect.

Arvieux et al. (125) investigated the effect of murine monoclonal anti-β_2GPI antibodies with LA activity on platelet activation. These monoclonal antibodies by themselves were unable to cause platelet aggregation and secretion but strongly potentiated these responses to subthreshold concentrations of epinephrine or ADP in the presence of appropriate amounts of β_2GPI. This effect was shown to be dependent upon binding to the platelet FcγRII receptor.

Effect of Antiphospholipid Antibodies on Endothelial Cells

Tannenbaum et al. (126) and Rustin et al. (127) showed several years ago that sera and

IgG from patients with an LA induce tissue factor activity in endothelial cells. This was further investigated by Hasselaar et al. (128) who demonstrated that aPL by themselves were unable to induce tissue factor expression in intact endothelial cells but strongly enhanced tissue factor activity induced by tumor necrosis factor. Applying this system to an in vitro thrombosis model, the same group observed a significantly higher procoagulant activity in the endothelial cell matrix formed in the presence of aPL (129). The role of β_2GPI in this "double-hit" model was not studied but it should be noted that the endothelial cells were cultured and stimulated in a medium supplemented with 20% human serum that would provide sufficient amounts of this cofactor.

β_2GPI binds to endothelial cells (130) and enhanced binding of affinity-purified aPL has been observed after membrane perturbation of endothelial cells (131). The need of cell activation for optimal binding of aPL is certainly plausible in view of the above-cited findings of Hasselaar et al. that aPL potentiate procoagulant expression by endothelial cells preactivated by tumor necrosis factor (128). In addition, Simantov et al. recently reported that aPL activate human endothelial cells in a β_2GPI dependent fashion (132).

Effect of Antiphospholipid Antibodies on Other Cells

Other cells to which aPL bind via β_2GPI include trophoblasts, neutrophils, and probably monocytes. Placentas obtained from patients with an APS have increased β_2GPI deposition (133), and immunofluorescence staining showed that these deposits were located at the trophoblast surfaces and were associated with a comparably increased deposition of IgG (134).

In 1994, Arvieux et al. reported on the β_2GPI-dependent binding of murine anti-β_2GPI with LA activity to human neutrophils resulting in their activation, degranulation, and adherence to endothelial cell monolayers (135). This was accompanied by proteolytic cleavage of heparin sulfate from the endothelial membrane. The observed effects were also dependent on binding of the antibodies to the neutrophil FcγRII receptor. The authors postulated that the interplay between neutrophils and endothelial cells in the presence of aPL would be prothrombotic.

Autoantibodies in the APS have been shown to induce tissue factor expression on monocytes (136). Since monocytes carry the FcγRII receptor, it is possible that this action occurs through antibody binding and receptor occupancy. Alternatively, complement activation could be involved, since C5a is known to induce tissue factor expression on monocytes (137).

Effect of β₂GPI and Antiphospholipid Antibodies on Apoptotic Cells

It has recently been shown that β_2GPI binds to apoptotic cells and therefore may play a role in their immune clearance (138). In addition, aPL has been shown to bind to apoptotic cells in a β_2GPI- dependent manner (139). One may speculate that aPL also might have a role in the immune clearance of apoptotica cells.

Proposed Pathogenic Scenario

From these results, the following scenario emerges: a small initial activation results in local exposure of anionic PL on the cell surface and binding of β_2GPI (or other PL-binding proteins) occurs; aPL subsequently bind to the cell surface via interaction with these PL-binding proteins; attachment of aPL to the cell membrane is further reinforced through interaction of its Fc portion with the surface FcγRII receptor; further cellular activation ensues that would create a vicious circle, ultimately leading to thrombosis.

One cannot help but be struck by the remarkable similarity of this scenario with the mechanism involved in the pathogenesis of heparin-induced thrombocytopenia and thrombosis, as recently emphasized by Arnout (140).

Clinical evidence is compatible with this proposed scenario. A few recent retrospective clinical studies on the APS clearly indicated that the recurrence rate for thrombosis is very high and that arterial events are almost always followed by arterial events and venous thrombosis most likely followed by another venous thrombosis (23,141). This is most compatible with a local trigger causing slight activation that is secondarily amplified by the antibody reaction.

LABORATORY DIAGNOSIS OF ANTIPHOSPHOLIPID ANTIBODIES

Detection of the Lupus Anticoagulant

General Guidelines for Lupus Anticoagulant Detection

In 1990, guidelines for LA detection based on minimal criteria have been proposed by the subcommittee for LAs of the International Society of Thrombosis and Haemostasis (142). These guidelines have recently been updated with emphasis on the preanalytic preparation of the sample, the exclusion of transient forms of LAs often seen in association with infectious disease, and the use of clotting factor assays in some difficult cases (143) (Table 46-3).

The laboratory diagnosis of an LA should follow a three-step procedure, verifying the following principles:

1. PL-dependent coagulation times of the test plasma should be prolonged. The APTT with a reduced phospholipid content, the dilute prothrombin time (dPT), the dilute Russell's viper venom time (dRVVT), and the kaolin clotting time (KCT) are currently the most often used screening tests for the detection of an LA (143).
2. The presence of an inhibitor should be demonstrated by use of mixing studies, i.e., clotting times of a mixture of test and normal plasmas should be significantly longer than those of normal plasma mixtures.

TABLE 46-3. *Laboratory diagnosis of lupus anticoagulants*

1. Screening tests
   Phospholipid-dependent clotting tests should be prolonged. Useful tests are:
   • activated partial thromboplastin time (APTT)
   • dilute prothrombin time (dPT)
   • dilute Russell viper venom time (dRVVT)
   • Kaolin clotting time (KCT)

2. Mixing studies
   The presence of anticoagulant is demonstrated when the clotting time remains prolonged upon addition of normal patient plasma.

3. Phospholipid dependency
   Lupus anticoagulants are differentiated from other coagulation inhibitors by correction in the presence of excessively high phospholipid concentrations. Phospholipids used for this purpose can be:
   • Platelet lysates
   • Platelet-derived microvesicles
   • Phospholipid liposomes
   • Hexagonal phospholipids

4. Distinction from other coagulopathies by specific factor assays.

Note: Special attention should be given to the pre-analytic variables, especially platelet contamination.

2. The antiphospholipid nature of the inhibitor should be confirmed by use of an LA neutralization procedure: There should be a relative correction of the clotting defect by the addition of lysed, washed platelets or PL liposomes. The most widely used test is the platelet neutralization procedure as described by Triplett et al. in 1983 (144). An LA- sensitive APTT or dRVVT is performed in the absence and the presence of activated platelets. The test is generally accepted to be quite specific for the presence of an LA. False-positive results, however, may be obtained with weak factor V inhibitors or when heparin is present in the sample. Another approach is the use of hexagonal phase PL for LA neutralization as described by Rauch et al. (145).

It is firmly recommended not to rely on a single screening test and to confirm a positive diagnosis on a second blood sample taken at least 8 weeks later. LA tests can only be performed on plasma samples that are as platelet-free as possible since the sensitivity of any screening procedure is inversely proportional to the residual number of platelets in the platelet-poor plasma, especially when the tests are performed on frozen plasma (143).

General Comments on LA Detection

The laboratory diagnosis of LAs is not easy considering the relatively poor results from interlaboratory surveys (146,147). To date, it is almost impossible to formulate precise recommendations on which assays or combination of assays to use. Only few comparative studies are available evaluating the differences in sensitivity among various tests. These studies have several limitations such as the small number of patients included, differences in inclusion criteria, instruments, reagents, plasma preparation, etc. There is no "gold standard" patient population available against which assays could be validated. There is an urgent need for internationally accepted quality control specimens.

The precise mechanism by which LAs prolong clotting in vitro is still not well understood although the antigens are already quite well characterized. Better insight in this will hopefully lead to the development of test systems with improved sensitivity and specificity.

Immunologic Assays for Antiphospholipid Antibodies

Detection of Anticardiolipin Antibodies

ACL are now usually measured with a very sensitive solid phase enzyme-linked immunosorbent assay (ELISA) using cardiolipin in solid phase (10,17). The results are usually expressed in IgG antiphospholipid (GPL) and IgM antiphospholipid (MPL) units when using the standards introduced by Harris et al. (17). Although relatively easy to perform, small variations in the assay conditions for aCL can lead to large variations in the results and the standardization is far from optimal, as recently demonstrated by a multicentric evaluation of nine commercial kits for the detection of aCL (148). It is therefore recommended to report titers in a semi- quantitative manner (17).

As for LAs, a positive result should have a repeat measurement several weeks later to discriminate between persistent and transient aPL.

Other PL solid phase immunoassays were developed employing partial thromboplastin or pure phosphatidylserine as the antigen with the aim of quantitatively detecting antibodies causing LA activity (149,150). Comparative studies, however, disclosed only a moderate agreement between clotting tests and ELISAs. In fact, with the development of sensitive tests for LA, many LA-positive patients are found who prove negative in the antiphospholipid ELISAs. In contrast, a close relationship between the presence and level of aCL and antibodies to other anionic PL is generally observed that can now be better understood in the light of the recent finding that aCL found in patients with the APS are directed against β_2GPI complexed with PL. The still moderate agreement between coagulation assays and immunologic assays may be related to the fact that many LAs act in a β_2GPI-dependent way.

Other Immunologic Assays to Detect Antiphospholipid Antibodies

Because aCL are directed to β_2GPI via which they bind to anionic PL, direct assays to measure anti-β_2GPI have been developed mostly using irradiated microtiter plates (100). Viard et al. reported that 36% of patients with SLE have anti-β_2GPI and a strong association was found with a history of

thrombosis when these antibodies were present together with an LA (101). Several other investigators found an excellent correlation between anti-β_2GPI antibody levels, aCL levels, and thrombosis in patients with the APS (102). From these results one might expect that direct anti-β_2GPI antibody assays should soon replace the aCL test. However, it is still uncertain as to whether both assays measure the same populations of autoantibodies (151).

Since the discovery that some LAs are directed against PL bound prothrombin (109), direct antiprothrombin antibody assays have also been developed (22,152). In the study of Arvieux et al. (152), antiprothrombin antibodies were present in approximately 70% of patients with SLE. Data on the association of anti-prothrombin antibodies and clinical manifestations of APS are very scarce. In the study of Horbach et al. (22) approximately 33% of patients with SLE had anti-prothrombin antibodies. Univariate analysis of risk factors for thrombosis showed a significant correlation between these antibodies and thrombosis. After multivariate analysis, LA and aCL IgM were found to be the strongest risk factors and the presence of anti-β_2GPI or antiprothrombin did not increase the risk for thrombosis. These data question the clinical need to develop direct anti-β_2GPI or antiprothrombin assays.

TREATMENT OF PATIENTS WITH THE ANTIPHOSPHOLIPID SYNDROME

Treatment of Patients with Thrombosis

Three recent studies underline the need for anticoagulation of patients with the APS and a history of thrombosis. The first study analyzed a retrospective survey of 70 consecutive patients, mostly with a primary APS (23). The authors conclude that the site of the first event tends to predict the site of subsequent events and that intermediate- to high-intensity (INR >2.6) anticoagulant prophylaxis should be used. They also advise indefinite anticoagulation for reliable patients who have had recur-

TABLE 46-4. *Treatment of the antiphospholipid syndrome (APS)*

1. Antiphospholipid antibodies (aPL) are a fortuitous finding.
   • These patients do not fulfill the criteria for APS.
   • Only careful follow-up is recommended.
2. Nonpregnant patients with thrombosis and aPL.
   • Acute venous thrombosis associated to a circumstantial predisposing factor, e.g., surgery.
     Standard treatment with heparin and warfarin (3 months) is recommended.
   • Acute spontaneous or recurrent thrombosis.
     Long-term warfarin INR 2.5–3.5 is recommended.
   • Recurrent thrombosis in patients under warfarin treatment.
     Warfarin INR 2–3 plus low-dose aspirin may be considered.
   • Arterial thrombosis.
     Low-dose aspirin is recommended.
     This can be associated with warfarin (INR 2–3) in patients with recurrent events
3. Pregnant patients with aPL and a history of previous thrombosis.
   Aspirin should be given, eventually together with prophylactic doses of heparin
4. Pregnant patients with aPL and acute thrombosis
   Therapeutic dose of low molecular weight heparin + aspirin
5. Patients with aPL and a history of fetal loss
   Nonpregnant
     No special treatment is recommended: the patient should be followed carefully.
   Pregnant
     Dependent on the number of fetal losses and failure of previous treatments, the patient should
     be treated with aspirin, aspirin plus heparin, heparin, or immunoglobulins.

Note: Most of these recommendations are derived from retrospective studies and anecdotal reports.

rent thrombosis. The second study analyzes a retrospective survey of 19 patients, mostly with SLE, with aPL and a history of venous thromboembolism (153). Using a Kaplan-Meier analysis, the authors calculated that patients receiving oral anticoagulants had a 100% probability of survival without recurrence at 8 years, whereas patients in whom anticoagulation was stopped had a 50% probability of a recurrent venous thromboembolic episodes at 2 years, and a 78% probability of recurrence at 8 years. The third study is a retrospective analysis of 147 patients with the APS (141). This study reports an annual recurrence rate of 0.29 for untreated patients, 0.18 for those receiving aspirin, and nearly 0 for those treated with high- dose oral anticoagulants (INR >3). However, this study was retrospective and had a nonrandomized design, which limits the validity of the conclusion that long-term anticoagulation (INR >3) is to be maintained. In a recent prospective cohort study, 11 patients with LAs and thrombosis treated with conventional warfarin (INR 2 to 3 for 3 months) had the same incidence of thrombotic recurrences as 49 patients without aPL (19). Because aPL are not associated with thrombosis in all patients and because they will probably be discovered more frequently as more sensitive tests are in common use, it would at present seem unwise to recommend anticoagulant therapy in all patients with aPL, also in view of the bleeding risk involved in long-term anticoagulation (Table 46-4). Furthermore, thrombocytopenia frequently seen in APS patients might augment the risk of bleeding associated with oral anticoagulants. Therefore, prospective clinical trials are needed to establish the proper treatment of these patients. Another problem that needs to be clarified is the validity of the INR values obtained in patients with LA treated with oral anticoagulants. A few recent reports show that different thromboplastins may be variably affected by the presence of LAs (154). Therefore, INR values obtained with LA-sensitive reagents might reflect both the effect of warfarin and the in vitro anticoagulant action of the antibodies and thus overestimate the oral anticoagulant effects. The monitoring of warfarin therapy in APS patients with a prolonged PT at baseline could be more accurately performed using the Thrombotest or the Owren P&P test.

Treatment of Patients with Stroke

Treatment regimens used in patients with aPL and cerebrovascular disease are multiple and have recently been reviewed (155). Although today no firm recommendations can be made, the use of low-dose aspirin for secondary prevention in patients with ischemic stroke seems reasonable. Warfarin therapy should be considered in patients with cardioembolic stroke.

Management of Patients with the Antiphospholipid Syndrome During Pregnancy

Corticosteroids

The rationale for the use of corticosteroid therapy is suppression of the aPL. After the first promising report by Lubbe et al. (156), many studies describing corticosteroid therapy, often in combination with acetylsalicylic acid, were published and a pooling of these usually small series yields a successful pregnancy outcome in about 60% (157). However, the enthusiasm concerning this therapy has been tempered after the report by Lockshin and colleagues, who described 10 fetal deaths in 13 pregnancies with steroids (158). In recent studies corticosteroids used in combination with low-dose aspirin did not result in a better fetal outcome than heparin in association with low-dose aspirin, but the frequency of preterm delivery and serious maternal morbidity was significantly higher among women randomly assigned to prednisone (159). Therefore, the routine use of prednisone in these patients can no longer be recommended.

Aspirin

Only few studies describe the effects of aspirin alone in patients with aPL and fetal loss, and they seem to indicate improvement of the pregnancy success rate (160,161). In a recent study of 60 patients, pregnancy outcome improved from 19% to 70% after treatment with low-dose aspirin (75 mg daily) in all patients

and subcutaneous heparin in those with previous thrombosis (162) (Table 46-4).

Heparin

The rationale of heparin is based on the evidence that fetal loss may be due to thrombosis within the uterine vessels leading to placental dysfunction. However, several studies, very limited in size, have reported a successful outcome in 75% to 93% of the cases with heparin dosages ranging from 10,000 to 36,000 IU (163). Two recently published prospective randomized trials on 50 and 90 patients have shown that heparin (5,000 U UFH bid) plus low-dose aspirin (75 mg daily) provides a significantly better pregnancy outcome than low-dose aspirin alone (164,165). Potential risks associated with heparin therapy are hemorrhage, osteoporosis, and heparin-induced thrombocytopenia. There is growing use of low molecular weight heparin for thrombosis prophylaxis in patients during pregnancy. From the available data one can reasonably speculate that it may be as effective and probably safer than unfractionated heparin, also in the treatment of pregnant APS patients (Table 46-4).

Immunoglobulins

Successful pregnancy outcome in women with the APS has been reported following treatment with high doses of intravenous immunoglobulins (166,167). Given the cost of this treatment and the lack of controlled prospective trials, immunoglobulin therapy should be reserved for women with failures using the previously mentioned therapies (Table 46-4).

CONCLUSION

Persistently elevated levels of antiphospholipid antibodies are associated with an increased risk for thrombosis, fetal loss, neurologic disorders, and thrombocytopenia. This association is known as the antiphospholipid syndrome.

It is now widely accepted that autoimmune antiphospholipid antibodies do not bind to phospholipid per se but to phospholipid-binding protein–phospholipid complexes. The major phospholipid- binding proteins involved are β_2-glycoprotein I and prothrombin.

In vitro experimental data, in vivo animal models, and epidemiologic evidence strongly suggest that antiphospholipid antibodies are involved in the pathogenesis of the antiphospholipid syndrome. However, the pathogenic mechanism remains to be elucidated.

Patients with thrombosis and the antiphospholipid syndrome have a high recurrency rate. Retrospective studies suggest that these patients need to be treated with long-term, high-intensity, oral anticoagulation.

REFERENCES

1. Moore JE, Mohr CF. Biologically false-positive serologic tests for syphilis: type, incidence, and cause. *JAMA* 1952;150:467–473.
2. Moore JE, Lutz WB. The natural history of systemic lupus erythematosus: an approach to its study through chronic biologic false-positive reactions. *J Chronic Dis* 1955;1:297–316.
3. Conley CL, Hartmann RC. A hemorrhagic disorder caused by circulating anticoagulant in patients with disseminated lupus erythematosus. *J Clin Invest* 1952;31:621–622.
4. Feinstein DI, Rapaport SI. Acquired inhibitors of blood coagulation. *Prog Hemost Thromb* 1972;1:75–95.
5. Bowie EJW, Thompson JH Jr, Pascuzzi CA, Owen CA Jr. Thrombosis in systemic lupus erythematosus despite circulating anticoagulants. *J Lab Clin Med* 1963;62:416–430.
6. Laurell AB, Nilsson IM. Hypergammaglobulinaemia, circulating anticoagulant, and biologic false positive Wassermann reaction: a study of 2 cases. *J Lab Clin Med* 1957;49:694–707.
7. Lechner K. Acquired inhibitors in nonhemophilic patients. *Haemostasis* 1974;3:65–93.
8. Thiagarajan P, Shapiro SS, De Marco L. Monoclonal immunoglobulin M coagulation inhibitor with phospholipid specificity. Mechanism of lupus anticoagulant. *J Clin Invest* 1980;66:397–405.
9. Harris EN, Gharavi AE, Boey ML, et al. Anticardiolipin antibodies: detection by radioimmunoassay and association with thrombosis in systemic lupus erythematosus. *Lancet* 1983;2:1211–1214.
10. Loizou S, McCrea JD, Rudge AC, Reynolds R, Boyle CC, Harris EN. Measurement of anticardiolipin antibodies by an enzyme-linked immunosorbent assay (ELISA): standardization and quantitation of results. *Clin Exp Immunol* 1985;62:738–745.
11. Hughes GRV, Harris EN, Gharavi AE. The anticardiolipin syndrome. *J Rheumatol* 1986;13:486–489.
12. Alarcon-Segovia D, Sanchez-Guerrero J. Primary antiphospholipid syndrome. *J Rheumatol* 1989;16:482–488.
13. Carreras LO, Vermylen JG. Lupus anticoagulant and thrombosis—possible role of inhibition of prostacyclin formation. *Thromb Haemost* 1982;48:38–40.
14. Lechner K, Pabinger-Fasching I. Lupus anticoagulants and thrombosis. A study of 25 cases and review of the literature. *Haemostasis* 1985;15:254–262.
15. Love PE, Santoro SA. Antiphospholipid antibodies: anticardiolipin and the lupus anticoagulant in systemic lupus erythematosus (SLE) and in non-SLE disorders. *Ann Intern Med* 1990;112:682–698.
16. Triplett DA, Brandt JT, Maas RL. The laboratory heterogeneity of lupus anticoagulants. *Arch Pathol Lab Med* 1985;109:946–951.
17. Harris EN, Gharavi AE, Patel SP, Hughes GRV. Evaluation of the anti-cardiolipin antibody test: report of an international workshop held 4 April 1986. *Clin Exp Immunol* 1987;68:215–222.
18. Ginsburg KS, Liang MH, Newcomer L, et al. Anticardiolipin antibodies and the risk for ischemic stroke and venous thrombosis. *Ann Intern Med* 1992;117:997–1002.
19. Ginsberg JS, Wells PS, Brill-Edwards P, et al. Antiphospholipid antibodies and venous thromboembolism. *Blood* 1995;86:3685–3691.
20. Finazzi G, Brancaccio V, Moia M, et al. Natural history and risk factors for thrombosis in 360 patients with antiphospolipid antibodies: a four-year prospective study from the italian registry. *Am J Med* 1996;100:530–536.
21. Vianna JL, Khamastha MA, Ordi-Ros J, et al. Comparison of the primary and secondary antiphospholipid syndrome: a European multicenter study of 114 patients. *Am J Med* 1994;96:3–9.
22. Horbach DA, Oort EV, Donders RCJM, Derksen RHWM, de Groot PhG. Lupus anticoagulant is the strongest risk factor for both venous and arterial thrombosis in patients with systemic lupus erythematosus. Comparison between different assays for the detection of antiphospholipid antibodies. *Thromb Haemost* 1996;76:916–924.
23. Rosove MH, Brewer PMC. Antiphospholipid thrombosis: Clinical course after the first thrombotic event in 70 patients. *Ann Intern Med* 1992;117:303–308.
24. Vermylen J, Blockmans D, Spitz B, Arnout J, Grillet B. Thrombosis as an immune phenomenon. *Baillière's Clin Immunol Allergy* 1987;1:619–641.
25. Asherson RA, Mackworth-Young CG, Boey ML, et al. Pulmonary hypertension in systemic lupus erythematosus. *Br Med J* 1983;287:1024–1025.
26. Moser KM, Auger WR, Fedullo PF, Jamieson SW. Chronic thromboembolic pulmonary hypertension: clinical picture and surgical treatment. *Eur Respir J* 1992;5:334–342.
27. Hamsten A, Norberg R, Björkholm M, de Faire U, Holm G. Antibodies to cardiolipin in young survivors of myocardial infarction: an association with recurrent cardiovascular events. *Lancet* 1986;1:113–116.
28. Sletnes KE, Smith P, Abedlnoor M, Arnesen H, Wisloff F. Antiphospholipid antibodies and myocardial infarction and their relation to mortality, reinfarction and nonhaemorrhagic stroke. *Lancet* 1992;339:451–453.

29. Vaarala O, Mänttäri M, Mannine V, et al. Anticardi-olipin antibodies and risk of myocardial infarction in a prospective cohort of middle-aged men. *Circulation* 1995;91:23–27

30. Morton KE, Gavaghan TP, Krilis SA, Daggard GE, Baron DW, Hickie JB. Coronary artery bypass graft failure—an autoimmune phenomenon? *Lancet* 1986; 2:1353–1357.

31. Englert HJ, Hawkes CH, Boey ML, et al. Degos' disease: association with anticardiolipin antibodies and the lupus anticoagulant. *Br Med J* 1984;289:576.

32. Finazzi G, Cortelazzo S, Viero P, Galli M, Barbui T. Maternal lupus anticoagulant and fatal neonatal thrombosis. *Thromb Haemost* 1987;57:238.

33. Sheridan-Pereira M, Porreco RP, Hays T, Burke MS. Neonatal aortic thrombosis associated with the lupus anticoagulant. *Obstet Gynecol* 1988;71;1016–1018.

34. Nilsson IM, Astedt B, Hedner U, Berezin D. Intrauterine death and circulating anticoagulant ("antithromboplastin"). *Acta Med Scand* 1975;197:153–159.

35. Soulier JP, Boffa MC. Avortements à répétition, thromboses et anticoagulant circulant antithromboplastine. Trois observations. *Nouv Presse Med* 1980;9:859–864.

36. Firkin BG, Howard MA, Radford N. Possible relationship between lupus inhibitor and recurrent abortion in young women. *Lancet* 1980;2:366.

37. Ginsberg JS, Brill-Edwards P, Johnston M, et al. Relationship of antiphospholipid antibodies to pregnancy loss in patients with systemic lupus erythematosus: a cross-sectional study. *Blood* 1992;80:975–980.

38. McNeil HP, Chesterman CN, Krilis SA. Immunology and clinical importance of antiphospholipid antibodies. *Adv Immunol* 1991;49:193–280.

39. Out HJ, Bruinse HW, Christiaens GCML, et al. A prospective, controlled multicenter study on the obstetric risk of pregnant women with antiphospholipid antibodies. *Am J Obstet Gynecol* 1992;167:26–32.

40. MacLean MA, Cumming GP, McCall F, Walker ID, Walker JJ. The prevalence of lupus anticoagulant and anticardiolipin antibodies in women with a history of first trimester miscarriages. *Br J Obstet Gynaecol* 1994;101:103–106.

41. Infante-Rivard C, David M, Gauthier R, Rivard GE. Lupus anticoagulants, anticardiolipin antibodies, and fetal loss. *N Engl J Med* 1991;15:1063–1066.

42. Branch DW, Andres R, Digre KB, Rote NS, Scott JR. The association of antiphospholipid antibodies with severe preeclampsia. *Obstet Gynecol* 1989;73:541–545.

43. Rai RS, Regan L, Clifford K, et al. Antiphospholipid antibodies and beta-2-glycoprotein I in 500 women with recurrent miscarriage; results of a comprehensive screening approach. *Hum Reprod* 1995;10:101–105.

44. Branch DW, Silver RM, Blackwell JL, Reading JC, Scott JR. Outcome of treated pregnancies in woman with the antiphospholipid syndrome: an update of the Utah experience. *Obstet Gynecol* 1992;80:614–620.

45. Lockshin MD, Druzin ML, Goei S, et al. Antibody to cardiolipin as a predictor of fetal distress or death in pregnant patients with systemic lupus erythematosus. *N Engl J Med* 1985;313:152–156.

46. Harris EN, Chan JKH, Asherson RA, Aber VR, Gharavi AE, Hughes GR. Thrombosis, recurrent fetal loss and thrombocytopenia: predictive value of the anti-cardiolipin antibody test. *Arch Intern Med* 1986;146: 2153–2159.

47. Harris EN. The Second International Anti-Cardiolipin Standardization Workshop/The Kingston Anti-Phospholipid Antibody Study (KAPS) Group. *Am J Clin Pathol* 1990;94:476–484.

48. Lubbe WF, Butler WS, Palmer SJ, Liggins GC. Lupus anticoagulant in pregnancy. *Br J Obstet Gynaecol* 1984;91:357–363.

49. De Wolf F, Carreras LO, Moerman P, Vermylen J, Van Assche A, Renaer M. Decidual vasculopathy and extensive placental infarction in a patient with repeated thromboembolic accidents, recurrent fetal loss and a lupus anticoagulant. *Am J Obstet Gynecol* 1982;142: 829–834.

50. Out HJ, Kooijman CD, Bruinse HW, Derksen RHWM. Histopathololological findings in placentae from patients with intra-uterine fetal death and anti-phospholipid antibodies. *Eur J Obstet Gynecol Reprod Biol* 1991;41:179–186.

51. Labarerre CA, Catoggio LJ, Mullen EG, Althabe OH. Placental lesions in maternal autoimmune disease. *Am J Reprod Immunol Microbiol* 1986;12:78–86.

52. Mari G, Wasserstrum N. Flow velocity waveforms of the fetal circulation preceding fetal death in a case of lupus anticoagulant. *Am J Obstet Gynecol* 1991;164: 776–778.

53. Greenspoon JS. Cerebral infarction, lupus anticoagulant and habitual abortion. *JAMA* 1986;255:2164.

54. Levine SR, Kim S, Deegan MJ, Welch KMA. Ischemic stroke associated with anticardiolipin antibodies. *Stroke* 1987;18:1101–1106.

55. Coull BM, Bourdette DN, Goodnight SH Jr, Briley DP, Hart R. Multiple cerebral infarctions and dementia associated with anticardiolipin antibodies. *Stroke* 1987; 18:1107–1112.

56. Hughson MD, McCarty GA, Sholer CM, Brumback RA. Thrombotic cerebral arteriopathy in patients with the Antiphospholipid Syndrome. *Mod Pathol* 1993;6: 644–653.

57. Digre KB, Durcan FJ, Branch DW, Jacobson DM, Varner MW, Baringer JR. Amaurosis fugax associated with antiphospholipid antibodies. *Ann Neurol* 1989; 25:228–232.

58. Levine SR, Langer SL, Albers JW, Welch KMA. Sneddon's syndrome: an antiphospholipid antibody syndrome? *Neurology* 1988;38:798–800.

59. Stephens CJM. Sneddon's syndrome. *Clin Exp Rheumatol* 1992;10:489–492.

60. Levine SR and Brey RL. Neurological aspects of antiphospholipid antibody syndrome. *Lupus* 1996;5: 347–353.

61. The Antiphospholipid Antibodies in Stroke Study (APASS) Group. Anticardiolipin antibodies are an independent risk factor for first ischemic stroke. *Neurology* 1993;43:2069–2073.

62. Shi W, Chong BH, Chesterman CN. Beta 2 glycoprotein I is a requirement for anticardiolipin antibodies binding to activated platelets: differences with lupus anticoagulants. *Blood* 1993;81:1255–1266.

63. Galli M, Finazzi G, Barbui T. Thrombocytopenia in the antiphospholipid syndrome. *Br J Haematol* 1996;93: 1–5

64. Stasi R, Stipa E, Masi M, et al. Prevalence and clinical significance of elevated antiphospholipid antibodies in patients with idiopathic thrombocytopenic purpura. *Blood* 1994;84:4203–8.

65. Libman E, Sacks B. A hitherto undescribed form of valvular and mural endocarditis. *Arch Intern Med* 1924;33:701–737.

66. D'Alton JG, Preston DN, Bormanis J, Green MS, Kraag GR. Multiple transient ischemic attacks, lupus anticoagulant and verrucous endocarditis. *Stroke* 1985;16:512–514.

67. Ford PM, Ford SE, Lillicrap DP. Association of lupus anticoagulant with severe valvular heart disease in systemic lupus erythematosus. *J Rheumatol* 1988;15:597–600.

68. Khamashta MA, Cervera R, Asherson RA, et al. Association of antibodies against phospholipids with heart valve disease in systemic lupus erythematosus. *Lancet* 1990;335:1541–1544.

69. Cervera R, Font J, Pare C, et al. Cardiac disease in sytemic lupus erythematosus: prospective study of 70 patients. *Ann Rheum Dis* 1992;51:156–159.

70. Hojnik M, George J, Ziporen L, Shoenfeld Y. Heart valve involvement (Libman-Sacks endocarditis) in the antiphospholipid syndrome. *Circulation* 1996;93:1579–1587.

71. Asherson RA, Piette JC. The catastrofic antiphospholipid syndrome 1996: acute multi-organ failure associated with antiphospholipid antibodies a review of 31 patients. *Lupus* 1996;5:414–417.

72. Stephens CJM. The antiphospholipid syndrome. Clinical correlations, cutaneous features, mechanism of thrombosis and treatment of patients with the lupus anticoagulant and anticardiolipin antibodies. *Br J Dermatol* 1991;125:199–210.

73. Carreras LO, Defreyn G, Machin SJ, et al. Arterial thrombosis, intrauterine death and `lupus' anticoagulant: detection of immunoglobulin interfering with prostacyclin formation. *Lancet* 1981;1:244–246.

74. Watson KV, Schorer AE. Lupus anticoagulant inhibition of in vitro prostacyclin release is associated with a thrombosis-prone subset of patients. *Am J Med* 1991;90:47–53.

75. Schorer AE, Duane PG, Woods VL, Niewoehner DE. Some antiphospholipid antibodies inhibit phospholipase A2 activity. *J Lab Clin Med* 1992;120:67–77.

76. Carreras LO, Maclouf J. Antiphospholipid antibodies and eicosanoids. *Lupus* 1994;3:271–273.

77. Hasselaar P, Derksen RHWM, Blokzijl L, de Groot PG. Thrombosis associated with antiphospholipid antibodies cannot be explained by effects on endothelial and platelet prostanoid synthesis. *Thromb Haemost* 1988;59:80–85.

78. Habib A, Martinuzzo ME, Carreras LO, Levy-Toledano S, Maclouf J. Increased expression of inducible cyclooxygenase-2 in human endothelial cells by antiphospholipid antibodies. *Thromb Haemost* 1995;74:770–777.

79. Comp PC, De Bault LE, Esmon NL, Esmon CT. Human thrombomodulin is inhibited by IgG from two patients with non specific anticoagulants. *Blood* 1983;62(suppl I):299.

80. Freyssinet JM, Cazenave JP. Lupus-like anticoagulants, modulation of the protein C pathway and thrombosis. *Thromb Haemost* 1987;58:679–81.

81. Cariou R, Tobelem G, Bellucci S, et al. Effect of lupus anticoagulant on antithrombogenic properties of endothelial cells—inhibition of thrombomodulin-dependent protein C activation. *Thromb Haemost* 1988;60:54–58.

82. Marciniak E, Romond EH. Impaired catalytic function of activated protein C: a new in vitro manifestation of lupus anticoagulant. *Blood* 1989;74:2426–2432.

83. Kordich LC, Forastiero RR, Basilotta E, Porterie P, Carreras LO. Natural inhibitors of blood coagulation and fibrinolysis in patients with lupus anticoagulant. *Blood Coagulat Fibrinol* 1992;3:765–771.

84. Smirnov MD, Triplett DA, Comp PC et al. On the role of phosphatidylethanolamine in the inhibition of activated protein C activity by antiphospholipid antibodies. *J Clin Invest* 1995;95:309–316.

85. Tsakiris DA, Yasikoff ML, Worf F, Marbet GA. Anticardiolipin antibodies do not seem to be associated with aPC resistance in vivo or in vitro. *Ann Hematol* 1995;71:195–198.

86. Cosgriff TM, Martin BA. Low functional and high antigenic antithrombin III level in a patient with the lupus anticoagulant and recurrent thrombosis. *Arthritis Rheum* 1981;24:94–96.

87. Shibata S, Harpel P, Gharavi A, Rand J, Fillit H. Autoantibodies to heparin from patients with antiphospholipid antibody syndrome inhibit formation of antithrombin III-thrombin complexes. *Blood* 1994;83:2532–2540.

88. Angles-Cano E, Sultan Y, Clauvel JP. Predisposing factors to thrombosis in systemic lupus erythematosus. Possible relation to endothelial cell damage. *J Lab Clin Med* 1979;94:312–323.

89. Francis RB Jr, Neely S. Effect of the lupus anticoagulant on endothelial fibrinolytic activity in vitro. *Thromb Haemost* 1989;61:314–317.

90. Tsakiris DA, Marbet GA, Makris PE, Settas L, Duckert F. Impaired fibrinolysis as an essential contribution to thrombosis in patients with lupus anticoagulant. *Thromb Haemost* 1989;61:175–177.

91. Sammaritano LR, Gharavi AE, Soberano C, Levy RA, Michael D, Lockshin MD. Phospolipid binding of antiphospholipid antibodies and placental anticoagulant protein. *J Clin Immunol* 1992;12:27–35.

92. McNeil HP, Simpson RJ, Chesterman CN, Krilis SA. Anti-phospholipid antibodies are directed against a complex antigen that includes a lipid-binding inhibitor of coagulation: beta-2-glycoprotein I (apolipoprotein H). *Proc Natl Acad Sci USA* 1990;87:4120–4124.

93. Galli M, Comfurius P, Maassen C, et al. Anticardiolipin antibodies (ACA) directed not to cardiolipin but to a plasma protein cofactor. *Lancet* 1990;335:1544–1547.

94. Pierangeli SS, Harris EN, Davis SA, DeLorenzo G. Beta2-glycoprotein 1 (beta 2GP1) enhances cardiolipin binding activity but is not the antigen for antiphospholipid antibodies. *Br J Haematol* 1992;82:565–570.

95. Matsuura E, Igarashi Y, Fujimoto M, Ichikawa K, Koike T. Anticardiolipin cofactor(s) and differential diagnosis of autoimmune disease. *Lancet* 1990;336:177–178.

96. Hunt JE, McNeil HP, Morgan GJ, Crameri RM, Krilis SA. A phospholipid-beta 2-glycoprotein I complex is an antigen for anticardiolipin antibodies occurring in autoimmune disease but not with infection. *Lupus* 1992;1:75–81.

97. Wagenknecht DR, McIntyre JA. Changes in beta 2-glycoprotein I antigenicity induced by phospholipid binding. *Thromb Haemost* 1993;69:361–5.
98. Ichikawa K, Khamashta MA, Koike T, Matsuura E, Hughes GR. β_2-Glycoprotein I reactivity of monoclonal anticardiolipin antibodies from patients with the antiphospholipid syndrome. *Arthritis Rheum* 1994,37:1453–61.
99. Pengo V, Biasiolo A, Fior MG. Autoimmune antiphospholipid antibodies are directed against a cryptic epitope expressed when β_2-glycoprotein I is bound to a suitable surface. *Thromb Haemost* 1995;73:29–34.
100. Arvieux J, Roussel B, Jacob MC, Colomb MG. Measurement of anti-phospholipid antibodies by ELISA using beta 2-glycoprotein I as an antigen. *J Immunol Meth* 1991;143:223–229.
101. Matsuura E, Igarashi Y, Yasuda T, Triplett DA, Koike T. Anticardiolipin antibodies recognize β_2-Glycoprotein I structure altered by interaction with an oxygen modified solid phase surface. *J Exp Med* 1994;179:457–462.
102. Viard JP, Amoura Z, Bach JF. Association of anti-beta 2-glycoprotein I antibodies with lupus-type circulating anticoagulant and thrombosis in systemic lupus erythematosus. *Am J Med* 1992;93:181–186.
103. Matsuda J, Saitoh N, Gohchi K, Gotoh M, Tsukamoto M. Detection of beta-2-glycoprotein-I-dependent antiphospholipid antibodies and anti-beta-2-glycoprotein-I antibody in patients with systemic lupus erythematosus and in patients with syphilis. *Int Arch Allergy Immunol* 1994;103:239–244.
104. Martinuzzo ME, Forastiero RR, Carreras LO. Anti beta 2 glycoprotein I antibodies: detection and association with thrombosis. *Br J Haematol* 1995;89:397–402.
105. Roubey RAS, Eisenberg RA, Harper MF, Winfield JB. "Anticardiolipin" autoantibodies recognize β_2-glycoprotein I in the absence of phospholipid. Importance of Ag density and bivalent binding. *J Immunol* 1995;154:954–960.
106. Oosting JD, Derksen RH, Entjes HT, Bouma BN, de Groot PG. Lupus anticoagulant activity is frequently dependent on the presence of beta 2-glycoprotein I. *Thromb Haemost* 1992;67:499–502.
107. Roubey RA, Pratt CW, Buyon JP, Winfield JB. Lupus anticoagulant activity of autoimmune antiphospholipid antibodies is dependent upon beta 2-glycoprotein I. *J Clin Invest* 1992;90:1100–1104.
108. Galli M, Comfurius P, Barbui T, Zwaal RF, Bevers EM. Anticoagulant activity of beta 2-glycoprotein I is potentiated by a distinct subgroup of anticardiolipin antibodies. *Thromb Haemost* 1992;68:297–300.
109. Bevers EM, Galli M, Barbui T, Comfurius P, Zwaal RF. Lupus anticoagulant IgG's (LA) are not directed to phospholipids only, but to a complex of lipid-bound human prothrombin. *Thromb Haemost* 1991;66:629–32.
110. Oosting JD, Derksen RH, Bobbink IW, Hackeng TM, Bouma BN, de Groot PG. Antiphospholipid antibodies directed against a combination of phospholipids with prothrombin, protein C, or protein S: an explanation for their pathogenic mechanism? *Blood* 1993;81:2618–2625.
111. Sugi T, McIntyre JA. Autoantibodies to phosphatidyle-thanolamine (PE) recognize a kininogen-PE complex. *Blood* 1995;86:3083–3089.
112. Vermylen J, Arnout J. Is the antiphospholipid syndrome caused by antibodies directed against physiologically relevant phospholipid-protein complexes? *J Lab Clin Med* 1992;120:10–12.
113. Roubey RA. Autoantibodies to phospholipid-binding plasma proteins: a new view of lupus anticoagulants and other "antiphospholipid" autoantibodies. *Blood* 1994;84:2854–2867.
114. Arvieux J, Pouzol P, Roussel B, Jacob MC, Colomb MG. Lupus-like anticoagulant properties of murine monoclonal antibodies to β 2-glycoprotein I. *Br J Haematol* 1992;81:568–573.
115. Branch DW, Dudley DJ, Mitchell MD, Creighton KA, Abbott TM, Hammond EH, Daynes RA. Immunoglobulin G fractions from patients with antiphospholipid antibodies cause fetal death in BALB/c mice: a model for autoimmune fetal loss. *Am J Obstet Gynecol* 1990;163:210–216.
116. Blank M, Cohen J, Toder V, Shoenfeld Y. Induction of anti-phospholipid syndrome in naive mice with mouse lupus monoclonal and human polyclonal anti-cardiolipin antibodies. *Proc Natl Acad Sci USA* 1991;88:3069–73.
117. Bakimer R, Fishman P, Blank M, Sredni B, Djaldetti M, Shoenfeld Y. Induction of primary antiphospholipid syndrome in mice by immunization with a human monoclonal anticardiolipin antibody (H-3). *J Clin Invest* 1992;89:1558–1563.
118. Gharavi AE, Sammaritano LR, Wen J, Elkon KB. Induction of antiphospholipid autoantibodies by immunization with β_2-glycoprotein I (apolipoprotein H). *J Clin Invest* 1992;90:1105–1109.
119. Blank M, Faden D, Tincani A, et al. Immunization with anticardiolipin cofactor (beta-2-glycoprotein I) induces experimental antiphospholipid syndrome in naive mice. *J Autoimmun* 1994;7:441–455.
120. Pierangeli SS, Liu XW, Anderson G, Barker JH, Harris EN. Thrombogenic properties of murine anti-cardiolipin antibodies induced by β_2 Glycoprotein I and human immunoglobulin G antiphospholipid antibodies. *Circulation* 1996;94:1746–1751.
121. Martinuzzo ME, Maclouf J, Carreras LO, Levy-Toledano S. Antiphospholipid antibodies enhance thrombin-induced platelet activation and thromboxane formation. *Thromb Haemost* 1993;70:667–671.
122. Lellouche F, Martinuzzo M, Said P, Maclouf J, Carreras LO. Imbalance of thromboxane/prostacyclin biosynthesis in patients with lupus anticoagulant. *Blood* 1991;78:2894–2899.
123. Arfors L, Vesterqvist O, Johnsson H, Grien K. Increased thromboxane formation in patients with antiphospholipid syndrome. *Eur J Clin Invest* 1990;20:607–612.
124. Lin YL, Wang CT. Activation of human platelets by the rabbit anticardiolipin antibodies. *Blood* 1992;80:3135–3143.
125. Arvieux J, Roussel B, Pouzol P, Colomb MG. Platelet activating properties of murine monoclonal antibodies to beta 2-glycoprotein I. *Thromb Haemost* 1993;70:336–341.
126. Tannenbaum SH, Finko R, Cines DB. Antibody and immune complexes induce tissue factor production by

human endothelial cells. *J Immunol* 1986;137: 1532–1537.

127. Rustin MH, Bull HA, Machin SJ, Isenberg DA, Snaith ML, Dowd PM. Effects of the lupus anticoagulant in patients with systemic lupus erythematosus on endothelial cell prostacyclin release and procoagulant activity. *J Invest Dermatol* 1988;90:744–748.

128. Hasselaar P, Derksen RH, Oosting JD, Blokzijl L, de Groot PG. Synergistic effect of low doses of tumor necrosis factor and sera from patients with systemic lupus erythematosus on the expression of procoagulant activity by cultured endothelial cells. *Thromb Haemost* 1989;62:654–660.

129. Oosting JD, Derksen RH, Blokzijl L, Sixma JJ, de Groot PG. Antiphospholipid antibody positive sera enhance endothelial cell procoagulant activity: studies in a thrombosis model. *Thromb Haemost* 1992;68: 278–284.

130. Meroni PL, Del Papa N, Beltrami B, Tincani A, Balestrieri G, Krilis SA. Modulation of endothelial cell function by antiphospholipid antibodies. *Lupus* 1996;5:448–450.

131. Del Papa N, Meroni PL, Tincani A, et al. Relationship between antiphospholipid and anti-endothelial cell antibodies: further characterization of the reactivity on resting and cytokine-activated endothelial cells. *Clin Exp Rheumatol* 1992;10:37–42.

132. Simantov R, LaSala JM, Lo SK, et al. Activation of cultured vascular endothelial cells by antiphospholipid antibodies. *J Clin Invest* 1995;96:2211–2219.

133. Chamley LW, Pattison NS, McKay EJ. Elution of anticardiolipin antibodies and their cofactor β2-glycoprotein I from placentae of patients with a poor obsteric history. *J Reprod Immunol* 1993;25:209–220.

134. La Rosa L, Meroni PL, Tincani A, et al. β2 glycoprotein I and placental anticoagulant protein I in placentae from patients with antiphospholipid syndrome. *J Rheumatol* 1994;21:1684–1693.

135. Arvieux J, Jacob MC, Roussel B, Bensa JC, Colomb MG. Neutrophil activation by anti-β2 glycoprotein I monoclonal antibodies via Fcg receptor II. *J Leuk Biol* 1995;57:387–394.

136. Atsumi T, Khamashta MA, Amengual O, Hughes GRV. Up-regulated tissue factor expression in antiphospholipid syndrome. *Thromb Haemost* 1997;77:222–223.

137. Muhlfelder TW, Niemetz J, Kreutzer D, Beebe D, Ward PA, Rosenfeld SI. C5 chemotactic fragment induces leukocyte production of tissue factor activity: a link between complement and coagulation. *J Clin Invest* 1979;63:147–150.

138. Chonn A, Semple SC, Cullis P. β2-Glycoprotein I is a major protein associated with very rapidly cleared liposomes in vivo, suggesting a significant role in the immune clearance of 'non-self' particles. *J Biol Chem* 1995;270:25845–25849.

139. Manfredi A, Rovere P, Heltai S, et al. Anti-phospholipid antibodies bind apoptotic cells in a b2-GPI dependent fashion [Abstract]. *Lupus* 1996;5:558.

140. Arnout J. The pathogenesis of the antiphospholipid syndrome: a hypothesis based on parallelisms with heparin-induced thrombocytopenia. *Thromb Haemost* 1996;75:536–541.

141. Khamashta MA, Cuadrado MJ, Mujic F, Taub NA, Hunt BJ, Hughes GR. The management of thrombosis in the antiphospholipid-antibody syndrome. *N Engl J Med* 1995;332:993–997.

142. Exner T, Triplett DA, Taberner D, Machin SJ. Guidelines for testing and revised criteria for lupus anticoagulants. *Thromb Haemost* 1991;65:320–322.

143. Brandt JT, Triplett DA, Alving B, Scharrer I. Criteria for the diagnosis of lupus anticoagulants: an update. *Thromb Haemost* 1995;74:1185–1190.

144. Triplett DA, Brandt JT, Kaczor D, Schaeffer J. Laboratory diagnosis of lupus inhibitors: a comparison of the tissue thromboplastin inhibition procedure with a new platelet neutralization procedure. *Am J Clin Pathol* 1983;79:678–682.

145. Rauch J, Tannenbaum M, Janoff AS. Distinguishing plasma lupus anticoagulants from anti-factor antibodies using hexagonal (II) phase phospholipids. *Thromb Haemost* 1989;62:892–896.

146. Roussi J, Roisin JP, Goguel A. Lupus anticoagulants. First French Interlaboratory Etalanorme Survey. *Am J Clin Pathol* 1996;105:788–793.

147. Jennings I, Kitchen S, Woods TAL, Preston FE, Greaves M. Clinically important inaccuracies in testing for the lupus anticoagulant: an analysis of results from three surveys of the UK national external quality assessment scheme (NEQAS) for blood coagulation. *Thromb Haemost.* 1997;77:934–937.

148. Reber G, Arvieux J, Comby, et al. Multicenter evaluation of nine commercial kits for the quantitation of anticardiolipin antibodies. *Thromb Haemost* 1995;73: 444–454.

149. Arnout J, Huybrechts E, Vanrusselt M, Falcon C, Vermylen J. Detection of lupus-like anticoagulants by an enzyme-linked immunosorbent assay using a partial thromboplastin as antigen: a comparative study. *Thromb Haemost* 1990;64:26–31.

150. Falcon CR, Foffer AM, Forastiero RR, Carreras LO. Clinical significance of various ELISA assays for detecting antiphospholipid antibodies. *Thromb Haemost* 1990;64:21–25.

151. Sorice M, Circella A, Griggi T, et al. Anticardiolipin and anti-B2-GPI are two distinct populations of autoantibodies. *Thromb Haemost* 1996;75:303.

152. Arvieux J, Darnige L, Reber, et al. Development of an ELISA for autoantibodies to prothrombin showing their prevalence in patients with lupus anticoagulants. *Thromb Haemost* 1995;74:1120–1125.

153. Derksen RHWM, de Groot PhG, Kater L, Nieuwenhuis HK. Patients with antiphospholipid antibodies and venous thrombosis should receive long term anticoagulant treatment. *Ann Rheum Dis* 1993;52:689–692.

154. Della Valle P, Crippa L, Safa O, et al. Potential failure of the international normalized ratio (INR) system in the monitoring of oral anticoagulation in patients with lupus anticoagulants. *Ann Med Interne* 1996;147 (suppl 1):10–14.

155. Babikian VL, Levine SR. Therapeutic considerations for stroke patients with antiphospholipid antibodies. *Stroke* 1993;23(suppl I):I-33–I-37.

156. Lubbe WF, Butler WS, Palmer SJ, Liggins GC. Fetal survival after prednisone suppression of maternal lupus anticoagulant. *Lancet* 1983;1:1361–1363.

157. Out HJ, Bruinse HW, Derksen HWM. Anti-phospholipid antibodies and pregnancy loss. *Hum Reprod* 1992;6:889–897.

158. Lockshin MD, Druzin ML, Qamar T. Prednisone does not prevent recurrent fetal death in women with antiphospholipid antibody. *Am J Obstet Gynecol* 1989; 160:439–443.

159. Silver RK, Macgregor SN, Sholl JS, Hobart JM, Neerhof MG, Ragin A. Comparative trial of prednisone plus aspirin versus aspirin alone in the treatment of anticardiolipin antibody positive obstetric patients. *Am J Obstet Gynecol* 1993;169:1411–1417.

160. Elder MG, de Swiet M, Robertson A, Elder MA, Floyd E, Hawkins DF. Low-dose aspirin in pregnancy. *Lancet* 1988;1:410.

161. Balasch J, Carmona F, Lopezsoto A, Font J, Creus M, Fabregues F, Ingelmo M, Vanrell JA. Low-dose aspirin for prevention of pregnancy losses in women with primary antiphospholipid syndrome. *Hum Reprod* 1993; 8:2234–2239.

162. Lima F, Khamashta MA, Buchanon NMN, Kerslake S, Hunt BJ, Hughes GRV. A study of sixty pregnancies in patients with the antiphospholipid syndrome. *Clin Exp Rheumatol* 1996;14:131–136.

163. Rosove MH, Tabsh K, Wasserstrum N, Howard P, Hahn BH, Kalunian KC. Heparin therapy for pregnant women with lupus anticoagulant or anticardiolipin antibodies. *Obstet Gynecol* 1990;75:630–634.

164. Kutteh WH. Antiphospholipid antibody-associated recurrent pregnancy loss: treatment with heparin and low-dose aspirin is superior to low-dose aspirin alone. *Am J Obstet Gynecol* 1996;174:1584–1589.

165. Rai R, Cohen H, Dave M, Regan L. Randomized controlled trial of spirin and aspirin plus heparin in pregnant women with recurrent miscarriage associated with phospholipid (or antiphospholipid antibodies). *Br Med J* 1997;314:253–257.

166. Carreras LO, Perez GN, Vega HR, Casavilla F. Lupus anticoagulant and recurrent fetal loss: successful treatment with gammaglobulin. *Lancet* 1988;2: 393–394.

167. Arnout J, Spitz B, Wittevrongel C, Vanrusselt M, Van Assche A, Vermylen J. High-dose intravenous immunoglobulin treatment of a pregnant patient with an antiphospholipid antibody syndrome: immunological changes associated with a succesful outcome. *Thromb Haemost* 1994;71;741–747.

*Cardiovascular Thrombosis: Thrombocardiology
and Thromboneurology, Second Edition,*
edited by M. Verstraete, V. Fuster, and E. J. Topol,
Lippincott–Raven Publishers, Philadelphia © 1998.

47

Disseminated Intravascular Coagulation

Gert Müller-Berghaus, *Hugo ten Cate, and †Marcel M. Levi

*Department of Hemostaseology and Transfusion Medicine,
Kerckhoff-Klinik, D-61231 Bad Nauheim, Germany;
*Department of Internal Medicine, Slotervaart Hospital, 1066 EC Amsterdam, The Netherlands; and
†Department of Hemostasis, Thrombosis, Atherosclerosis, and Inflammation Research,
Academic Medical Center, 1105 AZ Amsterdam, The Netherlands*

Since the first publication of *Disseminated Intravascular Coagulation* by McKay (1), a large body of information has been accumulated in detailed reviews and monographs (2–6). Although it is realized that disseminated intravascular coagulation (DIC) is an "intermediary mechanism of disease" (1) and although disseminated intravascular coagulation has been intensively studied during the last three decades, several aspects relating to the clinical problem of DIC are still under discussion. For example, a uniform and uncontradictory definition of disseminated intravascular coagulation has not yet been reached. The pathophysiology of DIC is in its main features reasonably well understood, although the trigger of the activation of intravascular coagulation has not yet been fully identified. The diagnosis can be precisely made if a specialized coagulation laboratory is available, but a general laboratory still has the problem of doing so in due time. Equally well, DIC might be prevented if the therapy is started early enough. Thus, effective treatment of a patient is highly dependent on the early diagnosis and monitoring of the dynamic process.

DEFINITION

A variety of expressions describing very similar clinical disease states has been used to define the events occurring in patients with DIC: defibrination syndrome (7,8), consumption coagulopathy (9), generalized intravascular coagulation (10), thrombohemorrhagic phenomenon (11), consumptive thrombohemorrhagic disorder (12), and, most recently, disseminated intravascular fibrin formation (13). These different delineations indicate the incomplete understanding of the pathophysiologic and pathobiochemical processes. A few essential aspects have to be taken into account to describe what is nowadays understood as disseminated intravascular coagulation (DIC).

DIC is a syndrome. DIC is not a disease or a symptom but a syndrome characterized by a dynamic process of intravascular coagulation. It has not yet been clarified as to whether the coagulation process is triggered locally (such as in Kasabach-Merritt syndrome) or in the entire vascular bed. It might also be conceivable that the coagulation process is triggered locally but extends to the entire microcirculation. Finally, it is possible that activation of coagulation takes place in the entire vascular bed but the formation of microclots is a local process. Thus, one can argue that the term "disseminated intravascular coagulation" is precise enough as it explains the coagulation process as an intravascular phenomenon that is not localized but disseminated.

DIC is an acquired disorder. It can be agreed that DIC is an acquired disorder in which the hemostatic system is activated followed by the activation of platelets and the conversion of fibrinogen to fibrin. Animal experiments indicate that the entire clinical picture of DIC can be mimicked by an infusion of tissue thromboplastin (tissue factor) (14,15), thrombin (16,17), or soluble fibrin (18). The velocity of the infusion of the procoagulant will result in different intensities of the intravascular coagulation process and determines whether soluble fibrin in plasma, fibrin-rich microclots, and a hemorrhagic diathesis, consecutive to the consumption of coagulation factors, occur. It is difficult to diagnose in a patient whether microclots have occurred but nowadays the generation of soluble fibrin in the plasma can be precisely determined. If the intravascular coagulation process is slow or not intensive, the amount of soluble fibrin circulating in the blood might be below a critical threshold. Such a situation might still be classified as DIC but it does not represent a clinical problem leading to microclot formation or a hemorrhagic diathesis. Preferably such a situation would not be termed DIC but rather hypercoagulability. If the concentration of soluble fibrin exceeds the critical threshold, it will form microclots in the peripheral circulation leading to multiple organ failure.

Consumption coagulopathy. The term consumption coagulopathy is used to describe the bleeding disorder that may occur in the course of DIC due to consumption of platelets and coagulation factors (9,19). Consumption coagulopathy is not always present in patients with DIC: In patients as well as in animal experiments, it has been shown that microclot formation can occur without a consumption coagulopathy.

Fibrinolysis. In the course of DIC the fibrinolytic system may be activated concurrently with intravascular coagulation (20). Animal experiments have demonstrated that the activation of fibrinolysis drastically intensifies the bleeding tendency. The activation of fibrinolysis in the course of intravascular coagulation is a secondary phenomenon as animal experiments demonstrate that the infusion of tissue factor or thrombin also causes activation of fibrinolysis and that the inhibition of intravascular coagulation might also interrupt fibrinolysis. Since the pathomechanism of intravascular coagulation leading to an hemorrhagic diathesis is different from that of primary fibrinolysis, primary fibrinolysis should not be included in the definition of DIC. Degradation of fibrinogen by other enzymes, e.g., elastase, should also not be termed DIC although a clinical entity such as consumption coagulopathy may occur.

Hypercoagulability. The demonstration of increased plasma levels of coagulation activation markers, e.g., an increase of prothrombin fragment 1+2 (F1+2) or thrombin–antithrombin (TAT) complexes, indicates an activation of the coagulation system and should preferably be called "hypercoagulable state" (see also Chapter 7) (21,22). This should not be termed DIC but may under certain conditions be a prodromal state of DIC. Equally well, an increase in fibrinopeptide A (FPA) may be an indication for DIC but does not prove its existence because proteolysis of fibrinogen by thrombin could have occurred in the extravascular space.

From the different aspects discussed the following definition may be deduced: "Disseminated intravascular coagulation is an acquired syndrome characterized by the activation of intravascular coagulation up to intravascular fibrin formation. The process may be accompanied by secondary fibrinolysis or inhibited fibrinolysis."

The definition of DIC implies that microclot formation and consecutive organ failure and/or a hemorrhagic diathesis may occur.

CLINICAL CONDITIONS ASSOCIATED WITH DISSEMINATED INTRAVASCULAR COAGULATION

A spectrum of clinical entities has been associated with DIC, and the major conditions are listed in Table 47-1. The frequency of DIC in these diseases varies considerably, ranging from rare or doubtful according to current criteria for DIC, to virtually obligatory (gram-negative sepsis). Here we will indicate some of the characteristic features of the listed diseases in relation to the development of DIC, indicating specific risk factors.

Obstetric Complications

Pre-eclampsia is the most common obstetric condition associated with activation of blood coagulation (23) resulting in macroscopic fibrin deposits in various organs in severe cases (24). Thrombocytopenia is an early indicator of DIC developing in the course of the HELLP syndrome (hemolysis, elevated liver enzymes, and low platelets), which complicates pregnancy-induced hypertension in

5% to 10% and preeclampsia in up to 50% of cases (25). The central pathophysiologic stimulus of DIC in this syndrome appears to be microangiopathic hemolytic anemia (MHA) accompanying vascular endothelial damage, and platelet adhesion and activation, facilitating fibrin formation.

In a retrospective survey of patients with acute fatty liver of pregnancy, a disorder mimicking the pre-eclampsia and HELLP syndromes, evidence of DIC was found in all of 28 patients and was probably related to the liver failure (see below) (26).

Acute DIC occurs in placental abruption and amniotic fluid embolism. In placental abruption the degree of placental separation appears to correlate with the extent of fibrin formation and thrombocytopenia, suggesting that local factors are responsible for initiating DIC (24).

Women surviving acute amniotic fluid embolism are at high risk (50% or more) of developing DIC within 4 hours after the insult. In vitro data confirm the potential of amniotic fluid to activate coagulation, involving a substance activating factor X in vitro (27,28).

Vascular Disorders

Hemolysis occurring in the course of the hemolytic uremic syndrome (HUS), or thrombotic thrombocytopenic purpura (TTP), or MHA as described for the HELLP syndrome, or after transfusion of incompatible blood initiates DIC (see also "Obstetric Complications") (29). Similarly, hemolysis in the course of sickle cell disease, or related to blood transfusion, may cause acute DIC. The mechanisms leading to thrombotic complications remain largely unknown. A possible scenario involves microvascular obstruction by fragmented erythrocytes, causing an inflammatory response with upregulation of adhesion molecules, adherence of leukocytes, generation of tissue factor at cell surfaces, and subsequent formation of fibrin. In addition, in sickle cell disease sickled red cells and membrane fragments contain prothrombin-converting enzyme properties, contributing to a hypercoagulability that is common in this disease (30).

TABLE 47-1. *Underlying diseases causing acute or chronic DIC*

Acute DIC	Chronic DIC
Medicine	
Septicemia/infections[a]	Solid tumors
Fulminant hepatic failure	Liver cirrhosis
Allergic reactions	Allergic reactions
Transplantation	Vasculitis
Heat stroke	Kasabach-Merrit syndrome
Hypothermia	Adult respiratory distress syndrome
Leukemia	Leukemia
Homozygous protein C deficiency	
Snake bites	
Surgery	
Polytrauma	Organ transplantations
Large operations	Aortic aneurysm
Brain injury	Vascular tumors
Septicemia[a]	
Extracorporeal circulation	
Thermal injury	
Hypothermia	
Fat embolism	
Cardiac bypass surgery	
Peritoneovenous shunt	
Obstetrics and Gynecology	
Amniotic fluid embolism	Late gestosis
Abruptio placentae	HELLP syndrome
Septic abortion	Retained dead fetus
Acute fatty liver	
Uterine rupture	
Toxemia of pregnancy	
Septicemia[a]	
Transfusion Medicine	
Acute hemolytic transfusion reaction	Artificial surfaces
Massive transfusion	

[a]Septicemia/infections: Bacterial: Gram-negative bacteria (endotoxin), gram-positive bacteria (membrane constituents).
Viral: Arboviruses, varicella, variola, rubella, paramyxoviruses, HIV, Marburg virus, Ebola virus.
Parasitic: Malaria, Kala-azar.
Rickettsial: Rocky Mountain spotted fever.
Mycotic: Acute histoplasmosis, *Candida albicans*.

Malignancy

Solid tumor cells can express different procoagulant molecules including tissue factor (TF), which assembles with factor VIIa to activate factors IX and X, and a cancer procoagulant (CP), a cysteine protease with factor X–activating properties (31). Recent studies show the occurrence of TF in vascular endothelial cells as well as tumor cells in breast cancer while not appearing in material from patients with benign fibrocystic breast disease, whereas TF was functionally active (32). It should be noted that the roles of TF in pathophysiology are only partly understood. Independent from its clotting cofactor function TF appears to be involved in tumor metastasis (33) and angiogenesis (34), factors that may directly influence the course of malignancy and affect the occurrence of thrombosis (see also Chapter 45).

Cellular factors presumably precipitate coagulation activation in patients with in most cases solid tumors. In addition, in a series of patients with malignant neoplasms, high endothelin plasma levels correlated well with progression of DIC, suggesting that this protein may influence the development of DIC in cancer (35).

Hematologic malignancies are associated with (chronic) DIC with incidences between 13% and 20% in patients with acute leukemia (36,37). It is currently believed that cellular TF is the main initiator of DIC in leukemias. A distinct form of DIC is encountered in acute promyelocytic leukemia, where clinically hemorrhagic phenomena predominate, but diffuse thrombosis is still found in 15% to 25% of cases at autopsy (38,39). Both thromboplastin-like material and profibrinolytic proteases were found in promyelocytic cellular components, and the enhanced level of fibrinolysis may help to explain the occurrence of hemorrhage and the observed beneficial effect of the fibrinolytic inhibitor ε-aminocaproic acid (40).

Hepatic Disease

Although there has been considerable debate about the interpretation of clotting abnormalities in patients with liver disease, particularly liver cirrhosis, current evidence favors chronic (low-grade) DIC in this disorder (41).

One factor influencing higher plasma levels of coagulation activation markers is reduced clearance. Furthermore, reduced levels of coagulation proteins reflect impaired synthesis by the diseased liver. The severity of DIC correlates with the degree of liver disease, and it is likely that the coagulopathy contributes to the hemorrhagic tendency in these patients. DIC is thus likely to be multifactorial in liver disease. Importantly, it has been shown that cirrhosis of the liver leads to enhanced circulating levels of endotoxin; this constituent of gram-negative bacteria is known to elicit a chain of events leading to enhanced coagulation activity in humans and correlates well with coagulation activity in patients with cirrhosis (42).

Trauma

Polytrauma by physical force, induced by burns or heat stroke, may result in DIC due to a combination of mechanisms including hemolysis, endothelial activation, release of tissue material in the circulation (fat, phospholipids), and acidosis following hypoperfusion. In addition, systemic infection frequently contributes to the development of DIC (43,44).

Infection

DIC occurs in a variety of systemic infections, including viruses (herpes, cytomegalovirus, human immunodeficiency virus, varicella, filovirus), parasites (malaria), and both gram-positive and gram-negative bacteria. Bacterial infections are the most common entity associated with DIC, and the incidence of sepsis due to gram-positive organisms varied from 27% to 74% in recent studies (reviewed in 45); gram-negative organisms are responsible for the majority of cases of sepsis and related DIC. Several factors are involved in the occurrence of DIC in gram-positive sepsis: Specific cell membrane components, including capsular polysaccharides, peptidoglycans, and lipoteichoic acid, activate the complement system, generate cytokine release, and may directly activate platelets and lead to DIC when administered to animals (peptidoglycans) (45). "Superantigens" directly interact with T cells, interfering with the immunologic response. Staphylococcal α-toxin activates platelets, generating prothrombinase activity that may induce DIC. Furthermore, in the majority of patients with gram-positive sepsis the plasma levels of cytokines, tumor necrosis factor (TNF), and interleukins-1 and 6 (IL-1 and IL-6) are elevated and not much different from those in gram-negative sepsis. These cytokines may enhance the procoagulant response leading to DIC as it does in gram-negative sepsis (see below).

PATHOGENESIS

DIC is characterized by widespread intravascular fibrin deposition, which appears to be a result of enhanced fibrin formation and impaired fibrin degradation. As outlined

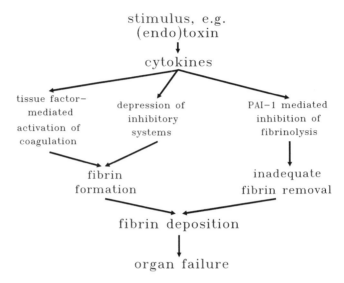

FIG. 47-1. Schematic representation of the pathogenetic pathways involved in disseminated intravascular coagulation (DIC).

in the following paragraphs and schematically represented in Fig. 47-1, enhanced fibrin formation is caused by tissue factor–mediated thrombin generation and simultaneously occurring depression of inhibitory mechanisms, such as the protein C and S system. The impairment of endogenous thrombolysis is mainly due to high circulating levels of PAI-1, the principal inhibitor of plasminogen activation. These derangements in coagulation and fibrinolysis are mediated by several cytokines, in particular in the case of DIC associated with infectious disease, but most probably also in the case of other clinical conditions associated with DIC.

As a result of the diffuse and ongoing activation of coagulation, platelets and coagulation factors become depleted, which may ultimately result in bleeding. Obviously, this complication mainly occurs in trauma patients or in patients in the early postoperative phase.

Pathogenesis of Thrombin Generation

Gram-negative sepsis is the most common disorder associated with DIC and also one of the best studied conditions. Most of our

knowledge of the pathogenesis of DIC comes from observations in septic patients or experimental sepsis models. Pivotal triggers in the sepsis syndrome are toxins, such as endotoxin lipopolysaccharide (LPS), a cellular membrane constituent of gram-negative bacteria, which is released into the circulation. Experimental studies of the biological effects of either live gram-negative bacteria (E. coli, Salmonella), or purified LPS, in experimental animals and in humans have clarified the chain of events leading to DIC in this condition (46,47). During gram-negative infection or after LPS infusion the cytokines (IL-1, IL-6, and TNF) are systemically detectable at an early stage. These cytokines trigger a host of biological responses including a procoagulant reaction. After LPS infusion in healthy human volunteers, thrombin formation measured as the plasma levels of prothrombin fragment F1 + 2 and thrombin–antithrombin complexes gradually occurs, peaking at 4 hours after injection of LPS. Recent data indicate evidence of an early activation of factor XI in this model, with a peak in free factor XIa in plasma at 1 hour (Minnema M, unpublished) and previous studies also provided evidence of early activation of factor X after infusion of the LPS induced mediator TNF (48). Thus, a twofold procoagulant response is observed, with an early short-lasting peak in activation of the intrinsic pathway, followed by a longer lasting generation of thrombin, which may lead to fibrin formation depending on additional factors (discussed below). The origin of coagulation activation in these models of LPS stimulation appeared to be TF. Coinfusion of LPS and either a monoclonal antibody blocking TF (49) or an antibody Fab fragment interfering with factor VIIa–TF complex formation (50) abolished thrombin formation in a primate model, demonstrating that under these conditions contact activation is not involved in activation of the intrinsic pathway. The current scenario of TF-induced coagulation activation assumes that the TF–factor VIIa complex activates both factors IX and X (51) and bypasses the classic contact factors. Activation of factor XI probably occurs due to thrombin feedback activation (52), although a contribution of factor XIIa in this reaction cannot be excluded yet. The progression of thrombin formation to overt DIC with fibrin deposition may be facilitated by the observed marked increment in PAI-1, which offsets initial fibrinolytic activity measured as increments in tissue plasminogen activator (t-PA) and plasmin–antiplasmin complexes (53).

The importance of TF as a component of the sepsis syndrome is illustrated by the fact that baboons subjected to a lethal infusion of live *E. coli* only survived when an antibody against TF or the natural inhibitor tissue factor pathway inhibitor (TFPI) was administered in conjunction with bacteria (46). This leaves open the question of the relevance of DIC for sepsis related mortality: Previous studies in the same baboon model showed that intervention in the coagulation cascade per se can reduce clotting activation but does not necessarily diminish mortality (46).

Another issue in the pathogenesis of DIC in gram-negative sepsis is the contribution of the contact pathway proteins. Studies in septic patients have provided direct evidence of contact activation in a given number of patients in some studies (54). In the lethal baboon model

of gram-negative sepsis it appeared that contact activation indeed occurred but did not contribute to activation of coagulation because an antibody that blocked factor XIIa did not reduce DIC in this animal model (55), although critics argue that the inhibitory effect was incomplete (56). These experiments did, however, reveal that blockade of the contact pathway had physiologic implications, i.e., mortality was reduced, probably due to a blunted secondary hypotensive response after *E. coli* infusion (55).

Inhibitors of Coagulation and Fibrinolysis in Disseminated Intravascular Coagulation

In the pathophysiology of DIC several inhibitors play an important role. Tissue factor, the trigger of coagulation, is inhibited by TFPI in vitro and in vivo experiments in lethal baboon models indicate that TFPI is a potent inhibitor of sepsis-related mortality (56,57). Whether this effect is solely the result of impaired clotting activity remains uncertain. In contrast to other coagulation inhibitors, acquired deficiencies of TFPI have not been observed, and DIC is in general associated with modestly reduced levels, or even increased concentrations, of TFPI (58,59). It is therefore uncertain as to whether administration of supranormal concentrations of TFPI are of benefit in preventing DIC.

Further activation of the coagulation pathway is influenced by the other coagulation inhibitors, of which antithrombin, protein C, and protein S are the best studied examples. Markedly reduced plasma levels of antithrombin and protein C have been repeatedly demonstrated in DIC, and particularly lowered protein C levels have been associated with a poor outcome of sepsis. In patients with a systemic inflammatory response syndrome, mostly due to sepsis, reductions in plasma levels of antithrombin and protein C were associated with more extensive disease (60). In meningococcal sepsis, reduced protein C levels predicted mortality (61). It has been speculated that protein C would play additional functions in mediating anti-inflammatory activity in vivo, which may explain its apparent physiologic significance as an inhibitor. Indeed, studies in the sublethal baboon model suggested that activated protein C reduced neutrophil activation and cytokine release (62). A direct association between coagulation inhibitors and inflammation came from a study in the same sepsis model in baboons, showing that enhanced inhibition of the protein C cofactor protein S, by coinfusing antibodies against protein S, or C4b-binding protein (C4bBP), increased the response to sublethal amounts of *E. coli.* In effect, blockade of the protein S system caused enhanced activation of neutrophils, elastase release, enhanced levels of TNF, and fibrinogen consumption (63).

As indicated earlier, the contact activation pathway proteins probably do not contribute to DIC, with the exception of factor XI, which may be feedback-activated by thrombin. In case of severe sepsis, however, factor XI activation may be the result of activation of the classic contact route, as suggested by the strong correlation between factor XII antigen levels and factor XIa–α_1-antitrypsin complexes in plasma from patients with meningococcal sepsis (64). In any case, the inhibition of factor XIa by its physiologically most relevant inhibitor, i.e., C1 inhibitor (65), becomes impaired during sepsis due to proteolytic cleavage of the inhibitor (66). Because minute amounts of factor XIa may be important for enhancing intrinsic coagulation activity, the reduced inhibitory potential of C1 inhibitor may bear pathophysiologic significance.

Finally, the formation of fibrin in the course of DIC is determined by the potential of the fibrinolytic mechanism to cleave polymerized fibrin. Clinical studies have demonstrated that evidence of enhanced fibrin cleavage is generally measurable in the form of D-dimer fragments in plasma. At the same time, fibrinolytic efficacy may be impaired by high levels of PAI-1 in septic patients, which have been associated with a poor clinical outcome (60,67,68). In specific situations enhanced cleavage of PAI-1 may occur, con-

tributing to hyperfibrinolysis and bleeding (69).

Overall, the actual rate and distribution of fibrin formed during DIC appears to depend not only on the extent of TF present but on the integrity of the inhibitory mechanisms available, which depends on the specific nature of the underlying disorder.

Cytokines

As indicated, several cytokines are involved in the LPS-induced inflammatory response. With regard to DIC, IL-1, IL-6, and TNF appear to be the most relevant stimuli. Although IL-1 is a potent agonist of TF synthesis under in vitro conditions, its role has not been clarified in the experimental studies described. Administration of a recombinant IL-1 receptor antagonist partly blocked the procoagulant response in a sepsis model in baboons (70) and treatment of patients with an IL-1 receptor inhibitor agent reduced the increase in thrombin–antithrombin complexes (71). However, most of the procoagulant changes after LPS infusion occurred well before IL-1 became detectable in the circulation, leaving open questions regarding its role in DIC.

Infusion of TNF in patients and in healthy volunteers has indicated that this cytokine induced a cascade of procoagulant and fibrinolytic changes with a similar pattern as compared to the LPS-induced reactions (48). These observations led us to speculate that TNF would be the critical mediator of the DIC syndrome in sepsis. However, later studies showed that blockade of TNF with monoclonal antibodies did not significantly reduce coagulation activation in animal models but rather markedly reduced the fibrinolytic response (72). Further studies indicated that blockade of IL-6 after LPS infusion in primates, resulted in attenuation of clotting activity, suggesting that not TNF but rather IL-6 was critical for generating the procoagulant activity of LPS in vivo (73). Recent studies indeed confirmed that infusion of IL-6 in patients caused enhanced thrombin formation (74).

DIAGNOSIS

According to the definition of DIC stated above, the determination of soluble fibrin appears to be crucial for the diagnosis of DIC. If the concentration of soluble fibrin has increased above a defined threshold, the diagnosis of DIC can definitely be made (75–78). The only problem so far is that a reliable test has up to now not been available for quantitatively measuring soluble fibrin in plasma. The semiquantitative assays that are commercially available can be used to support the data obtained by screening tests.

No single laboratory test or combination of tests are available that are sensitive or specific enough to allow a definite diagnosis. However, the diagnosis can reliably be made without ambiguity by taking into consideration the underlying disease and a combination of laboratory findings (79–83).

Underlying Diseases

The basis of the diagnosis is the knowledge of underlying diseases in which DIC can occur (see Table 47-1). Because patients suffering from acute DIC need urgent therapy, the underlying diseases associated with DIC should always be taken into consideration if a complex coagulation defect is observed.

Laboratory Tests

Because DIC is a continuously progressive process, it can be subdivided into three phases that might be helpful in the diagnosis and consequent therapy.

Phase I: Compensated activation of the hemostatic system. During this phase, no clinical findings are observed but the underlying disease may raise suspicion for the occurrence of DIC. Under these circumstances tests should be performed for demonstrating the activation of coagulation (Table 47-2).

Phase II: Decompensated activation of the hemostatic system. In contrast to phase I, the prothrombin time as well as the activated partial thromboplastin time (APTT) are pro-
longed during phase II. Under these circumstances the thrombin time may still be normal as the fibrinogen levels are still adequate and the level of fibrinogen degradation products (FDPs) is not very high. In this phase, frequent analyses are necessary to demonstrate the dynamics of the intravascular coagulation process. Repeated determinations will demonstrate a continuous drop in platelet count as well as in fibrinogen concentration and coagulation factor activities, especially factor V activity (Table 47-2).

Phase III: Full-blown DIC. Full-blown DIC is characterized by an extremely prolonged or even unclottable prothrombin time as well as APTT. Frequently, the thrombin time is pronouncedly prolonged or also unclottable. During this phase, the platelet counts are very low and the coagulation factor activities are <50% of normal values.

The continuous transition from phase I to phase II or even to phase III is typical for DIC. If in the course of DIC hemolysis and/or schistocytes are observed, this indicates microclot formation causing damage to the red cells.

Screening Tests

Although screening tests (Table 47-2) are always performed if a coagulation defect is assumed, prothrombin time, APTT, and thrombin time do not give any information in phase I of the syndrome. Normal prothrombin time and normal APTT do not exclude the activation of the hemostatic system. If, however, prothrombin time and APTT are prolonged, coagulation is already markedly activated causing a consumption of coagulation factors. This decrease in coagulation factors is responsible for the prolongation of the prothrombin time and APTT. Under these circumstances, it is helpful to determine the prothrombin time as well as the APTT frequently to judge the course of DIC and to monitor therapeutic approaches. For further assessment of the course of DIC, it is essential to determine the platelet count. Because the normal platelet count varies between 150,000 and 450,000/μl, a single determina-

TABLE 47-2. *Phases and laboratory data of acute disseminated intravascular coagulation (DIC)*

Phases	Laboratory data
Phase I: Compensated Activation of the Hemostatic System Clinical findings: No symptoms Laboratory analysis: No measurable consumption of hemostasis components Increased levels of activation markers Increased levels of enzyme–inhibitor complexes	PT, APTT, thrombin time: within normal limits platelet count: within normal limits F1 + 2, TAT: elevated FDPs: elevated antithrombin: slightly decreased Soluble fibrin: ±
Phase II: Decompensated Activation of the Hemostatic System Clinical findings: Bleedings from injuries and venous puncture sites as well as decreased organ function (e.g., kidneys, lung, liver) Laboratory analysis: Continuous decrease in platelet count and coagulation factors Continuous increase in activation markers Continuous increase in enzyme-inhibitor complexes	PT, APTT: prolonged or continuous prolongation, respectively thrombin time: mostly within normal limits, but sometimes prolonged platelet count, fibrinogen concentration, coagulation factor activities, antithrombin: decreased or continuously decreasing F1 + 2, TAT, FDPs: clearly increased Soluble fibrin: increased
Phase III: Full-blown DIC Clinical findings: Skin bleedings of different sizes as well as multiorgan failure Laboratory analysis: Clearly expressed consumption of hemostasis components	PT, APTT: extremely prolonged or unclottable thrombin time: very pronounced prolongation or unclottable platelet count: strongly diminished (<40% of the initial value) Fibrinogen, antithrombin, and coagulation factor activities: pronouncedly decreased (<50% of the initial values) F1 + 2, TAT, FDPs: pronouncedly increased Soluble fibrin: increased

APTT, activated partial thromboplastin time; PT, prothrombin time; F1 + 2, prothrombin fragment F1 + 2; TAT, thrombin–antithrombin complex; FDPs, fibrin degradation products (including D-dimer).

tion is not helpful. But a continuous drop in platelet count, determined in acute DIC patients at intervals between 1 and 4 hours, indicates the generation of thrombin causing intravascular platelet aggregation. A stable platelet count suggests that thrombin formation has stopped. If the first laboratory analysis is done in phase II of the disease, fibrinogen concentration as well as FDP concentration should always be determined in addition to the screening tests because elevated FDP titers in combination with thrombocytopenia and a decrease in clotting factor activities allow the diagnosis of DIC. An increased FDP level is almost always seen from the beginning of DIC where fibrinolysis is still accelerated, whereas in the course of DIC fibrinolysis activation may be exhausted. If, in the beginning of suspected DIC, FDPs are not elevated, one can reliably exclude DIC because experience has taught that activation of fibrinolysis is almost always present in patients with DIC (79,81,82,84,85).

The severity of DIC can be judged by determining plasma factor, antithrombin, and plasminogen activities. If the activities of these factors are <60% of normal, an acute and high-grade DIC can be assumed. On examining the relationship between outcome and hemostasis parameters, antithrombin activity (86,87), protein C levels (60,61), plasminogen activity (86), PAP complexes (86), and PAI-1 activity (88,89) were related to outcome.

Indicators of Activation of Coagulation

The dynamics of DIC can be judged by measuring activation markers such as fibrinopeptide A (90–93), prothrombin fragment F1 + 2 (22,94–97), and soluble fibrin (75–78, 98–100), although these tests may not be widely available in the routine laboratories. These three markers indicate the effect of thrombin on coagulation factors. Because coagulation can take place extravascularly, such as in pneumonia or peritonitis, fibrinopeptide A and F1 + 2 are not specific parameters for the diagnosis of DIC. In contrast to that, soluble fibrin in plasma can only be generated in-

travascularly and thus represents a specific test for the diagnosis of hypercoagulability. A drawback may be that fibrinopeptide A, F1 + 2, and soluble fibrin are very much dependent on optimal venous puncture. Relatively easy to perform is the determination of thrombin–antithrombin (TAT) complexes which, similar to the mentioned activation marker, indicate the generation of thrombin (78,101–103).

Indicators of Fibrinolysis Activation

As mentioned above, FDP is an important parameter for making the diagnosis in combination with other assays (81,104,105). In recent years, it has been shown that the determination of D-dimer is more sensitive than that of FDP and that this test has a high negative predictive value for the presence of fibrin degradation (79,82,84). Since fibrinogen is also degraded extravascularly, an elevated FDP or D-dimer level does not prove intravascular fibrinolysis. Because FDPs are metabolized by the liver and secreted by the kidneys, FDP levels are influenced by liver and kidney function. Different FDP assays, including D-dimer tests, are commercially available and measure different subpopulations of FDPs. These assays are not specific for a certain type of FDP because the different FDP populations form complexes with each other and even with soluble fibrin (74,106). Extreme hyperfibrinolysis does generally not occur until circulating α_2-antiplasmin has been depleted (107). Thus, the determination of α_2-antiplasmin is a helpful test for judging the dynamics of fibrinolysis (86,108–110). Specific tests are available for the determination of plasmin-induced fibrinogen (Bβ1-42) or fibrin (Bβ15-42) peptides (111).

MANAGEMENT OF PATIENTS WITH DISSEMINATED INTRAVASCULAR COAGULATION

General Remarks

Several issues regarding the proper management of patients with DIC remain controversial (112). These controversies are based on the fact that due to the complexity of the clinical presentation of the syndrome, the variable and unpredictable course, and the either subtle or catastrophic clinical consequences of the presence of DIC, properly conducted clinical trials on DIC treatment are virtually unavailable (12). Besides, the clinical picture of a patient with widespread thrombotic depositions in small vessels of various organs on the one hand, and bleeding due to consumption and subsequent depletion of platelets and coagulation factors on the other hand, does not directly guide the physician to specific therapies for this condition. However, despite all of these complicating circumstances, it is well established that the cornerstone of DIC treatment is the specific and vigorous treatment of the underlying disorder. In some cases, the DIC will completely resolve within hours after the resolution of the underlying condition (e.g., in case of DIC induced by abruptio placentae and amniotic fluid embolism) (113,114). However, in other cases, such as DIC in patients with sepsis and a systemic inflammatory response syndrome, DIC may be present for a number of days, even after proper treatment has been installed and supportive measures to manage the DIC may be necessary.

Based on our present knowledge of the pathogenesis of DIC (see above), therapeutic interventions aimed at the interruption of ongoing thrombin formation or at the inhibition of thrombin might have a beneficial effect. This might be further facilitated by administration of protease inhibitors, such as antithrombin, the levels of which may have been decreased dramatically in the course of a DIC, due to consumption and impaired synthesis. Alternatively, administration of coagulation factors and/or platelets may be useful, particularly in the case of bleeding.

Inhibition of Ongoing Coagulation Activation

Theoretically, strategies aimed at the inhibition of thrombin once it has been formed might be useful in patients with DIC. At present, heparin is administered to achieve this; however, there is theoretical concern that heparin might not be effective in these circumstances due to simultaneously occurring low levels of antithrombin (115) and the inability of the heparin–antithrombin complex to block thrombin at the surface of the clot (116), which particularly in DIC might play a crucial role. At this time, there is no well-controlled prospective study of the use of heparin in patients with DIC, and although advocated by some authors (117–120) its use remains controversial (121–123). Some authors propose to limit the use of heparin to DIC occurring in the framework of a small number of well-defined clinical conditions, such as giant hemangiomas, aortic aneurysm, or solid tumors, whereas heparin is not considered helpful (and might even be harmful) in the case of septicemia, complications of pregnancy, and liver disease (12). A more useful approach is probably to determine whether heparin may be helpful based on the severity and stage of the DIC. At an early stage of a developing DIC heparin might be helpful as a prophylactic agent. In addition, at this time the number of platelets and plasma levels of clotting factors are only slightly decreased, and the risk of bleeding complications is minimal. At a more advanced stage of the DIC, when levels of platelets and coagulation proteins are dropping, the use of heparin is debatable and the decision as to whether to use heparin or not may be dependent on circumstantial factors. In particular, if multiple organ failure develops and it is believed that intravascular fibrin formation might play an important role in this respect, the use of heparin might be helpful. Finally, in the presence of full-blown DIC, the use of heparin is probably not useful and might even result in serious bleeding complications. An exception should be made for patients with clinically evident thrombotic complications, such as venous thromboembolism or hemorrhagic ischemic skin lesions or even necrosis. The amount of heparin and its route of administration should be tailored to the clinical situation. Generally, the continuous intravenous use of relatively moderate doses of heparin (e.g., 300 to 500 U per hour) is advocated. Due to its pharmacokinetic properties, intravenous heparin therapy should always be initiated with a bolus dose (e.g., 2500 to 5000 U). Low molecular weight heparins (LMWHs) have been used in patients with DIC in some preliminary clinical trials but have never shown a beneficial effect over unfractionated heparin in this situation (124). A potential disadvantage might be the longer half-life of LMWHs, which might render interruption of heparin therapy in the case of bleeding more troublesome.

More directly, and independent of antithrombin, inhibition of thrombin activity might be achieved with hirudin or hirudin analogues. These agents have so far not been used in patients with DIC in well-controlled clinical trials but have been applied in single patients with DIC (125). Animal experiments have demonstrated a complete inhibition of DIC if hirudin was given prophylactically (126–129). Although hirudin or hirudin analogues are much more effective thrombin inhibitors than heparin, this potential advantage is (theoretically) probably offset by the relatively high incidence of bleeding complications with the use of these agents in DIC patients.

Based on the previously described knowledge that the initiation of coagulation activation in DIC is mediated by the tissue factor pathway, treatment strategies aimed at the blockade of this route might be useful. Indeed, it has been shown that antibodies directed against tissue factor or against factor VII/VIIa were able to block DIC in experimental models of DIC in primates (49,50). However, these agents, or newer peptide-based inhibitors of tissue factor, have so far not been tested in patients with DIC, and their efficacy and safety in this situation are completely unknown.

Administration of Protease Inhibitors

Since consumption and depletion of protease inhibitors appear to play a role in the pathogenesis of DIC, administration of these inhibitors might be useful in the management of patients with DIC (130). This concept has been most extensively studied for administration of antithrombin, which theoretically, on the one hand, could neutralize excess thrombin and factor Xa and, on the other hand, could make heparin therapy more effective. Although antithrombin concentrates appear to be useful to some extent in the amelioration of DIC laboratory parameters, no clinical studies have resulted in a reduction in mortality or morbidity of patients who were treated with antithrombin concentrates (131–133). However, a recent study with very high doses of antithrombin concentrate (90 to 120 IU per kg per day) and achieving supraphysiologic plasma concentrations (120% to 140%) showed a promising reduction in mortality, although the results were not statistically significant (134).

Replacement therapy with (activated) protein C concentrates appears to be a rational alternative, based on the pivotal role of this system in the pathogenesis of DIC (135). Protein C concentrates were shown to be effective in animal studies (63,136) but have so far not been tested in clinical trials. Theoretically, this treatment could be particularly useful in patients with a purpura fulminans type of DIC, such as in meningococcal septicemia (137–139).

Administration of Coagulation Factors and Platelets

If serious depletion of platelets and clotting factors occurs, replacement therapy could be considered. However, replacement should not be instituted on the basis of laboratory findings alone and is only required in patients who are actively bleeding, require an invasive procedure, or are at risk for bleeding complications (e.g., postoperative patients) (12). Replacement of platelets and clotting factors can be achieved by infusion of platelet concentrate and fresh frozen plasma, respectively. The argument that these infusions may "fuel the fire" and promote intravascular thrombus formation might theoretically be possible but has rarely been proved to occur, and simultaneous (low-dose) heparin might be useful to prevent this complication (140). Large volumes of plasma may be needed to sufficiently correct the coagulation system, and therefore some authors advocate the use of clotting factor concentrates. However, besides the fact that these concentrates usually contain only a selected number of the various clotting factors, concentrates may be contaminated with traces of activated coagulation factors and may therefore be particularly harmful for patients with DIC, further complicating the situation.

Fibrinolytic Inhibitors

Fibrinolytic inhibitors, such as ε-aminocaproic acid or tranexamic acid, are usually contraindicated in patients with DIC (12). Although these agents are generally useful in patients with severe bleeding, the use of antifibrinolytic agents is thought to further block the already depressed fibrinolytic system, thereby seriously promoting intravascular fibrin deposition. An exception can be made in patients with a rarely occurring syndrome, characterized by primary excessive fibrinolytic activation, most often associated with acute promyelocytic leukemia (AML-M3) or sometimes with prostate carcinoma. Treatment with tranexamic acid has shown to be highly effective and safe in these patients (40,141). However, this syndrome could, on the basis of laboratory tests, easily be distinguished from DIC and will not be further discussed here.

Aprotinin is a 58-amino-acid polypeptide, mainly derived from bovine lung, parotid gland, or pancreas. Aprotinin directly inhibits the activity of various serine proteases, including plasmin, but also of coagulation factors, as well as constituents of the kallikrein-kinin and angiotensin systems (142). Aprotinin might be used as an alternative fibrinolytic inhibitor in patients with excessive fibrinolysis, whereas the (relatively small) potential for thrombin generation might be useful in patients with DIC (143). However, the efficacy and safety of aprotinin in patients with DIC has never been proven.

Conclusion

The management of DIC is very complicated because of the variability in clinical presentation and underlying disease. A pivotal point in DIC management is proper treatment of the underlying disease. Supportive measures could be contemplated and may include strategies to block thrombin formation or thrombin action, administration of depleted protease inhibitors, and—in case of serious bleeding— administration of platelets and coagulation factors.

The lack of well-controlled studies concerning the optimal management of DIC in the various categories of patients that develop DIC will keep some issues regarding the most optimal DIC treatment controversial, but the improvement of the understanding of the pathogenesis of DIC may provide new means to come to more rational and specific treatment strategies in the near future.

GENERAL CONCLUSION

DIC is a syndrome characterized by systemic intravascular activation of coagulation, leading to widespread deposition of fibrin in the circulation. There is ample experimental and pathologic evidence that the fibrin deposition contributes to multiple organ failure. The massive and ongoing activation of coagulation may result in depletion of platelets and coagulation factors, which may cause bleeding (consumption coagulopathy).

DIC is not a clinical entity in itself but always occurs secondary to a broad spectrum of various diseases.

The pathogenesis of DIC is reasonably well understood, based on clinical observations and experimental studies. The trigger for the activation of the coagulation system depends on the underlying condition and is frequently mediated by several cytokines. Thrombin generation proceeds via the (extrinsic) tissue factor/factor VIIa route and simultaneously occurring depression of inhibitory mechanisms, such as the protein C and S system. Also, impaired fibrin degradation, due to high circulating levels of PAI-1, contributes to enhanced intravascular fibrin deposition.

The diagnosis of DIC is based on the presence of an underlying disease and a combination of laboratory tests, indicating activation of the coagulation system and fibrin formation, and consumption of platelets and coagulation factors (associated with prolongation of clotting times). At present, not a single laboratory test is available to definitively assess the presence or absence of DIC.

The cornerstone of the management of DIC is the specific and vigorous treatment of the underlying disorder. Strategies aimed at the inhibition of coagulation activation may theoretically be justified and have been found beneficial in experimental studies. However, there is in general no good clinical evidence for the use of anticoagulant agents for prevention and treatment of DIC. Novel, more potent, and specific anticoagulant regimens are currently being investigated. There are no clinical studies indicating that the use of protease inhibitors, such as antithrombin concentrates, result in a reduction of mortality and morbidity, although laboratory parameters of DIC may improve. An exception may possibly be made for the use of very high doses of antithrombin concentrate, which have shown to be potentially useful in preliminary, small, controlled clinical trials. Administration of platelets or plasma should be strictly limited to patients with bleeding or those who are at high risk for bleeding complications.

REFERENCES

1. McKay DG. *Disseminated Intravascular Coagulation. An Intermediary Mechanism of Disease.* New York: Hoeber, 1964;715–728.
2. Bick RL. Disseminated intravascular coagulation. Objective laboratory diagnostic criteria and guidelines for management. *Clin Lab Med* 1994;14:729–768.
3. Müller-Berghaus G. Pathophysiologic and biochemical events in disseminated intravascular coagulation: dysregulation of procoagulant and anticoagulant pathways. *Semin Thromb Hemost* 1989;15:58–87.
4. Baker WF Jr. Clinical aspects of disseminated intravascular coagulation: a clinician's point of view. *Semin Thromb Hemost* 1989;15:1–57.
5. Müller-Berghaus G, Madlener K, Blombäck M, ten Cate JW (eds). *DIC: Pathogenesis, Diagnosis and Therapy of Disseminated Intravascular Fibrin Formation.* Amsterdam: Elsevier, 1993.
6. Williams EC, Mosher DF. Disseminated intravascular coagulation. In: Hoffman R, Benz EJ Jr, Shattil SJ, Furie B, Cohen HJ, Silberstein LE (eds). *Hematology: Basic Principles and Practice.* New York: Churchill Livingstone, 1995;1758–1769.
7. Merskey C, Johnson AJ, Kleiner GJ, Wohl H. The defibrination syndrome: Clinical features and laboratory diagnosis. *Br J Haematol* 1967;13:528–549.
8. Schneider CL. "Fibrin embolism" (disseminated intravascular coagulation) with defibrination as one of the end results during placenta abruptio. *Surg Gynecol Obstet* 1951;92:27–34.
9. Lasch H-G, Heene DL, Huth K, Sandritter W. Pathophysiology, clinical manifestations and therapy of consumption-coagulopathy ("Verbrauchskoagulopathie"). *Am J Cardiol* 1967;20:381–391.
10. Müller-Berghaus G. Pathophysiology of generalized intravascular coagulation. *Semin Thromb Hemost* 1977;3:209–246.
11. *Selye H: Thrombohemorrhagic Phenomena.* Springfield, IL: Charles C Thomas, 1966.
12. Marder VJ, Martin SE, Francis CW, Colman RW. Consumptive thrombohemorrhagic disorders. In: Colman RW, Hirsh J, Marder VJ, Salzman EW (eds). *Hemostasis and Thrombosis: Basic Principles and Clinical Practice.* Philadelphia: Lippincott, 1987;975–1015.
13. Müller-Berghaus G, Blombäck M, ten Cate JW. Attempts to define disseminated intravascular coagulation. In: Müller-Berghaus G, Madlener K, Blombäck M, ten Cate JW (eds). *DIC: Pathogenesis, Diagnosis and Therapy of Disseminated Intravascular Fibrin Formation.* Amsterdam: Elsevier, 1993;3–8.
14. Schneider CL. Thromboplastin complications of late pregnancy. In: *Toxemias of Pregnancy, Human and Veterinary.* (A Ciba Foundation Symposium.) Philadelphia: Blakiston, 1950;163–181.
15. Ratnoff OD, Conley CL. Studies on afibrinogenemia. II. The defibrinating effect on dog blood of intravenous injection of thromboplastin material. *Bull Johns Hopk Hosp* 1951;88:414–424.
16. Quick AJ, Hussey CV, Harris J, Peters K. Occult intravascular clotting by means of intravenous injection of thrombin. *Am J Physiol* 1959;197:791–794.
17. Margaretten W, Zunker HO, McKay DG. Production of the generalized Shwartzman reaction in pregnant rats by intravenous infusion of thrombin. *Lab Invest* 1964;13:552–559.
18. Müller-Berghaus G, Róka L, Lasch HG. Induction of glomerular microclot formation by fibrin monomer infusion. *Thromb Diath Haemorrh* 1973;29:375–383.
19. Verstraete M, Vermylen C, Vermylen J, Vandenbroucke J. Excessive consumption of blood coagulation components as cause of hemorrhagic diathesis. *Am J Med* 1965;38:899.
20. Alkjaersig N, Fletcher AP, Sherry S. Pathogenesis of the coagulation defect developing during pathological plasma proteolytic ("fibrinolytic") states. II. The significance, mechanism and consequences of defective fibrin polymerization. *J Clin Invest* 1962; 41:917–934.
21. Nachman RL, Silverstein RL. Hypercoagulable states. *Ann Intern Med* 1993;119:819.
22. Bauer KA. Hypercoagulable states. In: Hoffman R, Benz EJ Jr, Shattil SJ, Furie B, Cohen HJ, Silberstein LE (eds). *Hematology: Basic Principles and Practice.* New York: Churchill Livingstone, 1995;1781–1795.
23. de Boer K, ten Cate JW, Sturk A, Borm JJJ, Treffers PE.

Enhanced thrombin generation in normal and hypertensive pregnancy. *Am J Obstet Gynecol* 1989;160: 95–100.

24. Weiner CP. The obstetric patient and disseminated intravascular coagulation. *Clin Perinatol* 1986;13: 705–717.

25. Martin JN, Stedman CM. Imitators of preeclampsia and HELLP syndrome. *Obstet Gynecol Clin North Am* 1991;18:181–198.

26. Castro MA, Goodwin TM, Shaw KJ, Ouzounian JG, McGehee WG. Disseminated intravascular coagulation and antithrombin III depression in acute fatty liver of pregnancy. *Am J Obstet Gynecol* 1996;174:211–216.

27. Philips LL, Davidson EC. Coagulant properties of amniotic fluid. *Am J Obstet Gynecol* 1972;113:911.

28. Weiner CP, Brandt J. A modified activated partial thromboplastin time with the use of amniotic fluid. *Am J Obstet Gynecol* 1982;144:234–238.

29. Krevans JR, Jackson DP, Conley CL, et al. The nature of the hemorrhagic disorder accompanying hemolytic transfusion reactions in man. *Blood* 1957;12:834–837.

30. Peters M, Plaat BE, ten Cate H, Wolters HJ, Weening RS, Brandjes DP. Enhanced thrombin generation in children with sickle cell disease. *Thromb Haemost* 1994;71:169–172.

31. Donati BM. Cancer and thrombosis: from phlegmasia alba dolens to transgenic mice. *Thromb Haemost* 1995;74:278–281.

32. Contrino J, Hair G, Kreutzer D, Rickles FR. In situ detection of expression of tissue factor in vascular endothelial cells: correlation with the malignant phenotype of human breast tissue. *Nature Med* 1996;2: 209–215.

33. Bromberg ME, Konigsberg WH, Madison JF, Pawashe A, Garen A. Tissue factor promotes melanoma metastasis by a pathway independent of blood coagulation. *Proc Natl Acad Sci USA* 1995;92:8205–8209.

34. Zhang Y, Deng Y, Luther T, Muller M, Ziegler R, Waldherr R, Stern DM, Nawroth PP. Tissue factor controls the balance of angiogenic and antiangiogenic properties of tumor cells in mice. *J Clin Invest* 1994; 94:1320–1327.

35. Ishibashi M, Ito N, Fujita M, Furue H, Yamaji T. Endothelin-1 as an aggravating factor of disseminated intravascular coagulation associated with malignant neoplasms. *Cancer* 1994;73:191–195.

36. Sletnes KE, Godal HC, Wisloff F. Disseminated intravascular coagulation (DIC) in adult patients with acute leukemia. *Eur J Haematol* 1995;54:34–38.

37. Nur S, Anwar M, Saleem M, Ahmad PA. Disseminated intravascular coagulation in acute leukaemias at first diagnosis. *Eur J Haematol* 1995;55:78–82.

38. Albarracin NS, Haust MD. Intravascular coagulation in promyelocytic leukemia: A case study including ultrastructure. *Am J Clin Pathol* 1971;55:677–679.

39. Gralnick HR, Sultan C. Acute promyeolocytic leukemia: haemorrhagic manifestation and morphologic criteria. *Br J Haematol* 1975;29:373–377.

40. Avvisati G, ten Cate JW, Buller HR, Mandelli F. Tranexaminic acid for control of haemorrhage in acute promyelocytic leukaemia. *Lancet* 1989;2:122–124.

41. Kelly DA, Tuddenham EGD. Haemostatic problems in liver disease. *Gut* 1986;27:339–349.

42. Violi F, Ferro D, Basili S, et al. Association between low-grade disseminated intravascular coagulation and

endotoxemia in patients with liver cirrhosis. *Gastroenterology* 1995;109:531–539.

43. Bick RL. Disseminated intravascular coagulation: a common complication of trauma and shock. In: Borris LC, Lassen MR, Bergqvist D (eds). *The Traumatized Patient*. Romer Grafik 1992;33–53.

44. Al-Mashhadani SA, Gader AGM, Al Harthi SS, et al. The coagulopathy of heat stroke: alterations in coagulation and fibrinolysis in heat stroke patients during the pilgrimage (Haj) to Makkah. *Blood Coag Fibrinol* 1994;5:731–736.

45. Bone RC. Gram-positive organisms and sepsis. *Arch Intern Med* 1994;154:26–34.

46. Taylor FB Jr. Role of tissue factor in the coagulant and inflammatory response to LD100 E. coli sepsis and in the early diagnosis of DIC in the baboon. In: Müller-Berghaus GM, Madlener K, Blomback M, ten Cate JW (eds). *DIC: Pathogenesis, Diagnosis and Therapy of Disseminated Intravascular Fibrin Formation.* Amsterdam: Excerpta Medica, 1993;19–32.

47. Levi M, van der Poll T, ten Cate H, van Deventer SJH. The cytokine-mediated imbalance between coagulant and anticoagulant mechanisms in sepsis and endotoxaemia. *Eur J Clin Invest* 1997;27:3–9.

48. van der Poll T, Buller HR, ten Cate H, et al. Activation of coagulation after administration of tumor necrosis factor to normal subjects. *N Engl J Med* 1990;322: 1622–1627.

49. Levi M, ten Cate H, Bauer KA, et al. Inhibiton of endotoxin-induced activation of coagulation and fibrinolysis by pentoxifylline or by a monoclonal anti-tissue factor antibody in a chimpanzee model. *J Clin Invest* 1994;93:114–120.

50. Biemond BJ, Levi M, ten Cate H, et al. Complete inhibition of endotoxin-induced coagulation activation in chimpanzees with a monclonal antibody to factor VII/VIIa. *Thromb Haemost* 1995;73:223–228.

51. ten Cate H, Bauer KA, Levi M, et al. The activation of factor IX and factor X by recombinant factor VIIa in vivo is mediated by tissue factor. *J Clin Invest* 1993; 92:1207–1212.

52. Broze GJ Jr, Gailani D. The role of factor XI in coagulation. *Thromb Haemost* 1993;70:72–74.

53. Biemond BJ, Levi M, ten Cate H, et al. Endotoxin-induced activation and inhibition of the fibrinolytic system: effects of various interventions in the cytokine and coagulation cascades in experimental endotoxemia in chimpanzees. *Clin Sci* 1995;88:587–594.

54. Kaufman N, Page JD, Pixley RA, Schein R, Schmaier AH, Colman RW. Alfa-2 macroglobulin-kallikrein complexes detect contact system activation in heriditary angioedema and human sepsis. *Blood* 1991;77:2660–2667.

55. Pixley RA, de la Cadena R, Page J, et al.The contact system contributes to hypotension but not disseminated intravascular coagulation in lethal bacteremia: in vivo use of a monclonal anti-factor XII antibody to block contact activation in baboons. *J Clin Invest* 1993;92:61–68.

56. Colman RW. Disseminated intravascular coagulation due to sepsis. *Semin Hematol* 1994;31:10–27.

57. Creasey AA, Chang ACK, Feigen L, Wun TC, Taylor FB Jr, Hinshaw LB. Tissue factor pathway inhibitor reduces mortality from Escherichia coli septic shock. *J Clin Invest* 1993;91:2850–2860.

58. Novotny WF, Brown SG, Miletich JP, Rader DJ,

Broze GJ Jr. Plasma antigen levels of the lipoprotein-associated coagulation inhibitor in patient samples. *Blood* 1991;78:387–393.

59. Saito M, Asakura H, Yoshida T, et al. Levels of activated factor VII in patients with disseminated intravascular coagulation. *Blood* 1995;85:3770–3771.

60. Gando S, Kameue T, Nanzaki S, Nakanishi Y. Disseminated intravascular coagulation is a frequent complication of systemic inflammatory response syndrome. *Thromb Haemost* 1996;75:224–228.

61. Fijnvandraat K, Derkx B, Peters M, et al. Coagulation activation and tissue necrosis in meningococcal septic shock: severely reduced protein C levels predict a high mortality. *Thromb Haemost* 1995;73:15–20.

62. Esmon CT, Taylor FB Jr, Snow TR. Inflammation and coagulation: linked processes potentially regulated through a common pathway mediated by protein C. *Thromb Haemost* 1991;66:160–165.

63. Taylor FB Jr, Chang A, Ferrell G, et al. C4b-binding protein exacerbates the host response to *Escherichia coli*. *Blood* 1991;78:357–363.

64. Wuillemin WA, Fijnvandraat K, Derkx BHF, et al. Activation of the intrinsic pathway of coagulation in children with menigococcal septic shock. *Thromb Haemost* 1996;74:1436–1441.

65. Wuillemin WA, Minnema M, Meijers JCM, et al. Inactivation of factor XIa in human plasma assessed by measuring factor XIa-protease inhibitor complexes: major role for C1-inhibitor. *Blood* 1995;85:1517–1526.

66. Nuijens JH, Eerenberg-Belmer AJM, Huijbregts CCM, et al. Proteolytic inactivation of plasma C1 inhibitor in sepsis. *J Clin Invest* 1989;84:443–450.

67. Brandtzaeg P, Joo GB, Brusletto B, Kierulf P. Plasminogen activator inhibitor 1 and 2, alpha-2-antiplasmin, plasminogen, and endotoxin levels in systemic meningococcal disease. *Thromb Res* 1990;57:271–278.

68. Gando S, Nakanishi Y, Tedo I. Cytokines and plasminogen activator inhibitor-1 in posttrauma disseminated intravascular coagulation: relationship to multiple organ dysfunction syndrome. *Crit Care Med* 1995;23:1835–1842.

69. Sakata Y, Murakami T, Noro A, Mori K, Matsuda M. The specific activity of plasminogen activator inhibitor-1 in disseminated intravascular coagulation with acute promyelocytic leukemia. *Blood* 1991;77:1949–1957.

70. Fischer E, Marano MA, van Zee KJ, et al. Interleukin-1 receptor blockade improves survival and hemodynamic performance in Escherichia coli septic shock but fails to alter host-responses to sublethal endotoxemia. *J Clin Invest* 1992;89:1551–1556.

71. Boermeester MA, van Leeuwen PAM, Coyle SM, et al. Interleukin-1 receptor blockade in patients with sepsis syndrome: evidence that interleukin-1 contributes to the release of interleukin-6, elastase and phospholipase A2, and to the activation of the complement, coagulation and fibrinolytic systems. *Arch Surg* 1995;130:739–48.

72. van der Poll T, Levi M, van Deventer SJH, et al. Differential effects of anti-tumor necrosis factor monoclonal antibodies on systemic inflammatory responses in endotoxemia in chimpanzees. *Blood* 1994;83:446–51.

73. van der Poll T, Levi M, Hack CE, et al. Elimination of interleukin-6 attenuates coagulation activation in experimental endotoxemia in chimpanzees. *J Exp Med* 1994;179:1253–9.

74. Stouthard J, Levi M, Hack CE, et al. Interleukin 6 stimulates coagulation but not fibrinolysis in humans. *Thromb Haemost* 1996;76:738–42.

75. Dempfle CE, Pfitzner SA, Dollman M, Huck K, Stehle G, Heene DL. Comparison of immunological and functional assays for measurement of soluble fibrin. *Thromb Haemost* 1995;74:673–679.

76. Bredbacka S, Blombäck M. Soluble fibrin: a predictor for development and outcome of multiple organ failure. In: Müller-Berghaus G, Madlener K, Blombäck M, ten Cate JW (eds). *DIC: Pathogenesis, Diagnosis and Therapy of Disseminated Intravascular Fibrin Formation*. Amsterdam: Excerpta Medica, 1993; 111–112.

77. Okajima K, Uchiba M, Murakami K, Okabe H, Takatsuki K. Determination of plasma soluble fibrin using a new ELISA method in patients with disseminated intravascular coagulation. *Am J Hematol* 1996;51:186–191.

78. Stibbe J, Gomes M, de Oude A. The value of the FM-test (KABI) and thrombin-antithrombin-III complexes (TAT) in the management of DIC in cancer. *Thromb Haemost* 1991;65:1238.

79. Bovill EG. Disseminated intravascular coagulation: pathophysiology and laboratory diagnosis. *Fibrinolysis* 1993;7(suppl 2):17–19.

80. Spero JA, Lewis JH, Hasiba U. Disseminated intravascular coagulation. Findings in 346 patients. *Thromb Haemost* 1980;43:28–33.

81. Williams EC, Mosher DF. Disseminated intravascular coagulation. In: Hoffman R, Benz EJ Jr, Shattil SJ, Furie B, Cohen HJ, Silberstein LE (eds). *Hematology: Basic Principles and Practice*. New York: Churchill Livingstone, 1995;1758–1769.

82. Bick RL. Disseminated intravascular coagulation: objective clinical and laboratory diagnosis, treatment, and assessment of therapeutic response. *Semin Thromb Hemost* 1996;22:69–88.

83. Cembrowski GS, Griffin JH, Mosher DF. Diagnostic efficacy of six plasma proteins in evaluating consumptive coagulopathies. Use of receiver operating characteristic curves to compare antithrombin III, plasminogen α_2-plasmin inhibitor, fibronectin, prothrombin, and protein C. *Arch Intern Med* 1986;146:1997–2002

84. Fukutake K, Kuroso K, Isogai N, Shinozawa K. Clinical evaluation of D-dimer testing in disseminated intravascular coagulation (DIC). *Fibrinolysis* 1993;7 (suppl 2): 20–22.

85. Takahashi H, Tatewaki W, Wada K, Niwano H, Shibata A. Fibrinolysis and fibrinogenolysis in disseminated intravascular coagulation. *Thromb Haemost* 1990;63:340–344.

86. Wada H, Wakita Y, Nakase T, et al. Outcome of disseminated intravascular coagulation in relation to the score when treatment was begun. *Thromb Haemost* 1995;74:848–852.

87. Mesters RM, Mannucci PM, Coppola R, Keller T, Ostermann H, Kienast J. Factor VIIa and antithrombin III activity during severe sepsis and septic shock in neutropenic patients. *Blood* 1996;88:881–886.

88. Mesters RM, Flörke N, Ostermann H, Kienast J. In-

crease of plasminogen activator inhibitor levels predicts outcome of leukocytopenic patients with sepsis. *Thromb Haemost* 1996;75:902–907.

89. Gando S, Kameue T, Nanzaki S, Nakanishi Y. Disseminated intravascular coagulation is a frequent complication of systemic inflammatory response syndrome. *Thromb Haemost* 1996;75:224–228.

90. Leeksma OC, Meijer-Huizinga F, Stoepman-van Dalen EA, van Ginkel CJW, van Aken WG, van Mourik JA. Fibrinopeptide A and the phosphate content of fibrinogen in venous thromboembolism and disseminated intravascular coagulation. *Blood* 1986; 67:1460–1467.

91. Nossel HL, Yudelman I, Canfield RE, et al. Measurement of fibrinopeptide A in human blood. *J Clin Invest* 1974;54:43–53.

92. Cronlund M, Hardin J, Burton J, Lee L, Haber E, Bloch KJ. Fibrinopeptide A in plasma of normal subjects and patients with disseminated intravascular coagulation and systemic lupus erythematosus. *J Clin Invest* 1976;58:142–151.

93. Neame PB, Kelton JG, Walker IR, Stewart IO, Nossel HL, Hirsh J. Thrombocytopenia in septicemia: the role of disseminated intravascular coagulation. *Blood* 1980; 56:88–92.

94. Bauer KA, Rosenberg RD. Thrombin generation in acute promyelocytic leukemia. *Blood* 1984;64: 791–796.

95. Teitel JM, Bauer KA, Lau HK, Rosenberg RD. Studies of the prothrombin activation pathway utilizing radioimmunoassays for the F2/F1 + 2 fragment and thrombin-antithrombin complex. *Blood* 1982;59: 1086–1097

96. Bruhn HD, Conard J, Mannucci M,et al. Multicentric evaluation of a new assay for prothrombin fragment F1 + 2 determination. *Thromb Haemost* 1992;68:413–417.

97. Stibbe J. Monitoring the anticoagulant treatment of DIC and recurrent thrombosis in patients with malignancies using the measurement of "soluble fibrin" (FM-test, Chromogenix), F1 + 2 and TAT complexes. In: Müller-Berghaus G, Madlener K, Blombäck M, ten Cate JW (eds). *DIC: Pathogenesis, Diagnosis and Therapy of Disseminated Intravascular Fibrin Formation.* Amsterdam: Excerpta Medica, 1993;113–123.

98. Nieuwenhuizen W, Hoegee-de Nobel E, Laterveer R. A rapid monoclonal antibody-based enzyme immunoassay (EIA) for the quantitative determination of soluble fibrin in plasma. *Thromb Haemost* 1992;68: 273–277

99. Scheefers-Borchel U, Müller-Berghaus G, Fuhge P, Eberle R, Heimburger N. Discrimination between fibrin and fibrinogen by a monoclonal antibody against a synthetic peptide. *Proc Natl Acad Sci USA* 1985;82: 7091–7095.

100. Nieuwenhuizen W, Creighton LC, Gaffney PJ, et al. A double blind comparative study of six monoclonal antibody-based plasma assays for fibrinogen derivatives. In: Lowe GDO, Douglas JT, Forbes CD, Henschen A (eds). *Fibrinogen 2. Biochemistry, Physiology and Clinical Relevance.* Amsterdam: Elsevier, 1987;181–186.

101. Boisclair MD, Lane DA, Wilde JT, Ireland H, Preston FE, Ofosu FA. A comparative evaluation of assays for markers of activated coagulation and/or fibrinolysis: thrombin-antithrombin complex, D-dimer and fibrinogen/fibrin fragment E antigen. *Br J Haematol* 1990; 74:471.

102. Kario K, Matsuo T, Kodama K, Matsuo M, Yamamoto K, Kobayashi H. Imbalance between thrombin and plasmin activity in disseminated intravascular coagulation. Assessment by the thrombin-antithrombin-complex/ plasmin-alpha-2-antiplasmin complex ratio. *Haemostasis* 1992;22:179–186.

103. Takahashi H, Wada K, Niwano H, Shibata A. Comparison of prothrombin fragment 1-2 with thrombin-antithrombin III complex in plasma of patients with disseminated intravascular coagulation. *Blood Coagul Fibrinol* 1992;3:813–818.

104. Mersky C, Johnson AJ, Kleiner GJ. The defibrination syndrome: clinical features and laboratory diagnosis. *Br J Haematol* 1967;13:528.

105. Lane DA, Preston FE, van Ross ME, Kakkar VV. Characterization of serum fibrinogen and fibrin fragments produced during disseminated intravascular coagulation. *Br J Haematol* 1978;40:609–615.

106. Pfitzner SA, Dempfle CE, Matsuda M, Heene DL. Fibrin detected in plasma of patients with disseminated intravascular coagulation by fibrin-specific antibodies consists primarily of high molecular weight factor XIIIa-crosslinked and plasmin-modified complexes partially containing fibrinopeptide A. *Thromb Haemost* 1997;78:1069–1078.

107. Williams EC. Plasma α_2-antiplasmin activity. Role in the evaluation and management of fibrinolytic states and other bleeding disorders. *Arch Intern Med* 1989; 149:1769–1772.

108. Harpel PC. α_2-plasmin inhibitor and α_2-macroglobulin-plasmin complexes in plasma. Quantitation by an enzyme-linked differential antibody immunosorbent assay. *J Clin Invest* 1981;68:46–55.

109. Brower MS, Harpel PC. α_1-antitrypsin-human leukocyte elastase complexes in blood: quantification by an enzyme-linked differential antibody immunosorbent assay and comparison with α_2-plasmin inhibitor–plasmin complexes. *Blood* 1983;59:842.

110. Holvoet P, de Boer A, Verstreken M, Collen D. An enzyme linked immunosorbent assay (ELISA) for the measurement of PAP complexes in human plasma: application to the detection of in vivo activation of the fibrinolytic system. *Thromb Haemost* 1986; 56:124.

111. Nieuwenhuizen W. Degradation of fibrinogen and its derivatives in the course of disseminated intravascular coagulation. In: Müller-Berghaus G, Madlener K, Blombäck M, ten Cate JW (eds). *DIC. Pathogenesis, Diagnosis and Therapy of Disseminated Intravascular Fibrin Formation.* Amsterdam: Excerpta Medica, 1993;117–123.

112. Corrigan JJ, Colman RW, Robboy SJ. Management of DIC. In: Inglefinger FJ, et al (eds). *Controversies in Internal Medicine II.* Philadelphia: Saunders, 1974.

113. Pritchard JA, Brekken AL. Clinical and laboratory studies on severe abruptio placentae. *Am J Obstet Gynecol* 1967;97:681.

114. Ginsberg J, Hirsh J, Marder VJ. Thrombotic and hemorrhagic complications in the obstetric patient. In: Colman RW, Hirsh J, Marder VJ, Salzman EW (eds). *Hemostasis and Thrombosis:* Basic Principles and Clinical Practice, 2nd ed. Philadelphia: Lippincott, 1987:981–988.

115. von Kries R, Stannigel H, Göbel U. Anticoagulant therapy by continuous heparin-ATIII infusion in newborns with DIC. *Eur J Pediatrics* 1985;144:191.

116. Weitz JI, Hudoba M, Massel D, Maraganore J, Hirsh J. Clot-bound thrombin is protected from inhibition by

heparin-antithrombin III but is susceptible to inactivation by antithrombin III-independent inhibitors. *J Clin Invest* 1990;86:385–391.

117. Colman RW, Robboy SW, Minna JD. DIC, A reappraisal. *Annu Rev Med* 1979;30:359–363.

118. Sack GH, Levin J, Bell WR. Trousseau's syndrome and other manifestations of chronic DIC in patients with neoplasms. *Medicine (Baltimore)* 1977;56:1.

119. Spicer TE, Rau JM. Purpura fulminans. *Am J Med* 1976;48:910.

120. Fischer DR Jr, Yawn DH, Crawford ES. Preoperative DIC associated with aortic aneurysms: a prospective study of 76 cases. *Arch Surg* 1983;118:1252.

121. Feinstein DI. Diagnosis and management of disseminated intravascular coagulation: the role of heparin therapy. *Blood* 1982;60:284–287.

122. Corrigan JJ Jr. Heparin therapy in bacterial septicemia. *J Pediatrics* 1977;91:695.

123. Heene DL. DIC: evaluation of therapeutic approaches. *Semin Thromb Hemost* 1977;3:291.

124. Oguma Y, Sakuragawa N, Maki M, Hasegawa H, Nakagawa M. Treatment of disseminated intravascular coagulation with low molecular weight heparin. Research Group of FR-860 on DIC in Japan. *Semin Thromb Hemost* 1990;16(suppl):34–40.

125. Saito M, Asakura H, Jokaji H, et al. Recombinant hirudin for the treatment of disseminated intravascular coagulation in patients with haematological malignancy. *Blood Coag Fibrinol* 1995;6:60–64.

126. Dickneite G, Czech J. Combination of antibiotic treatment with the thrombin inhibitor recombinant hirudin for the therapy of experimental *Klebsiella pneumoniae* sepsis. *Thromb Haemost* 1994;71:768–772.

127. Dickneite G, Czech J, Keuper H. Formation of fibrin monomers in experimental disseminated intravascular coagulation and its inhibition by recombinant hirudin. *Circ Shock* 1994;42:183–189.

128. Zawilska K, Zozulinska M, Turowiecka Z, Blauht M, Drobnik L, Vinazzer H. The effect of a long-acting recombinant hirudin (PEG-hirudin) on experimental disseminated intravascular coagulation (DIC) in rabbits. *Thromb Res* 1993;69:315–320.

129. Nowak G, Markwardt F. Hirudin in disseminated intravascular coagulation. *Haemostasis* 1991;21(suppl 1):142–148.

130. Fourrier F, Jourdain M, Tournois A, Caron C, Goudemand J, Chopin C. Coagulation inhibitor substitution during sepsis. *Intens Care Med* 1995;21(suppl 2): S264–8.

131. Blauhut W, Kramar H, Vinazzer H, Bergmann H. Substitution of ATIII in shock and DIC: a randomized study. *Thromb Res* 1985; 39:81–87.

132. van Beek EJ, von der Mohlen MA, ten Cate JW, Brandjes DP, Buller HR. Antithrombin III concentrate in the treatment of DIC: a retrospective follow-up study. *Neth J Med* 1994;45:206–210.

133. Lechner K, Kyrle PA. Antithrombin III concentrates: are they clinically useful? *Thromb Haemost* 1995;73: 340–348.

134. Fourrier F, Chopin C, Huart JJ, Runge I, Caron C, Goudemand J. Double-blind placebo-controlled trial of antithrombin III concentrate in septic shock with disseminated intravascular coagulation. *Chest* 1993; 104:882–888.

135. Esmon CT, Taylor FB Jr, Snow TR. Inflammation and coagulation: linked processes potentially regulated through a common pathway mediated by protein C. *Thromb Haemost* 1991;66:160–165.

136. Taylor FB, Chang A Jr, Esmon CT, D'Angelo A, Vigano-D'Angelo S, Blick KE. Protein C prevents the coagulopathic and lethal effects of *Escherichia coli* infusion in the baboon. *J Clin Invest* 1987; 79:918–925.

137. Okajima K, Imamura H, Koga S, Inoue M, Takatsuki K, Aoki N. Treatment of patients with disseminated intravascular coagulation by protein C. *Am J Hematol* 1990;33:277–278.

138. Rivard GE, David M, Farrell C, Schwarz HP. Treatment of purpura fulminans in meningococcemia with protein C concentrate. *J Pediatrics* 1995;126:646–652.

139. Rintala E, Seppala O, Kotilainen P, Rasi V. Protein C in the treatment of coagulopathy in meningococcal disease. *Lancet* 1996;347:1767.

140. Wong VK, Hitchcock W, Mason WH. Meningococcal infections in children: a review of 100 cases. *Pediatr Infect Dis* 1989;8:224.

141. Booth NA, Bennett B. Plasmin-α2-antiplasmin complexes in bleeding disorders characterized by primary or secondary fibrinolysis. *Br J Haematol* 1984;56: 545–547.

142. Verstraete M. Clinical application of inhibitors of fibrinolysis. *Drugs* 1985;29:236.

143. Milne AA, Drummond GB, Paterson DA, Murphy WG, Ruckley CV. Disseminated intravascular coagulation after aortic aneurysm repair, intraoperative salvage autotransfusion, and aprotinin. *Lancet* 1994; 344:470–471.

Cardiovascular Thrombosis: Thrombocardiology and Thromboneurology, Second Edition, edited by M. Verstraete, V. Fuster, and E. J. Topol, Lippincott–Raven Publishers, Philadelphia © 1998.

48

Special Aspects of Thrombosis in Diabetes

J. Andrew Davies and *Peter J. Grant

*Division of Medicine, University of Leeds School of Medicine, Leeds LS1 3EX, United Kingdom; and *Unit of Molecular Vascular Medicine, University of Leeds School of Medicine, Leeds LS1 3EX, United Kingdom*

Vascular Disorders in Diabetes Mellitus 801
Risk Factors for Thromboocclusive Disease in Diabetes 802
Coagulation and Fibrinolysis in IDDM 804
  Fibrinogen and Factor VII 804
  von Willebrand Factor 805
  Fibrinolysis in IDDM 805
Non-Insulin-Dependent Diabetes Mellitus 806
Coagulation and Fibrinolysis in NIDDM 806
  Fibrinogen and Factor VII 806
von Willebrand Factor 806
Fibrinolysis in NIDDM 806
Genetics of Coagulation and Fibrinolysis in Diabetes Mellitus 807
  Fibrinogen 807
  Factor VII 807
  von Willebrand Factor 807
  Plasminogen Activator Inhibitor Type 1 807
Platelet Function in Diabetes Mellitus 807
Conclusion 809

The identification and extraction of insulin by Banting and Best in 1922 lead to the availability of insulin for commercial use, transforming the prognosis of insulin-dependent diabetes (IDDM) from a few painful weeks to many years of near-normal life. However, the price paid has been a huge burden of vascular complications with associated morbidity and mortality. Within a few years of the discovery of insulin, the first clinical descriptions of insulin resistance emerged and in 1956 Vague identified the relationship between obesity and vascular disease. Such observations, coupled with the development of an assay for insulin, defined non-insulin-dependent diabetes (NIDDM) as a condition in which resistance to the action of insulin leads to hyperglycemia, whereas in IDDM an absolute deficiency of insulin occurs.

VASCULAR DISORDERS IN DIABETES MELLITUS

Although there are many differences between IDDM and NIDDM, they share the common features of fasting and postprandial hyperglycemia and a propensity to the development of both micro- and macrovascular complications. Microvascular complications principally affect the vessels in the retina (retinopathy), kidneys (nephropathy), and autonomic and peripheral nerves (neuropathy). A detailed discussion of this is outside the scope of this chapter, although it is worth noting that in IDDM, strict control of glycemia leads to marked attenuation of microvasculopathy. The microvascular complications account for much of the morbidity in the diabetic population, but ultimately it is the macrovascular complications (coronary artery,

801

cerebrovascular, and peripheral vascular disease) that mainly lead to early mortality.

The prevalence of diagnosed diabetes in the UK is 3% to 5%, approximately 70% of the total presenting as NIDDM. Although both types of diabetes share a high risk of cardiovascular disorders, most studies have been carried out in NIDDM because of the greater numbers available for investigation. The metabolic disturbance in subjects with NIDDM is related to decreased glucose uptake and resistance to the action of insulin in skeletal muscle, increased hepatic glucose output, and abnormalities in insulin secretion. This pattern of metabolism is commoner in the general population than NIDDM itself, with estimates of the prevalence of insulin resistance of 25%, depending on the definition employed. Diagnosed NIDDM is accordingly only the tip of an iceberg that comprises undiagnosed NIDDM, impaired glucose tolerance (IGT), and compensated normal glucose tolerance (NGT). The original World Health Organization (WHO) criteria for the diagnosis of diabetes were based on levels of glycemia associated with the development of microvascular complications. Evidence is accumulating that minor increases in blood glucose, previously thought to be harmless, are associated with subtle alterations in cardiac function and increase in mortality from ischemic heart disease. In the Honolulu Heart Study, subjects with a 1-hour blood glucose of >6.4 mmol/L had an increased 12-year coronary artery disease risk that was further increased in the groups with higher blood glucose levels at 1 hour (1). The Bedford Study reported increased cardiovascular mortality in subjects with IGT and a two- to threefold increase in 10- year mortality in NIDDM both being more marked in females (2). The Framingham Study reported that the incidence of cardiovascular disease was twice that seen in nondiabetic males and approaching threefold in females (3). Figures for other vascular conditions reveal a similar extent of morbidity and mortality. The Honolulu Heart Study showed diabetes to be associated with a twofold risk of stroke, and other studies have confirmed

that at all ages men and women have twice the risk of cerebral infarction compared to nondiabetic subjects (4). Framingham revealed a fourfold increase in peripheral vascular disease associated with diabetes and, again, a relatively greater increase in females.

RISK FACTORS FOR THROMBO-OCCLUSIVE DISEASE IN DIABETES

Patients with both IDDM and NIDDM have an increased risk of all forms of atherothrombotic vascular disease. The thrombotic component is most conspicuous in myocardial infarction, with thrombotic occlusion occurring at the site of plaque rupture in over 90% of cases of sudden cardiac death, irrespective of the presence of diabetes (5). Stroke is a heterogeneous disorder and in the majority of cases the nature of the vascular lesion is not characterized. In peripheral vascular disease the clinical syndrome results from increasing tissue ischemia due to progressive reduction in luminal diameter by encroaching atheroma. In all three disorders, however, activation of hemostatic mechanisms will invariably occur where plaques ulcerate. Thrombus may be incorporated into the plaque, accelerating luminal obliteration, or platelet-fibrin thrombi may embolize downstream resulting, for example, in transient ischemic attacks.

Diabetics are subject to risk factors for vascular diseases similar to the population in which they live, although these do not fully account for the higher prevalence of macrovascular disease in the diabetic population. The prevalence of smoking is similar to that in the general population (an indictment of the relative failure of prevention in high risk groups). Hypertension accounts for a significant proportion of the increase in myocardial infarction and stroke in diabetic patients. About 30% of patients are hypertensive, and hypertension is twice as common as it is in nondiabetics of similar age. In IDDM the risk of hypertension increases progressively with time, developing in about half of all patients with diabetes of 30 years duration. In diabetes, hypertension and renal disease are

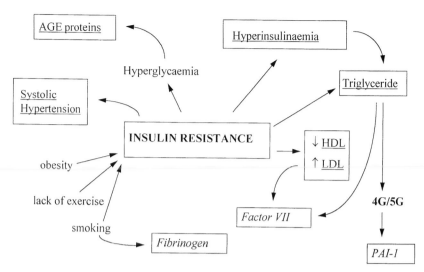

FIG. 48-1. Complex interrelationship between insulin resistance, atherogenic risk *(underlined)*, and thrombotic risk *(italics)* in the metabolic syndrome and NIDDM.

linked to atherothrombotic vascular disease through the development of albuminuria (6). In NIDDM hypertension is often present at diagnosis and is linked to the metabolic disturbances that accompany insulin resistance (the metabolic syndrome) (Fig. 48-1). Studies of the effects of treating hypertension and albuminuria on cardiac mortality in NIDDM are currently underway.

Profiles of lipid subclasses in patients tend to differ between IDDM and NIDDM patients. In well-controlled IDDM lipid levels are not dissimilar from those in the general population (7). Raised triglycerides are frequent, however, in patients with NIDDM and with poorly controlled IDDM (8). Synthesis of triglyceride-rich very-low- density lipoproteins (VLDLs) is increased in diabetes, and metabolism impaired, so that VLDL (and triglyceride) levels are higher than normal in many diabetics (8). In parallel, reduced catabolism of VLDL in poorly controlled diabetes leads to impaired production of high-density lipoproteins (HDLs). There is also an increase in atherogenic intermediate density lipoproteins (IDLs). The resultant high triglyceride, low HDL plasma is strongly associated with increased risk of vascular disease.

Hypercholesterolemia is less striking than hypertriglyceridemia in most diabetic patients. Insulin modulates uptake of low-density lipoproteins (LDLs) to a small extent, increase in insulin availability resulting in a small reduction in plasma LDL. The effect of high blood glucose, leading to glycation of plasma proteins, may also increase LDL concentrations through the reduced clearance of LDL carrying glycated apolipoprotein B.

Although hypertension and hyperlipidemia promote thromboocclusive vascular disease in diabetes, multiple additional mechanisms probably contribute. Small increases in blood glucose levels are associated with risk of vascular events even in the nondiabetic population. In NIDDM insulin resistance is associated with clustering of atherothrombotic risk factors leading to hypertension and vascular disease. Many proteins undergo glycation following prolonged exposure to high blood glucose levels leading to the formation of advanced glycosylation end-products (AGEs), or AGEs that bind to receptors on endothelial and other cells and may have deleterious effects on endothelial cell function (9).

In addition, patients with diabetes have abnormalities of hemostatic function that may

TABLE 48-1. *Major hemostatic changes in patients with diabetes mellitus*

	IDDM	NIDDM
Fibrinogen	Increased (13)	Increased (33)
Factor VII	Normal (15)	Increased (36)
Fibrinopeptide A	Increased (17)	Increased (17)
	Normal (18)	
vWF	Increased (20)	Increased (38)
Fibrinolytic activity	Normal (31)	Reduced (40)
PAI-1	Normal (31)	Increased (40)
Platelet aggregation	More sensitive to agonists (52)	
Plasma βTG	Increased (57)	
TXB$_2$	Increased (55)	Normal (65)

Reference numbers are in parentheses.

contribute both to atherogenesis and to a pro-thrombotic plasma in which the complications of advanced atheroma occur more readily (Table 48-1). Abnormalities of fibrinogen, factor VII, and plasminogen activator inhibitor type 1 (PAI-1) are particularly likely to contribute to the enhanced risk of vascular disease because these are risk factors in the general population (10–12). The contribution of platelet abnormalities is more conjectural. How the hemostatic abnormalities interact with other risk factors to render diabetics so susceptible to vascular disease is not yet established. If diabetes leads to thrombophilic plasma it would be expected that patients with diabetes were at higher risk of venous thromboembolism, but there is no evidence that this is the case (although the possibility has not been rigorously evaluated). It is more likely that the diabetic milieu enhances atherothrombotic risk by accelerating damage on the arterial side of the circulation. The subtle changes in hemostatic function in diabetes then further tip the balance toward arterial occlusion.

COAGULATION AND FIBRINOLYSIS IN IDDM

Fibrinogen and Factor VII

Plasma fibrinogen is significantly higher in patients with IDDM than in controls (13,14), and tends to be higher in those with estab-lished vascular disease (14). Increase in blood viscosity may be one mechanism whereby higher plasma fibrinogen contributes to vascular disease, although fibrinogen also has a crucial role in platelet aggregation as the ligand that binds aggregating platelets through glycoprotein IIb/IIIa receptors.

Fibrinogen and factor VII levels have been compared in patients with IDDM and microalbuminuria to those with normal albumin excretion (15,16). Fibrinogen levels were significantly higher in those with microalbuminuria in both studies, although levels of factor VII were found to be increased with microalbuminuria in one (16) though not in the other (15) series.

Measurements of fibrinopeptide A (FPA) concentrations are an indication of thrombin activity. In one study of 48 diabetic patients, mean plasma FPA values were twice as high as in controls (17) with no significant differences in plasma or urinary FPA concentrations between patients with IDDM and NIDDM. In our own studies (18), we were unable to detect higher levels of FPA in diabetic patients or evidence of activation of coagulation in response to hypo- or hyperglycemia. In IDDM subjects, levels of thrombomodulin (TM) have been related to both vascular complications in general and to the presence of albuminuria (19). As membrane-bound TM is a cofactor for protein C activation while inhibiting thrombin activation of factors V, VIII, and XIII, the significance of these findings are unclear. However, the presence of circulating TM may indicate underlying endothelial cell damage.

von Willebrand Factor

Many studies have shown higher than normal plasma concentrations of von Willebrand factor (vWF) in patients with IDDM (20–22). Though vWF levels fluctuate, daytime levels are characteristically higher in patients with IDDM. A study of 59 IDDM patients showed that increasing concentrations of plasma vWF were associated with deterioration of renal function over a 3-year follow-up (21). It was proposed that the increase in vWF indicated a damaging effect of poorly controlled diabetes on vascular endothelium (the source of vWF) and the kidney. Plasma vWF concentration has been shown to be significantly higher in IDDM patients with nephropathy than in patients with normal renal function who have levels similar to controls (22). Though higher plasma levels of vWF are associated with diabetic renal disease, vWF, unlike albuminuria, was not an independent predictor of symptomatic vascular disease over an 11-year period (23). Structure of vWF may be altered by the action of diabetic plasma on endothelial cells, resulting in release of vWF multimers with abnormalities of structure and function that are potentially reversible by improving glycemic control (24).

Fibrinolysis in IDDM

In an early study fibrinolysis was found to be depressed in an heterogeneous group of 100 patients with IDDM and NIDDM compared with controls (25). Patients with ischemic changes on electrocardiogram were more likely to have reduced fibrinolytic activity. Interest in fibrinolytic potential as a vascular risk factor increased after it was shown that reduced capacity to lyse clots in diluted whole blood (26) and raised levels of the fibrinolytic inhibitor PAI-1 in plasma (12) were associated with risk of myocardial infarction in nondiabetic patients.

In patients with IDDM, there is no consistent, major defect in fibrinolytic function. Review of the major studies of fibrinolysis (27,28) suggests there is an increase in basal fibrinolytic activity and tissue plasminogen activator (t-PA) concentrations, with normal or reduced levels of PAI-1 in IDDM patients. Studies have not been consistent, with some investigators finding fibrinolytic function to be similar to that in healthy volunteers.

Understanding the effects of fibrinolysis in IDDM is hampered by the limitations physiology imposes on clinical studies. The excess of inhibitors in plasma prevents measurement of fibrinolytic activity unless they are removed, and because t-PA and PAI-1 are complexed, immunologic assays do not directly equate with function. In addition, fibrinolysis is a dynamic system in which t-PA and PAI-1 are released by a variety of stimuli from the vessel wall. Investigators have approached this by studying response to changes in insulin and glucose levels, and to venous occlusion.

In our own study, uncomplicated IDDM was associated with normal responses to venous occlusion with a rise in t-PA, whereas PAI-1 remained unchanged (29). This response was progressively obtunded with increasing evidence of vascular disease, with PAI-1 remaining at a similar level but t-PA activity and antigen failing to rise (29). Similar results were found in a much smaller study of six IDDM patients (30).

Changes in levels of blood glucose affect fibrinolytic function in experimental systems and in vivo. Endothelial cells expressed PAI-1 and t-PA at about twice the rate in culture medium containing 30 mM as they did in 5 mM glucose, though overall fibrinolytic potential fell slightly (31). These in vitro data are consistent with findings in patients. We found that euglobulin clot lysis activity was increased in response both to hyper- and hypoglycemia in patients with IDDM (18) though there was no change in cross-linked fibrin-fibrinogen degradation products. In a similar study of response to hypoglycemia, fibrin plate lysis area increased slightly, as did t-PA antigen concentration, whereas PAI-1 activity fell and fibrinogen degradation products (FDPs) remained unchanged (30).

In a study of 31 patients with IDDM, euglobulin clot lysis, t-PA, and PAI-1 were found to be similar to levels in controls (32). However, with increasing degrees of renal disease there was a progressive reduction in euglobulin clot lysis activity and a significant increase in PAI-1 (32).

In summary, relatively minor differences exist in fibrinolytic capacity comparing IDDM patients with the healthy population. Based on the size of these differences alone, it does not seem likely that disturbance of fibrinolytic mechanisms is a major element in the vascular complications of IDDM.

NON-INSULIN-DEPENDENT DIABETES MELLITUS

Vague in 1956 recognized the association between male pattern or android obesity and the development of cardiovascular disease (33). In 1988 Reaven proposed that the clustering of cardiovascular risk around insulin resistance represents a syndrome of metabolic dysfunction (34) whose features include android obesity, insulin resistance and hyperinsulinemia, dyslipidemia, hypertension, and coronary artery disease. Initially described as syndrome X, this title has now been largely dropped in Europe in favor of the more descriptive "metabolic syndrome." Some (presently) nondiabetic subjects with increased insulin responses also exhibit similar clustering of cardiovascular risk.

COAGULATION AND FIBRINOLYSIS IN NIDDM

Fibrinogen and Factor VII

Levels of fibrinogen have been reported as high in insulin treated NIDDM, but normal in those treated with either diet or tablets (35). The Scottish Heart Study, in a younger group of subjects reported higher levels of fibrinogen in subjects with a personal history of diabetes mellitus and other cardiovascular risk

factors (36). In a study of relatives of NIDDM subjects there were higher levels of fibrinogen compared to controls with no family history of NIDDM, indicating the familial nature of this observation (37).

Levels of factor VII relate to some features of the insulin resistance syndrome in NIDDM subjects with strong correlations with total cholesterol, insulin, and triglyceride (38). Similar patterns occur in relatives of NIDDM subjects, with significant correlations between factor VII and body mass index, fasting insulin and triglyceride (37). Women have higher levels of factor VII than men and this is particularly marked in NIDDM (39).

von Willebrand Factor

Levels of vWF are increased in cerebrovascular disease and in NIDDM subjects, whereas high vWF concentrations have been related to risk of myocardial infarction and death in both diabetic and nondiabetic subjects (40). Levels of vWF do not appear to be related to features of the insulin resistance syndrome (41), though there is not total agreement on this issue.

Fibrinolysis in NIDDM

Marked differences exist in fibrinolytic activity comparing subjects with IDDM and NIDDM. Patients with NIDDM have profound suppression of fibrinolysis due to increased levels of PAI-1 (42). Several studies have noted the strong clinical relationship between features of the metabolic syndrome and elevated PAI-1 levels in NIDDM. In particular, PAI-1 is elevated in the presence of obesity and reduced by weight loss, increased in the presence of hypertension and strongly correlates with triglyceride concentrations (42,43). Many population studies have shown a relationship between fasting insulin concentrations and PAI-1 in diabetic and nondiabetic subjects and insulin has been shown to enhance PAI-1 synthesis and secretion in cells of hepatic origin (44). In humans, however, no study has yet demonstrated an increase in

PAI-1 in response to insulin, and it seems that insulin levels in population studies are probably acting as a surrogate for insulin resistance, which appears to be the major determinant of plasma PAI-1 concentrations.

GENETICS OF COAGULATION AND FIBRINOLYSIS IN DIABETES MELLITUS

Fibrinogen

The α, β, and γ chains of the fibrinogen molecule are coded by three genes in close proximity on chromosome 4, position q21–28. The α-fibrinogen gene is situated about 10 kb downstream of the γ and 13 kb upstream of the β chain. A number of important factors influence circulating levels of fibrinogen, including age, smoking, and gender. There is a strong genetic component determining fibrinogen levels, with as much as 51% of the variation in levels being ascribed to genetic factors (45). The fibrinogen β-chain Bcl I polymorphism is associated with the development of peripheral arterial disease (46). We have found the fibrinogen 448 G/A polymorphism to be associated with cerebrovascular disease in nondiabetic women (47), and the -455 G/A polymorphism to be independently associated with coronary artery disease in subjects with NIDDM (48). A number of additional polymorphisms on the beta chain and their relationship to coronary artery disease have recently been described (49).

Factor VII

The factor VII gene is composed of nine exons and is localized to the long arm of chromosome 13. Studies of the factor VII gene have demonstrated two sites in linkage disequilibrium that relate to circulating levels of factor VII: a promoter decanucleotide repeat and an Msp 1 cutting site in exon 8. Several studies have demonstrated a relationship between circulating factor VII and dyslipidemia. In a study of NIDDM patients, a strong relationship existed between circulating insulin and factor VII

concentrations, although the relationships did not appear to be genotype-specific (38).

von Willebrand Factor

The gene for vWF is situated on chromosome 12 and consists of a promoter of just under 3 kb and many introns and exons. There has been tremendous interest in the vWF gene because of the need to understand the genetics of von Willebrand's disease, but there is no published work on the gene in relation to vascular disorders. A study of a common vWF polymorphism, vWF levels, and insulin resistance in NIDDM demonstrated no relationships of note (41).

Plasminogen Activator Inhibitor Type 1

The PAI-1 gene is located on chromosome 7 in position 7q21–22, which codes for two distinct mRNA species of 2.4 and 3.2 kb. The gene for PAI-1 spans some 12 kb and is split into nine exons. A 4G/5G polymorphism 675Bp 5 of the start of transcription has been shown to be related to circulating PAI-1 levels with highest values in the 4G/4G subjects, lowest in 5G/5G, and intermediate in 4G/5G (41). It appears that there is genotype-specific regulation of PAI-1 by triglyceride at the 4G allele, which may explain the tight relationship between these components of the metabolic syndrome (43).

The 4G/4G genotype has been reported to occur more frequently in nondiabetic patients with myocardial infarction (50,51) and in NIDDM patients with a history of ischemic heart disease (52). In large populations of diabetic patients we were unable to find any difference in the prevalence of these mutations in relation to either peripheral vascular disease or retinopathy (53).

PLATELET FUNCTION IN DIABETES MELLITUS

Numerous studies have been carried out on the function of platelets in diabetes (54). In most, samples from patients with IDDM and

NIDDM have not been differentiated, and it is not clear as to whether there is any systematic difference in platelet behavior comparing the two types of disease. Most investigators have found platelets from diabetic subjects to react abnormally, with a lowered threshold to activation by aggregating agents, increased plasma concentrations of released α-granule proteins and platelet eicosanoids, altered platelet plasma membrane function, and reduced platelet survival. In general, abnormalities have been more marked in patients with overt vascular disease. As many of the changes seen in platelets from diabetic patients are similar to those observed in platelets from patients with atherosclerotic vascular disease, it is not clear as to whether they are related mainly to the metabolic disturbances or to the vascular disease in diabetes.

Platelets from diabetic subjects are more likely to aggregate when exposed to a range of platelet agonists. Many workers in the 1970s showed that diabetic platelets aggregated at lower concentrations of adenosine diphosphate (ADP) than controls (55). Aggregation is similarly induced more readily in response to collagen (56,57), sodium arachidonate (56–58), and platelet-activating factor (59). Use of platelet aggregation in whole blood (which avoids artifacts induced by processing) has shown platelets from diabetic subjects to be more susceptible to activation by shaking and stirring (60) the abnormality being greater in patients with IDDM who had vascular complications. In some studies, improved diabetic control and exposure of platelets to lower levels of plasma glucose restored the pattern of platelet activity toward control values (57), whereas in others it did not (56). Recent evidence indicates that platelet- dependent thrombi generation is enhanced in diabetic subjects, particularly in poorly controlled patients (61).

Platelets from patients with diabetes also exhibit more GpIIb/IIIa receptors on their surface (62) and bind greater amounts of fibrinogen (63) than platelets from nondiabetic subjects.

As might be expected, platelets that are more sensitive to agonists that induce aggregation will be more likely to release the contents of the α granules into plasma. Most observers have found increased levels in diabetic plasma of the released proteins β-thromboglobulin (TG) (59,64,65) and platelet factor 4 (PF4) (59,65). Minimal platelet activation and release can lead to increase in plasma TG during processing, but studies that circumvent this by using the ratio of TG:PF4 (65) or urinary TG levels (66) have similarly shown that plasma from diabetic subjects has higher concentrations of platelet release proteins, consistent with a low level of intravascular platelet activation in diabetes.

An early observation was that diabetic platelets produced increased amounts of metabolites of arachidonic acid following stimulation (67). Plasma from patients with diabetes has higher than normal levels of thromboxane B2 (TXB2), a metabolite of TXA2 that activates platelets and induces vasoconstriction (54,58). One study using gas chromatography–mass spectrometry to detect a stable metabolite of TXB2 in urine (though in small numbers of patients) failed to detect any increase in TXB2 production from platelets in patients with IDDM whether or not they had vascular disease (68). In contrast, using urine extraction and refined immunoassay, levels of 11-dehydro-TXB2 were increased in the urine of 50 patients with NIDDM and levels of the metabolite fell after a period of tight metabolic control (57).

Platelets activated by interaction with damaged blood vessels, artificial surfaces, or other platelets have a shortened life span in the circulation. A number of studies using different techniques to determine platelet survival have shown that platelets in the circulation of patients with diabetes survive for a shorter time than those in healthy controls (54,67).

Three broad explanations have been considered for the abnormalities of platelet function in diabetes: (a) abnormal platelets are synthesized; (b) platelets become abnormal when exposed to the metabolic environment of diabetic plasma; and (c) platelets are affected by interaction with damaged blood vessels. There is little evidence to suggest that diabetic platelets are inherently abnormal; it is more plausible that platelets become abnormal in diabetic plasma due to changes induced in platelet plasma membrane function. Glycation of membrane proteins occurs following chronic exposure of platelets to high blood glucose levels (54,67). High concentrations of cholesterol and triglycerides, particularly in NIDDM, can alter the fluidity of platelet membranes, leading to a lowered threshold for platelet activation. Finally, platelets from diabetic patients exist in a circulation in which they are exposed early in the disease to an endothelium that has subtly altered function and, later, to a highly abnormal microcirculation and to atherosclerotic large vessels. It has not yet been resolved as to whether platelets are significant contributors to the genesis of micro- and macrovascular disease, or largely innocent carriers of evidence of a damaged circulation.

CONCLUSION

IDDM and NIDDM are complex metabolic disorders characterized by hyperglycemia and the chronic development of micro- and macrovascular disorders. The pathogenesis of vascular complications of diabetes are similarly complex and, as yet, not fully elucidated. The Diabetes Control and Complications Trial (DCCT) demonstrated that the microvascular complications associated with IDDM are directly related to levels of glycemic control and, in particular, protein glycosylation.

The mechanisms linking poor metabolic control to microvascular disease are unclear, but it seems unlikely that the hemostatic mechanism has a direct role in this process. Two studies (DCCT) in IDDM and the United Kingdom Prospective Diabetes Study in NIDDM have attempted to unravel the relationships between metabolic control and macrovascular disease—so far with little success. It seems likely that the initiation of macrovascular disease in both IDDM and NIDDM is related in some way to the underlying metabolic defect, hyperglycemia and glycosylation being high on the list of suspects.

In IDDM variation in metabolic control early in life may be a major influence on vascular pathology with abnormalities in hemostasis having lesser effects.

Fluctuations in metabolic control are less severe in NIDDM and, of course, occur much later in life. The increase in vascular disease in this group is probably related to insulin resistance and the associated clustering of cardiovascular risks: android obesity, glucose intolerance, dyslipidemia, and hypertension.

Patients with NIDDM frequently have elevated levels of PAI-1 and this should be regarded as a feature of the metabolic syndrome. Elevated levels of PAI-1 have been linked to the development of myocardial infarction in nondiabetic subjects in prospective studies, providing evidence that it may have an important role in NIDDM. There is a small contribution to circulating levels from genetic variation and two small studies have demonstrated a relationship between a promoter polymorphism in the PAI-1 gene and cardiovascular disease.

Definition of the elements in the metabolic syndrome provides the first steps toward a global theory for the pathogenesis of vascular disease and explains how patients can be both at increased atherogenic risk (from dyslipidemia, hypertension, hyperglycemia) and increased risk of thrombus formation (from elevated PAI-1 and possibly factor VII), the two essential elements of acute myocardial infarction.

REFERENCES

1. Donahue RP, Abbott RD, Reed DM, Yano K. Postchallenge glucose concentration and coronary heart disease in men of Japanese ancestry: Honolulu heart program. *Diabetes* 1987;36:689–692.
2. Jarrett RJ, McCartney P, Keen H. The Bedford Survey: ten year mortality rates in newly diagnosed diabetics, borderline diabetics and normoglycaemic controls and risk indices for coronary heart disease in borderline diabetics. *Diabetologia* 1982;22:79–84.
3. Garcia MJ, McNamara PM, Gordon T, Kannel WB. Morbidity and mortality in diabetics in the Framingham population. Sixteen year follow-up study. *Diabetes* 1974;23:105–111.
4. Fuller JH, Shipley MJ, Rose G, Jarrett RJ, Keen H. Mortality from coronary heart disease and stroke I relation

to degree of glycaemia: the Whitehall Study. *Br Med J* 1983;287:867–870.

5. Davies MJ, Thomas A. Thrombosis and acute coronary artery lesions in sudden cardiac ischemic death. *N Engl J Med* 1984;310: 1137–1140.

6. Mogensen CE. Microalbuminuria predicts clinical proteinuria and early mortality in maturity-onset diabetes. *N Engl J Med* 1986;310:356–360.

7. Dubrey SW, Reaveley DA, Leslie DG, O'Donnell M, O'Connor BM, Seeds M. Effect of insulin-dependent diabetes mellitus on lipids and lipoproteins: a study of identical twins. *Clin Sci* 1993;84:537–542.

8. Abbate SL, Brunzell JD. Pathophysiology of hyperlipidaemia in diabetes mellitus. *J Cardiovasc Pharmacol* 1990;16(suppl 9):S1–S7.

9. Schmidt AM, Hori O, Chen JX, et al. Advanced glycation endproducts interacting with their endothelial receptor induce expression of vascular cell adhesion molecule–1 (VCAM-1) in cultured human endothelial cells and in mice. A potential mechanism for the acceleration of vasculopathy of diabetes. *J Clin Invest* 1995;96:1395–1403.

10. Heinrich J, Balleisen L, Schulte H, Assmann G, van de Loo J. Fibrinogen and factor VII in the prediction of coronary risk. *Arterioscler Thromb* 1994;14:54–59.

11. Ernst E, Resch KL. Fibrinogen as a cardiovascular risk factor: a met-analysis and review of the literature. *Ann Intern Med* 1993;118:956–963.

12. Hamsten A, De Faire U, Walldivis G, et al. Plasminogen activator inhibitor in plasma: risk factor for recurrent myocardial infarction. *Lancet* 1987;iv:3–9.

13. Ceriello A, Taboga C, Giacomello R, et al. Fibrinogen plasma levels as a marker of thrombin activation in diabetes. *Diabetes* 1994;43:430–432.

14. Lowe GDO, Lowe JM, Drummond MM, et al. Blood viscosity in young male diabetics with and without retinopathy. *Diabetologia* 1980;18:359–363.

15. Jones SL, Close CF, Mattock MB, Jarrett RJ, Keen H, Viberti GC. Plasma lipid and coagulation factor concentrations in insulin dependent diabetics with microalbuminuria. *Br Med J* 1989;298:487–490.

16. Gruden G, Cavallo-Perin P, Bazzan M, Stella S, Vuolo A, Pagano G. PAI-1 and factor VII activity are higher in IDDM patients with microalbuminuria. *Diabetes* 1994; 43:426–429.

17. Jones RL. Fibrinopeptide-A in diabetes mellitus. Relation to levels of blood glucose, fibrinogen disappearance, and hemodynamic changes. *Diabetes* 1985;34: 836–843.

18. Grant PJ, Stickland MH, Wiles PG, Gaffney PJ, Davies JA, Prentice CRM. Acute changes in blood glucose concentration do not promote thrombin generation or fibrin breakdown in type 1 diabetes. *Diab Med* 1988;5: 867–870.

19. Gabat S, Keller C, Kempe HP, et al. Plasma thrombomodulin: a marker for microvascular complications in diabetes mellitus. *Vasa* 1996;25:233–241.

20. Porta M, Maneschi F, White MC, Kohner EM. Twenty-four hour variations of von Willebrand factor and factor VIII-related antigen in diabetic retinopathy. *Metabolism* 1981;30:695–699.

21. Stehouwer CDA, Stroes ESG, Hackeng WHL, Mulder PGH, den Ottolander GJH. von Willebrand factor and development of diabetic nephropathy in IDDM. *Diabetes* 1991;40:971–976.

22. Jensen T. Increased plasma concentration of von Wille-brand factor in insulin dependent diabetics with incipient nephropathy. *Br Med J* 1989;298:27–28.

23. Deckert T, Yokoyama H, Mathieson E, et al. Cohort study of predictive value of urinary albumin excretion for atherosclerotic vascular disease in patients with insulin dependent diabetes. *Br Med J* 1996;312:871–874.

24. Pasi KJ, Enayar MS, Horrocks PM, Wright AD, Hill FGH. Qualitative and quantitative abnormalities of von Willebrand antigen in patients with diabetes mellitus. *Thromb Res* 1990;59:581–591.

25. Fearnley GR, Chakrabarti R, Avis PRD. Blood fibrinolytic activity in diabetes mellitus and its bearing on ischaemic heart disease and obesity. *Br Med J* 1963;i: 921–923.

26. Meade TW, Chakrabarti R, Haines AP, et al. Haemostatic function and cardiovascular death: early results of a prospective study. *Lancet* 1980;1:1050–1053.

27. Mansfield MW, Grant PJ. Fibrinolysis and diabetes mellitus. In: Glas-Greenwalt P (ed). *Fibrinolysis in Disease. Molecular and Hemovascular Aspects of Fibrinolysis.* Boca Raton: CRC Press, 1996;172–183.

28. Gough SCL, Grant PJ. The fibrinolytic system in diabetes mellitus. *Diab Med* 1991;8:898–905.

29. Walmsley D, Hampton KK, Grant PJ. Contrasting fibrinolytic responses in type 1 (insulin-dependent) and type 2 (Non-insulin-dependent) diabetes. *Diab Med* 1991;8: 954–959.

30. Fisher BM, Quin JD, Rumley A, et al. Effects of acute insulin-induced hypoglycaemia on haemostasis, fibrinolysis and haemorheology in insulin-dependent diabetic patients and control subjects. *Clin Sci* 1991;80: 525–531.

31. Maiello M, Boeri D, Podesta F, et al. Increased expression of tissue plasminogen activator and its inhibitor and reduced fibrinolytic potential of human endothelial cells cultured in elevated glucose. *Diabetes* 1992;41: 1009–1015.

32. Mahmoud R, Raccah D, Alessi MC, Aillaud MF, Juhan-Vague I, Vague P. Fibrinolysis in insulin dependent diabetic patients with or without nephropathy. *Fibrinolysis* 1992;6:105–109.

33. Vague J. The degree of masculine diffferentiation of obesities, a factor determining predisposition to diabetes, atherosclerosis, gout and uric calculous disease. *American Journal of Clin Nutr* 1956;4:20–34.

34. Reaven GM. Role of insulin resistance in human disease. *Diabetes* 1988;37:1595–1607.

35. Missov RM, Stolk RP, van der Bom JG, et al. Plasma Fibrinogen in NIDDM. The Rotterdam Study. *Diab Care* 1996;19:157–159.

36. Lee AJ, Lowe DO, Woodward M, Tunstall-Pedoe H. Fibrinogen in relation to personal history of prevalent hypertension, diabetes, stroke, intermittent claudication, coronary heart disease and family history: the Scottish Heart Health Study. *Br Heart J* 1993;69:338–342.

37. Mansfield MW, Heywood DM, Grant PJ. Circulating levels of factor VII, fibrinogen and von Willebrand factor and features of insulin resistance in first degree relatives of patients with NIDDM. *Circulation* 1996;94: 2171–2176.

38. Heywood D, Mansfield MW, Grant PJ. Factor VII gene polymorphisms, factor VII:C levels and features of insulin resistance in non-insulin-dependent diabetes mellitus: a link with vascular risk. *Thromb Haemost* 1996; 75:401–407.

39. Mansfield MW, Heywood DM, Grant PJ. Sex differences in coagulation and fibrinolysis in white subjects with non-insulin-dependent diabetes mellitus. *Arterioscler Thromb Vasc Biol* 1996;16:160–164.

40. Jansson JH, Nilsson T, Johnson O. von Willebrand factor in plasma: a novel risk factor for recurrent myocardial infarction and death. *Br Heart J* 1991;66:351–355.

41. Heywood DM, Mansfield MW, Grant PJ. Levels of von Willebrand factor with features of the metabolic syndrome and a common vWF gene polymorphism in type 2 diabetes mellitus. *Diab Med* 1996;13:720–725.

42. Juhan-Vague I, Alessi MC, Vague P. Increased plasma plasminogen activator inhibitor 1 levels: a possible link between insulin resistance and atherothrombosis. *Diabetologia* 1991;34:457–462.

43. Grant PJ. Polymorphisms of coagulation/fibrinolysis genes: gene-environment interactions and vascular risk. *Prostaglandins Leukotrienes and Essential Fatty Acids*. In press.

44. Grant P.J, Ruegg M, Medcalf RL. Basal expression and insulin mediated induction of PAI-1 mRNA in Hep G2 cells. *Fibrinolysis* 1991;5:81–86.

45. Hamsten A, Iselius L, De Faire U, Blomback M. Genetic and cultural inheritance of plasma fibrinogen concentration. *Lancet* 1987;2:988–990.

46. Fowkes FG, Connor JM, Smith FB, Wood J, Donnan PT, Lowe GD. Fibrinogen genotype and risk of peripheral atherosclerosis. *Lancet* 1992;339:693–696.

47. Carter A, Catto AJ, Bamford JM, Grant PJ. Gender specific associations of the fibrinogen Bβ 448 polymorphism, fibrinogen levels and acute cerebrovascular disease. *Arterioscler Thromb Vasc Biol* 1997;17:589–594.

48. Carter AM, Mansfield MW, Stickland MH, Grant PJ. Fibrinogen β gene -455 G/A polymorphism and fibrinogen levels: risk factors for coronary artery disease in subjects with non-insulin-dependent diabetes mellitus. *Diab Care* 1996;19:1265–1268.

49. Behague I, Poirier O, Nicaud V, et al. β fibrinogen gene polymorphisms are associated with plasma fibrinogen and coronary artery disease in patients with myocardial infarction. The ECTIM study. *Circulation* 1996;93: 440–449.

50. Erikkson P, Kallin B, van t Hooft FM, Båvenholm P, Hamsten A. Allele-specific increase in basal transcription of the plasminogen-activator inhibitor 1 gene is associated with myocardial infarction. *Proc Natl Acad Sci USA* 1995;92:1851–1855.

51. Ossei-Gerning N, Mansfield MW, Stickland MH, Wilson IJ, Grant PJ. Plasminogen activator inhibitor-1(PAI-1) promoter 4G/5G genotype and levels in relation to a history of myocardial infarction in patients characterised by coronary angiography. *Arterioscler Thromb Vasc Biol* 1997;17:33–37.

52. Mansfield MW, Stickland MH, Grant PJ. Plasminogen activator inhibitor-1 (PAI-1) promoter polymorphism and coronary artery disease in non-insulin-dependent diabetes. *Thromb Haemost* 1995;74:1032–1034.

53. Mansfield M.W, Stickland MH, Carter AM, Grant PJ. Polymorphisms of the plasminogen activator inhibitor-1 gene in type 1 and type 2 diabetes, and in patients with diabetic retinopathy. *Thromb Haemost* 1994;71:731–736.

54. Winocour PD. Platelet abnormalities in diabetes mellitus. *Diabetes* 1992;41:26–31.

55. Colwell JA, Halushka PV. Platelet function in diabetes mellitus. *Br J Haematol* 1980;40:521–526.

56. Jackson CA, Greaves M, Boulton AJM, Ward JD, Preston FE. Near-normal glycaemic control does not correct abnormal platelet reactivity in diabetes mellitus. *Clin Sci* 1984;67:551–555.

57. Daví G, Catalano I, Averna M, et al. Thromboxane biosynthesis and platelet function in type II diabetes mellitus. *N Engl J Med* 1990;322:1769–1774.

58. García Frade LJ, de la Calle H, Alava I, Navarro JL, Creighton LJ, Gaffney PJ. Diabetes mellitus as a hypercoagulable state: its relationship with fibrin fragments and vascular damage. *Thromb Res* 1987;47:53–540.

59. Fritschi J, Christe M, Lämmle B, Marbet GA, Berger W, Duckert F. Platelet aggregation, β-thromboglobulin and platelet factor 4 in diabetes mellitus and in patients with vasculopathy. *Thromb Haemost* 1984;52:236–239.

60. Cho NH, Becker D, Dorman JS, et al. Spontaneous whole blood platelet aggregation in insulin-dependent diabetes mellitus: an evaluation in an epidemiologic study. *Thromb Haemost* 1989;61:127–130.

61. Aoki I, Shimoyama K, Aoki N, et al. Platelet-dependent thrombin generation in patients with diabetes mellitus: effects of glycemic control on coagulability in diabetes. *J Am Coll Cardiol* 1966;27:560–566.

62. Tschoepe D, Roesen P, Kaufmann L, et al. Evidence for abnormal platelet glycoprotein expression in diabetes mellitus. *Eur J Clin Invest* 1990;20:166–170.

63. Lee M, Paton RC, Passa P, Caen JP. Fibrinongen binding and ADP-induced aggregation in platelets from diabetic subjects. *Thromb Res* 1981;24:143–150.

64. Burrows AW, Chavin SI, Hockaday TDR. Plasma-thromboglobulin concentrations in diabetes mellitus. *Lancet* 1978;1:235–237.

65. Zahavi J, Zahavi M. Platelet function in type 1 diabetes mellitus [Letter]. *N Engl J Med* 1988;319:1665–1666.

66. van Oost BA, Veldhuyzen B, Timmermans APM, Sixma JJ. Increased urinary β-thromboglobulin excretion in diabetes assayed with a modified RIA kit-technique. *Thromb Haemost* 1983;49:18–20.

67. Mustard JF, Packham MA. Platelets and diabetes mellitus. *N Engl J Med* 1984;311:665–667.

68. Alessandrini P, McRae J, Feman S, FitzGerald GA. Thromboxane biosynthesis and platelet function in type 1 diabetes mellitus. *N Engl J Med* 1988;319:208–212.

Cardiovascular Thrombosis: Thrombocardiology and Thromboneurology, Second Edition,
edited by M. Verstraete, V. Fuster, and E.J. Topol,
Lippincott–Raven Publishers, Philadelphia © 1998.

49

Thrombosis on Artificial Surfaces

Charles D. Forbes and *James McNiven Courtney

*Department of Medicine, University of Dundee, Ninewells Hospital and Medical School, Dundee DD1 9SY, United Kingdom; and *Bioengineering Unit, University of Strathclyde, Glasgow G4 0NW, United Kingdom*

Thrombus formation on artificial surfaces remains clinically relevant and the level of interest is certain to continue. This is understandable when consideration is given to the widespread use of biomaterials in blood-contacting applications (1,2) and the consequent need for artificial surfaces capable of providing an acceptable clinical performance in contact with blood (3). It is a general opinion that an improved utilization of current materials and the development of novel materials with enhanced properties require a better understanding of the reactions occurring when blood contacts an artificial surface.

The response of blood to contact with an artificial surface can be viewed in terms of blood–biomaterial interactions and the investigation of blood–biomaterial interactions has a broad objective of achieving a correlation between a characteristic property of the biomaterial and a representative feature of the blood response (4). While such a correlation is advantageous, its establishment is made difficult by the complexity of the blood response and the fact that clinical utilization often involves multimaterial contact. The investigation of biomaterials would benefit from greater knowledge of the biomaterial, particularly its surface characteristics, and improved methodologies for monitoring the levels of blood components.

Information on the interactions of blood with artificial surfaces is regarded as an essential prerequisite to the production of improved materials and consequent clinical benefit. Therefore, a clearer understanding of blood–biomaterial interactions is a key feature of successful material development.

The acquisition of information on blood–biomaterial interactions is dependent on assessment procedures. These range from in vitro methods to clinical evaluation and there is a general dependency on the mode of blood–biomaterial contact, the selection of a parameter as representative of the blood response, the methodology used to determine blood component levels, and the interpretation of data obtained.

On the basis of the points raised above, prior to describing clinical implications, it is relevant to consider thrombosis on artificial surfaces in terms of the following:

• Interactions of blood with artificial surfaces
• Improved biomaterial performance
• Preclinical evaluation procedures

INTERACTIONS OF BLOOD WITH ARTIFICIAL SURFACES

A consideration of blood interactions with artificial surfaces has to accept that the artificial surface cannot act in a manner similar to that of the endothelium. The nature of the endothelium ensures the ability to perform an active role in thromboresistance and the provision of a nonattractive surface. While modification of an artificial surface can lead to inhibition of thrombus formation, this does not compare with the action of the endothelium. Additionally, artificial surfaces, far from being nonattractive, promote the attachment of blood components. A striking example of the difference in behavior between the artificial surfaces and the endothelium is that of the influence on proteins. Under physiologic conditions, the endothelium does not appear to adsorb proteins, but protein adsorption onto artificial surfaces is considered to be an inevitable and important consequence of blood–biomaterial interactions (5,6).

The blood response to contact with an artificial surface can be viewed (3) as the involvement of protein adsorption; platelet adhesion, release, and aggregation; activation of the intrinsic coagulation; participation of the fibrinolytic, complement, and kallikrein-kinin systems; and the interaction of cellular elements. The response promotes the formation of thrombus and simultaneous therapy with anticoagulants, platelet aggregation inhibitors, or plasminogen activators is a general requirement for the clinical utilization of artificial surfaces.

Although the integrated nature of the blood response and the complexity of blood interactions with artificial surfaces should be borne in mind (3,7), examination of blood alterations induced by surface contact can be conveniently undertaken in terms of contributions from particular blood components. In this respect, relevant features are protein adsorption, platelet reactions, intrinsic coagulation, fibrinolytic activity, complement activation, and the presence of erythrocytes and leukocytes.

Protein Adsorption

The importance of protein adsorption comes from the fact that the adsorption of protein onto an artificial surface is regarded as the first major event resulting from blood–surface contact. Protein adsorption is rapid and the nature of the adsorbed protein layer has a strong influence on subsequent blood interactions (6). The significant role of the adsorbed protein has been long recognized (8–10) and supports the belief that information on protein adsorption is beneficial for biomaterial utilization and development. There have been studies of protein adsorption from solution (11,12), plasma (13,14), and blood (15,16), although there are problems in correlating laboratory performance with the clinical situation (17).

The spontaneity of protein adsorption onto artificial surfaces can be attributed to the amphipathic (polar/nonpolar) character of protein molecules providing a driving force for the concentration of proteins at interfaces, the limited solubility of proteins due to the high molecular weight of the macromolecules, and the tendency of protein adsorption to induce a reduction in free energy of the system (9). While there has been a general opinion that protein adsorption is greater and involves stronger attachment on hydrophobic than on hydrophilic surfaces (3), hydrophilicity does not eliminate the adsorption of protein.

Proteins that have been extensively investigated are fibrinogen, gammaglobulin, and albumin. There is a close relationship between fibrinogen and platelet reactions (3). Platelets are strongly attracted by fibrinogen and platelet reactivity is promoted by fibrinogen adsorption. Other features of fibrinogen adsorption are the replacement of adsorbed fibrinogen by high molecular weight kininogen (HMWK), a phenomenon referred to as the Vroman effect (13), and a possible interaction of fibrinogen with leukocytes (5). The importance of fibrinogen adsorption is emphasized by the view that the timing of fibrinogen adsorption and its removal from arti-

ficial surfaces may have important clinical consequences (18). Investigation of gamma-globulin indicates that the adsorption of this protein onto artificial surfaces promotes platelet adhesion and stimulates the platelet release reaction and gammaglobulin adsorption may be followed by leukocyte adhesion. The behavior of albumin contrasts with that of fibrinogen and gamma globulin, in that albumin adsorption reduces platelet and leukocyte adhesion and inhibits thrombus formation.

The importance of the adsorbed protein layer, the possible influence of even trace quantities of proteins, and the identification in the adsorbed layer of proteins other than fibrinogen, gammaglobulin and albumin combine to support further investigation. Adsorbed proteins identified include lipoproteins; fibronectin with a possible role in leukocyte adhesion; von Willebrand–factor VIII protein complex with a possible link to increased platelet adhesion; and plasminogen

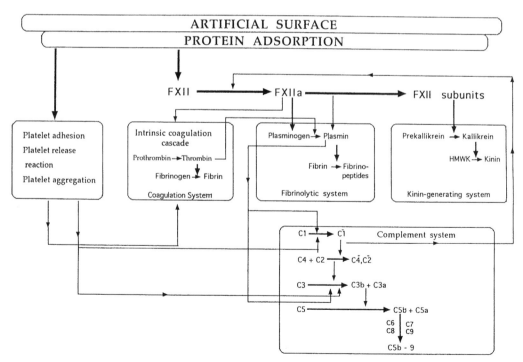

FIG. 49-1. Interaction of blood with an artificial surface showing the mechanisms of protein adsorption and activation. (From Courtney et al., ref. 128.)

with a possible effect on surface-associated fibrinolytic activity.

Other aspects of protein adsorption merit consideration. There is the role in the contact activation phase of the intrinsic pathway of the contact proteins factor XII, factor XI, HMWK, and prekallikrein (19). The adsorption of HMWK and factor XII initiates a sequence of enzymatic reactions. A complex is formed between bound HMWK and prekallikrein. This complex cleaves factor XII into factor XIIa, which catalyzes the conversion into kallikrein of the prekallikrein involved in the complex with HMWK. With the activation of factor XII by kallikrein, a cycle of reactions leads to the rapid availability of factor XII on or near the artificial surface. HMWK is also able to form a complex with factor XI, which makes factor XI available to factor XIIa and enables the progression of the coagulation cascade. With respect to the Vroman effect and the replacement of fibrinogen by HMWK, the relevance for artificial surfaces is that a low Vroman effect with fibrinogen retention should induce less activation of the intrinsic coagulation, whereas a high Vroman effect with fibrinogen displacement should induce less platelet reactivity (6).

Finally, it is important to distinguish between protein adsorption and protein activity. This is exemplified in contact activation, where a strong adsorption of factor XII onto an artificial surface does not always correlate with high factor XII activity (20), and in complement activation, where the extent of activation can be influenced by the ability of artificial surfaces to adsorb components such as C3a, which are normally released into plasma (21) (Fig. 49-1).

Platelet Reactions

In the interactions of blood with artificial surfaces, a general consequence of blood contact with the surface is the adhesion and aggregation of platelets (22,23), with the extent of platelet adhesion strongly influenced by the nature of the adsorbed protein layer.

The attachment of circulating platelets to the protein layer on an artificial surface produces a change in platelet shape from anucleate discs to spheres with long filiform pseudopodia, the coalescence of platelets into an irregular monolayer, and, with increasing platelet adhesion (Fig. 49-2),the formation of mounds with erythrocytes and leukocytes entrapped in fibrin (24) (Fig. 49-3).The sequence of platelet reactions is that platelet adhesion to an artificial surface is followed by the platelet release reaction taking place in the adherent platelets, with platelet aggregation occurring on the surface (25). Some of these platelet masses may be swept into the circulation (Fig. 49-4) and embolize in small downstream vessels.

As thrombus formation on the artificial surface proceeds, there is an interaction between platelets and the intrinsic coagulation (26). Initiation of the intrinsic coagulation is induced by procoagulants liberated from the platelets (27,28) or by factor XII activation caused by platelets stimulated by released adenosine diphosphate (ADP). Interaction is enhanced when intrinsic pathway activation causes thrombin formation, since the generation of thrombin leads to the rapid production of a fibrin monolayer on an artificial surface, thereby promoting platelet adhesion and aggregation (29,30) and also induces the platelet

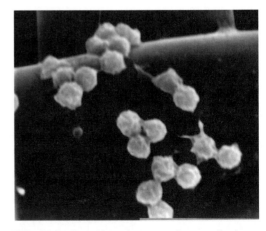

FIG. 49-2. Seaming electron micrograph showing the adhesion of platelets to an artificial surface with examples of viscous metamorphosis.

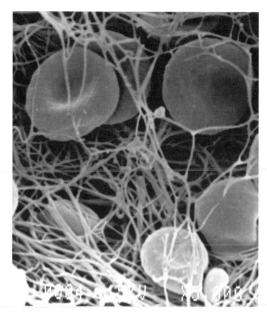

FIG. 49-3. Formed elements of the blood entrapped in a fibrin mesh that has formed on a cellulose membrane in the course of hemodialysis.

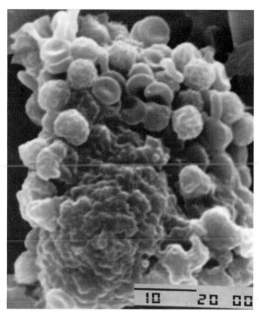

FIG. 49-4. An embolus of platelets, red cells, and white cells that has been dislodged from a membrane surface. If returned to the body it could produce clinical sequelae.

release reaction and the secretion of platelet factor 4, thromboxane B_2, and thrombospondin (31–33).

Platelet reactions resulting from blood–surface contact are influenced by diffusion (34) and shear forces (35), with the shear rate and contact time considered critical for platelet adhesion (36).

In some clinical situations, it is relevant that consideration of platelet reactivity be widened from a role in the mechanism of hemostasis to a participation in immunologic and inflammatory reactions (37).

Intrinsic Coagulation

Initiation of the intrinsic pathway by the contact activation phase as a consequence of blood–biomaterial interactions has been reported above. There is interest in the relationship between the nature of an artificial surface and its influence on the contact proteins (38,39), with interest promoted by the fact that contact proteins can induce major biological consequences because of the close con-

nection with biologically important proteolytic pathways.

Fibrinolytic Activity

While the relationship between artificial surfaces and fibrinolysis has not been a major topic of interest in blood–biomaterial interactions (6), the integrated nature of the different systems participating in the response of blood to artificial surfaces (7) makes it relevant to take into account fibrinolysis and fibrinolytic activity. Surface-induced fibrinolytic activity has been demonstrated by measurement of the levels of fibrin degradation products and activation of the fibrinolytic system has been reported for different clinical applications (40,41).

Complement Activation

The contact of blood with an artificial system can lead to activation of the complement system (42–44). In general, alternative pathway activation is considered relevant for artificial surfaces, although leucopheresis studies have indicated the possibility of classical pathway activation (45) and involvement of the classical pathway has been inferred in cardiopulmonary bypass (46).

A feature of complement activation by artificial surfaces is the release of the anaphylatoxins C3a and C5a. The significance of the ability of some artificial surfaces to bind C3a has been noted in the consideration of protein adsorption. The importance of C5a release is due to its role as a potent mediator of granulocyte responses, including adherence, aggregation, degranulation, chemotaxis, and toxic oxygen radical production. While C5a normally contributes to host defense by promoting leukocyte accumulation and activation at local sites of inflammation, systemic or intravascular complement activation and C5a formation are believed to induce granulocyte activation and damage to multiple organ systems (45).

Following blood contact with an artificial surface, platelet interactions with the complement system may be relevant and mediation of platelet and leukocyte adhesion to artificial surfaces has been reported (47).

Erythrocytes

When blood contacts an artificial surface, erythrocytes can adhere to the adsorbed protein layer (26). Under certain conditions, hemolysis occurs, with the platelet release reaction induced by liberated ADP and erythrocyte ghosts (48). The pattern of protein adsorption on an artificial surface can also be influenced by erythrocytes. There is the possibility that deposition of cell membrane components can result in a less adsorptive surface and a reduction in the amount of protein adsorbed (49,50). Another possibility is an effect arising from the competitive adsorption of released hemoglobin. The flow of blood over an artificial surface may induce hemolysis, thus increasing the local concentration of free hemoglobin in the plasma, and hemoglobin adsorption will be promoted by the high surface activity of hemoglobin (50,51).

In thrombosis on artificial surfaces, platelet adhesion can be enhanced by the hydrodynamic behavior of erythrocytes, a reduction in the adsorption of platelet-protective proteins, or the deposition by erythrocytes of an adhesive substance (9). Shear-induced hemolysis may occur and in coagulation under low shear forces, entrapped erythrocytes and fibrin form the red thrombus (52).

Leukocytes

The adhesion of leukocytes to artificial surfaces has been long recognized (53), with the preferential adsorption of polymorphonuclear leukocytes over that of lymphocytes supported by evidence from in vitro studies (54,55) and leucopheresis (56). The adsorbed protein layer influences leukocyte adhesion and enhanced adhesion of leukocytes has been reported for surfaces with deposition of thrombin and prothrombin (57). Leukocytes appear similar to platelets with respect to sensitivity to mechanical trauma (58). Leukocyte damage and aggregation are influenced by shear stress and leukocyte incorporation into platelet microaggregates has been reported (59).

In thrombosis on artificial surfaces, the action of leukocytes can be contrasted with the primarily passive role of the erythrocytes (5). Leukocytes are attracted to the thrombus and in the thrombosis process leukocytes may contribute to platelet recruitment and then participate in fibrinolysis. There is a direct role for leukocytes in thrombosis on artificial surfaces (60), arising from granulocyte possession of endogenous procoagulant activity (61,62) and proaggregatory activity (63).

An important aspect of the leukocyte response to blood contact with an artificial surface is that of changes in cell function. Cell damage induced by surface contact (53) causes an impairment in phagocytosis and a reduced ability to combat infection. Following leukocyte adhesion, there is often activation and the stimulation of cell functions such as protein synthesis, causing the production and release of substances, including superoxide and other free radicals, leukotrienes, interleukins, tumor necrosis factor, plasminogen activator, prostaglandins, histamine, and platelet-activating factor (64–66).

Investigation of the leukocyte response often examines the relationship between leukocytes and complement activation, with this relationship of particular relevance to extracorporeal applications.

IMPROVED BIOMATERIAL PERFORMANCE

In many clinical applications it is necessary to use an antithrombotic agent to avoid thrombus formation on the artificial surface of a biomaterial. Therefore, it is important to consider the possible interaction between biomaterial and antithrombotic agent because adsorption of the agent by the biomaterial can alter the pharmacologic activity. In the overall relationship between blood, biomaterial, and antithrombotic agent, an improved blood response can result from alteration to the biomaterial, the antithrombotic agent, or both (67), and for a given biomaterial, improvement has been reported by replacement of heparin by a low molecular weight heparin (68) or hirudin (69).

There have been numerous attempts to improve the performance of a biomaterial by modification of the artificial surface to enhance its blood compatibility. Relevant approaches may be considered in terms of the following: surface physical properties, hydrophilicity increase, chemical modification, antithrombotic agent attachment, surface treatment with protein, and biomembrane-mimetic surface preparation (70,71).

Surface Physical Properties

The physical nature of an artificial surface can strongly influence the blood response. An unsatisfactory blood response can result from excessive surface roughness causing mechanical damage or producing adverse effects on blood flow due to material shape and presentation. Therefore, an initial step in the improvement of blood compatibility may be the achievement of a smoother surface. However, in certain applications smoothness is avoided and a porous surface is produced in order to induce neointima formation. Porous surfaces can be achieved by the use of expanded polymers (72), textured polymers (73), and woven or knitted fabric structures (74,75). The relevance of the physical nature of an artificial surface means that surface texture should be considered with surface chemistry because surface texture may have an important influence.

Hydrophilicity Increase

The basis for producing artificial surfaces with greater hydrophilicity is the view that protein adsorption and cellular adhesion will decrease with increasing hydrophilicity. Hydrophilic artificial surfaces are obtained with polymeric hydrogels (76,77), which swell extensively in aqueous media while remaining insoluble. However, the poor mechanical strength of hydrogels limits the applicability and procedures for increasing hydrophilicity may require coating or copolymerization.

Techniques for increasing hydrophilicity often utilize polymers based on hydroxyethyl methacrylate (HEMA), but in some applications the utilization of poly(ethylene oxide) (PEO) is preferable. Polymers containing HEMA may reduce the platelet response but activate complement through hydroxyl groups (78), whereas PEO can reduce the platelet response and complement activation (79).

Chemical Modification

An improved blood response with a polymeric biomaterial can be achieved by chemical modification, where a functional group undergoes replacement or substitution. The influence of chemical modification is dependent on both the nature of the substituting group and the degree of substitution, whereas the integrated nature of the blood response means that an improvement with respect to a particular blood component may be offset by an increased adverse effect on another (80).

Antithrombotic Agent Attachment

The attachment of anticoagulants, platelet aggregation inhibitors, or plasminogen activators to artificial surfaces is intended to be an alternative or supplement to the administration of antithrombotic agents. Efforts have been dominated by the utilization of heparin. Heparin attachment to an artificial surface can be achieved by ionic or covalent bonding (70,71). The strong anionic nature of heparin means that ionic binding takes place readily on cationic surfaces or on surfaces rendered cationic by pretreatment. However, the simplicity of ionic attachment is offset by the ease of heparin removal in contact with blood or plasma (81). The long-term retention of heparin and the preparation of more stable surfaces require covalent binding. Covalent attachment is more complex than ionic binding. The effectiveness of covalent binding depends on the possible utilization of the functional groups in the active sites of the heparin molecule during the attachment procedure and inhibition of blood–heparin contact by protein adsorption (82), as well as the mobility of the heparin chain on the artificial surface. In order to preserve the ability of heparin to bind and activate antithrombin III, procedures for covalent attachment have taken into account the effect of the attachment process on antithrombin III binding sites. In this respect, protection of the antithrombin III binding sites during heparin immobilization has been accomplished by a technique producing endpoint attachment of heparin (82). As a means of achieving more controlled covalent attachment, polymer chains have been used as spacers between the heparin molecule and the artificial surface (83–85). Covalent attachment to an artificial surface of an albumin-heparin conjugate has been employed to obtain the benefits of both heparin attachment and albumin adsorption (86).

Surface attachment of platelet aggregation inhibitors improves the blood compatibility of a biomaterial by reducing platelet adhesion and aggregation. Examples of agents utilized are prostaglandins (87,88) and dipyridamole (89). Covalent binding is the preferred approach to the attachment of platelet aggregation inhibitors and options for functionalization and the selection of coupling agents have been reported (88,90).

The attachment of plasminogen activators is intended to provide artificial surfaces that are fibrinolytically active and capable of reducing thrombus formation by dissolution. There has been a focus on the attachment of urokinase (91–96), with attachment achieved by ionic binding (95) or covalent binding (94).

Surface Treatment with Protein

The deposition of protein onto an artificial surface in order to improve blood compatibility has taken advantage of the ability of adsorbed albumin to reduce platelet adhesion. This property of albumin has encouraged the identification of polymers capable of albumin adsorption (97) and the preparation of polymers with enhanced albumin adsorption (98,99).

A particular utilization of protein is in *biolization* (100), a term applied to the chemical and thermal treatment of proteins either coated onto a polymer or blended with a polymer (101).

Biomembrane–Mimetic Surface Preparation

Biomembrane-mimetic surfaces are intended to mimic the biological membrane of blood cells and thereby avoid recognition of the artificial surface by the blood as foreign. A fundamental step is the utilization on an artificial surface of the phosphorylcholine (PC) head group, a major component of erythrocyte and platelet outer membrane surfaces (102). Approaches include coating polymers containing PC groups onto polymer surfaces (103), covalent attachment of functionally active PC-containing compounds to polymer surfaces (104), and use of a monomer containing PC in copolymerization (105) or grafting (106). Biomembrane-mimetic surfaces are reported to reduce protein adsorption, platelet reactions, thrombogenicity, and complement activation.

PRECLINICAL EVALUATION PROCEDURES

While the establishment of procedures capable of promoting the quality control and development of materials is considered to be an important objective (10), it has to be accepted that test procedures for predicting the clinical performance of artificial surfaces in blood-contacting applications are subject to limitations (107).

Test procedures range from those intended to provide an initial screening of materials to those designed for a detailed investigation (3,108). The basic features of a test procedure are the nature of the blood, the method for achieving blood–material contact, and parameter selection. The nature of the blood is determined by species selection, the presence of antithrombotic or pharmaceutical agents, and the possible influence of a disease state. The method chosen for contacting the material with blood should ensure that the blood response is dependent on the material surface rather than the contact procedure. Parameter selection is based on blood components representative of features of the blood response. Selection may involve a compromise between the advantages of multiparameter assessment and the benefit of determining a single parameter by a consistent methodology.

In Vitro Evaluation

In vitro test procedures generally use human blood and have been designed to evaluate materials in the form of sheet, tubing, or hollow fiber. Test procedures range from the use of incubation cells relevant to rapid screening to circuits with closely controlled blood flow and wall shear rates appropriate for more detailed investigation of blood–material interactions (3,108).

With respect to the blood response, features studied in vitro include protein adsorption, platelet adhesion, release and aggregate for-mation, thrombogenicity, contact activation, and complement activation.

Ex Vivo Evaluation

Single-pass human ex vivo procedures designed for the evaluation of hollow fiber hemodialysis membranes (109,110) can be adapted for the evaluation of sheet or tubing. These systems ensure control of blood flow but each test may require a donation of 500 ml blood.

In animal-based ex vivo systems, arteriovenous shunts have been utilized in the dog, sheep, and baboon, with an emphasis on monitoring the deposition of radiolabeled proteins and platelets. Materials in sheet form have been assessed in the dog and pig with flow-through cells. Miniaturized rat extracorporeal circuits have been designed to mimic hemoperfusion, hemodialysis, membrane plasma separation, and cardiopulmonary bypass.

In Vivo Evaluation

In vivo test procedures are based on the implantation of materials in animals for selected periods, as in the vena cava ring test (111) and renal embolus test (112).

There are difficulties in linking the evaluation of a material to its potential clinical performance. In vitro test procedures allow the use of human blood but cannot take into account the inter-relationships between the patient and the clinical utilization of the material (113–115). Ex vivo procedures using human blood require evaluation in a clinical environment. The data obtained from animal experiments must be interpreted with the recognition of species-related differences for blood components (116,117).

CLINICAL CONSEQUENCES OF BLOOD CONTACT WITH ARTIFICIAL SURFACES

Emergency admission of most patients to hospital now results in exposure of the patients blood to some form of artificial surface.

TABLE 49-1. *Chronology of blood–surface interactions*

Within hours of contact	Protein absorption
	Cell adhesion/activation
	Coagulation factor activation
	Fibrin production
	Complement activation
	Embolization
Days	Consumption:
	(a) coagulation factors
	(b) cells
	Multiple recurrent platelet-fibrin emboli
	Inflammatory response
Months/Years	Fibrosis/calcification
	Continuing embolization
	Neointimal growth
	Changes in physical properties of implant

The most common of these exposures results from the insertion of an intravenous cannula or catheter, usually to maintain venous access for sampling or for administration of drugs or fluids, and this is of trivial consequence for the patient despite there being local activation of coagulation and platelets on the surface of the cannula. However many other invasive processes take place in which there is a substantial and prolonged exposure of patients blood to an artificial surface. These include hemodialysis, cardiopulmonary bypass, arterial and venous indwelling cannulae, vascular prostheses, stenting of arteries, arterial grafting, artificial heart and left ventricular assist devices, and the insertion of valves. Changes in the blood resulting from blood–material interaction may be acute in the first few hours of exposure, become more chronic over the next few days, and in the long term produce a different profile of effects (see Table 49-1). Interaction with blood coagulation proteins, platelets, white cells, and complement may be substantially avoided by the use of anticoagulants and antiplatelet agents.

ARTERIAL STENTING
(SEE ALSO CHAPTER 34)

In a situation where an artery has become severely occluded by the development of atheromatous plaque, it may not be possible to bypass the blockage or to perform angioplasty. In such cases an arterial stent may be im-

planted to maintain the patency of the lumen of the artery. Such stents are implanted via an intra-arterial catheter and expand at the site of application to push back and hold in place the friable atheromatous lesion. While these stents are made from different materials that may be coated or uncoated, they act as an artificial surface and the deposition of platelets and activation of platelets is greater when a stent is used than for a standard balloon angioplasty alone (118). The combination of arterial wall damage, disruption of atheromatous plaque, and a foreign body is a powerful prothrombotic stimulus and over the years several anti-thrombotic regimes have been tried, mainly involving combinations of antiplatelet agents and anticoagulants (119,120). As yet there is no agreement on the individual drugs that provide the best mixture of antiplatelet and anticoagulant effect. However, a preliminary release of information (121) suggests that a combination of aspirin and ticlopidine was more effective than aspirin and warfarin in combination or aspirin alone. The measurement here was the composite clinical event rate, which included death, Q-wave, myocardial infarction, emergency surgery, subacute closure, and repeat angioplasty (121). The evidence is now becoming clearer in favor of antiplatelet therapy than anticoagulants, especially when used in combination (121). Newer antiplatelet regimes using inhibitors of the adhesive proteins (GpIIb:IIIa) are currently under trial and are exciting options.

ARTIFICIAL HEARTS

There can be no doubt about the importance of transplantation of a human heart on the recipient's quality of life. Despite the problems of chronic immunosuppression with subsequent opportunistic infections and the longer term problems of arterial disease affecting the coronary arteries of the transplanted heart, this is undoubtedly the best treatment option for selected patients (122). However, there will always be a shortage of supply and a transplantable organ may not become available in the time frame of the patient's need. Such patients may, however, be kept alive with an artificial heart used as a bridge to transplantation. A variety of pumping devices have been used and the first successful device was the intra-aortic balloon pump (123). Thereafter a series of mechanical devices was prepared. All had variable success but suffered from the problems of thrombosis in the blood chamber and also infection. The first fully portable electric system was used in 1990 and depended on a pneumatically powered pump (124). With advancing technology and design, the complication rate (in particular the instance of neurologic complications and hemolysis) was substantially reduced so that the duration of use of such devices increased exponentially and patients were kept alive for up to 2 years with such a device. This is important as the median waiting time for patients who require heart transplantation was approximately 200 days in the United States and up to half of patients on the waiting list died before transplantation (125). With more appropriate materials being used in such devices and a higher flow rate, the incidence of thromboembolism from the device diminished with the introduction of various antithrombotic regimes including aspirin and other antiplatelet agents and anticoagulants that were tightly controlled by International Normalized Ratio (INR) checks (126).

HEMODIALYSIS AND RELATED PROCEDURE

With the advent of an increasing number of elderly in the populations of the Western

world, end-stage renal failure has become common and methods of renal support are now widely used in hospital settings. Chronic ambulatory peritoneal dialysis (CAPD) has become extremely popular and uses the physiologic membrane of the peritoneum, whereas membrane-based hemodialysis uses a series of artificial membranes to which blood is exposed and which allows the products of metabolism, electrolytes, and water to pass. Hemodialysis lasts for several hours and blood from the patient is therefore exposed to vascular catheters, plastic tubing, and the material of the membrane itself (127). The commonest material used for these dialysis membranes remains cellulose because of its low cost, despite the fact that there is evidence that newer membranes are more biocompatible, less likely to interact with blood components, and less likely to induce activation of coagulation platelets, white cells, and complement. In the absence of any anticoagulant, blood components, mainly proteins, coagulation factors, white cells, and platelets, rapidly adhere to the membrane and tubing (128,129). Coagulation and complement factors that adhere and are activated and these activated and adherent white cells and platelets are returned to the patient's body where they may induce pulmonary dysfunction following the procedure. Arterial hypoxemia is associated with pulmonary basal constriction and also with small vessel embolization by platelet and white cell/fibrin aggregates. The formation of such activated products can be inhibited by standard unfractionated heparin or by the use of low molecular weight heparin. In addition, aspirin, dipyridamole, and prostacyclin may also be used as an adjunct to standard heparin anticoagulation and also with use of low molecular weight heparins (130).

VALVE PROSTHESES (SEE ALSO CHAPTER 22)

Severe disease of heart valves requires replacement with a prosthesis as the only practical option. Over the past 30 years, major improvements have been made in the available heart valve so that reasonably good physiologic valve function devoid of the risk of major complications, such as thromboembolism and hemolysis, is now available (131). There are two broad groups of valves: (a) biological and (b) mechanical. Biological valves are made from human or animal tissue and have the advantage of having a reduced incidence of thromboembolic events but suffer from the disadvantage of long-term failure of function and therefore may require replacement at a future date. Mechanical valves are made from a variety of materials and consist essentially of a case containing a ball or disc that opens a valve in systole and obstructs the return of blood in diastole. The long-term risk is of thrombosis on the artificial surfaces and subsequent thromboembolism. Such valves have a good reputation for long-term function and the risk of thromboembolism can be significantly reduced by the use of anticoagulation, often in association with the concurrent use of antiplatelet agents. The initiating factor in mechanical valves seems to be localized trauma to red cells on the moving parts. This release of adenosine diphosphate induces platelet aggregation as shown by the measurement of levels of circulating β-thromboglobulin (bTG), and this increased consumption of platelets is shown by a dramatically diminished platelet half-life in the circulation. Aspirin and dipyridamole significantly reduce this risk (131,132). The optimal dose of anticoagulation is still under debate as it is important to strike a balance between prevention of thrombo-embolism and bleeding risk (133). The INR should be kept between 3 and 4 (134,135).

ARTERIAL GRAFTS

Atheroma formation in the central arteries and the larger peripheral vessels remains a major problem in our aging population. Replacement of occluded or damaged vessels using prosthetic grafting material is a daily occurrence. Materials such as porous woven Dacron, expanded microporous polytetrafluo-

roethylene, and glutaraldehyde-treated human femoral artery have been used for such grafts. The incidence of major thromboembolism in these grafts is not particularly high due to the velocity of the blood flow and they have a low incidence of complications in both the short and the long term. Arterial grafts for small-diameter vessels (below 6 mm) have a high incidence of thrombotic occlusion due to the significant reduction in arterial flow. Antithrombotic regimens such as antiplatelet agents and anticoagulants are often used in these situations and significantly enhance the long-term viability of small grafts. A variety of regimes with low- and medium-dose aspirin plus other antiplatelet agents combined with long-term warfarin are used. INR should be kept in the 3 to 4 range.

Cardiopulmonary Bypass

This is a commonly used procedure in cardiac surgery in which cardiac standstill is a requirement and the pumping and oxygenation function of the heart and lungs is replaced with membrane oxygenation by means of an extracorporeal circuit (136). Blood that is removed from the superior vena cava is passed through a heat exchanger that regulates temperature. The blood is pumped then through an oxygenator and returned to a reservoir where it is filtered and eventually returned at arterial pressure to the heart. Blood is therefore in contact with the tubing, membranes, pumps, and gases. During this time red cells and white cells are damaged whereupon the released ADP stimulates platelet and white cell activation and contact with the surfaces initiates the coagulation and complement activation (115,137). During the process, heparin is used as an anticoagulant and prostacyclin, aspirin, and other related antiplatelet agents may also be used. The amount of heparin required is usually monitored using the activated partial of a thromboplastin time. Numerous other physical factors must also considered including temperature and mechanical trauma and blood flow. The use of priming fluids also dilutes coagulation factors and may compound the tendency to bleed. After cardiopulmonary bypass, there is commonly evidence of neurologic deficits of a minor nature and these may be related to platelet -fibrin thromboemboli as well as materials and bubbles coming from the circuit.

ARTERIAL AND VENOUS ACCESS LINE

In modern medicine, it is extremely common for most patients admitted for acute medical procedures to have arterial or venous catheters inserted for blood sampling, parenteral nutrition, or the administration of chemotherapeutic agents or long-term antibiotics, as well as for appropriate imaging of arteries and veins. It is inevitable that if a catheter is left in an artery or vein it will stimulate damage to the endothelium resulting in local thrombosis. In addition, use of infusions of various chemicals may further irritate and desquamate endothelium, and the presence of the foreign surface results in adhesion of proteins, coagulation factors, platelets, and white cells to the cannula itself. It is usual to infuse and leave a small amount of heparin in the cannula to inhibit the clotting of blood that has refluxed into the cannula, but this does little to stop thrombosis on the arterial or venous wall or on the outside of the cannula. This requires the systemic administration of anticoagulants and/or antiplatelet agents, which must be done with caution if there are additional potential sites of bleeding from other surgical procedures in individual patients. Despite long-term warfarin usage with good INR control thrombosis still limits long-term intravenous cannula usage.

CONCLUSION

Biocompatibility of materials used in clinical medicine has changed dramatically over the last 20 years, so that there is much less interaction between blood components and materials. The optimal implant should be nonthrombogenic, nontoxic, and should not interact with blood in the short or long term. No material so far devised achieves all of these conditions. It is therefore necessary to use a variety of pharmacologic agents to reduce the tendency to coagulation and complement, platelet, and white cell activation. Antithrombotic measures have significantly enhanced the long-term survival of indwelling devices. However, our future research into blood compatibility for clinical applications should involve a continued search for a more compatible surface to prevent these interactions and also better use of existing antithrombotics and a search for new and more effective antithrombotic agents.

REFERENCES

1. Szycher M (ed). *Biocompatible Polymers, Metals, and Composites.* Lancaster, PA: Technomic, 1983.
2. Sharma CP, Szycher M (eds). *Blood Compatible Materials and Devices.* Lancaster, PA: Technomic, 1991.
3. Forbes CD, Courtney JM. Thrombosis and artificial surfaces. In: Bloom AL, Forbes CD, Thomas DP, Tuddenham EGD (eds). *Haemostasis and Thrombosis, 3rd ed,* vol 2. Edinburgh: Churchill Livingstone, 1994; 1301–1324.
4. Courtney JM, Lamba NMK, Sundaram S, Forbes CD. Biomaterials for blood-contacting applications. *Biomaterials* 1994;15:737–744.
5. Syzycher M. Thrombosis, hemostasis, and thrombolysis at prosthetic interfaces. In: Szycher M (ed). *Biocompatible Polymers, Metals, and Composites.* Lancaster, PA: Technomic, 1983;1–33.
6. Brash JL. Role of plasma protein adsorption in the response of blood to foreign surfaces. In: Sharma CP, Szycher M (eds). *Blood Compatible Materials and Devices.* Lancaster, PA: Technomic, 1991;3–24.
7. Murabayashi S, Nosé Y. Biocompatibility: bioengineering aspects. *Artif Organs* 1986;10:114–121.
8. Baier RE. The organization of blood components near interfaces. *Ann NY Acad Sci* 1977;283:17–36.
9. Brash JL. Protein adsorption and blood interactions. In: Szycher M (ed). *Biocompatible Polymers, Metals, and Composites.* Lancaster, PA: Technomic, 1983: 35–52.
10. Klinkmann H. The role of biomaterials in the application of artificial organs. In: Paul JP, Gaylor JDS, Courtney JM, Gilchrist T (eds). *Biomaterials in Artificial Organs.* London: Macmillan, 1984;1–8.
11. Bagnall RD. Adsorption of plasma proteins on hydrophobic surfaces. II. Fibrinogen and fibrinogen-containing protein mixtures. *J Biomed Mater Res* 1978; 12:203–217.
12. Chan BMC, Brash JL. Adsorption of fibrinogen on glass: reversibility aspects. *J Colloid Interf Sci* 1981; 82:217–225.
13. Horbett TA. Mass action effects on the adsorption of fibrinogen from hemoglobin solutions and from plasma. *Thromb Haemost* 1984;51:174–181.

14. Brash JL, Thibodeau JA. Identification of proteins adsorbed from human plasma to glass bead columns: plasmin-induced degradation of adsorbed fibrinogen. *J Biomed Mater Res* 1986;20:1263–1275.

15. Seifert LM, Greer RT. Evaluation of in vivo adsorption of blood onto hydrogel-coated silicone rubber by scanning electron microscopy and Fourier transform infrared spectroscopy. *J Biomed Mater Res* 1985;19: 1043–1071.

16. Horbett TA. The kinetics of baboon fibrinogen adsorption to polymers: in vitro and in vivo studies. *J Biomed Mater Res* 1986;20:739–772.

17. Courtney JM, Irvine L, Jones C, et al. Compatibility aspects of biomaterials in artificial organs and assist devices. In: Paul JP, Rappelsberger P, Schütz PW (eds). *The Influence of New Technologies on Medical Practice.* Vienna: Verlag für medizinische Wissenschaften Wilhelm Maudrich, 1991;154–162.

18. Vroman L. Protein/surface interaction. In: Szycher M (ed). *Biocompatible Polymers, Metals, and Composites.* Lancaster, PA: Technomic, 1983;81–88.

19. Griffin JG, Cochrane CG. Recent advances in the understanding of contact activation reactions. *Semin Thromb Hemost* 1979;5:254–273.

20. Matata BM, Courtney JM, Lowe GDO. Contact activation with haemodialysis membranes. *Int J Artif Organs* 1994;17:432.

21. Mahiout A, Matata BM, Vienken J, Courtney JM. Ex vivo complement protein adsorption on positively and negatively charged cellulose dialyser membranes. *J Mater Sci: Mater in Med* 1997;8:287–296.

22. Mason RG. The interaction of blood hemostatic elements with artificial surfaces. *Prog Hemost Thromb* 1972;1:141–164.

23. Mason RG, Mohammad SF, Chuang HYK, Richardson PD. The adhesion of platelets to subendothelium, collagen and artificial surfaces. *Semin Thromb Hemost* 1976;3:98–116.

24. Salzman EW, Lindon J, Brier D, Merrill EW. Surface-induced platelet adhesion, aggregation and release. *Ann N Y Acad Sci* 1977;283:114–127.

25. Baumgartner HR, Muggli R, Tschopp TB, Turitto VT. Platelet adhesion, release and aggregation in flowing blood: effects of surface properties and platelet function. *Thromb Haemost* 1976;35:124–138.

26. Feijen J. Thrombogenesis caused by blood-foreign surface interaction. In: Kenedi RM, Courtney JM, Gaylor JDS, Gilchrist T (eds). *Artificial Organs.* London: Macmillan, 1977;235–247.

27. Walsh PN. Platelet—coagulant protein interactions. In: Colman RW, Hirsh J, Marder VJ, Salzman EW (eds). *Hemostasis and Thrombosis: Basic Principles and Clinical Practice.* Philadelphia: Lippincott, 1982; 404–420.

28. Needleman SW, Hook JC. Platelets and leukocytes. In: Colman RW, Hirsh J, Marder VJ, Salzman EW (eds). *Hemostasis and Thrombosis: Basic Principles and Clinical Practice.* Philadelphia: Lippincott, 1982;716–725.

29. Waugh DF, Baughman DJ. Thrombin adsorption and possible relations to thrombus formation. *J Biomed Mater Res* 1969;3:145–164.

30. Chuang HYK, Crowther PE, Mohammad SF, Mason RG. Interactions of thrombin and antithrombin III with artificial surfaces. *Thromb Res* 1979;14:273–282.

31. Patrono C, Ciabattoni G, Pinca E, et al. Low dose aspirin and inhibition of thromboxane B_2 production in healthy subjects. *Thromb Res* 1980;17:317–327.

32. Phillips DR, Jennings LK, Prasanna HR. Ca^2-mediated association of glycoprotein G (thrombin-sensitive protein, thrombospondin) with human blood. *J Biol Chem* 1980;255:11629–11632.

33. Shuman MA, Levine SP. Relationship between secretion of platelet factor 4 and thrombin generation during in vitro blood clotting. *J Clin Invest* 1980;65: 307–313.

34. Feuerstein IA, Brophy JM, Brash JL. Platelet transport and adhesion to reconstituted collagen and artificial surfaces. *Trans Am Soc Artif Intern Organs* 1975;21: 427–434.

35. Richardson PD, Mohammad SF, Mason RG. Flow chamber studies of platelet adhesion at controlled, spatially varied shear rates. *Proc Europ Soc Artif Organs* 1977;4:175–188.

36. Rieger H. Dependency of platelet aggregation (PA) in vitro on different shear rates. *Thromb Haemost* 1980; 44:166.

37. Henson PM, Ginsberg MH. Immunological reactions of platelets. In: Gordon JL (ed). *Platelets in Biology and Pathology.* Amsterdam: Elsevier, 1981;265–308.

38. Matata BM, Wark S, Sundaram S, et al. In vitro contact phase activation with haemodialysis membranes: role of pharmaceutical agents. *Biomaterials* 1995;16: 1305–1312.

39. Matata BM, Courtney JM, Sundaram S, et al. Determination of contact phase activation by the measurement of the activity of supernatant and membrane surface—adsorbed factor XII (FXII): its relevance as a useful parameter for the in vitro assessment of haemodialysis membranes. *J Biomed Mater Res* 1996; 31:63–70.

40. Kurz H, Lerner RG, Weseley S, Nelson JC. Changes in fibrinolytic activity during the course of a single hemodialysis session. *Clin Nephrol* 1985;24:1–4.

41. Paramo JA, Rifon J, Llorend R, Casures J, Paloma AJ, Rocha E. Intra and postoperative fibrinolysis in patients undergoing cardiopulmonary bypass surgery. *Haemostasis* 1991;21:58–64.

42. Herzlinger GA. Activation of complement by polymers in contact with blood. In: Szycher M (ed). *Biocompatible Polymers, Metals, and Composites.* Lancaster, PA: Technomic, 1983;89–101.

43. Chenoweth DE. Complement activation produced by biomaterials. *Trans Am Soc Artif Intern Organs* 1986; 32:226–232.

44. Kazatchkine MD, Carreno MP. Activation of the complement system at the interface between blood and artificial surfaces. *Biomaterials* 1987;9:30–35.

45. Nusbacher J, Rosenfeld SJ, MacPherson JL, Thiem PA, Leddy JP. Nylon fiber leukapheresis: associated complement component changes and granulocytopenia. *Blood* 1978;51:359–365.

46. Jones HM, Mathews N, Vaughan RS, Stark JM. Cardiopulmonary bypass and complement activation. Involvement of classical and alternative pathways. *Anaesthesia* 1982;37:629–633.

47. Herzlinger GA, Cumming RD. Role of complement activation in cell adhesion to polymer blood contact surfaces. *Trans Am Soc Artif Intern Organs* 1980;26: 165–170.

48. Stormorken H. Platelets, thrombosis and hemolysis. *Fed Proc* 1971;1551–1555.

49. Brash JL, Uniyal S. Adsorption of albumin and fibrinogen to polyethylene in presence of red cells. *Trans Am Soc Artif Intern Organs* 1976;22:253–259.

50. Uniyal S, Brash JL, Degterev IA. Influence of red blood cells and their components on protein adsorption. *Am Chem Soc Adv Chem* 1982;199:277–292.

51. Horbett TA, Weathersby PK, Hoffman AS. The preferential adsorption of hemoglobin to polyethylene. *J Bioeng* 1977;1:61–77.

52. Bruck SD. *Properties of Biomaterials in the Physiological Environment.* Boca Raton: CRC Press, 1980.

53. Kusserow B, Larrow R, Nichols J. Perfusion- and surface-induced injury in leucocytes. *Fed Proc* 1971;30:1516–1520.

54. Lederman DM, Cumming RD, Petschek HE, Levine PH, Krinsky NI. The effect of temperature on the interaction of platelets and leukocytes with materials exposed to flowing blood. *Trans Am Soc Artif Intern Organs* 1978;24:557–560.

55. Absolom DR, Neumann AW, Zingg W, van Oss CJ. Thermodynamic studies of cellular adhesion. *Trans Am Soc Artif Intern Organs* 1979;25:152–156.

56. Wright DG, Kauffman JC, Terpstra GK, Graw RG, Deisseroth AB, Gallin JJ. Mobilization and exocytosis of specific (secondary) granules by human neutrophils during adherence to nylon wool infiltration leukapheresis (FL). *Blood* 1978;52:770–782.

57. Altieri CD, Edgington TS. Sequential receptor cascade for coagulation proteins on monocytes. *J Biol Chem* 1989;264:2969–2972.

58. Dewitz TS, Hung TC, Martin RR, McIntire LV. Mechanical trauma in leukocytes. *J Lab Clin Med* 1977;90:728–736.

59. Dewitz TS, Martin RR, Solis RT, Hellums HD, McIntire LV. Microaggregate formation in whole blood exposed to shear stress. *Microvasc Res* 1978;16: 263–271.

60. Cumming RD. Important factors affecting initial blood-material interactions. *Trans Am Soc Artif Intern Organs* 1980;26:304–308.

61. Niemitz J. Coagulant activity of leukocytes. Tissue factor activity. *J Clin Invest* 1971;51:307–313.

62. Saba H J, Herion JC, Walker RI, Roberts HR. The procoagulant activity of granulocytes. *Proc Soc Exp Biol Med* 1973;142:614–620.

63. Harrison MJ, Emmons PR, Mitchell JR. The effect of white cells on platelet aggregation. *Thromb Diathes Haemorrh* 1966;16:105–121.

64. Bourne HR. Immunology. In: Ramwell PW (ed). *The Prostaglandins,* vol 2. New York: Plenum, 1974; 277–291.

65. Ringoir S, Vanholder R. An introduction to biocompatibility. *Artif Organs* 1986;10:20–27.

66. Tetta C, Segoloni G, Carnussi G, et al. In vitro complement-independent activation of neutrophils by haemodialysis membranes. *Int J Artif Organs* 1987; 12:502–504.

67. Courtney JM, Lamba NMK, Gaylor JDS, Ryan CJ, Lowe GDO. Blood-contacting biomaterials: bioengineering viewpoints. *Artif Organs* 1995;19:852–856.

68. Courtney JM, Travers M, Douglas JT, et al. Blood-membrane interations: in vitro evaluation of the influence of membrane structure and antithrombotic agents. In: Barbenel JC, Gaylor JDS, Angerson WJ, Sheldon CD (eds). *Blood Flow in Artificial Organs and Cardiovascular Prostheses.* Oxford: Clarendon, 1989;104–112.

69. Robertson LM, Courtney JM, Irvine L, Jones C, Lowe GDO. Modification of the blood compatibility of hemodialysis membranes. *Artif Organs* 1990;14(suppl 2):41–43.

70. Engbers GH, Feijen J. Current techniques to improve the blood compatibility of biomaterial surfaces. *Int J Artif Organs* 1991;14:199–215.

71. Courtney JM, Yu J, Sundaram S. Immobilisation of macromolecules for obtaining biocompatible surfaces. In: Sleytr UB, Messner P, Pum D, Sàra M (eds). *Immobilised Macromolecules: Application Potentials.* London: Springer, 1993;175–193.

72. Baker LD Jr, Johnson JM, Goldfarb D. Expanded polytetrafluoroethylene (PTFE) subcutaneous arteriovenous conduit: an improved vascular access for chronic hemodialysis. *Trans Am Soc Artif Intern Organs* 1976;22:382–385.

73. Szycher M, Poirier V, Bernhard WF, Franzblau C, Haudenschild CC, Toselli P. Integrally textured polymeric surfaces for permanently implantable cardiac assist devices. *Trans Am Soc Artif Intern Organs* 1980;26: 493–498.

74. Snyder RW, Botzko KM. Woven, knitted and externally supported Dacron vascular prostheses. In: Stanley JC (ed). *Biologic and Synthetic Vascular Prostheses.* New York: Grune and Stratton, 1982;488–489.

75. Hood RG, Pollock JG, Guidoin R. The knitted structure and its interaction with tissue and blood. In: Paul JP, Gaylor JDS, Courtney JM, Gilchrist T (eds). *Biomaterials in Artificial Organs.* London: Macmillan, 1984;269–276.

76. Hoffman AS. Hydrogels—a broad class of biomaterials. In: Kronenthal RL, Oser Z, Martin E (eds). *Polymers in Medicine and Surgery.* New York: Plenum, 1975;33–44.

77. Ratner BD. Biomedical applications of hydrogels: review and critical appraisal. In: Williams DF (ed). *Biocompatibility of Clinical Implant Materials.* Boca Raton: CRC Press, 1981;145–175.

78. Payne MS, Horbett TA. Complement activation by hydroxyethylmethacrylate-ethylmethacrylate copolymers. *J Biomed Mater Res* 1987;21:843–859.

79. Yu J, Sundaram S, Weng D, Courtney JM, Moran CR, Graham NB. Blood interactions with novel polyurethaneurea hydrogels. *Biomaterials* 1991;12:119–120.

80. Courtney JM, Robertson LM, Jones C, et al. Blood compatibility of biomaterials in artificial organs. In: Paul JP, Barbenel JC, Courtney JM, Kenedi RM (eds). *Progress in Bioengineering.* Bristol: Adam Hilger, 1989;21–27.

81. Falb RD, Takahashi MT, Grode GA, Leininger RI. Studies on the stability and protein adsorption characteristics of heparinized polymer surfaces by radioisotope labelling techniques. *J Biomed Mater Res* 1967;1:239–251.

82. Larm O, Larsson R, Olsson P. Surface-immobilized heparin. In: Lane DA, Lindahe U (eds). *Heparin: Chemical and Biological Properties, Clinical Applications.* London: Edward Arnold, 1989;597–608.

83. Park KD, Okano T, Nojiri C, Kim SW. Heparin immobilization onto segmented polyurethaneurea surfaces: effect of hydrophilic spacers. *J Biomed Mater Res* 1988;22:977–992.

84. Grainger DW, Kim SW. Poly (dimethylsiloxane)–poly (ethylene oxide)–heparin block copolymers. 1. Synthe-

sis and characterisation. *J Biomed Mater Res* 1988; 22:231–249.

85. Vulic I, Okano T, Kim SW, Feijen J. Synthesis and characterization of polystyrene–poly (ethylene oxide)–heparin block copolymers. *J Polym Sci Polym Chem* 1988;26:381–391.

86. Hennink WE, Dost L, Feijen J, Kim SW. Interaction of albumin-heparin conjugate preadsorbed surfaces with blood. *Trans Am Soc Artif Intern Organs* 1983;29: 200–205.

87. Grode GA, Pitman J, Crowley JP, Leininger RI, Falb RD. Surface-immobilized prostaglandin as a platelet protective agent. *Trans Am Soc Artif Intern Organs* 1974;20:38–41.

88. Ebert CD, Lees ES, Kim SW. The antiplatelet activity of immobilized prostacyclin. *J Biomed Mater Res* 1982;16:629–638.

89. Marconi W, Bartoli F, Mantovani E, et al. Development of new antithrombogenic surfaces by employing platelet antiaggregating agents: preparation and characterization. *Trans Am Soc Artif Intern Organs* 1979;25: 280–285.

90. Bamford CH, Middleton I. Studies on functionalizing and grafting to poly (ether-urethanes). *Eur Polym J* 1983;19:1027–1035.

91. Kusserow BK, Larrow RW, Nichols JE. The surface bonded covalently crosslinked urokinase surface. In vitro and chronic in vivo studies. *Trans Am Soc Artif Intern Organs* 1973;19:8–12.

92. Ohshiro T, Kosaki G. Urokinase immobilized on medical polymer materials: fundamental and clinical studies. *Artif Organs* 1980;4:58–64.

93. Sugitachi A, Tanaka M, Kawahara T, Takagi K. Antithrombogenicity of UK-immobilized polymer surfaces. *Trans Am Soc Artif Intern Organs* 1980;26: 274–278.

94. Watanabe S, Shimuzu Y, Teramatsu T, Mirachi T, Hino T. The in vitro and in vivo behaviour of urokinase immobilized onto collagen-synthetic polymer composite material. *J Biomed Mater Res* 1981;15:553–563.

95. Aoshima R, Kand Y, Takada A, Yamashita A. Sulfonated poly (vinylidene fluoride) as a biomaterial: immobilization of urokinase and biocompatibility. *J Biomed Mater Res* 1982;16:289–299.

96. Senatore F, Bernard F, Meisner K. Clinical study of urokinase-bound fibrocollagenous tubes. *J Biomed Mater Res* 1986;20:177–188.

97. Lyman DJ, Knutson K, McNeill B, Shibatani K. The effects of chemical structure and surface properties of synthetic polymers on the coagulation of blood. IV. The relation between polymer morphology and protein adsorption. *Trans Am Soc Artif Intern Organs* 1975; 21:49–53.

98. Munro MS, Eberhart RC, Maki NJ, Brink BE, Fry WJ. Thromboresistant alkyl derivatized polyurethanes. *Am Soc Artif Intern Organs J* 1983;6:65–75.

99. Frautschi JR, Munro MS, Lloyd DR, Eberhart RC. Alkyl derivatized cellulose acetate membranes with enhanced albumin affinity. *Trans Am Soc Artif Intern Organs* 1983;29:242–244.

100. Nosé Y, Tajima K, Imai Y, et al. Artificial heart constructed with biological material. *Trans Am Soc Artif Intern Organs* 1971;17:482–487.

101. Kambic HE, Murabayashi S, Nosé Y. Biolized surfaces as chronic blood compatible interfaces. In: Szycher M (ed). *Biocompatible Polymers, Metals, and Composites.* Lancaster, PA: Technomic, 1983;179–198.

102. Chapman D, Charles CA. A coat of many lipids—in the clinic. *Chemistry in Britain* 1992;28:253–256.

103. Durrani AA, Chapman D. Modification of polymer surfaces biomedical applications. In: Feast WJ, Munro HS (eds). *Polymer Surfaces and Interfaces.* New York: Wiley, 1987;189–200.

104. Hall B, Bird R, Kojima M, Chapman D. Biomembranes as models for polymer surfaces. V. Thromboelastographic studies of polymeric lipids and polyesters. *Biomaterials* 1989;10:219–224.

105. Ishihara K, Ziats NP, Tierney BP, Nakabayashi N, Anderson JM. Protein adsorption from human plasma is reduced on phospholipid polymers. *J Biomed Mater Res* 1991;25:1397–1407.

106. Ishihara K, Takayama R, Nakabayashi N. Improvement of blood compatibility on cellulose dialysis membranes. *Biomaterials* 1992;13:235–239.

107. Bruck SD. On the evaluation of medical plastics in contact with blood. *Biomaterials* 1982;3:121–123.

108. Forbes CD, Courtney JM. Thrombosis on foreign surfaces. *Br Med Bull* 1994;50:966–981.

109. Bosch T, Schmidt B, Spencer PC, et al. Ex vivo biocompatibility evaluation of a new modified cellulose membrane. *Artif Organs* 1987;11:144–148.

110. Mahiout A, Meinhold H, Kessel M, Baurmeister U. Dialyzer membranes: effect of surface area and chemical modification of cellulose on complement and platelet activation. *Artif Organs* 1987;11: 149–154.

111. Gott VL, Furuse A. Antithrombogenic surfaces, classification and in vivo evaluation. *Fed Proc* 1971;30: 1679–1685.

112. Kusserow B, Larrow R, Nichols J. Observations concerning prosthesis-induced thromboembolic phenomena made with an in vivo embolus test system. *Trans Am Soc Artif Intern Organs* 1970;16:58–62.

113. Lindsay RM, Mason RG, Kim SW, Andrade JD, Hakim RM. Blood surface interactions. *Trans Am Soc Artif Intern Organs* 1980;26:603–610.

114. Klinkmann H, Falkenhagen D, Courtney JM. Clinical relevance of biocompatibility—the material cannot be divorced from the device. In: Gurland HJ (ed). *Uremia Therapy.* Berlin: Springer, 1987;125–138.

115. Courtney JM, Sundaram S, Forbes CD. Extracorporeal situations: biocompatibility of biomaterials. In: Forbes CD, Cushieri A (eds). *Management of Bleeding Disorders in Surgical Practice.* Oxford: Blackwell Scientific, 1993;236–276.

116. Henson PM. The adhesion of leukocytes and platelets induced by fixed IgG antibody or complement. *Immunology* 1969;16:107–121.

117. Grabowski EF, Didisheim P, Lewis JC, Franta JT, Stropp JQ. Platelet adhesion to foreign surfaces under controlled conditions of whole blood flow: human vs. rabbit, dog, calf, sheep, macaque, and baboon. *Trans Am Soc Artif Intern Organs* 1977;23:141–149.

118. Inoue T, Sakai Y, Fugimota T, et al. Expression of activation dependent platelet membrane protein after coronary stenting. A comparison with balloon angioplasty. *Circulation* 1996;94(suppl 1):Abstract 1523.

119. Jordan C, Carvalho H, Fagadet J, et al. Reduction of subacute thrombosis rate after coronary stenting using a new anticoagulant protocol. *Circulation* 1994;90 (suppl 1);5–125.

120. Brunnel P, Jordan C, Fagadet J, Cassagneau D, Marco J. Successive steps in the management of coronary stenting. *Circulation* 1995;92(suppl 1):1–87.

121. Moore RS, Chauhan E. Antiplatelet rather than anticoagulant therapy with coronary stenting. *Lancet* 1997; 349:146–147.

122. Oz MC, Rose EA, Levin HR. Selection criteria for placement of left ventricular assist devices. *Am Heart J* 1995;129:173–177.

123. Reemtsma K, Krusin R, Edie R, Bregman D, Dobell EW, Hardy M. Cardiac transplantation for patients requiring mechanical circulatory support. *N Engl J Med* 1978;298:670–676.

124. McCarthy PM. Heart made implantable left ventricular assist device: bridge to transplantation and future applications. *Ann Thorac Surg* 1995;59:S46–51.

125. Smith WM. Epidemiology of congestive heart failure. *Am J Cardiol* 1985;55:3.

126. Westaby S. The need for artificial hearts. *Heart* 1996; 76:200–206.

127. Basile C, Drucke T. Dialysis membrane biocompatibility. *Nephron* 1989;52:113–118.

128. Courtney JM, Sundaran S, Lamba NMK, et al. Monitoring of the blood response in blood purification. *Artif Organs* 31993;17:260–266.

129. Courtney JM, Sundaran S, Forbes CD. Biocompatibility-haematological aspects. *EDTA-ERCA J* 1993; 19(suppl 1) 29–34.

130. Bambauer R, Rucker S, Weber U, et al. Comparison of low molecular weight heparin and standard heparin in haemodialysis. *Trans Am Soc Artif Intern Organs* 1990;36:646–649.

131. Jamieson WRE. Modern cardiac valve devices—bioprostheses and mechanic prostheses: state of the art. *J Card Surg* 1993;8:89–98.

132. Chesebro JH, Fuster V, Elveback LR. Trial of combined warfarin plus dipyridamole or aspirin therapy is prosthetic heart valve replacement: danger of aspirin compared with dipyridamole. *Am Heart J Cardiol* 1983;51:1537–1541.

133. Turpie AGG, Gent M, Laupacis A, et al. A comparison of aspirin with placebo in patients treated with warfarin after heart valve replacement. *N Engl J Med* 1993;329:524–529.

134. Saour JN, Sieck JO, Mamo LAR, et al. Trial of different intensities of anticoagulation in patients with prosthetic heart valves. *N Engl J Med* 1990;322:428–432.

135. Cannogieter SC, Rosendaal FR, Wintzen AR, et al. Optimal oral anticoagulant therapy in patients with mechanical heart valves. *N Engl J Med* 1995;333: 11–17.

136. Courtney JM, Sundaram S, Matada BM, Gaylor GDS, Forbes CD. Biomaterials in cardiopulmonary bypass. *Perfusion* 1994;9: 3–10.

137. Courtney JM, Matada BM, Yin HY, et al. The influence of biomaterials on inflammatory responses to cardiopulmonary bypass. *Perfusion* 1996;11:220–228.

Cardiovascular Thrombosis: Thrombocardiology and Thromboneurology, Second Edition,
edited by M. Verstraete, V. Fuster, and E. J. Topol,
Lippincott–Raven Publishers, Philadelphia © 1998.

50

Hemorrhagic Complications of Long-Term Antithrombotic Treatment

Gary E. Raskob and *C. Seth Landefeld

*Departments of Biostatistics, Epidemiology, and Medicine, University of Oklahoma Health Sciences Center, Oklahoma City, Oklahoma 73190; and *Division of Geriatrics, Veterans Administration Medical Center, San Francisco, California 94121*

Bleeding is the most common complication of long-term antithrombotic treatment. The incidence of bleeding during long-term anticoagulant treatment and the risk factors predisposing to bleeding have been extensively reviewed recently by a committee of the American College of Chest Physicians (ACCP) Consensus Conference on Antithrombotic Therapy (1).

This chapter will review the incidence and risk factors for bleeding during long-term antithrombotic treatment with oral anticoagulants, aspirin, or combined therapy with these agents. The emphasis will be on new information published since the ACCP Consensus Conference findings were reported in late 1995 (1). The conclusions and recommendations in this chapter are linked to the strength of the evidence from clinical trials. In defining the incidence of bleeding and identifying risk factors, conclusions are based on data from either prospective cohort studies or randomized clinical trials. Conclusions about the

influence of intensity of anticoagulant treatment, and about the relative risks of bleeding for different regimens of antithrombotic treatment, are based on randomized clinical trials that evaluated sufficient patients to make valid conclusions (level I evidence).

The severity of bleeding during long-term antithrombotic treatment may range from minimal bleeding (e.g., minimal epistaxis) to fatal hemorrhage. To document the severity of bleeding, investigators in clinical trials have usually categorized bleeding as major or minor. However, the definitions of major and minor bleeding have not been consistent across clinical trials (1). This has led to significant variation in the reported incidences of major and minor bleeding. For this chapter, we have used the definition used by the ACCP Consensus Conference. Bleeding was classified as major if it was intracranial or retroperitoneal, if it led directly to death, or if it resulted in hospitalization or transfusion (1). All other bleeding episodes were classified as minor. A key recommendation of the ACCP committee was to standardize the criteria for defining the severity of bleeding in clinical trials.

Although the focus of this chapter is on bleeding, the risk of bleeding should not be considered in isolation, and clinicians must balance the benefit of treatment (decrease in thromboembolism) against the risk of bleeding.

BLEEDING DURING LONG-TERM ORAL ANTICOAGULANT THERAPY

The key factors that influence the risk of bleeding during long-term oral anticoagulant treatment are (a) the intensity of the anticoagulant effect (1–5) and (b) the indication for treatment and other patient characteristics (e.g., comorbid conditions) (1,6–8). The cumulative risk of bleeding increases with increasing duration of treatment (6,9), but this increase in risk over time may be most rapid early in the course of therapy when the monthly risk of anticoagulant-related bleeding is likely highest.

The intensity of anticoagulant effect is a major determinant of the risk of bleeding (2–5). This has been established by level I randomized trials in patients with deep vein thrombosis (2), bioprosthetic heart valves (3), and mechanical heart valves (4,5). The clinical trial data also strongly suggest that the intensity of anticoagulant effect is a key determinant of the incidence of bleeding, including intracranial bleeding, in patients with atrial fibrillation (9,10).

The indication for oral anticoagulant treatment influences the risk of bleeding in two ways. First, the indication determines the intensity of anticoagulant treatment. For example, patients with mechanical prosthetic heart valves are treated with a higher intensity of anticoagulant effect than patients with atrial fibrillation. Second, patient characteristics that predispose to bleeding vary among the different patient groups for which oral anticoagulant treatment is indicated. Patients with established cerebrovascular disease are at high risk of fatal bleeding, usually due to intracranial he-

morrhage (1). This appears to be the case even at less intense levels of anticoagulant intensity, such as an International Normalized Ratio (INR) of 2.0 to 3.0. The high risk for intracranial bleeding in patients with cerebrovascular disease may be due to the vascular disease per se and is contributed to by hypertension. Patients with venous thromboembolism commonly have underlying conditions that may predispose them to major bleeding (e.g., recent surgery, peptic ulcer disease, etc.).

Recent large prospective studies have provided new data on the incidence of bleeding complications during long-term oral anticoagulant treatment and the factors that contribute to an increased risk of bleeding. Palareti and colleagues performed a prospective cohort study of 2,745 consecutive patients who were followed from the start of their oral anticoagulant treatment among 34 anticoagulation clinics in Italy (6). The indications for treatment among these patients were venous thromboembolism in 32%, non-ischemic heart disease (including atrial fibrillation) in 24%, ischemic heart disease in 15%, cerebral or peripheral vascular disease in 10%, artificial heart valve in 11%, and miscellaneous conditions in the remaining 8%. The target anticoagulant intensities were an INR of 2.0 to 3.0 for patients with venous thromboembolism, atrial fibrillation, cardiomyopathy, or bioprosthetic heart valve, and 2.5 to 4.5 for patients with ischemic heart disease, cerebral or peripheral vascular disease, and mechanical heart valves. The overall rate of bleeding among this cohort of patients with a mean follow-up of 267 days was 5.6% (153 bleeding complications); major bleeding occurred in 23 patients (0.8%), minor bleeding in 125 patients (4.5%), and fatal bleeding in 5 patients (0.2%, all cerebral hemorrhages). The annualized rates of bleeding based on 2,011 patient-years of follow-up were 7.6% per year for total bleeding, 1.1% for major bleeding, 6.2% for minor bleeding, and 0.25% for fatal bleeding (6).

This study also documented two important findings on factors that contribute to bleeding. The rate of bleeding was higher in older patients: 10.5% per year for those age 70 or more, compared to 6.0% for those under 70 (p < 0.001, relative risk 1.75, 95% confidence interval 1.3 to 2.4) (6). The risk of bleeding was higher during the first 90 days of treatment compared with later (11.0% versus 6.3%, p < 0.001, relative risk 1.75, 95% confidence interval 1.3 to 2.4). The bleeding rate was also higher for the indications of cerebrovascular or peripheral arterial disease than for the indication of venous thromboembolism or other indications (12.5% per year compared with 6.0% per year, p < 0.01, relative risk 1.8, 95% confidence interval 1.2 to 2.7) (6). This finding is probably explained by the higher intensity of anticoagulant effect (INR 2.5 to 4.5) used for patients with the former indications than in those with venous thromboembolism or other indications (INR 2.0 to 3.0). This is supported by the finding in this study of a gradient of bleeding risk associated with increasing anticoagulant intensity. The annual rates of bleeding were 4.8%, 9.5%, and 40.5% associated with INR ranges of 2.0 to 2.9, 3.0 to 4.4, and 4.5 to 6.9, respectively. These findings are consistent with the observation from randomized trials that the risk of bleeding is increased by higher intensities of anticoagulant effect (2–5).

Fihn and colleagues have evaluated the relation of age to the risk of bleeding during warfarin treatment in a combined prospective and retrospective cohort of patients (7). The 2,376 patients analyzed were identified from six anticoagulation clinics in the United States. These patients were receiving warfarin for a variety of indications: venous thromboembolism in 27%, atrial fibrillation in 17%, valvular heart disease in 17%, cerebrovascular disease in 10%, other systemic embolism in 7%, and miscellaneous reasons in 22%. After adjustment for the intensity of anticoagulant effect using Cox regression methods, age was not generally associated with the occurrence of bleeding. The exception, however, was life-threatening and fatal bleeding complications among patients 80 years of age or older (relative risk 4.6, 95% confidence interval 1.2 to 18.1). Overall, the intensity of anticoagulant

effect was a much stronger predictor of bleeding risk than age (7).

The independent contribution of age to the risk of bleeding during long-term oral anticoagulant treatment has been controversial, with several studies either reporting a positive association or lack of an association (1). The reasons for these conflicting results include different patient populations, differences in study design, and the difficulty of separating the confounding effect of anticoagulant intensity from the contribution of age itself. Based on the current data, when oral anticoagulant treatment is indicated, this therapy should not be withheld on the basis of age alone. The elderly are often at high risk for thromboembolism, such as those over age 75 who have atrial fibrillation (10). In patients who have an indication for oral anticoagulant treatment, the clinician must determine whether the expected benefit of decreased risk of thromboembolism exceeds the risk of bleeding. The patient's age should not be considered in isolation as a reason to withhold anticoagulant treatment.

White and colleagues reported a combined prospective and retrospective study that evaluated the incidence of life-threatening bleeding during warfarin treatment, the site of bleeding, risk factors for life-threatening bleeding, and the risk of subsequent bleeding among patients who continued to receive treatment (8). The study was performed in five anticoagulation clinics and included 1,999 patients followed-up for a total of 3,865 patient-years. Life-threatening bleeding was defined as bleeding that led to cardiopulmonary arrest, a surgical or angiographic intervention, irreversible sequelae, or any two of either transfusion of three or more units, hypotension (systolic blood pressure <90 mm Hg), or hematocrit ≤0.20 (8). There were 4 patients who had fatal bleeding among the 1,999 patients. The incidence of life-threatening bleeding was 0.8% per year (95% confidence interval 0.54% to 1.12%). The gastrointestinal tract was the site of bleeding in two-thirds of the patients with life-threatening bleeding, and approximately one-half of the patients had a history of peptic ulcer disease

TABLE 50-1. *Ranges in reported incidences of bleeding from clinical trials of long-term oral anticoagulant treatment*

Indication	Target INR	Time frame	Bleeding (%)		
			Total	Major	Fatal
Venous thromboembolism	2.0 to 3.0	3 to 6 months (2,14,15–17)	4%–5%	2%–5%	0–0.9%
	3.0 to 4.5	3 months (1,2,12,13)	17%–37%	4%–17%	0
	2.0 to 3.0	4 years (16)	Not reported	9%	2%
Atrial fibrillation	2.0 to 3.0	Annualized rate (1,9,10,18,19)	1.3%–14%	1.7%–2.1%	0.2%–0.8%
Mechanical heart valves	3.0 to 4.5	Annualized rate (1,4,5,24,25)	1.6%–10.4%	0.8%–6.6%	0–2.3
Bioprosthetic heart valves	3.0 to 4.5	3 months (3)	14%	5%	0
	2.0 to 3.0	3 months (3)	6%	0	0

or gastrointestinal bleeding. Among 25 patients in whom warfarin treatment was restarted or continued, 8 had an additional life-threatening bleeding event after a median of 11.5 months. The findings indicate that when life-threatening bleeding occurs, the gastrointestinal tract is a common site, and most patients who experience life-threatening bleeding have multiple risk factors for bleeding. The data also suggest that patients who have life-threatening bleeding are at high risk for a recurrence of this outcome during continued oral anticoagulant treatment.

Hart and colleagues have reviewed the risk factors and prognosis of patients with intracranial hemorrhage during oral anticoagulant treatment (11). Most (70%) anticoagulant related intracranial hemorrhages are intracerebral hematomas and approximately 60% of these events are fatal. Most of the remaining intracranial bleeding events are subdural hematomas. Risk factors for intracerebral hematoma include advanced age, prior ischemic stroke, hypertension, and the intensity of anticoagulant effect. In approximately 50% of the patients with intracerebral hematoma, the bleeding evolves slowly over 12 to 24 hours, and emergency reversal of the anticoagulant effect may be key in patient management.

INCIDENCE OF BLEEDING FOR DIFFERENT CLINICAL INDICATIONS

The reported incidences of bleeding for the different clinical indications for oral anticoag-

ulant treatment are summarized in Table 50-1. The range of incidences are provided for the rates of all bleeding, major bleeding, and fatal bleeding, according to the target INR ranges.

Venous Thromboembolism

The intensity of anticoagulant effect is the key factor which determines the risk of bleeding during oral anticoagulant treatment in patients with venous thromboembolism (2). The risk of bleeding can be markedly reduced (from >20% to <5%), without loss of effectiveness for preventing recurrent venous thromboembolism, by dose titration to maintain the anticoagulant effect within the INR range of 2.0 to 3.0 (2), compared to the more intense range of an INR of 3.0 to 4.5 (2,12,13). The incidence of bleeding during oral anticoagulant treatment for 3 to 6 months, using a target INR of 2.0 to 3.0, is 4% to 5%, and the incidence of major bleeding ranges from 2% to 5% (2,14–16). Most patients who have major bleeding during oral anticoagulant treatment have underlying predisposing factors or lesions, such as peptic ulcer disease, unsuspected carcinoma, and so forth (1,2,14–17).

A recent randomized trial (16) provides important new information on the risk of bleeding during extended treatment with oral anticoagulants in patients with venous thromboembolism. Schulman et al. reported a multicenter randomized open-label trial evaluating oral anticoagulant therapy given for either

6 months or continued indefinitely in patients with a second episode of venous thromboembolism (16). A total of 227 patients were enrolled; 111 were allocated to 6 months of treatment and 116 patients to receive indefinite treatment. The target INR was 2.0 to 2.85. The duration of follow-up was 4 years. The endpoints were recurrent venous thromboembolism, major bleeding, and death.

The rates of major bleeding were 2.7% (3 of 111 patients) in the 6-month group and 8.6% (10 of 116 patients) in the indefinite group (p = 0.084). Two of the major bleeding events in the indefinite treatment group were fatal (a fatal subarachnoid hemorrhage and a patient with fatal hemorrhagic pancreatitis). None of the major bleeding events in the 6-month group were fatal. Recurrent venous thromboembolism occurred in 20.7% of patients in the 6-month group (23 of 111 patients) as compared with 2.6% (3 of 116 patients) in the indefinite treatment group (p < 0.001). None of the recurrent venous thromboembolic events were fatal. There was a total of 16 deaths in the 6-month group (14.4%) compared with 10 in the indefinite duration group (8.6%) (p = 0.21; relative risk of death with 6 months of treatment 1.7, 95% confidence interval 0.8% to 3.5%) (16).

The results of this study suggest that extending the duration of warfarin treatment is effective for reducing recurrent venous thromboembolism, but at a cost of increased major bleeding. The risk-to-benefit ratio of extended warfarin treatment remains incompletely resolved in this context. Although there were fewer thromboembolic events with indefinite treatment, these were not fatal events, whereas there were two fatal bleeding events in the indefinite treatment group. Although there were overall fewer deaths in the indefinite treatment group, this did not achieve statistical significance and the relative risk has a wide 95% confidence interval that crosses 1.0 (16). Unfortunately, this study does not provide a definitive conclusion with respect to total mortality.

Further clinical trials are required to more precisely define the risk-to-benefit ratio of extended or indefinite treatment in patients with venous thromboembolism and to assess the risk-to-benefit ratio in key subgroups of patients (such as those with idiopathic recurrent venous thrombosis versus thrombosis occurring postoperatively, and patients with genetic predisposition to recurrence such as the factor V Leiden gene mutation).

Atrial Fibrillation

There have been seven randomized trials evaluating long-term warfarin treatment in patients with atrial fibrillation (10,18). Among the trials in which the target intensity of treatment was an INR of 1.4 to 3.0, the annual rates of major bleeding ranged from 0.9% to 4.2% per year and fatal bleeding from 0 to 1.3% per year (10,18). In the Stroke Prevention in Atrial Fibrillation (SPAF) II trial, the rate of major bleeding (2.3% per year) exceeded that of the other trials (9). This may have been a chance finding or due to the higher upper limit of anticoagulant intensity targeted in the SPAF II study (upper INR limit 4.5), or due to differences in the patients, particularly the inclusion of more elderly patients (age >75 years), in whom the rate of major bleeding was 4.2% per year (9). In the SPAF II trial, the rate of major bleeding was 1.7% per year in patients 75 years or less, compared with 4.2% per year in patients older than 75 years (p < 0.05, relative risk 2.6). The corresponding rates for intracranial bleeding were 0.6% per year in patients 75 years of age or younger and 1.8% per year in older patients (p = 0.05). It is not possible based on the SPAF II data to definitively separate out the contribution of age from the effect of anticoagulant intensity. The high rate of intracranial bleeding in the elderly patients in the SPAF II trial was the key factor in offsetting the benefit of oral anticoagulant treatment in these patients. In an analysis (19) of the pooled data from 223 patients older than 75 years of age in the other trials of anticoagulant treatment in atrial fibrillation, most of which used a tighter and less intense anticoagulant range with an upper INR limit of 3.0, the rate of intracranial bleeding was 0.3% per year (95% confidence interval 0.04% to 2.1%). The overall data suggest that the more intense anticoagulant effect allowed in the SPAF II trial combined with an increasing proportion of elderly patients resulted in higher rates of major bleeding and intracranial hemorrhage.

The recently completed SPAF III trial provides further data on the risk of bleeding in patients with atrial fibrillation who receive oral anticoagulant treatment (18). All of the patients enrolled in this study were high risk for stroke based on the presence of at least one risk factor in addition to atrial fibrillation. The study compared adjusted dose warfarin targeted to an INR of 2.0 to 3.0, with a combined regimen of fixed dose warfarin (after initial titration to an INR of 1.2 to 1.5) and aspirin 325 mg per day. The study was discontinued early by the safety monitoring committee after a mean follow-up of 1.1 years due to an excess of thromboembolic stroke among patients receiving the combination therapy (7.9% per year) compared to those given adjusted dose warfarin (1.9% per year) (p <0.0001) (18). This represents an absolute reduction in stroke incidence of 6.0% per year (95% confidence interval 3.4% to 8.6%) using adjusted dose warfarin. The rates of major bleeding were similar and low in the two treatment groups. Major bleeding occurred at a rate of 2.1% per year in the adjusted warfarin group (12 of 523 patients) and 2.4% per year for the combination regimen (13 of 521 patients). Only 3 of the 523 patients (0.5% per year) given adjusted dose warfarin had intracranial bleeding. Of the 12 patients who had major bleeding during the one year of treatment with adjusted dose warfarin (INR 2.0 to 3.0), the INR was greater than 3.0 at the time of bleeding in 7 of these patients.

The SPAF III trial results have been very important in clarifying the role of adjusted dose warfarin in patients with atrial fibrillation. The aggregate data from the clinical trials indicate that when warfarin is adjusted to an INR of 2.0 to 3.0, the rate of major bleeding is about 2% per year, and the rate of intracranial hemorrhage is about 0.3% to 0.5%

per year (9,10,18). These risks are markedly outweighed by the benefit of adjusted warfarin based on an absolute reduction in stroke incidence of 6.0% per year compared with the use of no antithrombotic treatment or ineffective antithrombotic treatment (10,18). This includes a major benefit for preventing disabling stroke (absolute reduction of 3.9% per year). Thus, with warfarin treatment targeted to the appropriate intensity, the clinical trials indicate a major net benefit. It is important that this information is communicated effectively to the health care community and acted on because recent data document a significant underutilization of oral anticoagulant treatment in patients with atrial fibrillation (20–23). This underutilization is due at least in part to a fear of bleeding complications, particularly in the elderly (age >75 years) (20–23). The elderly (>75 years) are also at highest risk of stroke, and adjusted dose warfarin is the only proven effective treatment for preventing this devastating complication in these patients (10). The appropriate implementation of adjusted dose warfarin treatment in patients with atrial fibrillation can be expected to have a major impact on the disease burden of stroke in the community. The clinician must use prudent judgment in the individual patient about the risks and benefit of warfarin treatment. A fear of intracranial bleeding based on age alone should not be a reason for withholding warfarin treatment because the clinical trials indicate that when targeted to an appropriate intensity of anticoagulant effect, the benefit outweighs the risk of treatment. It is prudent to closely monitor warfarin treatment in the elderly and to maintain the INR below 3.0.

Prosthetic Heart Valves

The risk of bleeding in patients with artificial heart valves is considered separately for patients with bioprosthetic valves and for those with mechanical valves. Patients with bioprosthetic valves can be effectively treated using a less intense anticoagulant effect (INR

2.0 to 3.0) (3) than patients with mechanical valves (INR 3.0 to 4.5). Furthermore, in patients with bioprosthetic valves, treatment can be usually discontinued at 3 months if the patient is in sinus rhythm, whereas patients with mechanical valves require indefinite treatment. These differences in the management of patients with bioprosthetic and mechanical valves impact the risk of bleeding.

Turpie and colleagues have demonstrated in a level I randomized trial (3) that for patients with bioprosthetic valves the risk of bleeding can be reduced, without loss of effectiveness, by adjusting the warfarin dose to achieve an INR of 2.0 to 3.0, rather than the traditional more intense range of 3.0 to 4.5. The risk of bleeding during the 3 months of treatment was reduced from 14% (15 of 108 patients) to 6% (6 of 102 patients) (p = 0.043), and major bleeding was reduced from 5% to none (p = 0.034).

In patients with mechanical valves in whom oral anticoagulant treatment is targeted to an INR range of 3.0 to 4.5, the annual incidence of bleeding ranges from 1.6% to 10%, major bleeding from 0.9% to 6.6%, and fatal bleeding from 0 to 2.3% (1,24,25).

Turpie and colleagues performed a randomized double-blind trial to evaluate the effectiveness and safety of adding 100 mg of aspirin daily to warfarin treatment (target INR 3.0 to 4.5) (24). In the control group receiving warfarin only, the annual incidence of major bleeding was 6.6%. Further details of this trial are outlined under the heading "Combined Warfarin and Aspirin Therapy."

Cannegieter and colleagues followed a total of 1,608 patients treated at four anticoagulant clinics in the Netherlands (25). These patients were followed during a total of 6,475 patient-years. The target INR range for oral anticoagulant treatment was 3.6 to 4.8. Major bleeding (extracranial) occurred with an incidence of 2.1% per year, and intracranial bleeding occurred with an incidence of 0.57% per year. The incidence of fatal bleeding was 0.3% per year. The investigators also related the occurrence of events to the time spent at different levels of anticoagulant intensity as indicated

by INR ranges. The incidence of hemorrhagic stroke increased with increasing intensity of anticoagulant effect (25). The incidence of hemorrhagic stroke increased steeply to >4% per year at INR values of >5.0. The descriptive data of Cannegieter et al. (25) support the results from level I randomized trials that higher intensities of anticoagulant effect result in increased rates of bleeding. However, this descriptive study design (25) does not allow definitive conclusions about the optimal intensity of anticoagulant effect to maximize antithrombotic effectiveness while minimizing bleeding risk. This can only be determined by direct randomized comparisons of treatment targeted to different anticoagulant intensities.

Ischemic Heart Disease

The incidence of bleeding complications in patients with ischemic heart disease has been reported from several randomized trials evaluating oral anticoagulant treatment (1). The target INR range for these trials has varied, but more recent trials have targeted ranges of 2.8 to 4.8 (26,27). These large trials have provided more precise estimates of the risk of bleeding with long-term oral anticoagulant treatment.

In the WARIS trial, more than 600 patients treated with warfarin sodium were followed an average of 37 months (26). Bleeding occurred in 52 patients, and major bleeding occurred in 13 patients (2.1%). Intracranial bleeding occurred in 5 patients (0.8%) and fatal bleeding occurred in 3 patients (0.5%) (all were intracranial events). These risks were more than offset by a 24% risk reduction in all-cause mortality (26).

The ASPECT trial evaluated 1,700 patients treated with oral anticoagulation using nicoumalone or phenprocoumon (27,28). The target INR was 2.8 to 4.8 and the average follow-up was 37 months. Major bleeding occurred in 51 patients (4.3%), compared with 6 (1.1%) receiving placebo. Intracranial bleeding occurred in 14 patients, compared with 1 patient receiving placebo, and 7 patients given anticoagulation had fatal bleeding (0.6%). The annual rate of major bleeding in the anticoagulated group was 1.5% per year compared with 0.2% per year in placebo-treated patients (p < 0.05) (26). This risk was offset by a greater than 50% risk reduction in the incidence of myocardial reinfarction (from 14.2% to 6.7%) and a greater than 40% risk reduction in the incidence of stroke (from 3.6% to 2.1%) (p < 0.01 for both comparisons). After adjustment for anticoagulant intensity (INR), increased age (≥60), and higher levels of systolic blood pressure (>120 mm Hg) were associated with increased bleeding risk (relative risks of 1.5 and 2.0, respectively) (28).

The major issue to be resolved by clinical trials is to determine the relative roles of long-term oral anticoagulant treatment and aspirin, either alone or in combination, in patients with ischemic heart disease. This will require additional randomized trials comparing these approaches, alone and in combination, and at different intensities of anticoagulant effect, to optimize the benefit and minimize the risk of bleeding.

Cerebrovascular Disease

Patients with cerebrovascular disease are at high risk of major bleeding with oral anticoagulant treatment, which is usually manifested as intracranial bleeding (1). The risk of major bleeding (usually intracerebral) has been >7% in several studies, and fatal hemorrhage ranged from 2% to 7% (1). The studies that have evaluated long-term oral anticoagulant treatment in patients with cerebrovascular disease have utilized varying and wide target INR ranges. However, even when the INR was targeted to a range of 2.0 to 2.5, the incidence of fatal bleeding was high (7.0%, 5 of 71 patients, 95% confidence interval 2.3% to 15.7%) (1).

The available data indicate that patients with ischemic cerebrovascular disease are at high risk of major bleeding and fatal intracranial bleeding. The benefit of long-term anticoagulant treatment in patients with cerebrovascular disease is uncertain. Given the demonstrated effectiveness of aspirin,

ticlopidine, and, more recently, clopidogrel, long-term oral anticoagulant treatment is not indicated at the present time for most patients with cerebrovascular disease. Ongoing trials may clarify the role of less intense oral anticoagulant regimens, either alone or in combination with antiplatelet therapy, in patients with cerebrovascular disease.

The exception are patients who present with symptoms of cerebral ischemia and are also shown to have atrial fibrillation. In these patients, who are at very high risk for stroke and vascular death, oral anticoagulant treatment was much more effective than aspirin at decreasing the stroke and vascular events (29,30). Oral anticoagulant treatment reduced the annual incidence of all of strokes from 12% per year to 4% per year (p < 0.01, risk reduction 66%, 95% confidence interval 43% to 80%), whereas the incidence of stroke in patients treated with aspirin 325 mg per day was 10% per year (p = 0.31, risk reduction 14%, 95% confidence interval -15% to 34%). After adjustment for intensity of anticoagulant effect (INR), age (>75) was independently associated with increased risk of bleeding (relative risk 3.1, 95% confidence interval 1.5% to 6.4%) (30).

BLEEDING DURING LONG-TERM ASPIRIN TREATMENT

The risk of important bleeding is much less with aspirin treatment than with oral anticoagulant treatment at currently recommended therapeutic ranges. In patients with ischemic heart disease, the risk of bleeding with aspirin is more than offset by the major benefit in reducing mortality and reinfarction. The risk of bleeding with aspirin becomes a more important consideration in the setting of primary prevention of myocardial infarction, where the risk of thromboembolic events is lower than in patients receiving treatment for secondary prevention and the absolute reductions in the incidences of myocardial infarction are much lower (31,32).

The recently completed Coumadin Aspirin Reinfarction Study (CARS) provides new data on the incidence of bleeding in a large group of patients with myocardial infarction who received long-term aspirin treatment (33). The average follow-up was 1.2 years. Among the 3,393 patients treated with aspirin 160 mg per day, the incidence of spontaneous major bleeding was 0.7% at 1 year. In this double-blind trial, only 3.3% of patients had aspirin treatment interrupted for bleeding. Intracranial bleeding occurred in only one patient (0.03%).

The incidence of bleeding during aspirin treatment for primary prevention has been documented in two completed trials: the U.S. Physicians' Health Study (31) and the British Doctors Study (32). The incidence of hemorrhagic stroke in these studies was 0.42 and 0.69 per 1,000 patients per year, respectively. This represents an absolute increase in hemorrhagic stroke per 1,000 subjects per year of 0.22 for the Physicians' Health Study and 0.06 in the British Doctors Study, neither of which achieved statistical significance. In the U.S. Physicians' Health Study, the incidence of overall bleeding was 54.0 per 1,000 subjects per year, compared to 40.8 for patients receiving placebo (p < 0.0001). Bleeding requiring transfusion occurred in 0.81 per 1,000 subjects per year, compared with 0.5 for patients given placebo (p < 0.02) (31). This represents an absolute increase of 0.3 per 1,000 patients per year in the incidence of bleeding requiring transfusion. In contrast, the absolute reduction in the incidence of all myocardial infarction was 1.9 per 1,000 patients per year with aspirin treatment (from 4.40 to 2.55, p < 0.0001) (31).

BLEEDING DURING COMBINED WARFARIN AND ASPIRIN TREATMENT

The risk of bleeding during combined warfarin and aspirin treatment is considered in three settings: (a) the addition of aspirin to intensive oral anticoagulant treatment (INR 3.0 to 4.5) in patients with mechanical valves; (b) the combined use of fixed low doses of warfarin and aspirin in patients with coronary

heart disease or atrial fibrillation; and (c) primary prevention of ischemic heart disease events in high-risk patients. The data come from large level I randomized trials.

Turpie and colleagues evaluated the effectiveness and safety of adding 100 mg of aspirin per day to treatment with warfarin (INR 3.0 to 4.5) in patients with mechanical valves (24). This study was a randomized double-blind trial. The main outcome events evaluated were death, major systemic embolism, death from vascular causes, and bleeding. There were approximately 180 patients in each treatment group followed for an average of 2.5 years. The incidence of clinically important bleeding was increased from 22% per year with warfarin treatment alone to 35% per year in the combined warfarin and aspirin group (p = 0.02). This difference was accounted for primarily by minor bleeding events such as minor hematuria, epistaxis, and bruising. Major bleeding occurred at a rate of 6.6% per year in the warfarin-alone group and 8.5% per year in the group given combined warfarin and aspirin treatment. This represents a risk increase of 27% (95% confidence interval -30% to 132%), which was not statistically significant. This wide confidence interval does not allow a definitive conclusion about whether major bleeding is increased by the addition of aspirin to intense warfarin treatment. The bleeding risk was more than offset by the considerable benefit of adding aspirin to warfarin. The annual rate of death from all causes was reduced from 7.4% for warfarin alone to 2.8% with combined warfarin and aspirin (p = 0.01, a risk reduction of 63%, 95% confidence interval 19% to 83%). The incidence of major systemic embolism or death was reduced from 11.6% per year to 4.2% (p < 0.001, risk reduction 65%, 95% confidence interval 33% to 82%). Finally, for the composite outcome of major systemic embolism, nonfatal intracranial bleeding, death from bleeding, or death from vascular causes—an outcome that reflects both the potential benefits and harms of treatment—there was a net reduction in incidence of this outcome from 9.9% per year to 3.9% per year in favor of adding aspirin to warfarin (p = 0.005, risk reduction 61%, 95% confidence interval 24% to 80%). Thus, although the absolute rates of bleeding with combined warfarin and aspirin treatment are high, even when a low dose of aspirin is added to intense warfarin treatment, the major benefits in mortality and thromboembolic events more than offset this risk. Ongoing clinical trials in these patients are evaluating whether the risk of major bleeding can be reduced without loss of antithrombotic effectiveness, by reducing the intensity of warfarin treatment utilized in combination with aspirin.

Three recently completed randomized trials have evaluated the effectiveness and safety of fixed low doses of warfarin used in combination with aspirin in the setting of secondary prevention after myocardial infarction (33), prevention of stroke in atrial fibrillation (18), and antithrombotic treatment following coronary artery bypass grafting (34). These studies evaluated either fixed low doses of warfarin (such as 1 to 3 mg) or doses titrated to a minimal INR effect (1.2 to 1.5) in combination with aspirin treatment.

These studies have documented a low rate of major bleeding among patients treated with these combined regimens (18,33). In the CARS trial, the incidence of major bleeding at 1 year was 1.4% among 3,382 patients treated with warfarin 3 mg and aspirin 80 mg, compared to 0.7% among 3,039 patients who received aspirin alone (160 mg per day) (p = 0.014). Intracranial bleeding occurred in 5 patients (0.2%) who received combined warfarin and aspirin (3 mg and 80 mg, respectively), compared with 1 patient (0.03%) who received aspirin alone (p = 0.10).

In the SPAF III trial (18) in patients with atrial fibrillation, major bleeding during the 1-year follow-up occurred in 13 of 521 patients (2.4%) who received combined warfarin (INR 1.2 to 1.5) plus aspirin (325 mg), compared with 12 of 523 patients (2.1%) who received adjusted dose warfarin without aspirin (INR 2.0 to 3.0). The respective rates on intracranial bleeding were 5 patients (0.9%) and 3 patients (0.5%).

The data document low rates of major and intracranial bleeding among patients treated with low doses of warfarin combined with aspirin. Unfortunately, these combined regimens were either ineffective (in the case of atrial fibrillation) (18) or no more effective than aspirin alone in the setting of secondary prevention after myocardial infarction (33).

The key issue now is whether modest intensities of warfarin treatment (INR 1.5 to 3.0) combined with aspirin will provide antithrombotic benefit without increased bleeding risk.

Meade and colleagues have reported interim safety data from a large randomized trial of warfarin and aspirin in the primary prevention of ischemic heart disease in high-risk patients (35). Patients are randomized to low-dose warfarin (target INR 1.5), the same regimen combined with 75 mg of aspirin, aspirin alone, or placebo. The interim safety results in a total of 3,667 patients followed for 1.1 years have been reported. The incidences of major bleeding were 2 of 917 patients (0.2%) receiving low-dose warfarin, 2 of 911 patients (0.2%) receiving combined low-dose warfarin and aspirin, 2 of 907 patients receiving aspirin alone, and none of 932 patients receiving placebo. The currently unresolved issue is whether these low risks of major bleeding will be offset by benefit in the primary prevention of ischemic heart disease events.

CONCLUSION

Bleeding is the most common complication of long-term antithrombotic therapy. The incidence of bleeding varies according to several treatment and patient characteristics that determine the risk for bleeding in individual patients treated with antithrombotic agents. In patients treated with oral anticoagulants, the most important determinant of bleeding is the intensity of the anticoagulant effect, with rates of major bleeding generally <2% per year when the INR is <3.0. The risk of bleeding also probably varies over time during the course of treatment, with risk for bleeding highest during the first month of treatment. Several patient characteristics also increase risk for bleeding during antithrombotic therapy, including previous bleeding during antithrombotic therapy, serious comorbid illness, older age, and the indication for treatment, with the highest rates of bleeding observed in patients with cerebrovascular disease and venous thromboembolism. These risk factors for bleeding may be useful in discriminating among patients according to their relative risks for bleeding and the intensity with which therapy should be monitored. Nonetheless, for indications such as venous thromboembolism, prosthetic heart valves, and atrial fibrillation, the risk of bleeding is outweighed in most patients by the efficacy of anticoagulant therapy in preventing thromboembolism.

REFERENCES

1. Levine MN, Raskob G, Landefeld S, Hirsh J. Hemorrhagic complications of anticoagulant treatment. *Chest* 1995;108:(Oct suppl):276s–290s.
2. Hull R, Hirsh J, Jay R, et al. Different intensities of oral anticoagulant therapy in the treatment of proximal-vein thrombosis. *N Engl J Med* 1982;307:1676–1681.
3. Turpie ACG, Gunstensen J, Hirsh J, et al. Randomized comparison of two intensities of oral anticoagulant therapy after tissue heart valve replacement. *Lancet* 1988;1:1242–1245.
4. Saour JN, Sieck JO, Mamo LAR, et al. Trial of different intensities of anticoagulation in patients with prosthetic heart valves. *N Engl J Med* 1990;322:428–432.
5. Altman R. Rouvier J, Gurfinkel E. Comparison of two levels of anticoagulant therapy in patients with substitute heart valves. *J Thorac Cardiovasc Surg* 1991;101:427–431.
6. Palareti G, Leali N, Coccheri S, et al., on behalf of the Italian Study on Complications of Oral Anticoagulant Therapy. Bleeding complications of oral anticoagulant treatment: an inception-cohort, prospective collaborative study (ISCOAT). *Lancet* 1996;348:423–428.
7. Fihn SD, Callahan CM, Martin DC, McDonell MB, Henikoff JG, White RH for The National Consortium of Anticoagulation Clinics. The risk for and severity of bleeding complications in elderly patients treated with warfarin. *Ann Intern Med* 1996;124:970–979.
8. White RH, McKittrick T, Takakuwa J, Callahan C, McDonell M, Fihn S, and the National Consortium of Anticoagulation Clinics. Management and prognosis of life-threatening bleeding during warfarin therapy. *Arch Intern Med* 1996;156:1197–1201.
9. The Stroke Prevention in Atrial Fibrillation Investigators. Bleeding during antithrombotic therapy in patients with atrial fibrillation. *Arch Intern Med* 1996;156:409–416.
10. Laupacis A, Albers G, Dalen J, Dunn M, Feinberg W, Jacobson A. Antithrombotic therapy in atrial fibrillation. *Chest* 1995;108:(Oct suppl):352s–359s.
11. Hart RG, Boop BS, Anderson DC. Oral anticoagulants and intracranial hemorrhage. Facts and hypotheses. *Stroke* 1995;26:1471–1477.
12. Hull R, Delmore T, Genton E, et al. Warfarin sodium versus low-dose heparin in the long-term treatment of venous thrombosis. *N Engl J Med* 1979;301:855–858.
13. Hull R, Delmore T, Carter C, et al. Adjusted subcutaneous heparin versus warfarin sodium in the long-term treatment of venous thrombosis. *N Engl J Med* 1982;306:189–194.
14. Brandjes DPM, Heijboer H, Büller HR, de Rijk M, Jagt H, ten Cate JW. Acenocoumarol and heparin compared with acenocoumarol alone in the initial treatment of proximal-vein thrombosis. *N Engl J Med* 1992;327:1485–1489.
15. Schulman S, Rhedin AS, Lindmarker P, et al, and the Duration of Anticoagulation Trial Study Group. A comparison of six weeks with six months of oral anticoagulant therapy after a first episode of venous thromboembolism. *N Engl J Med* 1995;332:1661–1665.
16. Schulman S, Granqvist S, Holmström M, et al, and the Duration of Anticoagulation Trial Study Group. The duration of oral anticoagulant therapy after a second episode of venous thromboembolism. *N Engl J Med* 1997;336:393–398.
17. Levine MN, Hirsh J, Gent M, et al. Optimal duration of oral anticoagulant therapy: a randomized trial comparing four weeks with three months of warfarin in patients with proximal deep vein thrombosis. *Thromb Haemost* 1995;74:606–611.
18. Stroke Prevention in Atrial Fibrillation Investigators. Adjusted-dose warfarin versus low-intensity, fixed-dose warfarin plus aspirin for high-risk patients with atrial fibrillation: Stroke Prevention in Atrial Fibrillation III randomised clinical trial. *Lancet* 1996;348:633–638.
19. Connolly S for the Atrial Fibrillation Investigators. Stroke Prevention in Atrial Fibrillation II study. *Lancet* 1994;343:1509.
20. Stafford RS, Singer DE. National patterns of warfarin use in atrial fibrillation. *Arch Intern Med* 1996;156:2537–2541.
21. Whittle J, Wickenheiser L, Venditti LN. Is warfarin underused in the treatment of elderly persons with atrial fibrillation? *Arch Intern Med* 1997;157:441–445.
22. Antani MR, Beyth RJ, Covinsky KE, et al. Failure to prescribe warfarin to patients with nonrheumatic atrial fibrillation. *J Gen Intern Med* 1996;11:713–720.
23. Beyth RJ, Antani MR, Covinsky KE, et al. Why isn't warfarin prescribed to patients with nonrheumatic atrial fibrillation? *J Gen Intern Med* 1996;11:721–728.
24. Turpie AGG, Gent M, Laupacis A, et al. A comparison of aspirin with placebo in patients treated with warfarin after heart-valve replacement. *N Engl J Med* 1993;329:524–429.
25. Cannegieter SC, Rosendaal FR, Wintzen AR, van der Meer FJM, Vandebroucke JP, Briët E. Optimal oral anticoagulant therapy in patients with mechanical heart valves. *N Engl J Med* 1995;333:11–17.
26. Smith P, Arnesen H, Holme I. The effect of warfarin on mortality and reinfarction after myocardial infarction. *N Engl J Med* 1990;323:147–152.

27. ASPECT Research Group. Effect of long-term oral anticoagulant treatment on mortality and cardiovascular morbidity after myocardial infarction. *Lancet* 1994;343: 499–503.

28. Azar AJ, Cannegieter SC, Deckers JW, et al. Optimal intensity of oral anticoagulant therapy after myocardial infarction. *J Am Coll Cardiol* 1996;27:1349–1355.

29. EAFT (European Atrial Fibrillation Investigators) Study Group. Secondary prevention in non-rheumatic atrial fibrillation after transient ischemic attack or minor stroke. *Lancet* 1993;342:1255–1262.

30. The European Atrial Fibrillation Trial Study Group. Optimal oral anticoagulant therapy in patients with non-rheumatic atrial fibrillation and recent cerebral ischemia. *N Engl J Med* 1995;333:5–10.

31. The Steering Committee of the Physicians' Health Study Research Group. Final report on the aspirin component of the ongoing Physicians' Health Study. *N Engl J Med* 1989;321:129–135.

32. Peto R, Gray R, Collins R, et al. Randomized trial of prophylactic daily aspirin in British male doctors. *Br Med J* 1988 296:313–316.

33. The CARS Investigators. Randomized, double-blind trial of fixed low-dose warfarin plus aspirin after myocardial infarction. *Lancet* 1997;350:389–396.

34. Ferguson JJ. Meeting highlights: American College of Cardiology 45th annual scientific session, Orlando, Florida, March 24 to 27, 1996. *Circulation* 1996;94:1–9.

35. Meade T, Roderick P, Brennan P, et al. Extra-cranial bleeding and other symptoms due to low-dose aspirin and low intensity oral anticoagulation. *Thromb Haemost* 1992;68:1–6.

Cardiovascular Thrombosis: Thrombocardiology
and Thromboneurology, Second Edition,
edited by M. Verstraete, V. Fuster, and E. J. Topol,
Lippincott–Raven Publishers, Philadelphia © 1998.

51

Computer-Assisted Anticoagulation

Hamsaraj Gundal Mahabala Shetty and *Philip A. Routledge

*Department of Integrated Medicine, University Hospital of Wales, Cardiff CF4 4XN, United Kingdom;
and *Departments of Pharmacology, Therapeutics, and Toxicology, University of Wales
College of Medicine, Cardiff CF4 4XN, United Kingdom*

Advances in cardiac surgery and the discovery of newer indications for anticoagulation (e.g., chronic nonrheumatic atrial fibrillation) have resulted in a progressive increase in the number of patients on long-term anticoagulant therapy. In the United States in 1994, warfarin was the thirteenth most prescribed drug and the fifth most prescribed cardiovascular drug (1). Anticoagulants need careful monitoring if serious and potentially fatal hemorrhages are to be prevented. With the rapidly increasing use of warfarin to prevent embolic strokes in nonrheumatic atrial fibrillation the burden of monitoring anticoagulation is gradually shifting to primary care and thus to family practitioners in some countries, although many do not have the experience or training in managing long-term warfarin therapy. Hematologists or physicians may also run hospital-based anticoagulation clinics, but these are sometimes delegated to relatively inexperienced junior doctors and therefore it is not surprising that anticoagulant control is often less than ideal. There is obviously a need for the development of a system for optimizing control of anticoagulant ther-apy in a cost-effective manner. Computer-assisted anticoagulation systems are aimed at assisting toward this goal.

Since the mid-1980s computers have gradually crept into all aspects of patient management. With the ubiquitous availability of powerful and affordable computers, "computer-assisted therapy" has become a reality. Computers have been used to assist anticoagulant therapy over the past 15 years. In this chapter we review how computers have been used in clinical practice and speculate about their potential future uses for optimizing anticoagulation.

DATABASE MANAGEMENT

All the essential background data about a given patient, such as date of birth, address, identification number, and anticoagulant therapy (indication, duration, and intended intensity of anticoagulation), coexistent medical conditions, and concurrent drug therapy, can be stored in a computer and accessed with ease whenever needed. With networking facilities, it is possible to access such information in several distant centers. Having such data available in an easily accessible format saves time, reduces administrative and secretarial work, and facilitates audit. In addition, some of the currently available programs can produce letters to the family practitioners and allocate clinic appointments for patients.

IDENTIFICATION OF RISK SITUATIONS

Several factors affect response to warfarin therapy (2), including drug interactions (3). As the number of new drugs increases, it is not always possible for doctors to be aware of a given drug's potential for interaction with warfarin. Computer programs can be set to trigger alerts about potential interactions with any of the concurrently prescribed medications. Reminder about the coexistence of risk situations, such as liver or heart disease, should alert doctors to the potential problems and the need for meticulous control of anticoagulant therapy. Availability of information about coexisting medical conditions and drug interactions will help doctors to explain sudden changes in anticoagulant control and may enable them to adjust the dose to prevent such changes.

PREDICTION OF DOSE

Initiation of Therapy

In most centers empirical methods are used to choose warfarin dose. This can cause problems in the initiation of anticoagulant therapy because requirements vary up to 10- to 20-fold between patients. When 10 mg is given on three successive days, for example, the International Normalized Ratio (INR) is in the therapeutic range in only about one third of patients (4). Another third is above the range, and the remainder are inadequately anticoagulated on day 4. Excessive anticoagulation owing to large doses of warfarin at this time can increase the risk of bleeding. Avoidance of large loading doses may also reduce the risk of skin necrosis, one of the rarer complications of warfarin therapy (5).

The first attempt at predicting warfarin requirements was based on Thrombotest measurements. It was found that the daily warfarin requirement was correlated with the Thrombotest value on the fourth day after a fixed induction dose of 10 mg on three successive days (4). This relationship was sufficiently close to be predictive and was not affected by whether or not the patients had concomitant heparin therapy during the first 3 days (6). However, with the changeover to INR measurement, the induction dose was adjusted daily to prevent excessive initial anticoagulation (7). The INR was not affected by heparin infusion provided the activated partial thromboplastin time was within the recommended range of 1.5 to 2.5 times control (8). It was therefore possible to adjust the induction dose and still predict the maintenance requirements of warfarin with some accuracy. This semiempirical approach (Table 51-1) either can be made available to the prescribing doctor in printed form (e.g., on the reverse of the anticoagulation form) or can be used as a computer algorithm.

More sophisticated computer-assisted pharmacokinetic/pharmacodynamic models have been developed for induction of therapy. Some of these models have been evaluated clinically. White et al. evaluated a program that used a pharmacokinetic/pharmacodynamic model and Bayesian forecasting methods to predict warfarin dose for initiation of anticoagulation therapy (9). Bayesian methods combine population pharmacokinetic parameters with actual observations in individual patients. A prospective randomized study showed that the computer-assisted warfarin dosing was better than those by house staff physicians who did not routinely manage warfarin therapy. A stable therapeutic dose was achieved 3.7 days earlier using the computer ($p = 0.002$). Only 10% of patients were over-anticoagulated using the computer method (versus 41% by the house staff). Following the predicted maintenance dose resulted in anticoagulation within the therapeutic range in 85% with computer-assisted dosing compared with 42% by house staff physicians ($p < 0.02$).

TABLE 51-1. *An example of a widely used empirical Warfarin induction schedule*

Warfarin day	International Normalized Ratio (preferably measured at 9–10 a.m.)	Warfarin dose (preferably given at 5–6 p.m.) (mg)
1	<1.4	10.0
2	<1.8	10.0
	1.8	1.0
	>1.8	0.5
3	<2.0	10.0
	2–2.1	5.0
	2.2–2.3	4.5
	2.4–2.5	4.0
	2.6–2.7	3.5
	2.8–2.9	3.0
	3.0–3.1	2.5
	3.2–3.3	2.0
	3.4	1.5
	3.5	1.0
	3.6–4.0	0.5
	>4.0	0

		Predicted maintenance dose (mg)
4	<1.4	>8.0
	1.4	8.0
	1.5	7.5
	1.6–1.7	7.0
	1.8	6.5
	1.9	6.0
	2–2.1	5.5
	2.2–2.3	5.0
	2.4–2.6	4.5
	2.7–3.0	4.0
	3.1–3.5	3.5
	3.6–4.0	3.0
	4.1–4.5	Miss out next day's dose then give 2 mg
	>4.5	Miss out 2 day's doses then give 1 mg

1. Caution in patients with heart failure, liver disease, or immediately postoperative because their sensitivity to warfarin may vary with time.
2. If International Normalized Ratio (INR) on day 4 is <2.0, heparin can be used until the INR is within the desired range.
3. If the INR on day 1 is 1.4 or greater, the initial dose of warfarin should be reduced and the schedule is no longer relevant.
4. If KCCT is above 2.5 while the patient is receiving heparin, neutralize heparin's effect on INR by adding protamine (0.4 µg/ml plasma) to sample.

From Fennerty et al., ref. 7.

Abbrecht et al. evaluated a program based on a maximum drug-induced effect pharmacodynamic model to initiate warfarin therapy (10). A prospective study comparing 10 patients with a control group of 10 patients showed that computer-assisted patients required fewer days (4.8 versus 6.8) to first reach prothrombin complex activity values in the 20% to 30% therapeutic range. The delay in achieving therapeutic ranges in computer-assisted patients was attributed to the conservative upper limits set for warfarin dosage in the first few days of therapy. Once the therapeutic range was achieved, however, computer-assisted patients remained within it for 83% of the time (compared with 60% in controls) and they were much less over-anticoagulated.

Vadher and coworkers have used a method based on simple proportional derivative control, an approach using feedback control, to initiate warfarin (11,12). Although the time to reach the therapeutic range was comparable to the results obtained by trainee doctors provided with guidelines based on the method shown in Table 51-1, the time to stable dosing was significantly shorter (7 versus 9 days, p < 0.01, n = 148). Its performance during maintenance therapy is discussed below.

Maintenance Therapy

Computer-assisted methods, both empirical and model-based, have been used for predicting warfarin doses during long-term administration. Wilson and James obtained suggestions for changes in dosing from doctors who prescribed warfarin and used this to construct a relationship between the difference from the target INR and the change in dosage. This was incorporated into a computer program that provided recommended doses in terms of previous dose and the current prothrombin time. The program also maintained and updated data file on each patient, recommended the interval before next visit, produced clinic and ambulance lists, and alerted doctors about the decisions regarding continuation or otherwise of anticoagulant therapy. The anticoagulation control achieved by the program was found to be as effective as that obtained by manual methods (13). Kubie and colleagues used this program and found that better anticoagulant control could be achieved than they had obtained by other means, with only about 10% (range 7% to 19%) being under-anticoagulated and about 4% (range 0.9% to 8.5%) being over-anticoagulated (14). Wyld et al. used the same program with minor alterations and showed that it reduced the number of under-anticoagulated patients from 14% to 6% in the first 13 months. The number of over-anticoagulated patients did not increase in the same period (15).

Using a program similar to that of Wilson and James, Ryan et al. after 6 months noted an increase in the mean INR from 2.98 to 3.45 and an increase in the proportion of patients in the therapeutic range from 45.3% to 62.9%. They also found that the number of patients below the therapeutic range had dropped to 25.9% from 42.5% and those who were above it had fallen from 12.3% to 11.3% (16).

Poller et al. compared the effectiveness of the Hillingdon System AC Version 3.1 (derived from programs used by Wilson et al. and Wyld at al.), the Charles Anticoagulant Clinic Manager (used by the Department of Hematology, St Thomas's Hospital, London), and the Coventry Program (derived from Ryan et al.) with customary dosing by experienced medical staff. They found no significant difference in the control achieved by the four methods overall (p = 0.57) and all methods were more likely to undertreat than overtreat. Computerized dosing maintained INRs in the therapeutic range more frequently (on 56% and 58.6% of visits for the Charles and Coventry systems, respectively, versus 36.8% of visits with customary dosing) in patients assigned therapeutic ranges of INR between 3 and 4.5. Patients in this group were twice as likely to be over-anticoagulated by the Coventry system compared with other methods. For those assigned therapeutic INR ranges between 2 and 3 no significant difference was noted between the four methods. They concluded that computer-assisted anticoagulation is as good as that achieved by medical staff in most patients but significantly better than the latter in those assigned higher therapeutic INR ranges (3 to 4.5) (17).

Galloway and coworkers (18) used the program developed by Ryan et al. (16) in a general practice setting in the United Kingdom. Only 46% of patients had INRs within the therapeutic range prior to the introduction of the computerized system. At that time, 55% of those with assigned therapeutic INR ranges between 2 and 3 were within the range but only 13% of those assigned higher therapeutic ranges between 3 and 4.5 were within the therapeutic range. With computer-assisted anticoagulation the proportion of patients within the therapeutic ranges for the two groups increased to 72% and 57%, respectively. The improvement in the higher intensity group was statistically significant.

Warfarin 2.0 program, which is being used at the University Hospital in Montevideo, is claimed to be comparable to other similar programs that are in clinical use (19). Recently, Vadher et al. have evaluated a computer-based algorithm for initiation and maintenance control of oral anticoagulation (11,12). This relatively simple decision support system resulted in patients spending a greater proportion of time in the therapeutic range both as inpatients (59% versus 52%) and as outpatients (64% versus 51%) and it deserves wider evaluation in the hospital and primary care setting.

Model-based methods for long-term control of warfarin therapy have been evaluated clinically but are not widely available. Sawyer and Finn compared a log-linear pharmacodynamic model with a linear pharmacodynamic model and found that in 12 hospitalized patients a stable dose prediction could be achieved after 6.1 doses with the former and 8 doses with the latter. The mean of the average prediction error for maintenance dose was 0.25 mg for both models (error ±12%) (20). Svec et al. compared the predictive performance of a Bayesian computer program when given between 0 and 5 measured prothrombin ratios. They found that the predictions based on population parameters and one prothrombin ratio feedback were significantly biased, but when four and five prothrombin ratios were provided the predictive performance improved significantly to enable them to provide clinically useful dosage guidelines early in the course of warfarin therapy (21). This study highlighted the need for further delineation of true population parameter estimates if meaningful dose predictions are to be made.

White and Mungall in a prospective randomized trial involving 50 patients evaluated a computer program based on a pharmacokinetic/ pharmacodynamic model plus Bayesian forecasting methods for prediction of steady-state warfarin dose. They found the accuracy of computer-assisted dosage adjustments to be comparable to that of an experienced nurse-specialist (22). Model-based methods may be time consuming and complex, however, and have not achieved widespread use.

HOME AND NEAR-PATIENT MONITORING OF WARFARIN

Several workers have investigated the feasibility of patients measuring and adjusting their own anticoagulant therapy. A battery-powered portable laser photometer to rapidly measure prothrombin time on a fingerstick capillary blood sample has been used to assess the possibility of home monitoring. There was a close relationship (r = 0.96) between this approach and that using venous blood samples (23). Another small prospective randomized study showed the feasibility of home monitoring with this equipment, and better control was achieved than by a conventional anticoagulant clinic. This was largely due to a significant reduction in the proportion of patients who were under-anticoagulated with equivalent proportions being above the therapeutic range (24). Another small study has shown that patients can self-manage their anticoagulant therapy with the aid of this same home prothrombin time monitor together with appropriate dose adjustment guidelines (25).

The laser-photometer method described above performed best at INR values around 3, but it underestimated the INR by up to 0.5 in the range of INR values between 3 and 4.5 and overestimated values by around 0.3 between INR values of 2 and 3.26 The results also correlated poorly with those obtained using capillary Thrombotest reagents and this was thought to be in part related to the relative poor sensitivity of the thromboplastin used (27). Other workers have confirmed the feasibility of home monitoring using a conventional coagulometer and capillary blood samples (28).

The value of home monitoring is likely to be greatest in situations where access to anticogulant clinics is difficult or venous access is poor, but it requires well-motivated and informed individuals to use the equipment correctly and regularly. Certain groups such as the elderly may also have difficulties in attending distant hospitals but some may also find it difficult to learn the skills needed to use technical equipment. In some countries, "near-patient" monitoring facilities have therefore been developed using general practices and other sites in the community that are closer to, and therefore more convenient for, the patient. The monitoring is performed by the general practitioner, pharmacist, or nurse-practitioner, and measurement of prothrombin time may been made more simple and convenient by the development of capillary blood testing and test strips (29). Computerized decision-support systems may also be helpful in the primary care setting (12,30) and in one study resulted in better control than by the hospital clinic (30).

STRATEGIES FOR THE FUTURE

With the availability of portable prothrombin time monitors, it is now possible for patients to monitor their own anticoagulant therapy. This approach requires considerable input of time and training and may not be suitable for all patients. Some portable prothrombin time monitors employ relatively insensitive thromboplastins but are easy to use. With wider use, they may become more affordable and more sensitive and reliable thromboplastins may become available (31). If one of the models of computer-assisted anticoagulation therapy were programmed into a hand-held calculator or home computer, it could be used at home along with portable prothrombin time monitors. The computers could also be used to communicate with a family practitioner or a hematologist if the patient needs further specialist advice.

CONCLUSION

Computers are playing an important role in the management of anticoagulant therapy in many centers. They save time, reduce secretarial work, provide important background information about patients, identify risk situations, and may improve control, particularly in those who require higher intensity of anticoagulation. With refinements in home prothrombin monitoring and availability of computer programs, anticoagulation could be largely managed at home by some patients. Because of the potential risk for serious hemorrhage with anticoagulant therapy, appropriate patient selection for such modes of treatment will be of paramount importance.

Although computers can free health care professionals from repetitive and time-consuming tasks to concentrate on patient education and other developments, they are no substitute for well-trained and motivated people. Unless artificial intelligence systems are developed much more rapidly than they have been to date, it will be many years before computers can rival human skills such as serendipity (the faculty of making unexpected discoveries by accident), which still allow people to contribute more than machines to improvements in anticoagulant therapy.

In conclusion, key points are as follows:

1. Computer programs have been shown to contribute to improvements in initiation and maintenance of warfarin therapy.
2. Computerized decision support systems can also optimize recall periods, give advice on potential risk situations such as drug or food interactions, and improve administration and audit of the anticoagulant service.
3. Self-monitoring is still a relatively new approach but may become increasingly valuable in suitable patients. Computer-assisted dosing also shows potential in this situation.
4. Computer-assisted anticoagulation is applicable both in the hospital setting and in the increasing number of community-based clinics run by family practitioners, pharmacists, and other health care professionals.
5. In all of these circumstances, computers are an adjunct to, and not a substitute for, the advice, experience, and support of a well-trained health care professional.

REFERENCES

1. Ansell JE, Hughes R. Evolving models of Warfarin management: anticoagulation clinics, patients self-monitoring and patient self management. *Am Heart J* 1996;132:1095–1100.

2. Shetty HGM, Fennerty AG, Routledge PA. Clinical Pharmacokinetic considerations in the control of oral anticoagulant therapy. *Clin Pharmacokinet* 1989;16: 238–253.

3. Serlin MJ, Breckenridge AM. Drug interactions with warfarin. *Drugs* 1983;25:610–620.

4. Routledge PA, Davies DM, Bell SM, Cavanagh JS, Rawlins MD. Predicting patients' warfarin requirements. *Lancet* 1977;2:854–855.

5. Cole MS, Minifee PK, Wolma FJ. Coumarin necrosis—a review of literature. *Surgery* 1988;103:271–276.

6. Sharma NK, Routledge PA, Rawlins MD, Davies DM. Predicting the dose of warfarin for therapeutic anticoagulation. *Thromb Haemost* 1982;47:230–231.

7. Fennerty A, Dolben J, Thomas P, et al. Flexible induction dose regimen for warfarin and prediction of maintenance dose. *Br Med J* 1984;288:1268–1270.

8. Thomas P, Fennerty A, Backhouse G, Bentley DP, Campbell IA, Routledge PA. Monitoring oral anticoagulant therapy during heparin therapy. *Br Med J* 1984;188–191.

9. White RH, Hong R, Venook AP, et al. Initiation of warfarin therapy: comparison of physician dosing with computer-assisted dosing. *J Gen Intern Med* 1987;2:141–148.

10. Abbrecht PH, O'Leary TJ, Behrendt DM. Evaluation of a computer-assisted method for individualised anticoagulation: retrospective and prospective studies with a pharmacodynamic model. *Clin Pharmacol Ther* 1982; 32:129–136.

11. Vadher BD, Patterson DLH, Leaning MS. Validation of an algorithm for oral anticoagulant dosing and appointment scheduling. *Clin Lab Haematol* 1995;17:339–345.

12. Vadher B, Patterson DLH, Leaning M. Evaluation of a decision support system for initiation and control of anticoagulation in a randomised trial. *Br Med J* 1997;314: 1252–1256.

13. Wilson R, James AH. Computer-assisted management of warfarin treatment. *Br Med J* 1984;423–424.

14. Kubie A, James AH, Timms J, Britt RP. Experience with a computer-assisted anticoagulation clinic. *Clin Lab Haematol* 1989;11:385–913.

15. Wyld PJ, West D, Wilson TH. Computer dosing in anticoagulant clinics—the way forward? *Clin Lab Haematol* 1988;10:235–236.

16. Ryan PJ, Gilbert M, Rose PE. Computer control of anticoagulant dose for therapeutic management. *Br Med J* 1989;299:1207–1209.

17. Poller L, Wright D, Rowlands M. Prospective comparative study of computer programs used for management of warfarin. *J Clin Pathol* 1993;46:299–303.

18. Galloway MJ, Foggin JJ, Dixon S. Introduction of computer assisted control of oral anticoagulation in general practice. *J Clin Pathol* 1995;48:1144–1146.

19. Margolis A, Flores F, Kierszenbaum M, et al. Warfarin 2.0—a computer program for warfarin management. Design and clinical use. *Proc Annu Symp Computer Appl Med Care* 1994;18M:846–850.

20. Sawyer WT, Finn AL. Digital computer-assisted warfarin therapy: comparison of two models. *Comp Biomed Res* 1979;12:221–231.

21. Svec JM, Coleman RW, Mungall DR, Ludden TM. Bayesian pharmacokinetic/pharmacodynamic forecasting of prothrombin response to warfarin therapy: preliminary evaluation. *Ther Drug Monit* 1985;7: 174–180.

22. White RH, Mungall D. Outpatient management of warfarin therapy: comparison of computer-predicted dosage adjustment to skilled professional care. *Ther Drug Monit* 1991;13:46–50.

23. Lucas FV, Duncan A, Jay R, et al. A novel whole blood capillary technic for measuring the prothrombin time. *Am J Clin Pathol* 1987;88:442–446.

24. White RH, McCurdy SA, von Mansdorff H, Woodruff DE, Leftgoff L. Home prothrombin time monitoring after the initiation of warfarin therapy. A randomised, prospective study. *Ann Intern Med* 1989;111:730–737.

25. Ansell J, Holden A, Knapic N. Patient self-management of oral anticoagulation guided by capillary (fingerstick) whole blood prothrombin times. *Arch Intern Med* 1989;149:2509–2511.

26. McCurdy SA, White RH. Accuracy and precision of a portable anticoagulation monitor in a clinical setting. *Arch Intern Med* 1992;152:589–592.

27. Jennings I, Luddington RJ, Baglin T. Evaluation of the Ciba Corning Biotrack 512 coagulation monitor for the control of oral anticoagulation. *J Clin Pathol* 1992;44: 950–953.

28. Bernado A, Halhuber C, Horstkotte D. Home prothrombin estimation. In: Butchart EG, Bodnar E (eds). *Current Issues in Heart Valve Disease: Thrombosis, Embolism and Bleeding.* London: ICR, 1992.

29. Kapiotis S, Quehenberger P, Speiser W. Evaluation of the new method Coaguchek R for the determination of prothrombin time from capillary blood: comparison with Thrombotest on KC-1. *Thromb Res* 1995; 77:563–567.

30. Fitzmaurice DA, Hobbs FD, Murray ET, Bradley CP, Holder R. Evaluation of computerized decision support for oral anticoagulation management in primary care. *Br J Gen Prac* 1996;46:533–535

31. Tripodi A, Arbini AA, Chantarangkul V, Bettega D, Mannucci PM. Are capillary whole blood coagulation monitors suitable for the control of oral anticoagulant treatment by the international normalized ratio? *Thromb Haemost* 1993;70:921–924.

Subject Index

Note: Main entries appear in **boldface**; page numbers in **boldface** refer to major discussions of subjects; page numbers in *italics* refer to illustrations; and page numbers followed by t refer to tables.

A

Abciximab, 132–135
  in myocardial infarction, *519–520*
  in percutaneous transluminal coronary angioplasty, 576—578, *577*
  in unstable angina, 446, *447*
  with heparin, 197
Abdominal surgery
  danaparoid after, 227
  venous thrombosis and, 95, 665
Acenocoumarol, 289
Acetylsalicylic acid. See *Aspirin.*
Activated partial thromboplastin time, for heparin monitoring, 190–191, 196
Activated protein C resistance, 699
  in pregnancy, 722
Adenocarcinoma, venous thrombosis and, 94, 94t, 97–98
Adenosine diphosphate
  in platelet activation, 32
  in platelet thrombus formation, 11
Afibrinogenemia, platelet aggregation in, 36
Age
  prosthetic valve—related thromboembolism and, 371
  thrombolytic agent—induced hemorrhage and, 534, *534, 535,* 536, 536t, *538*
  venous thrombosis and, 93–94, 94t, 97
Allergy
  dextran, 243–244
  streptokinase, 540
Alteplase, hemorrhage with, 529t, 530–531, 530t
ε-Aminocaproic acid, in hemorrhage management, 540
Amniotic fluid embolism, disseminated intravascular coagulation and, 783
Anaphylactoid reaction, with dextran, 243–244
Ancrod
  in ischemic stroke, 612
  in plasma viscosity reduction, 329–330
Anesthesia, venous thrombosis and, 99
Angina
  stable
    atherosclerotic plaques in, 54–55
    desirudin in, 145–146
    hemodilution in, 327
    iloprost in, 272–273
    percutaneous transluminal coronary angioplasty in, 145–146
    taprostene in, 276
  unstable, **439–456.** See also *Myocardial infarction.*
    angiography in, 23, 454–455
    Chlamydia pneumoniae in, 52
    classification of, 439–440, 440t

coronary anatomy in, 444
fibrinopeptide A levels and, 109–111, *110*
flow variation in, 444
incidence of, 439, *440*
myocardial infarction with, 456
pathophysiology of, 440–444, 441t, *442, 443*
plaque disruption in, 441–444, *442*
prevention of, **461–468**
  anticoagulant therapy in, 464–465
  antiplatelet therapy in, 461–464, 462t, *463,* 465–467, 466t
  fibrates in, 328
prothrombin activation fragment 1+2 levels and, 109–111, *110*
supply demand mismatch in, 440–441, 441t
thrombosis in, 441–444, *443*
treatment of, 444–455
  ancrod in, 329
  angiography in, 454–455
  antianginals in, 451–453
  antiplatelet agents in, 445–447, 445t, *447, 448*
  antithrombin agents in, 448–450, *449, 450*
  argatroban in, 158–159
  beta-adrenergic blockers in, 452, *453*
  bleeding with, 455
  calcium channel blockers in, 452–453, *453*
  heparin in, 111–112, *112, 113,* 193, 208–209, 208t, 209t
  hypolipidemic agents in, 453–454, *454*
  inogatran in, 164–165
  low molecular weight heparin in, 208–209, 208t, 209t
  outcome of, 455–456
  percutaneous transluminal coronary angioplasty in
    bivalirudin in, 154–155
    desirudin in, 145–146
    preoperative, 568–569
    prostacyclin in, 274
    roxithromycin in, 52
    thrombolytic therapy in, 113–114, *114, 115,* 450–451, *451, 452*
    tirofiban in, 135
    vasoconstriction in, 448
Angiography
  in myocardial infarction, 503–504, *504*
  in unstable angina, 23, 454–455
AngioJet, 341–345
  clinical application of, 343–345, *344-345*
  description of, 341–343, *342*
  technique of, 343
AngioJet LF140 catheter, 342, *342*